THE COLOR ATLAS
OF FAMILY MEDICINE

NOTICE

Medicine is an ever-changing science. As new research and clinical experience broaden our knowledge, changes in treatment and drug therapy are required. The authors and the publisher of this work have checked with sources believed to be reliable in their efforts to provide information that is complete and generally in accord with the standards accepted at the time of publication. However, in view of the possibility of human error or changes in medical sciences, neither the editors nor the publisher nor any other party who has been involved in the preparation or publication of this work warrants that the information contained herein is in every respect accurate or complete, and they disclaim all responsibility for any errors or omissions or the results obtained from use of the information contained in this work. Readers are encouraged to confirm the information contained herein with other sources. For example and in particular, readers are advised to check the product information sheet included in the package of each drug they plan to administer to be certain that the information contained in this work is accurate and that changes have not been made in the recommended dose or in the contraindications for administration. This recommendation is of particular importance in connection with new or infrequently used drugs.

THE COLOR ATLAS OF FAMILY MEDICINE

EDITORS

Richard P. Usatine, MD

Professor of Family and Community Medicine
Professor of Dermatology and Medicine
Assistant Director, Medical Humanities Education
University of Texas Health Science Center at San Antonio
Medical Director, Skin Clinic, University Health System
San Antonio, Texas

Mindy A. Smith, MD

Professor of Family Medicine
Michigan State University, College of Human Medicine
East Lansing, Michigan
Associate Editor, Family Medicine
Associate Medical Editor, FP Essentials
American Academy of Family Physicians

Heidi Chumley, MD

Associate Professor of Family Medicine
Associate Chair for Undergraduate
    Medical Education
Department of Family Medicine
Kansas University School of Medicine
Kansas City, Kansas

E.J. Mayeaux, Jr., MD

Professor of Family Medicine
Professor of Obstetrics and Gynecology
Associate Family Medicine Residency Program Director
Louisiana State University Health Sciences Center
Shreveport, Louisiana

James Tysinger, PhD

Professor of Family and Community Medicine
Deputy Chair for Faculty Development
Department of Family & Community Medicine
University of Texas Health Science Center at San Antonio
San Antonio, Texas

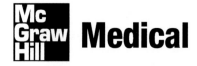

New York   Chicago   San Francisco   Lisbon   London   Madrid   Mexico City
New Delhi   San Juan   Seoul   Singapore   Sydney   Toronto

The **McGraw·Hill** Companies

The Color Atlas of Family Medicine

1 2 3 4 5 6 7 8 9 0 CTP/CTP 12 11 10 9 8

MHID: 978-0-07-147464-1

ISBN: 0-07-147464-1

This book was set in Perpetua by Aptara®, Inc.
The editors were Jim Shanahan, Karen G. Edmonson.
The production manager was Phil Galea.
The cover designer was Pehrsson Design.
The indexer was Kathy Unger.
China Translation & Printing Service, Ltd., was printer and binder.

This book is printed on acid-free paper.

Library of Congress Cataloging-in-Publication Data

The color atlas of family medicine / editors, Richard P. Usatine . . . [et al.].
        p. ; cm.
    Includes bibliographical references and index.
    ISBN-13: 978-0-07-147464-1 (alk. paper)
    ISBN-10: 0-07-147464-1 (alk. paper)
  1. Family medicine—Atlases.   I. Usatine, Richard.
    [DNLM: 1. Family Practice—Atlases.   WB 17 C719 2009]
    R729.5.G4C58 2009
    610—dc22
                                                    2008034328

DEDICATION

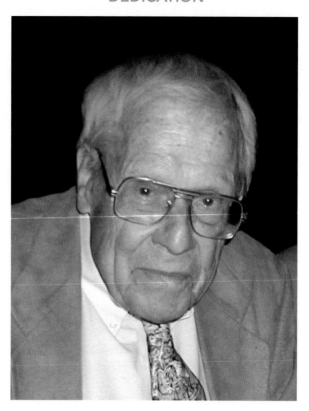

This book is dedicated to the memory of Leonard G. Paul, MD. Leonard was a family physician in rural practice before becoming a mentor and teacher for many family doctors across the country. Leonard was the epitome of the warm-hearted, kind, and compassionate family physician. He cared for his patients, staff, nurses, and doctors in training. Leonard was loved by everyone and practiced medicine until he was 82 years of age. His patients were saddened when he retired, but they knew he had given everything to them and the practice of medicine. Leonard Paul was the chair of the Department of Family and Community Medicine at the University of Texas Health Sciences Center at San Antonio for 12 years. During that time he fought to establish a family medicine inpatient service and enabled family physicians to deliver babies in delivery rooms controlled by obstetrics. Leonard loved his family, staff, and animals. He was a loving husband, father, grandfather, and man. He treated his staff to generous holiday dinners and brought food to the clinic each day. His favorite pastime was feeding deer. Every morning and evening scores of deer waited patiently for him to scatter corn on his driveway. He spoiled his dogs with steaks and people food.

Leonard was a self-directed learner. He graduated at the top of his class at Stanford School of Medicine. Despite being told multiple times that he should pursue other specialties, Leonard was steadfast in his determination to become a true family doctor. He read his journals, including the *New England Journal of Medicine*, every day throughout his career and even after he retired. He clipped interesting articles and put them in his colleagues' mailboxes. He was one of the best-read family physicians.

Leonard had a busy private practice for years in which he delivered babies and did a full range of family medicine. It was only in his later years that he practiced family medicine exclusively in the ambulatory setting. In his last year of practice he could no longer drive. Some evenings I would take Leonard home in my car. We had wonderful conversations about the world and shared our lives and visions. He knew that we were working on this book and was very supportive of this endeavor. He stopped practicing medicine only when his health made it difficult for him to get around the clinic without falling. Leonard passed away one week before I had the chance to tell him of our decision to dedicate this book to him. His humanism and caring will be passed down for generations of family physicians to come.

PART 1

LEARNING WITH IMAGES AND DIGITAL PHOTOGRAPHY

PART 2

THE ESSENCE OF FAMILY MEDICINE

PART 3

PHYSICAL AND SEXUAL ABUSE

PART 4

OPHTHALMOLOGY

Section 1: External Eye

Section 2: Internal Eye

PART 5

EAR, NOSE AND THROAT

Section 1: Ear

Section 2: Nose and Sinus

Section 3: Mouth and Throat

PART 6

ORAL HEALTH

PART 7

THE HEART AND CIRCULATION

Section 1: Central

Section 2: Peripheral

CONTENTS

CONTENTS

CONTENTS

Cathleen M. Abbott, MD

Assistant Professor
Department of Family Medicine
College of Human Medicine
Michigan State University
East Lansing, Michigan

Anna M. Allred, MD

Resident Physician
Department of Neurological Surgery
University of Texas Southwestern
Dallas, Texas

James Anderst, MD, MS

Assistant Professor of Pediatrics
Division of Child Abuse Pediatrics
The University of Texas Health Science Center at San Antonio
Christus Santa Rosa Center for Miracles
San Antonio, Texas

Hend Azhary, MD

Assistant Professor
Department of Family Medicine
Michigan State University College of Human Medicine
East Lansing, Michigan

Michael Babcock, MD

Chief Resident, Dermatology
Division of Dermatology
Department of Medicine
University of Texas Health Science Center at San Antonio
San Antonio, Texas

Lesa V. M. Brookes, MD, FAAP

Associate Director, Pediatrics Education
Director of Student Education
Oakwood Hospital and Medical Center
Department of Pediatrics
Dearborn, Michigan

Pierre P. Chanoine, MD

Drexel University School of Medicine
Philadelphia, Pennsylvania
St. Christopher's Hospital for Children
Philadelphia, Pennsylvania

Beth A. Choby, MD

Assistant Professor
Department of Family Medicine
University of Tennessee—Chattanooga College of Medicine
Chattanooga, Tennessee

Heidi Chumley, MD

Associate Professor of Family Medicine
Associate Chair for Undergraduate Medical Education
Department of Family Medicine
Kansas University School of Medicine
Kansas City, Kansas

Thomas J. Corson, D.O.

Emergency Medicine Resident
University of Connecticut School of Medicine
Hartford Hospital
Hartford, Connecticut

Zoe Diana Draelos, MD

Dermatology Consulting Services
High Point, North Carolina

Cristina Fernandez, MD

Clinical Assistant Professor
Department of Pediatrics
College of Human Medicine
Michigan State University
East Lansing, Michigan

Damian Flowers, MD

Emergency Medicine Resident
University of Connecticut School of Medicine
Farmington, Connecticut

Jeremy A. Franklin, MD, FAAP

Assistant Professor
Department of Pediatrics
Chief, Division of Pediatric Infectious Diseases
Texas Tech University Health Sciences Center
Lubbock, Texas

Linda M. French, MD

Professor and Chair
Department of Family Medicine
University of Toledo College of Medicine
Toledo, Ohio

Radha Raman Murthy Gokula, MD, CMD

Geriatrician & Palliative Medicine Consultant
University of Toledo Medical Center
Assistant Professor
Department of Family Medicine
University of Toledo
Toledo, Ohio

Wanda C. Gonsalves, MD

Associate Professor
Department of Family Medicine
Medical University of South Carolina
Charleston, South Carolina

James Haynes, MD

Lieutenant Colonel
United States Air Force
Program Director
Family Medicine Residency Clinic
Eglin Air Force Base, Florida

Jimmy H. Hara, MD, FAAFP

Clinical Professor of Family Medicine
David Geffen School of Medicine at UCLA
Family Medicine Residency Program Director
Kaiser Permanente Center for Medical Education
Los Angeles, California

Kelli D. Hejl, MS

Research Coordinator
Trauma Services Department
University Medical Center Brackenridge
Austin, Texas

David D. Henderson, MD

Assistant Professor
Department of Family Medicine
University of Connecticut School of Medicine
Farmington, Connecticut

Nathan Hitzeman, MD

Clinical Faculty
University of California at Davis
Sacramento, California
Sutter Health Family Medicine Physician
Sutter Medical Group
Sacramento, California

Karen A. Hughes, MD, FAAFP

Associate Director
North Mississippi Center Family Medicine Residency Program
Tupelo, Mississippi

Khalilah Hunter-Anderson, MD

University of Connecticut School of Medicine
Residency Administration
University of Connecticut Health Center
Farmington, Connecticut

Jennifer A. Keehbauch, MD, FAAFP

Clinical Assistant Professor of Family Medicine
Florida State University Medical School
Tallahassee, Florida
Assistant Director
Family Medicine Residency
Florida Hospital
Orlando, Florida

Nancy D. Kellogg, MD

Professor of Pediatrics
Division Chief of Child Abuse
University of Texas Health Science Center at San Antonio
San Antonio, Texas

J. Michael King, MD

Fellow
University of Texas Health Science Center at San Antonio
Department of Otolaryngology--Head and Neck Surgery
Attending Physician
University HealthCare System
San Antonio, Texas

Amor Khachemoune, MD, CWS

Assistant Professor of Dermatology
New York University School of Medicine
New York, New York

Robert Kraft, MD

Assistant Clinical Professor of Family and Community Medicine
University of Kansas School of Medicine Wichita, KS,
Associate Director,
Smoky Hill Family Medicine
Residency Program Salina, KS

Andreas Kuhn, MD, MBA

Clinical Assistant Professor
Department of Family Medicine
College of Human Medicine
Michigan State University
East Lansing, Michigan

Javier La Fontaine, MD

Assistant Professor
Director, Podiatric Residency Training Program
Departments of Orthopedics
University of Texas Health Science Center at San Antonio
San Antonio, Texas

Megha Madhukar, BA

University of Texas Health Science Center at San Antonio
School of Medicine
San Antonio, Texas

Ashfaz A. Marghoob, MD

Memorial Sloan Kettering Cancer Center
Associate Professor of Dermatology
Stony Brook University Hospital
Stony Brook, New York
Memorial Sloan Kettering Cancer Center
Associate Member
Division of Dermatology
New York, New York

E.J. Mayeaux, Jr., MD, DABFP, FAAFP

Professor of Family Medicine
Professor of Obstetrics and Gynecology
Associate Family Medicine Residency Program Director
Louisiana State University Health Sciences Center
Shreveport, Louisiana

Maria D. McColgan, MD, MEd

Assistant Professor
Departments of Pediatrics and Emergency Medicine
Director, Child Protection Program
Drexel University College of Medicine
Philadelphia, Pennsylvania

Carolyn Milana, MD

Associate Director, Division of General Pediatrics
Assistant Professor of Pediatrics
State University of New York Stony Brook
Department of Pediatrics
Stony Brook, New York

Shashi Mittal, MD
Faculty Director of Research
Baylor Family Medicine Residency at Garland
Garland, Texas

Asad Mohmand, MD
Assistant Professor
Department of Medicine
Lead Clerkship Director Advanced Medicine College of Human
    Medicine Michigan State University
East Lansing, Michigan

Melissa Muszynski, BS
University of Texas Health Science Center at San Antonio
School of Medicine
San Antonio, Texas

Anjeli K. Nayar, MD, Capt, USAF, MC
Wright State University Internal Medicine
Wright-Patterson Air Force Base, Ohio

Richard A. Paulis, MD
Attending Physician
Department of Emergency Medicine
Frankford Hospital
Philadelphia, Pennsylvania

Brian Z. Rayala, MD
Assistant Professor of Family Medicine
Michigan State University College of Human Medicine
East Lansing, Michigan

Suraj G. Reddy, MD
The University of Texas Health Science Center at San Antonio
San Antonio, Texas

Michelle J. Rowe, MD
Farmington Hills, Michigan

Mark Jason Sanders, MD
Department of Pediatrics
Assistant Professor of Pediatrics
The University of Texas Medical School at Houston
Houston, Texas

Khashayar Sarabi, MD
Loma Linda Medical Center
Department of Physical Medicine and Rehabilitation
Loma Linda, California

Ana Trevino Sauceda, MD
Chief Resident, Dermatology
Division of Dermatology
Department of Medicine
University of Texas Health Science Center at San Antonio
San Antonio, Texas

Andrew D. Schechtman, MD, FAAFP
Adjunct Clinical Instructor
Stanford University School of Medicine
Department of Family and Community Medicine
Stanford, California
Faculty, San Jose-O'Connor Hospital Family Medicine Residency
    Program
San Jose, California

Angela D. Shedd, BA
University of Texas Health Science Center at San Antonio
School of Medicine
San Antonio, Texas

Andrew Shedd, MD
Emergency Medicine Resident
Department of Emergency Medicine
Advocate Christ Medical Center
Oak Lawn, Illinois

Maureen K. Sheehan, MD, FACS
Assistant Professor of Vascular Surgery
University of Texas Health Science Center at San Antonio
San Antonio, Texas

Naohiro Shibuya, DPM, MS, AACFAS
Clinical Instructor
Department of Orthopaedics
Division of Podiatry
University of Texas Health and Science Center at San Antonio
San Antonio, Texas

Leslie A. Shimp, PharmD, MS
Professor of Pharmacy
University of Michigan
Clinical Pharmacist
Integrative Family Medicine
Briarwood Family Practice
Ann Arbor, Michigan

C. Blake Simpson, MD
Professor and Director University of Texas Voice Center
University of Texas Health Science Center at San Antonio
Department of Otolaryngology—Head and Neck Surgery
San Antonio, Texas

Mindy A. Smith, MD
Professor of Family Medicine
Michigan State University, College of Human Medicine
East Lansing, Michigan
Associate Editor, Family Medicine
Associate Medical Editor, FP Essentials, American Association of
    Family Physicians

James Tysinger, PhD
Professor of Family and Community Medicine
Deputy Chair for Faculty Development
Department of Family & Community Medicine
University of Texas Health Science Center at San Antonio
School of Medicine
San Antonio, Texas

Richard P. Usatine, MD, FAAFP
Professor of Family and Community Medicine
Professor of Dermatology and Medicine
Assistant Director, Medical Humanities Education
University of Texas Health Science Center at San Antonio
Medical Director, Skin Clinic, University Health System
San Antonio, Texas

Alejandra Varela, MD
Family Medicine Resident
Austin Medical Education Program
Austin, Texas

Christopher J. Wenner, MD
Associate Director
University of Minnesota/St. Cloud Hospital Family Medicine
    Residency Program
St. Cloud, Minnesota
Assistant Professor of Family Medicine
University of Minnesota
Minneapolis, Minnesota

Shehnaz Aysha Zaman, MD
Internal Medicine Resident
Northwestern Memorial Hospital
Chicago, Illinois

Family physicians probably see a wider variety of rashes, eye conditions, foot disorders, lumps, and bumps than any other specialty. In speaking with health care providers and medical students over the years it became clear that a comprehensive atlas that aided the diagnosis of outwardly appearing signs and manifestations would be of tremendous value. We have assembled more than 1500 outstanding clinical images for this very purpose, and are proud to present what is to our knowledge the first comprehensive atlas of family medicine ever produced. Some photographs will amaze you, and all will inform you about the various conditions that befall our patients.

It took many people many years to create *The Color Atlas of Family Medicine*. For me it has been a life work that started with little notebooks I kept in my white coat pocket to take notes during my residency. It then took on color and images as I kept a camera at work and took photographs of any interesting clinical finding that I might use to teach medical students and residents the art and science of medicine. I was inspired by many great family physicians including Dr. Jimmy Hara who had the most amazing 35-mm slide collection I had seen. His knowledge of medicine is encyclopedic and I thought that taking photographs might have something to do with that. Also, I realized that these photographs would be great to enhance my teaching. As I began to do more dermatology, my photograph collection skyrocketed. Digital photography made it more affordable and practical to take and catalogue many new images.

This book is written for family physicians, but can be invaluable to medical students, residents, and health care providers in primary care. It certainly has much to offer internists, pediatricians, and dermatologists. It is especially for anyone who loves to look at clinical photographs for learning, teaching, and practicing medicine. The first chapter begins the adventure with an introduction to learning with images and digital photography. The core of the book focuses on medical conditions organized by anatomic and physiological systems. Both adult and childhood conditions are included as this book covers health care from birth to death. There are special sections on the essence of family medicine, physical/sexual abuse, women's health and substance abuse.

The collection of clinical images is supported by evidence-based information that will help the health care provider diagnose and manage common medical problems. The text is concisely presented with many easy to access bullets as a quick point of care reference. Each chapter begins with a patient story that ties the photographs to the real life stories of our patients. The photographic legends are also designed to connect the images to the people and their human conditions. Strength of recommendation ratings are cited throughout so that the science of medicine can be blended with the art of medicine for optimal patient care.

We have created three special indexes to help you find information and diagnoses quickly and efficiently. The topic index printed on the front inside cover allows for quick access to major topic areas. The regional index for diagnosis in the appendix can be used when you have an unknown condition and want to search for possible diagnoses by region of the body. Finally, the morphology index is to aid in the diagnosis of conditions which you can describe morphologically but the actual diagnosis remains uncertain.

Since knowledge continues to advance after any book is written, use the online resources presented in many chapters to keep up with the newest changes in medicine. Care deeply about your patients and enjoy your practice, it is an honor to be a health care provider and healer.

This book could not have been completed without the contributions of many talented physicians, health-care professionals, and photographers. We received photographs from people who live and work across the globe. Most of the photographs have never been published before and are coming from a wide range of people. Each photograph is labeled and acknowledges the photographer and contributor. Some photographs were previously published in the Photo Rounds column of the *Journal of Family Practice*. For these we thank Dowden publishers for generously sharing these photographs with our readers. Being the founding editor of this column gave me the opportunity to see a great collection of clinical photographs over the years.

In the year 2000, I began giving every medical student a digital camera as they rotated through the family medicine clerkship at UCLA. We have continued this process at University of Texas Health Sciences Center at San Antonio (UTHSCSA). Some of the best of these photographs are incorporated into our book. What could be better than to have our medical students record the clinical images that they see while rotating on family medicine? Not only do the students teach each other using these photographs but they now will help educate our readers on the vast breadth and scope of family medicine.

There are some people who contributed so many photographs it is appropriate to acknowledge them upfront in the book. Paul Comeau is the professional ophthalmology photographer at UTHSCSA. His beautiful photographs of the external and internal eye make the ophthalmology section of this book so rich and valuable. The dermatology division at UTHSCSA contributed much of their expertise in photography, writing, and reviewing to the extensive dermatology section. During the last few years, I was fortunate to work closely with the dermatology faculty and residents and they all contributed generously to our book. Dr. Eric Kraus, the program director, gave us many wonderful photographs, especially for the section on bullous diseases. He also gave us open access to the 35-mm slides collected by the Division of Dermatology. Dr. Jeff Meffert also contributed photographs to many chapters. Many dermatology residents wrote chapters and contributed photographs. Dr. Jack Resneck, Sr, from Louisiana, scanned his slides from over 40 years of practice and gave them to Dr. EJ Mayeaux, Jr., for use. Dr. Resneck's vast dermatologic experiences add to our atlas.

The UTHSCSA Head and Neck Department contributed many photographs for this book. We especially thank Dr. Frank Miller and Dr. Blake Simpson for their contributions. UTHSCSA pediatrics faculty contributed to our chapters on child abuse and otitis media. We are fortunate to have Dr. Nancy Kellogg contribute her photographs and expertise in caring for abused children to the book. Dr. Dan Stulberg, a family physician from New Mexico, with a passion for photography and dermatology, contributed many photographs throughout our book. Dr. Ellen Eisenberg, an oral pathologist was generous in sharing her vast collection of images with us.

We thank our learners, many of whom co-authored chapters with us. Dr. Mindy A. Smith worked with many of her fellows in the Michigan State University Primary Care Faculty Development Fellowship Program and Dr. Susan Dufel worked with her emergency medicine residents to write chapters for the book. UTHSCSA medical students co-authored chapters and contributed photographs with great enthusiasm to the creation of this work. It was a pleasure to mentor these young writers and experience with them the rewards of authorship.

We want to thank the specialty reviewers who reviewed their respective sections. This included Drs. Malvinder Hoonjan for ophthalmology, Heidi Tonken for musculoskeletal, Marvin Derezin for gastroenterology, Chris McMains for ENT, Aaron Liddell for oral health and Michelle Hamilton for cardiology. Dr. Suraj Reddy reviewed all 97 dermatology chapters during his last months as chief resident in dermatology at UTHSCSA.

Of course, we would have no book without the talented writing and editing of my co-editors, Drs. Mindy A. Smith, EJ Mayeaux, Heidi Chumley, and Jim Tysinger. They each bring years of clinical and educational experience to the writing of the Atlas. Dr. Mayeaux contributed many of his own photographs, especially in women's health care, to our Atlas. One family physician from University of South Carolina, Dr. Wanda Gonsalves, wrote the entire oral health section. Two podiatrists at UTHSCSA wrote the podiatry section. To these prolific writers, many thanks are due.

Most of all we need to thank our patients who generously gave their permission for their photographs to be taken and published in this book. While some photos are not recognizable, we have many photos of the full face that are very recognizable and were generously given to us by our patients with full written permission to be published as is. For photographs that were taken decades ago in which written consents were no longer available, we have used bars across the eyes to make the photos less recognizable—verbal consent was always obtained for these images.

The last section of this book is dedicated to understanding substance abuse (chemical dependency) and its treatment. This could not have been done without the generous contributions of the dedicated staff and the women residents at Alpha Home, nonprofit alcohol and drug treatment program in San Antonio. The medical students from UTHSCSA and I spend one to two evenings a week providing free health care to these women bravely facing their addictions and fighting to stay sober one day at a time. Their pictures have been generously added to our book with their permission.

I (Dr. Richard Usatine) thank my family for giving me the support to see this book through. It has taken much time from my family life and my family has supported me through the long nights and weekends it takes to write a book while continuing to practice and teach medicine. I am fortunate to have a loving wife and two beautiful children who add meaning to my life and allowed me to work hard on the creation of this Color Atlas.

Dr. Mindy Smith adds, "I wish to thank an old family friend, Isadore Berger, for triggering my interest in photography as a form of learning about the world around us, my husband, Gary, and daughter, Jenny, for putting up with my constant photo opportunities, and my brother-in-law Rus Benson for demonstrating the artistry and warmth that photography holds. The use of images as teaching tools provides a unique view into family medicine and the lives of many of our patients; I thank them all for their generosity."

Dr. EJ Mayeaux adds, "I would like to thank my wife and son for understanding the many hours of work and computer time in my meager efforts to leave the world a better place. I would also thank my family for teaching me to see the world as a beautiful, joyous, photogenic, beckoning, fascinating place. I hope this book helps each reader see the world this way."

ACKNOWLEDGEMENTS

Dr. Heidi Chumley adds, "I want to thank my husband, John Delzell, who has brought love and peace to my often chaotic life, and my children, Cullen, Sierra, David, Selene, and Jack, who give me joy and provide the incentive to stay on task. Each one, in turn, has cheerfully pitched in to help a grumpy and tired mom who stayed up most of the night working on one of many chapters. I have been very blessed."

Dr. James Tysinger adds, "I appreciate the support my wife, Sylvia, has given me throughout my career and life. I also recognize my many colleagues who have supported my career and encouraged me to develop as a person and a professional."

Finally, we all thank James Shanahan and Karen Edmonson from McGraw-Hill for believing in this project and never giving up as the book grew larger and more comprehensive over time.

THE COLOR ATLAS
OF FAMILY MEDICINE

PART 1

LEARNING WITH IMAGES AND DIGITAL PHOTOGRAPHY

1 AN ATLAS TO ENHANCE PATIENT CARE, LEARNING, AND TEACHING

Richard P. Usatine, MD

"People only see what they are prepared to see."

—Ralph Waldo Emerson

Whether you are viewing **Figure 1-1** in a book, in an aquarium, or from under the sea, you immediately recognize this image as that of a fish. Those of you who are more schooled in the classification of fish might recognize that this is an angelfish with the tail being the head of the angel and the posterior fins being the wings. If you are truly prepared to see this fish in all her splendor, you would see the blue circle above her eye as the crown of the queen angelfish.

Making a diagnosis in medicine often involves the kind of pattern recognition needed to identify a queen angelfish. This is much the same as recognizing a beautiful bird or the painting of a favorite artist. If you are prepared to look for the clues that lead to the identification (diagnosis), you will see what needs to be seen. What are the best ways to become prepared to see? There is nothing more valuable than seeing an image or a patient who has the condition in question at least once before you encounter it on your own. The memory of a powerful visual image can become hard wired into your brain for ready recall.

In medicine it also helps to know where and how to look to find the clues you may need when the diagnosis cannot be made at a single glance. For example, a patient with inverse psoriasis may present with a rash under the breast that has been repeatedly and unsuccessfully treated with antifungal agents for candidiasis or tinea (**Figures 1-2** and **1-3**). The prepared clinician knows that not all erythematous plaques under the breast are fungal and looks for clues such as nail changes (**Figures 1-2** and **1-4**) or the subtle plaques of the elbows, knees, or umbilicus (**Figure 1-3**) to make the diagnosis of psoriasis.

USING OUR SENSES

As physicians we collect clinical data through sight, sound, touch, and smell. While physicians in the past used taste to collect data, such as tasting the sweet urine of a diabetic patient, this sense is rarely if ever used in modern medicine. We listen to heart sounds, lung sounds, bruits, and percussion notes to collect information for diagnoses. We touch our patients to feel lumps, bumps, thrills, and masses. We occasionally use smell for diagnosis. Unfortunately, the smells of disease are rarely pleasant. Even the fruity odors are not like the sweet fruits of a farmers' market. Of course, we also use the patient's history, laboratory data, and more advanced imaging techniques to diagnose and manage patients' illnesses.

It is our belief in the great value of visual imagery that led to the development of *The Color Atlas of Family Medicine*. Changes in the appearance of the body can give us clues to diseases of almost any

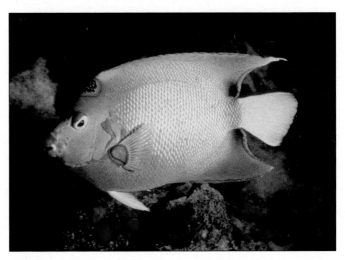

FIGURE 1-1 Queen Angelfish. (*Courtesy of Al Grotel.*)

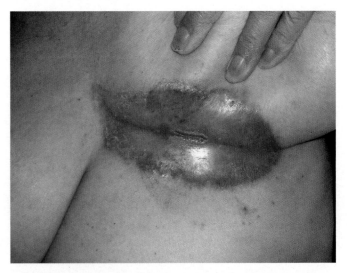

FIGURE 1-2 Inverse psoriasis under the breast that might appear to be a fungal infection to the untrained eye. Note the splinter hemorrhages in the nail of the third digit that provide a clue that the patient has psoriasis. (*Courtesy of Richard P. Usatine, MD.*)

organ system. We use clues such as changes of skin color and areas of body swelling to help us diagnose our patients. Some of the more common changes that we see are erythema, jaundice, edema, joint swelling, petechiae, purpura, purulence, papules, macules, plaques, and ulcers. Use the "Morphology Index for Diagnosis" to help find conditions by the morphological changes that you are observing. (See pages xx–xx)

EXPANDING OUR INTERNAL IMAGE BANKS

The larger our saved image bank in our brain, the better clinicians and diagnosticians we can become. The expert clinician has a large image bank stored in memory to call on for rapid pattern recognition. Our image banks begin to develop in medical school when we view pictures in lectures and textbooks. We then begin to develop our own clinical image bank by our clinical experiences. Our references are printed color atlases and those color atlases available on the Internet and electronically.

Studying and learning the patterns from any atlas can enhance your expertise by enlarging the image bank stored in your memory. An atlas takes the clinical experiences of clinicians over decades and gives it to you as a single compact reference. We offer you, for the first time in the United States, a comprehensive family medicine color atlas including areas, such as oral health, dermatology, podiatry, and the eye.

USING IMAGES TO MAKE A DIAGNOSIS

We all see visible clinical findings on patients that we do not recognize. When this happens, open this book and look for a close match. Use the Appendix, Index, or Table of Contents to direct you to the section with the highest yield photos. If you find a direct match, you may have found the diagnosis. Read the text and see if the history and physical examination match your patient. Perform or order tests to confirm the diagnosis, if needed.

If you cannot find the image in our book try the Internet and the Google search engine. Try a Google image search and follow the leads. Of course this is easiest to do if you have a good differential diagnosis and want to confirm your impression. If you don't have a diagnosis in mind, you may try putting in descriptive words and look for an image that matches what you are seeing. If the Google image search does not work, try a Web search and look at the links for other clues.

Finally, there are dedicated atlases on the Internet for organ system, which can help you find the needed image. Most of these atlases have their own search engines, which can help direct you to the right diagnosis.

Table 1-1 lists some of the best resources currently available online:

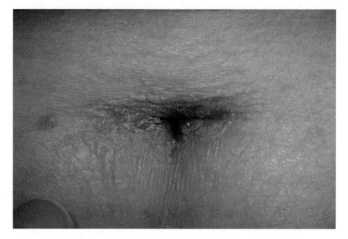

FIGURE 1-3 The patient in **Figure 1-2** with inverse psoriasis had a typical psoriatic plaque in the umbilicus. This was the only other area involved besides the breasts and the nails but easily could have been missed without the knowledge of where to look for the clues needed to make the diagnosis. (*Courtesy of Richard P. Usatine, MD.*)

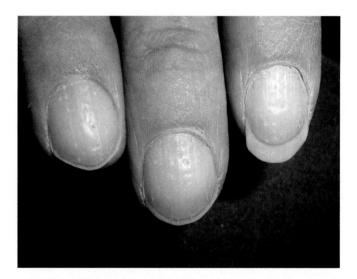

FIGURE 1-4 When the diagnosis of psoriasis is being considered, look at the nails for pitting or other nail changes such as splinter hemorrhages, onycholysis, or oil spots. This is a good example of nail pitting in a patient with psoriasis. (*Courtesy of Richard P. Usatine, MD.*)

TABLE 1-1 Best Free Clinical Image Collections on the Internet

DermAtlas	www.dermatlas.org/	Johns Hopkins University
DermIS	www.dermis.net	Derm Information Systems from Germany
Dermnet	www.dermnet.com/	Skin Disease Image Atlas
Interactive Derm Atlas	www.dermatlas.net/	From Richard P. Usatine, MD
ENT	www.entusa.com	From an ENT physician
Eye	www.eyerounds.org	From University of Iowa
Infectious Diseases	www.phil.cdc.gov/	CDC Public Health Image Library
VisualDxHealth	www.visualdxhealth.com/	From Logical Images

USING IMAGES TO BUILD TRUST IN THE PATIENT—PHYSICIAN RELATIONSHIP

If you are seeing a patient with a mysterious illness that remains undiagnosed and you figure out the diagnosis, you can often bridge the issue of mistrust and anxiety by showing the patient the picture of another person with the diagnosis. Use our atlas for that purpose and supplement this with the Internet. This is especially important for a patient who has gone undiagnosed or misdiagnosed for some time. "Seeing is believing" for many patients. Ask first if they would want to see some pictures of other persons with a similar condition and most will be very interested. The patient can see the similarities between their condition and the other images and feel reassured that your diagnosis is correct. Write down the name of the diagnosis for your patient and use your patient education skills.

Do be careful when searching for images on the Web in front of patients. Sometimes what pops up is not "pretty" (or for that matter G or PG rated). I turn the screen away from the patients before initiating the search and then screen out what I will show them.

If you teach, model this behavior in front of your students. Show them how reference books and the Internet at the point of care can help with the care of patients.

TAKING YOUR OWN PHOTOGRAPHS

Images taken by you with your own camera of your own patients complete with their own stories are more likely to be retained and retrievable in your memory because they have a context and a story to go with them. We encourage our readers to use a digital camera and consider taking your own photos. Of course, always ask permission before taking any photograph of a patient. Explain how the photographs can be used to teach other doctors and to create a record of the patient's condition at this point in time. If the photograph will be identifiable, ask for written consent; for patients under age 18, ask the parent to sign. Store the photos in a manner that avoids any HIPAA privacy violations such as on a secure server or on your own computer with password protection and data encryption. These photographs can directly benefit the patient, for example, when following nevi for changes.

Digital photography is a wonderful method for practicing, teaching, and learning medicine. You can show patients pictures of conditions on parts of their bodies that they could not see without multiple mirrors and some unusual body contortions. You can also use the zoom view feature on the camera to view or show a segment of the image in greater detail. Children generally love to have their photos taken and will be delighted to see themselves on the screen of your camera.

The advent of digital photography makes the recording of photographic images less expensive, easier to do, and easier to maintain. Also, digital photography gives you immediate feedback and a sense of immediate gratification. No longer do you have to wait for a roll of film to be completed and processed before finding out the results of your photography. Not only does this give you immediate gratification to see your image displayed instantaneously in the camera, but also alerts you to poor-quality photographs that can be repeated while the patient is still in the office. This speeds up the learning curve of the beginning photographer in a way that could not happen with film photography.

OUR GOALS

Many of the images in this atlas are my collected works over the past 23 years of my practice in family medicine. My patients have generously allowed me to photograph them so that their photographs would help the physicians and patients of the future. To these photos, we have added images that represent decades of experiences by other family physicians and specialists. Family physicians who have submitted their images to Photo Rounds in the *Journal of Family Practice* are also sharing their photos with you. Finally, 8 years of providing students with cameras during their Family Medicine clerkships at UCLA and UTHSCSA has allowed our students to add their experiences to our atlas.

It is the goal of this atlas to provide you with a wide range of images of common and uncommon conditions and provide you with the knowledge you need to make the diagnosis and initiate treatment. We want to help you be the best diagnostician you can be. We may aspire to be a clinician like Sir William Osler and have the detective acumen of Sherlock Holmes. The images collected for this atlas can help move you in that direction by making you prepared to see what you need to see.

PART 2

THE ESSENCE OF FAMILY MEDICINE

2 PATIENT—PHYSICIAN RELATIONSHIP

Mindy A. Smith, MD, MS

Humor is one way through which patients and physicians relate to each other on a human level. Even politics is not off-limits in the patient–physician relationship.

PATIENT STORY

Patient stories, particularly if we listen attentively and nonjudgmentally, provide us with a window into their lives and experiences. These stories help us to know our patients in powerful ways and that knowledge about the patient, as someone special, provides the context, meaning, and clues about their symptoms and illnesses that can lead to healing. At our best, we serve as witness to their struggles and triumphs, supporter of their efforts to change and grow, and guide through the medical maze of diagnostic and therapeutic options. And sometimes, their stories become our own stories—those patients who we will never forget because their stories have changed our lives and the way we practice medicine (**Figure 2-1**).

WHAT PATIENTS WANT FROM THEIR PHYSICIAN

As part of the future of family medicine (FFM) initiative, telephone interviews of the general public ($N = 1,031$) were conducted in 2002.[1] Most patients strongly agreed that they wanted to take an active role in their health care (82% and 91%, patients with family physicians and patients with general internists, respectively), they wanted their physicians to treat a wide variety of medical problems but refer to a specialist when necessary (88% and 84%), and they wanted a physician who looks at the whole person—emotional, psychological, and physical (73% and 74%). In addition, of 39 possible attributes of physicians, most patients (68%–97% stated extremely or very important) viewed the following as the most important attributes/services that drive overall satisfaction with their physician:

- Does not judge; understands and supports.
- Always honest, direct.
- Acts as partner in maintaining health.
- Treats both serious and nonserious conditions.
- Attends to emotional and physical health.
- Listens to me.
- Encourages healthier lifestyle.
- Tries to get to know me.
- Can help with any problem.
- Someone I can stay with as I get older.

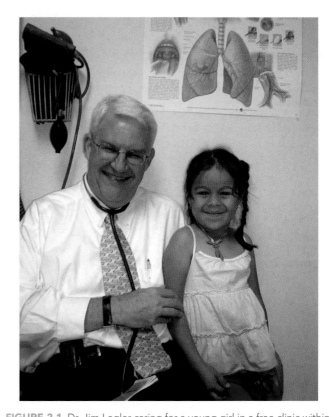

FIGURE 2-1 Dr. Jim Legler caring for a young girl in a free clinic within a transitional housing village for homeless families. He is a family physician who volunteers every week to care for the 40 families working their way out of homelessness. He has been caring for Kimberly and her family for many months at the time this photograph was taken. Dr. Legler serves as a role model for students interested in primary care of the underserved. He is known for his kindness and compassion to all his patients.

WHAT PHYSICIANS WANT FROM AND FOR PATIENTS

Although the types and intensity of relationships with patients differ, our positive and negative experiences with patients shape us as clinicians, influence us in our personal relationships, and shape the character of our practices. Arthur Kleinman, in his prologue to *Patients and Doctors: Life-Changing Stories from Primary Care*, wrote, "We all seem to want (or demand) experiences that matter, but maybe what is foremost is that we want experiences in which *we* matter." There is perhaps no greater satisfaction than the beliefs that what we do and who we are matters to those we care for in both our personal and professional lives.[2] A positive relationship with a patient then is one of mutual growth. This concept of physician–patient reciprocity is not a new one and can be found in the writings of Erasmus over 500 years ago, arising from a classical conception of friendship.[3]

As clinicians we want patients to be healthier, and improved in some meaningful way after our encounter with them. Meaningful elements common to healing practices across cultures include[4]

- Providing a meaningful explanation for the sickness.
- Expressing care and concern.
- Offering the possibility of mastery and control over the illness or its symptoms.

Family physicians ($N = 300$) who were interviewed as part of the FFM initiative stated that the following things completely captured the essence of what they found as most satisfying about being a family physician[1]:

- The deep relationships developed with patients over the years (54%).
- The variety—no day is ever the same (54%).
- Offers me a strong sense of purpose because I can make a real difference in people's lives (48%).
- Don't spend their days taking care of illness, but take care of the whole patient (**Figure 2-2**) (46%).

LEARNING FROM PATIENTS

In order to learn from patients, clinicians must

- Move outside of their worldview and accept the patient's point of view and belief system.
- Let go of stereotypes, biases, and dogma.
- Use active empathic listening, see the patient in context, and adopt reflective and reflexive practice.[5]
- Emphasize patient dignity and control within a supportive team, which may include family, friends, aids, and community resources.
- Graciously accept differences of opinion or patient refusal without abandoning the patient.
- Look at each patient encounter as a cross-cultural event.[4] Western medical training acculturates clinicians into a world seen in large part as one of problems and solutions; this is often at odds with patients' needs to find meaning in the illness episode, be heard and acknowledged, and learn to live a quality life with chronic illness.

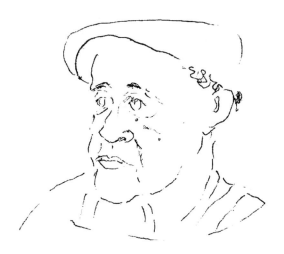

FIGURE 2-2 Dr. Alan Blum is a family physician who has been doing sketches of his patients for decades now. When he presents his drawings of his patients, he reads his poetic stories that go with the drawings. Some of his drawings have been published in *JAMA*. Here is the poem that goes with this man's story:

"Gov'ment gave me a chance
to get a hearin' aid for free.
But when I went to th' doctor,
he say,
'Well, cap'n,
there gonna be a lot o' things
you don't want to hear!'"

BENEFITS OF A GOOD PATIENT–PHYSICIAN RELATIONSHIP

Beyond the benefit of enhancing the medical experience for both clinicians and patients, data that support developing a good patient–physician relationship include the following:

- Patients who are satisfied with their physicians are three times more likely to follow a prescribed medical regimen.[6]

- There is a direct link between patient satisfaction and the amount of information that physicians provide.[7]

- Provision of health information to patients influences patient decision-making in important ways.

ESSENTIALS OF GOOD PATIENT–PHYSICIAN RELATIONSHIP

Although the patient–physician relationship may be viewed as a contract for providing services, Dr. Candib argues that this view does not fit well with developing healing relationship that must be based on "unconditional positive regard," beneficence, caring, and a moral basis of conduct.[8] Further, contracts fail to deal with the unpredictable and fail to acknowledge the power inequality between physicians and patients. To counter this power imbalance, Candib emphasizes the need for clinicians to use that power to empower the patient. Following are the requirements of empowerment of patients[9]:

- Recognition of oppression—acknowledging the patient's contextual problems (e.g., poverty, race, religion, sexual preference) and the sources of inequality and oppression that contribute to their health status for the purpose of naming and supporting the patient's reality.

- Expressing empathy—a characteristic of being with the patient that leads to empowerment by confirming the worthiness of the other.

- Respecting the patient as a person (particularly those who are cognitively or otherwise impaired).

- Responding to the changing abilities of the patient—using flexibility, timing, and a shifting of skills to advance the movement of the patient in a positive stronger direction.

- Using language that increases patient's power—solicit and legitimize the patient's explanations and experience. This may include using questions about what patients want from the encounter, what they think about their problem, what they think the clinician should do about the problem, and what they have tried that has worked for them in the past.

- Taking the patient seriously—this includes respecting the patients' fears, not trivializing their concerns, and allowing the truth to unfold over time to prevent patient harm or embarrassment.

- Supporting choice and control—accepting patient priorities, even if health is not the top one, and allowing patients to choose, even if their choice is to relinquish control.

- Eliciting the patient's story, often over time, to be able to put the illness experience into historical and social context.

- Providing patient education in a context in which the clinician asks what the patient already knows, what they want and need to know, and whether they have any questions. Health educators should discuss risks and benefits of a proposed diagnostic or treatment plan that are meaningful to the patient and provide patients with the tools and information to make their own decisions.

Some patients prefer to delegate authority to the physician to make medical decisions—the challenge then is for the physician to find out the patient's preferences.

Caring is also an essential feature of a good patient–physician relationship. Caring, as connectedness with a patient, evolves from the relationship. Within the context of this relationship, the clinician makes the patient feel known, pays attention to the meaning that a symptom or illness has in the patient's life, expresses real feeling (separate from reflecting back the patient's feelings), and practices devotion (e.g., a willingness at times to do something extra for the patient).[10] To provide caring to patients, clinicians must take care of themselves.

SKILLS FOR BUILDING GOOD PATIENT–PHYSICIAN RELATIONSHIPS

- One strategy for improving communication with patients is the use of the patient-centered interview.[11] This technique focuses on eliciting the patient's agenda in order to address their concerns more promptly.

- Use of self-disclosure for the purposes of role modeling and guiding, showing empathy, building trust, and developing a stronger relationship in the context of shared assumptions about the relationship. Self-disclosure, however, must be balanced with the obligation not to take advantage of patients by using such disclosure as an appeal for help or intimacy.[12] In addition, it may be prudent to avoid disclosure of unresolved issues and to avoid repetitiousness (as when disclosure predominates over inquiry).

MAXIMIZING THE EFFECTIVENESS OF PATIENT EDUCATION

Steps for maximizing patient education for behavior change[13]:

- Understanding the power of the clinician's expertise as a motivator toward behavior change.

- Being patient centered and patient responsive (e.g., assess readiness to change, patient wishes for autonomy or assistance in decision making).

- Encouraging the patient to choose one or at most two behavior goals at a time.

- Being specific in the advice given.

- Obtaining commitment from the patient for change.

- Using multiple educational strategies often over time and from a team of providers.

- Using social support when possible.
- Assuring appropriate follow-up.

Some guidance can be found in the literature for discussing clinical evidence with patients in the process of making medical decisions. Despite lack of clinical outcomes from this research, authors of a systematic review found the following[14]:

- Methods for communicating clinical evidence to patients include nonquantitative general terms, numerical translation of clinical evidence, graphical representations, and decision making aids.
- Focus-group data suggested that clinicians present options and/or equipoise before asking patients about preferred decision-making roles or formats for information.
- Absolute risk reduction is preferred.
- The order of information presented and time frame of outcomes can bias patient understanding.
- Limited evidence supports use of human stick figure graphics or faces for single probabilities and vertical bar graphs for comparative information.
- Less-educated and older patients preferred proportions to percentages and did not appreciate confidence intervals.

PROVIDER RESOURCES

- Borkan J, Reis S, Steinmetz D, Medalie JH, eds. *Patients and Doctors: Life-Changing Stories from Primary Care*. Madison, WI: University of Wisconsin Press, 1999.
- Candib LM. *Medicine and the Family—A Feminist Perspective*. New York: Basicbooks, 1995.

REFERENCES

1. www.futurefamilymed.org/x14818.html. Accessed December 6, 2008.
2. Kleinman A. Prologue. In: Borkan J, Reis S, Steinmetz D, Medalie JH, eds. *Patients and Doctors: Life-Changing Stories from Primary Care*. Madison, WI: University of Wisconsin Press, 1999:ix.
3. Albury WR, Weisz GM. The medical ethics of Erasmus and the physician—patient relationship. *Med Humanit*. 2001;27(1):35–41.
4. Brody H. Family and community—reflections. In: Borkan J, Reis S, Steinmetz D, Medalie JH, eds. *Patients and Doctors: Life-Changing Stories from Primary Care*. Madison, WI: University of Wisconsin Press, 1999:67–72.
5. Medalie JH. Leaning from patients—reflections. In: Borkan J, Reis S, Steinmetz D, Medalie JH, eds. *Patients and Doctors: Life-changing Stories from Primary Care*. Madison, WI: University of Wisconsin Press, 1999:50.
6. Rosenberg EE, Lussier MT, Beaudoin C. Lessons for clinicians from physician-patient communication literature. *Arch Fam Med*. 1997;6:279–283.
7. Blanchard CG, Labrecque MS, Ruckdeschel JC, Blanchard EB. Physician behaviors, patient perceptions, and patient characteristics as predictors of satisfaction of hospitalized adult cancer patients. *Cancer*. 1991;65:186–192. Hall JA, Roter KL, Katz NR. Meta-analysis of correlates of provider behavior in medical encounters. *Med Care*. 1988;26:657–675.
8. Candib LM. *Medicine and the Family—A Feminist Perspective*. New York: Basicbooks, 1995:119–145.
9. Candib LM. *Medicine and the Family—A Feminist Perspective*. New York: Basicbooks, 1995:246–273.
10. Candib LM. *Medicine and the Family—A Feminist Perspective*. New York: Basicbooks, 1995:206–239.
11. Brown J, Stewart M, McCracken E, et al. The patient-centered clinical method. 2. Definition and application. *Family Practice*. 1986;3:75–79.
12. Candib LM. *Medicine and the Family—A Feminist Perspective*. New York: Basicbooks, 1995:181–205.
13. Jaques LB, Curtis P, Goldstein AO. Helping your patients stay healthy. In: Sloane PD, Slatt LM, Ebell MH, Jacques LB, eds. *Essentials of Family Medicine*. Baltimore, MD: Lippincott Williams & Wilkins, 2002:117–125.
14. Epstein RM, Alper BS, Quill TE. Communicating evidence for participatory decision making. *JAMA*. 2004;291(19):2359–2366.

3 FAMILY PLANNING

E.J. Mayeaux, Jr., MD

PATIENT STORY

Your patient is a 25-year-old married woman who wants to postpone having children for another 2 years while she finishes graduate school. She and her husband are currently using condoms, but would like to change to something different. She is in good health and does not smoke. It is now your opportunity to discuss with her about all the available methods to prevent pregnancy. First, you determine what she knows about the methods and if she has any preferences. She tells you that she is specifically interested in either the *hormonal vaginal ring* (NuvaRing) (**Figure 3-1**) or the newest *intrauterine device* that releases a hormone (**Figure 3-2**). Then you participate in shared decision making as she comes up with the method that best fits her lifestyle and health issues.

EPIDEMIOLOGY

- Approximately one-half of pregnancies in the United States are unintended.[1] Although some methods of contraception have side effects, morbidity and mortality rates are significantly higher for pregnancy and childbirth than for the use of any contraceptive method alone.[2]

- The most commonly used contraceptive methods in the United States are oral contraceptive pills (OCPs), male condoms, and female sterilization.[3]

- In addition to the desire to become pregnant, women stop using contraception because of the side effects, difficulty of use, safety concerns, and lack of access to health care.

- Newer contraceptives often have improved side effect profiles or have more convenient delivery systems that may not require daily patient adherence. Having a wide range of contraceptive options helps patients find a method that will work best for them.

- This chapter focuses on newer contraceptive methods available in the United States.

CONSIDERATIONS

- No contraception method is perfect. Each individual or couple must balance the advantages and disadvantages of each method and decide which offers the best choice. See **Table 3-1**.

- One important consideration in choosing a contraceptive method is its potential to prevent sexually transmitted diseases (STDs). Combining more effective contraception with condoms, which protect against STDs, is a good choice for many patients.

- Smoking increases the risks of the most dangerous side effects of estrogen-containing contraceptives. This is an important issue in helping a patient choose the safest and the best method. Encouraging smoking cessation is always a good intervention but one might

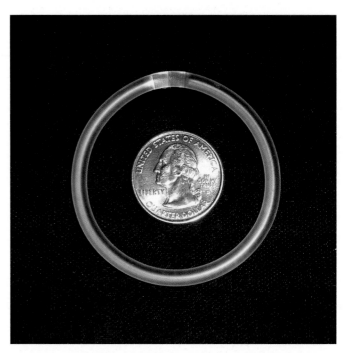

FIGURE 3-1 NuvaRing is a combined hormonal intravaginal contraceptive ring. The flexible material of the ring allows for easy insertion and removal. Note the size in comparison to a quarter. (*Courtesy of Richard P. Usatine, MD.*)

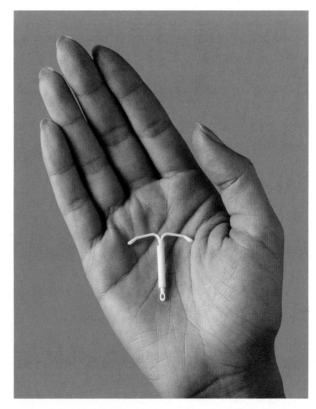

FIGURE 3-2 Mirena (levonorgestrel-releasing intrauterine system) provides effective contraception for at least 5 years. (*Printed with Permission from Bayer HealthCare Pharmaceuticals Inc.*)

TABLE 3-1 Contraceptive Options Available in the United States in 2008

| Method | Unintended Pregnancies with 1 Year of Use (%) | | Frequency of Use | Use with Breast-Feeding |
	Typical Use	Theoretical		
None	85	85	—	—
Spermicide	29	18	Each time	Yes
Withdrawal	27	4	Each time	Yes
Periodic abstinence (fertility awareness)	25	3–5	Each time	Yes
Diaphragm with spermicide	16	6	Each time	Yes
Female condom	21	5	Each time	Yes
Male condom	15	2	Each time	Yes
OCPs–combined & progestin-only	8	0.3	Taken daily	No
Contraceptive patch	8	0.3	Applied weekly	No
Vaginal ring	8	0.3	Inserted Q4 weeks	No
Depo-provera	3	0.3	Injected Q3 months	Yes
Copper-containing IUD	0.8	0.6	Inserted Q10 years	Yes
Levonorgestrel IUD	0.2	0.2	Inserted Q5 years	Yes
Female sterilization	0.5	0.5	Once	Yes
Male sterilization	0.15	0.10	Once	Yes
Etonogestrel implant	0.05	0.05	Inserted Q3 years	Safety conditional

OCP, oral contraceptive pill; IUD, intrauterine device.
Data from Trussell J. Contraceptive efficacy, In Hatcher RA, Trussell J, Nelson AL, Cates W, Stewart FH, Kowal D. *Contraceptive Technology: Nineteenth Revised Edition.* New York NY: Ardent Media, 2007. Herndon EJ, Zieman M. New contraceptive options. *Am Fam Physician* 2004;69:853–860; Herndon EJ, Zieman M. *Improving Access to Quality Care in Family Planning: Medical Eligibility Criteria for Contraceptive Use,* 2nd ed. Geneva: Reproductive Health and Research, World Health Organization, 2000. Available at: http://whqlibdoc.who.int/publications/2004/9241562668.pdf (accessed July 4, 2006).

avoid prescribing an estrogen-containing contraceptive until the patient can truly quit smoking.

- Avoid estrogen containing contraceptives in women with hypertension or migraine and aura. In both cases, the theoretical or proven risk of stroke outweigh the advantages.

NEW CONTRACEPTIVE CHOICES

- In addition to the traditional 20–35 mcg ethinyl estradiol (EE) OCPs, 30 and 20 mcg EE in combination with the new progestogen *drospirenone* (Yasmin, YAZ) are available. Drospirenone has some antimineralocorticoid activity and has been shown to decrease the water retention, negative effect, and appetite changes that are commonly associated with menstrual cycle changes.[4] Serum potassium levels should be monitored when women are at a risk for hyperkalemia. The progesterone in these pills often helps in decreasing the severity of acne.

- *Extended OCP* regimens with 84 days of levonorgestrel-ethinyl estradiol pills and 7 days of nonhormonal pills (Seasonale) are available. Seasonique has the same pills for the first 84 days but uses 10 mcg ethinyl estradiol pills for the last 7 days to make up the 91 day cycle. They have similar advantages to other OCPs except that the patient has only four periods a year. Another extended OCP regimen combining levonorgestrel and ehinyl estradiol has been released in which there are no nonhormonal pills at all (Lybrel).

- The *hormonal vaginal ring* (NuvaRing) has similar active ingredients of OCPs, but does not require daily attention (**Figure 3-1**). It is placed in the vagina for 3 weeks at a time (with 1 week off) and releases ethinyl estradiol and etonogestrel. Withdrawal bleeding occurs during the ring-free week. The vaginal ring is associated with a lower incidence of breakthrough bleeding than standard OCPs.

- There is a newer form of Depo-Provera given every 3 months, but give SQ instead of IM. The SQ version provides 30% less hormone, 104 versus 150 mg per injection. It works at least as well as Depo-Provera IM does as a contraceptive, and also works as well as Lupron Depot for endometriosis pain with fewer hot flashes and less bone loss. If long term use is considered, it may be prudent to select another contraceptive, discuss the risk of possible bone loss, or consider monitoring bone density in women using either version of Depo-Provera for more than 2 years. These medications can increase the incidence of acne and weight gain in some women as a result of the androgenic effects of the progesterone.

- The newest *intrauterine device* releases levonorgestrel (Mirena) and provides effective contraception for at least 5 years (**Figure 3-2**). Pregnancy rates are comparable with those occurring with surgical sterilization. While copper-containing IUDs may increase dysmenorrhea, the levonorgestrel system usually decreases painful periods. Twenty percent of women have amenorrhea after 1 year of use, and as with the copper-containing IUDs, there is a risk of expulsion. The absolute risk of ectopic pregnancy with IUP use is extremely low due to the high effectiveness of IUDs. However, if a woman becomes pregnant during IUD use, the relative likelihood of ectopic pregnancy is greatly increased.[5]

- Implanon (etonogestrel implant) is an *etonogestrel-containing single rod implant* for subdermal use (**Figure 3-3**). It is a long-acting (up to 3 years), reversible, contraceptive method. It must be removed or replaced by the end of the third year. The implant is 4 cm in length with a diameter of 2 mm and contains 68 mg of the synthetic progestin etonogestrel (ENG). It does not contain estrogen or latex and is not radiopaque. The contraceptive effect of the etonogestrel implant involves suppression of ovulation, increased viscosity of the cervical mucus, and alterations in the endometrium. The effectiveness of Implanon in women who weigh more than 130% of their ideal body weight has not been studied. Because ENG is metabolized by the liver, its use in patients with active liver disease is contraindicated. It should not be used in women with any history of thrombosis or thromboembolic disorders, undiagnosed abnormal genital bleeding, or suspected carcinoma of the breast. Other problems are similar to other progestin-only contraceptives (acne and gaining weight).

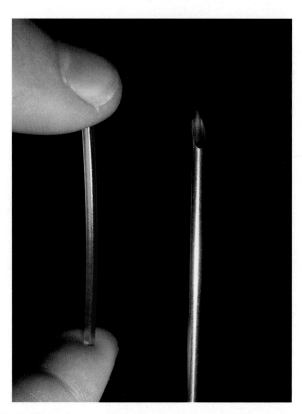

FIGURE 3-3 Implanon implantable subcutaneous contraceptive system. Note the insertion device is a sharp trochar and the implant is made of a soft silastic tube. The actual implant is white and the practice implant is blue. (*Courtesy of Richard P. Usatine, MD.*)

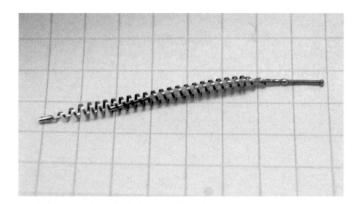

FIGURE 3-4 Essure tubal occlusion device for permanent sterilization. It is placed within the fallopian tubes using a vaginal approach and a hysteroscope. (*Courtesy of Jay Berman, MD.*)

- Sterilization is a common and very effective form of contraception that should be considered permanent.

- Hysteroscopic tubal occlusion (Essure) is a newer technique (**Figures 3-4** to **3-6**). The device is a flexible microcoil designed to promote tissue growth in the fallopian tubes. It does not require any incisions and can be performed without general anesthesia, typically in less than 30 minutes. There is a 3-month waiting period after the device is placed when an alternative birth control must be used. At the 3-month follow-up visit, a hysterosalpingogram is performed to document that the tubes have been blocked.

- The *combination contraceptive patch* (Ortho Evra) releases ethinyl estradiol and norelgestromin and has the same mechanism of action as OCPs (**Figure 3-7**). It is applied weekly for 3 weeks, followed by a patch-free week during which menses occur. Recommended application sites include the upper arm, buttocks, and torso (excluding the back and breasts). It has similar efficacy to OCPs but may be less effective in women weighing more than 90 kg (198 lb). In a rare instance of patch detachment, it must be replaced. The progesterone in the patch may decrease the severity of acne.

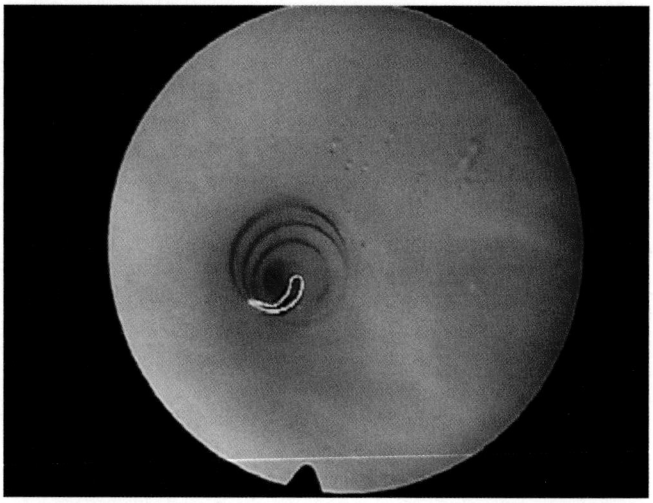

PATIENT EDUCATION

For some contraceptive methods to be effective, the patient must be willing to use them consistently and correctly. Other methods do not require any action on the part of the patient. Patients will need to understand the benefits and risks of the method they choose and how to be best assure that the method is working for them. If patients are aware of the possible side effects, they can address any such effect with their physician if an adverse effect occurs.

FOLLOW-UP

Monitor for side effects, level of usage, and tolerability. The contraceptive choice should be periodically reexamined since the patient may want to switch to a different method of contraception as needs and circumstances change.

PATIENT RESOURCES

- Managing Contraception website has a choices section that is good for patients, **http://managingcontraception.com/**.
- ACOG Patient Resources, **http://www.medem.com/MedLB/article_detaillb.cfm?article_ID=ZZZ48OI527C&sub_cat=5.**
- NuvaRing Web site, **http://www.nuvaring.com/**.
- Mirena Web site, **http://www.mirena-us.com/**.
- Essure Web site, **http://www.essure.com/**.
- Implanon Web site, **http://www.implanon.com/**.

FIGURE 3-5 Hysteroscopic view showing the coiled Essure device within a fallopian tubes immediately after it was implanted. (*Courtesy of Jay Berman, MD.*)

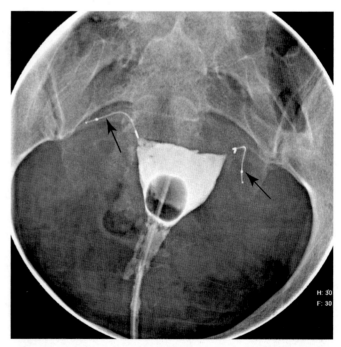

FIGURE 3-6 Hysterosalpingogram (HSG) with bilateral Essure devices within the fallopian tubes (arrows). Contrast material distends the uterine cavity but does not enter the cornua, fallopian tubes or peritoneal cavity, indicating successful occlusion. The black/grey bubble in the white-appearing uterus is the HSG catheter balloon. (*Courtesy of Samuel Johnson, MD.*)

PROVIDER RESOURCES

- Contraceptive Technology Table of Contraceptive Efficacy: **http://www.contraceptivetechnology.org/table.html.**

- USFDA, **http://www.fda.gov/fdac/features/1997/ babytabl.html.**

- Am Fam Physician New Contraceptive Options, **http://www.aafp.org/afp/20040215/853.html.**

- Medical Eligibility Criteria for Contraceptive Use. Third edition — 2004 from the World Health Organization. Available at: **http://www.who.int/reproductive-health/ publications/mec/.**

- Contraception On-line, **http://www.contraceptiononline. org/** includes patient handouts and PowerPoint presentations and clinical cases for providers.

REFERENCES

1. Henshaw SK. Unintended pregnancy in the United States. *Fam Plann Perspect.* 1998;30:24–29, 46.

2. Kost K, Forrest JD, Harlap S. Comparing the health risks and benefits of contraceptive choices. *Fam Plann Perspect.* 1991;23:54–61.

3. Piccinino LJ, Mosher WD. Trends in contraceptive use in the United States: 1982–1995. *Fam Plann Perspect.* 1998;30:4–10, 46.

4. Herndon EJ, Zieman M. New contraceptive options. *Am Fam Physician.* 2004;69:853–860.

5. Medical Eligibility Criteria for Contraceptive Use. Third edition —2004 from the World Health Organization. Available at: http://www.who.int/reproductive-health/publications/mec/ Accessed June 5, 2008.

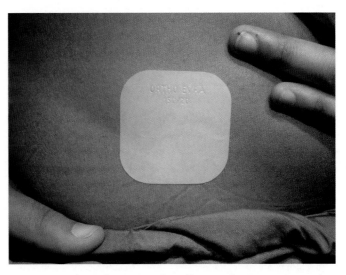

FIGURE 3-7 The Ortho Evra combined hormonal contraceptive patch. The patch is changed weekly for 3 weeks then left off for 1 week per cycle. (*Courtesy of E.J. Mayeaux, Jr., MD.*)

4 PREGNANCY AND BIRTH

Mindy A. Smith, MD, MS
Beth Choby, MD
Leslie Shimp, PharmD, MS

PATIENT STORY

As a longtime pregnancy care provider, it was difficult to choose a single story as representative of pregnancy and birth. Most of the stories are meaningful because of the context of the relationship with the woman and the family, a few are tragic and yet filled with grace and the amazing strength displayed by even the very young, some are truly epic tales, and all are learning opportunities. Pregnancy experiences are filled with consternation at the myriad of changes, discomforts, and worries. They are filled with laughter as women's bodies alter in amazing ways; we waddle, unconsciously rest plates on our bellies, and lose sight of our feet (**Figure 4-1**). Our partners and/or supportive others alternate between reassurance and befuddlement. And then a child appears, miraculously from a space that seems far too small to accommodate, and (regardless of the outcome) a new journey begins.

EPIDEMIOLOGY

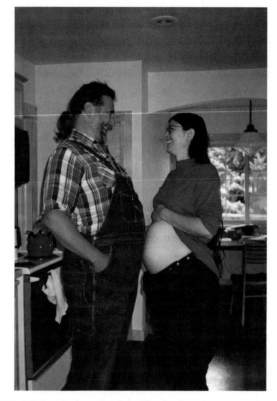

FIGURE 4-1 Dr. Mindy A. Smith and her husband, Gary, touching bellies during Mindy's pregnancy with Jenny.

- Planned pregnancy—Approximately 85% of sexually active women not using a contraceptive method will become pregnant over the course of a year. The probability of conception is 15% to 33% per cycle, depending upon the frequency of sexual intercourse.[1]
- Unplanned pregnancy—Half of all pregnancies in the United States are unintended.[2]
  - Unintended pregnancy (defined as a pregnancy mistimed or not wanted at the time conception occurred) is the result of lack of use of a contraceptive or failure of the contraceptive.
  - Unintended pregnancy occurs among women of all ages, socioeconomic status, and marital status. While unintended pregnancies are often associated with teens, 41% of pregnancies among women 35 to 39 years of age and 51% of those among women older than 40 years are unintended.[3]
  - Some unintended pregnancies end in abortions. A total of 1.29 million legally induced abortions occurred in the United States in 2002 (16 per 1000 women aged 15–44 years).[4]

    The highest percentages of reported abortions were for women who were unmarried (82%), white (55%), and aged <25 years (51%). Of all abortions for which gestational age was reported, 60% were performed at ≤8 weeks' gestation.[4]

- Maternal mortality—In the 1990s, 11.8 per 100,000 U.S. women died annually of pregnancy-related causes.[5] The leading causes of pregnancy-related death were embolism (20%), hemorrhage (17%), and pregnancy-induced hypertension (16%). Major racial disparities continue to exist.
  - Maternal mortality in African American women is 12 per 100,000 compared with 8.1 per 100,000 in whites. African

American women have three to four times the risk of pregnancy-related death compared to whites.

- Care delivery by family physicians—Twenty four percent of family physicians perform deliveries as a regular part of their practice, 18% perform vacuum extraction, 6.4% do forceps deliveries, 6.5% offer trial of labor after cesarean delivery, and 4.3% perform cesarean deliveries (up to 27% in some rural areas) (**Figure 4-2**).[6]

- Care outcomes by family physicians—Numerous studies were conducted during the mid-1980s to mid-1990s comparing outcomes between family physicians and obstetricians, primarily for comparable patients at low maternal risk (although proportions of high-risk patients are frequently similar across disciplines). Findings were consistent in demonstrating no differences in neonatal outcomes with fewer interventions (e.g., induction, augmentation, episiotomy, forceps)[7–9] and fewer births by cesarean section. In the later two studies, cesarean section rates were 15.4% for family physicians compared with 26.5% for obstetricians[8] and 9.3% for family physicians compared with 16% for obstetricians.[9]

ETIOLOGY AND PATHOPHYSIOLOGY

- The most fertile period for women is the several days prior to ovulation and ends 24 hours after ovulation.[10] The ovum is able to be fertilized for only 12 to 24 hours after ovulation.[10]

- Sperm usually remain viable for 3 days after intercourse.

- Once the egg is fertilized, it is transported to the uterine cavity in approximately 2 to 3 days. Implantation occurs approximately 6 to 7 days after fertilization following cell division that forms a blastocyst.[10]

- Pregnancy is defined by the National Institutes of Health, the American College of Obstetricians and Gynecologists, and the Food and Drug Administration as implantation of the blastocyst in the endometrium.[11]

- The precise cause of labor is not known but the physiologic changes prior to labor onset include decreased placental progesterone secretion and stimulation of prostaglandin production (E_2 and $F_{2\alpha}$) from the decidua, uterine endometrium, and fetal membranes.

- Labor is defined as progressive dilation of the cervix with uterine contractions. Bloody show (blood-tinged mucous from the vagina), indicating extrusion of the mucus plug, is helpful in predicting impending labor onset.

DIAGNOSIS

A detailed menstrual history should be obtained with one goal of accurately determining the first day of the most recent menstrual cycle. This date is traditionally used to calculate the estimated date of delivery (EDD) by using Naegele's rule (EDD = [first day of last menstrual period minus 3 months] plus 7 days). The rule is most useful in women who have regular 28-day cycles followed by an abrupt cessation of menses.

CLINICAL FEATURES

- Common early symptoms include amenorrhea, nausea, fatigue, and breast tenderness.

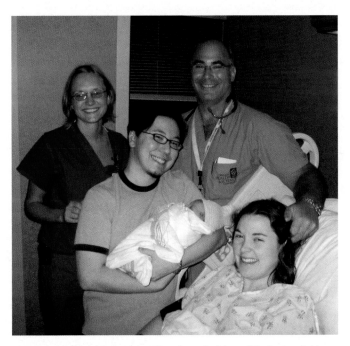

FIGURE 4-2 Family physicians Drs. Scott Fields and Katherine Schlessman have just delivered Jennifer Kam's baby. Dr. Fields knows Jennifer (Dr. John Saultz's daughter—Oregon's Chair of Family Medicine) since she was 6 years old. This is a happy event for all.

- Signs of pregnancy include the following:
  - Alterations in the skin (e.g, a hyperpigmented streak appearing below the umbilicus [linea nigra] and a reddish hyperpigmentation over the bridge of the nose and cheeks [chloasma]) (**Figure 4-3**).
  - Alterations in the vulva, vagina, and cervix (i.e., bluish discoloration [Chadwick's sign] caused by vascular engorgement of the pelvic organs and softening of the cervix [Hegar's sign]).

LABORATORY

- Pregnancy tests are an accurate marker for pregnancy and use urine (qualitative) or serum (quantitative) to check for beta human chorionic gonadotropin (B-HCG).
  - Urine tests are generally positive around the time of the first missed period. B-HCG concentrations in the range of 25 to 50 mIU/mL are detectable in qualitative urine samples.
  - Home pregnancy test kits detect HCG in the urine. HCG is detectable within 1 to 2 weeks after fertilization, but a pregnancy cannot be detected prior to implantation. The highest sensitivity (97%) of home pregnancy tests is at 1 week after the first day of the missed period.
  - Serum pregnancy tests detect B-HCG at levels as low as 10 to 15 mIU/mL and mean levels closely correspond with gestational age during the first trimester. In healthy gestations, B-HCG levels double every 1.4 to 2 days, increasing exponentially until the fetus is 8 to 10 weeks old and then declining somewhat and remaining steady throughout the pregnancy. A minimum increase of 66% is expected every 48 hours. An appropriate rise in B-HCG levels on two quantitative (serum) pregnancy tests drawn 48 hours apart is reassuring for normal pregnancy development.

IMAGING

- Transvaginal ultrasound may be used to confirm and date a pregnancy. Sonographic landmarks such as the gestational sac and fetal pole correlate highly with B-HCG levels.
  - The gestational sac is generally seen when the pregnancy is 4.5 to 5 weeks along and the B-HCG level is greater than 1000 mIU/mL.
  - The double decidual sign is the thick, hyperechoic (white) ring that surrounds the gestational sac. The yolk sac is the early nourishment for the embryo, seen at 6 weeks when HCG levels are greater than 2500 mIU/mL.
  - The fetal pole is seen at 7 weeks gestation with HCG levels more than 5000 mIU/mL.
  - Ultrasound measurements of the gestational sac and the crown to rump length (**Figure 4-4**) of the fetus are a very accurate means of establishing the EDD. First trimester transvaginal ultrasound confirms gestational age within +/− 4 days.

DIFFERENTIAL DIAGNOSIS

The differential diagnosis of pregnancy includes several gynecologic and nongynecologic conditions. Conditions presenting with an enlarged uterus or abdominal mass include the following:

- Uterine leiomyomas are benign tumors that arise from uterine smooth muscle cells. While most women with symptomatic

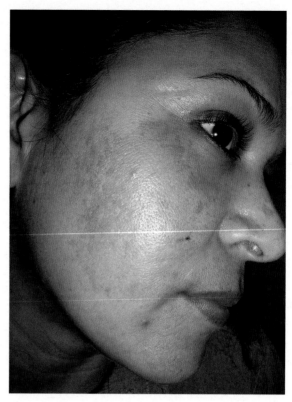

FIGURE 4-3 Chloasma (melasma) in a young woman after having children. This hyperpigmentation over the cheeks and nose is sometimes called the mask of pregnancy. (*Courtesy of Richard P. Usatine, MD.*)

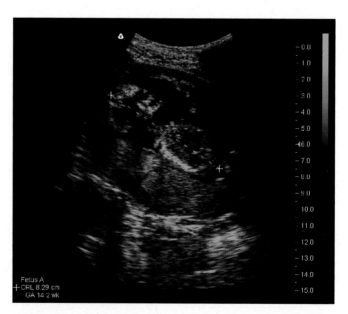

FIGURE 4-4 First trimester ultrasound showing crown to rump length. (*Courtesy of Richard P. Usatine, MD.*)

leiomyomas are in the age range of 30 to 40 years, tumors are occasionally found in adolescents. Myomas occur as single or multiple tumors and range in size from microscopic to large masses. A 20-cm myoma often mimics pregnancy with increased abdominal girth and fullness, but can be distinguished on ultrasound.

- Large adnexal masses and tuboovarian abscesses—The bimanual examination often distinguishes between an adnexal mass and an enlarged uterus. Tuboovarian abscess is associated with cervical motion tenderness and abdominal pain. Both conditions can be further evaluated by transvaginal ultrasonography.

Conditions that can present with amenorrhea include the following:

- Hyperthyroidism—Reproductive symptoms can include hypomenorrhea, irregular menses, infertility, and decreased libido. Graves disease is the most common cause among younger patients and common symptoms are nervousness, fatigue, heat intolerance, and tachycardia. Hyperthyroidism is confirmed by a subnormal or undetectable thyroid-stimulating hormone (TSH) and elevated thyroxine (T_4).

- Sheehan's syndrome is a form of acquired hypopituitarism; pituitary apoplexy (sudden neurologic impairment resulting from cerebrovascular disorder) can occur in the postpartum period and may result in severe hypoglycemia and hypotension. Acute symptoms can include severe headache and bilateral visual changes and long-term symptoms depend on which hormones are lost (i.e., TSH, FSH and luteinizing hormone [LH], prolactin, adrenocorticotroptin hormone [ACTH], and growth hormone [GH]) and the extent of the hormone deficiency. Diagnosis is made with low levels of trophic hormones in conjunction with low levels of target hormones.

- Premature menopause—menopause, defined as permanent amenorrhea in a previously cycling woman—is considered premature when it occurs before the age of 40; approximately 10% of women are menopausal by the age of 46. Vasomotor symptoms (e.g., hot flashes) and menstrual irregularity usually precede cessation of menses, the latter by approximately 4 years. An follicle-stimulating hormone level (FSH) more than 40 mIU/mL helps to confirm, but may drop again if the ovulatory cycles return.

Conditions that can present with symptoms of pregnancy include the following:

- Ectopic pregnancy is an important diagnosis to exclude in women with a positive pregnancy test, abdominal pain, or vaginal bleeding. Transvaginal ultrasound is useful to delineate between intrauterine and ectopic gestations in combination with serial β-HCGs. Heterotopic pregnancies (i.e., concomitant intrauterine and ectopic pregnancies) are seen in 1 out of 30,000 gestations.

- Pseudopregnancy is a psychiatric condition in which a woman thinks she is pregnant when she is actually not. She may have symptoms and behaviors consistent with a diagnosis of pregnancy, including weight gain, abdominal pain, and sensations of fetal movement. Confirmatory labwork is negative, although the woman often cannot be convinced of these results.

MANAGEMENT

- Decision making—Many women and their partners find themselves facing an unplanned pregnancy. Options include continuing the pregnancy and caring for the infant, continuing the pregnancy and placing the infant with an adoptive family, or ending the pregnancy via medical or surgical abortion. Couples need support and information to assist them with this decision.

- Methods to prevent or terminate an unwanted pregnancy include the following:
  - Emergency contraceptives (EC)—two oral methods can be used within 72 hours after unprotected intercourse (or failed contraceptive) to prevent pregnancy. EC, like other hormonal contraceptives, has the potential to inhibit implantation of a fertilized egg.[11] These agents are not abortifacients and prevent pregnancy before implantation occurs. They do not disrupt an already established pregnancy and there are no evidence-based medical contraindications to their use. The agents are most effective when the first dose is taken within 12 hours of unprotected intercourse; each 12-hour delay in beginning use reduces efficacy by 50%.

    The levonorgestrel product Plan B (reduces the likelihood of pregnancy by 89%). Side effects include nausea (approximately 25%) and vomiting (10%). The standard dosing regimen for Plan B is one 0.75 mg tablet as soon as possible within 72 hours of unprotected intercourse followed by a second tablet 12 hours later. It can also be taken as a single dose (1.5 mg).

    Use of OCs containing ethinyl estradiol plus either levonorgestrel or norgestrel (reduces the likelihood of pregnancy by 75%).[8] Approximately 50% of users experience nausea and 20% experience vomiting. Use of oral contraceptives as ECs requires a regimen that includes two doses—one dose taken as soon as possible within 72 hours of unprotected intercourse and the second dose taken 12 hours later. Each dose must include at least 100 mcg of ethinyl estradiol and either 1 mg of norgestrel or 0.5 mg of levonorgestrel.
  - Medical abortion (i.e., use of medications to induce an abortion)—Medical abortions account for 5% to 6% of the abortions performed in the United States.[12] Medical abortion is an option for women who wish to terminate a pregnancy up to 63 days gestation (calculated from the first day of the last menstrual period). The efficacy of the various regimens ranges from 88% to 99%. Regimens including 200 mg of oral mifepristone followed by 800 micrograms of misoprostol vaginally from 6 to 8 hours to 72 hours afterwards been shown to be most effective with fewer side effects and lower cost.[13] SOR Ⓐ Side effects of medical abortion using mifepristone and misoprostol include nausea (20%–52%), thermoregulatory dysfunction (i.e., warmth, fever, chills, hot flash; 9%–56%), dizziness (12%–37%), headache (10%–37%), vomiting (5%–30%), and diarrhea (1%–27%).[13]
  - Surgical (aspiration) abortion—this method can be performed in the office up to 13 weeks gestation and has a rate of major complications of <1 in 200 cases.[4] Other surgical options are available and described elsewhere.[4]

- Pregnancy care—Despite the widespread use of prenatal care, evidence of its effectiveness is limited. Prenatal care offered by family physicians likely benefits both maternal and infant health by encouraging long-term health maintenance within a continuity relationship and increasing the likelihood that those infants receive timely care. Future research must explore whether enhanced prenatal care benefits certain groups of women, i.e., the young, the uninsured, and women in high-risk ethnic groups. Routine visits provide opportunities for screening, management of complications, anticipatory guidance, and educational activities.[14]
  - First trimester care includes a detailed history to identify medical, health habit, and prior pregnancy problems requiring management (e.g., use of safer medications for pregnancy, smoking cessation, prior gestational diabetes).

    An initial pelvic examination is completed to detect anatomic defects of the reproductive tract and to screen for gonorrhea and chlamydia.

    Screening laboratory tests include blood type (D (Rh) factor), hepatitis B surface antigen, VDRL (syphilis), urine culture, and HIV for high-risk women. SOR **A**

    Blood pressure and weight are monitored.

    Folic acid fortified multivitamin supplements once daily are recommended. SOR **A** In a recent meta-analysis, use of multivitamin supplements provided consistent protection against neural tube defects, cardiovascular defects, and limb defects in multiple types of studies, including randomized controlled trials.[15] Folic acid (400–800 mcg/day) ideally should be started in the preconception period and continued during pregnancy.

    Iron supplementation of at least 30 mg of elemental iron is recommended orally daily (may start in the second trimester). SOR **C** Although demonstrated to increase hemoglobin levels in maternal blood in both the antenatal and postnatal periods, there is limited information related to clinical maternal and infant outcomes.[16]

    Common chronic medical conditions that may require treatment modification or more intense monitoring include asthma (e.g., lowest dose of steroids and stress-dose coverage in labor), hypertension (e.g., safer medication such as alpha-methyldopa and consideration of discontinuing diuretics [metabolic abnormalities] and angiotensin-converting enzyme inhibitors [adverse fetal effects]), thyroid disease (e.g., adjust medication), and seizure disorders (e.g., possible teratogenesis of phenytoin, 50% have worsening seizures).
  - Second trimester care includes continued monitoring, support, and education. Women should be queried about new symptoms and fears, including direct questions about intimate partner violence (present in up to 20% of pregnant women).

    Routine measurement of maternal weight, blood pressure, fundal height, and fetal heart tones are conducted. SOR **C**

    Second trimester screening can include maternal serum tests (e.g., quadruple test combines serum markers of maternal serum alpha-fetoprotein, estriol, B-HCG, and inhibin A and detects 86% of infants with Down's syndrome [trisomy 21] with a false positive rate of 8.2%), amniocentesis, 1-hour glucola (gestational diabetes), and an antibody screen for Rh-negative women.

    Ultrasound at 18 to 20 weeks' gestation is the standard of care in many regions; however, current evidence fails to correlate routine ultrasound screening in pregnancy with improved fetal outcomes.[17]

    Counseling to encourage a healthful diet and moderate exercise.
  - Third trimester care includes preparation for birth and newborn care, monitoring, and support.

    Evidence-based recommendations include repeat screening for hepatitis B, syphilis, gonorrhea, and chlamydia in high-risk populations (i.e., women younger than age 25 years with two or more sexual contacts, women who are prostitutes, and women with prior history of syphilis or gonorrhea) and screening for GBS at 35 to 37 weeks' gestation.

    Breast-feeding for 6 months should be encouraged and birth preferences discussed (**Figure 4-5**).

    Childbirth classes are often recommended, but evidence supporting their benefit is lacking.
  - Labor and birthing:

    Labor—True labor is defined as progressive cervical dilation with uterine contractions. Effacement, the process of thinning of the cervix, occurs before and during labor. Traditionally, labor has been defined as occurring in three stages:

    a. First stage is divided into latent (1–20 hours) characterized by milder and less frequent contractions and active (averaging 5 hours in multiparas and 8 hours in primaparas), where the cervix dilates from 4 cm to complete (10 cm) characterized by stronger, regular contractions lasting 60 seconds or more.

    b. Second stage begins when dilation is complete and ends with the birth of the baby and averaging 20 minutes in multiparas and 50 minutes in primaparas.

    c. Third stage is from the delivery of the baby to delivery of the placenta (up to 30 minutes is considered normal).

    Birthing requires flexibility and patience. Traditional labor interventions such as withholding food and drink, giving enemas, and perineal shaving have no evidence to support their routine use. Many options are available to increase comfort and ease the process of labor and birth. For example:

    a. Ambulation and frequent changes in position (e.g., side, upright) during labor.

    b. The presence of a supportive labor companion (e.g., partner, doula).

    c. Pain control options include supportive others, physical contact, massage, warm showers, inhaled nitrous oxide, narcotic pain control, and regional analgesia (e.g., blocks and epidurals). With respect to epidural blocks, excellent pain control can be achieved but at the risk of increased use of oxytocin augmentation, forceps, and cesarean section.[18]

    There is no evidence to support routine electronic fetal monitoring,[19] episiotomy,[20] and supine birth positions.[21]

    Women who are culture positive for GBS should receive antibiotic prophylaxis when in labor (e.g., intravenous penicillin G (PCN G) in nonallergic women).

PATIENT EDUCATION

- Pregnancy detection with home pregnancy test kits—The urine tested is the first morning urine. The most accurate results will be obtained by waiting at least 1 week after the date of the expected period to test, using the urine collection container in the kit, and testing the urine immediately after collection or, if urine is refrigerated, allowing it to come to room temperature (20–30 minutes) prior to testing. Common reasons for a test to be read as negative when a woman is actually pregnant include testing too early (i.e., on or before the first day of a missed period), using a waxed cup for urine collection, soap residue in the container used to collect urine, or testing refrigerated urine.

- Pregnancy prevention—Use of contraceptives dramatically reduces the likelihood of unplanned pregnancy (only 8% of women per year using the oral contraceptive become pregnant and of women whose partners are using a condom only 15% become pregnant).[1] Many pregnancies occur when a woman discontinues a contraceptive method and does not begin use of another method prior to intercourse; women should be encouraged to know about a second method they can use if the first chosen method proves unsatisfactory and about the availability of the emergency contraceptive.

- Abortion choices—Approximately 6% of abortions are performed using medication and approximately 90% of abortions are performed using surgical curettage.[13]
  - Benefits of medical abortion include earlier implementation, avoidance of surgery for most, and increased privacy. Medical abortion does cause more bleeding than surgical abortion and cramping may be severe. With all medical regimens, there is some degree of waiting and uncertainty (expulsion may take days to weeks) and an extra clinic visit is required. Additional side effects of medical abortion using mifepristone and misoprostol include nausea; fever, chills, or hot flashes; dizziness; headache; vomiting; and diarrhea.[10]
  - Benefits of surgical abortion are immediate resolution, termination of pregnancy is completed in a predictable period of time, bleeding is usually light, and one visit is often sufficient. The rate of major complications is <1 in 200 cases;[4] potential complications include infection, intrauterine blood clots, and cervical or uterine trauma.

- Pregnancy planning begins with preconception care, ideally occurring 3 to 6 months prior to the conception to discuss health promotion, risk assessment, and medical intervention.
  - Environmental exposures that adversely affect the fetus should be minimized (e.g., pesticides, paint thinner/strippers, fertilizers, and heavy metals). Women who work in hospital settings should avoid exposure to ionizing radiation, chemotherapeutic agents, and misoprostol.
  - Intake of 400 mcg/day of folic acid prior to and during the early part of pregnancy reduces the risk of neural tube defects. SOR **A**
  - Certain heritable genetic diseases can be diagnosed in individuals prior to becoming pregnant (e.g., sickle cell disease, cystic fibrosis).

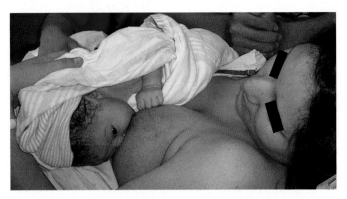

FIGURE 4-5 We are privileged to observe this newborn baby breastfeeding for the first time immediately after the delivery performed by Dr. Richard P. Usatine. (*Courtesy of Richard P. Usatine, MD.*)

- ○ Treatment of chronic medical conditions (e.g., diabetes, epilepsy, hypertension) can be optimized to reduce fetal loss and adverse effects, including possible change to safer medications for pregnancy.
- ○ Smoking cessation and eliminating alcohol consumption can be attempted.
- ○ Immunizations (e.g., rubella, varicella) can be provided.

- Patients should be encouraged to discuss their birthing preferences and their practitioner's practice style with respect to the routine use of technology.

PATIENT RESOURCES

- **http://womenshealth.gov/pregnancy/.**
- **http://www.childbirth.org/** (includes birth planning forms).

PROVIDER RESOURCES

- **http://www.nlm.nih.gov/medlineplus/ pregnancy.html.**
- **http://www.cdc.gov/doc.do/id/0900f3ec802286e6.**

REFERENCES

1. Smith MA, Shimp LA. Family planning. In: Smith MA, Shimp LA, eds. *20 Common Problems in Women's Health Care*. New York: McGraw-Hill, 2000:21–64.

2. Issues in Brief. *Preventing Unintended Pregnancy in the U.S.* New York: The Alan Guttmacher Institute, 2004.

3. Seibert C, Barbouche E, Fagan J, et al. Prescribing oral contraceptives for women older than 35 years of age. *Ann Intern Med.* 2003;138:54–64.

4. Stewart FH, Ellertson C, Cates W. Abortion. In: Hatcher RA, Trussell J, Stewart FH, et al. eds. *Contraceptive Technology*, 18th ed.. New York: Ardent Media, 2004:673–700.

5. Chang J, Elam-Evans LD, Berg CJ. Pregnancy-related mortality surveillance—United States 1991–1999. *MMWR.* 2003;52(SS02): 1–8. Available at http://www.cdc.gov/mmwr/preview/ mmwrhtml/ss5202a1.htm#fig2. Accessed March 5, 2007.

6. American Academy of Family Physicians; AAFP-ACOG Liaison Committee, 2005.

7. Reid AJ, Carroll JC, Ruderman J, Murray MA. Differences in intrapartum obstetric care provided to women at low risk by family physicians and obstetricians. *CMAJ.* 1989;140(6):625–633.

8. Deutchman ME, Sills D, Connot PD. Perinatal outcomes: A comparison between family physicians and obstetricians. *J Am Board Fam Pract.* 1995;8(6):440–447.

9. Hueston WJ, Applegate JA, Mansfield CJ, et al. Practice variations between family physicians and obstetricians in the management of low-risk pregnancies. *J Fam Pract.* 1995;40(4):345–351.

10. Hatcher RA, Namnoun AB. The menstrual cycle. In: Hatcher RA, Trussell J, Stewart FH, et al. eds. *Contraceptive Technology*, 18th ed. New York: Ardent Media, 2004:63–72.

11. Stewart FH, Trussell J, Van Look PFA. Emergency contraception. In: Hatcher RA, Trussell J, Stewart FH, et al. eds. *Contraceptive Technology*, 18th ed. New York: Ardent Media, 2004:279–303.

12. Finer LB, Henshaw SK. Abortion incidence and services in the United States in 2000. *Perspect Sex Reprod Health.* 2003;35:6–15.

13. ACOG Practice Bulletin. Clinical management guidelines of obstetrician-gynecologists. Number 67, October 2005. Medical management of abortion. *Obstet Gynecol.* 2005;106(4):871–882.

14. Choby B. Prenatal care. In: Sloane PD, Slatt LM, Ebell MH, Jacques LB, Smith MA, eds. *Essentials of Family Medicine 5th ed.* Baltimore, MD: Lippincott William & Wilkins, 2008:51–72, Chap 4.

15. Goh YI, Bollano E, Einason TR, Koren G. Prenatal multivitamin supplementation and rates of congenital anomalies: A meta-analysis. *J Obstet Gynaecol Can.* 2006;28(8):680–689.

16. Pena-Rosas JP, Viteri FE. Effects of routine oral iron supplementation with or without folic acid for women during pregnancy. *Cochrane Database Syst Rev.* 2006;3:CD004736.

17. Ewigman BG, Crane JP, Frigoletto FD, et al. Effect of prenatal ultrasound screening on perinatal outcome. RADIUS Study Group. *N Engl J Med.* 1993;329:821–827.

18. Howell CJ. Epidural vs. nonepidural analgesia in labour. *Cochrane Database Syst Rev.* 1993; Review No. 03399.

19. Graham EM, Patersen SM, Christo DK, Fox HE. Intrapartum electronic fetal heart rate monitoring and the prevention of perinatal brain injury. *Obstet Gynecol.* 2006;108(3 Pt 1):656–666.

20. Hartmann K, Viswanathan M, Pamlmieri R, et al. Outcomes of routine episiotomy: A systematic review. *JAMA* 2005;293(17):2141–2148.

21. Gupta JK, Hofmeyr GJ. Position for women during second stage of labour. *Cochrane Database Syst Rev.* 2004;(1):CD002006.

5 END OF LIFE

Mindy A. Smith, MD, MS
Radha Ramana Murthy Gokula, MD

PATIENT STORY

An 89-year-old frail woman presents with Alzheimer's dementia, hypothyroidism, depression, congestive heart failure and macular degeneration. Her functional status was gradually declining. It was difficult for the family to provide 24-hour care and she was admitted to a nursing facility. Her dementia worsened over a period of 2 years in the nursing facility and she became incontinent of urine and feces while developing limitations in speech and ambulation. She could not sit up without assistance and lost her ability to smile and hold her head up independently. The facility was very supportive and a hospice consult was initiated. **Figure 5-1** shows Dr. Gokula along with the hospice nurse visiting the patient for admission to hospice care.

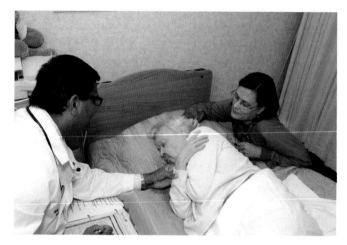

FIGURE 5-1 Family physician Dr. Murthy Gokula and hospice nurse Chris Emch are comforting and examining a terminally-ill patient nearing the end-of-life in Heartland Hospice.

EPIDEMIOLOGY

- According to National Health Center statistics, there were approximately 2.4 million deaths in the United States in 2003; most were attributed to cardiovascular disease (28%) and cancer (22.7%).[1] Additional causes of death were stroke (6.4%), chronic obstructive pulmonary disease (5.2%), accidents (4.5%), diabetes (3.0%), and pneumonia/influenza (2.7%).
  - Among patients aged 1 to 14 years, the major causes of death were unintentional injuries; cancer; homicide; heart disease; and congenital malformations, deformations, and chromosomal abnormalities.
  - The major causes of death in the population aged 15 to 34 years were unintentional injuries, cancer, homicide, intentional self-harm (suicide), and heart disease.
  - HIV was among the top 10 leading causes of death in patients aged 20 to 54 years.
  - Heart disease and cancer were the first and second leading causes of death, respectively, of both men and women. Rankings were similar for death from diabetes (6th) and kidney disease (9th), but men were more likely to die from unintentional injuries (3rd vs. 7th) and women were more likely to die from Alzheimer's disease (5th vs. 10th).
  - Heart disease and cancer were the top two causes of death among whites, blacks, Native Americans, and Hispanics. For the Asian/Pacific Islander population, cancer was the leading cause of death. There were unique causes within the top 10 leading causes of death by racial group. Among Native American populations, chronic liver disease and cirrhosis ranked 5th, homicide ranked 6th, and HIV disease 9th for the black population, whereas Alzheimer's disease ranked 6th for the white population.
- In 2000, in-patients deaths in the hospital occurred in 40% of cases (decreased from 60% in the 1980s).[2]
- Hospice services were involved in approximately 20% of dying patients.[2] More than 70% of hospice patients had cancer and 90% of hospice patients died outside the hospital.[2]

- The use of hospice and other end-of-life services varies among different racial groups in the United States[3]:
  - Caucasians are more aware of advanced directives when compared to the non-white racial or ethnic groups.
  - The use of life-sustaining treatments is more common among African Americans when compared to other racial groups.
  - Cultural differences are also seen for disclosure of information about a terminal illness. Korean, Mexican, Japanese, and Native American populations are more likely to discourage discussion of terminal illness and patient prognosis and prefer families to be informed.
  - The involvement of family in the decision-making process with end-of-life care was seen among all racial groups, but Asian and Hispanic Americans prefer family-centered decision making when compared to other racial and ethnic groups.

ETIOLOGY AND PATHOPHYSIOLOGY

Causes of death are multifactorial. Following are the major modifiable contributors:

- Tobacco use—20.9% of all the adults in the United States smoke cigarettes; the highest rates are among 18- to 24-year-olds (24.4%) and American Indians/Alaska Natives (32.0%).[4] It is estimated that nearly one of every five deaths each year in the United States is attributed to smoking. Smoking increases the risk of developing emphysema (10–13-fold), heart and cardiovascular disease (2–4-fold), and many cancers (1.4–3-fold).

- Poor diet—Diets that are high in fat (>40% of calories consumed) are associated with increased risk of breast, colon, endometrial, and prostate cancer. Diet is important in controlling diabetes, heart disease, obesity, and chronic renal disease.

- Physical inactivity—Those who exercise regularly live longer and are healthier; exercise reduces the risk of cardiovascular disease and hypertension and improves function in those with depression, osteoarthritis, and fibromyalgia.

- Alcohol consumption—Alcohol is consumed by 80% of the population, and 10% to 15% of men and 5% to 8% of women are alcohol dependent. Excess alcohol consumption (>3 drinks per day) is associated with mood disorders (10%–40%), cirrhosis (15%–20%), and neuropathy (5%–15%); it increases the risk of pancreatitis (3-fold) as well as cancers of the breast (1.4-fold), esophagus (3-fold), and rectum (1.5-fold).[5]

- Motor vehicle accidents and incidents involving firearms—According to data from 1990, motor vehicles and firearms cause more than half of all injury-related deaths.[6] The age-adjusted death rate from motor-vehicle crashes was highest for black and white males (26.2 per 100,000 population and 24.2 per 100,000, respectively); 2.5 times that for white females (10.4 per 100,000), and 3 times that for black females (8.7 per 100,000). The age-adjusted death rate for firearms also was highest for black males (66.4 per 100,000). This rate was 3.2 times that for white males (20.7 per 100,000), 8.3 times that for black females (8.0 per 100,000), and 17.9 times that for white females (3.7 per 100,000).[6]

- Sexual behaviors—Sexually transmitted diseases (STDs) are among the most common infectious diseases and affect approximately 13 million people in the United States each year; most of these people are younger than age 25. Although some infections (e.g., syphilis, gonorrhea, and human immunodeficiency virus [HIV]) are most common among those engaging in high-risk sexual behaviors, others (e.g., chlamydia, human papillomavirus [HPV], genital herpes) are distributed across low-risk population groups. STDs are associated with increased risk of HIV/AIDS; approximately 950,000 adults and adolescents are living with HIV/AIDS in the United States. Causes of death from AIDS include infections (especially, pulmonary and central nervous system), cancer (especially, Kaposi sarcoma and non-Hodgkin lymphoma), cardiomyopathy, and nephropathy.

- Illicit use of drugs—Drug addiction remains a major problem in the United States. According to data from the National Institute on Drug Abuse, more than 40% of the U.S. population have used an illicit drug at least once, including approximately 37% who have used marijuana and 12% who have used cocaine.[7] Cocaine is associated with death from respiratory depression, cardiac arrhythmias, and convulsions; methamphetamine use is associated with life-threatening hypertension, cardiac arrhythmia, subarachnoid and intracerebral hemorrhage, ischemic stroke, convulsions, and coma.

- Microbial agents—Microbial agents remain a major cause of death and disability with continued discovery of new agents (e.g., Ebola, retroviruses) and increasing drug resistance. Although it is difficult to ascertain whether an infectious agent caused death or was incidental to death, the expert panel of the investigators in New Mexico, on the basis of autopsy data between late 1994 and mid-1996, found that 85% (106/125) of the deaths were identified as infectious disease-related.[8]

- Toxic agents—Toxic agents include poisons and environmental toxins. In the United States in 2003, there were 28,700 poisoning deaths; 5543 (19.3%) were intentional with 5462 suicides and 81 homicides (CDC 2005).[9] Drugs caused 94.3% of the unintentional and undetermined poisoning deaths with opioid pain medications most commonly involved, followed by cocaine and heroin. The most commonly used drugs identified in drug-related suicides were psychoactive drugs.

DIAGNOSIS

It is estimated that approximately 70% of all deaths are preceded by a disease/condition such that it is reasonable to plan for dying in the near future.[2] These diseases/conditions are as follows:

- Cancer that is widespread and for patients who no longer seek curative care.

- Dementia with:
  - The inability to ambulate or dress without assistance.
  - Life-threatening infections.
  - Multiple stage 3 or 4 skin ulcers.
  - Inability to maintain sufficient fluid and calorie intake.

- Failure to thrive:
  - Patients confined to bed or who require assistance with all the basic activities of daily living.
  - Patients with a body mass index <22 and/or those who refuse or do not respond to enteral or parenteral nutritional support.

- Heart disease:
  - Poor response or intolerance to optimal medical treatment.
  - NYHA class IV.
  - Congestive heart failure, especially with ejection fraction $\leq$20%.
- HIV/AIDS with CD4 count <25, especially with major AIDS-defining refractory infections or significant functional decline in the activities of daily living.
- Neurologic diseases, e.g., Parkinson's disease, amyotrophic lateral sclerosis, multiple sclerosis, muscular dystrophy, and myasthenia gravis:
  - Rapid disease progression and/or critical nutritional state.
  - Life-threatening infections in the preceding 12 months.
  - Stage 3 or 4 skin ulcers.
  - Critically impaired breathing capacity and declined ventilator support.
- Pulmonary disease:
  - Disabling dyspnea at rest or with minimal exertion.
  - Increase in emergency department visits and/or hospitalizations.
  - Hypoxemia on room air (oxygen saturation <88%).
  - Forced expiratory volume in 1 second (FEV1) <30%.
- Renal failure:
  - Not seeking dialysis or not a candidate.
  - Calculated creatinine clearance <10 (<15 for patients with diabetes).
  - Serum creatinine >8 (>6 for patients with diabetes).
- Stroke:
  - Coma in the acute phase.
  - Dysphagia and insufficient intake of fluids and calories.
  - Post-stroke dementia.
- Nonspecific terminal illness:
  - Rapid decline, disease progression, or progressive weight loss.
  - Dysphasia with aspiration.
  - Increase in emergency department visits and/or hospitalizations.
  - Worsening pressure ulcers despite optimum care.
  - Decline in systolic blood pressure below 90 mm Hg.

Unfortunately, physicians are often reluctant to make this determination, resulting in palliative and hospice care not being offered until very late in the course of the illness. In addition, physicians often feel that they must be able to predict a life expectancy of less than 6 months with certainty to institute hospice care.

The National Hospice and Palliative Care Organization has evidence-based guidelines on determining prognosis for a number of non cancer conditions.[10] This information can assist clinicians in working with patients at the end of life on advanced care decisions and planning.

CLINICAL FEATURES

- Common physical symptoms reported by dying patients[2]:
  - Constipation (90%).
  - Fatigue and weakness (90%).
  - Dyspnea (75%) and other cardiopulmonary symptoms such as cough.
  - Pain (36–90%).
  - Insomnia.
  - Other gastrointestinal symptoms, including dry mouth, anorexia, nausea, vomiting, constipation, diarrhea, and dysphagia.
  - Fecal and urinary incontinence.
  - Dizziness.
  - Swelling and numbness of the extremities.
- Common mental and psychological symptoms reported by dying patients[2]:
  - Depression (75% symptomatic; <25% with major depression) and feelings of hopelessness.
  - Anxiety.
  - Irritability.
  - Confusion and delirium (up to 85% at the end stage).
- A population-based survey of family members, friends, and care givers in six U.S. communities found that[11]
  - 71% of terminally ill patients had shortness of breath.
  - 50% had moderate to severe pain.
  - 36% were incontinent of urine or feces.
  - 18% were fatigued enough to spend more than 50% of their waking hours in bed.

MANAGEMENT

The five basic principles of palliative care are as follows[12]:

- Respect the goals, preferences, and choices of the person.
- Look after the medical, emotional, social, and spiritual needs.
- Support the needs of family members.
- Help patients and their families access needed medical health care providers and appropriate care settings.
- Provide excellence in care at the end of life (**Figure 5-1**).

The quality-of-care domains for a person at the end of life are as follows[13]:

- Physical and emotional symptom management.
- Support of function, autonomy, personal dignity, and self-respect.
- Advanced care planning.
- Aggressive symptom control near death.
- Patient and family satisfaction.
- Patient's assessment of overall quality of life and well-being.
- Family burden—emotional and financial.
- Survival time.
- Provider continuity and skill.
- Bereavement services.

Management often begins with communicating bad news to patients and families about likely or imminent death. This task can be extremely difficult. In cases where the patient is not deemed legally competent, make sure that the legal decision maker is present. In addition, if the patient is a non-English speaker, consider obtaining a skilled medical interpreter rather than relying on a family member. Providers may find the following P-SPIKES approach useful[14]:

- Preparation—Review information to be presented and practice.
- Setting—Arrange time and place, ensure privacy, and include important support persons.

- Perception of patient—Inquire about the patient's and the family's understanding of the illness.

- Information needs—Find out about what the patient and family need to be told and in how much detail.

- Knowledge of the condition—Provide bad news sensitively and slowly, warning them any bad news is imminent and checking to see whether there is understanding.

- Empathy and exploration—Acknowledge the feelings expressed, give the patient and family time to react, and remind them that you are not abandoning them.

- Summary/strategic planning—Discuss next steps or schedule follow-ups to do this if more time is needed.

Roles for the primary care provider include consultation, providing anticipatory guidance, providing support and comfort, and assisting with identifying and managing symptoms (including pain control) (**Figure 5-2**).

In assisting dying patients and their families/caregivers with making decisions about their care, clinicians should be prepared to discuss the following:

- Realistic treatment options for cure or palliation of the primary disease process.

- Advance directives and withholding of life-sustaining treatment.

- Cultural beliefs and preferences (e.g., truth-telling vs. protecting the patient, religious beliefs).

- Preferences for place of care for those dying, involvement of others, and symptom management.

A number of factors are important in providing optimal care to the dying. In a study of factors considered important to seriously ill patients, recently bereaved family members, and physicians involved in end-of-life care, investigators found the following[15]:

- There was a general agreement on the items relating to having preferences in writing, symptom control, being kept clean, experiencing physical touch, good communication and knowing what to expect, getting one's affairs in order and achieving a sense of completion, and maintaining dignity and a sense of humor.

- Patients reported wanting to remain mentally aware, not be a burden, and noted the importance of prayer and being at peace with God. They were not as concerned about dying at home.

- Family members reported wanting to use all the treatment options and to help patients avoid pain, shortness of breath, and suffering.

Advance directives and advance care planning:

- Introduce the concept and the goals of empowering the patient and understanding the patient's preferences if they are too sick to speak for themselves. Possible scenarios can be discussed such as recovery from an acute event (specifying acceptable interventions) and persistent vegetative state (preferences for life-sustaining interventions).

- Documents—These are of two broad types:
  - Instructional directives such as living wills that describe decisions about care and health care. These can be general or specific. Although 80% of Americans endorse completing living wills,

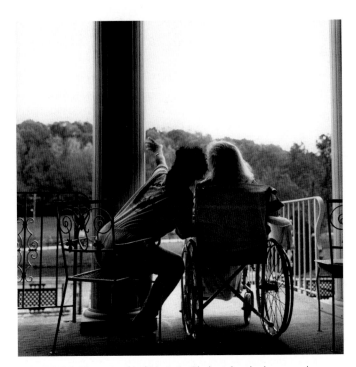

FIGURE 5-2 Photograph of Marjorie Clarke taken by her grandson. She suffered from Alzheimer's disease that left her depressed and frustrated. In this picture, taken in 1996, Marjorie listens to her nurse describe the scene and explain that they are on the front porch of her home. She died in January, 1997. (*Courtesy of Marshall Clarke*).

only 20% (and fewer than 1/3 of health care providers) have completed them.[2] Specific forms do not have to be used and oral directives may be enforceable.[16]

- Proxy designations—Appointing an individual or individuals to make medical decisions (i.e., durable power of attorney for health care).

• Legal aspects—The United States Supreme Court has ruled that patients have a right to decide about refusing or terminating medical interventions. Many states have their own statutory forms for living wills.

- The American College of Physicians and the American Society of Internal Medicine End-of-Life Care Consensus Panel note that life-sustaining treatment may be withheld for patients unable to speak for themselves if it is believed to be the patient's wish, the surrogate decision maker states that it is the patients wish, and/or it is in the patient's best interests to do so.[16]

- The prescription of high-dose opioids to relieve pain in terminally ill patients that result in death will not lead to criminal prosecution provided it was the physician's intent to relieve suffering.[16]

Hospice care and services:

• Hospice care refers to care when curative interventions have been judged to be no longer beneficial. This type of care can be delivered in many settings including home, hospital, or special residential facilities.

• The types of services include physician and nursing care, home health aides, pastoral care, counseling, respite care, and bereavement programs (**Figure 5-3**).

• Hospice eligibility general guidelines include the following:
  - Fulfilling the criteria for end-stage disease as outlined above.
  - Patient and family deciding on palliative care rather than curative care.
  - Documented rapid disease progression.
  - Significant functional decline documented by validated instruments like FAST (Functional Assessment Staging), PPS (Palliative performance scale), BADLs (Basic Activities of Daily Living), and/or NYHA class IV heart disease.
  - Weight loss of 7.5% or 10% in the preceding 3 to 6 months, respectively, or serum albumin <2.5 g/dL.

• Physicians should be aware of the Medicare Hospice Benefit (MHB) covered under Medicare Part A (physician services are billed under Medicare Part B).[17] In the United States, the MHB pays for 80% of all hospice care including medical, nursing, counseling, and bereavement services to terminally ill patients and their families.
  - Medicare beneficiaries who choose hospice care receive noncurative medical and support services for their terminal illness. Home care may be provided along with inpatient care if needed and a variety of other services that are not covered by Medicare.
  - Eligibility criteria:
    ▪ Patient eligible for Medicare Part A or Medicaid.
    ▪ Patient is terminally ill, i.e., patient's physician and medical director of hospice certify that the patient is terminally ill and has a life expectancy of 6 months or less if the disease runs its normal course. If the medical director is the patient's physician only one signature is required.

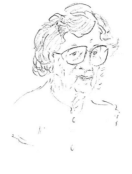
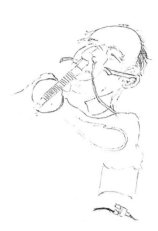

FIGURE 5-3 Dr. Alan Blum is a family physician who has been doing sketches of his patients for decades now. When he presents his drawings of his patients, he reads his poetic stories that go with the drawings. Some of his drawings have been published in *JAMA*.

The wife maintained a weeklong vigil over her comatose husband in the ICU and wouldn't let us change his code status to let him go. She explained why:

"When he had his automobile accident
29 years ago in Louisiana,
15 inches of plastic aorta,
punctured lung, and all this stuff...
The Lord performed three miracles:
He lived.
He was able to walk.
He went back to work.
I'll be there.
I been there
48 years."

- Patient chooses hospice care and signs a Medicare hospice benefits form. This process is reversible and patients may at a future time elect to return to Medicare Part A.
- Hospice care is provided by a Medicare-certified hospice program.
- Under Medicare, DNR status cannot be used as a requirement for admission.
  - Length of benefits:
    - Entitled to receive hospice care as long as he or she meets the eligibility criteria.
    - Hospice benefit consists of two 90-day benefit periods, followed by an unlimited number of 60-day benefit periods.
    - Benefit periods may be used consecutively or at intervals.
    - Patient needs to be certified terminally ill at the beginning of each period.
    - No life time limit to hospice care for Medicare beneficiaries.
    - If patient experiences remission of the disease and is discharged from hospice, he or she can be eligible for hospice care in the future without any regard to the previous use of hospice services.
    - Same rules apply for Medicaid patients.
  - Services covered include physician, nurse, dietician, and medical social services, medical supplies and equipment, outpatient drugs for symptom management and pain relief, and home care (e.g., aids, physical, occupational, and speech therapy). Other services included are as follows:
    - Short-term general inpatient care for problems that cannot be managed at home—most commonly intractable pain or delirium.
    - Short-term respite care—up to 5 days to permit family caregivers to take a break (can incur a 5% copayment).
    - Counseling in home for patient and family.
    - Bereavement, pastoral, and spiritual support for patient and family.
    - Payment of consulting physician fees at 100% of Medicare allowance.
    - Physician, nurse, social worker, and counselor on-call availability 24 hours a day, 7 days a week.
  - Services not covered include active treatment of terminal illness (except for symptom management and pain control of the terminal illness), care provided by a physician or facility that has not contracted with the patient's hospice agency, and continuous nursing assistant or nursing home room and board charges.

Palliative care is care focused on preventing, relieving, reducing, or soothing symptoms of disease without affecting a cure.[18] As such, it is not restricted to patients who are dying but can be used along with a curative therapy. Many hospitals now have inpatient palliative care services to assist patients, families, and primary care providers in delivering this type of care.

- General approach focuses on four broad domains:
  - Managing physical symptoms.
  - Managing psychological symptoms.
  - Addressing social needs.
  - Understanding spiritual needs.
- Needs assessment—Clinicians should focus on the four domains and try to understand the degree of difficulty and how much the identified problem interferes with the patient's life.

- Setting goals and continuous reassessment—Goals for care include improving symptoms, delaying disability, finding peace, and providing for the loved ones. Plan times to review these goals as the course of the illness changes or progresses.

Pain management: There is no reason that patients need to suffer, particularly at the end of life. Barriers to managing pain successfully include limited ability of providers to assess pain severity, fear of sanction/prosecution, and lack of knowledge (including awareness of guidelines).

- Assessment of pain—Important aspects include periodicity (e.g., continuous), location, intensity, modifying factors, effects of treatments, and impact on the patient.
- Intervention—This includes nonpharmacologic treatment (e.g., massage, positioning, transcutaneous electrical nerve stimulation [TENS], physical therapy), pain medications, and other palliative procedures (e.g., nerve blocks, radiotherapy, acupuncture).
  - Pain medications may be approached in a stepwise fashion from nonopiods (e.g., acetaminophen [4 g/d], ibuprofen [1600 mg/d]), to mild opioids (e.g., codeine [30 mg every 4 hours] or hydrocodone [5 mg every 4 hours]) to stronger opioids (e.g., morphine 5–10 mg every 4 hours).[19] Doses should be titrated as needed. Side effects (e.g., constipation, nausea, and drowsiness) should be anticipated and prevented (e.g., laxatives and antiemetic) or treated. Patients may become tolerant to these side effects after approximately 1 week.
  - Specific pain syndromes may require additional consideration. These include:
    - Continuous pain, which requires round-the-clock dosing, rescue medication, and regular assessment and readjustment. If rescue medication has been needed, increase the daily opioid dose by the total dose of rescue medication the next day. For longer duration of action, transdermal fentanyl may be considered (100 mcg/hour is equianalgesic to morphine 4 mg/hour and has a duration of 48–72 hours).
    - Neuropathic pain (arising from disordered, ectopic nerve signals), which is typically shock-like or burning. Medications to consider in addition to opioids are gabapentin (100–300 mg daily or up to three times daily), 5% lidocaine patch (three patches daily for a maximum of 12 hours), tramadol (50–100 mg one to three times daily), and tricyclic antidepressants (10–25 mg at bedtime titrated to 75–150 mg).[20]
    - Adjunctive analgesic medications are those that potentiate the effects of opioids. These include the above treatments for neuropathic pain, glucocorticoids (e.g., dexamethasone once daily), clonidine, and baclofen.
- Legal concerns—Physicians may be unwilling or uncomfortable providing high-dose opioids out of fear that they would be hastening the patient's death. However, the assumption that opioids appropriately titrated to control pain hasten death is not supported by medical evidence. In addition, as noted above, the physician's intent to relieve suffering, despite the risk of death, is ethical and unlikely to result in prosecution.

Control of common symptoms:[2]

- Constipation—Secondary to medications, inactivity, and poor nutritional/hydration status. Options include increasing fiber, stool softeners (e.g., Sodium docusate [colace] 300–600 mg/day oral), stimulant laxatives (e.g., prune juice 1/2 to 1 glass/day, senna [Senekot] 2–4 tablet/day, bisacodyl 5–15 mg/day orally or per rectum), and osmotic laxatives (e.g., lactulose 15–30 mL every 4–8 hours, magnesium hydroxide [milk or magnesia] 15–30 mL/day).

- Dyspnea—When possible, treat reversible causes (e.g., infection, hypoxia). Options include opioids (e.g., codeine 30 mg every 4 hours, morphine 5–10 mg every 4 hours) and anxiolytics (e.g., lorazepam 0.5–2 mg oral/sublingual/intravenous [IV], diazepam 5–10 mg oral/IV).
  - For patients with a history of respiratory disease consider bronchodilators and/or glucocorticoids.
  - For patients with excessive secretions, scopolamine may be considered.
- Fatigue—Secondary to disease factors (e.g., heart failure, tumor necrosis factor), cachexia, dehydration, anemia, hypothyroidism, and medications. Options include decreasing activity, increasing exercise as tolerated, changing medications, glucocoticoids (e.g., dexamethasone once daily), or stimulants (e.g., dextroamphetamine 5–10 mg oral).
- Depression—Because many of the somatic symptoms used to diagnose depression in healthy individuals are present in patients who are dying, psychological criteria become more important in making treatment decisions. Options include counseling, exercise, and medications (e.g., selective serotonin reuptake inhibitor [SSRI]); low doses should be used initially (e.g., fluoxetine 10 mg/d) and increased as needed. Psychostimulants (e.g., dextroamphetamine or methylphenidate 2.5–5 mg twice daily) may be considered if rapid onset of action is needed; these may be used in conjunction with traditional antidepressants.
- Delirium—Secondary to metabolic abnormalities (liver failure, electrolyte disturbance, vitamin B12 deficiency), infection, brain tumors, medications, and multiple other causes. Options include treating reversible causes and medications including neuroleptics (e.g., haloperidol 0.5–5 mg oral/subcutaneous/intramuscular [IM]/IV every 1–4 hours, risperidone 1–3 mg every 12 hours), anxiolytics (e.g., lorazepam 0.5–2 mg oral/IM/IV), and anesthetics (propofol 0.3–2 mg/hour continuous infusion).

Addressing social needs: Considerations include economic burden and caregivers.

- The U.S. health insurance system is neither universal nor comprehensive and many patients and their families find themselves under tremendous financial strain.
  - Twenty percent of terminally ill patients spend >10% of the family income on health care costs beyond insurance premiums.[2]
  - Ten to thirty percent of families need to secure additional monies by means such as selling assets or taking out a second mortgage to cover health care costs.[2]
  - Twenty percent of caregivers stop work to provide care for a terminally ill family member.[2]
- Families/caregivers often need outside help such as providing personal care for the patient such as bathing, psychological or spiritual counseling, respite care, or making arrangements for the body after death.

- Primary care providers can facilitate encounters with family and friends by offering their presence and suggestions about easing the visits (e.g., reading to the patient, sharing music, or creating a videotape, audiotape, or scrapbook).
- Hospice and social workers can offer great assistance to patients and families in addressing these needs.

Understanding spiritual needs:

- Approximately 70% of dying patients become more religious or spiritual at the end of life.
- As noted by Steinhauser et al., patients noted the importance of prayer and being at peace with God.[15]
- Physicians should ask about and support patient and family expressions of spirituality and consider encouraging pastoral care, as desired.

Physician-assisted suicide (PAS):

- PAS is legal in the Netherlands, Belgium, and in the state of Oregon in the United States.
- Less than 10% to 20% of patients consider PAS.[2]
- Patients who request PAS may not be aware of the extent to which palliative and hospice care can alleviate symptoms and other concerns. Providers should explore the patient's reasons for this request and make every attempt to address remediable factors and provide support and comfort.

PATIENT AND FAMILY EDUCATION

- It is very important to involve patients and their families in discussion at an early stage as most want to know their diagnosis and prognosis.
- The role of the primary care physician should be discussed, particularly if other providers are involved in the care of the patient. Possible roles include consultation about care needs, anticipatory guidance on prognosis and expected symptoms, provision of support and comfort, and assistance with managing symptoms.
- Families usually suffer emotionally, spiritually, and financially as they care for the patient.[21] Family members often experience a sense of hopelessness, anger, guilt, and powerlessness when they cannot relieve the suffering of their terminally ill family member.
- Families which need to provide care for a terminally ill patient should be made aware of community resources and the provisions in the Family Medical Leave Act.[22]
- It is not unusual to see hidden family conflicts resurface in the face of a terminal illness and any emotional tension that exists between the caregivers and patient can impede care. Physicians should be sensitive to the conflicts and cultural influences and closely observe how patients and their families are communicating so that they can better support them, allowing them to express their emotions and concerns and referring them to appropriate counselors or support groups when needed.[23,24]
- Children should not be excluded from this process and the physician, with permission, can help in determining what children

already know about the illness and in providing accurate information about the diagnosis, prognosis, and treatment expectations for the dying family member. Other advice for the patient and family may be as follows:

- Try to maintain the children's daily schedule and routines of the family as much as possible.
- Ask about the child's specific concerns and whether they are experiencing problems in school or at home.
- Encourage the child to ask questions but do not force discussions. Make sure you understand the real question before answering; take your time to think about how you want to answer.
- Avoid euphemisms (e.g., lump, boo-boo, or sickness) that may confuse children.
- Encourage visiting the terminally ill family member at the end of life and provide activities to keep them busy such as painting or reading a story at the bedside.
- Inform the teachers and counselors at school about the family situation and request that the teachers let the parent know if the child is having any difficulty or talks about worries.
- Consider counseling for the child if any of the following occur:
  - Symptoms of depression or anxiety that interfere with school, home, or peers.
  - Risk-taking behavior.
  - Significant discord between the child and the terminally ill or surviving parent.
  - Significant discord between the parents.
  - The child says he or she wants to talk to someone outside of the family.
- The following are processes that many dying persons go through:
  - Social withdrawal—Initial withdrawal is from the surroundings and then worldly interests decline and finally withdrawal from family, ultimately leading to loss of communication.
  - Decreasing nutritional requirements—There is a decreased need for fluids and solids; fluids are usually preferred and should follow what the patient wants rather than force-feeding.
  - Disorientation—There is increased confusion with time, place, and person. Usually patients talk about seeing people who have already died or state that their death is nearing. Redirecting the patient is necessary only if asked for or if the patient is distressed.
  - Decreased senses—Hearing and vision decrease. Using soft lights helps with decreasing visual hallucinations. Speak softly and gently as patients hear even at the end of life. Hearing is the last of the five senses to be lost.
  - Restlessness—Also called "terminal restlessness" is caused by the change in the body's metabolism. Reassurance is important and appropriate symptom management with medications may be helpful.
  - Sleep—There is increased time spent in sleep that may be as a result of changes in the body's metabolism or natural to the underlying disease process. Spending time at the bedside can help capture the time when the patient is most alert.
  - Incontinence of urine and bowel movements is often not a problem until death is very near. Absorbent pads can be placed under the patient for greater comfort and cleanliness or a urinary catheter may be used for comfort care. The amount of urine will decrease and becomes darker at the end of life.

- Physical changes to be expected include the following:
  - Skin color changes including flushing, bluish hue to the skin, and cold sensation of the skin. Skin may have a jaundiced look when the patient is approaching death. The arms and legs of the body may become cool to the touch. The hands and feet become purplish. The knees, ankles, and elbows are blotchy. These symptoms are a result of decreased circulation.
  - Blood pressure decreases; the pulse may increase or decrease.
  - Body temperature can fluctuate; fever is common.
  - Increased perspiration along with clamminess.
  - Respirations may increase, decrease, or become irregular; there may be periods of cessation of breathing (apnea).
  - Congestion can present as a rattling sound in the lungs and/or upper throat. This occurs because the patient is too weak to clear the throat or cough. The congestion can be affected by positioning, may be very loud, and sometimes just comes and goes. Elevating the head of the bed and swabbing the mouth with oral swabs may be helpful.
  - The patient may enter a coma before death and not respond to verbal or tactile stimuli. Signs of death include the following:

    No breathing and heartbeat.
    Loss of bowel or bladder control.
    No response to verbal commands or gentle shaking.
    Eyelids are slightly open; eyes fixed on a certain spot.
    Jaw relaxed and mouth slightly open.

FOLLOW-UP

- Withdrawal of life-sustaining treatment:
  - Evidence-based criteria for guiding physicians through this process is lacking; however, general consensus exists based on ethical and clinical principles in the care of these patients.[25,26]
    - Withdrawal of life-sustaining treatment can be considered when curative care is not possible and supportive or other treatment is no longer desired and does not provide comfort to the patient.
    - Withholding life-sustaining treatment is morally, ethically, and legally equivalent to withdrawing life support.
    - When the goal is to hasten death, there are moral and legal complications.
    - Any kind of treatment that is given to the patient can be withdrawn or withheld.
    - Treat withdrawal of life-sustaining treatment equivalent to a medical procedure and all formalities (e.g., informed consent) should be fulfilled prior to the procedure.
    - If withdrawal of one life-sustaining treatment is indicated, then consider withdrawing all existing treatments for the patient.
  - A general consensus should be reached with the health care team and family members that is in the best interest of the patient. Following are the steps that should be taken for withdrawal of life support[26]:
    - Informed consent.
    - Appropriate setting and monitoring.
    - Sedation and analgesia.
    - Having a plan for withdrawal (information about the protocol can be found in fast facts at www.eperc.mcw.edu).

- Pastoral, nursing, and emotional support.
- Documentation.
- Interventions to improve care during withdrawal of life-sustaining treatment should be considered:[27]

    ethics consultation

    palliative care consultation

    a standardized order form for withdrawing life-sustaining therapies

    family conferences

    informational leaflet for the families consisting of patient's illnesses and treatments and family satisfaction

- Grief and bereavement follow-up:
  - Manifestations of grief consist of both psychological symptoms (e.g., sadness, anxiety, emotional lability, apathy, impaired concentration) and physical symptoms (anorexia, change in weight, trouble initiating or maintaining sleep, fatigue, headache). In the first month following a death, it is important to reassure surviving family members and friends that these manifestations of grief are normal and to offer support, suggestions for symptom management, and coping resources.
  - Subsequent follow-up visits should be used to assess the progress of mourning and to identify depression; if the latter is identified, consider pharmacotherapy and counseling.
- Usually, the primary physician is notified of the death and may be required to make the pronouncement (based on lack of vital signs and lack of response to noxious stimulus) and complete the death certificate (noting cause of death and contributing medical conditions).
- Following the death of the patient, personal expressions of condolence from the primary care provider(s) and staff should be encouraged and range from cards to attending visitation and the funeral; based on personal experience, the latter can assist with grieving and closure for the physician.

PATIENT RESOURCES

- **http://www.caringinfo.org.**
- **www.HospiceCare.com.**
- **www.getpalliativecare.org.**
- **http://www.adec.org/.**
- **http://www.nfcacares.org/.**
- **http://www.nhpco.org.**

SUGGESTED READINGS

- Callanan M, Kely, P. *Final Gifts: Understanding the Special Awareness, Needs and Communications of the Dying.* Bantam Books, 1992. [ISBN: 0-553-37876-7.]
- Ray MC. I Am Here to Help: A Hospice Workers Guide to Communicating with Dying People and Their Loved Ones. Hospice Handouts, McRay Company. [ISBN:0-963611-0-1.]
- Lattanzi-Licht M, Mahoney JJ, Miller GW. The National Hospice Organization Guide to Hospice Care: The Hospice Choice: In Pursuit of A Peaceful Death. Simon & Schuster. [ISBN:0-684-82269-5.]

- Hanson W. The Next Place. Waldman House Press, 1997. [ISBN: 0-931674-32-8.]
- Baugher R, Calija M. A Guide to the Bereaved Survivor Newcastle, WA 1998. [ISBN:0-9635975-0-7.]
- Brown LK, Brown M. When Dinosaurs Die: A Guide to Understanding Death. Little Brown & Company. [ISBN:0-316-11955-5.]
- Sameul-Traisman E. Fire in My Heart, Ice in My Veins: A Journey for Teenagers Experiencing a Loss. Centering Corporation. [ISBN:1-56123-056-1.]
- Heegaard M. When Someone Special Dies: Children Can Learn to Cope with Grief. Minneapolis: Woodland Press, 1988. [ISBN:0-9620502-0-2.]

PROVIDER RESOURCES

- American Academy of Hospice and Palliative Medicine— **http://www.aahpm.org/.**
- American Board of Hospice and Palliative Medicine (ABHPM)—**http://www.abhpm.org.**
- National Hospice and Palliative Care Organization— **http://www.nhpco.org.**
- American Pain Society—**http://www.ampainsoc.org.**
- American Society for Bioethics and Humanities— **http://www.asbh.org.**
- American Society of Law, Medicine and Ethics— **http://www.aslme.org.**
- End-of-Life Care Consensus Panel—American College of Physicians-American Society of Internal Medicine— **http://www.acponline.org/ethics/papers.htm.**
- The EPEC Project (Education resource online)— **www.epec.net.**
- The End of Life Palliative care education resource center (helpful titles include Delivering Bad News, Grief in Children and Developmental Concepts of Death, Teaching the Family What to Expect When the Patient is Dying, and What Do I Tell the Children?)—**http://www.eperc.mcw.edu/.**
- Palliative Care Matters—**http://www.pallcare.info.**
- American Hospice Foundation—**http://www.americanhospice.org/.**

REFERENCES

1. Heron MP, Smith, BL. Deaths: Leading Causes for 2003. *National Vital Statistics Reports* 55(10):1–93. Available at: www.cdc.gov/nchs/data/nvsr/nvsr55/nvsr55_10.pdf. Accessed April 20, 2007.

2. Emanuel EJ, Emanuel LL. Palliative and end-of-life care. In: Kasper DL, Braunwald E, Fauci AS, et al., eds. *Harrison's Principles of Internal Medicine*, 16th ed. New York: McGraw-Hill, 2005:53–66.

3. Kwak J, Healy WE. Current research findings on end-of-life decision making among racially or ethnically diverse groups. *Gerontologist* 2005;45(5):634–641.

4. Surgeon General Report on Smoking. http://www.cdc.gov/tobacco/data_statistics/Factsheets/index.htm. Accessed April 20, 2007.

5. Schuckit MA. Alcohol and alcoholism. In: Kasper DL, Braunwald E, Fauci AS, eds. *Harrison's Principles of Internal Medicine*, 16th ed. New York: McGraw-Hill, 2005:2562–2566.

6. Deaths Resulting from Firearm- and Motor-Vehicle-Related Injuries—United States, 1968–1991. *MMWR.* 1994;43(3):37–42.

7. National Institute on Drug Abuse. http://www.nida.nih.gov/DrugPages/DrugsofAbuse.html. Accessed April 9, 2007.

8. Wolfe MI, Nolte KB, Yoon SS. Fatal Infectious Disease Surveillance in a Medical Examiner Database. Available at: http://www.cdc.gov/ncidod/eid/vol10no1/02-0764.htm. Accessed April 9, 2007.

9. National Center for Injury Prevention and Control. http://www.cdc.gov/health/poisoning.htm. Accessed April 9, 2007.

10. National Hospice and Palliative Care Organization. www.nhpco.org (for members). Accessed April 20, 2007.

11. Emanuel EJ, Fairclough DL, Slutsman J, et al. Assistance from family members, friends, paid care givers, and volunteers in the care of terminally ill patients. *N Engl J Med.* 1999;341(13):956–963.

12. Von Gunten CF. Interventions to manage symptoms at the end of life. *J Palliat Med.* 2005;8(Suppl 1):S88–S94.

13. Lynn J. Measuring quality of care at the end of life: A statement of principles. *J Am Geriatr Soc.* 1997;45:526–527.

14. Buckman R. *How to Break Bad News: A Guide for Health Care Professionals.* Baltimore, MD: Johns Hopkins University Press; 1992.

15. Steinhauser KE, Christakis NA, Clipp EC, et al. Factors considered important at the end of life by patients, family physicians, and other care providers. *JAMA.* 2000;284(19):1476–1482.

16. Meisel A, Snyder L, Quill T American College of Physicians—American Society of Internal Medicine End-of-Life Care Consensus Panel. Seven legal barriers to end-of-life care: Myths, realities and grains of truth. *JAMA.* 2000;284(19):2495–2501.

17. Turner R. Fast Facts and Concepts No. 82 and 83. Medicare Hospice Benefit Part 1. January 2003. End-of-Life Physician Education Resource Center, www.eperc.mcw.edu. Accessed April 20, 2007.

18. Field MJ, Cassel CK, eds. *Approaching Death: Improving Care at the End of Life.* Washington, DC: National Academy Press; 1997.

19. World Health Organization. Pain Ladder. Available at: www.who.int/entity/cancer/palliative/painladder/en/. Accessed March 1, 2007.

20. Dworkin RH, Backonja M, Rowbotham MC, et al. Advances in neuropathic pain: Diagnosis, mechanisms, and treatment recommendations. *Arch Neurol.* 2003;60:1524–1534.

21. Rabow M, Hauser J, Adams J. Supporting family caregivers at the end of life: "They don't know what they don't know". *JAMA.* 2004;291:483–491.

22. U.S. Department of Labor. WHO's Pain Ladder Available at: http://www.dol.gov/esa/whd/fmla/. Accessed April 7, 2007.

23. Larson DG, Tobin DR. End of life conversations: Evolving practice and theory. *JAMA.* 2000;284:1573–1578.

24. Della Santina C, Bernstein RH. Whole patient assessment, goal planning, and inflection points: Their role in achieving quality end-of life care. *Clin Geriatr Med.* 2004;20:595–620.

25. Jonsen AR, Seigler M, Winslade WJ. *Clinical Ethics: A Practical Approach to Ethical Decisions in Clinical Medicine*, 4th ed. New York: McGraw-Hill, 1998.

26. Gordon DR. Principles and practice of withdrawing life-sustaining treatments. *Crit Care Clin.* 2004;20:435–451.

27. Curtis JR. Interventions to improve care during withdrawal of life-sustaining treatments. *J Palliat Med.* 2005;8(Suppl 1):S116–S131.

6 SOCIAL JUSTICE

Mindy A. Smith, MD, MS
Richard P. Usatine, MD

The first question which the priest and the Levite asked was "If I stop to help this man, what will happen to me?" But . . . the Good Samaritan reversed the question: "If I do not stop to help this man, what will happen to him?"

—Martin Luther King, Jr.

PATIENT STORIES

At only 5.5 pounds (10 pounds less than the 5th percentile for weight on the World Health Organization's growth chart), this 8-month-old boy suffered from severe malnutrition. In the summer of 2003, amidst the height of Liberia's civil war, his aunt brought him to the "Médecins sans Frontières/Doctors without Borders" hospital for treatment. Because of the war, his family had been forced to flee from their home, leaving behind their usual methods of getting food. Dr. Andrew Schechtman was there to help the day the child was brought to the clinic in Liberia (**Figure 6-1**). Despite the best available treatment for the malnutrition and concurrent pneumonia, he died on his third hospital day.

OUR STORIES AS CARING CLINICIANS

Those of us who become family physicians and other health care providers do so for many reasons. One of them is because of a desire to help someone else. Along the way, we sometimes lose ourselves in the day-to-day struggles, the disappointments, the obligations, the fatigue, and the profound helplessness that descends upon us after a particularly bad day. But we are still here and, if we listen with our hearts, we are still capable of great and small things. We are privileged in so many ways and we must recognize our power over ourselves and over the communities that we serve. It is easy to become overwhelmed by the problems that we face as clinicians and as fellow human beings. Our health care system is in shambles, our natural world is being poisoned, our nations are continually at war, and yet, as this chapter highlights, there is so much that we can do—we can listen, we can observe, we can witness, we can bring aid, we can touch, we can love, and we can lead.

The text that follows highlights just a few examples of the ways in which our colleagues are challenging themselves to find creative solutions to the many problems faced by those who are underserved, displaced, or suffering.

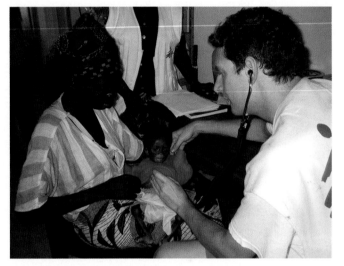

FIGURE 6-1 Dr. Andrew Schechtman was there to help the day a severely malnourished child was brought to the clinic in war-torn Liberia. Despite the best available treatment that could be provided in the "Doctors without Borders" hospital, the child died of complications of malnutrition and pneumonia—a casualty of war and poverty. (*Courtesy of Andrew Schechtman, MD.*)

DOCTORS WITHOUT BORDERS (ANDREW SCHECHTMAN, MD)

EPIDEMIOLOGY

The United Nations High Commissioner for Refugees reported that in 2006 there were 8.4 million refugees (those displaced across an international border) and 23.7 million internally displaced persons (those displaced within their own country).[1] During times of a complex humanitarian emergency (defined as a humanitarian crisis in a country, region, or society where there is a breakdown of authority resulting from internal or external conflict and which requires an international response that goes beyond the mandate or capacity of any single agency and/or the ongoing UN country program), the following usually occur:

- Civilian casualties.

- Populations besieged or displaced.

- Serious political or conflict-related impediments to delivery of assistance.

- Inability of people to pursue normal social, political, or economic activities.

- High security risks for relief workers.

ETIOLOGY

People can be displaced from their homes by man-made (war, persecution) or natural disasters (tsunami, earthquake, or hurricane). War is responsible for most of the displacement. Some of the source countries accounting for the most refugees are Afghanistan, Sudan, Somalia, the Palestinian territories, and Iraq.

- Communicable diseases usually cause the most illness and deaths in humanitarian emergencies in less-developed countries. Children younger than 5 years of age are the most vulnerable.[2] Other priority areas include provision of adequate, safe water, food, shelter, and protection from violence.

- In addition to the usual causes of illness and death in emergency-affected populations in less-developed countries (measles, malaria, pneumonia, and diarrhea), crowded settlements may be prone to outbreaks of cholera, meningitis, and other diseases, which can be rapidly spread. Such outbreaks may be explosive and cause many deaths in a relatively short period of time. For example, in 1994, within 6 weeks of their arrival in Goma, Zaire, there were around 1000 cholera-related deaths per day amongst the 500,000 to 800,000 Rwandan refugees.[3]

PROBLEM IDENTIFIED

In times of stability, writes Dr. Andrew Schechtman, many of the poorest people in the world succeed in their struggle to meet basic needs for shelter, food, and water. When displaced from their homes by war or natural disaster, communities and extended families are disrupted, access to food and water are lost, and marginal circumstances become desperate. Displaced people are often dependent on the support of the international aid community to meet their basic needs.

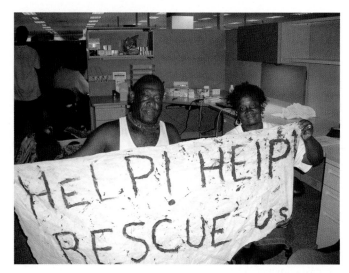

FIGURE 6-2 A husband and wife displaying the banner they made while being stranded on their roof during hurricane Katrina in New Orleans. The husband, who had an above-the-knee amputation, managed to climb with his crutches on the roof of their flooded home. After 2 days they were saved from the floodwaters. In a shelter in San Antonio they display the sign that helped save their lives. (*Courtesy of Richard P. Usatine, MD.*)

BEING PART OF THE SOLUTION

When infrastructure collapses as a result of man-made or natural disasters, access to health care can be limited or nonexistent. Serving as a volunteer physician with Medecins sans Frontieres(Doctors Without Borders) allowed Dr. Schechtman to provide medical care to people in desperate circumstances who had nowhere else to turn for assistance. Bearing witness to tragedies such as the case described in **Figure 6-1** gave him another means to help, i.e., the authority to speak out on behalf of victims like this child, to focus public attention on the situation, and encourage political pressure to bring the fighting to an end.

DISASTER RELIEF (MARIELOS VEGA, RN)

EPIDEMIOLOGY

Hurricane Katrina was the deadliest hurricane to strike the United States since 1928.[2] Katrina made initial landfall on August 25, 2005, in south Florida as a category 1 hurricane increasing rapidly in strength to category 5 upon reaching the Gulf of Mexico. On September 24, 2005, a second category 3 hurricane, Rita, forced the cessation of response activities in New Orleans and prompted the evacuation of Louisiana and Texas cities near the Gulf. In the days after the hurricane struck, displacement of persons living in these areas resulted in more than 200,000 in evacuation centers in at least 18 states (**Figures 6-2** to **6-4**). There were more than 1800 deaths reported in Louisiana, Mississippi, Florida, Alabama, and Georgia.

Eight hospitals and nine acute care facilities in New Orleans reported on 17,446 visits (including 8997 [51.6%] for illness; 4579 [26.2%] for injury) during the days after Hurricane Rita and during repopulation of the city.[4]

- 1500 people (10.9%) were admitted to a hospital. The most common reasons for hospital admission were heart disease (26.6%), gastrointestinal illness (12.3%), mental health condition (6.7%), and heat-related illness (6.1%).

- Of the 25 deaths occurring in this period (0.2%), 23 occurred in patients who were seen for an illness (92%) and 2 occurred in patients seen for an injury (8%).

- 1235 (9.1%) visits for injuries and illnesses were reported among relief workers (e.g., paid military, paid civilian, self-employed, or volunteer).

ETIOLOGY

When hurricanes move onto land, the resulting storm surges, violent winds, heavy rains, and flooding can cause extensive damage. Hurricanes Katrina and Rita caused devastating storm-surge conditions for coastal Mississippi, Louisiana, and Alabama and damage as far east as the Florida panhandle. Storm-induced breaches in the New Orleans levee system resulted in the catastrophic flooding of approximately 80% of that city.[5]

- Hurricane Katrina disrupted basic utilities, food-distribution systems, health care services, and communications in large portions of Louisiana and Mississippi.

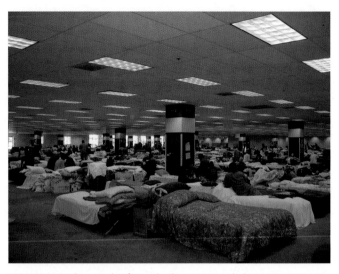

FIGURE 6-3 Thousands of people sleeping in a shelter in San Antonio after being evacuated from New Orleans. These evacuees experienced the horrors of the hurricane, the flood, and the Super Dome. (*Courtesy of Richard P. Usatine, MD.*)

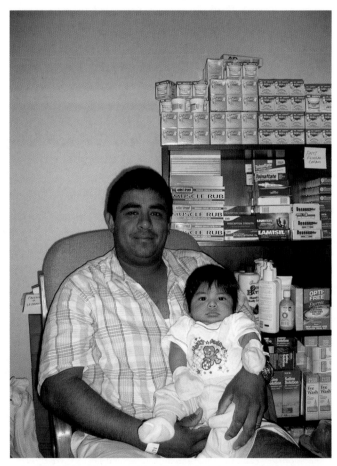

FIGURE 6-4 This father and daughter were evacuated from New Orleans to Houston after hurricane Katrina. Shortly thereafter, they were evacuated from Houston to San Antonio as hurricane Rita was about to hit. They are being seen for free health care in a shelter clinic in San Antonio. (*Courtesy of Richard P. Usatine, MD.*)

- Before 1990, the majority of hurricane-related deaths in the United States resulted from drowning caused by sudden storm surges.[6] Since 1990, advances in warning technology and timely evacuation have increased the proportion of indirect causes of death and injury from hurricanes, such as electrocutions, clean-up injuries, and carbon monoxide poisonings. During and after Hurricane Katrina, the majority of deaths resulted from storm surges along the Mississippi and Louisiana coastlines and flooding in the New Orleans area.

PROBLEM IDENTIFIED

Marielos Vega, a research nurse with the New Jersey Medical School, Department of Family Medicine, reported that with the recent natural disasters, including the tsunami and hurricanes Katrina and Rita, she felt a moral obligation to do something to help victims of these disasters. The eye of Hurricane Rita hit hardest in Orange County, a region 100 miles outside of Huston with a population of 84,966 that was already overwhelmed by the influx of evacuees a few weeks earlier from Hurricane Katrina. The storm tore off roofs and smashed windows of homes and businesses all over the county and knocked out power, water, and sanitation to all Orange County residents. Many governmental, medical, and public infrastructures in the county had suffered damage and had to close temporarily—the need for personnel was urgent.

BEING PART OF THE SOLUTION

Although she was already involved at the local level in fund raising with the Board of Concerned Citizens ("Backpacks of Hope for Children Victims of Hurricane Katrina" involving the collection of school backpacks with supplies for the children to continue with their education), Ms. Vega felt compelled to do more. She received training through her local American Red Cross chapter in mass care, shelter operations, and disaster health services and was deployed soon after to Texas to assist with Health Services Disaster Relief Efforts. She describes her 3-week experience this way:

- Household after household, we knocked on doors with first-aid supplies. At first, we were afraid not knowing what we were going to encounter behind the closed doors. Many houses were completely destroyed or had strong odors emanating from them. Cats and dogs were outside all over searching for food with no place to go.

- We provided first aid to those with minor cuts, abrasions, and burns. Public health education became a core duty—we taught people about proper hand washing, use of disinfectant gels, food safety, injury prevention, use of insect repellent, proper waste disposal, and proper removal of mold from their homes.

- We made mental and social services referrals as we found along our daily journey cases of elder and child abuse and neglect. We disbursed emergency supplies of prescription medications, diapers, formula, water, construction gloves, facial masks, cleaning kits, and blue tarps to cover the holes in the roofs caused by the fallen trees. We also had to ensure as much as possible that animals left behind were fed and had water to drink.

REFUGE ASYLUM (LUCY CANDIB, MD)

EPIDEMIOLOGY

The U.S. Committee for Refugees estimates that in 2001 there were approximately 15 million refugees and likely hundreds of thousands of asylum seekers in the world. Much of the data on asylum seekers comes from England.

- From more than 2000 applications for asylum from Turkish nationals (primarily Kurds) to the United Kingdom in 2003, investigators interviewed and examined 97 individuals requiring medical evaluation for evidence of torture.[7] A wide variety of injuries and psychological disorders were documented including posttraumatic stress disorder and major depression.

- A 2003 study from three community clinics in Los Angeles found that only 3% of torture victims told their physicians about their experience.[8]

ETIOLOGY

In a study of 89 asylum seekers from 30 countries, commonly reported reasons for abuse were political activity (59%), ethnicity (42%), and religion (32%).[9]

- Types of abuse in this population included punching/kicking (79%), genital electrical shock (8%), and rape (7%) (**Figure 6-5**).

- Persistent psychological symptoms were common; 40% had posttraumatic stress disorder.

PROBLEM IDENTIFIED

Dr. Lucy Candib is a family physician working at a community health center in Worcester, MA, a city of 168,000 people that has been a home to immigrants for hundreds of years. She has always been committed to cross-cultural medicine and has cared for patients and families from all over the world since her early training. She has a longstanding commitment to work with women survivors of physical and sexual violence but had never been involved in a formal way in working with immigrants seeking political asylum. She writes, "I started about 5 years ago with an evaluation of a woman from Kenya fleeing severe physical violence from her husband. Her story was emblematic of everything I had ever learned about battered women, including marital rape, the abduction of the children, and threats and harm against the woman's own parents."

BEING PART OF THE SOLUTION

Dr. Candib attended a 1-day training for medical professionals offered by Physicians for Human Rights and studied their materials, focusing on how to write a coherent and effective evaluation for asylum hearings. She began to work regularly with the local refugee and immigrant settlement organizations to conduct physical examinations and provide medical documentation for their clients who were seeking political asylum in the United States. She describes the process as follows:

- The asylum lawyer contacts me to schedule an evaluation and sends me the materials relevant to his/her client's case and to the country of origin about once every 2 or 3 months.

- I meet with a man or woman, often from a country in West Africa. I usually start with situating the person in their family and their region, and then move slowly into eliciting a history of the events that unfolded in their experiences of persecution, imprisonment, torture, and flight. I include a full medical history and review of their current symptoms. This detailed process may take one to three sessions depending on the person's ability to tell his/her story and tolerate the feelings that always emerge when recounting it.

- Afterwards, I do a physical examination, carefully documenting scars by measurement and photographs and describing any physical injuries resulting in pain or limitation of movement. I include an assessment of their mental and emotional condition. I do these assessments at the health center on my days off, as these long sessions do not fit in the short medical appointments in my regular schedule.

- Drawing on my notes, I then provide a narrative history and examination in a formal document for the asylum hearing and attach any relevant photographs. Some pictures leave no room for doubt: the photographs of the scars on the perineum of a man subjected to torture by having weights hung from his penis (**Figure 6-5**), or the symmetrical scars on both sides of the scalp of a man who had been clubbed by police wielding truncheons. Often I do some research on the Internet to understand how my clients' experiences fit into the overall political history of their country. This documentation work takes anywhere from 5 to 10 hours for each individual. The lawyers tell me that my assessments weigh heavily in their clients' favor at the hearings.

Dr. Candib concludes saying, "This work has changed me as a human being. After thirty years of clinical practice with low-income families, moments come when I feel that I have not accomplished much. But this work—engaged in advocacy that directly affects a person's future—reaffirms that I *can* make a difference, one person at a time. This is also humbling work. These individuals teach me not only about what unspeakable pain humans inflict on each other, but also what amazing strengths each person carries inside. These patients teach me about myself and how much I don't understand or know about any given person in front of me in the examination room, and, at the same time, teach me about the world. Without leaving Worcester, I become a doctor without a border, acting on behalf of others while growing myself."

CARING FOR THOSE WITH DISABILITIES (LAURIE WOODARD, MD)

EPIDEMIOLOGY

Approximately 54 million Americans currently live with at least one disability and the vast majority (52 million) live in their communities (**Figure 6-6**).[10]

- According to data from 1999, the prevalence rate of disability was 24% among women and 20% among men.[11] Approximately 32 million adults had difficulty with one or more functional activities and approximately 16.7 million adults had a limitation in the ability to work around the house. Two million adults used a wheelchair and seven million used a cane, crutches, or a walker.

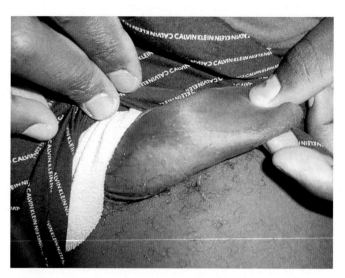

FIGURE 6-5 This man suffered torture in an African prison, wherein rocks were suspended from his penis. The image shows a hypopigmented scar at the base of his penis where he had an avulsion injury that healed slowly because of infection. This picture was essential in the process of gaining this man asylum. Images of scars resulting from torture and persecution combined with medical affidavits are instrumental in assisting other applicants in obtaining asylum in the United States. (*Courtesy of Lucy Candib, MD.*)

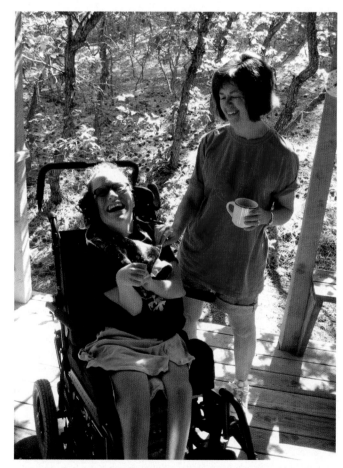

FIGURE 6-6 Dr. Laurie Woodard and her daughter Anika share a good laugh following breakfast while on vacation in New Mexico. Although Anika is dependent for all her activities of daily living and is nonverbal because of spastic quadriparetic cerebral palsy, she loves to travel and has a wonderful sense of humor.

- 4.9 million children aged 3 to 17 years were told that they have some type of learning disability and 12.8% (9.4 million) have special health care needs.[10]

- Racial and ethnic minorities have higher rates of disabilities than whites or Asian Americans; 7.3 million individuals (aged 15–65 years) with disabilities are of racial or ethnic minorities.

- In 2005, the surgeon general issued a Call to Action to improve the health and wellness of persons with disabilities underscoring the need in this population.[10]

ETIOLOGY

Challenges to a person's health can happen at any age and at any time. Disabilities are not illnesses, rather they are limitations related to a medical condition that have an influence on essential life functions such as walking, seeing, or working.[10] Further, disabilities do not affect all people in the same way.

- Of all the adults with disabilities, 41.2 million (93.4%) reported that their disability was associated with a health condition including arthritis and rheumatism (17.5%), back or spine problems (16.5%), heart trouble/hardening of the arteries (7.8%), lung or respiratory problems (4.7%), deafness or hearing problems (4.2%), mental or emotional problems (3.7%), blindness or visual problems (3.4%), and intellectual disability (2%).[11]

- Rates of disability are increasing in part because of the aging population, better survival of catastrophic illnesses and trauma, and advances in preventing infant and child mortality.

PROBLEM IDENTIFIED

As a mother of a child with profound disabilities, Dr. Laurie Woodard found that her medical training did little to prepare her for caring for her child or finding help (**Figure 6-6**). She became acutely aware that people with disabilities had great difficulty finding physicians and those who provided care often seemed afraid of them. She said, "I couldn't imagine someone not wanting to care for her because she had a disability." Physicians tend to focus on the medical condition and not the whole person and their families; when confronted with the patient's health care needs and functional issues, the feeling of acting more like a social worker than a physician caused them to fall back into medical model framework. In addition, societal support for those with disabilities, particularly disabilities acquired as an adult, are fragmented and the primary care physician needs to become the link.

BEING PART OF THE SOLUTION

Dr. Woodard began to care for increasing numbers of patients with disabilities, training herself through reading, experience, and asking patients what worked. As she worked with individual students she planned for a time when she could break into the medical student curriculum to provide this training. Two years ago, when the curriculum for third-year students underwent major reform, she saw her opportunity. Within the primary care 16-week experience, a curriculum on special populations was planned and Laurie made sure that it included teaching about persons with disabilities. Her curriculum, implemented in 2005 with goals ranging from sensitivity training to understanding both the capabilities and needs of individuals with disabilities, contains the following components:

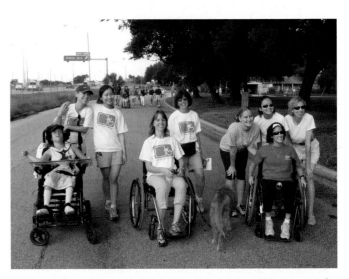

FIGURE 6-7 Dr. Woodard, daughter Anika, and dog Nikki are part of a team of University of South Florida medical students, faculty, and family who participated in a "wheel-a-thon" to raise money for Tampa's first fully accessible playground. Teaching medicals students the therapeutic value of sports and recreation for people with disabilities is an important aspect of the USF curriculum.

- Group experience with high-school students having intellectual disability including a "speed dating" technique of rapid introductions allows students to discover that these young adults are "just like us."
- Clinic-like experience with four to six model patients with physical disabilities (e.g., cerebral palsy, communication issues, wheelchair users) where pairs of students complete brief interview and physical examination under video monitoring. The session ends with a debriefing circle wrap up with students and patients.
- Panel discussion with patients with varying abilities and their advocates with an emphasis on community services and opportunities including the arts and sports.
- Home visits where student pairs (two medical students or a medical student and physical therapy student) receive a preparation sheet and checklist and learn how disability affects individuals and their family. Following the visit, students prepare reflection plus research reports that are posted on blackboard; part of the assignment is to read and comment on all the papers.
- Service learning project where students give presentations on topics (e.g., first aid, influenza) selected by staff at an adult day facility for individuals with intellectual disabilities or the high-school group noted above. Students also assist in the recreational activities for individuals with disabilities and at times perform sports physicals.
- Sensitivity training session, run by Parks and Recreation where students are randomly assigned a disability and complete tasks followed by watching the movie *Murderball* (an informative and proactive documentary about the paralympic sport, quadriplegic rugby, and its players).

"The students learn to see the patient first," she says, "that caring for these individuals requires recognizing the patient's expertise about their disability and problem solving together." (**Figure 6-7**)

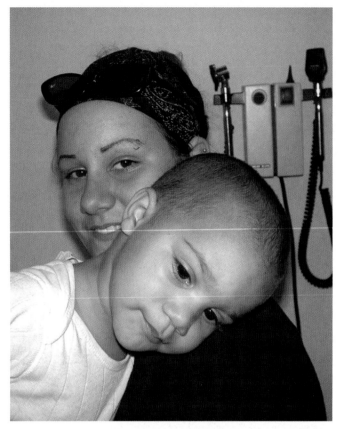

FIGURE 6-8 This mother and child are being cared for in the UCLA/Salvation Army free clinic run by medical students for homeless families in a transitional housing village. The boy had a bacterial infection on his leg and required antibiotics. The computer system in a pharmacy rejected his name and number and the child almost did not receive the antibiotic. Fortunately, the family doctor advocated for this child and the medicine was obtained. (*Courtesy of Richard P. Usatine, MD.*)

CARE FOR THE UNINSURED (CARYL HEATON, DO)

EPIDEMIOLOGY

- According to figures from the U.S. Census Bureau, 44.8 million individuals in the United States (15.9% of the population) are uninsured.[12]
  - The largest increase was in families with incomes more than $50,000 per year (17 million).
  - The number of uninsured children also rose to 8.3 million.
  - Lack of insurance disproportionately affects Hispanics (32.7% are uninsured), followed by blacks (19.6%), Asians (17.9%), and non-Hispanic whites (11.3%). (**Figures 6-8** and **6-9**)
  - According to the American College of Physicians,[13]
    - uninsured Americans may be up to three times as likely as privately insured individuals to experience adverse health outcomes.
    - uninsured patients have been found to be up to four times as likely as insured patients to require both avoidable hospitalizations and emergency hospital care.
  - Health outcomes are worse for those who have financial barriers to health care services and medications. For example, in a follow-up

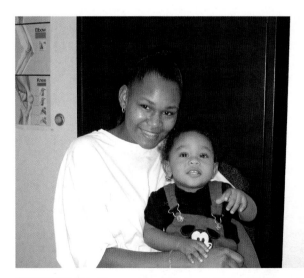

FIGURE 6-9 This 18-year-old mother has had type I diabetes since age 13. As a single mom she qualified for one of the living units within the Salvation Army transitional housing village. The week before this photo was taken, she presented to the student-run free clinic with diabetic ketoacidosis secondary to running out of her insulin. She knew that she needed her insulin but the pharmacy would not fill it because her insurance appeared to have lapsed in the computer system. After many calls to many pharmacies with no luck, her needed insulin was obtained from another free clinic in town. She survived without hospitalization and was feeling much better at the time of this photograph. (*Courtesy of Richard P. Usatine, MD.*)

study of patients with an acute myocardial infarction, at one year, those with financial barriers to services were more likely to have lower quality of life and to be rehospitalized (49.3% vs. 38.1%) and those with financial barriers to medications were more likely to have angina (34.9% vs. 17.9%) and to be rehospitalized (57% vs. 37.8%).[14]

○ Uninsured adults have a 25% greater mortality risk than adults with coverage; approximately 18,000 excess deaths among people <65 years are attributed to lack of coverage every year.[15]

ETIOLOGY

Included among the uninsured are those who have part-time jobs and do not qualify for benefits and those who work for employers who do not provide health insurance benefits.

• The percentage of Americans covered by employee-sponsored health insurance fell to 59.5% (2005) from 63.6% in 2000.[16] This puts the responsibility on individuals to find coverage.

• Between 2003 and 2005, 89% of Americans looking for health insurance never bought a plan; 58% reported that it was "very difficult or impossible" to find affordable coverage[17]; 21% were turned down or charged a higher premium because of preexisting conditions.

PROBLEM IDENTIFIED

As a practicing family physician in downtown Newark, NJ, Caryl Heaton witnessed the patchwork of coverage offered to the poor and working poor in her community. At the same time that she was excited by the prospect of a "new model" of family medicine, she was also deeply troubled by the concern that the "system" was too dysfunctional to allow it to work. She has written "no one sees the inadequacies of the system with more aching clarity than the family physician. We are asked to prioritize medications for a patient when they admit that they can't afford them all. We see the waste in a system that repeats 3 recent studies on a patient because they were admitted to a hospital across town. We see patients come and go from our practices based on the yearly deals made in their employer's health care negotiations."

BEING PART OF THE SOLUTION

Dr. Heaton was motivated to speak out on system-wide health care reform and to advocate for the adoption of universal single-payer health coverage for all Americans. She began to learn as much as she could about the subject of the uninsured and the approaches to a solution. She was convinced that teachers of family medicine must educate themselves, their patients, and their communities on the need for change in the American health care system. She joined Physicians for a National Health Plan (PNHP) as the only medical organization dedicated to a view of the health care system that was inclusive, equitable, and affordable. PNHP provided training, networking, and an avenue toward political action. Recently, Dr. Heaton (in her role as president of the Society of Teachers of Family Medicine [STFM]) organized a health care forum at their annual meeting, bringing together family physician experts in health policy to discuss the key issues and possible solutions for meaningful national reform. She is now a key contact for her state legislators

and makes "visits" to the legislative delegation from her state to advocate for her vision of social justice.

CARING FOR THE HOMELESS (RICHARD P. USATINE, MD)

EPIDEMIOLOGY

As many as 3.5 million people (approximately 1% of the U.S. population) are homeless over the course of a year; roughly one-third of them are children.[18,19] Of those who are homeless, 3% report having HIV/AIDS and 26% report other acute health problems, including tuberculosis and other sexually transmitted infections.[19]

Causes of death were investigated in one study of 40 homeless people for more than a 1-year period (1985-86) conducted by the Fulton County Medical Examiner in Georgia. It was thought at that time that between 4000 and 7000 individuals were homeless and so the crude death rate for that year was estimated at 5.7 to 10.0 per 1000.[18]

• Black males accounted for 19 (48%) of the 40 deaths, white males for 18 (45%), and black females for 3 (8%). The median age for 36 individuals whose age was known was 44 (range = 21–70 years).

• Twenty-two individuals (55%) died or were found dead outdoors. Of the 18 persons who died indoors, 7 were found in vacant buildings and 5 died at shelters.

• Cause of death, based on the medical history, investigation scene information, circumstances of death, and autopsy and toxicologic studies (when performed) was classified as either natural (16), accidental (19), or homicide (4) or suicide (1). Natural deaths included alcohol related (9 including 3 with seizures likely from alcohol withdrawal), heart disease (4), and lung disease (3). Accidental deaths were primarily a result of acute alcohol toxicity (7), fire (6), hypothermia (2), and pedestrian-motor vehicle incidents (2). No deaths were attributed to drugs other than alcohol.

ETIOLOGY

Homeless persons are often extremely poor and socially isolated, the latter considered a significant contributor to being homeless.[18] Many medical conditions are caused by or exacerbated by the adverse living conditions and lack of health care experienced by the homeless. These include

• Psychiatric illnesses (as many as 40% of homeless persons).

• Physical health problems, including injuries from trauma, respiratory disease (e.g., tuberculosis), scabies and pediculosis infestations, and chronic illnesses such as diabetes.

PROBLEM IDENTIFIED

Dr. Usatine has worked with homeless individuals and families for more than 24 years. Their stories and lives have touched his heart and soul in profound ways. He writes, "the homeless in America are at the bottom of our society in dire poverty and lacking a stable living environment. Losing a job and a home and suffering with mental illness and addictions make the homeless one of the most vulnerable populations in our wealthy country."

BEING PART OF THE SOLUTION

In 1984, Dr. Usatine began to provide health care to homeless people at the Venice Family Clinic, a free clinic in Venice, CA. Along with Mary Smith NP, a seasoned nurse practitioner who had years of experience working with the homeless, he delivered health care to the homeless of Los Angeles both in the free clinic and in the surrounding shelters. Dr. Usatine was also the medical director of a nurse-practitioner-run full-time free clinic in the largest homeless shelter on skid row of LA. Working with Aaron Strehlow, NP, PhD, they made care accessible to the approximately thousand homeless persons staying in that shelter on a daily basis.

He first established two student-run clinics for homeless families and individuals with the medical students of UCLA. He states that the "passion and motivation of the students to serve this vulnerable population has been a tremendous inspiration to him throughout his career." After moving to San Antonio, Dr. Usatine worked with medical students to establish two more student-run clinics: one for homeless families and another for women in a residential drug and alcohol treatment home (**Figures 6-10** to **6-12**).

- Dr. Usatine has made it easier for medical students to volunteer their time in the student-run clinics by creating approved courses that give students credit for their work with the homeless.

- Currently he is running a "Humanism Fellowship" in which fourth-year medical students work throughout their fourth year to take leadership roles in managing and directing the student-run clinics under faculty supervision. The elective supports and nourishes the inherent altruism of the students.

- As part of these experiences, students are asked to reflect on their work with the homeless. This comment from one student perhaps best expresses what many students have written about providing care to this vulnerable population, "Seeing how difficult it is to get back on your feet has greatly impacted how I treat those who are struggling. It has taught me that I am blessed with such a gift of providing healthcare that I should give back without any expectations of reimbursements or praise. I realize what a difference I can make in the lives of those who are homeless by providing them not only with healthcare but encouragement. It has taught me to be blind to those with and without insurance and to treat everyone equally regardless of their social background. It has made me more appreciative of the comforts that I take for granted and how easily we can be living in a bubble."

Dr. Usatine strongly believes that these students will be better physicians for the experiences in these student-run clinics. He states, "It is wonderful to be part of the solution to help people who have slipped through the cracks of the health care system get the health care they need. It is especially rewarding to see medical students put their hearts and souls into caring for this population." Students learn compassion and are inspired by the efforts being made by their patients to get their lives back together. They are always amazed by the tragic stories of abuse, violence, poverty, and deprivation that many of their patients have lived through.

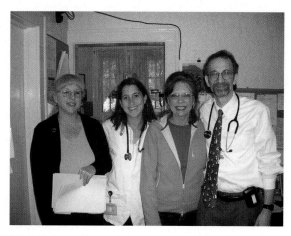

FIGURE 6-10 In an effort to help women recovering from substance abuse, the students and faculty of University of Texas Health Sciences Center San Antonio partnered with Alpha Home to open a free clinic on site. Alpha home is a residential treatment unit with a 40-year track record of helping women become clean and sober. Prior to the opening of this clinic within the home in which the women reside, most of these uninsured women would go to the crowded university emergency department for health care. Many went without health care for fear that a 36-hour wait would drive them back to drugs and alcohol. The photograph shows (from left to right) Melanie Lane, the head counselor; Amy Cantor, the student founder; Julie Wisdom-Wild, the CEO; and Richard P. Usatine, the faculty founder and advisor.

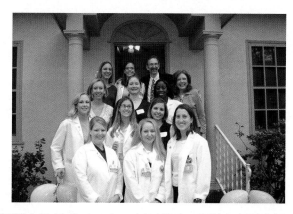

FIGURE 6-11 Medical students Julie Wisdom-Wild and Richard P. Usatine on the day of the clinic dedication at Alpha Home. The medical students derive great satisfaction from giving to the community. (*Courtesy of Richard P. Usatine, MD.*)

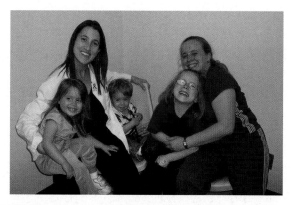

FIGURE 6-12 Amy Cantor as a fourth-year medical student in the Humanism Fellowship caring for a family at the second student-run clinic established in San Antonio. The mom and her four children have been reunited at the San Antonio Metropolitan Ministries Transitional Living and Learning Center. We saw this family almost weekly in our clinic and helped them make the transition from homelessness to independence. (*Courtesy of Richard P. Usatine, MD.*)

DISPARITY IN CAREERS IN MEDICINE (CRYSTAL CASH, MD)

EPIDEMIOLOGY

According to data from the American Association of Medical Colleges (AAMC),[20] few U.S. physicians practicing in 2004 were of minority race; blacks comprised only 3.3%, 2.8% were Hispanic, and 5.7% were Asian. Of black physicians, the vast majority (64.7%) are in office-based practice and 23.7% are in hospital-based practice (includes residents and fellows); the percentages are similar for physicians of other minority races. Only 1% of black physicians are in medical teaching (compared with 0.9% of Hispanics, 0.4% of Asians, and 0.4% of Native Americans). This lack of diversity is problematic for many reasons including workforce distribution; minority physicians are more likely to provide care for minority and indigent patients and to practice in underserved areas (51% of black, 41% of Native American, and 34% of Hispanic graduates in 2004 intended to practice in underserved areas compared with 18.4% of whites).[21]

- After steady declines in the number of applicants to medical schools since 1997, the number increased 2.7% from 2003 to 2004.[BC] In 2004, 15% of the applicants were of minority race including 7.8% black and 7.1% Hispanic. Between 41.3% and 48.8% of applicants were accepted.

- There are increasing numbers of minority physicians graduating from medical schools but the percentage remains small at 6.4%.[20]
  - Over the past two decades, the percentage of white physicians graduating from U.S. allopathic medical schools has decreased by 13.9% (12,916 in 1980 to 11,117 in 2004) while, over the same period, black physician graduates increased from 704 to 1063, Hispanics from 473 to 1050, Asians from 336 to 3554, and Native Americans from 40 to 112.
  - In 2004, black women comprised 62% of all the black graduates while Hispanic women comprised 52.7% of Hispanic graduates and white women comprised 47% of white graduates.

- Of 114,087 medical school faculty, 71.9% were white, 12.6% were Asian, 4.0% were Hispanic, and 3.1% were blacks. Minority faculty were primarily at the rank of assistant professor with 9% to 19% at full professor compared to whites where nearly 30% were at the rank of full professor.

ETIOLOGY

- Lack of representation of minorities in medicine is likely mulifactorial and includes lack of educational opportunity and encouragement, prejudice, and lack of mentoring.

- Problems in the pipeline from kindergarten to grade 12 play an essential role in hindering the numbers of ethnic and racial minorities from applying to medical school.[21]
  - Blacks and Hispanics have lower rates of graduating from high school than whites.
  - Only 39.9% of blacks and 34% of Hispanic high-school graduates enrolled in college from 2000 to 2002 compared to 45.5% of whites.

PROBLEM IDENTIFIED

In an attempt to improve test scores in a failing Chicago public school, the school was divided into three institutes, one of which is the Daniel Hale Williams Prep School for Medicine. Dr. Cash was one of the several physicians from Provident Hospital (also founded by Dr. Daniel Hale Williams) who were invited to an open house called "Doctor's Day." The idea for a mentoring program sprang from the days' activities to provide access for kids to practicing physicians.

BEING PART OF THE SOLUTION

- The Future Doctors of America Club (**Figure 6-13**) proposes that through leadership training and skills development, the students themselves can become resources and will mentor other students.
  - The program is based on principles similar to the school's mission—to have the students become physicians through improved resources and hands-on activities.
  - Mentors are assigned one to three mentees and mentor–student experiences include shadowing, tutoring, advising, volunteer activities, and social interaction.
- "In our first year," writes Dr. Cash, "we inducted 27 students into the club, and this year we added another 54 students. We developed guidelines for mentors, students, and for parent participation. The students developed their organizational structure, vision, and mission statements as well as a schedule of desired activities. Activities all are associated with service learning hours and skills development."

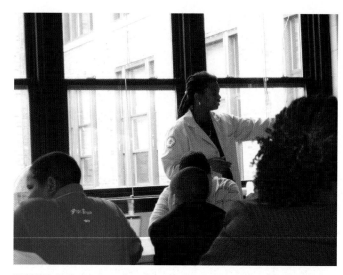

FIGURE 6-13 Dr. Crystal Cash working with inner-city students in The Future Doctors of America Club. This peer education session was held at a Chicago Public School (Daniel Hale Williams Preparatory School for Medicine).

PROVIDER RESOURCES

- Refugee information
  - United Nations High Commissioner for Refugees, **www.unhcr.ch;**, the U.S. Committee on Refugees, **www.refugees.org;** and Relief Web, **www.reliefweb.org.**
  - Doctors Without Borders, **www.doctorswithoutborders.org.**
- Disaster relief
  - Information on disaster relief agencies, **www.disastercenter.com/agency.htm.**
  - Red Cross, **www.redcross.org.**
  - International relief efforts, **www.ri.org** and **www.imcworldwide.org.**
- Asylum seekers
  - Refugees do have legal rights protected by international law. The 1951 Refugee Convention defines the rights of refugees. The United Nations High Commissioner for Refugees (UNHCR) is the UN agency responsible for refugee protection.
  - Ann Intern Med 1995;122(8):607–13. (Describes the current state of physician involvement in the prevention of international torture and in the treatment of victims; in addition, the authors

propose ways that individual physicians can become involved by caring for survivors and providing expert testimony.)

- Disabled
  - U.S. Department of Justice, **www.usdoj.gov/crt/ada/cguide.htm.**
  - Social Security Administration, **www.ssa.gov/disability/** (information on benefits).
  - Information on sports events for the disabled, **www.dsusa.org.**
  - **www.disabilityinfo.gov** and **www.direct.gov.uk.**
- Uninsured
  - Physicians for a National Health Plan, **www.pnhp.org.**
  - Kaiser Family Foundation, **http://www.kff.org/uninsured/index.cfm.**
  - Robert Wood Johnson Foundation, **http://www.kff.org/uninsured/index.cfm.**
- Homeless
  - National Coalition for the Homeless, **http://www.nationalhomeless.org/.**
  - National Alliance to End Homelessness, **http://www.naeh.org/.**
  - U.S. Department of Housing and Urban Development, **http://www.hud.gov/homeless/index.cfm.**
  - Veterans Affairs, **http://www1.va.gov/homeless/.**
- Underrepresented minorities in health care
  - **www.aamc.org/students/minorities/start.htm.**
  - 12th Report on Minorities in Medicine **www.cogme.gov/rpt12_2.htm.**
  - **www.amsa.org/div/.**

REFERENCES

1. United Nations High Commissioner for Refugees (UNHCR): www.unhcr.org. Accessed April 20, 2007.

2. Center for Disease Control (CDC): http://www.cdc.gov/nceh/ierh/FAQ.htm. Accessed April 20, 2007.

3. http://www.refugeecamp.org/learnmore/cholera/.

4. Daley WR. Public Health Response to Hurricanes Katrina and Rita—Louisiana, 2005: http://www.cdc.gov/mmwr/preview/mmwrhtml/mm5502a1.htm. CDC. Accessed May 1, 2007.

5. Injury and Illness Surveillance in Hospitals and Acute-Care Facilities After Hurricanes Katrina and Rita—New Orleans Area, Louisiana, Sept 25 to Oct 15, 2005: http://www.cdc.gov/mmwr/preview/mmwrhtml/mm5502a4.htm. Accessed May 1, 2007.

6. Hanzlick R. Office of the Fulton County Medical Examiner. Surveillance and Programs Br, Div of Environmental Hazards and Health Effects, Center for Environmental Health, CDC. *MMWR.* 1987;36(19):297–299.

7. Bradley L, Tawfig N. The physical and psychological effects of torture in Kurds seeking asylum in the United Kingdom. *Torture* 2006;16(1):41–47.

8. Eisenman DP, Gelberg L, Liu H, et al. Mental health and health-related quality of life among adult Latino primary care patients living in the United States with previous exposure to political violence. *JAMA* 2003;290(5):627–634.

9. Asgary RG, Metalios EE, Smith CL, et al. Evaluating asylum seekers/torture survivors in urban primary care: A collaborative approach at the Bronx Human Rights Clinic. *Health Hum Rights* 2006;9(2):164–179.

10. Department of Health and Human Services. The Surgeon General's call to action to improve the health and wellness of persons with disabilities. Rockville, MD: Public Health Service, 2005. http://www.surgeongeneral.gov/library/disabilities/calltoaction/calltoaction.pdf. Accessed April 25, 2007.

11. Prevalence of disabilities and associated health conditions among adults—United States, 1999. *MMWR.* 2001;50(07):120–125. http://www.cdc.gov/mmwr/preview/mmwrhtml/mm5007a3.htm.

12. Income, Poverty and Health Insurance coverage in the United States; 2005. Current population report, U.S. Census Bureau, August 2006.

13. No health insurance? It's enough to make you sick. www.acponline.org/uninsured/lack-contents.htm. Accessed May 12, 2007.

14. Rahimi AR, Spertus JA, Reid KJ, et al. Financial barriers to health care and outcomes after acute myocardial infarction. *JAMA.* 2007;297:1063–72.

15. Institute of Medicine: Fact Sheet 5. Uninsurance Facts and Figures. www.iom.edu/CMS/17645.aspx. Accessed May 12, 2007.

16. Kaiser foundation. *Changes in Employee's Health Insurance Coverage*, 2001–2005. Oct 2006.

17. Collins, et al. Squeezed: Why rising exposure to health care costs threatens the health and financial well-being of American families. Commonwealth Fund, Sept. 2006.

18. http://www.cdcnpin.org/scripts/population/homeless.asp. Accessed May 12, 2007.

19. http://www.cdcnpin.org/scripts/population/#1. Accessed May 12, 2007.

20. Diversity in the Physician Workforce: Facts & Figures 2006. https://services.aamc.org/Publications/index.cfm?fuseaction=Product.displayForm&prd_id=161&prv_id=191. Accessed May 7, 2007.

21. Minorities in Medical Education: Facts & Figures 2005. https://services.aamc.org/Publications/index.cfm?fuseaction=Product.displayForm&prd_id=133&prv_id=154. Accessed May 7, 2007.

PART 3

PHYSICAL AND SEXUAL ABUSE

7 CHILD PHYSICAL ABUSE

Maria D. McColgan, MD
James Anderst, MD, MS

PATIENT STORY

A 15-month-old child is brought to the emergency department by the police after a relative called 911. The child and his mother attended a family gathering where concerned relatives viewed the mother's story that the child "falls a lot" with suspicion. On examination there were many signs of physical abuse (**Figures 7-1** to **7-3**). His face was covered with bruises especially around the right eye and cheek (**Figure 7-1**). His axilla showed signs of being gouged with fingernails (**Figure 7-2**). While an initial skeletal survey did not show any fractures, a repeat skeletal survey and oblique views of the ribs were done 2 weeks later. The second skeletal series showed eight healing rib fractures. Repeat skeletal surveys are recommended in children younger than 4 years, who are confirmed or suspected victims of abuse (**Figure 7-3**). The child was admitted to the hospital and the police, hospital social workers, and child protective services were notified. In the emergency department, the child was evaluated by a forensic nurse examiner trained in child-abuse photodocumentation. The child was then referred to a child abuse pediatrician who assessed mechanisms of injuries, reexamined the child, and interpreted the initial and follow-up skeletal survey. Since the American Board of Pediatrics approved child abuse as a subspecialty in 2006, it is anticipated that many regions of the United States will have child abuse pediatricians available for consultation.

EPIDEMIOLOGY

- Occurs in 12.1/1000 children with highest rate of victimization in the 0 to 3 year age group (16.5/1000).
- The Department of Health and Human Services compilation of State Child Protective Services (CPS) Child Maltreatment 2005 had 3.3 million CPS reports filed in 2005 with 899,000 confirmed as abuse.[1] Of these,
  - More than 62% were neglected.
  - 17% were physically abused.
  - 9% were sexually abused.
  - 7% were emotionally abused.
- Nearly 80% of victims were abused by a parent acting alone or with another person.
- Medical personnel made only 8.1% of the referrals to CPS.

ETIOLOGY AND PATHOPHYSIOLOGY

Caregiver factors associated with child abuse include the following[2–4]:

- Inappropriate parental expectations of the child.
- Lack of empathy toward the child's needs.

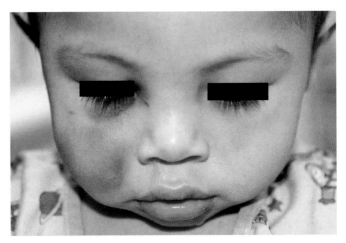

FIGURE 7-1 The sad face of a 15-month-old boy who has been physically abused by his mother's boyfriend for several weeks. There is bruising under both eyes, with the greatest degree of bruising seen under the right eye and on the right cheek. The boy is in the emergency department after concerned relatives called the police. (*Courtesy of James Anderst, MD, MS.*)

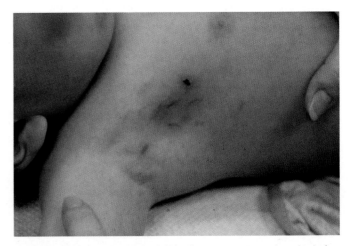

FIGURE 7-2 Same 15-month-old boy from Figure 7-1 with multiple fingernail gouges in his right axilla. Some are fresh and one appears to be older and somewhat crusted. Injuries in different stages of healing may indicate chronicity of abuse. (*Courtesy of James Anderst, MD, MS.*)

- The parent's belief in physical punishment.
- Parental role reversal.
- Personal history.
  ◦ Was abused during childhood.
  ◦ Parents' rearing practices modeled.
  ◦ Mental illness or substance abuse.

Factors specific to the child that are associated with abuse[2]:

◦ Prematurity.
◦ Disabilities.
◦ Difficult temperament.

Environmental factors associated with abuse:

◦ Domestic violence.
◦ Financial, family, or work stressors.
◦ Housing issues.

DIAGNOSIS

CONCERNING HISTORY

- History inconsistent with child's developmental stage.
- Injuries inconsistent with history given.
- History changes over time.
- Delay in seeking medical care (must consider families access to care and availability of transportation).
- Sibling blamed.
- Magical injury—no one knows how it happened.

CLINICAL FEATURES

- Pattern of lesion—loop marks (**Figure 7-4**), parallel lines consistent with hand print (**Figure 7-5**), bilateral black eyes, double marks of a pinch, ligature marks, petechiae on the face from strangulation (can also be caused by vomiting or severe coughing).
- Burn marks inconsistent with history (**Figure 7-6**). Liquid burns that are—well demarcated with a stocking glove distribution, and lack of splash marks can be more suspicious for intentionally inflicted burns.
- Oral lesions—torn frenula, palatal petechiae, contusions, or lacerations (typically from a bottle, finger, or other object forced into the child's mouth).[5]
- Failure to thrive and signs of malnutrition.
- Typical distribution—Location of bruises on upper arms, anterior thigh, trunk, genitalia, buttocks, face, ears, or neck (**Figures 7-4 to 7-8**).

LABORATORY STUDIES AND IMAGING[6]

- Bleeding diathesis screening—prothrombin time/partial thromboplastin time (PT/PTT), complete blood count (CBC).
- Abdominal trauma—Liver function tests (LFTs), amylase, lipase, urinalysis; computed tomography (CT) of abdomen recommended if laboratory results are elevated or urinalysis positive for blood.
- Fractures—Skeletal survey (including oblique views of the ribs) in children younger than 3 years or nonverbal children; consider

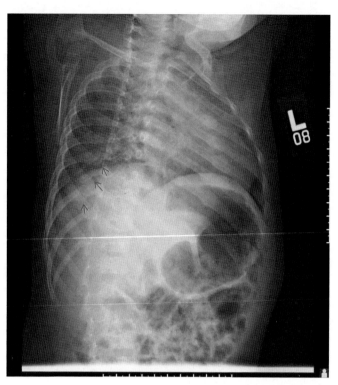

FIGURE 7-3 Same boy from Figure 7-1 with oblique x-ray showing healing rib fractures with callus in eight different locations as marked by the arrows. The degree of callus formation shows that these rib fractures are not new. Oblique radiographs should be requested in addition to a "skeletal survey" because lateral rib fractures are best seen with this view. (*Courtesy of James Anderst, MD, MS.*)

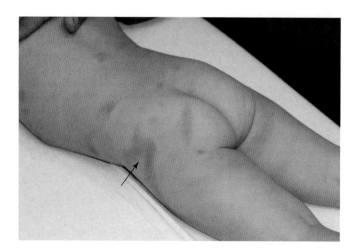

FIGURE 7-4 Young girl with linear bruising on the back, buttocks, and thigh from being hit with a belt. One bruise appears to have a loop-like form (see arrow) and was likely caused by blows with a cord or a looped belt. Blows with flexible objects produce patterns that tend to conform to the curved surfaces of the body whereas inflexible objects may produce a discontinuous pattern over curved surfaces. (*Courtesy of Nancy Kellogg, MD.*)

radionuclide bone scan to look for acute fractures, or a follow-up skeletal survey 2 weeks after initial presentation.

- Intracranial injury—CT/MR of head in all young children, even if there are no clinical signs of intracranial injury; ophthalmology examination for retinal hemorrhages.

DIFFERENTIAL DIAGNOSIS

- Bruises
  - Accidental bruises: Any bruising in an infant or precruiser is very concerning for abuse. Accidental bruising is much more common in cruising or walking children.[7] Any inflicted bruising or skin markings (including those from spanking or other punishment) lasting more than 24 hours constitutes abuse.[8] Ear bruising is very specific for abuse (**Figure 7-7**).[9] It is not possible to accurately date bruises.[10] Accidental bruising is typically located on the shins, lower arms, under chin, forehead, hips, elbows, ankles, and bony prominences. Loop-like bruising is suspicious for blows with a cord or a looped belt (**Figure 7-4**).
  - Bruising with tracking of blood can be seen with severe injuries to the head when a child is lifted up from the ground by their hair (**Figure 7-8**). Bleeding disorders: Familial history, abnormal coagulation laboratory test results, vitamin K deficiency.
  - Other rare diseases associated with bruising: Type 1 Ehlers-Danlos, Henoch Schönlein Purpura, phytophotodermatitis (skin reaction to psoralens, most commonly found in limes), osteogenesis imperfecta (brittle bones).
- Skin discoloration: Common examples are allergic shiners (dark, puffy lower eyelids) and Mongolian spots (macular blue-gray pigmentation usually on the sacral area of normal infants, usually present at birth or appears within the first weeks of life; see Chapter 102).
- Burns and skin lesions with similar appearance: Accidental burns (splash marks usually seen), sunburn, bullous impetigo, cellulitis, scalded skin syndrome, diaper rash, chemical burn caused by senna containing laxatives, and drug reaction.
- Cultural practices: Coining (**Figure 7-9**), cupping, Moxibustion (cultural practice of burning herbs on skin).
- Fractures from other diseases occurring in infants and young children.
  - Osteogenesis imperfecta: A congenital disorder with bone fragility; patients may have repeated fractures after mild trauma that heal readily. Other features include blue sclera, easy bruising, and deafness.
  - Rickets: Usually from vitamin D deficiency, consider in exclusively breastfed infants, dark skinned children, children with little sun exposure. The metaphyses show widening and cupping with irregular calcification due to poor calcification of osteoid.
- Failure to thrive from other causes including improper mixing of formula, breastfeeding difficulty, organic diseases such as cystic fibrosis, HIV, metabolic disorders, celiac disease, and renal disease.[11]

MANAGEMENT

- Emergent care first; treat injuries, burns, failure to thrive accordingly.
- Careful examination of the skin and oral cavity, palpation for bony tenderness or callous formation, signs of abdominal trauma or

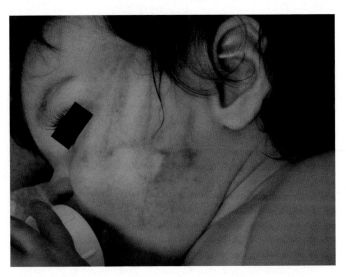

FIGURE 7-5 Linear ecchymosis on the cheek of a baby who was slapped in the face by an abusive parent. (*Courtesy of James Anderst, MD, MS.*)

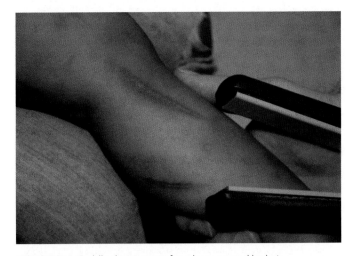

FIGURE 7-6 Toddler being seen for a burn caused by hair straightener. The family claimed the iron fell onto the leg but further investigation seemed to indicate that the iron was applied to the child by an angry parent to control a crying child. While the iron falling could explain the injury on the calf it does not explain the additional injury higher up on the leg. (*Courtesy of James Anderst, MD, MS.*)

neurologic abnormalities, ophthalmologic evaluation for retinal hemorrhages.

- Document the history provided by caregivers and physical findings accurately, including pictures.
- Consider consultation with a child abuse pediatrician or a family physician with additional training or expertise. Child abuse pediatrics is a new subspecialty requiring additional fellowship training.
- In cases where the injury was truly caused by an accidental mechanism, the role of neglect must be considered.
- Mandated reporting:
  - All 50 states require that all professionals who work with children report suspected child abuse and neglect.
  - Reporter of abuse is granted legal immunity.
  - Once the case is reported, further collaboration with Child Protective Services or law enforcement is usually necessary to ensure appropriate outcomes.

PATIENT EDUCATION

- Prevention programs: Universal screening for domestic violence, community education and awareness such as having parents of newborns view a video on shaken baby syndrome.[12]
- Home visitation programs and parenting skills classes.

FOLLOW-UP

- If there is suspicion of fractures, obtain repeat skeletal x-ray in 2 weeks to look for evidence of healing fractures.
- Siblings of abused children should be interviewed and examined for findings concerning for abuse.
- Counseling for child and family as appropriate.
- Frequent follow up with primary care provider to evaluate for signs of abuse and neglect.
- Report to Child Protective Services.

PATIENT RESOURCES

- Child Help, http://childhelp.org/.
- Prevent Child Abuse America, http://www.preventchildabuse.org/index.shtml.

PROVIDER RESOURCES

- The American Academy of Pediatrics
  - When Inflicted Skin Injuries Constitute Child Abuse, http://aappolicy.aappublications.org/cgi/content/full/pediatrics;110/3/644.
  - Evaluation of Suspected Child Physical Abuse, http://pediatrics.aappublications.org/cgi/content/full/119/6/1232.
  - The American Professional Society on the Abuse of Children, www.apsac.fmhi.usf.edu/index.asp.
  - Child Abuse Evaluation & Treatment for Medical Providers, http://www.childabusemd.com/index.shtml.

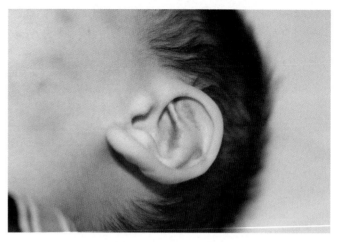

FIGURE 7-7 Bruising of the ear in a young boy who was physically abused by a parent. Ear bruising is rarely accidental. The additional bruising on the cheek suggests this child was hit with a hand or another object to produce the bruising seen in this photo. (*Courtesy of James Anderst, MD, MS.*)

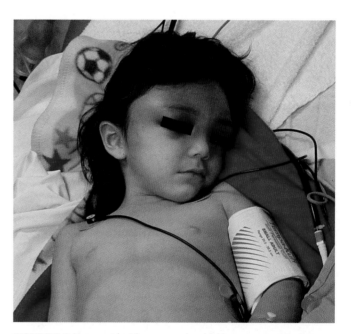

FIGURE 7-8 Young girl with severe subgaleal hematoma with extensive blood tracking into the upper face after being lifted off the ground by her hair. Blood tracking after significant injury is most commonly seen on the face although some injuries to the genitals may also track into the perineum. (*Courtesy of James Anderst, MD, MS.*)

REFERENCES

1. Gateway CWI. *Child Maltreatment 2005.* U.S. Department of Health and Human Services, Administration on Children, Youth and Families, 2007.

2. Giardino AP, Alexander R. *Child Maltreatment: A Clinical Guide and Reference.* G.W. Medical Publishing, 2005.

3. Bavolek, S. *The Nuturing Parent Programs.* Washington DC: Office of Juvenile Justice and Delinquency Prevention, U.S. Department. of Justice, 2000.

4. Helfer RM. The etiology of child abuse. *Pediatrics.* 1973;51 (Suppl 4):777–779.

5. Kellogg ND, American Academy of Pediatrics, Committee on Child Abuse and Neglect. Oral and dental aspects of child abuse and neglect. *Pediatrics.* 2005;116(6):1565–1568.

6. Kellogg ND, American Academy of Pediatrics, Committee on Child Abuse and Neglect. Evaluation of suspected child physical abuse. *Pediatrics.* 2007;119(6):1232–1241.

7. Sugar NF, Taylor JA, Feldman KW. Bruises in infants and toddlers: Those who cruise rarely bruise. *Arch Pediatr Adolesc Med.* 1999;153:399–403.

8. American Academy of Pediatrics, Committee on Child Abuse and Neglect. When inflicted skin injuries constitute child abuse. *Pediatrics.* 2002;110(3):644–645.

9. Dunstan FD, Guildea ZE, Kontos K, Kemp AM, Sibert JR. A scoring system for bruise patterns: A tool for identifying abuse. *Arch Dis Child.* 2002;86:330–333.

10. Maguire S, Mann MK, Sibert J, Kemp A. Can you age bruises accurately in children? A systematic review. *Arch Dis Child.* 2005;90: 187–189.

11. Block RW, Krebs NF. Failure to thrive as a manifestation of child neglect. *Pediatrics.* 2005;116(5):1234–1237.

12. Dias MS, Smith K, DeGuehery K, et al., Preventing abusive head trauma among infants and young children: A hospital-based, parent education program. *Pediatrics.* 2005;115(4):470–477.

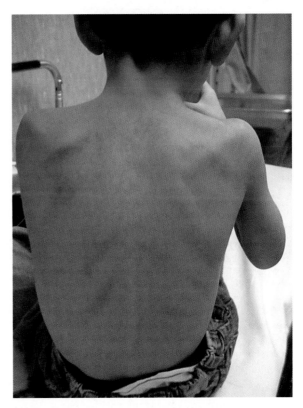

FIGURE 7-9 Young boy with the marks of coining on his back. A coin was rubbed across his back leaving ecchymoses over bony prominences with the intent to help the child heal from an acute illness. This cultural practice is more common among Asian immigrants to this country and mimics child abuse. (*Courtesy of Maria McColgan, MD.*)

8 CHILD SEXUAL ABUSE

Maria D. McColgan, MD
Nancy D. Kellogg, MD

PATIENT STORY

A 12-year-old girl is being seen for chronic abdominal pain by her family physician. The physician asks the mother to step out of the room and does a complete history including the HEADSS questions. The girl tearfully reports that her stepfather has been touching her in her private areas when her mother is not home. On examination with a female nurse chaperone in the room, the physician finds that the girl's hymen appears normal (**Figure 8-1**). However, when the girl is more carefully examined with a cotton-tip applicator, a hymenal cleft is seen (**Figure 8-2**). When the girl is asked whether any other types of sexual abuse occurred with her stepfather, she admits to repeated penile penetration. Although rare, sometimes the examination reveals more than what the child is willing to disclose about the abuse. Partial disclosures of abuse are common in children. In addition, the findings of sexual abuse tend to be subtle and are easily missed if a careful examination and special techniques are not used. Attempts are made to reassure the girl that this should never happen and that this is not her fault. Her mother is brought back into the room and after a sensitive discussion, the police is called and Child Protective Services notified.

HEADSS is an acronym that provides a framework for interviewing adolescents and children about health risks. The questions start from easiest and least sensitive to more sensitive questions that need to be asked:

  H—home
  E—education
  A—activities
  D—depression and drugs
  S—sex and sexual abuse
  S—suicide

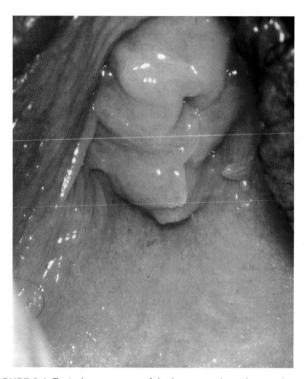

FIGURE 8-1 Typical appearance of the hymen and peri-hymenal tissues in a 12-year-old girl. Once females have entered puberty, the hymen becomes redundant with overlapping folds and is more difficult to examine for subtle signs of acute or healed injury. (*Courtesy of Nancy D. Kellogg, MD.*)

EPIDEMIOLOGY

- The Department of Health and Human Services compilation of State Child Protective Services (CPS) Child Maltreatment 2005 had 3.3 million CPS reports filed in 2005 with 899,000 confirmed as of abuse.[1] Of these, 9% were of sexual abuse. Not included in these numbers are several thousand additional victims who are sexually assaulted by nonfamily members; these cases are reported to law enforcement but not CPS.

- Sexual abuse of girls occurs at much higher rate than boys: 2.3 per 1000 females versus 0.6 per 1000 males.[2]

- Types of abusive sexual acts and relative frequencies, based on a population study of 191 consecutive cases, include the following[3]:
  ○ Touching, fondling, 100 (86%).
  ○ Vulvar coitus, 29 (25%).
  ○ Vaginal penetration, 6 (5%).
  ○ Anal penetration, 20 (20%).

○ Oral–genital contact, 15 (13%).
○ Insertion of foreign body, 8 (8%).
○ Unknown, 13 (11%).

ETIOLOGY AND PATHOPHYSIOLOGY

Child sexual abuse (CSA) occurs when a child is involved in sexual activities that he or she cannot comprehend, for which he or she is developmentally unprepared and cannot or does not give consent, and/or that violate laws. State laws vary considerably in what professionals are required to report; some are based on the professional's judgment that the activity was abusive whereas others are based on age-only criteria (i.e., report any sexual acts involving a minor).

Most sexual abuse involves an adult perpetrator the child knows and is expected to trust who uses deception and position of authority to gain the child's acquiescence and accommodation to the abuse,[4] generally progressing from less to more severe and intrusive sexual acts.

DIAGNOSIS

CLINICAL FEATURES

- Child victims of sexual abuse may have behavior changes, depression, increased sexual behaviors, somatic complaints (e.g., headaches or abdominal pain, constipation, enuresis/encopresis, genital/anal pain), or may be asymptomatic.
- Child may present to a medical provider for the following reasons:
  ○ Child has disclosed abuse (most common) or abuse was witnessed—most common scenario.
  ○ Caregiver suspects abuse because of behavioral or physical symptoms.
  ○ Child is brought for routine care and sexual abuse is suspected based on clinical findings (e.g., physical examination findings, behavioral concerns).
- Recent studies show that <5% of CSA victims have physical examination findings indicative of penetrative trauma because the type of sexual act either does not result in tissue damage or because when tissue damage occurs, healing starts and injuries heal quickly and completely.[5–7] In a study of 36 pregnant adolescents, only 2 had evidence of penetrative trauma.[8] The medical diagnosis relies predominantly on the child's history and clinicians should remember that "normal" does not mean "nothing happened."
- Tips for doing the physical examination:
  ○ The ano-genital examination should entail optimal direct light source, magnification, and appropriate examination positions and techniques.
  ○ Recommended examination positions include supine frog-leg or lithotomy and prone knee-chest; the latter position is particularly important to confirm any clefts viewed in supine position.
  ○ Various examination techniques include labial separation and traction, gluteal lifting in prone knee-chest and using cotton-tipped applicator for separating tissues.
  ○ In some cases, it may help to have an assistant gently squirt a small amount of nonbacteriostatic saline onto the hymen as the examiner uses gentle labial traction to view the hymen.

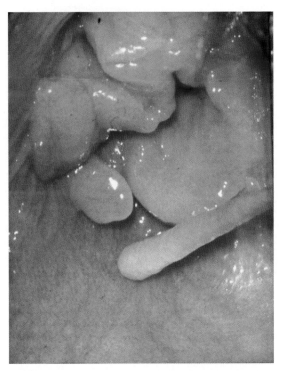

FIGURE 8-2 Hymenal cleft visible when the girl in **Figure 8-1** is more carefully examined using a saline moistened cotton-tip applicator to gently separate and demonstrate the edges of the hymen. This injury was caused by sexual abuse and may have been missed without the more careful examination. (*Courtesy of Nancy D. Kellogg, MD.*)

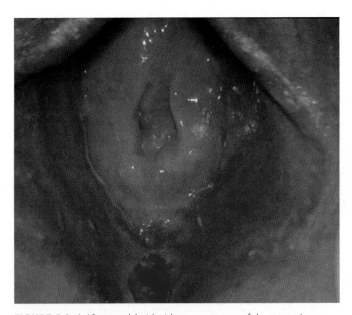

FIGURE 8-3 A 10-year-old girl with an acute tear of the posterior vestibule after recent sexual assault by a stranger. The posterior vestibule is the most common location for acute penetrative trauma in females. (*Courtesy of Nancy D. Kellogg, MD.*)

- A speculum examination and use of a cotton-tipped applicator to separate hymenal edges are traumatic procedures for prepubertal females and should not be used except under specific, rare circumstances.
  - Most findings of anal trauma can be visualized by gently spreading the anal folds.
- Physical findings concerning for abuse[9]:
  - Abrasions or bruising of the genitalia (**Figures 8-3** and **8-4**).
  - Acute or healed tear in the posterior aspect of the hymen extending to or nearly to the base or to the posterior fourchette or a complete hymen transection (**Figure 8-2**).
  - Markedly decreased hymenal tissue.
  - Anal bruising or lacerations (**Figure 8-5**).
  - Petecchiae or brusing on the soft palate.

LABORATORY TESTS AND IMAGING

- Forensic evidence collection if sexual assault occurred <72–96 hours prior to clinical presentation (consider referring to an emergency department or rape crisis center skilled in performing forensic evidence collection on children).
- Approximately 5% of sexually abused children and adolescents acquire a sexually transmitted infection (STI) from the abuse[9] (**Figure 8-6**).
- Consider STI testing in all postpubescent patients and in prepubescent children with a history of genital contact with any orifice.
  - HIV, hepatitis B&C, RPR (for syphilis), cultures for chlamydia, and gonorrhea and trichomonas.
  - Culture for HSV1 and 2 if ulcers or vesicles are present (**Figure 8-6**).
  - Condylomata acuminata is a clinical diagnosis and biopsy is required only if lesions are atypical or resistant to treatment.
- Pregnancy testing in postpubescent children; consider prophylaxis (e.g., plan B) if the event occurred <96 hours prior to evaluation.
- Follow up examinations 2–3 weeks after an acute assault to complete testing for STIs with prolonged incubation periods (especially HPV), assess resolution of injuries, and ensure emotional recovery.

DIFFERENTIAL DIAGNOSIS

In females, the following may be confused with abuse:

- Straddle injury (or other accidental trauma)—This occurs when a child falls onto an object. Bruising or lacerations to the labia majora, labia minora, or posterior fourchette may be seen. Although rare, accidental penetrating injury involving perihymenal tissues occurs, but rarely.
- Anatomic variants of normal, including shallow notches, anterior clefts, midline vestibule white lines, perineal defects, and narrow hymenal rims.
- Vulvar dermatitis—This may be caused by atopy, contact irritation, or seborrhea.
- Vulvovaginitis (e.g., nonspecific, shigella, streptococcus, poor hygiene, candidiasis)—Complaints include vaginal irritation or itching and vaginal discharge; wet prep and/or culture may be helpful.

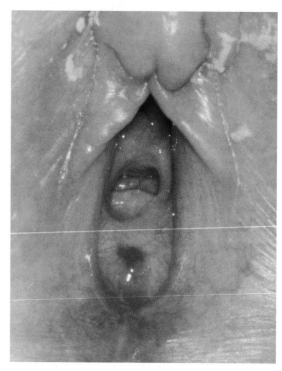

FIGURE 8-4 Acute hymenal hematoma in a prepubertal girl from penile penetration/contact. One reason why the considerable majority of examinations are normal may be that contact is more common than complete penetration and injuries resulting from penile contact are uncommon or are minor injuries that heal quickly and completely within days. (*Courtesy of Nancy D. Kellogg, MD.*)

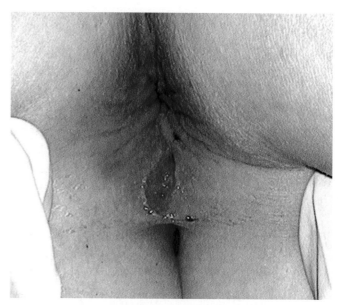

FIGURE 8-5 Acute rectal laceration in a young boy who was sexually abused by a relative. More than 95% of anal examinations in children with a history of anal penetration are normal or nonspecific. (*Courtesy of Nancy D. Kellogg, MD.*)

- Lichen sclerosus et atrophicus is a cutaneous disease not caused by sexual abuse. It may presents with bleeding, vulvar itching, or discomfort and the examination shows subepidermal hemorrhages and/or atrophic changes with areas of hypopigmentation over the vulva, perineum, and/or anus (**Figure 8-7**).

- Anogenital irritation or bleeding—This may be caused by shigella vaginitis, urethral prolapse, anal fissures, vulvar excoriations, lichen sclerosus et atrophicus, candidiasis, or dehiscence of a labial adhesion (**Figure 8-8**).

- Normal physiologic leukorrhea—Scant whitish discharge with a normal appearing vulvovaginal area. Wet mount normal.

  In males, the following may be confused with abuse:

- Accidental trauma (e.g., penis caught in zipper)—History should support pattern of injury. Most inflicted injuries of male genitals are physical, not sexual, abuse.

- Phimosis—unretractable foreskin. Irritation and redness as a result of trapped debris.

  In both male and female patients, the following rectal findings maybe confused with abuse:

- Anal fissure, which is a superficial excoriation or tear that extends from the anal verge into the anal canal; may or may not cause pain or bleeding during bowel movements. Sometimes, but not always, associated with diarrhea or constipation.

- Perianal venous pooling is sometimes mistaken for bruising.

- Hemorrhoids—Sometimes seen as a rectal protrusion or mass associated with itching and bleeding; a history of constipation is usually present.

- Pinworm or scabies infestation—Both can cause intense pruritus and excoriation; can be identified with microscopy (see Chapters 207 and 137.)

MANAGEMENT

- Children may present with nonspecific behavioral and physical symptoms (but no disclosure of abuse) that include chronic stomachaches or headaches, school difficulties, mood changes, and sleeping difficulties. These children should be questioned in a careful and nonleading manner about the possibility of sexual abuse. For example, the clinician may state: "I treat other children who have problems like you do with school and headaches. Some of these children have told me about things that have happened to their body or feelings that made them sad, scared, or confused. Has anything happened that has made you sad, scared, or confused?"

- Take a history from the child if necessary to make a medical diagnosis and to determine appropriate testing, treatment, and the need to file a report of suspected abuse. The clinician may opt not to take a history if the child was or will be interviewed elsewhere; in this case, information necessary to determine what type of medical assessment and testing should be obtained from other sources.
  ○ Ensure that the parent is not in the room for the history. Parents may be present for the physical examination.

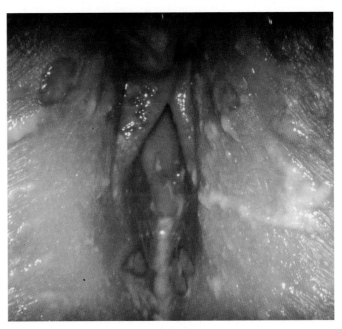

FIGURE 8-6 Herpes simplex virus (HSV) type 1 infection on the vulva of the prepubertal girl caused by sexual abuse. HSV type 1 of the genitals from sexual contact is increasing in prevalence relative to HSV type 2 infections of the genitals. (*Courtesy of Nancy D. Kellogg, MD.*)

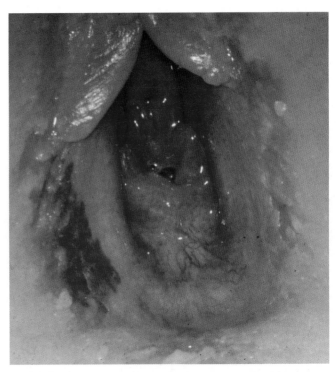

FIGURE 8-7 Lichen sclerosus et atrophicus in a young girl. This is a cutaneous disease, but commonly confused with sexual abuse because of the subepidermal hemorrhages. (*Courtesy of Nancy D. Kellogg, MD.*)

○ Use open-ended questions, such as "What happened?" or "Tell me more" as opposed to suggestive questions such as "Did daddy touch your private parts?"

○ Take careful notes and document with quotations whenever possible.

• Conduct a full physical examination including genitalia. Elicit cooperation from the child by explaining all procedures and earning his or her trust.

• Consider STI and pregnancy prophylaxis for postpubertal patients.

• Withhold STI treatment in asymptomatic prepubescent children until cultures are confirmed positive, as the incidence of STI in asymptomatic prepubertal children is relatively low.

• Consult with infectious disease specialist regarding HIV prophylaxis. If HIV prevalence is high in local regions, assailant risk factors are unknown or high for HIV, and if the child is evaluated within 72 hours of a high-risk exposure, then HIV prophylaxis may be appropriate.

• Examine closely for signs of physical and emotional abuse and neglect.

PATIENT EDUCATION

At well child visits, provider should discuss touches that make children sad, scared or confused, or that give them an "uh oh" feeling inside and encourage parents to reinforce these themes at home.

FOLLOW-UP

• Laws vary by state; however, all states have mandated reporting laws (see Child Welfare Information Gateway, http://www.childwelfare.gov/).

• All victims of sexual abuse and their families should be referred to local counseling agencies and to a Children's Advocacy Center, or other child abuse agency if available in the community.

PATIENT RESOURCES

• Child Help, **http://childhelp.org/.**

• Prevent Child Abuse America, **http://www.preventchildabuse.org/index.shtml.**

• National Center for Missing and Exploited Children, **http://www.missingkids.com/.**

PROVIDER RESOURCES

• The American Academy of Pediatrics Guidelines for the Evaluation of Sexual Abuse of Children, **http://aappolicy aappublications.org/cgi/content/full/pediatrics; 110/3/186.**

• National Guideline Clearing House—The evaluation of sexual abuse in children, **http://www.guideline.gov/summary/summary.aspx?doc_id=7583.**

• National Clearinghouse on Child Abuse and Neglect provides state statutes on child abuse and neglect, **http://nccanch.acf.hhs.gov/general/legal/statutes/define.cfm.**

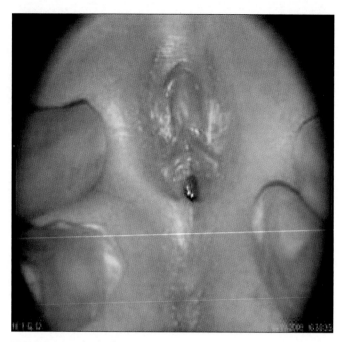

FIGURE 8-8 Labial adhesion can be confused with scarring secondary to child sexual abuse. This acquired condition is common in prepubertal girls and thought to be related to hygiene, irritation, and possibly trauma. (*Courtesy of Maria D. McColgan, MD.*)

REFERENCES

1. Gateway CWI. *Child Maltreatment: 2005.* U.S. Department of Health and Human Services. Administration of Children, Youth and Families. Washington, DC: Government Printing Office, 2007.

2. *Child Maltreatment 1998.* U.S. Department of Health and Human Services, Youth and Families. Washington, DC: Government Printing Office, 1999.

3. Emans SJ, Woods ER, Flagg NT, Freeman A. Genital findings in sexually abused, symptomatic and asymptomatic, girls. *Pediatrics.* 1987;79(5):778–785.

4. Summit R. Child sexual abuse accommodation syndrome. *Child Abuse Negl.* 1983;7(2):177–193.

5. Berenson AB, Chacko MR, Weimann CM, et al. A case-control study of anatomic changes resulting from sexual abuse. *Am J Obstet Gynecol.* 2000;182(4):820–831.

6. Heger A, Ticson L, Velasquez O, et al. Children referred for possible sexual abuse: Medical findings in 2384 children. *Child Abuse Negl.* 2002;26(6–7):645–659.

7. Adams JA, Harper K, Knudson S, Revilla J. Examination findings in legally confirmed child sexual abuse: It's normal to be normal. *Pediatrics.* 1994;94(3):310–317.

8. Kellogg ND, Menard SW, Santos A. Genital anatomy in pregnant adolescents: "Normal" does not mean "nothing happened." *Pediatrics.* 2004;113(1):e67–e69.

9. Kellogg ND. The evaluation of sexual abuse in children. *Pediatrics.* 2005; 116(2):506–512.

9 INTIMATE PARTNER VIOLENCE

Mindy A. Smith, MD, MS

PATIENT STORY

A woman who fled her abusive boyfriend is observed sitting at a table with other women in a residential chemical dependency treatment program. Her bruised face could not be missed (**Figure 9-1**). The program physician asked to speak with her and found out that her boyfriend beat her when she told him that she was voluntarily entering this program. The boyfriend was also an addict and had been physically abusive to her before. The violence escalated when she said that she needed help to stop the alcohol and drugs. She left him and did not believe that he would follow her. The program management assured her that they would not let him on the premises and would do all they could to keep her safe while she was recovering. **Figure 9-2** was taken 2 months later, when her face was healing along with her mind and spirit. She completed the 90-day program and is currently working and actively following a 12-step program.

EPIDEMIOLOGY

- Intimate partner violence (IPV), defined as an intimate partner's physical, emotional, or sexual abuse, affects up to half of the women in the United States during their lifetime.[1]
- Nearly 5.3 million IPV incidents occur each year among U.S. women (18 and older) and 3.2 million occur among men. Most of these assaults include pushing, grabbing, shoving, slapping, and hitting and do not result in major injury.[2]
- According to a national survey, 29% of women and 22% of men had experienced physical, sexual, or psychological IPV.[3]
- In the family practice setting, the lifetime prevalence of abuse of women was 38.8% with current abuse reported by 2% to 48% of women.[1]
- More than 1 million women and 371,000 men are stalked by intimate partners each year.[2]
- Clinicians identify only a small number of victims (1.5%–8.5%).[1] Only approximately 20% of IPV rapes or sexual assaults, 25% of physical assaults, and 50% of stalkings directed toward women are reported; fewer events against men are reported.[4]
- Battery, defined as the unlawful beating of another person or any threatening touch to clothes or body, is the greatest cause of injury.[1]
  - Up to 35% of women who visit an emergency department are battered; the lifetime prevalence of battering in this setting is 11% to 54%.
  - Almost 4% to 8% of women are battered during pregnancy.[4]
- According to the National Violence Against Women Survey, more than 200,000 women 18 years and older were raped by intimate partners in the 12 months preceding the survey.[5]

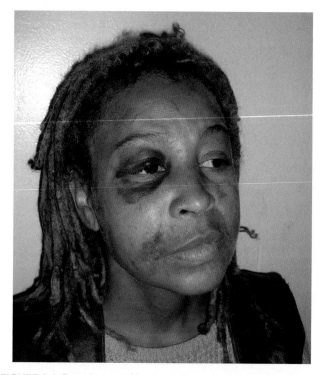

FIGURE 9-1 Bruising caused by intimate partner violence in a woman who fled her abusive boyfriend. (*Courtesy of Richard P. Usatine, MD.*)

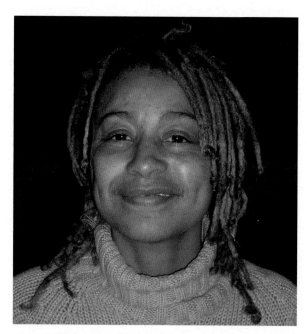

FIGURE 9-2 Photograph of the woman in Figure 9-1 taken 2 months later. Her facial and psychological wounds are healing. (*Courtesy of Richard P. Usatine, MD.*)

- IPV results in nearly 2 million injuries and 1300 deaths nationwide every year.
  - Approximately 11% of homicide victims were killed by an intimate partner (1976–2002).[6] The number of homicides from IPV, however, has been decreasing for the past 20 years.
  - In 2002, 76% of IPV homicide victims were female and 24% were male.[6]
- Annually, 10 million children witness wife-battering.[1] Children may become injured themselves. One study found that children of abused mothers were 57 times more likely to have been harmed because of IPV between their parents, compared to children of nonabused mothers.[7]

PATHOPHYSIOLOGY

Risk factors for IPV include the following:[4]

- Individual factors—Prior history of IPV or witnessing or experiencing violence as a child, being female, young, less educated, unemployed, heavy use of alcohol or illicit drugs, and engaging in high-risk sexual behavior.
  - For women, having a greater education level than their partner, being American Indian/Alaska Native or African American, and having a verbally abusive, jealous, or possessive partner increased risk. In addition, a risk of IPV by either a past or a new offender was almost double for women who had recently changed residence compared with those who had not moved.[8]
  - For men, having a different ethnicity from their partner's increased the risk of IPV.
- Relationship factors—Couples with income, educational, or job status disparities or in which there is dominance and control of the relationship by the male.
- Community factors—Poverty and associated factors or weak community sanctions against IPV (e.g., police unwilling to intervene).

DIAGNOSIS

Asking patients directly about violence at routine visits or when presenting with clues (as below) is recommended for identifying patients suffering from IPV,[1,2] SOR **C** although data are lacking that identification produces positive outcomes. It is important to use patient-centered approaches.

- Questions that may be asked include general questions about how things are going at home or more specific questions about experiences of nonviolent (e.g., insulting, threatening) or violent (e.g., grabbing, punching, beating, forced sex) abusive acts.
- Several self-administered instruments are available for detecting IPV including the Woman Abuse Screening Tool (WAST).[9] In a study of screening tools, women preferred self-completed approaches (vs face-to-face), although no differences on prevalence were found for method or screening instrument.[10] In a predominantly Hispanic population, investigators found the Spanish version of the 4-question instrument HITS (Hurt-Insult-Threaten-Scream) to be moderately reliable with good validity compared with WAST for

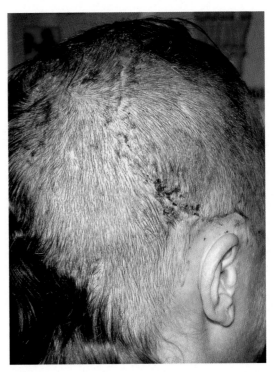

FIGURE 9-3 A woman with a large craniotomy wound that was needed to evacuate her intracranial bleeding secondary to being beaten over the head with a board by her fiancé. (*Courtesy of Richard P. Usatine, MD.*)

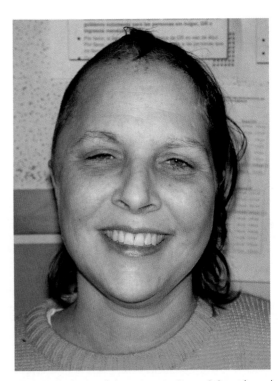

FIGURE 9-4 Frontal view of the woman in Figure 9-3 at a homeless shelter. She was putting her life back together again with the help of the shelter and the providers at the clinic. (*Courtesy of Richard P. Usatine, MD.*)

Spanish-speaking patients;[11] HITS has also been validated with male victims.[12]

CLINICAL FEATURES

Clues on patient history include the following:

- Chronic pain syndromes (e.g., headache, backache, stomach, or pelvic pain).
- Depression.
- Drug and alcohol abuse.

At least 42% of women and 20% of men who were physically assaulted as adults sustained injuries during their most recent victimization.[4] Clues on physical examination:

- Physical injury—Most physical injuries are minor (e.g., contusions, lacerations, abrasions) but include broken bones, traumatic brain injury, and knife wounds (**Figures 9-1 to 9-3**).
  - Ocular injuries can include soft tissue injuries, corneal abrasions, orbital fractures, lens dislocation, retinal detachment, visual field loss, double vision, and blindness (**Figure 9-1**).
  - Trauma to the mouth and lips may be accompanied by fractures, broken teeth, tongue lacerations, and altered taste and smell.
  - Injuries suspicious for abuse are those only in areas covered by clothing, injuries in different stages of healing, and injuries that show a defensive wound pattern particularly on the hands or arms.
  - Upper torso injury carries a high risk of injury to cervical spine, large vessels of the neck and chest and lungs.
- Depression or symptoms of posttraumatic stress disorder (e.g., emotional detachment, sleep disturbances, flashbacks, replaying assault in mind).
- Evidence of forced sexual assault.
- Presence of sexually transmitted infections.

MANAGEMENT

- Initial evaluation, following identification of abuse, is to assess for immediate danger to the woman and any children (e.g., do you feel safe to go home tonight, where is your partner?). If danger is perceived, assist the woman in finding a safe place to go (**Figures 9-4 and 9-5**).
- Document all findings and include photographs (with date), if possible (**Figure 9-6**).
- Develop a safety plan. This should include
  - a safe physical location that is not known to the abuser,
  - transportation to that location, and
  - a list of items to take or a packed suitcase—clothes, keys, cash, valuable documents, telephone numbers, prescriptions, something meaningful for each child.
- Address the needs of any children—30% to 40% of children are also injured physically.[1]
- Data on effective intervention programs are scarce.
  - In a community intervention program in rural South Africa, providing loans to poor women combined with a participatory learning and action curriculum integrated into loan meetings every 2 weeks reduced IPV.[13]

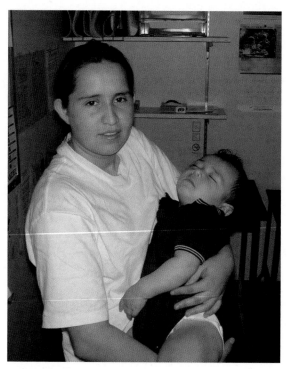

FIGURE 9-5 A young, Hispanic mom with her baby at a clinic in a homeless shelter. She had fled her abusive husband with her child. (*Courtesy of Richard P. Usatine, MD.*)

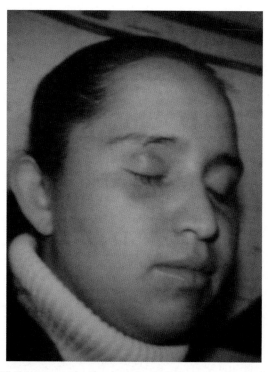

FIGURE 9-6 A copy of a photograph, which the woman had in her purse, showing her black eyes after being beaten by her husband the month before. Out of fear for her life and the well-being of her child, she left her husband. (*Courtesy of Richard P. Usatine, MD.*)

○ Women residents in a domestic violence shelter showed improvement in psychological distress symptoms and less health care utilization following a social support intervention.[14]

PATIENT EDUCATION

- Assist patients in recognizing the cycle of abuse, i.e., violence followed by remorse/apology, tension-building period (patient may experience fear, isolation, forced dependency, intermittent reward), followed by another episode of violence.

- Provide victim education and information on community resources (see Patient Resources).

- Acknowledge that leaving may take time.

- Recovery from abuse may include shame and guilt, but often leads to an improved sense of self and self-worth.

- In a follow-up study of women exiting a shelter, women who were employed, reported higher quality of life, and had people in their networks who provided practical help and/or were available to talk about personal matters were less likely to be re-victimized.[15]

FOLLOW-UP

- Plan for the next visit and provide ongoing support. Recognize that many women are not ready to leave the abusive relationship for a variety of reasons. In one study, duration of abuse was <1 year to 5 median years, and in 5% to 3% of the instances, IPV persisted for >20 years.[16]

- Monitor for depression (one in six abused women will attempt suicide[1]), insomnia, nightmares, and alcohol (16-fold risk of alcohol use[1]) and drug abuse (9-fold risk over nonabused patient[1]).

- If pregnant, monitor for miscarriage (twofold risk) and low birth weight (fourfold risk).[1] In one study, women reporting IPV in the year prior to pregnancy were at increased risk for high blood pressure or edema (adjusted odds ratio 1.37–1.40), vaginal bleeding (adjusted odds ratio 1.54–1.66), severe nausea, vomiting or dehydration (adjusted odds ratio 1.48–1.63), kidney infection or urinary tract infection (adjusted odds ratio 1.43–1.55), in addition to preterm delivery (adjusted odds ratio 1.37), low-birth-weight infant (adjusted odds ratio 1.17), and an infant requiring intensive care unit care (adjusted odds ratio 1.31–1.33) compared with those not reporting IPV.[17]

- Children exposed to IPV also should be monitored because they are at risk of behavioral problems including aggression, anxiety/depression, and inattention/hyperactivity; especially, if maternal mental health disorders or substance abuse are also present.[18]

PATIENT RESOURCES

National Domestic Violence Hotline connects individuals to help in their area by using a nationwide database that includes detailed information about domestic violence shelters, other emergency shelters, legal advocacy and assistance programs, and social service programs. Help is available in English or Spanish, 24 hours a day, 7 days a week. Interpreters are available to translate an additional 139 languages.

> Hotline: 800-779-SAFE (7233)
> TTY: 800-787-3224
> Administrative phone: 512-453-8117
> **www.ndvh.org.**

- National Coalition Against Domestic Violence—A membership organization that includes service programs, reading lists, advocacy, educational materials, and coordinates a national collaborative effort to assist battered women in removing the physical scars of abuse. **www.ncadv.org.**

PROVIDER RESOURCES

- **http://www.cdc.gov/ncipc/factsheets/ipvfacts.htm.**
- **http://www.cdc.gov/ncipc/factsheets/ipvlinks.htm.**
- Family Violence Prevention Fund, **http://www.endabuse.org.**
- Institute on Domestic Violence in the African American Community, **http://www.dvinstitute.org.**

REFERENCES

1. Gilchrest VJ. Abuse of women. In: Smith MA, Shimp LA, eds. *20 Common Problems in Women's Health Care*. New York: McGraw-Hill, 2000:197–224.

2. Tjaden P, Thoennes N. *Extent, Nature, and Consequences of Intimate Partner Violence: Findings from the National Violence Against Women Survey*. Washington, DC: Department of Justice (US), 2000. Publication No. NCJ 181867. www.ojp.usdoj.gov/nij/pubs-sum/181867.htm. Accessed January 12, 2007.

3. Coker AL, Davis KE, Arias I, et al. Physical and mental health effects of intimate partner violence for men and women. *Am J Prev Med*. 2002;23(4): 260–268.

4. IPV fact sheet. http://www.cdc.gov/ncipc/factsheets/ipvfacts.htm. Accessed January 12, 2007.

5. www.cdc.gov/ncipc/fact_book/24_Sexual_Violence.htm. Accessed January 4, 2007.

6. Fox JA, Zawitz MW. *Homicide Trends in the United States*. Washington, DC: Department of Justice, 2004. www.ojp.usdoj.gov/bjs/homicide/homtrnd.htm. Accessed January 12, 2007.

7. Parkinson GW, Adams RC, Emerling FG. Maternal domestic violence screening in an office-based pediatric practice. *Pediatrics*. 2001;108(3):E43.

8. Waltermaurer E, McNutt LA, Mattingly MJ. Examining the effect of residential change on intimate partner violence risk. *J Epidemiol Community Health*. 2006;60(11):923–927.

9. Fogarty CT, Burge S, McCord EC. Communicating with patients about intimate partner violence: Screening and interviewing approaches. *Fam Med*. 2002;34(5):369–375.

10. MacMillan HL, Wathen CN, Jamieson E, et al. Approaches to screening for intimate partner violence in health care settings: A randomized trial. *JAMA*. 2006;296(5):530–536.

11. Chen PH, Rovi S, Vega M, et al. Screening for domestic violence in a predominantly Hispanic clinical setting. *Fam Pract*. 2005; 22(6):617–623.

12. Shakil A, Donald S, Sinacore JM, Krepcho M. Validation of the HITS domestic violence screening tool with males. *Fam Med*. 2005;37(3):193–198.

13. Pronyk PM, Hargreaves JR, Kim JC, et al. Effect of a structural intervention for the prevention of intimate-partner violence and HIV in rural South Africa: A cluster randomised trial. *Lancet*. 2006;368(9551):1973–1983.

14. Contantino R, Kim Y, Crane PA. Effects of a social support intervention on health outcomes in residents of a domestic violence shelter: A pilot study. *Issues Ment Health Nurs*. 2005;26(6): 575–590.

15. Bybee D, Sullivan CM. Predicting re-victimization of battered women 3 years after exiting a shelter program. *Am J Community Psychol*. 2005;36(1–2):85–96.

16. Thompson RS, Bonomi AE, Anderson M, et al. Intimate partner violence: Prevalence, types, and chronicity in adult women. *Am J Prev Med*. 2006;30(6):447–457.

17. Silverman JG, Decker MR, Reed E, Raj A. Intimate partner violence victimization prior to and during pregnancy among women residing in 26 U.S. states: Associations with maternal and neonatal health. *Am J Obstet Gynecol*. 2006;195(1):140–148.

18. Whitaker RC, Orzol SM, Kahn RS. Maternal mental health, substance use, and domestic violence in the year after delivery and subsequent behavior problems in children at age 3 years. *Arch Gen Psychiatry*. 2006;63(5):551–560.

10 ADULT SEXUAL ASSAULT

Mindy A. Smith, MD, MS

PATIENT STORIES

A 19-year-old college girl presents to the office after being raped on a date 3 weeks ago. She went out on a date and was forced to have sex against her will. She states that she had been a virgin and that he made her bleed by penetrating her vagina with his penis. She tried to stop him, but was afraid to fight too hard because he was a strong man and was drunk. She is in tears as she tells her story. She waited so long to come in for help because she did not know where to turn. She took emergency contraception (EC) immediately and a home pregnancy test last night was negative. She is not worried about pregnancy, but she does want to be checked for any sexually transmitted infections (STI). Upon examination, there is a tear of her hymen at 5-o'clock position that has healed (**Figure 10-1**). There are no signs of infection, but STI screening is still performed. She is afraid to prosecute but would like to be referred to a rape-counseling program.

A 47-year-old woman is seen in follow-up for depression. She admits to being raped in a parking lot several months prior but did not report to police. She is continuing to have intrusive nightmares and flashbacks of the event. She is having difficulty concentrating at work and does not feel comfortable in social situations.

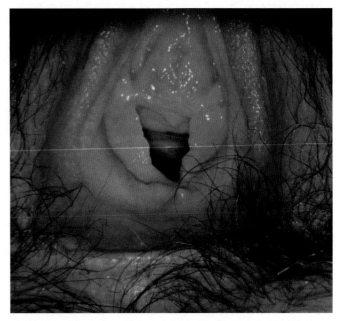

FIGURE 10-1 External genitalia of a 19-year-old college girl showing the tear of her hymen at approximately 5-o'clock position. This was the result of date rape 3 weeks before the photograph was taken. (*Courtesy of Nancy D. Kellogg, MD.*)

EPIDEMIOLOGY

- Between 13% and 25% of women in the United States will experience a rape in their lifetime.[1]
- Overall, an estimated 683,000 rapes occur each year in the United States.[2]
- Victims are more likely to be women than men (78% vs 22%).[3]
- Most victims of sexual assault are young[3]:
  - More than half of all rapes of women (54%) occur in those younger than 18 years, and of these, 22% occur in those younger than 12 years.
  - For men, 75% of all rapes occur in those younger than 18 years, and of these, 48% occur in those younger than 12.
- In surveys of college students, annually 10% of women described a rape, 17% reported an attempted rape, 26% reported unwanted sexual coercion, and 63% experienced unwanted sexual contact.[4]
- Women in substance abuse treatment are a particularly high-risk group for having experienced violence. In one study, 89% reported a history of interpersonal violence and 70% reported a history of sexual assault.[5]
- Men are most often the perpetrators of sexual violence[6]:
  - Among acts committed against women since the age of 18, 100% are of rapes, 92% are of men-perpetrated physical assaults, and 97% of stalking acts.
  - Among male victims, 70% are of men-perpetrated rapes, 86% of physical assaults, and 65% of stalking acts.

- Friends or acquaintances commit nearly half of the rapes and sexual assaults reported to police by women of all ages.[2] As many as 95% of the rapes that occur on college campuses are committed by someone the victim knows.
- According to the FBI Uniform Crime Reports, 70 per 100,000 women reported rape.[7] Most women, however, do not report to police:
  - According to the CDC, 84% of victims do not report the rape to the police.[2]
  - Reasons for failing to report include fear of reprisal, shame, fear of the justice system, and failure to define the act as rape.[1]

ETIOLOGY AND PATHOPHYSIOLOGY

- Sexual violence is a sex act completed or attempted against a victim's will or when a victim is unable to consent because of age, illness, disability, or the influence of alcohol or other drugs.[2]
  - It may involve actual or threatened physical force, use of guns or other weapons, coercion, intimidation, or pressure.
  - Sexual violence includes intentional touching of the genitals, anus, groin, or breast against a victim's will or when a victim is unable to consent, as well as voyeurism, exposure to exhibitionism, or undesired exposure to pornography.
- Two types of factors are believed to contribute to sexual violence: Vulnerability factors that increase the likelihood that a person will suffer harm and risk factors that increase the likelihood that a person will cause harm. Neither vulnerability nor risk factors are direct causes of sexual violence.[3]
- Vulnerability factors for sexual assault, in addition to young age and female gender, include[3]:
  - Prior history of sexual violence.
  - Poverty.
  - Those college women who use drugs, attend a university with high drinking rates, belong in a sorority, and drink heavily in high school are all at greater risk for rape.
- Factors that appear to be consequences of sexual violence and factors that increase a person's vulnerability to repeated victimization are[3]:
  - Engaging in high-risk sexual behavior, including unprotected sex, early sexual initiation, multiple sex partners, and trading sex for food, money, or other items.
  - Using or abusing harmful substances (e.g., cigarettes, alcohol, illicit drugs).
- Risk factors for perpetration[3]:
  - Childhood history of physical or sexual abuse and or witnessed family violence as a child.
  - Coercive sexual fantasies.
  - Preference for impersonal sex.
  - Hostility toward women.
  - Association with sexually aggressive and delinquent peers.
  - Family environment that is unsupportive, characterized by physical violence, and/or has a strong patriarchal relationship.
  - Poverty and lack of employment opportunities.

- Societal norms that support violence and contribute to sexual assault[8]:
  - Limited roles for and objectification and oppression of women.
  - Value placed on claiming and maintaining power (manifested as power over).
  - Tolerance of aggression and attribution of blame to victims.
  - Traditional constructs of manhood, including domination and control.
  - Notions of individual and family privacy that foster secrecy and silence.

DIAGNOSIS

It is recommended that patients are asked directly about violence during routine visits, when seen in the emergency department, or when presenting with substance abuse, depression, physical clues (as listed below) so as to identifying those who are suffering from the aftermath of sexual or physical violence.

CLINICAL FEATURES

- Twenty to forty percent of women have physical injuries, including 5% presenting with major nongenital injuries, 1% presenting with genital injury requiring surgery, and 0.1% presenting with fatal injuries.[1]
- Women who experience sexual as well as physical abuse are significantly more likely to have STIs.[9]
- Long-term consequences include chronic pain syndromes (e.g., pelvic, back, head), gastrointestinal disorders, and gynecologic and pregnancy complications.[3]
- Many women suffer psychological trauma following sexual assault such as posttraumatic stress disorder (PTSD); a similar constellation of symptoms has also been described as the rape trauma syndrome[1]:
  - Acute phase—Haunting, intrusive recollections, numbing constriction of feelings, heightened arousal.
  - Chronic phase—Sexual dysfunction (25%–40% at 1–6 years after the event); depression (50% within the first 6 months with 22% attempting suicide, especially among adolescents); increased risk of substance abuse (2.5-fold).
- Depression is common among rape victims (**Figure 10-2**).
  - Victims of marital or date rape are 11 times more likely than nonvictims to be clinically depressed and 6 times more likely to experience social phobia.[2]
  - Some victims experience psychological problems as long as 15 years after the assault.[2]
- Some victims may attempt suicide after being raped (**Figure 10-2**).

MANAGEMENT

Most women following a sexual assault report that they thought they were going to be killed.[1] The survivor may be terrified and unable to provide a complete history of the assault. It is important to provide support, reassurance of immediate safety, and obtain informed consent for examination, procedures, and contact of others. With permission, the

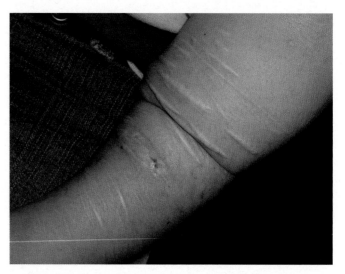

FIGURE 10-2 The mutilated arm of a 26-year-old woman who was raped 5 years prior to this photograph. After being raped, she became suicidal and began cutting her arm repeatedly. The additional malformation of the arm is secondary to osteomyelitis from previous intravenous drug use. (*Courtesy of Richard P. Usatine, MD.*)

clinician should contact a rape crisis worker and the police, although the survivor decides whether or not to file criminal charges.[1]

- History to include details of the assault (e.g., date, time, location, descriptors of assailant(s)), type of bodily and sexual contact, and presence of weapons.[1]
- Treat traumatic injuries—Physical examination should include observations of emotional state and descriptions of clothing and stains. Gently, and with permission, examine for lacerations, abrasions, ecchymoses, and bites. A genital examination should be preformed and a detailed examination of any area directed by history.
- Test and treat for STI—A guideline for managing STI following sexual assault is available through the CDC.[10]
  - Trichomoniasis, bacterial vaginosis (BV), gonorrhea, and chlamydial infection are the most frequently diagnosed infections. As the prevalence of these infections is high among sexually active women, their presence after an assault does not necessarily signify acquisition during the assault.
  - Test for *N. gonorrhoeae* and *C. trachomatis* from specimens collected from any sites of penetration or attempted penetration. Culture or FDA-cleared nucleic acid amplification tests (NAATs) for either *N. gonorrhoeae* or *C. trachomatis*; NAATs offer the advantage of increased sensitivity in detection of *C. trachomatis*.
  - Wet mount and culture of a vaginal swab specimen for *T. vaginalis* infection. If vaginal discharge, malodor, or itching is evident, the wet mount also should be examined for evidence of BV and candidiasis.
  - Collect a serum sample for immediate evaluation for HIV, hepatitis B, and syphilis.
  - The following prophylactic regimen is suggested as preventive therapy:
    - Hepatitis B vaccination, without HBIG, is administered to sexual assault victims at the time of the initial examination if they have not been previously vaccinated. Follow-up doses of vaccine should be administered 1 to 2 and 4 to 6 months after the first dose.
    - An empiric antimicrobial regimen for chlamydia, gonorrhea, trichomonas, and BV is ceftriaxone 125 mg IM in a single dose **plus** metronidazole 2 g orally (single dose) **plus** azithromycin 1 g orally (single dose) **or** doxycycline 100 mg orally twice daily for 7 days. Clinicians should counsel patients about the possible benefits and toxicities associated with these treatment regimens, such as gastrointestinal side effects.
  - HIV seroconversion has occurred in persons whose only known risk factor was sexual assault or sexual abuse, but the risk is probably low (in consensual sex, the risk for HIV transmission from vaginal intercourse is 0.1–0.2%, for receptive rectal intercourse is 0.5–3%, and for oral sex is substantially lower.).[10]
    - The health care provider should assess available information concerning HIV-risk behaviors of the assailant(s) (e.g., a man who has sex with other men and or injecting-drug or crack cocaine use), local epidemiology of HIV AIDS, and exposure characteristics of the assault. Specific circumstances of an assault that might increase risk for HIV transmission are trauma, including bleeding, with vaginal, anal, or oral penetration; exposure to ejaculate to mucous membranes; viral load in ejaculate (e.g., multiple assailants); and the presence of an STD or genital lesions in the assailant or survivor.

- If HIV postexposure prophylaxis (PEP) is offered, the following information should be discussed with the patient: (1) the unproven benefit and known toxicities of antiretrovirals; (2) the close follow-up that will be necessary; (3) the benefit of adherence to recommended dosing; (4) the necessity of early initiation to optimize potential benefits (as soon as possible after and up to 72 hours after the assault). Providers should emphasize that PEP appears to be well-tolerated and that severe adverse effects are rare.
  - Specialist consultation on PEP regimens is recommended. If the survivor and clinician decide that PEP is warranted, the survivor should be offered a 3- to 5-day supply with a follow-up visit scheduled for additional counseling after several days.
  - If PEP is started, perform CBC and serum chemistry at baseline (initiation of PEP should not be delayed, pending results).
  - Perform HIV antibody test at original assessment; repeat at 6 weeks, 3 months, and 6 months.
- Collect samples for legal evidence. Most emergency department have rape or sexual assault kits containing instructions for gathering material to support legal charges; all samples must be carefully labeled and kept under supervision. Details of these procedures may be found elsewhere.[1,11]
- Reproductive-aged female survivors should be evaluated for pregnancy, if appropriate, and offered EC if desired. Providers might also consider antiemetic medications, particularly if EC containing estrogen is provided.
- Arrange for safety.
- Provide written information about the visit and any instructions given to the patient.

PATIENT EDUCATION

- Recovery from sexual assault is a slow process. In one study, one-third of survivors reported recovery within 1 year but one-quarter felt that they had not recovered after 4 to 6 years.[12]
- Counseling and sometimes medication is available to help control symptoms and treat depression and posttraumatic stress syndrome (as discussed below) and patients should be encouraged to report and seek help for continuing difficulties.
- Women who have been physically assaulted as adolescents are at greater risk for revictimization during their college years.[13] Although dating violence prevention/intervention programs have not been uniformly successful, women should be counseled about strategies for avoiding future victimization (e.g., recognition of dangerous situations, limiting use of alcohol, safety with friends).

FOLLOW-UP

Follow-up visits provide an opportunity to (1) provide support and advocacy, (2) detect new infections acquired during or after the assault, (3) complete hepatitis B immunization, if indicated, (4) complete counseling and treatment for other STDs, and (5) monitor side effects and adherence to PEP, if prescribed.[10]

- Initial follow-up should be within 1 to 2 weeks following the assault.
  - Provide ongoing support—Survivors of sexual abuse report strained relationships with family, friends, and intimate partners including less emotional support and less frequent contact with friends and relatives.[3] In addition, only about half of victims keep this appointment and so outreach efforts may be needed.
  - Review results of tests and discuss the plan for redraw of VDRL in 4 to 6 weeks and HIV in 6 weeks and 3 and 6 months (if initial test results were negative).
- Long-term support, monitoring, and treatment:
  - For women suffering from PTSD, medications that may be useful include selective serotonin reuptake inhibitors and risperdal.[14]
  - In one study it was found that cognitive-processing therapy was useful in treating posttraumatic guilt in female rape victims.[15]
  - Imagery rehearsal therapy appears useful in decreasing chronic nightmares, improving sleep quality, and decreasing PTSD symptom severity.[16]

PATIENT RESOURCES

- National Sexual Violence Resource Center serves as a comprehensive collection and distribution center for information, statistics, and resources related to sexual violence, **www.nsvrc.org.**
- **http://www.cdc.gov/ncipc/factsheets/svfacts.htm.**
- **www.vawnet.org/SexualViolence/ServicesAnd ProgramDev/ServiceProvAndProg/.**
- National Domestic Violence Hotline, 1-800-799-SAFE; National Sexual Assault Hotline, 1-800-656-HOPE.

PROVIDER RESOURCES

- Williams A. Managing adult sexual assault. *Aust Fam Physician.* 2004;33(10):825–828. (This article outlines the process of a forensic medical examination as well as providing a management flowchart for practitioners who are caring for a victim of sexual assault.)
- National Criminal Justice Reference System—A National Protocol for Sexual Assault Medical Forensic Examinations, U.S. Department of Justice, Office on Violence Against Women. **www.ncjrs.gov.** Accessed Sept 6, 2004.
- Assistance with postexposure prophylaxis decisions can be obtained by calling the National Clinician's Post-Exposure Prophylaxis Hotline (PEPLine), 1-888-448-4911.
- National Sexual Violence Resource Center serves as a comprehensive collection and distribution center for information, statistics, and resources related to sexual violence, **www.nsvrc.org.**
- The American College of Obstetricians and Gynecologists provides publications about violence against women, intimate partner violence, sexual violence, adolescent dating violence, and patient education materials in both English and Spanish, **www.acog.org.**
- A directory of sexual assault centers in the United States can be obtained from the following URL: **www.nsvrc.org/ publications/SADirectoryOrderForm.pdf.**

- Communities Against Violence Network enhances collaboration among rape crisis centers, law enforcement, prosecutors, advocates, and others, **www.cavnet2.org.**
- Health providers can also become involved in prevention activities at multiple levels:[17]
  - Strengthening individual knowledge and skills through skill-building programs in high schools or training bystanders to safely interrupt sexist and harassing behavior.
  - Promoting community education by sponsoring activities such as plays that reinforce positive cultural norms and portray responsible sexual behavior or developing awards to recognize responsible media coverage.
  - Educating other community leaders and providers, such as little league coaches, prison guards, nursing home providers.
  - Fostering coalitions and networks to promote community understanding and strategies to prevent sexual violence.
  - Changing organizational practices such as implementation and enforcement of sexual harassment policies in schools and workplaces, implementing environmental safety measures such as adequate lighting and emergency call boxes.
  - Influencing policies and legislation such as offering comprehensive sex education programs in middle and high schools, including violence prevention.

REFERENCES

1. Gilchrest VJ. Abuse of women. In: Smith MA, Shimp LA eds. *20 Common Problems in Women's Health Care.* New York: McGraw-Hill, 2000:197–224.

2. www.cdc.gov/ncipc/fact_book/24_Sexual_Violence.htm. Accessed February 4, 2007.

3. www.cdc.gov/ncipc/factsheets/svfacts.htm. Accessed February 4, 2007.

4. Koss MP. Detecting the scope of rape: A review of prevalence research methods. *J Interpers Violenc.* 1993;8:198–222.

5. Lincoln AK, Liebschutz JM, Chernoff M, et al. Brief screening for co-occurring disorders among women entering substance abuse treatment. *Subst Abuse Treat Prev Policy.* 2006;1:26.

6. Tjaden P, Thoennes N. *Full Report of the Prevalence, Incidence, and Consequences of Violence Against Women: Findings from the National Violence Against Women Survey.* Washington, DC: National Institute of Justice, 2000. Report NCJ 183781.

7. *Uniform Crime Reports for the United States.* Federal Bureau of Investigation. Washington, DC: U.S. Department of Justice, 1997.

8. New Sexual Assault Forensic Examination Technical Assistance (SAFE TA) Project. www.nsvrc.org/. Accessed February 5, 2007.

9. Wingood G, DiClemente R, Raj A. Adverse consequences of intimate partner abuse among women in non-urban domestic violence shelters. *Am J Prev Med.* 2000;19:270–275.

10. www.cdc.gov/std/treatment/2006/sexual-assault.htm. Accessed February 4, 2007.

11. Williams A. Managing adult sexual assault. *Aust Fam Physician.* 2004;33(10):825–828.

12. Burgess AW, Holmstrom LL. Adaptive strategies and recovery from rape. *Am J Psychiatry*. 1979;136:1278–1282.

13. Smith PH, White JW, Holland LJ. A longitudinal perspective on dating violence among adolescent and college-age women. *Am J Public Health*. 2003;93(7):1104–1109.

14. Padala PR, Madison J, Monnahan M, et al. Risperidone monotherapy for post-traumatic stress disorder related to sexual assault and domestic abuse in women. *Int Clin Psychopharmacol*. 2006;21(5):275–280.

15. Nishith P, Nixon RD, Resick PA. Resolution of trauma-related guilt following treatment of PTSD in female rape victims: A result of cognitive processing therapy targeting comorbid depression? *J Affect Disord*. 2005;86(2–3):259–265.

16. Krakow C, Hollifield M, Johnston L, et al. Imagery rehearsal therapy for chronic nightmares in sexual assault survivors with posttraumatic stress disorder: A randomized controlled trial. *JAMA*. 2001;286(5):537–545.

17. Cohen L, Swift S. The spectrum of prevention: Developing a comprehensive approach to injury prevention. *Inj Prev*. 1999; 5:203–207.

PART 4

OPHTHALMOLOGY

SECTION 1   EXTERNAL EYE

11 PTERYGIUM

Heidi Chumley, MD

PATIENT STORY

A 50-year-old man had spent most of his adult life working outdoors in southern Texas near the Mexico border. He denies any problems with his vision, but wonders what is growing on his eye and if it should be removed (**Figure 11-1**). He is diagnosed with a pterygium and instructed that it does not need to be removed unless it interferes with his vision.

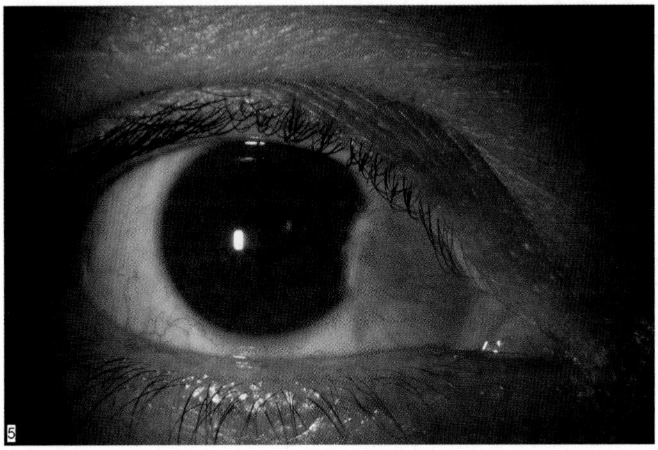

EPIDEMIOLOGY

- The frequency of pterygium increases with sun exposure and age. In the only population-based study (Indonesia), it was found that the prevalence ranged from 3% (in 21–29-year-olds) to 18% (older than 50 years).[1]

- In one study carried out in Australia, it was found that sun exposure is consistently the greatest risk factor attributing 43% of risk.[2]

ETIOLOGY AND PATHOPHYSIOLOGY

- A pterygium is a proliferation of fibrovascular tissue on the surface of the eye, which extends onto the cornea.

- The etiology of pterygium is incompletely understood; however, chronic UV exposure is accepted as a causative agent.

DIAGNOSIS

Pterygia are diagnosed clinically by their distinctive appearance (**Figures 11-1 to 11-4**).

DIFFERENTIAL DIAGNOSIS

- Pinguecula is a yellowish patch or nodule on the conjunctiva and does not extend onto the cornea.

- Conjunctivitis is conjunctival injection with discomfort and eye discharge (see Chapter 15).

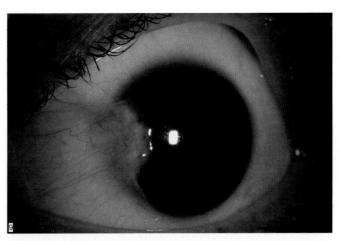

FIGURE 11-1 A medial pterygium extending to the cornea. (*Courtesy of Paul D. Comeau.*)

FIGURE 11-2 Pterygium that has grown onto the cornea but not covered the pupil. This fibrovascular tissue has the shape of a bird's wing (literal definition of pterygium). The small vessels are prominent in this view. (*Courtesy of Paul D. Comeau.*)

MANAGEMENT

- Pterygia are usually treated only when they interfere with vision (**Figure 11-3**). The standard therapy is surgical removal.

- Pterygia affect astigmatism[3,4] and are associated with increased rates of macular degeneration; however, it is unclear whether treatment reduces this risk.

- Eyes with a pterygium or previous pterygium surgery (but not pinguecula) have a higher risk of incident late age-related maculopathy (ARM) (OR 3.3, 95% CI 1.1–10.3) and early ARM (OR 1.8, 95% CI 1.1–2.9).[5]

PATIENT EDUCATION

Pterygia do not require treatment unless they interfere with vision.

FOLLOW-UP

No specific follow-up is needed; however, consider monitoring vision during annual examinations because of the increased risk of age-related macular degeneration.

REFERENCES

1. Gazzard G, Saw SM, Farook M, et al. Pterygium in Indonesia: Prevalence, severity and risk factors. *Br J Ophthalmol.* 2002; 86(12):1341–1346.

2. McCarty CA, Fu CL, Taylor HR. Epidemiology of pterygium in Victoria, Australia. *Br J Ophthalmol.* 2000;84(3):289–292.

3. Ashaye AO. Refractive astigmatism and size of pterygium. *Afr J Med Med Sci.* 2002;31(2):163–165.

4. Kampitak K. The effect of pterygium on corneal astigmatism. *J Med Assoc Thai.* 2003;86(1):16–23.

5. Pham TQ, Wang JJ, Rochtchina E, Mitchell P. Pterygium/pinguecula and the five-year incidence of age-related maculopathy. *Am J Ophthalmol.* 2005;139(3):536–537.

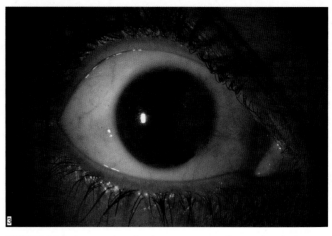

FIGURE 11-3 A pterygium that has grown over the pupil and is interfering with the person's vision. The patient plans to undergo surgery. (*Courtesy of Paul D. Comeau.*)

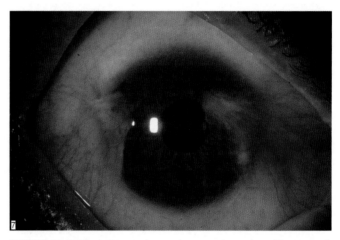

FIGURE 11-4 Bilateral pterygia growing over the cornea. (*Courtesy of Paul D. Comeau.*)

12 HORDEOLUM AND CHALAZION

Heidi Chumley, MD

PATIENT STORY

A 35-year-old woman presented with a tender nodule on the upper eyelid, which was diagnosed clinically as a hordeolum. She applied a warm, moist cloth to her eyelid four times a day for the next several days. Her hordeolum resolved within 3 days.

EPIDEMIOLOGY

- Unclear incidence or prevalence in the United States, but often stated to be more common in school-aged children and adults 30 to 50 years old.
- In one study in school-aged children in Brazil, the prevalence of chalazion was found to be 0.2% and that of hordeolum was 0.3%.[1]

ETIOLOGY AND PATHOPHYSIOLOGY

HORDEOLUM (ACUTELY TENDER NODULE IN THE EYE)

- Infection in the meibomian gland (internal hordeolum), often resolves into a chalazion (**Figure 12-1**).
- Infection in the Zeiss or Moll's glands (externdal hordeolum).
- *Staphylococcus aureus* is the causative agent in most cases.

CHALAZION

- Meibomian gland becomes blocked, often by blepharitis.
- Blocked meibomian gland's duct releases gland contents into the soft tissue of eyelid.
- Gland contents cause a lipogranulomatous reaction.
- Reaction can cause acute tenderness and erythema, which then resolves into a chronic nodule.

DIAGNOSIS

CLINICAL FEATURES

Chalazion and hordeolum are clinical diagnoses.

- Chalazion is a nontender nodule on the eyelid.
- Hordeolum
  - Tenderness and erythema localized to a point on the eyelid (**Figures 12-2** and **12-3**).
  - Conjunctival injection may be present.
  - Fever, preauricular nodes, and vision changes should be absent.
- Laboratory tests are generally not indicated.

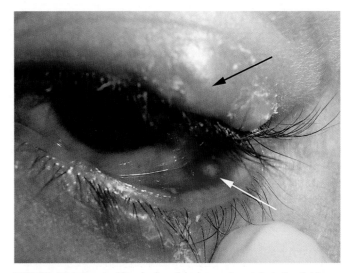

FIGURE 12-1 External hordeolum (black arrow) and chalazion (white arrow), which developed from an internal hordeolum. (*Courtesy of Richard P. Usatine, MD.*)

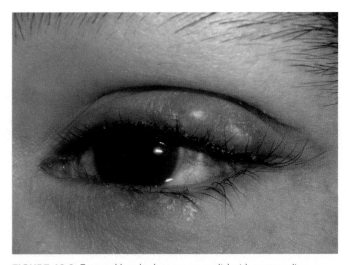

FIGURE 12-2 External hordeolum on upper lid with surrounding erythema. (*Courtesy of Richard P. Usatine, MD.*)

DIFFERENTIAL DIAGNOSIS

- Seborrheic keratosis—Pigmented, "stuck-on" lesions, can appear anywhere on the body including the eyelid; more common in elderly patients.

- Nevus—Pigmented or nonpigmented; flat or raised; generally present since birth.

- Actinic keratosis—Irregular, often erythematous with flaky white scale; seen in sun-exposed areas including eyelids.

- Xanthelasma—Yellowish plaques, generally near medial canthus.

- Molluscum contagiosum—Waxy nodules with central umbilication; generally multiple.

- Sebaceous cell carcinoma—More common in middle-age and elderly patients; difficult to distinguish from recurrent chalazion or unilateral chronic blepharitis but rare.

- Basal cell carcinoma—Pearly nodule, often with telangiectasias or central ulceration; more common on lower medial eyelid; seen in older patients.

- Rarely squamous cell carcinoma or malignant melanoma.

MANAGEMENT

- Hordeolum
  - Warm soaks, three to four times a day for 15 minutes, will elicit drainage in most cases.
  - Topical antibiotics (e.g., bacitracin ointment) may be beneficial for recurrent or spontaneously draining hordeolum.
  - Cases that do not respond to warm soaks or are extremely painful and swollen may be incised and drained with a stab incision. Make the incision on either the internal or external eyelid depending on where the hordeolum is pointing.
  - Antibiotics do not provide benefit after incision and drainage.[2]
  - Systemic antibiotics are usually not needed unless patient has preseptal cellulitis.

- Chalazion
  - Can be treated conservatively with lid hygiene and warm compresses. One study demonstrated a 58% response rate with conservative treatment along with 1% topical chloramphenicol.[3]
  - Higher percentages of resolution can be achieved with either incision and curettage or injection with steroid (e.g., 0.3 mL triamcinolone acetonide) (80%–92%).[3,4]
  - One study demonstrated a better response to incision and curettage in the following situations: Patients 35.1 years or older of age, with lesion duration ≥8.5 months and size ≥11.4 mm.[5]

PATIENT EDUCATION

Hordeolum commonly responds to warm soaks and topical antibiotics. It often recurs and can develop into a chronic chalazion, which may need to be treated with surgical removal or a steroid injection.

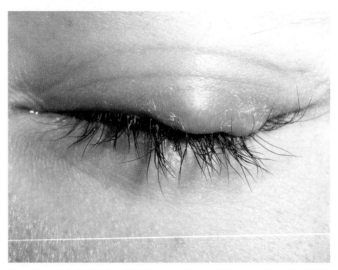

FIGURE 12-3 External hordeolum with eye closed. As can be seen the normal contour of the eyelid is disrupted. (*Courtesy of Richard P. Usatine, MD.*)

FOLLOW-UP

Patients who do not respond to conservative treatment in 2 to 3 days should be reevaluated or referred to a specialist.

PATIENT RESOURCES

- The American Academy of Ophthalmology has a patient education handout on chalazion available through Medem at **www.medem.com.**
- The American Academy of Family Physicians has a useful algorithm for eye problems located at **www.familydoctor.org.**

PROVIDER RESOURCES

The American Family Physician has a review article on eyelid disorders available at **www.aafp.org.**

REFERENCES

1. Garcia, Carlos Alexandre de Amorim, et al. Prevalence of biomicroscopic findings in the anterior segment and ocular adnexa among schoolchildren in Natal, Brazil. *Arq Bras Oftalmol São Paulo*. 2005;68(2):167–170.

2. Hirunwiwatkul P, Wachirasereechai K. Effectiveness of combined antibiotic ophthalmic solution in the treatment of hordeolum after incision and curettage: A randomized, placebo-controlled trial: A pilot study. *J Med Assoc Tha*. 2005;88(5):647–650.

3. Chung CF, Lai JS, Li PS. Subcutaneous extralesional triamcinolone acetonide injection versus conservative management in the treatment of chalazion. *Hong Kong Med J*. 2006;12(4):278–281.

4. Ahmad S, Baig MA, Khan MA, Khan IU, Janjua TA. Intralesional corticosteroid injection vs surgical treatment of chalazia in pigmented patients. *J Coll Physicians Surg Pak*. 2006;16(1):42–44.

5. Dhaliwal U, Bhatia A. A rationale for therapeutic decision-making in chalazia. [Journal Article] *Orbit*. 2005;24(4):227–230.

13 SCLERAL AND CONJUNCTIVAL PIGMENTATION

Heidi Chumley, MD

PATIENT STORY

A 40-year-old white man came to see his physician about a brown spot in his eye (**Figure 13-1**). He noticed this spot many years ago, but after recently reading information on the Internet about brown spots in the eye became concerned about ocular melanoma. He thinks the spot has changed in size. He denies any eye discomfort or visual changes. He was referred for a biopsy, and the pathology showed a benign nevus that did not require further treatment.

EPIDEMIOLOGY

Although there is little information on the prevalence of ocular pigmentation other than physiologic (racial) melanosis, in a study of pigmented lesions referred for biopsy, investigators reported that 52% were nevi, 21% were primary acquired melanosis, and 25% were melanoma.[1]

- Scleral and conjunctival nevi are the most common cause of ocular pigmentation in light-skinned races. The pigmentation is generally noticeable by young adulthood, and is more common in Caucasians.[2]

- Physiologic (racial) melanosis is seen in 90% of black patients.[3] It can be congenital, and often presents early in life.

- Primary acquired melanosis is generally noted in middle to older adults[4,5] and is also more common in Caucasians.

- Conjunctival melanoma is rare, occurring in 0.000007% (7 per 1,000,000) of Caucasians, and is even less common in other races.[5]

ETIOLOGY AND PATHOPHYSIOLOGY

The etiology of scleral or conjunctival nevi is not well understood. Racial melanosis is genetically determined.

DIAGNOSIS

Definitive diagnosis of pigmented ocular lesions is by biopsy.

CLINICAL FEATURES

- Benign nevi (**Figures 13-1** and **13-2**) and physiologic or racial melanosis (**Figure 13-3**) are stable over time, whereas primary acquired melanosis and melanoma change.

- Eighty-seven percent of biopsy proven nevi do not change over time.[4]

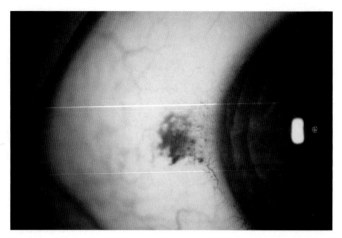

FIGURE 13-1 Scleral nevus—Unilateral localized distinct area of dark pigmentation on sclera. (*Courtesy of Paul D. Comeau.*)

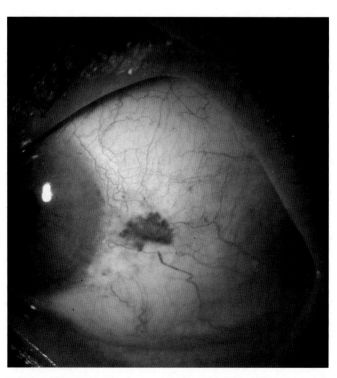

FIGURE 13-2 Conjunctival nevus—Unilateral localized distinct area of dark pigmentation on conjunctiva. (*Courtesy of Paul D. Comeau.*)

- Features seen higher in malignancy: Ulceration, hemorrhage, change in color, and formation of new vessels around the lesion.
- Pathological factors of conjunctival melanoma with a higher mortality rate include increased tumor thickness, location on the palpebral, caruncular or forniceal conjunctiva, increased mitotic activity, lymphocytic invasion, and association with primary acquired melanosis.[6]

DIFFERENTIAL DIAGNOSIS

Pigmented areas on the sclera or conjunctiva include

- Benign nevi—Unilateral and stable over time (**Figures 13-1** and **13-2**).
- Physiologic or racial melanosis—Bilateral and symmetric, most common circumlimbally, and relatively consistent throughout patient's life (**Figure 13-3**).
- Primary acquired melanosis—Typically unilateral, often multifocal indistinct areas of dark pigmentation, and can progress to malignancy over time (**Figure 13-4**).
- Secondary acquired melanosis—Seen with hormonal changes or after trauma to the conjunctiva with irradiation, chemical irritation, or chronic inflammation.
- Conjunctival melanoma—Unilateral, nodular, with variegated color and size changes (**Figures 13-5** to **13-7**).
- Alkaptonuria—Rare disease accompanied by dark urine and arthritis.
- Nevus of ota (also known as oculodermal melanocytosis)—Unilateral blue-grey lesions, often involves periorbital skin, more common in Asian population (**Figure 13-8**).

MANAGEMENT

- Refer any changing pigmented lesion in the eye to a specialist who can perform a biopsy.
- Two lesions can be monitored for changes without a biopsy: racial melanosis and nevi.
- Biopsy-proven primary acquired melanosis without atypia does not require excision, but must be monitored for stability.
- Melanosis with atypia is generally removed with large margins because of its potential for conversion into melanoma.[4]
- The primary treatment for conjunctival melanoma is surgical removal. Cryotherapy, radiotherapy, and chemotherapy may be used as adjunct therapy.

PATIENT EDUCATION

Most pigmentation in the eye is benign and does not change over time. Discuss the importance of reporting any changing pigmented lesion, even in the eye.

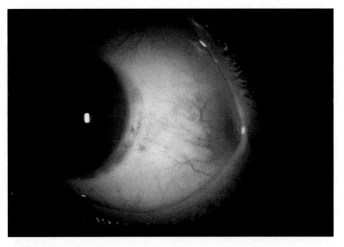

FIGURE 13-3 Physiologic (racial) melanosis—Flat conjunctival pigmentation present bilaterally starting at the limbus and most prominent in the interpalpebral zone is likely to be racial melanosis in a darkly pigmented patient. (*Courtesy of Paul D. Comeau.*)

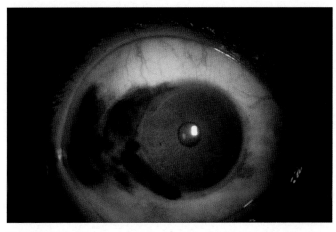

FIGURE 13-4 Primary acquired melanosis—Multiple unilateral indistinct areas of dark pigmentation. (*Courtesy of Paul D. Comeau.*)

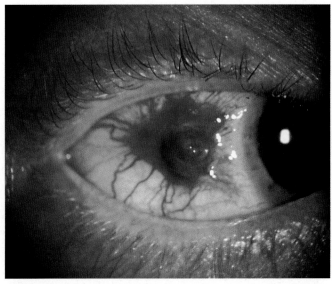

FIGURE 13-5 Conjunctival melanoma—Unilateral, nodular lesion with irregular contours and colors, and surrounded by hyperemic vessels. (*Courtesy of Paul D. Comeau.*)

FOLLOW-UP

Follow-up is based on the type of lesion. Nevi and physiologic melanosis that have not changed can be monitored without biopsy. Primary acquired melanosis requires close follow-up because of its potential conversion to melanoma.

REFERENCES

1. Shields CL, Demirci H, Karatza E, Shields JA. Clinical survey of 1643 melanocytic and nonmelanocytic conjunctival tumors. *Ophthalmology.* 2004;111(9):1747–1754.

2. Shields CL, Fasiudden A, Mashayekhi A, Shields JA. Conjunctival nevi: Clinical features and natural course in 410 consecutive patients. *Arch Ophthalmol.* 2004;122(2):167–175.

3. Singh AD, Campos OE, Rhatigan RM, Schulman JA, Misra RP. Conjunctival melanoma in the black population. [Review] *Surv Ophthalmol.* 1998;43(2):127–133.

4. Folberg R, Mclean IW, Zimmerman LE. Conjunctival melanosis and melanoma. *Ophthalmology.* 1984;91(6):673–678.

5. Seregard S, AFTE, Mansson-Brahme E, Kock E, Bergenmar M, Ringborg U. Prevalence of primary acquired melanosis and nevi of the conjunctiva and uvea in the dysplastic nevus syndrome. A case-control study. *Ophthalmology.* 1995;102(10):1524–1529.

6. Shields CL, Shields JA, Gunduz K, et al. Conjunctival melanoma: Risk factors for recurrence, exenteration, metastasis, and death in 150 consecutive patients.[comment]. *Arch Ophthalmol.* 2000;118(11):1497–1507.

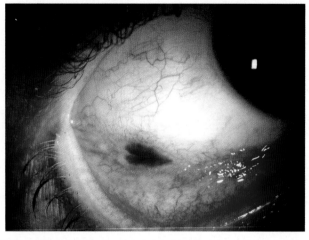

FIGURE 13-6 Early photo of conjunctival melanoma with irregular borders and variations in color. (*Courtesy of Paul D. Comeau.*)

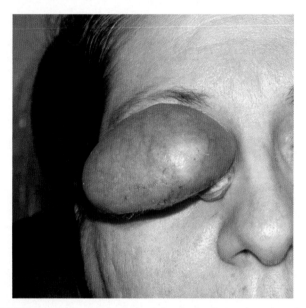

FIGURE 13-7 Conjunctival melanoma, 1 year after the previous photo, in a patient who initially declined treatment. (*Courtesy of Paul D. Comeau.*)

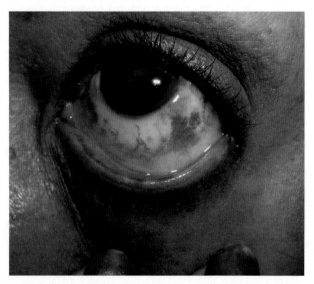

FIGURE 13-8 Nevus of Ota (also known as oculodermal melanocytosis). Unilateral blue-grey ocular pigmentation with periorbital hyperpigmentation. (*Courtesy of Richard P. Usatine, MD.*)

14 CORNEAL FOREIGN BODY/ABRASION

Heidi Chumley, MD

PATIENT STORY

A 28-year-old man felt something fly into his eye while he was using a table saw without wearing protective eye gear. He presented with pain, tearing, photophobia, and felt that something was still in his eye. On examination with a slit lamp, the physician noted that he had a wood chip that had perforated the cornea (**Figures 14-1** and **14-2**). He was referred to an ophthalmologist who successfully removed the foreign body. He was treated with a short course of topical NSAIDs for pain relief and had complete healing.

EPIDEMIOLOGY

- Corneal abrasions with or without foreign bodies are common; however, the prevalence or incidence of corneal abrasions in the general population is unknown.
- Corneal abrasions accounted for 85% of closed eye injuries to adults presenting to an emergency department.[1]

ETIOLOGY AND PATHOPHYSIOLOGY

- The cornea overlies the iris and provides barrier protection, filters ultraviolet light, and refracts light onto the retina.
- Abrasions in the cornea are typically caused by direct injury from a foreign body, resulting in an inflammatory reaction.
- The inflammatory reaction causes the symptoms and can persist for several days after the foreign object is out.

DIAGNOSIS

CLINICAL FEATURES

- History of ocular trauma or eye rubbing (although corneal abrasions can occur with no trauma history).
- Symptoms of pain, eye redness, photophobia, and a foreign body sensation.
- Foreign body seen with direct visualization or a slit lamp (**Figure 14-3**).
- Fluorescein application demonstrates green area under cobalt-blue filtered light (**Figure 14-4**).

DIFFERENTIAL DIAGNOSIS

- Uveitis or iritis—360 degrees perilimbal injection, which is most intense at the limbus; eye pain, photophobia, and vision loss (see Chapter 17).

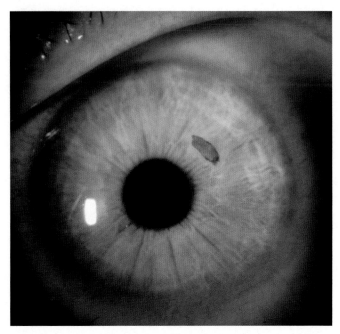

FIGURE 14-1 Wood chip is visible over the cornea on close inspection of the eye. (*Courtesy of Paul D. Comeau.*)

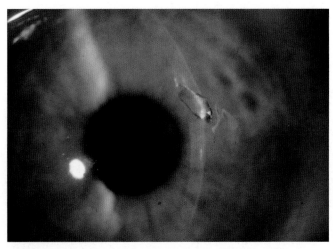

FIGURE 14-2 Slit lamp examination reveals this wood chip has perforated the cornea. (*Courtesy of Paul D. Comeau.*)

- Keratitis or corneal ulcerations—Diffuse erythema with ciliary injection often with pupillary constriction; eye discharge; pain, photophobia, and vision loss depending on the location of ulceration (**Figures 14-5** and **14-6**).
- Conjunctivitis—Conjunctival injection; eye discharge; gritty or uncomfortable feeling; no vision loss (see Chapter 15).
- Acute-angle closure glaucoma—Cloudy cornea and scleral injection; eye pain with ipsilateral headache; severe vision loss (see Chapter 18).

MANAGEMENT

- Confirm diagnosis with fluorescein (for abrasion) if no foreign body is readily visible (**Figure 14-4**).
- Carefully inspect for a foreign body. Invert the upper eyelid for full visualization. Slit-lamp visualization may be needed to determine if the cornea has been penetrated (**Figure 14-2**).
- Remove (or refer for removal) nonpenetrating foreign bodies. Apply a topical anesthetic, such as proparacaine or tetracaine. Remove with irrigation, a wet-tipped cotton applicator, or a fine gauge needle.
- Refer penetrating foreign bodies to an experienced eye surgeon.
- Prescribe ophthalmic NSAIDs for pain if needed.[2] SOR **A**
- Consider topical antibiotics. SOR **C** Chloramphenicol ointment reduced the risk of recurrent ulcer in a prospective, nonplacebo controlled trial.[3] While chloramphenicol is rarely used in the United States, other ophthalmic antibiotics such as erythromycin ointment are used for corneal abrasions.
- Remove contact lenses until corneal is healed.[4] SOR **C**
- Avoid patching, it does not help.[5] SOR **A**

PATIENT EDUCATION

- Advise patients in specific professions (i.e., woodworking, metal working) and those who play sports such as racquetball or hockey to wear eye protection for primary prevention.
- Advise patients with corneal abrasions that healing usually occurs within 2 to 3 days, and they should report persistent pain, redness, and photophobia.

FOLLOW-UP

See all patients in 24 hours for reassessment. If there is no improvement, look for an initially overlooked foreign body or a full thickness injury.

PATIENT RESOURCES

Patient education handout on corneal abrasion is available at **www.familydoctor.org.**

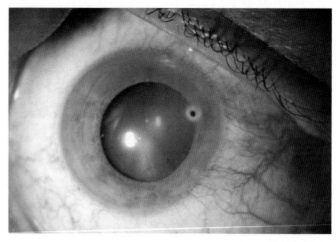

FIGURE 14-3 Metallic foreign body with rust ring within the corneal stroma and conjunctival injection. (*Courtesy of Paul D. Comeau.*)

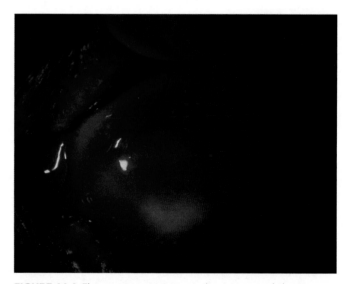

FIGURE 14-4 Fluorescein stains green indicating corneal abrasion. (*Courtesy of Paul D. Comeau.*)

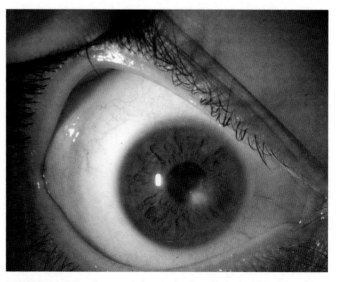

FIGURE 14-5 Small corneal ulcer in the line of vision. (*Courtesy of Paul D. Comeau.*)

REFERENCES

1. Oum BS, Lee JS, Han YS. Clinical features of ocular trauma in emergency department. *Korean J Ophthalmol.* 2004;18(1):70–78.

2. Weaver CS, Terrell KM. Evidence-based emergency medicine. Update: Do ophthalmic nonsteroidal anti-inflammatory drugs reduce the pain associated with simple corneal abrasion without delaying healing? [Review] *Ann Emerg Med.* 2003;41(1):134–140.

3. Upadhyaya MP, Karmacharyaa PC, Kairalaa S, et al. The Bhaktapur eye study: Ocular trauma and antibiotic prophylaxis for the prevention of corneal ulceration in Nepal. *Br J Ophthalmol.* 2001; 85:388–392.

4. Weissman BA. *Care of the Contact Lens Patient: Reference Guide for Clinicians.* St Louis: American Optometric Association, 2000.

5. Turner A, Rabiu M. Patching for corneal abrasion. *Cochrane Database Syst Rev.* 2006;2.

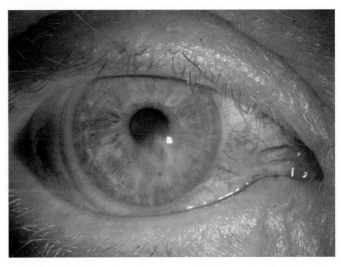

FIGURE 14-6 Larger corneal ulcer partially covering pupil. (*Courtesy of Paul D. Comeau.*)

15 CONJUNCTIVITIS

Heidi Chumley, MD

PATIENT STORY

A 35-year-old woman presents with 2 days of redness and tearing in her eyes (**Figure 15-1**). She has some thin matter in eyes, but neither eye has been glued shut when she awakens. She does not have any trouble seeing once she blinks to clear any accumulated debris. Both eyes are uncomfortable and itchy, but she is not having any severe pain. She does not wear contact lenses and has not had this problem previously. The patient was diagnosed with viral conjunctivitis and scored −1 on the clinical scoring system (see "Diagnosis"). She was instructed about eye hygiene and recovered in 3 days.

EPIDEMIOLOGY

Conjunctivitis is common and often occurs in outbreaks making the prevalence difficult to estimate.

- Between 1997 and 2001, approximately 2 per 1000 visits to the emergency department or hospital outpatient clinics were for conjunctivitis.[1]

- Conjunctivitis is estimated to be higher in children 0 to 4 years old with an incidence of 5.3 per 1000; among 15- to 24-year-olds the incidence is estimated to be 2.3 per 1000 and among 25- to 35-year-olds it is estimated to be 2.5 per 1000.

ETIOLOGY AND PATHOPHYSIOLOGY

Conjunctivitis is predominately infectious (bacterial or viral) or allergic, and the most common etiologies vary by age.

- Neonatal conjunctivitis is often caused by *Chlamydia trachomatis* and *Neisseria gonorrhoeae.*[2]

- Children younger than 6 years are more likely to have a bacterial than viral conjunctivitis.

- Haemophilus influenzae was the most common infectious agent, cultured from 40% to 50% of children with conjunctivitis and 74% of children with concurrent otitis media prior to extensive use of HIB vaccination.[3]

- Adenovirus was cultured from 13% to 20% of children with conjunctivitis and 65% of children with concurrent pharyngitis.[3]

- Children older than 6 years are more likely to have viral or allergic causes for conjunctivitis.[3,4]

DIAGNOSIS

- To distinguish conjunctivitis from other causes of a red eye, ask about pain and check for vision loss. Patients with a red eye and

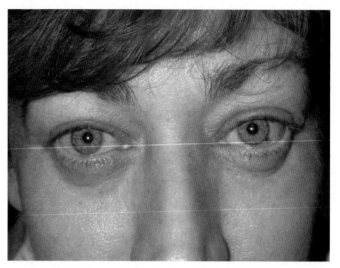

FIGURE 15-1 Viral conjunctivitis demonstrating bilateral conjunctival injection with little discharge. The patient has an incidental left eye conjunctival nevus. (*Courtesy of Richard P. Usatine, MD.*)

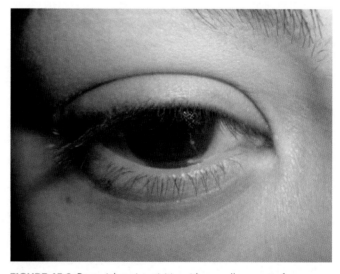

FIGURE 15-2 Bacterial conjunctivitis, with a small amount of discharge. The patient was unable to clean her contacts while being evacuated from a hurricane-threatened Houston. (*Courtesy of Richard P. Usatine, MD.*)

intense pain or vision loss that does not clear with blinking are unlikely to have conjunctivitis and should undergo further evaluation.

- To differentiate bacterial (**Figures 15-2** and **15-3**) from viral and allergic conjunctivitis, use the clinical prediction rule. Allergic conjunctivitis is typically bilateral and accompanied by eye itching. Giant papillary conjunctivitis is a type of allergic reaction, most commonly to soft contact lenses (**Figure 15-4**).

CLINICAL FEATURES

Typical clinical features are conjunctival injection, eye discharge, gritty or uncomfortable feeling, and no vision loss. A clinical scoring system has been developed to distinguish bacterial from other causes of conjunctivitis in healthy adults who did not wear contact lenses.

A score of $+5$ to -3 is determined as follows:

- Two glued eyes ($+5$); one glued eye ($+2$); history of conjunctivitis (-2); eye itching (-1).

- A score of $+5$, $+4$, or $+3$ is useful in ruling in bacterial conjunctivitis with specificities of 100%, 94%, and 92%, respectively.

- Scores of -1, -2, or -3 are useful in ruling out bacterial conjunctivitis with sensitivities of 98%, 98%, and 100%, respectively.[5]

DIFFERENTIAL DIAGNOSIS

- Episcleritis—Segmental or diffuse inflammation of episclera (pink color), mild or no discomfort but can be tender to palpation, and no vision disturbance (see also Chapter 16).

- Scleritis—Segmental or diffuse inflammation of sclera (dark red, purple, or blue color), severe boring eye pain often radiating to head and neck, and photophobia and vision loss (see also Chapter 16).

- Uveitis or iritis—360 degrees perilimbal injection, which is most intense at the limbus, eye pain, photophobia, and vision loss. Usually treated as conjunctivitis without resolution (see also Chapter 17).

- Keratitis or corneal ulcerations—Diffuse erythema with ciliary injection often with pupillary constriction, eye discharge, pain, photophobia, and vision loss depending on the location of ulceration. Herpes keratitis is a diagnosis that should not be missed (**Figures 15-5** and **15-6**). The use of fluorescein and an ultraviolet light can pick up dendritic ulcers or other corneal damage and prompt an emergent referral to an ophthalmologist (**Figure 15-6**).

- Acute-angle closure glaucoma: Cloudy cornea and scleral injection, eye pain with ipsilateral headache, and severe vision loss (see also Chapter 18).

- A foreign body in the eye can cause conjunctival injection and lead to a bacterial superinfection. If the foreign body is not easily dislodged with conservative measures or appears to be superinfected with ulceration or leucocyte infiltrate, prompt referral to an ophthalmologist is required (**Figure 15-7**).

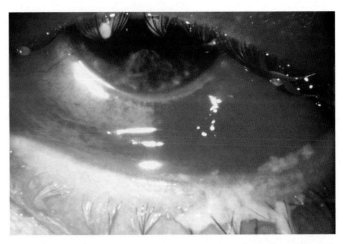

FIGURE 15-3 Gonococcus conjunctivitis has a copious discharge. This severe case resulted in partial blindness. (*Courtesy of CDC.*)

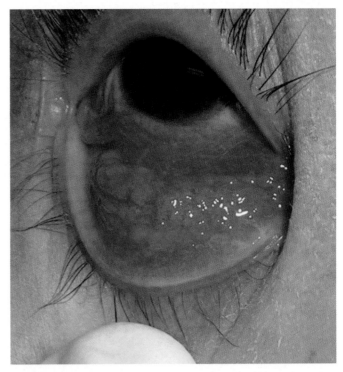

FIGURE 15-4 Giant papillary conjunctivitis in a contact lens wearer. (*Courtesy of Mike Johnson, MD.*)

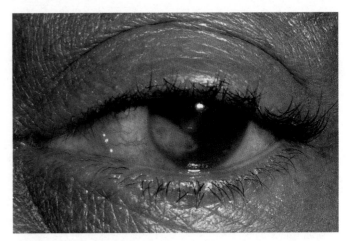

FIGURE 15-5 Herpetic keratitis in a 56-year-old woman staying in a shelter after Hurricane Katrina. (*Courtesy of Richard P. Usatine, MD.*)

MANAGEMENT

Most episodes are viral infections and resolve without treatment. Following are the categories of patients who have a high probability of bacterial conjunctivitis and who are treated with topical antibiotics:

• Children younger than age 6 (unless they have accompanying pharyngitis).

• Adults who score +3 or above on the clinical scoring system for bacterial conjunctivitis.

Studies have shown that more than 80% of patients show improvements with 0.3% ciprofloxacin, tobramycin, norfloxacin, or gentamicin.[6,7] Refer patients who have vision loss, severe pain, lack of response to therapy, or a history of herpes simplex or zoster eye disease to an ophthalmologist.

PATIENT EDUCATION

• Most adults and children older than 6 years have a nonbacterial cause of conjunctivitis.

• Remove contact lens until conjunctivitis has resolved.

• Avoid touching the face or rubbing the eyes and wash hands immediately afterwards.

• Do not share face towels, eye make-up, or contact lens cases.

• For appropriate contact precautions, stop working until the symptoms have resolved.

• Inform your physician immediately if you experience eye pain or vision loss.

FOLLOW-UP

Routine follow-up is generally not needed if symptoms resolve in 3 to 5 days.

PATIENT RESOURCES

An "Information from your Family Doctor" patient handout is available at **www.aafp.org.**

PROVIDER RESOURCES

An extensive guideline on conjunctivitis is available at the National Guideline Clearinghouse at **www.guidelines.gov.**

REFERENCES

1. Center for Disease Control, National Center for Health Statistics. NHAMCS Data. http://www.cdc.gov/nchs/. Accessed February 3, 2007.

2. Wald ER. Conjunctivitis in infants and children. *Pediatr Infect Dis J.* 1997;16(2 Suppl):S17–S20.

3. Gigliotti F, Williams WT, Hayden FG, et al. Etiology of acute conjunctivitis in children. *J Pediatr.* 1981;98(4):531–536.

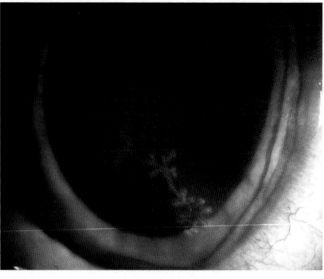

FIGURE 15-6 Slit-lamp view of a dendritic ulcer with fluorescein uptake from herpetic keratitis. (*Courtesy of Paul D. Comeau.*)

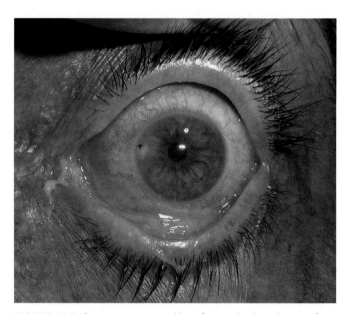

FIGURE 15-7 Conjunctivitis caused by a foreign body in the eye of a machinist. The ground metal speck is seen on the cornea and the purulent discharge indicates a bacterial superinfection. (*Courtesy of Richard P. Usatine, MD.*)

4. Weiss A, Brinser JH, Nazar-Stewart V. Acute conjunctivitis in childhood. *J Pediatr.* 1993;122(1):10–14.

5. Rietveld RP.. Predicting bacterial cause in infectious conjunctivitis: Cohort study on informativeness of combinations of signs and symptoms. *BMJ.* 2004;329:206–210.

6. Gross RD, Hoffman RO, Lindsay RN. A comparison of ciprofloxacin and tobramycin in bacterial conjunctivitis in children. *Clin Pediatr.* 1997;36(8):435–444.

7. Miller IM, Vogel R, Cook TJ, Wittreich J. Topically administered norfloxacin compared with topically administered gentamicin for the treatment of external ocular bacterial infections. The Worldwide Norfloxacin Ophthalmic Study Group. *Am J Ophthalmol.* 1992;113(6):638–644.

16 SCLERITIS AND EPISCLERITIS

Heidi Chumley, MD

PATIENT STORY

A 45-year-old woman presents with 1 day of increasing eye pain, eye redness, and difficulty in seeing. On exam there was scleral injection and exquisite globe tenderness (**Figure 16-1**). Her review of systems is positive for morning stiffness and swelling in both of her hands. She was diagnosed with scleritis and additional testing revealed rheumatoid arthritis. Her scleritis resolved on treatment with oral NSAIDs, and she began therapy for rheumatoid arthritis.

EPIDEMIOLOGY

- Scleritis is uncommon, but often occurs with systemic disorders, specifically autoimmune diseases and infections.
- Forty-four percent of patients presenting with scleritis to specialty health centers were found to have an associated systematic disease (37% rheumatic, 7% infection), most commonly (15%) rheumatoid arthritis.[1]

ETIOLOGY AND PATHOPHYSIOLOGY

- Scleritis and episcleritis are inflammatory conditions causing congestion of the deeper two of the three vascular layers (conjunctival, episcleral, and scleral plexi) overlying the sclera.
  - Scleritis often occurs with episcleritis; episcleritis does not involve the sclera.
  - Scleritis disrupts vascular architecture and may have avascular areas; episcleritis does not.
- Causes of scleritis:
  - Systemic autoimmune diseases (rheumatoid arthritis, Wegener's granulomatosis, seronegative spondyloarthropathies, relapsing polychondritis, systemic lupus erythematosus).
  - Infections (Pseudomonas, tuberculosis, syphilis, herpes zoster).
  - Less common causes include gout and sarcoidosis.
  - Idiopathic.
- Episcleritis is most often idiopathic, but may also be associated with any of the conditions listed above.
- Scleritis can be posterior or anterior:
  - Posterior scleritis can produce retinal detachments and subretinal exudates and is often associated with uveitis (inflammation of the iris, ciliary body, or choroid).
  - Anterior scleritis can be either necrotizing or nonnecrotizing; non-necrotizing can be diffuse or nodular.
  - Anterior scleritis can result in loss of sight.
- Episcleritis is often segmental, but can be diffuse, and is typically benign.

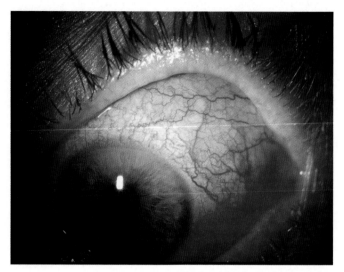

FIGURE 16-1 Scleritis in a patient with eye pain and exquisite globe tenderness. Untreated this can result in loss of vision. (*Courtesy of Paul D. Comeau.*)

DIAGNOSIS

CLINICAL FEATURES

- Scleritis
  - Segmental or diffuse inflammation of sclera (dark red, purple, or blue color), with overlying episclera and conjunctival inflammation (**Figures 16-1** and **16-2**).
  - Severe boring eye pain often radiating to head and neck.
  - Photophobia and vision loss.
- Episcleritis
  - Segmental or diffuse inflammation of episclera (pink color) and overlying conjunctival vessel injection (**Figure 16-3**).
  - Mild if any discomfort but can be tender to palpation.
  - No vision disturbance.

Scleritis and episcleritis are often distinguished by history and physical examination features; however, when scleritis has extensive overlying episcleritis, the diagnosis becomes more difficult. Scleritis must be differentiated from episcleritis because scleritis requires treatment and an evaluation for underlying medical conditions.

- Ten percent phenylephrine bleaches inflamed episcleral and conjunctival vessels, but not scleral vessels; in scleritis, this can reveal a focus of scleral engorgement covered by episcleral engorgement.
- Scleritis and episcleritis, as opposed to iritis with overlying episcleral injection, often have areas of focal tenderness to palpation. These can be elicited with a sterile cotton swab after applying a topical anesthetic.
- Clinical features cannot distinguish among underlying systemic illnesses in scleritis.

BIOPSY

Histology can be used to distinguish among scleritis caused by rheumatic diseases, infections, or sarcoidosis, but this is not often needed.

- Rheumatic—Zonal necrotizing granulomatous scleral inflammation with loss of anterior scleral tissue.
- Infectious—Necrotizing scleritis with microabscesses.
- Sarcoid—Sarcoidal granulomatous inflammation can be identified in cases of sarcoidosis.

DIFFERENTIAL DIAGNOSIS

Causes of red eye, other than scleritis and episcleritis:

- Uveitis or iritis—360 degrees perilimbal injection, which is most intense at the limbus; eye pain, photophobia, and vision loss (see also Chapter 17, Uveitis and Iritis).
- Keratitis or corneal ulcerations—Diffuse erythema with ciliary injection often with pupillary constriction; eye discharge; pain, photophobia, and vision loss depending on location of ulceration.
- Conjunctivitis—Conjunctival injection, eye discharge, gritty or uncomfortable feeling, no vision loss (see Chapter 15, Conjunctivitis).

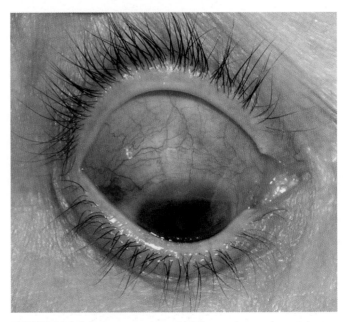

FIGURE 16-2 Scleritis in a patient with Wegener's granulomatosis. Deep vessels are affected giving the eye a purplish or blue hue. (*Courtesy of Everett Allen, MD.*)

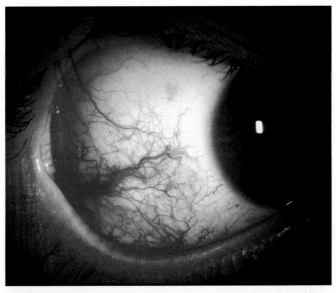

FIGURE 16-3 Episcleritis showing inflammation of the conjunctival and episcleral tissue with associated vascular engorgement. A sector of this eye is involved and that is typical. Vessels were blanched with 2.5% phenylephrine, which helped distinguish this from scleritis. (*Courtesy of Paul D. Comeau.*)

- Acute-angle closure glaucoma—Cloudy cornea and scleral injection; eye pain with ipsilateral headache; severe vision loss (see Chapter 18, Glaucoma).

MANAGEMENT

- Episcleritis often resolves spontaneously. Eye redness and irritation improve by 50% in less than a week. Treatment with topical NSAIDs was no better than artificial tears on measures of redness and comfort.[2] SOR **B**

TREAT SCLERITIS

- Scleritis is initially treated with systemic NSAIDs and/or topical steroids; however, in one study only 47% of patients responded to two drops of 1% prednisolone every 2 hours for up to 2 weeks.[3]
- Refer patients who do not respond to initial therapy to ophthalmologist. Other treatments include systemic steroids, subconjunctival steroids, and immune modulators.

EVALUATE FOR UNDERLYING CAUSES WITH SCLERITIS

- Evaluate for signs and symptoms of rheumatoid arthritis, Wegener's granulomatosis (respiratory or renal symptoms), relapsing polychondritis (vasculitis around ear or nose cartilage or trachea), and seronegative spondyloarthropathies (inflammatory back pain, arthritis, and inflammatory bowel symptoms).
- Evaluate for signs, symptoms, and risk factors for infection including eye trauma, recent ocular surgery, recurrent herpes simplex or varicella zoster, or risk factors for tuberculosis.
- Evaluate for history of gout or symptoms of sarcoidosis.
- Consider the following ancillary tests depending on the patient's presentation:
  ○ Chest radiograph (Wegener's granulomatosis, tuberculosis, sarcoidosis).
  ○ Rheumatoid factor, antinuclear antibodies, syphilis serology, antinuclear cytoplasmic antibody testing (c-ANCA for Wegener's granulomatosis).
  ○ Other tests based on clinical suspicion (i.e., PPD for tuberculosis, HLA-B27 for seronegative spondyloarthropathies such as ankylosing spondylitis, or uric acid for gout.)

  Patients who smoke may take longer to recover from episcleritis or scleritis. One retrospective trial demonstrated that patients who smoked and had episcleritis or scleritis were 5.4 times more likely to have a delayed response of more than 4 weeks to any medication (95% CI=1.9–15.5).[4]

PATIENT EDUCATION

- Reassure patients with episcleritis of its generally benign nature and that oral NSAIDs may be used for discomfort.
- Advise patients with scleritis of its association with systemic illnesses and the need for further work-up.

FOLLOW-UP

- Advise patients with episcleritis to return for any increases in eye pain, changes in vision, or no improvement in 1 week.

- Advise patients with scleritis to follow-up testing for underlying systemic illnesses. If none is found, consider retesting as patients with idiopathic scleritis develop a systemic illness at a 4% annual rate.[1]

REFERENCES

1. Akpek EK, Thorne JE, Qazi FA, Do DV, Jabs DA. Evaluation of patients with scleritis for systemic disease. *Ophthalmology*. 2004;111(3):501–506.

2. Williams CP, Browning AC, Sleep TJ, Webber SK, McGill JI. A randomised, double-blind trial of topical ketorolac vs artificial tears for the treatment of episcleritis. *Eye*. 2005;(7):739–742.

3. McMullen M, Kovarik G, Hodge WG. Use of topical steroid therapy in the management of nonnecrotizing anterior scleritis. *Can J Ophthalmol*. 1999;34(4):217–221.

4. Boonman ZF, de Keizer RJ, Watson PG. Smoking delays the response to treatment in episcleritis and scleritis. *Eye*. 2005;19(9):945–955.

SECTION 2   INTERNAL EYE

17 UVEITIS AND IRITIS

Heidi Chumley, MD

PATIENT STORY

A 28-year-old man presented with sudden onset of a right red eye, severe eye pain, tearing, photophobia, and decreased vision. He denied eye trauma. His review of systems was positive for lower back pain and stiffness over the past year. On examination, he had a ciliary flush (**Figure 17-1**) and decreased vision. He was referred to an ophthalmologist who confirmed the diagnosis of acute anterior uveitis. He was found to be HLA-B27 positive with characteristics of ankylosing spondylitis. His uveitis was treated with topical steroids.

EPIDEMIOLOGY

Uveitis, inflammation of structures in the uveal tract, includes iritis and can be traumatic or nontraumatic.

- Annual incidence of uveitis is 17 to 52 per 100,000 and prevalence is 38 to 714 per 100,000.[1]

- Occurs at any age, most commonly between 20 and 59 years.[1]

- Anterior uveitis (iritis) accounts for approximately 90% of uveitis as seen in primary care settings.[1]

- Eighty percent of uveitis cases seen in children are caused by juvenile rheumatoid arthritis.[2]

ETIOLOGY AND PATHOPHYSIOLOGY

- The uveal tract contains the iris (anterior), ciliary body (intermediate), and choroids (posterior).

- Uveitis refers to inflammation of any part of the uveal tract and is classified as anterior, intermediate, or posterior depending on the structures involved.

- Uveitis can be caused by trauma, infections, inflammation, or rarely neoplasms. Most likely causes differ by location.[3]
  - Anterior (iritis)—Trauma is common (**Figure 17-2**). In nontraumatic cases, causes include idiopathic (50%); seronegative spondyloarthropathies, i.e., ankylosing spondylitis, reactive arthritis, psoriatic arthritis, inflammatory bowel disease, (20%); and juvenile idiopathic arthritis (10%). Infections are less common and include herpes, syphilis, and tuberculosis.[3]
  - Intermediate—Most are idiopathic[3] (**Figure 17-3**).
  - Posterior—Toxoplasmosis is the most common, followed by idiopathic.[3]
  - Panuveitis (affecting all layers)—Idiopathic (22%–45%) and sarcoidosis (14%–28%).[3]

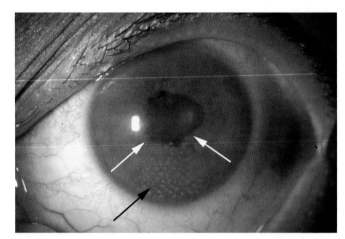

FIGURE 17-1 Acute anterior uveitis with corneal endothelial white cell aggregates (black arrow) and posterior synechiae formation (*iris adhesions to the lens, white arrows*). (*Courtesy of Paul D. Comeau.*)

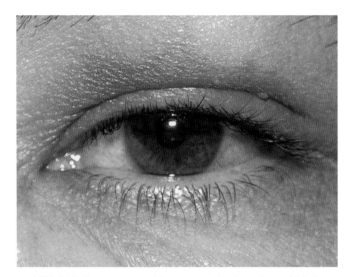

FIGURE 17-2 A young man with traumatic iritis (anterior uveitis) after being hit in the eye with a baseball. He has photophobia and eye pain. (*Courtesy of Richard P. Usatine, MD.*)

DIAGNOSIS

CLINICAL FEATURES

Anterior acute uveitis presents with:

- Unilateral eye pain, redness, tearing, photophobia, and decreased vision.
- 360 degrees perilimbal injection, which is most intense at the limbus (**Figures 17-1, 17-2,** and **17-4**).
- History of eye trauma, an associated systemic disease, or risk factors for infection.
- Severe anterior uveitis may cause a hypopyon from layering of leukocytes and fibrous debris in the anterior chamber (**Figure 17-4**).

Intermediate and posterior uveitis:

- Presents with altered vision or floaters.
- Often have no pain, redness, tearing, or photophobia.

Sarcoid uveitis presents with:

- Panuveitis (anterior, intermediate, and posterior).
- Gradual and usually a bilateral onset.
- Few vision complaints unless cataracts or glaucoma develops.
- Characteristic findings on slit lamp examination (i.e., mutton-fat keratic precipitates, posterior iris synechiae).[4]

DIFFERENTIAL DIAGNOSIS

Causes of red eye, other than uveitis:

- Scleritis—Segmental or diffuse inflammation of sclera (dark red, purple, or blue color), severe boring eye pain often radiating to head and neck, and photophobia and vision loss (see Chapter 16, Episcleritis/Scleritis).
- Episcleritis—Segmental or diffuse inflammation of episclera (pink color), mild or no discomfort but can be tender to palpation, and no vision disturbance (see Chapter 16, Episcleritis/Scleritis).
- Keratitis or corneal ulcerations—Diffuse a erythema with ciliary injection often with constricted pupils; eye discharge; and pain, photophobia, and vision loss depending on the location of ulceration.
- Conjunctivitis—Conjunctival injection, eye discharge, gritty or uncomfortable feeling, and no vision loss (see Chapter 15, Conjunctivitis).
- Acute-angle closure glaucoma—Cloudy cornea and scleral injection, eye pain with ipsilateral headache, and severe vision loss (see Chapter 18, Glaucoma).

MANAGEMENT

Refer patients for any red eye along with loss of vision to ophthalmologist. Patients with uveitis warrant additional examinations by the ophthalmologist.

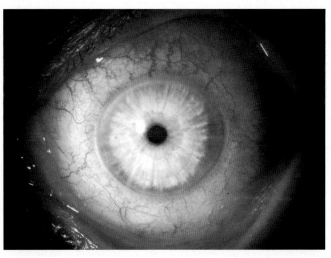

FIGURE 17-3 Idiopathic intermediate uveitis. The ciliary flush is perilimbal injection from dilation of blood vessels adjacent to the cornea, extending 3 mm into the sclera. Perilimbal injection may appear as a violet hue around the limbus with blurring of individual vessels. (*Courtesy of Paul D. Comeau.*)

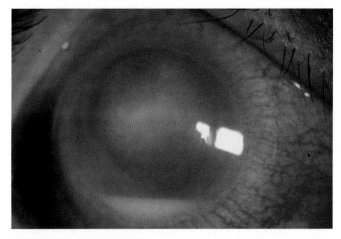

FIGURE 17-4 Hypopyon with severe anterior uveitis, showing layering of leukocytes and fibrous debris in the anterior chamber. May be sterile or infectious. An intense ciliary flush is seen. Most commonly seen in HLA-B27-positive patients with uveitis. Hypopyon may also be a presenting sign of malignancy (*retinoblastoma and lymphoma*). (*Courtesy of Paul D. Comeau.*)

- Traumatic uveitis—Dilated funduscopy for other ocular trauma, gonioscopy to evaluate intraocular pressure, and treatment may include cycloplegics for comfort.

- Non-traumatic uveitis—Slit lamp examination and laboratory tests to assist with diagnosis of underlying cause; treatment is based on underlying cause but is usually topical steroid drops.

- Therapeutic dilation is used to break up the synechiae that can occur (**Figure 17-5**).

PATIENT EDUCATION

- See a physician immediately for a red eye with loss of vision.

- A series of tests may be performed to determine the cause of the uveitis; however, the underlying cause is often elusive.

FOLLOW-UP

Appropriate follow-up is based on the underlying cause.

PATIENT RESOURCES

www.familypractice.org has a flowchart to assist patients with eye problems to determine if they can provide initial treatment or should see a physician.

REFERENCES

1. Wakefield D, Chang JH. Epidemiology of uveitis. *Int Ophthalmol Clin.* 2005;45(2):1–13.

2. Foster CS. Diagnosis and treatment of juvenile idiopathic arthritis-associated uveitis. *Curr Opin Ophthalmol.* 2003;14(6):395–398.

3. Brazis PW, Stewart M, Lee AG. The uveo-meningeal syndromes. *Neurologist.* 2004;10(4):171–184.

4. Uyama M. Uveitis in sarcoidosis. *Int Ophthalmol Clin.* 2002; 42(1):143–150.

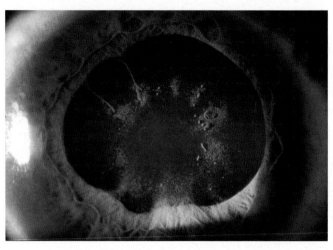

FIGURE 17-5 This patient with uveitis had posterior synechiae that are attachments of the iris to the anterior capsule of the lens. Therapeutic dilation broke up the synechiae, but left residual pigment on the anterior capsule. (*Courtesy of Paul D. Comeau.*)

18 GLAUCOMA

Heidi Chumley, MD

PATIENT STORY

A 50-year-old black man was noted to have a large cup-to-disc ratio during a funduscopic examination by his primary care provider (**Figure 18-1**). The patient reported no visual complaints. Further evaluation revealed elevated intraocular pressure and early visual field defects. He was started on medication to lower his intraocular pressure. He remained asymptomatic, and his visual field defects did not progress for the next several years.

EPIDEMIOLOGY

- Approximately 2.5 million persons in the United States have glaucoma.

- Glaucoma is the second leading cause of blindness in the United States and the leading cause of blindness among African Americans.[1]

- Population studies predict there will be 60.5 million people worldwide with glaucoma by 2010, and of these 74% will have open-angle glaucoma.[2]

- Women comprise approximately 60% of all glaucoma cases, but 70% of patients with acute angle-closure glaucoma.[2]

- Asians comprise approximately 47% of all glaucoma cases, but 87% of acute angle-closure glaucoma.[2]

- The incidence of primary open-angle glaucoma was 8.3 per 100,000 in people older than 40 years in a Minnesota population study.[3]

- According to a population-based study, a family history of glaucoma increased the risk of having glaucoma (OR = 3.08).[4]

ETIOLOGY AND PATHOPHYSIOLOGY

- Glaucoma is acquired optic nerve atrophy, after associated with increased intraocular pressure.

- Increased intraocular pressure occurs from impaired outflow of aqueous humor as either:
  - Open-angle—Dysfunction of the aqueous humor drainage system with no visible pathology to the anterior chamber angle.
  - Angle-closure—Occlusion of the anterior chamber angle.

- Impaired outflow of aqueous humor elevates intraocular pressure in some patients, but many patients with open-angle glaucoma have normal intraocular pressures.

- Optic nerve atrophy is seen as optic disc cupping and irreversible visual field loss. Compare **Figures 18-1** and **18-2** to see the difference between abnormal and normal optic disc cupping.

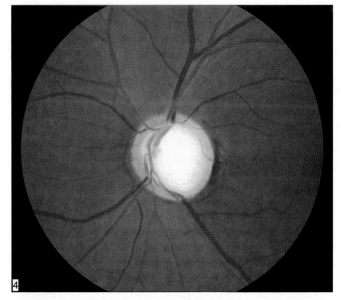

FIGURE 18-1 A 50-year-old man with glaucoma has an increased optic cup-to-disc ratio of 0.8. Median cup-to-disc ratio is 0.2–0.3, but varies considerably among individuals. (*Courtesy of Paul D. Comeau.*)

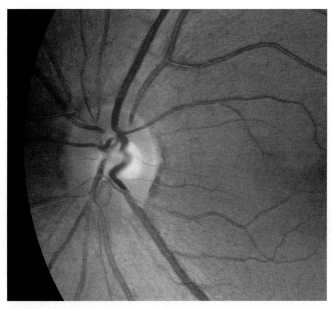

FIGURE 18-2 Normal eye with a normal cup-to-disc ratio of 0.4. A cup-to-disc ratio of more than 0.5 requires further evaluation. (*Courtesy of Paul D. Comeau.*)

DIAGNOSIS

CLINICAL FEATURES

- Open-angle glaucoma:
  - Risk factors—Older than 50 years, African descent, first-degree family history, high intraocular pressures.
  - History—Often asymptomatic, occasionally "tunnel vision."
  - Physical examination—Optic cupping and/or elevated intraocular pressure (glaucomatous changes can occur with intraocular pressures in the normal range), loss of peripheral vision by automated perimetry (typically bilateral, but may be asymmetric).

- Acute closed-angle glaucoma:
  - Risk factors—Asian race, women.
  - History—Painful red eye (unilateral), vision loss, headache, nausea, and vomiting (**Figure 18-3**).
  - Physical examination—Shallow anterior chamber, optic cupping and elevated intraocular pressure, injection of the conjunctiva, and cloudy cornea (**Figure 18-3**).

DIFFERENTIAL DIAGNOSIS

Glaucoma is the most common cause of optic disc cupping and is sometimes accompanied by elevated intraocular pressure.

- Optic disc cupping without elevated intraocular pressure can be caused by[5]:
  - Physiologic cupping (**Figure 18-2**).
  - Congenital optic-disc anomalies (i.e., coloboma or tilted discs).
  - Ischemic (i.e., compression by tumors), traumatic (closed-head injury), or hereditary optic neuropathies.

- Glaucomatous optic disc cupping compared to other causes has[5]:
  - Larger cup-to-disc ratios (compare **Figure 18-1** to **Figure 18-2**).
  - Vertical (as opposed to horizontal) elongation of the cup.
  - Disc hemorrhages.

MANAGEMENT

- Emergently refer patients with suspected angle-closure glaucoma to an ophthalmologist (**Figure 18-3**).

- Evaluate (or refer for evaluation) patients with abnormal optic nerve cupping (cup-to-disc ratio of >0.5; difference in cup-to-disc ratio of 0.2 or greater between eyes; asymmetric cup) or increased intraocular pressure measured by tonometry or visual field deficits.

- Refer patients with shallow anterior chambers, severe far-sightedness (hyperopia) or previous history of acute angle closure glaucoma to an ophthalmologist.

- Document the location and extent of visual field deficits with automated perimetry.

- Treat with topical agents to decrease intraocular pressure by 20% to 40%, which has been demonstrated to decrease glaucoma progression.[6] SOR **Ⓐ** Many medications are available including:
  - Nonspecific beta-blockers (e.g., levobunolol 0.5%, once or twice a day).

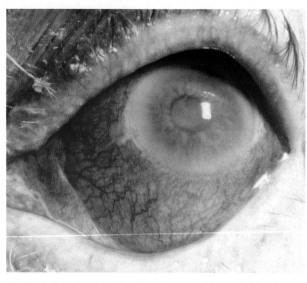

FIGURE 18-3 Acute closed-angle glaucoma with a painful red eye, vision loss, headache, nausea, and vomiting. This is a phacomorphic (i.e. lens induced) secondary acute angle closure. The mature cataract increased in AP diameter thus moving the lens-iris diaphragm forward and closing off the angle as well as the pupil thus resulting in high intraocular pressure, injected conjunctiva, and a cloudy cornea. (*Courtesy of the American Academy of Ophthalmology.*)

- Prostaglandin analogs (e.g., latanoprost 0.005%, once a day).
- Carbonic anhydrase inhibitors (e.g., dorzolamide 2%, three times a day).
- Alpha agonists (e.g., apraclonidine 0.5–1.0%, three times a day).

- Refer for surgical evaluation if you are unable to medically reduce the intraocular pressure.

- Screening—According to the U.S. Preventive Services Task Force update in 2005 (http://www.ahrq.gov/clinic/uspstf/uspsglau.htm), there is insufficient evidence to recommend for or against population screening for open-angle glaucoma. However, African Americans have been underrepresented in trials. Previously screening has been recommended for African Americans older than 40, whites older than 65, and patients with a family history of glaucoma.[7] SOR **C**

PATIENT EDUCATION

Advise patients that glaucoma is a progressive disease requiring continued therapy to prevent vision loss.

FOLLOW-UP

Patients with glaucoma should have regular measurements of their intraocular pressure and visual fields to follow treatment efficacy.

PATIENT RESOURCES

- A glaucoma handout is available in English or Spanish at **http://familydoctor.org/216.xml** (accessed Sept. 18, 2006).
- Information about glaucoma is available at the National Eye Institute Web site: English: **http://www.nei.nih.gov/health/glaucoma/glaucoma_facts.asp** and Spanish: http://www.nei.nih.gov/health/espanol/glaucoma_paciente.asp. Both accessed Sept. 18, 2006.

PROVIDER RESOURCES

An in-depth review of open-angle glaucoma is available full-text online at **http://www.aafp.org/afp/20030501/1937.html.**[11] Accessed Sept. 18, 2006.

REFERENCES

1. Distelhorst JS, Hughes GM. Open-angle glaucoma. *Am Fam Physician.* 2003; 67(9):1937–1944.

2. Quigley HA, Broman AT. The number of people with glaucoma worldwide in 2010 and 2020. *Br J Ophthalmol.* 2006;90(3):262–267.

3. Erie JC, Hodge DO, Gray DT. The incidence of primary angle-closure glaucoma in Olmsted County, Minnesota. *Arch Ophthalmol.* 1997;115(2):177–181.

4. Leske MC, Warheit-Roberts L, Wu SY. Open-angle glaucoma and ocular hypertension: the Long Island Glaucoma Case-control Study. *Ophthalmic Epidemiol.* 1996;3(2):85–96.

5. Piette SD, Sergott RC. Pathological optic-disc cupping. *Curr Opin Ophthalmol.* 2006;17(1):1–6.

6. Heijl A, Leske MC, Bengtsson B, et al. Reduction of intraocular pressure and glaucoma progression: results from the Early Manifest Glaucoma Trial. *Arch Ophthalmol.* 2002;120(10):1268–1279.

7. Distelhorst JS, Hughes GM. Open-angle glaucoma. *Am Fam Physician.* 2003;67(9):1937–1944.

19 DIABETIC RETINOPATHY

Heidi Chumley, MD

PATIENT STORY

A 38-year-old man saw a physician for the first time in 10 years after noticing visual loss in his left eye. His history revealed many risk factors for and symptoms of diabetes mellitus. On an undilated fundoscopic examination, his physician was able to see some hemorrhages and hard exudates. A fingerstick in the office showed a blood glucose level of 420 mg/dL. He was treated for diabetes mellitus and referred to an ophthalmologist to be evaluated for his diabetic retinopathy (**Figure 19-1**).

EPIDEMIOLOGY

- In developed nations, diabetic retinopathy is the leading cause of blindness among people younger than 40 years.[1]
- Twenty-one percent of patients diagnosed with type 2 diabetes mellitus already have retinopathy.[2]
- More than 60% of patients with type 2 diabetes mellitus have retinopathy within 20 years of diagnosis.[2]
- Most patients with type 1 diabetes mellitus as children develop retinopathy in their 20s or 30s.[2]

ETIOLOGY AND PATHOPHYSIOLOGY

- Hyperglycemia results in microvascular complications including retinopathy.
- Several biochemical pathways linking hyperglycemia and retinopathy have been proposed.[2]
- In nonproliferative retinopathy, microaneurysms weaken vessel walls. Vessels then leak fluid, lipids, and blood resulting in macular edema, exudates, and hemorrhages (**Figures 19-1** and **19-2**).
- Cotton wool spots result when small vessel occlusion causes focal ischemia to the superficial nerve fiber layer of the retina.
- In proliferative retinopathy, new blood vessels form in response to ischemia (**Figure 19-3**).

DIAGNOSIS

Definitive diagnosis is made by an eye specialist:

- Gold standard is grading of stereoscopic color fundus photographs in seven standard fields.[2]
- In comparison to the gold standard, a single monochromatic digital photo through a nondilated eye holds promise for large population

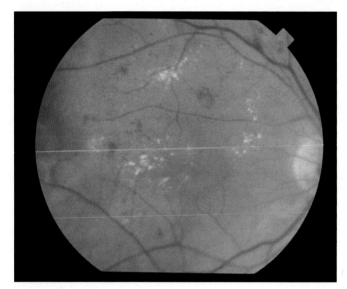

FIGURE 19-1 Dilated fundoscopic photograph demonstrating microaneurysms (small red swellings attached to vessels), which are often the first change in diabetic retinopathy. Also present are hemorrhages and hard exudates (yellow). (*Courtesy of Paul D. Comeau.*)

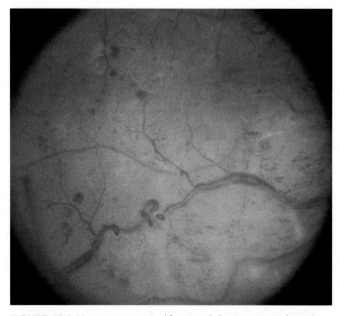

FIGURE 19-2 Very severe nonproliferative diabetic retinopathy with multiple blot hemorrhages, venous beading, and looping. This patient may benefit from panretinal photocoagulation. (*Courtesy of Paul D. Comeau.*)

screening with a sensitivity and specificity of 78% and 86%, respectivey.[3] SOR Ⓑ

- Dilated fundoscopic examination by an ophthalmologist has a sensitivity of only 34%.[3]

CLINICAL FEATURES

- Central vision loss as a result of macular edema.
- Nonproliferative retinopathy—Microaneurysms are seen initially, followed by macular edema, cotton wool spots, superficial (flame) or deep (dot-blot) hemorrhages, and exudates (**Figures 19-1** and **19-2**).
- Proliferative retinopathy—Neovascularization, i.e., growth of new blood vessels on the optic disc, the retina, or iris (**Figure 19-3**).

DIFFERENTIAL DIAGNOSIS

Retinopathy is also seen with other systemic illnesses and infections including:

- Hypertensive retinopathy—arterial narrowing or AV nicking in addition to cotton wool spots (see Chapter 20, Hypertensive Retinopathy).
- HIV retinopathy—cotton wool spots and infections such as cytomegalovirus.

MANAGEMENT

Refer all patients with diabetes mellitus to an eye specialist for an yearly dilated eye examination. Control diabetes and vascular risk factors:

- Glycemic control lowers the risk of retinopathy (35% risk reduction per 1 point HgbA1C reduction).[2] SOR Ⓐ
- Blood pressure control improves visual outcomes (34% risk reduction in retinopathy progression; 47% risk reduction risk for declines in visual acuity).[2] SOR Ⓐ
- Patients with high lipids have more hard exudates and a higher risk of vision loss, but it is unclear if lipid control changes outcomes. SOR Ⓒ

Work with an ophthalmologist to prevent vision loss:

- Complications of diabetic retinopathy are vitreous hemorrhage, retinal detachment, and neovascular glaucoma. All these complications can result in devastating vision loss (**Figure 19-4**).
- Ophthalmologists will determine when peripheral photocoagulation is indicated (**Figure 19-5**). Photocoagulation reduces the risk of severe visual loss by more than 50% with side effects of peripheral and night vision loss.[4] SOR Ⓐ Other surgical treatments, including vitrectomy have been less successful.[2]

PATIENT EDUCATION

Preventing retinopathy by controlling diabetes and hypertension leads to better vision outcomes than any available treatment.[2,4]

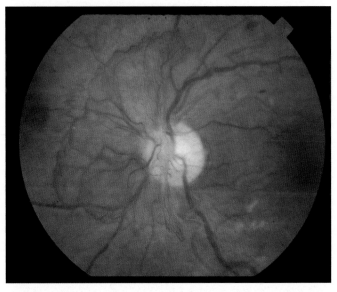

FIGURE 19-3 Proliferative diabetic retinopathy (PDR) showing newly developed, porous, friable blood vessels. New vessels can be seen on the optic disc and peripheral retina. Panretinal photocoagulation may help prevent vitreous hemorrhage, retinal detachment, and neovascular glaucoma. (*Courtesy of Paul D. Comeau.*)

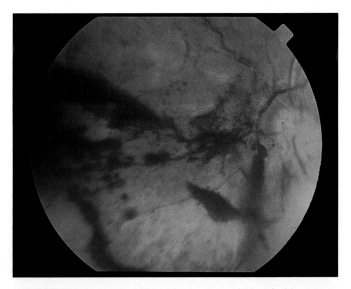

FIGURE 19-4 This vitreous hemorrhage occurred when friable neovascular membranes broke spontaneously. The patients described a "shower of red dots" obscuring the vision and then loss of vision in that eye. (*Courtesy of Paul D. Comeau.*)

FOLLOW-UP

National guidelines recommendations:[5]

- Type 1 diabetes mellitus—Screen for retinopathy 3 to 5 years after diagnosis and at regular intervals as recommended by an eye specialist.

- Type 2 diabetes mellitus—Screen for retinopathy at diagnosis and then annually.

PATIENT RESOURCES

- National Eye Institute's information for patients can be found at **http://www.nei.nih.gov/health/diabetic/retinopathy.asp.**

- American Diabetes Association information about eye complications can be found at **http://www.diabetes.org** (in both English and Spanish).

PROVIDER RESOURCES

Information about diabetes and retinopathy is available at **http://www.diabetes.org.**

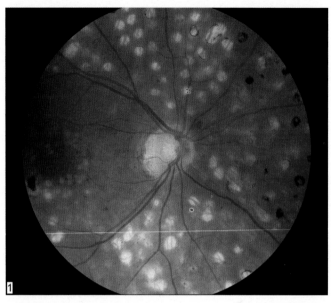

FIGURE 19-5 Panretinal photocoagulation is the application of laser burns to the peripheral retina. The ischemic peripheral retina is treated with thousands of laser spots to presumably eliminate vasogenic factors responsible for the development of neovascular vessels. Laser spots cause scarring of the retina and choroid and scars may be hypotrophic (white spots) or hypertrophic (black spots). (*Courtesy of Paul D. Comeau.*)

REFERENCES

1. Congdon NG, Friedman DS, Lietman T. Important causes of visual impairment in the world today. *JAMA.* 2003;290(15):2057–2060.

2. Fong DS, Aiello LP, Ferris FL, III, Klein R. Diabetic retinopathy. *Diabetes Care.* 2004;27(10):2540–2553.

3. Lin DY, Blumenkranz MS, Brothers RJ, Grosvenor DM. The sensitivity and specificity of single-field nonmydriatic monochromatic digital fundus photography with remote image interpretation for diabetic retinopathy screening: A comparison with ophthalmoscopy and standardized mydriatic color photography. *Am J Ophthalmol.* 2002;134(2):204–213.

4. Photocoagulation treatment of proliferative diabetic retinopathy: The second report of diabetic retinopathy study findings. *Ophthalmology.* 1978;85(1):82–106.

5. American Diabetes Association. http://www.diabetes.org. Accessed January 16, 2006.

20 HYPERTENSIVE RETINOPATHY

Heidi Chumley, MD

PATIENT STORY

A 65-year-old man comes in for a physical examination and is noted to have a blood pressure of 194/102. He has no symptoms at the time. During his examination, the physician notes hard exudates and flame hemorrhages on his funduscopic examination (**Figure 20-1**). The physician treats his hypertension and evaluates him for other cardiac risk factors. He is also referred to ophthalmology for a more comprehensive eye examination because of his age and risk factors.

EPIDEMIOLOGY

- Prevalence of 7.7% (black) versus 4.1% (white) in a population study of men and women between 49 and 73 years of age without diabetes.[1]
- Multiple studies show that patients with moderate hypertensive retinopathy are two to three times more likely to have a stroke than those without at the same level of blood pressure control independent of other risk factors.[2]

ETIOLOGY AND PATHOPHYSIOLOGY

High blood pressure results in these retinal findings:[3]

- Retinal vessels become narrow and straighten at diastolic blood pressure (DBP) of 90 to 110 mm Hg.
- Arteriovenous "nicking" (**Figure 20-1**) occurs when the arteriolar wall enlarges from arteriosclerosis, compressing the vein.
- Microaneurysms (**Figures 20-1** and **20-2**) result from the increased intravascular pressure.
- DBP 110 to 115 mm Hg causes leakage of plasma proteins and blood products resulting in cotton wool patches, retinal hemorrhages, or hard exudates (**Figures 20-1 to 20-4**).
- Optic nerve swelling occurs at DBP of 130 to 140 mm Hg (**Figure 20-3**).

DIAGNOSIS

The diagnosis is made clinically from typical retinal findings in a patient with hypertension.

CLINICAL FEATURES

Microaneurysms and retinal hemorrhages, arteriolar narrowing, and AV nicking.

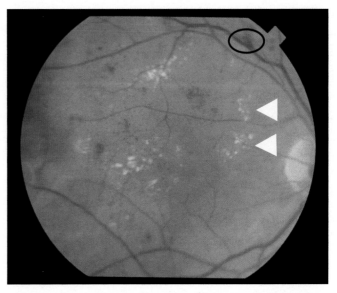

FIGURE 20-1 Hypertensive retinopathy with microaneurysms (black circle) and hard exudates (white arrowheads). (*Courtesy of Paul D. Comeau.*)

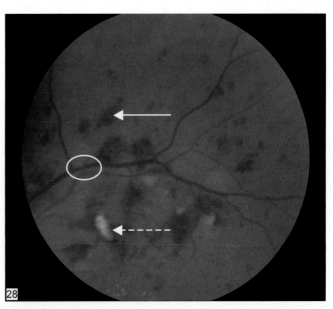

FIGURE 20-2 More advanced hypertensive retinopathy with flame hemorrhages (white arrow), arteriovenous nicking (white circle), and cotton wool spots (dashed arrow). (*Courtesy of Paul D. Comeau.*)

DIFFERENTIAL DIAGNOSIS

Retinal vessel narrowing, AV nicking, microaneurysms, retinal hemorrhages, hard exudates, and cotton wool spots are also seen in other conditions that impair blood flow, including:

- Diabetic retinopathy (see Chapter 19, Diabetic Retinopathy).
- Radiation retinopathy.
- Venous or carotid artery occlusive disease.
- Systemic illnesses such as collagen vascular disease.

Optic nerve swelling and a macular star (blurring of the macula in a star-like pattern) also occur in:

- Neuroretinitis.
- Diabetic papillopathy.
- Radiation optic retinopathy.
- Optic neuritis.
- Intracranial disease.

MANAGEMENT

Patients with funduscopic findings of hypertensive retinopathy should have their blood pressure measured and treated to reduce the risk of heart and cerebrovascular disease.[4] SOR Ⓐ

- Assist patients in smoking cessation. This will result in the greatest benefit in morbidity and mortality.
- Reduce weight or maintain normal BMI.
- Eat a diet rich in fruits and vegetables and low in saturated fats.
- Reduce sodium to less than 6 g of sodium chloride per day.
- Engage in regular physical activity for 30 minutes most days of the week.
- Limit alcohol to two drinks per day in men and one drink per day in women.
- Start a thiazide diuretic to achieve blood pressure of less than 140/90 unless contraindicated; a blood pressure goal of 130/80 should be used for patients with diabetes. Consider an ACEI as an initial medication for patients with diabetes. Consider other medications only for patients with compelling indications.
- Although the largest benefit in outcomes is seen with the first medication, additional medications should be considered to achieve blood pressure less than 140/90 after weighing the risks and benefits with the patient.
- Evaluate and manage other risk factors for cardiovascular disease including high cholesterol and diabetes.

Patients with hypertension do not require routine funduscopic examination, unless they also have diabetes mellitus.[5] SOR Ⓐ Patients experiencing acute visual disturbances should be referred for evaluation of hemorrhage or optic nerve edema (**Figures 20-3** and **20-4**).

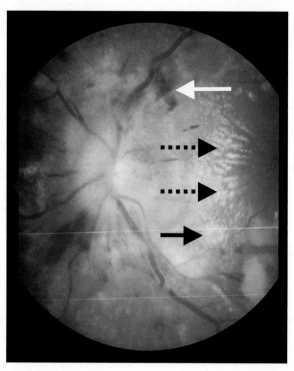

FIGURE 20-3 Malignant hypertensive retinopathy with optic nerve head edema (papilledema), flame hemorrhages (white arrow), cotton wool spots (black arrow), and macular edema with exudates (dashed arrows). The patient was admitted to hospital to treat malignant HTN aggressively. (*Courtesy of Paul D. Comeau.*)

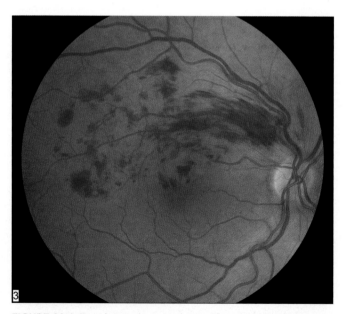

FIGURE 20-4 Branch retinal vein occlusion of a major retinal vein associated with hypertension. The patient noted new onset of blurred vision and visual field constriction. Flame hemorrhages are seen along the course of the obstructed vein. (*Courtesy of Paul D. Comeau.*)

PATIENT EDUCATION

- Hypertensive retinopathy does not require treatment other than lowering blood pressure unless acute vision changes occur.
- Control of blood pressure typically reverses hypertensive retinopathy findings, except for optic nerve edema, which may result in permanent vision loss.
- Control of blood pressure also reduces the risk of heart attack and stroke.

FOLLOW-UP

Once diagnosed with hypertension, patients should be seen every month until blood pressure is controlled and then every 3 to 6 months.[4] SOR ◉

PATIENT AND PROVIDER RESOURCES

The seventh report of the Joint National Committee on the Prevention, Detection, Evaluation, and Treatment of High Blood Pressure has patient information and handouts and provider guidelines and information, which can be downloaded to PalmOS or PocketPC operating systems, **http://www.nhlbi.nih.gov/guidelines/hypertension/.**

REFERENCES

1. Wong TY, Klein R, Duncan BB, et al. Racial differences in the prevalence of hypertensive retinopathy. *Hypertension.* 2003; 41(5):1086–1091.

2. Grosso A, Veglio F, Porta M, Grignolo FM, Wong TY. Hypertensive retinopathy revisited: Some answers, more questions. *Br J Ophthalmol.* 2005;89(12):1646–1654.

3. Luo BP, Brown GC. Update on the ocular manifestations of systemic arterial hypertension. *Curr Opin Ophthalmol.* 2004; 15(3):203–210.

4. NIH, NHLBI, and National High Blood Pressure Education Program. *The Seventh Report of the Joint National Committee on the Prevention, Detection, Evaluation, and Treatment of High Blood Pressure,* 2004. U.S. Department of Health and Human Services, 2006.

5. van den Born BJ, Hulsman CA, Hoekstra JB, Schlingemann RO, van Montfrans GA. Value of routine funduscopy in patients with hypertension: Systematic review. *BMJ.* 2005;331(7508):73.

21 PAPILLEDEMA

Heidi Chumley, MD

PATIENT STORY

A 29-year-old obese woman presented with chronic headaches that were worse in the morning or while lying down. She denied nausea or other neurological symptoms. She had no other medical problems and took no medications. On examination, she had a visual acuity of 20/20 in both eyes, bilateral papilledema (**Figure 21-1**), no spontaneous venous pulsations (SVP), and no other neurologic signs. She had a normal brain MRI and elevated intracranial pressure measured by lumbar puncture. She was diagnosed with idiopathic intracranial hypertension and was followed closely for any changes in her vision. She was started on acetazolamide and assisted with a weight loss program. Her symptoms resolved spontaneously over the course of 18 months.

EPIDEMIOLOGY

Idiopathic intracranial hypertension (IIH), formerly pseudotumor cerebri or benign intracranial hypertension, occurs in:

- 1 per 100,000 people.[1]
- 20 per 100,000 obese females aged 15 to 44 years.[1]

ETIOLOGY AND PATHOPHYSIOLOGY

The optic disc swells because of elevated intracranial pressure. Typically, both discs are swollen; however, unilateral optic disc swelling has been rarely noted with elevated intracranial pressure. Patients with papilledema should undergo imaging, preferably MRI, followed by lumbar puncture. IIH is a diagnosis of exclusion with the following criteria:[3]

- No symptoms and signs (if present), except those of increased intracranial pressure (headaches, nausea/emesis) or papilledema (transient visual problems, loss of SVP, decreased visual acuity, and visual field defect). Unilateral or bilateral sixth nerve palsy may be present.
- Elevated intracranial pressure is present, as measured by lumbar puncture opening pressure over 250 mm of water in the lateral decubitus position with normal cerebral spinal fluid.
- No evidence of mass, hydrocephalus, or vascular lesions by MRI.
- No other identifiable cause of increased intracranial hypertension.

CLINICAL FEATURES

- Over 90% of patients with IIH are obese women of childbearing age. Look for a different diagnosis in children, men, and older patients.[3]
- Papilledema is present and bilateral in the overwhelming majority of cases (**Figures 21-1** and **21-2**).

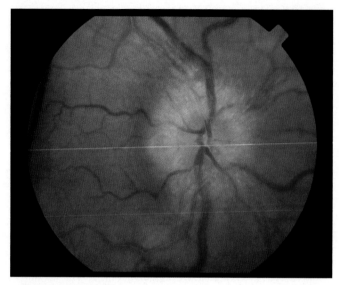

FIGURE 21-1 Papilledema from increased intracranial pressure. The optic disc is elevated and hyperemic with engorged retinal veins. The entire optic disc margin is blurred. Optic neuropathies can also have blurring of the entire disc margin, but often, only part of the disc is blurred. (*Courtesy of Paul D. Comeau.*)

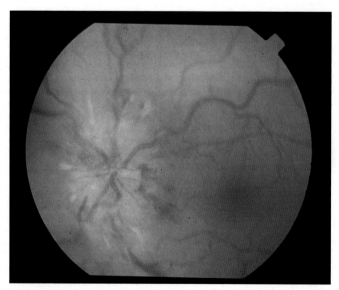

FIGURE 21-2 Severe acute papilledema with papillary flame hemorrhages and cotton wool spots that obscure the disc vessels. The blurred edges of the optic disc appear as a starburst. (*Courtesy of Paul D. Comeau.*)

- SVP are retinal vein pulsations at the optic disc and are typically absent in IIH patients. SVP are seen in 90% of patients with normal intracranial pressure, and are absent when the CSF pressure is above 190 mm Hg. As the CSF pressure may be transiently normal in IIH, the presence of SVP does not preclude IIH, but indicates that the CSF pressure is normal at that moment.[4]

DIFFERENTIAL DIAGNOSIS

Papilledema can be confused with:

- Pseudopapilledema or optic disc drusen, an optic nerve anomaly that elevates the optic disc surface and blurs the disc margins, which can be caused by calcifications in the optic nerve head.
- Optic neuropathies, swelling of all or parts of one or both discs, which can be caused by ischemia or demyelination (as in multiple sclerosis), and may be seen in 1% to 2% of patients with diabetes mellitus type 1 or 2.[2]

  Elevated intracranial pressure can also be caused by obstructing lesions, medical conditions, or medications[3]:

- Mass lesions, hydrocephalus, venus sinus or jugular venus thrombosis, and meningeal infections.
- Addison's disease, hypoparathyroidism, COPD, sleep apnea, renal failure, pulmonary hypertension, and severe anemia.
- Antibiotics in the tetracycline family, vitamin A, anabolic steroids, lithium, and corticosteroid withdrawal.

MANAGEMENT

In many cases, IIH is self-limiting, presents without visual symptoms, and will resolve over several years without loss of vision. However, when patients present with persistent or worsening visual disturbances, treatment is required to lower the intracranial pressure to prevent optic nerve damage and irreversible loss of vision. Management includes the following:

- Careful observation (often by an ophthalmologist) with documentation of any visual changes.
- Weight loss of 15% of body weight is beneficial but will not decrease intracranial pressure quickly enough if visual compromise is present.[1] SOR Ⓒ

- Acetazolamide 1000 to 2000 mg/day; early studies indicate that topiramate may also be effective; other diuretics such as furosemide are less effective.[5] SOR Ⓒ
- High-dose corticosteroids for short time periods for rare cases of rapidly advancing vision loss.[1,5] SOR Ⓒ
- Surgical interventions for severe, recalcitrant cases include optic nerve sheath fenestration or lumbar peritoneal shunt. Surgery is also considered in special populations such as pregnant women and dialysis patients.[1,5] SOR Ⓒ

PATIENT EDUCATION

Advise patients with new papilledema of the need for an evaluation for dangerous causes of increased intracranial pressure, such as intracranial masses or underlying medical illnesses. Also advise patients that IIH often resolves spontaneously over several years, but they should report any visual changes immediately.

FOLLOW-UP

Patients should be followed every 3 to 6 months by a physician who can adequately view the entire optic disc and document visual acuity. They should be seen immediately for any visual changes.

REFERENCES

1. Mathews MK, Sergott RC, Savino PJ. Pseudotumor cerebri. *Curr Opin Ophthalmol.* 2003;14(6):364–370.
2. Bayraktar Z, Alacali N, Bayraktar S. Diabetic papillopathy in type II diabetic patients. *Retina.* 2002;22(6):752–758.
3. Friedman DI, Jacobson DM. Diagnostic criteria for idiopathic intracranial hypertension. *Neurology.* 2002;59(10):1492–1495.
4. Jacks AS, Miller NR. Spontaneous retinal venous pulsation: Aetiology and significance. *J Neurol Neurosurg Psychiatry.* 2003;74(1):7–9.
5. Friedman DI, Jacobson DM. Idiopathic intracranial hypertension. *J Neuroophthalmol.* 2004;24(2):138–145.

22 AGE-RELATED MACULAR DEGENERATION

Heidi Chumley, MD

PATIENT STORY

A 78-year-old white woman presents with loss of central vision that has gradually worsened over the last 6 months. Fully independent before, she can no longer drive and has difficulty with activities of daily living. Her peripheral vision remains normal. Fundoscopic examination reveals macular depigmentation and drusen (yellowish-colored subretinal deposits on the macula) (**Figure 22-1**). She is diagnosed with dry age-related macular degeneration. After her physician discusses the available information about antioxidants and therapeutic options, she decides to start antioxidants and see an ophthalmologist to discuss laser, surgical, or medical treatments.

EPIDEMIOLOGY

Age-related macular degeneration (AMD) is the leading cause of severe vision loss in the elderly.

- Prevalence of AMD is 9.2%; prevalence of significant vision loss with AMD is 1.2% to 1.8%, increasing to 7.1% for those older than 75 years.[1]

- At age 75, the 5-year incidence rate is estimated to be 10.8%.[1]

- AMD that causes significant vision loss is more common in whites than blacks or Hispanics.[1]

- Smoking increases risk in women (RR 2.5 for current smokers; 2.0 for former smokers).[1]

- AMD aggregates in families, but the specific genetic and familial risk factors are not clear.[1]

ETIOLOGY AND PATHOPHYSIOLOGY

AMD affects central but not peripheral vision. Environment and genetic attributes increase risk of these pathologic changes with aging.[2]

- Oxidative stress from the buildup of free oxygen radicals causes retinal pigment epithelial (RPE) injury.

- RPE injury evokes a chronic inflammatory response.

- RPE injury/inflammation forms an abnormal extracellular matrix (ECM), with altered diffusion of nutrients to the retina and RPE.

- The abnormal ECM and diffusion leads to retina atrophy and new vessel growth.

MAKING THE DIAGNOSIS

CLINICAL FEATURES

Diagnosis is made by ophthalmoscopy. AMD can be dry (early, intermediate, or advanced) or wet (always considered advanced).

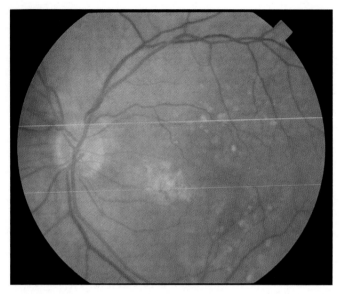

FIGURE 22-1 Intermediate dry age-related macular degeneration with macular depigmentation and drusen (yellowish-colored subretinal deposits on the macula). This patient has central vision distortion. (*Courtesy of Paul D. Comeau.*)

- Early dry—May have no vision change; drusen present (**Figure 22-2**).
- Intermediate dry—Distortion in the center of vision; multiple-medium size drusen (**Figure 22-1**).
- Advanced dry—Significant central vision loss from breakdown of support tissues around the macula.
- Advanced wet—(Exudative) gradual or sudden significant loss of vision; new onset of distortion in vision (straight lines appear wavy); abnormal blood vessels grow under the macula and can cause hemorrhage (**Figure 22-3**). Late changes include subretinal scarring and retinal atrophy (**Figure 22-4**).

DIFFERENTIAL DIAGNOSIS

Vision loss in the elderly can also be caused by any of the following:[3]

- Glaucoma (open angle)—Often asymptomatic until late in the disease, but then has visual field defects instead of central vision loss; fundoscopic examination may reveal a large cup-to-disc ratio (see Chapter 18, Glaucoma).
- Diabetic retinopathy—May have central vision loss with macular edema; fundoscopic examination demonstrates microaneurysms, cotton wool spots, hemorrhages, and exudates (see Chapter 19, Diabetic Retinopathy).
- Cataracts—Blurred vision or glare; lens opacities seen when examining the red reflex.

MANAGEMENT

- Refer to ophthalmologist to evaluate for treatments such as laser photocoagulation or photodynamic therapy, intraocular injections, or surgery.[3,4] Intraocular injections are performed with antagonists of vascular endothelial growth factor (anti-VGEF) agents.[4] Acute changes in vision (distortion of lines, objects) in a patient with a history of dry AMD is an indication for urgent referral to an ophthalmologist for evaluation and possible anti-VEGF treatments such as bevacizumab (Avastin) or ranibizumab (Lucentis) to prevent further vision loss.[4] SOR **C**
- Consider antioxidants (vitamin C, 500 mg; vitamin E, 400 IU; and beta carotene, 15 mg) plus 80 mg zinc per day to decrease the risk of worsening vision loss in patients with intermediate to advanced AMD.[5] SOR **B** These antioxidants are available in single tablet formulations. Avoid beta carotene for smokers or people who have smoked in the last 10 years.

PATIENT RESOURCES

The National Eye Institute has information for patients at **http://www.nei.nih.gov.**

REFERENCES

1. Seddon JM, Chen CA. The epidemiology of age-related macular degeneration. *Int Ophthalmol Clin.* 2004;44(4):17–39.

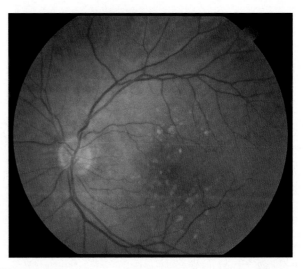

FIGURE 22-2 Early dry age-related macular degeneration demonstrating drusen, yellowish-colored subretinal deposits on the macula. Patients may have no visual complaints at this stage. (*Courtesy of Paul D. Comeau.*)

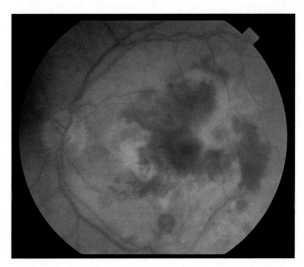

FIGURE 22-3 Late wet age-related macular degeneration (exudative) with subretinal hemorrhages. Patients usually have significant central vision loss. (*Courtesy of Paul D. Comeau.*)

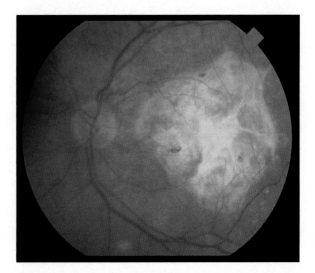

FIGURE 22-4 Late wet age-related macular degeneration (exudative) with subretinal scarring. Patients usually have significant central vision loss resulting from destruction of tissue around the macula. (*Courtesy of Paul D. Comeau.*)

2. Zarbin MA. Current concepts in the pathogenesis of age-related macular degeneration. *Arch Ophthalmol.* 2004;122(4):598–614.

3. Kroll P, Meyer CH. Which treatment is best for which AMD patient? *Br J Ophthalmol.* 2006;90(2):128–130.

4. Avery RL, Pieramici DJ, Rabena MD, Castellarin AA, Nasir MA, Giust MJ. Intravitreal bevacizumab (Avastin) for neovascular age-related macular degeneration. *Ophthalmology.* 2006;113(3): 363–372.

5. Age-Related Eye Disease Study Research Group. A randomized, placebo-controlled, clinical trial of high-dose supplementation with vitamins C and E, beta carotene, and zinc for age-related macular degeneration and vision loss: AREDS Report No. 8. *Arch Ophthalmol.* 2001;119(10):1417–1436.

23 EYE TRAUMA—HYPHEMA

Heidi Chumley, MD

PATIENT STORY

A 22-year-old man was hit in the eye with a baseball and presented to the emergency department with eye pain and redness and decreased visual acuity. There was a collection of blood in his anterior chamber (**Figure 23-1**) and he was diagnosed with a hyphema. He was given an eye shield for protection, advised to take acetaminophen for pain, and counseled not to engage in sporting activities until his hyphema resolved. He saw his physician daily for the next 2 days, during which his vision improved. His hyphema resolved in 5 days.

EPIDEMIOLOGY

- Severe eye injuries, such as hyphema, account for approximately 5% of patients presenting to emergency departments with eye complaints.[1]

- One study found that 60% of hyphemas result from sports injuries.[1]

ETIOLOGY AND PATHOPHYSIOLOGY

- A hyphema is a collection of blood, mostly erythrocytes, that layer within the anterior chamber.

- Trauma is the most common cause, often a direct blow from a projectile object such as a ball, air pellet or BB, rock, or fist.

- Direct force to the eye (blunt trauma) forces the globe inward, distorting the normal architecture.

- Intraocular pressure rises instantaneously causing the lens/iris/ciliary body to move posteriorly, thus disrupting the vascularization with resultant bleeding.

- Intraocular pressure continues to rise and bleeding stops when this pressure is high enough to compress the bleeding vessels.

- A fibrin-platelet clot forms and stabilizes in 4 to 7 days; this is eventually broken down by the fibrinolytic system and cleared through the trabecular meshwork.

DIAGNOSIS

The diagnosis of hyphema is clinical, depending on the classic appearance of blood layering in the anterior chamber.

CLINICAL FEATURES

- Layered blood in the anterior chamber.
- History of eye trauma or risk factor for nontraumatic hyphema.
- Increased intraocular pressure (32%).
- Decreased vision.

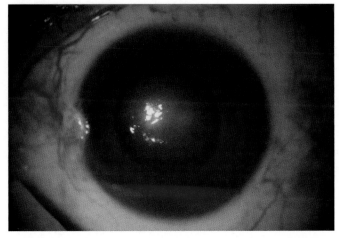

FIGURE 23-1 Layering of red blood cells in the anterior chamber following blunt trauma. This grade 1 hyphema has blood filling in less than one-third of the anterior chamber. (*Courtesy of Paul D. Comeau.*)

CLASSIFICATION

Hyphemas are classified according to the amount of blood in the anterior chamber:

- Grade 1: Less than ⅓ of the anterior chamber (**Figure 23-1**); 58% of all hyphemas.
- Grade 2: ⅓ to ½ of the anterior chamber; 20% of all hyphemas.
- Grade 3: ½ to almost completely filled anterior chamber; 14% of all hyphemas.
- Grade 4: Completely filled anterior chamber; 8% of all hyphemas.

Eye trauma without hyphema (**Figure 23-2**) can be conjunctivitis, anterior uveitis, and/or distortion of the normal architecture.

DIFFERENTIAL DIAGNOSIS

Hyphema is an unmistakable physical examination finding that can be caused by any of the following:

- Trauma—History of trauma, including nonaccidental trauma (i.e., child abuse).
- Blood clotting disturbances—Personal or family history of bleeding disorder, little or no trauma, and black race (increased incidence of sickle trait and disease).
- Medication-induced anticoagulation—Chronic use of aspirin or warfarin and little or no trauma.
- Neovascularization—Diabetes mellitus or history of prior eye surgery (cataract); without trauma, often painless, sudden, blurry vision.
- Melanoma or retinoblastoma—Variety of presentations depending on the size and location; hyphema occurs when mass effect sheers the lens/iris/ciliary body causing bleeding.
- Abnormal vasculature, i.e., juvenile xanthogranuloma—Red to yellow papules and nodules in the eyes, skin, and viscera, most often present by 1 year of age.

MANAGEMENT

- Most hyphemas resolve in 5 to 7 days; management strategies protect the eye and decrease complications, including rebleeding.
- Evaluate or refer for evaluation for elevated intraocular pressure and other associated injuries. Signs of a violated globe, such as a perforation of the cornea, conjunctiva or sclera, distorted ocular architecture, or exposed and/or distorted uveal tissue such as the iris (causing a peaked pupil), require immediate surgical evaluation and repair (**Figure 23-2**).
- Patch and shield the injured eye and restrict activity to quiet ambulatory with head elevated as much as possible.[2] SOR **B**
- Outpatient management is acceptable for adults and children if patient is likely to be able to follow treatment plan.[2,3] SOR **B**
- Although controversy remains about the best treatment, each of the following has been demonstrated to lower the risk of rebleeding in randomized-controlled trials:

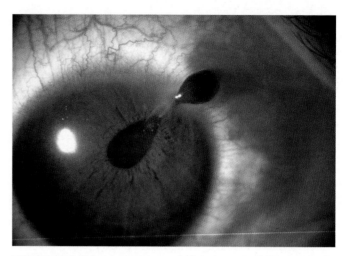

FIGURE 23-2 This young patient was hit in the eye with the corner of a laminated name card. The sharp edge perforated the cornea and pulled a portion of the iris out of the wound. Note the abnormal configuration of the pupil (dyscoria). No hyphema noted. This patient required emergent surgical repair. (*Reprinted with permission from, Lo MW, Chalfin S. Retrobulbar anesthesia for repair of ruptured globes. Am J Ophthalmol. 1997;123(6):833–835. Photo by Paul D. Comeau.*)

- Oral antifibrinolytic agents (Aminocaproic acid 50 mg/kg every 4 hours for 5 days, not to exceed 30 g/day; or Tranexamic acid 75 mg/kg/day divided into three doses).[2] SOR **C**
- Topical aminocaproic acid (30% in a gel vehicle four times a day) as effective as oral.[2] SOR **C**
- Topical cycloplegics and corticosteroids have also been recommended.[2] SOR **B**
- Surgical intervention has been recommended for patients with persistent total hyphema or prolonged elevated intraocular pressure.
- Avoid aspirin and NSAIDs, which have been associated with higher rates of rebleeding.
- Use acetaminophen, if needed, for pain.
- Consider laboratory tests to evaluate for bleeding disorders: Bleeding time, electrophoresis for sickle cell trait, platelet count, prothrombin and partial thromboplastin time, and liver tests.

PATIENT EDUCATION

- Complications include rebleeding, decreased visual acuity, posterior or peripheral anterior synechiae, corneal bloodstaining, glaucoma, and optic atrophy. Patients may need surgical or medical management for glaucoma.
- Patients who are more likely to rebleed include black patients (irrespective of sickle cell/trait status),[4,5] patients with a grade 3 or 4 hyphema, and patients with high initial intraocular pressure.
- Most patients (80%) will regain visual acuity of 20/50 or better.[6]
- Warn patients that they may have angle recession from traumatic causes of the hyphema. This will predispose the patient to a lifetime risk of traumatic glaucoma, which can cause blindness without any symptoms. These patients need to be monitored regularly for increased pressure and glaucomatous nerve changes.

FOLLOW-UP

Patients should be monitored daily for the first 5 or more days by a provider familiar with caring for hyphemas. Patient with a hyphema should be followed subsequently for signs of angle recession and high intraocular pressure, which predisposes the patient to traumatic glaucoma, an insidious cause of blindness in patients with a history of trauma.

PROVIDER RESOURCES

Emedicine has an excellent review of the management of traumatic hyphema, **www.emedicine.com.**[6]

REFERENCES

1. Schein OD, Hibberd PL, Shingleton BJ, et al. The spectrum and burden of ocular injury. *Ophthalmology.* 1988;95(3):300–305.
2. Walton W, Von HS, Grigorian R, Zarbin M. Management of traumatic hyphema. *Surv Ophthalmol.* 2002;47(4):297–334.
3. Rocha KM, Martins EN, Melo LA, Jr., Moraes NS. Outpatient management of traumatic hyphema in children: Prospective evaluation. *J AAPOS.* 2004;8(4):357–361.
4. Lai JC, Fekrat S, Barron Y, Goldberg MF. Traumatic hyphema in children: Risk factors for complications. *Arch Ophthalmol.* 2001;119 (1):64–70.
5. Spoor TC, Kwitko GM, O'Grady JM, Ramocki JM. Traumatic hyphema in an urban population. *Am J Ophthalmol.* 1990;109(1): 23–27.
6. Sheppard J, Williams P, Crouch P. Hyphema. *emedicine.* 2005.

24 THE RED EYE

Heidi Chumley, MD
Richard P. Usatine, MD

PATIENT STORY

A 41-year-old man wakes up with eyes that are reddened bilaterally (**Figure 24-1**). He has some burning and itching in the eyes, but no pain. He describes minimal crusting on his eyelashes. Examination shows no loss of vision, no foreign bodies, and pupils that are equal, round, and reactive to light. He is diagnosed with viral conjunctivitis, which does not require antibiotic treatment. He is advised about methods to prevent spreading conjunctivitis to others and is asked to notify the physician immediately if he experiences eye pain or loss of vision. He recovers spontaneously without complications after a few days.

EPIDEMIOLOGY

- An acute red eye or eyes is a common presentation in ambulatory and emergency departments.
- Conjunctivitis is the most common cause of a nontraumatic red eye in primary care.

ETIOLOGY/PATHOPHYSIOLOGY

Red eye is caused by any of the following:

- Infectious or noninfectious inflammation of any layer of the eye (conjunctivitis, episcleritis, scleritis, uveitis, keratitis).
- Eyelid pathology (blepharitis, entropion, i.e., inward turning of eyelash).
- Acute glaucoma (usually angle closure).
- Trauma.
- Subconjunctival hemorrhage (**Figure 24-2**).

DIAGNOSIS

CLINICAL FEATURES

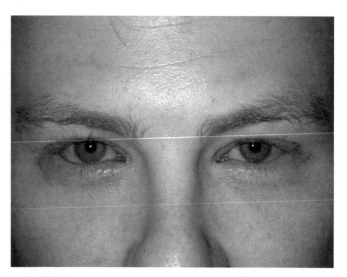

FIGURE 24-1 Bilateral viral conjunctivitis in a 41-year-old man. (*Courtesy of Richard P. Usatine, MD.*)

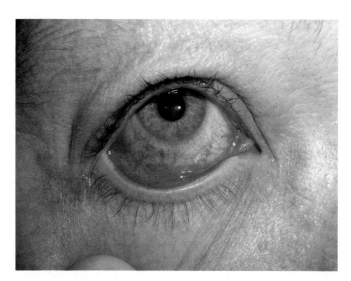

FIGURE 24-2 Bacterial conjunctivitis in a contact lens user. (*Courtesy of Richard P. Usatine, MD.*)

	Conjunctivitis	Episcleritis	Scleritis	Uveitis	Keratitis	Closed-Angle Glaucoma	Sub-Conjunctival Hemorrhage	Ocular Rosacea
Redness	Diffuse	Segmental; pink	Segmental or diffuse; dark red, purple or blue	360° perilimbal (worse at limbus)	Diffuse, ciliary injection	Diffuse, scleral	Blotchy, outside vessels	Diffuse
Eye pain	No	Mild, may be tender to touch	Severe, boring	Sometimes	Usually	Yes	No, unless due to trauma	No
Vision loss	No	No	Sometimes	Sometimes	Maybe, depending on location	Yes	No	In severe cases
Discharge	Usually	No	No	No	Maybe	No	No	No
Photophobia*	No	No	Yes	Yes, if anterior	Yes	Yes	No	Sometimes
Pupil	Normal	Normal	Normal	Constricted	Normal to constricted	Mild dilation, less responsive	Normal; unless affected by trauma	Normal
Cornea	Clear	Clear	Clear	Clear to hazy	Hazy	Usually hazy	Clear	Clear or neovascular-ization, cloudy
Assoc.	URI, allergy, exposure	Occasional systemic disease	Systemic disease	Systemic disease, id-iopathic	Contact lenses, HSV or varicella, rosacea	Causes headaches, nausea, vomiting, GI symptoms	HTN, trauma, Valsalva, cough, blood thinners	Acne rosacea (can exist with-out also), blepharitis

*For identifying serious causes of red eye, the presence of photophobia elicited with a penlight in a general practice had a positive predictive value of 60% and a negative predictive value of 90%.[1] HSV, herpes simplex virus.

DIFFERENTIAL DIAGNOSIS

An acute red eye can be caused by any of the following:

- Conjunctivitis—Conjunctival injection, eye discharge, gritty or uncomfortable feeling, and no vision loss (**Figures 24-1** to **24-5**) (see also Chapter 15, Conjunctivitis).

- Episcleritis—Segmental or diffuse inflammation of episclera (pink color), mild or no discomfort, but can be tender to palpation, and no vision disturbance (**Figure 24-6**) (see also Chapter 16, Episcleritis/Scleritis).

- Scleritis—Segmental or diffuse inflammation of sclera (dark red, purple, or blue color), severe boring eye pain often radiating to head and neck, and photophobia and vision loss (**Figure 24-7**) (see also Chapter 16, Episcleritis/Scleritis).

- Uveitis or Iritis—360 degrees perilimbal injection, which is most intense at the limbus and eye pain, photophobia, and vision loss (**Figures 24-8** and **24-9**) (see also Chapter 17, Uveitis and Iritis).

- Keratitis or corneal ulcerations—Diffuse erythema with ciliary injection often with pupillary constriction; eye discharge; and pain, photophobia, vision loss depending on the location of ulceration (**Figure 24-10**).

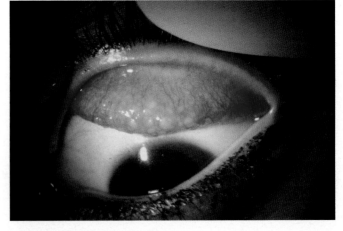

FIGURE 24-3 Giant papillary conjunctivitis secondary to contact lens use. (*Courtesy of Paul D. Comeau.*)

- Ocular rosacea—Eye findings present in more than 50% of people with rosacea. Can present as blepharitis, conjunctivitis, or episcleritis or cause corneal ulcerations and neovascularization (**Figures 24-8** and **24-11**).

- Trauma causing iritis, globe injury, or hemorrhage (**Figures 24-12, 24-13** and **24-14**) (see Chapter 23, Eye Trauma–Hyphema).

- Atraumatic subconjunctival hemorrhage (**Figure 24-2**).

- Acute-angle closure glaucoma—Cloudy cornea and scleral injection, shallow anterior chamber, eye pain with ipsilateral headache, and severe vision loss (see also Chapter 18, Glaucoma).

- Pterygium—Fibrovascular tissue on the surface of the eye extending onto the cornea (**Figure 24-15**) (see also Chapter 11, Pterygium).

- Eyelid pathology—Blepharitis (inflammation of the eyelid) (**Figure 24-16**). Entropion is a turning inward of the eyelid and can cause irritation to the conjunctiva and cornea.

MANAGEMENT

Refer patients with any of the following to an ophthalmologist[2]: SOR C

- Visual loss.
- Moderate or severe pain.
- Severe, purulent discharge.
- Corneal involvement.
- Conjunctival scarring.
- Lack of response to therapy.
- Recurrent episodes.
- Open globe or perforation.
- History of herpes simplex virus (HSV) eye disease.

Treatment for specific causes is discussed in the corresponding chapters.

PATIENT EDUCATION

Advise patients to notify their physician immediately for eye pain (other than gritty discomfort) and/or loss of vision.

FOLLOW-UP

Timing of follow-up and need for further testing is determined by the underlying cause (see corresponding chapters).

REFERENCES

1. Yaphe J, Pandher K. The predictive value of the penlight test for photophobia for serious eye pathology in general practice. *Fam Pract.*, 2003;20(4):425–427.

2. American Academy of Ophthalmology Cornea/External Disease Panel, Preferred Practice Patterns Committee. *Conjunctivitis*. San Francisco, CA: American Academy of Ophthalmology; 2003:25 p.

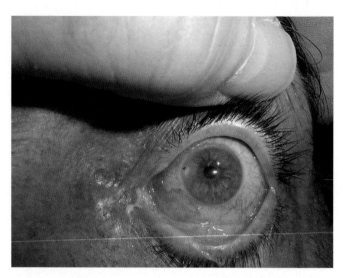

FIGURE 24-4 Conjunctival irritation due to a fleck of metal (at 9-o'clock position) that was embedded in the eye of a man who was grinding steel. (*Courtesy of Richard P. Usatine, MD.*)

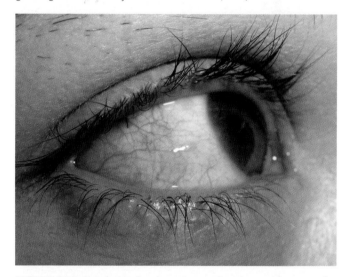

FIGURE 24-5 Episcleritis showing a sector of erythema. (*Courtesy of Richard P. Usatine, MD.*)

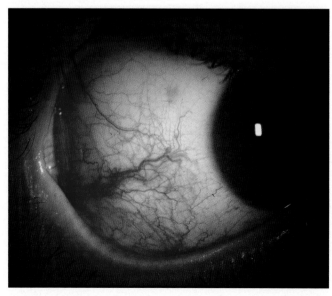

FIGURE 24-6 Scleritis with deeper darker vessels than the episcleritis. (*Courtesy of Paul D. Comeau.*)

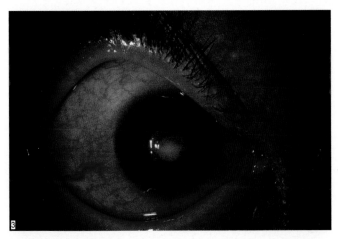

FIGURE 24-7 Diffuse ciliary injection and cloudy cornea demonstrating keratitis with corneal ulcer formation and a leucocyte infiltrate. (*Courtesy of Paul D. Comeau.*)

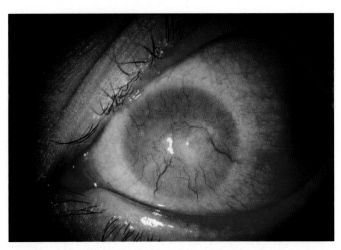

FIGURE 24-10 Severe occular rosacea with a blood vessels growing over the cornea leading to blindness. (*Courtesy of Paul D. Comeau.*)

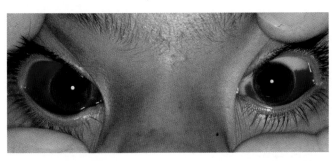

FIGURE 24-8 Subconjunctival hemorrhage secondary to trauma or hypertension. (*Courtesy of Paul D. Comeau.*)

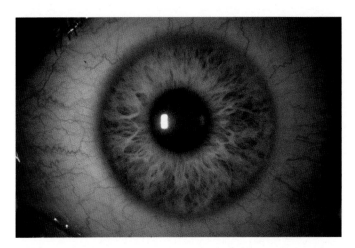

FIGURE 24-11 Iritis (anterior uveitis) with a limbal flair, red to purple perilimbal ring. For contrast, note the perilimbal area is not involved in conjunctivitis best seen in **Figure 24-2**. This patient has eye pain and vision loss, which are also absent in conjunctivitis. (*Courtesy of Paul D. Comeau.*)

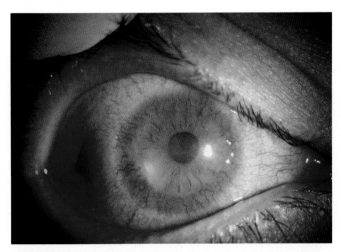

FIGURE 24-9 Ocular rosacea with new vessels growing onto the cornea. Many patients with rosacea have some ocular findings including blepharitis (inflammation of the eyelid), conjunctivitis (most common), episcleritis (rare), keratitis, or corneal ulceration/neovascularization. (*Courtesy of Paul D. Comeau.*)

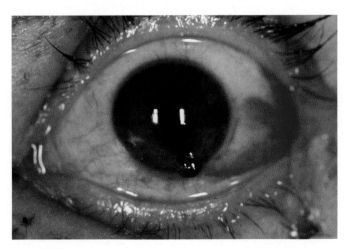

FIGURE 24-12 Trauma to the eye resulting in an open globe injury with extrusion of some of the iris through the cornea and an abnormal pupil. There is conjunctival injection and hemorrhage causing this red eye. (*Courtesy of Paul D. Comeau.*)

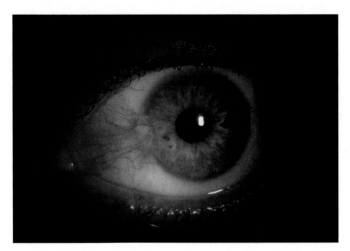

FIGURE 24-13 Pterygium that often becomes irritated and erythematous. (*Courtesy of Paul D. Comeau.*)

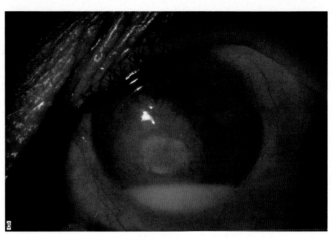

FIGURE 24-15 Hypopyon with white cells layered in the anterior chamber. (*Courtesy of Paul D. Comeau.*)

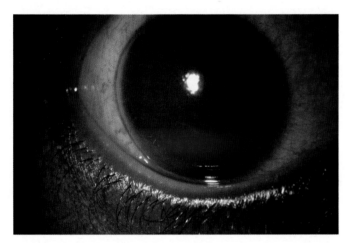

FIGURE 24-14 Hyphema with red cells in the anterior chamber and an inferior blood clot. (*Courtesy of Paul D. Comeau.*)

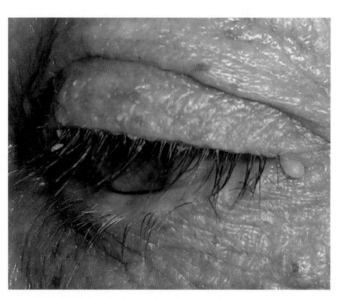

FIGURE 24-16 Blepharitis showing erythema of the eyelids and flaking in the eyelashes. Note the scale that has accumulated in the eyelashes. (*Courtesy of Richard P. Usatine, MD.*)

PART 5

EAR, NOSE, AND THROAT

SECTION 1   EAR

25 ACUTE OTITIS AND OTITIS MEDIA WITH EFFUSION

Brian Z. Rayala, MD

PATIENT STORY

A 15-month-old boy was brought by his parents to their family physi-cian with a 2-day history of fever, irritability, and frequent tugging of his left ear. This was preceded by a 1-week history of nasal congestion, cough, and rhinorrhea. On otoscopy, his left tympanic membrane (TM) appears erythematous, cloudy, bulging, and exudative (**Figure 25-1**). The diagnosis of acute otitis media was explained to his parents and the pros and cons of antibiotic use discussed. The parents choose to go ahead with a 10-day course of amoxicillin and the child gets well.

In the follow up, 2 months later, the child appeared healthy and was meeting all his developmental milestones. On otoscopic examina-tion, air–fluid levels were seen in the right ear (**Figure 25-2**). The di-agnosis of otitis media with effusion was explained to the parents and they chose to watch and wait rather than administering additional an-tibiotics at this time. Three months later the effusion was completely resolved.

EPIDEMIOLOGY

Acute otitis media (AOM) is the most common diagnosis for acute office visits of children.

- It accounted for $5 billion of the total national health expenditure in 2000, with more than 40% for children between 1 and 3 years of age.[1]

- It is estimated that 60% to 80% of children in the United States de-velop AOM by 1 year of age and that 80% to 90% develop AOM by age 2 to 3 years.

- The highest incidence occurs between 6 and 24 months of age.[2,3]

- AOM is the most common reason for outpatient antibiotic treatment in the United States[4] A national survey in 1992 revealed that 30% of all antibiotics prescribed for those younger than 18 years was for the treatment of AOM.[5]

- It is estimated that each year in the United Kingdom, approximately 30% of children younger than 3 years of age visit their general practitioner with AOM and 97% receive antimicrobial treatment.[6]

Otitis media with effusion (OME) is also very common in childhood:

- It is diagnosed in 2.2 million children every year in the United States.[7]

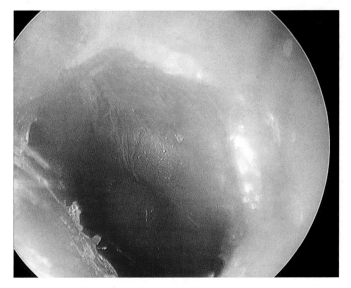

FIGURE 25-1 AOM in the left ear of a 15-month-old child with marked erythema and bulging of the TM. The malleus and light reflex are not visible. (*Courtesy of William Clark, MD.*)

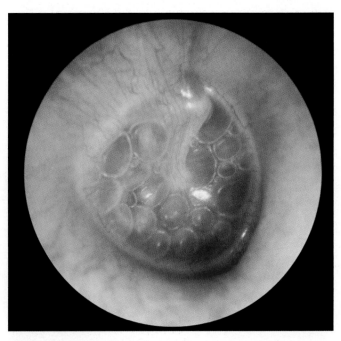

FIGURE 25-2 OME in the right ear. Note multiple air–fluid levels in this slightly retracted, translucent, nonerythematous TM. (*Courtesy of Frank Miller, MD.*)

- Approximately 90% of children (80% of individual ears) have OME at some time before school age, most often between ages 6 months and 4 years.[7]

- The combined direct and indirect health care costs amount to $4 billion annually.[7]

- Risk factors include age 6 years or younger, large number of siblings, low socioeconomic group, frequent upper respiratory tract infection, tobacco exposure, staying at daycare center, and bottle-feed.[8]

ETIOLOGY AND PATHOPHYSIOLOGY

AOM is characterized by middle ear effusion (MEE) in a patient with signs and symptoms of acute illness (e.g., fever, irritability, otalgia). It is often preceded by upper respiratory symptoms such as cough and rhinorrhea.

- Pathogenesis:[9]
  - Eustachian tube dysfunction (usually because of upper respiratory infection) and subsequent tube obstruction.
  - Increased negative pressure in the middle ear.
  - Accumulation of middle ear fluid.
  - Microbial growth.
  - Suppuration (that leads to clinical signs of AOM).
- Most common pathogens in the United States and United Kingdom:[10]
  - *Streptococcus pneumoniae.*
  - *Haemophilus influenzae.*
  - *Moraxella catarrhalis.*
- Viruses account for 16% of cases. RSV, rhinoviruses, influenza viruses, and adenoviruses have been the most common isolated viruses.[11]
- Most important risk factors include young age and staying at daycare centers. Other risk factors include the following:[6]
  - White race.
  - Male.
  - History of enlarged adenoids, tonsillitis, or asthma.
  - Multiple previous episodes.
  - Bottle-feed.
  - History of ear infections in parents or siblings.
  - Use of a soother or pacifier.
  - Passive smoking (when parents smoke at home).
- OME is a disorder characterized by fluid in the middle ear, but without signs and symptoms of acute ear infection.
- OME most commonly follows AOM; it may also occur spontaneously.
- Fluid limits sound conduction through the ossicles and results in decreased hearing.
- Reasons for the persistence of fluid in otitis media remain unclear, although potential etiologies include allergies, biofilms, or physiologic features.
- "Glue ear" refers to extremely viscous mucoid material within the middle ear and is a distinct subtype of OME.

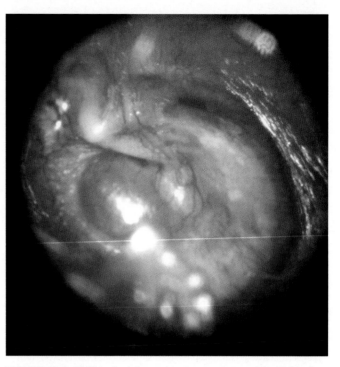

FIGURE 25-3 OME in the left ear showing retraction of the TM and straightening of the handle of the malleus as the retraction pulls the bone upward. (*Courtesy of Glen Medellin, MD.*)

DIAGNOSIS

CLINICAL FEATURES OF AOM

To diagnose AOM, the clinician should confirm a history of acute onset, identify signs of MEE, *and* evaluate for the presence of signs and symptoms of middle ear inflammation.[12] SOR **C**

Elements of the definition of AOM are *all* of the following:[12]

- Recent, usually abrupt, onset of signs and symptoms of middle ear inflammation and MEE.
- The presence of MEE, which is indicated by any of the following:
  ○ Bulging of the TM (**Figure 25-1**).
  ○ Limited or absent mobility of the TM (often seen as retraction of the TM).
    ■ The hallmark of establishing the diagnosis of AOM is the demonstration of fluid by pneumatic otoscopy. That is, the TM does not move when the air pressure is changed in the external ear.
  ○ Air–fluid level behind the TM.
  ○ Otorrhea.
- Signs or symptoms of middle ear inflammation, which maybe indicated by either of the following:
  ○ Distinct erythema of the TM (**Figure 25-1**) in contrast to the normal TM (**Figure 25-6**).

or

  ○ Distinct otalgia (discomfort, clearly referable to the ear[s], that results in interference with or precludes normal activity or sleep).

CLINICAL FEATURES OF OME

- The most common symptom, present in more than half of the patients, is mild hearing loss. This is usually identified when parents express concern regarding their child's behavior, performance at school, or language development.[8]
- Absence of signs and symptoms of acute illness assists in differentiating OME from AOM.
- Common otoscopic findings:
  ○ Air–fluid level or bubble (**Figures 25-2** and **25-3**).
  ○ Cloudy TM (**Figures 25-4** and **25-5**) in contrast to the normal TM (**Figure 25-6**).
  ○ Redness of the TM may be present in ~5% of ears with OME.
- Clinicians should use pneumatic otoscopy as the primary diagnostic method for OME.[13] SOR **A**
  ○ *Impaired mobility of the TM is the hallmark of middle ear effusion.*
  ○ According to a meta-analysis, impaired mobility on pneumatic otoscopy has a pooled sensitivity of 94% and specificity of 80%, and the positive likelihood ratio of 4.7 and negative likelihood ratio of 0.075.[13]

LABORATORY TESTS AND IMAGING

Since AOM and OME are clinical diagnoses, diagnostic testing has a limited role. When clinical presentation and physical examination (including otoscopy) do not establish the diagnosis, the following can be used as adjunctive techniques:

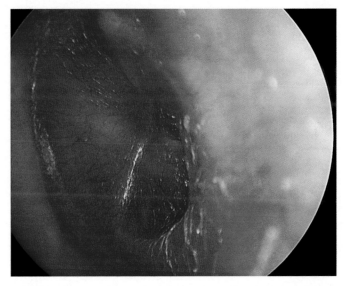

FIGURE 25-4 Early AOM, stage of eustachian tube obstruction. Note the slight retraction of the TM, the more horizontal position of the malleus, and the prominence of the lateral process. (*Courtesy of William Clark, MD.*)

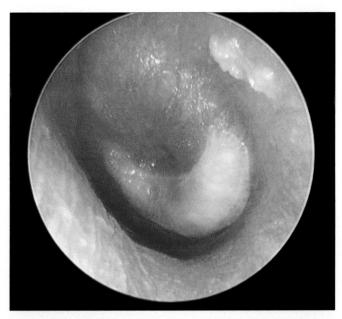

FIGURE 25-5 AOM, stage of suppuration. Note the presence of purulent exudate behind the TM, the outward bulging of the TM, prominence of the posterosuperior portion of the drum, and generalized TM edema. The white area is tympanosclerosis from a previous infection. (*Courtesy of William Clark, MD.*)

- Tympanometry—a procedure that records compliance of the TM by measuring reflected sound. AOM and OME will plot as a reduced or flat waveform. This technique requires patient's cooperation. This is a great way to confirm or question your clinical examination by providing more objective data.

- Acoustic reflectometry—a procedure, very similar to tympanometry, that measures sound reflectivity from the middle ear. With this test, the clinician is able to distinguish air- or fluid-filled space without requiring an airtight seal of the ear canal.

- Middle ear aspiration—for patients with AOM, aspiration may be warranted if patient is toxic, is immunocompromised, or has failed prior courses of antibiotics.

DIFFERENTIAL DIAGNOSIS

The key-differentiating feature between AOM and OME is the absence of signs and symptoms of acute illness in OME (e.g., fever, irritability, otalgia). Otoscopic findings may be similar. Other clinical entities that may be confused with AOM and OME include the following:

- Otitis externa—presents with otalgia, otorrhea, and mild hearing loss, all of which can be present in AOM. Tragal pain on physical examination and signs of external canal inflammation on otoscopic examination differentiate it from AOM. Careful ear irrigation, if tolerated, may be helpful to visualize the TM to differentiate otitis externa from AOM. Tympanometry can be used here if the canal is not fully blocked. The presence of a normal curve would make otitis externa more likely than AOM.

- Otitic barotrauma—often presents with severe otalgia. Key historical features include recent air travel, scuba diving, or ear trauma, preceded by an upper respiratory infection.

- Cholesteatoma—unlike AOM, is a clinically silent disease in its initial stages. Presence of white keratin debris in the middle ear cavity (on otoscopy) is diagnostic (**Figures 25-7** and **25-8**).

- Foreign body—may present with otalgia. Otoscopy reveals presence of foreign body (see Chapter 27, Ear: Foreign Body).

- Bullous myringitis—often associated with viral or mycoplasma infection as well as usual AOM pathogens. In approximately one-third of patients, there is a component of sensorineural hearing loss. Otoscopy shows serous-filled bulla on the surface of the TM (**Figure 25-9**). Patients present with severe otalgia.

- Chronic suppurative otitis media (CSOM)—otoscopy shows TM perforation and otorrhea. History reveals a chronically draining ear and recurrent middle ear infections with or without hearing loss.

- Referred otalgia—rare in children and in cases of bilateral otalgia. Should be considered in cases of otalgia that do not fit clinical features of AOM. Referred pain usually from other head and neck structures (e.g., teeth, jaw, cervical spine, lymph and salivary glands, nose and sinuses, tonsils, tongue, pharynx, meninges).

- Mastoiditis—may be differentiated from simple AOM by the presence of increasing pain and tenderness over mastoid bone in a patient with AOM who has not been treated by antibiotics or recurrence of mastoid pain and tenderness in patients treated with antibiotics. Recurrence or persistence of fever as well as progressive

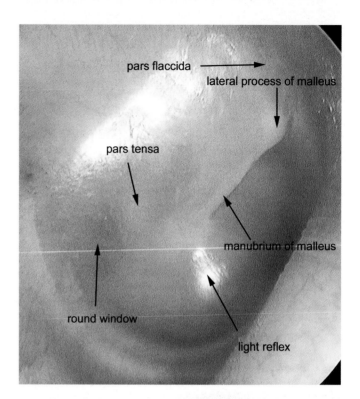

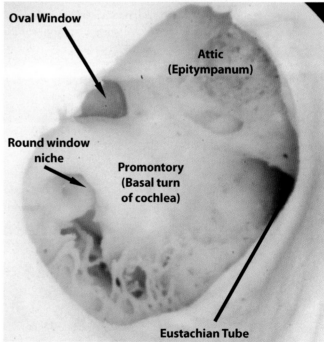

FIGURE 25-6 Normal right TM with comparison using normal bony landmarks of the inner ear. The ossicles were removed in this dissection. (*Courtesy of William Clark, MD.*)

otorrhea are other historical clues. The mastoid swelling may cause the pinna to protrude further than normal (**Figure 25-10**).

- Traumatic perforation of the TM (**Figure 25-11**)—a hole in the TM is seen without purulent drainage.

MANAGEMENT

Without antibiotics, AOM resolves within 24 hours in about 60% of children and within 3 days in about 80% of children. Rate of suppurative complications if antibiotics are withheld is 0.13%.[14] Other treatment options may include the following:

- Oral acetaminophen (paracetamol) and ibuprofen may reduce earache when given with antibiotics.[15] There is insufficient data to evaluate the effectiveness of topical analgesics in AOM.[16] SOR Ⓑ

- Antibiotics may lead to more rapid reduction in symptoms of AOM, but increase the risk of adverse effects, including diarrhea, vomiting, and rash.[15] SOR Ⓑ
  - Antibiotics seem to reduce pain in 2 to 7 days and may prevent development of contralateral AOM, but increase the risks of adverse effects compared with placebo.[13]
  - There is insufficient effectiveness data on which antibiotic regimen is better than another.[15] Antibiotics that have been found to be effective in AOM include amoxicillin, amoxicillin/clavulanic acid, ampicillin, penicillin, erythromycin, azithromycin, trimethoprim–sulfamethoxazole, and cephalosporins.[15] Therefore, amoxicillin is a good first-line treatment because it is very inexpensive and children tolerate the bubblegum taste well.
  - Longer (8–10 day) courses of antibiotics reduce short-term treatment failure, but have no long-term benefits compared with shorter regimens (5-day courses).[15]
  - Antibiotics seem to be most beneficial in children younger than 2 years of age with bilateral AOM, and in children with both AOM and otorrhea. For most other children with mild disease, an observational policy seems justified.[17]
  - An observational approach substantially reduces unnecessary use of antibiotics in children with AOM and may be an alternative to routine use of antimicrobials for treatment of such children.[18]

- Immediate antibiotic treatment (i.e., given at initial consultation) may reduce the duration of symptoms of AOM, but increases the risk of vomiting, diarrhea, and rash compared with delayed treatment (i.e., given after 72 hours).[15] SOR Ⓑ

- Treatment of AOM with decongestants and antihistamines is not recommended.[19] SOR Ⓑ

- Myringotomy appears to be less effective than antibiotics in reducing symptoms. Tympanostomy with ventilation tube insertion leads to short-term reduction in the number of episodes of AOM, but increases the risk of complications (i.e., tympanosclerosis)[15] SOR Ⓑ (**Figures 25-12 to 25-13**).

- Long-term antibiotic prophylaxis may reduce recurrence rates, but increases the risks of vomiting, diarrhea, and rash. There are insufficient data regarding which antibiotic regimen should be used in preference to another to prevent recurrent attacks.[15] SOR Ⓑ

- In children aged 2 months to 7 years, large-scale pneumococcal vaccination strategies are unlikely to be effective.[15] SOR Ⓑ

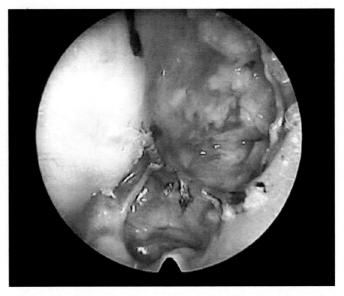

FIGURE 25-7 Cholesteatoma. (*Courtesy of Vladimir Zlinsky, MD, in Roy F. Sullivan, PhD: Audiology Forum: Video Otoscopy www.rcsullivan.com*)

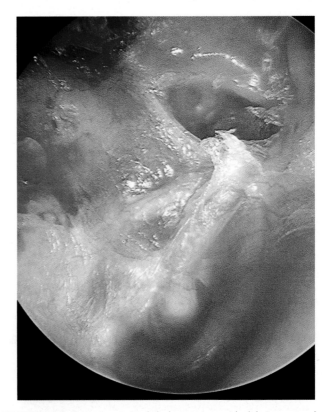

FIGURE 25-8 Primary-acquired cholesteatoma with debris removed from the attic retraction pocket. (*Courtesy of William Clark, MD.*)

Management of OME primarily consists of watchful waiting. Most cases resolve spontaneously within 3 months; only 5% to 10% last 1 year or longer. Treatment depends on duration and associated conditions. The following options should be considered:

- Document the laterality, duration of effusion, and the presence and severity of associated symptoms at each assessment of the child with OME.[7] SOR Ⓒ

- Distinguish the child with OME who is at risk for speech, language, or learning problems from other children with OME and more promptly evaluate hearing, speech, language, and need for intervention in children at risk.[7] SOR Ⓒ Risk factors for developmental difficulties may include the following:
  ○ Permanent hearing loss independent of OME.
  ○ Suspected or diagnosed speech and language delay or disorder.
  ○ Autism-spectrum disorder and other pervasive developmental disorders.
  ○ Syndromes (e.g., Down syndrome) or craniofacial disorders that include cognitive, speech, and language delays.
  ○ Blindness or uncorrectable visual impairment.
  ○ Cleft palate with or without associated syndrome.
  ○ Developmental delay.

- Manage the child with OME who is not at risk with watchful waiting for 3 months from the date of effusion onset (if known) or diagnosis (if onset is unknown).[7] SOR Ⓑ

- Hearing testing is recommended when OME persists for 3 months or longer or at any time if language delay, learning problems, or significant hearing loss is suspected in a child with OME.[7] SOR Ⓑ

- Autoinflation with nasal balloon, in one systematic review, provided short-term benefits, although 12% of children aged 3 to 10 years were unable to use it.[8]

- Antihistamines and decongestants are not effective for OME.[7] SOR Ⓐ

- Antimicrobials and corticosteroids are not recommended.[7] SOR Ⓐ

- Insertion of tympanostomy tubes in young children with persistent middle ear infection does not improve cognitive development, language acquisition, or speech development compared with waiting 6 to 9 months for the effusion to resolve before placing the tubes.[20] Moreover, delayed insertion of tubes helps children avoid getting tubes altogether and does not result in worse developmental outcomes.[21] SOR Ⓐ

- When a child becomes a surgical candidate, tympanostomy tube insertion is the preferred initial procedure; adenoidectomy should not be performed unless a distinct indication exists (e.g., nasal obstruction, chronic adenoiditis).[7] SOR Ⓑ

- Repeat surgery consists of adenoidectomy plus myringotomy, with or without tube insertion. Tonsillectomy alone or myringotomy alone should not be used to treat OME.[7] SOR Ⓑ

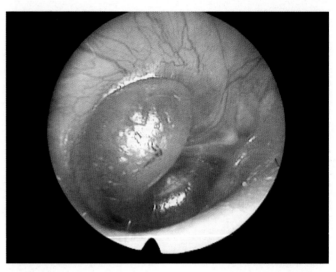

FIGURE 25-9 Bullous myringitis can be differentiated from OME by identifying serous-filled bulla on the surface of the TM. (*Courtesy of Vladimir Zlinsky, MD in Roy F. Sullivan, PhD: Audiology Forum: Video Otoscopy.www.rcsullivan.com*)

PATIENT EDUCATION

- Patient education should focus on identification, prevention, and control of risk factors (see above).

- Parents should be made aware of the high rates of spontaneous resolution of AOM and potential adverse effects of antibiotics.

Providing a prescription for an antibiotic at the initial visit, but advising delay of initiation of medication (i.e., observational approach for up to 48 hours) is an alternative to immediate treatment and is associated with lower antibiotic use.[18]

- Patients should be informed that the natural history of OME is spontaneous resolution.

- Periodic follow-up to monitor resolution of middle ear effusion is extremely important.

- If middle ear effusion is persistent and signs and symptoms of hearing loss, language difficulties, and learning problems arise, additional treatment may be considered.

FOLLOW-UP

For patients with AOM, follow-up consists of the following:

- If the patient fails to respond to the initial management option within 48 to 72 hours, the clinician must reassess the patient to confirm AOM and exclude other causes of illness. If AOM is confirmed in a patient initially managed with observation, the clinician should begin antibacterial therapy. If the patient was initially managed with an antibacterial agent(s), the clinician should change the antibacterial agent(s).[12] SOR Ⓑ

- Potentially serious complications, such as mastoiditis or facial nerve involvement, require urgent referral.

- There is no consensus in the medical community regarding the timing of posttreatment follow-up of AOM or who should be receiving follow-up. There is some evidence that parents can be reliable predictors in the resolution or persistence of AOM following antibiotic treatment.[22]

For patients with OME, effusion will recur in 30% to 40%:

- Children with persistent OME who are not felt to be at significant risk should be reexamined at 3- to 6-month intervals until the effusion is gone, significant hearing loss is identified, or structural abnormalities of the eardrum or middle ear are suspected.[7] SOR Ⓑ

- Refer to specialist (otolaryngologist, audiologist, or speech-language pathologist)[7] SOR Ⓒ if
  ○ Persistent fluid ≥4 months with persistent hearing loss.
  ○ Associated speech delay.
  ○ Structural damage to TM or middle ear.

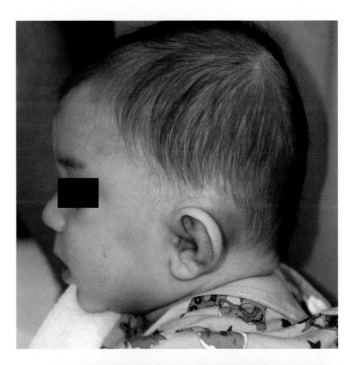

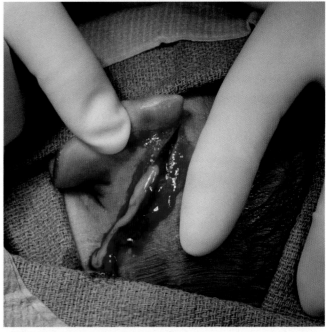

FIGURE 25-10 Mastoiditis in a young boy with recurrent otitis media. Note the erythema and swelling behind the ear. The ear is sticking out more than the other side. Surgical drainage was performed. (*Courtesy of William Clark, MD.*)

PROVIDER RESOURCES

AOM

- American Academy of Family Physicians, American Academy of Otolaryngology-Head and Neck Surgery, and American Academy of Pediatrics Subcommittee on Management of Acute Otitis Media. Diagnosis and management of acute otitis media. *Pediatrics.* 2004;113:1451–1465.

- http://www.npc.co.uk/MeReC_Bulletins/pdfs/Acute_otitis_media_Final.pdf.

- http://www.healthservices.gov.bc.ca/msp/protoguides/gps/otitaom.pdf.

- http://www.prodigy.nhs.uk/otitis_media_acute/view_whole_guidance.

- http://www.gpnotebook.co.uk/simplepage.cfm?ID=1926234161.

OME

- American Academy of Family Physicians, American Academy of Otolaryngology-Head and Neck Surgery, and American Academy of Pediatrics Subcommittee on Otitis Media with Effusion. Otitis media with effusion. *Pediatrics.* 2004;113:1412–1429.

REFERENCES

1. Bondy J, Berman S, Glazner J, Lezotte D. Direct expenditures related to otitis media diagnoses: extrapolations from a pediatric medicaid cohort. *Pediatrics.* 2000;105:72.

2. Teele DW, Klein JO, Rosner BA, et al. Epidemiology of otitis media during the first seven years of life in children in greater Boston: a prospective, cohort study. *J Infect Dis.* 1989;160:83.

3. Paradise JL, Rockette HE, Colborn DK, et al. Otitis media in 2253 Pittsburgh-area infants: prevalence and risk factors during the first two years of life. *Pediatrics.* 1997;99:318.

4. Del Mar C, Glasziou P, Hayem M. Are antibiotics indicated as initial treatment for children with acute otitis media? A meta-analysis. *BMJ.* 1997;314:1526–1529.

5. Nyquist AC, Gonzales R, Steiner JF, Sande MA. Antibiotic prescribing for children with colds, upper respiratory tract infections, and bronchitis. *JAMA.* 1998;279:875.

6. Froom J, Culpepper L, Jacobs M, et al. Antimicrobials for acute otitis media? A review from the International Primary Care Network. *BMJ.* 1997;315:98–102.

7. American Academy of Family Physicians, American Academy of Otolaryngology-Head and Neck Surgery, and American Academy of Pediatrics Subcommittee on Otitis Media with Effusion. Otitis media with effusion. *Pediatrics.* 2004;113:1412–1429.

8. Williamson I. Otitis media with effusion. *Clin Evid.* 2006;15:814–821.

9. Rovers MM, Schilder AG, Zielhuis GA, Rosenfeld RM. Otitis media. *Lancet.* 2004;363:465.

10. Berman S. Otitis media in developing countries. *Pediatrics.* 1995;96:126–131.

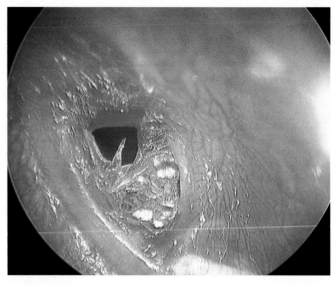

FIGURE 25-11 Traumatic perforation of the left TM. (*Courtesy of William Clark, MD.*)

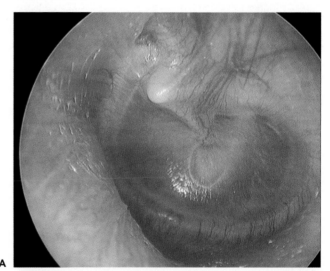

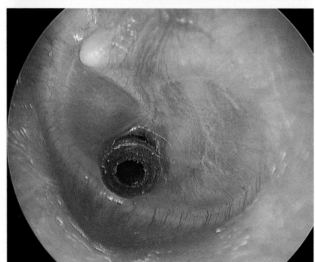

FIGURE 25-12 (**A**) Left TM of a 9-year-old girl with recurrent AOM and chronic TM retractions prior to PE tube placement. The circular area near the center of the TM is owing to the TM being retracted against the promontory of the medial wall of the middle ear. (**B**) A fluoroplastic PE tube is placed in the anteroinferior quadrant of the TM of a 9-year-old girl with recurrent AOM. It is black because it is impregnated with silver oxide to retard the growth of bacterial microfilms. (*Courtesy of William Clark, MD.*)

11. Ruuskanen O, Arola M, Heikkinen T, Ziegler T. Viruses in acute otitis media: increasing evidence for clinical significance. *Pediatr Infect Dis J*. 1991;10:425–429.

12. American Academy of Family Physicians, American Academy of Otolaryngology-Head and Neck Surgery, and American Academy of Pediatrics Subcommittee on Management of Acute Otitis Media. Diagnosis and management of acute otitis media. *Pediatrics*. 2004; 113;1451–1465.

13. Takata GS, Chan LS, Morphew T, et al. Evidence assessment of the accuracy of methods of diagnosing middle ear effusion in children with otitis media with effusion. *Pediatrics*. 2003;112: 1379–1387.

14. Rosenfeld RM. Natural history of untreated otitis media. *Laryngoscope*. 2003;113:1645–1657.

15. O'Neill P, Roberts T, Bradley Stevenson C. Otitis media in children (acute). *Clin Evid*. 2006;15:500–510.

16. Foxlee R, Johansson A, Wejfalk J, Dawkins J, Dooley L, Del Mar C. Topical analgesia for acute otitis media. *Cochrane Database Systc Rev*. 2006;3:CD005657. [Review]

17. Rovers MM, Glasziou P, Appelman CL, et al. Antibiotics for acute otitis media: a meta-analysis with individual patient data. *Lancet*. 2006;368:1429–1435.

18. Spiro DM, Tay KY, Arnold DH, Dziura JD, Baker MD, Shapiro ED. Wait-and-see prescription for the treatment of acute otitis media: a randomized controlled trial. *JAMA*. 2006;296:1235–1241.

19. Flynn CA, Griffin GH, Schultz JK. Decongestants and antihistamines for acute otitis media in children. *Cochrane Database Syst Rev*. 2004;3:CD001727. [Review]

20. Paradise JL, Dollaghan CA, Campbell TF, et al. Otitis media and tympanostomy tube insertion during the first three years of life: developmental outcomes at the age of four years. *Pediatrics*. 2003; 112:265–277

21. Paradise JL, Feldman HM, Campbell TF, et al. Tympanostomy tubes and developmental outcomes at 9 to 11 years of age. *N Engl J Med*. 2007;356:300–302.

22. Raimer PL. Parents can be reliable predictors in the resolution or persistence of acute otitis media following antibiotic treatment. Evidence-Based Pediatrics Web site, Department of Pediatrics, University of Michigan. Available at http://www.med.umich.edu/pediatrics/ebm/cats/omparent.htm. Accessed 2005.

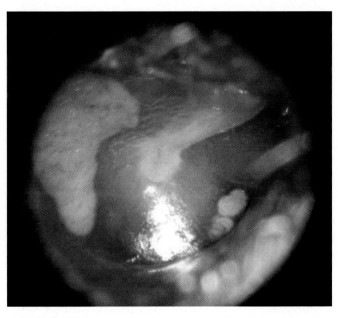

FIGURE 25-13 Tympanosclerosis as the result of previous recurrent episodes of otitis media and PE tube placement. (*Courtesy of Glen Medellin, MD.*)

26 OTITIS EXTERNA

Brian Z. Rayala, MD

PATIENT STORY

A 40-year-old woman with type 2 diabetes presents to her family physician with a 2-day history of bilateral otalgia, otorrhea, and hearing loss. Symptoms started in the right ear and then rapidly spread to the left ear. She had a low-grade fever and was systemically ill. The external ear was swollen with honey-crusts. (**Figures 26-1** and **26-2**). The external auditory canal (EAC) was narrowed and contained purulent discharge. ENT was consulted and she was admitted to the hospital for the presumptive diagnosis of malignant otitis externa (OE). The magnetic resonance imaging (MRI) showed some destruction of the temporal bone. She was started on intravenous (IV) ciprofloxacin and the ear culture grew out *Pseudomonas aeruginosa* sensitive to ciprofloxacin. The patient responded well to treatment and was able to go home on oral ciprofloxacin 5 days later.

EPIDEMIOLOGY

- Common in all parts of the world.
- Incidence of otitis externa is not known precisely; its lifetime incidence has been estimated at 10% in one study.[1]
- Occurs more in adults than in children.

ETIOLOGY AND PATHOPHYSIOLOGY

- Otitis externa is defined as inflammation, often with infection, of the EAC.[2]
- Common pathogens, which are part of normal EAC flora, include aerobic organisms predominantly (*P. aeruginosa* and *S. aureus*) and, to a lesser extent, anaerobes (*bacteroides* and *Peptostreptococcus*). Up to a third of infections is polymicrobial. A small proportion (2%–10%) of otitis externa is caused by fungal overgrowth (e.g., *Aspergillus niger* usually occurs with prolonged antibiotic use[2]; candida is common in hearing aid users[3]).
- Pathogenesis of otitis externa include the following[3]:
  ○ Initial breakdown of the skin–cerumen barrier (cotton swabs and other trauma can start this).
  ○ Skin inflammation and edema that leads to pruritus and obstruction of adnexal structures (e.g., cerumen glands, sebaceous glands, and hair follicles).
  ○ Pruritus leads to scratching, which in turn leads to further skin injury.
  ○ The above sequence of events leads to alteration in the milieu of the EAC (quality and quantity of cerumen produced, pH of the canal, and epithelial migration).
  ○ Finally, the EAC becomes a dark, warm, alkaline, and moist environment—ideal for growth of different pathogens.

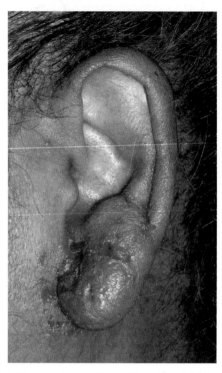

FIGURE 26-1 Malignant/Necrotizing otitis externa in a 40-year-old woman with diabetes. Note the swelling and honey-crusts of the pinna. The EAC and temporal bone were involved. (*Courtesy of E.J. Mayeaux, Jr., MD.*)

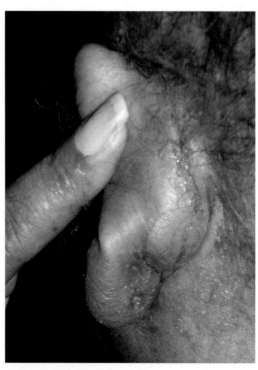

FIGURE 26-2 Another view of the malignant/necrotizing otitis externa. (*Courtesy of E.J. Mayeaux, Jr., MD.*)

- Etiology/risk factors[2]:
  - Local or generalized eczema of the EAC has been associated with otitis externa.
  - Swimming (otitis externa in swimmers is called swimmers' ear).
  - Humid environments.
  - People with an absence of ear wax or narrow external ear canals.
  - Devices that occlude the ear canal (hearing aids, headphones, diving caps).
  - Mechanical trauma.

DIAGNOSIS

CLINICAL FEATURES

- Otitis externa can either be localized, like a furuncle, or generalized. The latter is known as "diffuse otitis externa," or simply otitis externa. Seborrheic dermatitis of the external ear and ear canal can be diffuse or generalized (**Figure 26-3**).
- Forms of (diffuse) otitis externa[2]:
  - Acute—less than 6 weeks (**Figures 26-4** and **26-5**).
  - Chronic—greater than or equal to 3 months; may cause hearing loss and stenosis of the EAC (**Figure 26-6**).
  - Necrotizing or malignant form—defined by destruction of the temporal bone, usually in diabetics or immunocompromised people; often life-threatening (**Figure 26-1** and **26-2**).
- Key historical features include:
  - Otalgia, including pruritus.
  - Otorrhea (**Figures 26-4 to 26-7**).
  - Mild hearing loss.
- Key physical findings include[3]:
  - Pain with tragal pressure or pain when the auricle is pulled superiorly—this may be absent in very mild cases.
  - Signs of EAC inflammation (edema, erythema, aural discharge) (**Figures 26-4 to 26-6**).
  - Fever, periauricular erythema and lymphadenopathy point to severe disease.
  - Complete obstruction of EAC occurs in advanced otitis externa.
- Establishing the integrity of the tympanic membrane (TM) (through direct visualization) and the absence of middle ear effusion (through pneumatic otoscopy) is crucial in differentiating otitis externa from other diagnoses (e.g., suppurative otitis media, cholesteatoma).

LABORATORY STUDIES AND IMAGING

- Since otitis externa is mostly a clinical diagnosis, diagnostic testing has a limited role. When patient fails to respond to empiric treatment, obtaining a culture of aural discharge may help guide proper choice of treatment (antibacterial vs antifungal agents).
- If necrotizing or malignant otitis externa is suspected, computed tomography (CT) or MRI of the ear/skull base is warranted.

DIFFERENTIAL DIAGNOSIS

- Chronic suppurative otitis media—otoscopy shows TM perforation, history reveals a chronically draining ear and recurrent middle ear infections with or without hearing loss (**Figure 26-7**).

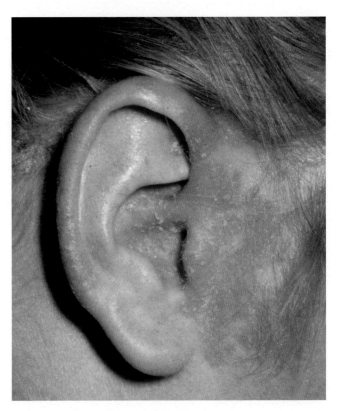

FIGURE 26-3 Seborrheic dermatitis causing erythema and greasy scale of the external ear and ear canal. The seborrheic dermatitis itself causes breaks in the skin and the coexisting pruritus may lead the patient to damage their own ear canal. All this can become secondarily infected. (*Courtesy of Eric Kraus, MD.*)

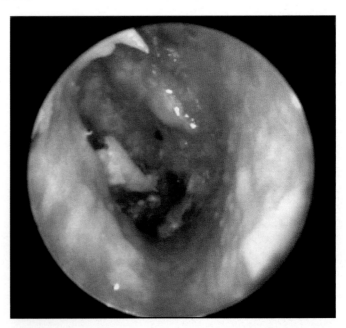

FIGURE 26-4 Acute otitis externa showing purulent discharge and narrowing of the ear canal. (*Courtesy of Roy F. Sullivan, Ph.D: Audiology Forum: Video Otoscopy www.rcsullivan.com*)

- Seborrheic dermatitis involving the external ear and ear canal can lead to inflammation and breaks in the skin (**Figure 26-3**). The co-existing pruritus may lead the patient to damage their own ear canal. All this can become secondarily infected and become an infected otitis externa.

- Acute otitis media with perforated TM—presents with purulent drainage from the canal in the setting of ear pain and clinical signs or symptoms of acute illness such as fever. If the TM is visible, it will be red with a perforation.

- Foreign body in the EAC—otoscopy, with or without aural toilet, confirms presence of foreign body (that incites an inflammatory response, leading to otalgia and otorrhea). (See Chapter 27, Ear: Foreign Body).

- Otomycosis—pruritus is generally more prominent and EAC inflammation (otalgia and otorrhea) is less pronounced; fungal organisms have a characteristic appearance in the EAC.

- Contact Dermatitis—usually because of ototopical agents (e.g., neomycin, benzocaine, propylene glycol); seen in patients with poor response to empiric otitis externa treatment; prominent clinical features include pruritus, erythema of conchal bowl, crusting, and excoriations.

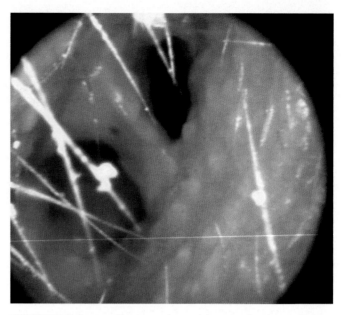

FIGURE 26-5 Acute otitis externa in an older man who wears a hearing aide. Note the viscous purulent discharge and narrowing of the ear canal. (*Courtesy of Roy F. Sullivan, Ph.D: Audiology Forum: Video Otoscopy www.rcsullivan.com*)

MANAGEMENT

- Acute otitis externa often resolve within 6 weeks and can recur.

- The management of acute otitis externa should include an assessment of pain. The clinician should recommend analgesic treatment based on the severity of pain.[4] SOR **B**

- Topical aluminum acetate drops are as effective as topical antibiotics.[2] SOR **B**

- Topical anti-infective agents may improve symptoms and signs of otitis externa.[2] SOR **B**
  - Methylprednisolone–neomycin drops are probably more effective than placebo in reducing signs and symptoms of otitis externa in approximately 28 days.
  - We do not know whether any one regimen should be used in preference to other possible treatments.
  - There is no evidence on the use of antifungal agents in otitis externa.

- Topical corticosteroids may reduce signs and symptoms of otitis externa, but this evidence is also limited.[2] SOR **B**
  - Topical budesonide is probably more effective than placebo in reducing signs and symptoms of otitis externa.
  - Low potency corticosteroids maybe as effective as higher potency corticosteroids after 1 week.
  - There is no evidence to compare topical corticosteroids with topical anti-infective agents.

- Oral antibiotics have not been shown to be beneficial.[2] SOR **C**

- Topical acetic acid may increase cure when used with topical anti-infective agents and corticosteroids, but is less effective than this combination when used alone.[2] SOR **C**

- Prophylactic treatments to prevent otitis externa (topical acetic acid, topical corticosteroids or water exclusion), and specialist aural toilet, have not been evaluated in clinical trials.[2]

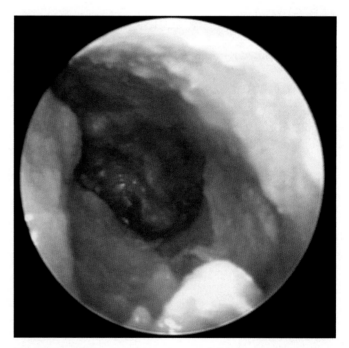

FIGURE 26-6 Chronic otitis externa in an older woman who wears a hearing aide. The ear canal is not narrowed but is coated with a purulent discharge. (*Courtesy of Roy F. Sullivan, Ph.D: Audiology Forum: Video Otoscopy www.rcsullivan.com*)

PATIENT EDUCATION

- To avoid recurrent infections:
  - Recommend that patients not use cotton swabs inserted into the ear canal.
  - Avoid frequent washing of the ears with soap as this leaves an alkali residue neutralizing the normal acidic pH of the ear canal.[5]
  - Avoid swimming in polluted waters.[5]
  - Ensure that the canals are emptied of water after swimming or bathing—this can be done by turning the head or holding a facial tissue on the outside of the ear to act like a wick.
- Consider ear drops for swimmers who get frequent otitis externa: A combination of a 2:1 ratio of 70% isopropyl alcohol and acetic acid may be used after each episode of swimming to assist in drying and acidifying the ear canal.[5]
- Do not use earplugs while swimming because they may cause trauma to the ear canal leading to otitis externa.[5]

FOLLOW-UP

- If the patient fails to respond to empiric therapy within 48 to 72 hours, the clinician should reassess the patient to confirm the diagnosis of otitis externa and to exclude other causes of illness.[4] SOR ○

PATIENT RESOURCES

- **http://familydoctor.org/657.xml.**

PROVIDER RESOURCES

- **http://www.emedicine.com/sports/topic161.htm.**
- **http://www.emedicine.com/emerg/topic350.htm.**

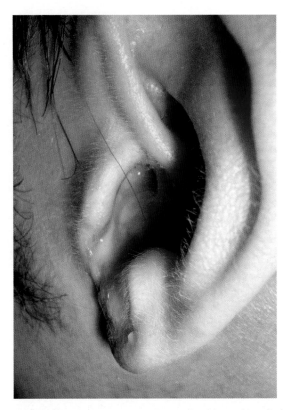

FIGURE 26-7 Chronic suppurative otitis media with purulent discharge chronically draining from the ear of this 25-year-old man. This image could be seen in acute otitis media with perforation of the TM or in a purulent otitis externa. (*Courtesy of Richard P. Usatine, MD.*)

REFERENCES

1. Raza SA, Denholm SW, Wong JC. An audit of the management of otitis externa in an ENT casualty clinic. *J Laryngol Otol.* 1995;109:130–133.

2. Hajioff, D. Otitis externa. *BMJ Clinical Evidence Online.* September 2006. http://clinicalevidence.bmj.com.proxy2.cl.msu.edu:2047/ceweb/conditions/ent/0510/ 0510_keypoints.jsp. Accessed January 28, 2008.

3. Goguen, L. External otitis. UpToDate Online 15.3. August 2007. http://www.utdol.com/utd/content/topic.do?topicKey=pc_id/2947&selectedTitle=2~45&source= search_result. Accessed January 28, 2008.

4. Rosenfeld RM, Brown L, Cannon CR, et al. American academy of Otolaryngology–Head and Neck Surgery Foundation. Clinical Practice guideline: Acute otitis externa. *Otolaryngol Head Neck Surg.* 2006;134(4 Suppl):S4–S23.

5. Garry, J. Otitis externa. Updated Dec 16, 2005. http://www.emedicine.com/sports/topic161.htm. Accessed September 30, 2007.

27 EAR: FOREIGN BODY

Brian Z. Rayala, MD

PATIENT STORY

A 3-year-old girl is brought by her parents to an urgent care facility after a day of crying, irritability, scant otorrhea, and frequent pulling of her right ear. Otoscopy reveals an erythematous, swollen external auditory canal (EAC) where a bead is wedged (**Figure 27-1**).

EPIDEMIOLOGY

- Ear foreign bodies (FBs) are commonly seen in children aged 1 to 6 years.[1-3]
- Equal male-to-female ratio.[4]
- Several retrospective studies from urban emergency departments showed that emergency physicians successfully removed most FBs (53%–80%) with minimal complications, and there was no need for operative removal.[5-9]

ETIOLOGY AND PATHOPHYSIOLOGY

- Most common FBs in children include[10]:
  - Inanimate objects such as beads, cotton tips, paper, toy parts, eraser tips, or natural products food, or organic matter including sand (**Figure 27-3**), sticks, or stones.
  - Insects (**Figure 27-4**).
- Pathogenesis include some of the key elements of otitis externa:
  - Initial breakdown of the skin–cerumen barrier (caused by presence of FB).
  - Skin inflammation and edema leading to subsequent obstruction of adnexal structures (e.g., cerumen glands, sebaceous glands, and hair follicles).
  - Foreign-body reaction leading to further skin injury.
  - In the case of alkaline battery electrochemical reaction, severe alkaline burns may occur.

DIAGNOSIS

CLINICAL FEATURES

- Key historical features include:
  - Otalgia.
  - Otorrhea or otorrhagia.
  - Mild hearing loss.
  - Irritability, crying.
  - History suspicious for FB insertion or witnessed FB insertion.
- Some children may be asymptomatic.
- Hallmark of diagnosis includes visualization of FB on otoscopy (**Figures 27-1** to **27-4**).

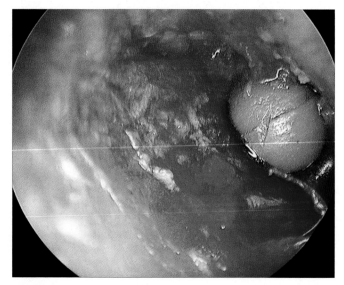

FIGURE 27-1 Foreign body (bead) in the ear canal of a 3 year-old girl with reactive tissue around it. (*Courtesy of William Clark, MD.*)

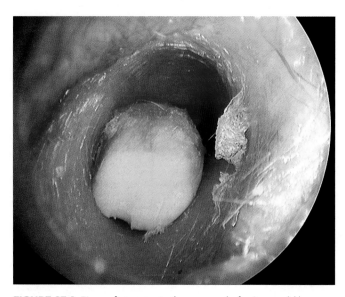

FIGURE 27-2 Piece of a crayon in the ear canal of a 4 year-old boy. (*Courtesy of William Clark, MD.*)

- Otoscopy may reveal signs of EAC inflammation (e.g., edema, erythema, aural discharge) (**Figure 27-3**).

LABORATORY STUDIES AND IMAGING

- Aural FB is a clinical diagnosis. Laboratory and imaging studies have very limited use.

DIFFERENTIAL DIAGNOSIS

- Otitis externa—presents with otalgia, otorrhea, and mild hearing loss, all of which can be present in aural FB. Absence of FB (on otoscopic exam) is the key differentiating factor (see Chapter 26, Otitis Externa).

- Acute otitis media (with or without perforated tympanic membrane [TM])—otoscopy shows absence of FB and presence of middle ear inflammation and effusion (i.e., bulging, erythematous, cloudy, and immobile TM). Patients present with clinical signs or symptoms of acute illness like fever (see Chapter 25, Acute Otitis Media and Otitis Media with Effusion).

- Chronic Suppurative Otitis Media—otoscopy shows absence of FB and presence of TM perforation; history reveals a chronically draining ear and recurrent middle ear infections with or without hearing loss (see Chapter 25, Acute Otitis Media and Otitis Media with Effusion).

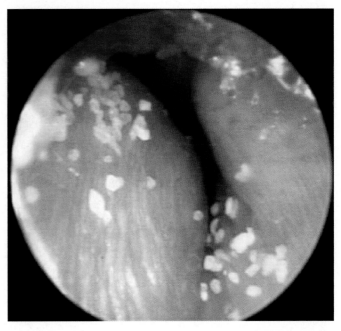

FIGURE 27-3 Beach sand granules with exostosis in the ear of a cold water surfer. The exostoses are common in cold water swimmers and surfers. (*Courtesy of Roy F. Sullivan, PhD: Audiology Forum: Video Otoscopy. www.rcsullivan.com*)

MANAGEMENT

- Adequate immobilization of the child (sedation if necessary) and proper instrumentation allow the uncomplicated removal of many EAC FBs in the pediatric population.[6] SOR **C**
  - The use of general anesthesia is preferred in very young children and in children of any age with aural FBs whose contour, composition, or location predispose to traumatic removal in the ambulatory setting.[6] SOR **C**

- Aural FBs can be removed by irrigation, suction, or instrumentation. The type of procedure depends on the type of FB being removed.[11]
  - Small inorganic objects can be removed from the EAC by irrigation. Contraindication to irrigation includes:
    - Perforated TM.
    - Vegetable matter—irrigation causes swelling of the vegetable matter which leads to further obstruction.
    - Alkaline (button) battery—irrigation enhances leakage and potential for liquefaction necrosis and severe alkaline burns.
  - Objects with protruding surfaces or irregular edges may be removed with alligator forceps underneath direct visualization.
  - Objects that are round or breakable can be removed using a wire loop, a curette, or a right-angle hook that is slowly advanced beyond the object and carefully withdrawn.
  - Cyanoacrylate adhesive (e.g., "superglue") has been used to remove tightly wedged, smooth, round FBs.
  - Live insects should be killed before removing them (by irrigation or forceps). Instilling alcohol or mineral oil into the auditory canal can kill them.

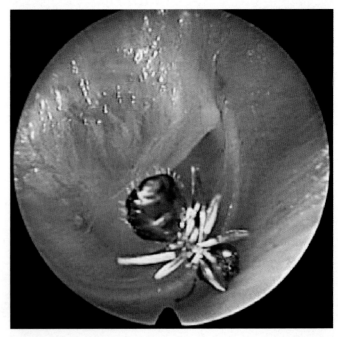

FIGURE 27-4 Ant in the ear canal. (*Courtesy of Vladimir Zlinsky, MD in Roy F. Sullivan, PhD: Audiology Forum: Video Otoscopy. www.rcsullivan.com*)

- Referral to otolaryngology should be considered if:
  - More than 1 attempt has been carried out without success.[5]
  - More than 1 instrument is needed for removal.[5]
  - Patients who have firm, rounded FBs (**Figures 27-1** and **27-2**).[8]
  - Patients who have FBs with smooth (nongraspable) surfaces (**Figure 27-1**).[9]

PATIENT EDUCATION

- Efforts should focus on preventing small children from having access to tiny objects (e.g., beads, small toys, etc.).
- Parents should be informed that successful removal depends a great deal on the length of time the FB has remained in the EAC.

FOLLOW-UP

- Follow-up is very important especially in cases where EAC inflammation or infection is likely (e.g., numerous attempts, use of numerous instruments, protracted exposure to the FB).

PATIENT RESOURCES

- http://www.emedicinehealth.com/foreign_body_ear/article_em.htm.
- http://www.aboutkidshealth.ca/ofhc/Article.asp?articleID=2040.

PROVIDER RESOURCES

- http://www.entusa.com/external_ear_canal.htm.
- http://www.nhshealthquality.org/nhsqis/files/Best%20Practice%20Statement%20-%20Ear%20Care.pdf.

REFERENCES

1. Balbani AP, Sanchez TG, Butugan O, et al. Ear and nose foreign body removal in children. *Int J Pediatr Otorhinolaryngol.* 1998; 46:37.

2. Mishra A, Shukla GK, Bhatia N. Aural foreign bodies. *Indian J Pediatr.* 2000;67:267.

3. Ansley JF, Cunningham MJ. Treatment of aural foreign bodies in children. *Pediatrics.* 1998;101:638.

4. Baker, MD. Foreign bodies of the ears and nose in childhood. *Pediatr Emerg Care.* 1987;3:67.

5. Marin JR, Trainor JL. Foreign body removal from the external auditory canal in a pediatric emergency department. *Pediatr Emerg Care.* 2006;22:630–634.

6. Ansley JF, Cunningham MJ. Treatment of aural foreign bodies in children. *Pediatrics.* 1999;103:857–858.

7. Ngo A, Ng KC, Sim TP. Otorhinolaryngeal foreign bodies in children presenting to the emergency department. *Singapore Med J.* 2005;46:172–178.

8. Thompson SK, Wein RO, Dutcher PO. External auditory canal foreign body removal: Management practices and outcomes. *Laryngoscope.* 2003;113:1912–1915.

9. DiMuzio J, Jr., Deschler DG. Emergency department management of foreign bodies of the external ear canal in children. *Otol Neurotol.* 2002;23:473–475.

10. Ryan C, Ghosh A, Wilson-Boyd B, et al. Presentation and management of aural foreign bodies in two Australian emergency departments. *Emerg Med Australas.* 2006;18:372–378.

11. Ojo A. Foreign bodies: Ears and nose. UpToDate Online 15.3. August 2007. http://www.utdol.com/utd/content/topic.do?topicKey=ped_proc/5375&selectedTitle=1~3&source=search_result. Accessed January 28, 2008.

28 CHONDRODERMATITIS NODULARIS HELICIS AND PREAURICULAR TAGS

Linda French, MD

PATIENT STORY

A 44-year-old white man presents with a painful nodule on his right ear for 1 year (**Figure 28-1**). The patient has a long history of occupational sun exposure but no skin cancers. He states that it is too painful to sleep on his right side because of the painful nodule on his ear. He tried to remove it once with nail clippers but it bled too much. The patient is told that this is likely to be a benign condition called chondrodermatitis nodularis helicis. A shave biopsy is performed that confirms the diagnosis. The patient is counseled to use sun protection. Cryotherapy is performed but in 2 months the painful nodule has regrown. Curettage and electrodesiccation is then chosen resulting in a full cure.

EPIDEMIOLOGY

Chondrodermatitis nodularis helicis (also known as chondrodermatitis nodularis chronica helicis).

- The incidence of chondrodermatitis nodularis has not been determined.
- Occurs most commonly in males more than 40 years of age.
- Older women can also be affected.

Preauricular tags are malformations of the external ear.

- Occurs in approximately 1 out of 12,500 births without predilection for gender or race.
- Ear malformations may occur in isolation or as part of a constellation of abnormalities, often involving the renal system.
- Several chromosomal abnormalities include preauricular tags as one of the phenotypic expressions.
- The Goldenhar syndrome is a rare syndrome that includes preauricular skin tags, bilateral limbal dermoids of the eye, and eyelid colobomas.

ETIOLOGY AND PATHOPHYSIOLOGY

Chondrodermatitis nodularis helicis:

- Benign neoplasm of the cartilage of the ear commonly believed to be related to excessive pressure, for example, during sleep and sun exposure. The result is a localized overgrowth of cartilage, and subsequent skin changes.

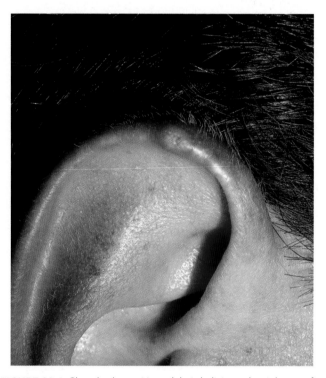

FIGURE 28-1 Chondrodermatitis nodularis helicis on the right ear of a 44-year-old man. (*Courtesy of Richard P. Usatine, MD.*)

- In rare cases, especially when occurring at younger ages, the lesion may be related to an underlying disease associated with microvascular injury such as vasculitis or other necrobiotic collagen disease.[1]

Preauricular tags arise from remnants of supernumerary brachial hillocks (**Figures 28-2** to **28-4**).[2]

- Early stage embryology involves the formation of several slit-like structures on the side of the head, the branchial clefts.

- The three hillocks between the first four clefts eventually form the structure of the outer ear. Preauricular tags are generally minor malformations arising from remnants of supernumerary branchial hillocks.[3,4]

DIAGNOSIS

CLINICAL FEATURES OF CHONDRODERMATITIS

- Firm, painful nodule 3 to 20 mm in size (**Figure 28-1**).

- The helix is most often affected; the antihelix is affected more often in women than men.

- Overlying skin normal in color or erythematous, a central ulcer may be present.

CLINICAL FEATURES OF PREAURICULAR TAGS

- Fleshy knob in front of the ear (**Figures 28-2** to **28-4**).

- Present from the time of birth.

- Generally asymptomatic.

TYPICAL DISTRIBUTION

- Chondrodermatitis is located at the helix or antihelix of the ear. The right ear is more often affected than the left (**Figure 28-1**).

- Preauricular tags may be unilateral or bilateral, more often present on the left.[5] Note that two of three of our patients depicted in this chapter had unilateral left preauricular tags (**Figures 28-2** and **28-3**).

Biopsy—often required for chondrodermatitis nodularis to rule out malignancy, especially when occurring in individuals with actinic damage and/or history of other skin cancers. Not indicated for preauricular tag.

DIFFERENTIAL DIAGNOSIS

- Chondrodermatitis nodularis helicis may be confused with skin cancer, especially squamous cell carcinoma. In squamous cell carcinoma, the overlying skin is often ulcerated and the tumor has poorly defined margins. (See Chapter 164, Squamous Cell Carcinoma.)

- The key issue in diagnosis of preauricular tags is whether the ear tags are an isolated anomaly or part of a syndrome involving vital organs, especially the kidneys. There is no consensus whether children with ear tags who otherwise appear to be healthy should be evaluated with renal ultrasound.[3,4]

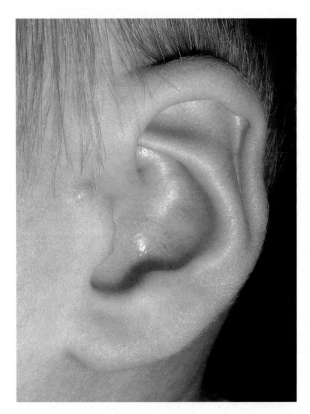

FIGURE 28-2 Small preauricular tag present since birth in a healthy one-year old boy. It is unilateral and on the left. Mother was reassured that surgical removal was not needed. Mother had a preauricular pit.

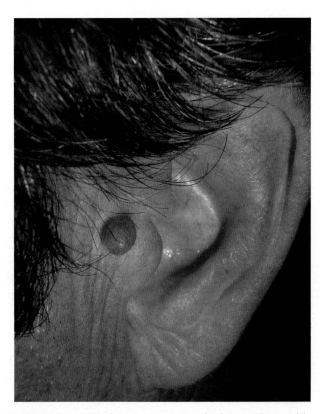

FIGURE 28-3 Preauricular tag present since birth in an 59-year-old man. The patient has never had any renal abnormalities or related medical problems. He wants it removed for cosmetic purposes. (*Courtesy of Richard P. Usatine, MD.*)

MANAGEMENT

Chondrodermatitis nodularis is treated with the following:

- Shave biopsy can be used to make the diagnosis and may relieve symptoms temporarily. SOR Ⓒ

- Cryotherapy, intralesional steroids, or curettage and electrodesiccation can be performed after the result from the shave biopsy is known and there is no malignancy. SOR Ⓒ

- If it grows back then a wedge excision or small elliptical excision with removal of excess cartilage is a more complicated and definitive treatment.[6,7] SOR Ⓒ

- Other options include a pressure-relieving prosthesis.[8] SOR Ⓒ

- A pressure-relieving prosthesis can be created by cutting a hole from the center of a bath sponge. The sponge can then be held in place with a headband if needed. A special prefabricated pillow is available from http://www.cnhpillow.com/

Preauricular tags can be left alone or surgically excised for cosmetic reasons. SOR Ⓒ

PATIENT EDUCATION

- Chondrodermatitis nodularis is a benign lesion that tends to recur; therapeutic options can be discussed.

- There is a low risk of urinary tract abnormalities in children who have preauricular tags.

FOLLOW-UP FOR CHONDRODERMATITIS NODULARIS

- Recurrences are common and may require further treatment.

PATIENT RESOURCES

A special prefabricated pillow is available that helps relieve pressure on the ear—**http://www.cnhpillow.com/** For more information: CNH Pillow, P.O. Box 1247, Abilene, TX 79604, Tel: 800-255-7487.

Preauricular tags—**http://nlm.nih.gov/medlineplus/ency/article/003304.htm**

PROVIDER RESOURCES

Marks VJ, Papa CA. **http://www.emedicine.com/derm/topic76.htm.** Accessed September 29, 2007.

Zuber TJ, Jackson E. Chondrodermatitis nodularis chronica helicis. *Arch Fam Med.* 1999;8:445–447.

Preauricular tags—**http://nlm.nih.gov/medlineplus/ency/article/003304.htm;http://www.emedicine.com/ent/topic200.htm**

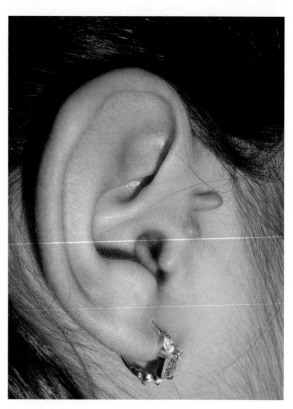

FIGURE 28-4 Two preauricular tags in a 4-year-old girl. Each is a remnant of supernumerary brachial hillock. (*Courtesy of Richard P. Usatine, MD.*)

REFERENCES

1. Magro CM, Frambach GE, Crowson AN. Chondrodermatitis nodularis helices as a marker of internal disease associated with microvascular injury. *J Cutan Pathol*. 2005;32:329–333.

2. Austin M. Prearicular cysts, pits, and fissures. http://www.emedicine.com/ent/topic200.htm. Accessed August 28, 2006.

3. Deshpande SA, Watson H. Renal ultrasound not required in babies with isolated minor ear abnormalities. *Arch Dis Child Fetal Neonatal Ed*. 2006;91:F29–F30.

4. Kohelet D, Arbel E. A prospective search for urinary tract abnormalities in infants with isolated preauricular tags. *Pediatrics*. 2000;105:E61.

5. Paulozzi LJ, Lary JM. Laterality patterns in infants with external birth defects. Teratology 1999;60:265–271.

6. Rex J, Ribera M, Bielsa I, Mangas C, Xifra A, Ferrandiz C. Narrow elliptical skin excision and cartilage shaving for treatment of chondrodermatitis nodularis. *Dermatol Surg*. 2006;32:400-404.

7. Hudson-Peacock MJ, Cox NH, Lawrence CM. The long-term results of cartilage removal alone for the treatment of chondrodermatitis nodularis. *Br J Dermatol*. 1999;141:703–705.

8. Moncrieff M, Sassoon EM. Effective treatment of chondrodermatitis nodularis chronica helices using a conservative approach. *Br J Dermatol*. 2004;150:892–894.

SECTION 2 NOSE AND SINUS

29 NASAL POLYPS

Linda French, MD

PATIENT STORY

A 35-year-old man complains of unilateral nasal obstruction for the past several months of gradual onset. On examination of the nose, a nasal polyp is found (**Figure 29-1**).

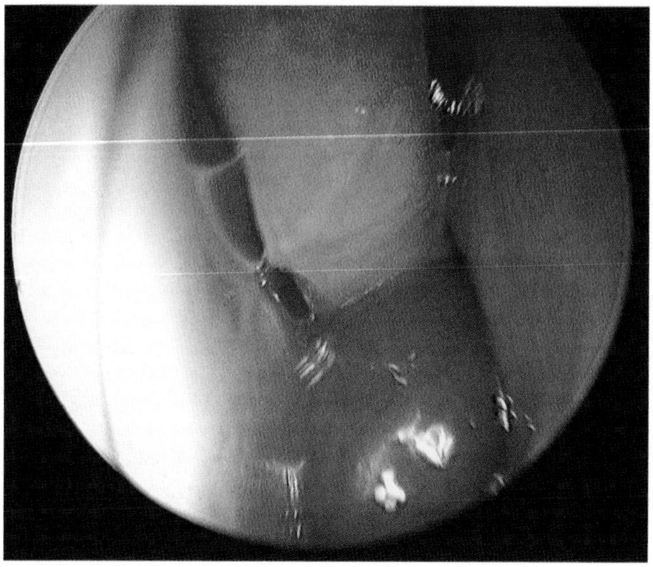

EPIDEMIOLOGY[1]

- Prevalence of 1% to 4% of adults, 0.1% of children of all races and classes.[1]
- The male-to-female ratio in adults is approximately 2:1.[1]
- Peak age of onset is 20 to 40 years old; rare in children less than 10 years old.[1]
- Associated with the following conditions:
  - Non-allergic and allergic rhinitis and rhinosinusitis.
  - Asthma—in 20% to 50% of patients with polyps.
  - Cystic fibrosis.
  - Aspirin intolerance—in 8% to 26% of patients with polyps.
  - Alcohol intolerance—in 50% of patients with polyps.[1]

ETIOLOGY AND PATHOPHYSIOLOGY

- The precise cause of nasal polyp formation is unknown.
- Infectious agents causing desquamation of the mucous membrane may play a triggering role.[2]
- Activated epithelial cells appear to be the major source of mediators that induce an influx of inflammatory cells, including eosinophils prominently; these in turn lead to proliferation and activation of fibroblasts.[3] Cytokines and growth factors play a role in maintaining the mucosal inflammation associated with polyps.
- Food allergies are also strongly associated with nasal polyps.[4]

DIAGNOSIS

CLINICAL FEATURES

- The appearance is usually smooth and rounded (**Figures 29-1** and **29-2**).
- Moist, and semi-translucent (**Figures 29-1** and **29-2**).
- Variable size.
- Color ranging from nearly none to pale blue-grey to deep erythema.

FIGURE 29-1 Nasal polyp in left middle meatus with normal surrounding mucosa. (*Courtesy of William Clark, MD.*)

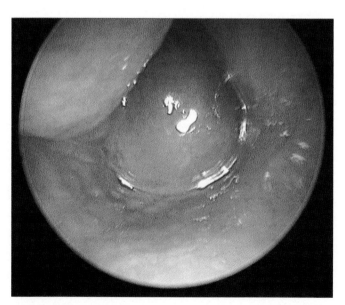

FIGURE 29-2 Nasal polyp in right nasal cavity in a patient with inflamed mucosa from allergic rhinitis. (*Courtesy of William Clark, MD.*)

LABORATORY STUDIES AND IMAGING

• Consider allergy testing.

• In children with multiple polyps, order sweat test to rule out cystic fibrosis.

• CT of the nose and paranasal sinuses may be indicated to evaluate extent of lesion(s) (**Figure 29-3**).

Typical distribution—The middle meatus is the most common location (**Figure 29-1**).

Biopsy—not usually indicated. Histology typically shows pseudostratified ciliary epithelium, edematous stroma, epithelial basement membrane, and pro-inflammatory cells with eosinophils present in 80% to 90% of cases.

DIFFERENTIAL DIAGNOSIS

Many relatively rare conditions can cause an intranasal mass in adults including:

• Papilloma—approximately 1% of nasal tumors, affecting 1/100,000 adults per year. Locally invasive, these tend to recur especially if excision is not complete. Papillomas are of unknown etiology but are associated with chronic sinusitis, air pollution, and viral infections. They are irregular and friable in appearance and bleed easily.[5]

• Meningoencephalocele —Grayish gelatinous appearance.[6]

• Nasopharyngeal carcinoma—firm, often ulcerated.

• Pyogenic granuloma—relatively common benign vascular neoplasm of skin and mucous membranes.[7] Not commonly seen where nasal polyps are found.

• Chordoma—locally invasive neoplasms with gelatinous appearance that arise from notochordal (embryonic) remnants. Occur in all age groups with mean age 48.[8]

• Glioblastoma—Rare manifestation of the most common kind of brain tumor in adults.

Conditions that may mimic nasal polyp in children include:

• Rhabdomyosarcoma—malignant tumor of childhood originating from striated muscle.

• Dermoid tumor—inclusion cysts of ectodermal epithelial elements, usually manifest before 20 years of age. May grow slowly.

• Hemangioma—congenital, abnormal proliferation of blood vessels that may occur in any vascularized tissue. Commonly seen on the skin but rare in the nose.

• Neuroblastoma—unusual presentation of relatively common malignancy of childhood.

• Meningoencephalocele—grayish gelatinous appearance.[6]

• Juvenile nasopharyngeal angiofibroma—Locally invasive neoplasm that appears as a firm grayish mass. Occurs in adolescent males age 14 to 18 years. Presents with frequent nosebleeds and nasal obstruction.[9]

• Pyogenic granuloma—common on the skin but rare up high in the nose where nasal polyps tend to form.[7]

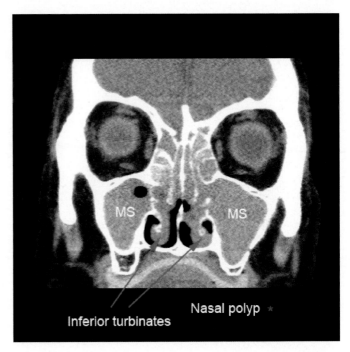

FIGURE 29-3 CT scan showing single nasal polyp (asterisk) and bilateral opacified maxillary sinuses (MS). Note the nasal polyp appears to be coming from the left maxillary sinus and is above the inferior turbinate. (*Courtesy of Richard P. Usatine, MD.*)

MANAGEMENT

- Medical treatment consists of intranasal corticosteroids.[10,11] SOR **B** An initial short course of oral steroids may be considered in severe cases.[12] Steroid treatment reduces polyp size, but does not generally resolve them.[13] Corticosteroid treatment is also useful preoperatively to reduce polyp size.
- Topical nasal decongestants may provide some symptom relief, but do not reduce polyp size.[14] SOR **B**
- Surgical excision is often required to relieve symptoms.
- Consider immunotherapy for patients with allergies.

PATIENT EDUCATION

Patients should be informed regarding the benign nature of nasal polyps and their tendency to recur.

FOLLOW-UP

Periodic re-evaluation is recommended because recurrence rates are high.[15]

PATIENT RESOURCE

http://www.mayoclinic.com/health/ nasal-polyps/DS00498.

PROVIDER RESOURCE

http://www.emedicine.com/ped/topic1550.htm.

REFERENCES

1. McClay JE. Nasal polyps. http://www.edmedicine.com/ ped/topic1550.htm. Accessed March 20, 2007.

2. Norlander T, Bronnegard M, Stierna P. The relationship of nasal polyps, infection, and inflammation. *Am J Rhinol*. 1999;13: 349–355.

3. Pawliczak R, Lewandowska-Polak A, Kowalski ML. Pathogenesis of nasal polyps: An update. *Curr Allergy Asthma Rep*. 2005;5: 463–471.

4. Pang YT, Eskici O, Wilson JA. Nasal polyposis: Role of subclinical delayed food hypersensitivity. *Otolaryngol Head Neck Surg*. 2000;122:298–301.

5. Sadeghi N. Sinonasal papillomas. http://www.emedicine.com/ ent/topic529.htm. Accessed September 26, 2006.

6. Kumar KK, Ganapathy K, Sumathi V, et al. Adult meningoencephalocele presenting as a nasal polyp. *J Clin Neurosci*. 2005;12:594–596.

7. Hoving EW. Nasal encephaloceles. *Childs Nerv Syst*. 2000;16: 702–706.

8. Palmer CA. Chordoma. Emedicine. http://www.emedicine.com/med/topic2993.htm. Accessed September 26, 2006.

9. Mansfield E. Angiofibroma. http://www.emedicine.com/med/topic2758.htm. Accessed September 26, 2006.

10. Jankowski R, Schrewelius C, Bonfils P, et al. Efficacy and tolerability of budesonide aqueous nasal spray treatment in patients with nasal polyps. *Arch Otoloaryngol Head Neck Surg.* 2001; 127:447–452.

11. Stjarne P, Mosges R, Jorissen M, et al. A randomized controlled trial of mometasone furoate nasal spray for the treatment of nasal polyposis. *Arch Otolaryngol Head Neck Surg.* 2006;132: 179–185.

12. Alobid I, Benitez P, Pujols L, et al. Severe nasal polyposis and its impact on quality of life: The effect of a short course of oral steroids followed by long-term intranasal steroid treatment. *Rhinology.* 2006;44:8–13.

13. Tuncer U, Soylu L, Aydogan B, Karakus F, Akcali C. The effectiveness of steroid treatment in nasal polyposis. *Auris Nasus Larynx.* 2003;30:263–268.

14. Johansson L, Oberg D, Melem I, Bende M. Do topical nasal decongestants affect polyps? *Acta Otolaryngol.* 2006:126:288–290.

15. Vento SI, Ertama LO, Hytonen ML, Wolff CYH, Malmberg CH. Nasal polyposis: Clinical course during 20 years. *Ann Allergy Asthma Immunol.* 2000;85:209–214.

30 SINUSITIS

Mindy A. Smith, MD, MS

PATIENT STORY

A 55-year-old woman complains of sinus pressure for the last 2 weeks along with headache, rhinorrhea, postnasal drip, and cough. This all started with a cold 3 weeks ago. She has chronic allergic rhinitis but now the pressure on the right side of her face has become intense and her right upper molars are painful. The nasal discharge has become discolored and she feels feverish. She is diagnosed clinically with right maxillary sinusitis and amoxicillin is prescribed. Two weeks later when her symptoms have persisted, a CT is ordered and she is found to have air-fluid levels in both maxillary sinuses and loculated fluid on the right side. (**Figures 30-1** and **30-2.**) The antibiotic is changed to amoxicillin/clavulanate and she is referred to ENT for further evaluation.

EPIDEMIOLOGY

- Rhinosinusitis is common in the United States with an estimated prevalence of 16% of the adult population annually.[1] The prevalence is increased in women and in individuals living in the southern United States.

- Only one-third to one-half of primary care patients with symptoms of sinusitis actually has bacterial infection.[2]

- Sinusitis is the 5th leading diagnosis for which antibiotics are prescribed in the United States.[3]

- On average children have six to eight colds per year. Of those, 0.5% to 5% will develop a sinus infection.[4]

- This problem is responsible for millions of office visits to primary care physicians each year.[3]

ETIOLOGY AND PATHOPHYSIOLOGY

- Sinus cavities are lined with mucus-secreting respiratory epithelium. The mucus is transported by ciliary action through the sinus ostia (openings) to the nasal cavity. In normal conditions, the paranasal sinuses are sterile cavities and there is no mucus retention.

- Bacterial sinusitis occurs when ostia become obstructed or ciliary action is impaired, causing mucus accumulation and secondary bacterial overgrowth.

- The causes of sinusitis include[3]:
  - Infection—most commonly viral (e.g., rhinovirus, parainfluenza, and influenza) followed by bacteria infection (e.g., community-acquired acute cases—approximately half from *S. pneumoniae* and Haemophilus influenzae followed by *Moraxella catarrhalis*). In immunocompromised patients, fulminant fungal sinusitis may occur (e.g., rhinocerebral mucormycosis).

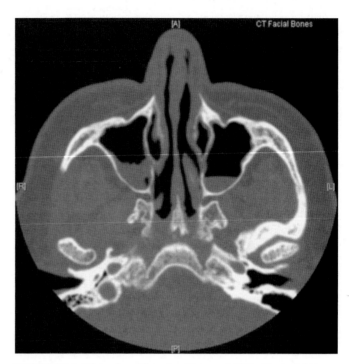

FIGURE 30-1 Bilateral maxillary sinusitis on axial CT with air–fluid levels; note fluid greater on the right. (*Courtesy of Kevin Chris McMains, MD.*)

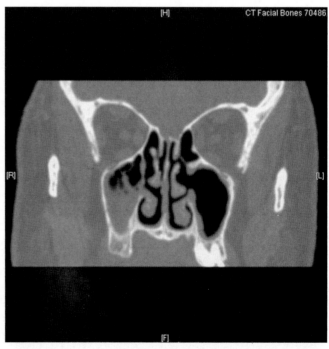

FIGURE 30-2 Maxillary sinusitis on coronal CT of same patient with loculated fluid in the right maxillary sinus. (*Courtesy of Kevin Chris McMains, MD.*)

- ○ Noninfectious obstruction—allergic, polyposis, barotrauma (e.g., deep sea diving, and airplane travel), chemical irritants, tumors (e.g., squamous cell carcinoma, granulomatous disease, and inverting papilloma), and conditions that alter mucus composition (e.g., cystic fibrosis).

- Sinusitis is further classified by duration into acute (less than 4 weeks), subacute (lasting between 4 and 12 weeks), or chronic (i.e., more than 12 weeks).

DIAGNOSIS

The diagnosis is based on the clinical picture with typical symptoms listed below. Symptoms arising from viral infection generally peak by day 5 or before. If symptoms are present for more than 7 days, bacterial infection becomes more likely (40%–50%).

CLINICAL FEATURES

- Most cases are seen in conjunction with viral upper respiratory infections and represent sinus inflammation rather than infection.[3]

- Nonspecific symptoms include cough, sneezing, fever, nasal discharge (may be purulent or discolored), congestion, and headache.

- Localizing symptoms include facial pain or pressure (especially severe if bending over or supine) over the involved sinus (i.e., forehead in frontal sinusitis, cheek with maxillary sinusitis, between the eyes with ethmoid sinusitis, and neck and top of the head with sphenoid sinusitis) and maxillary tooth pain, most commonly the upper molars; the latter is seen more often with bacterial sinusitis. Halitosis is also attributed to bacterial causes.

- "Double sickening" (improvement of symptoms before acute worsening) is often seen in acute rhinosinusitis caused by bacterial superinfection.

- In a study of patients with chronic rhinosinusitis, diagnosis based on symptoms was problematic and only dysosmia (impairment in the sense of smell) and the presence of polyps could distinguish between radiographically normal and abnormal/patients with disease.[5]

- Potentially life-threatening complications include subperiosteal orbital abscess, meningitis, epidural or cerebral abscess, and cavernous sinus thrombosis.

- In immunocompromised patients, fulminant fungal sinusitis may cause orbital swelling, cellulitis, proptosis, ptosis, impairment of extraocular motion, nasopharyngeal ulceration, and epistaxis. Bony erosion may be evident.[3] Nasal mucosa may appear black, blanched white, or erythematous.

- In hospitalized patients, patients may be critically ill and without localizing symptoms. Infections in these patients are often polymicrobial including *S. aureus*, *Pseudomonas aeruginosa*, *Serratia marcescens*, *Klebsiella pneumoniae*, and *Enterobacter*.[3]

TYPICAL DISTRIBUTION

- Most sinus infections involve the maxillary sinus followed in frequency by the ethmoid (anterior), frontal, and sphenoid sinuses; however, most cases involve more than one sinus.[3]

- Children are more likely to have inflammation in the posterior ethmoid and sphenoid sinuses.[6]

LABORATORY STUDIES AND IMAGING

- If culture is needed as a result of suspected bacterial resistance or persistence of infection, a recent meta-analysis found endoscopically-directed middle meatal cultures to be reasonably sensitive (80.9%), specific (90.5%), and accurate (87.0%; 95% confidence interval, 81.3%–92.8%) compared with maxillary sinus taps.[7]

- Radiography is not necessary for routine diagnosis. Plain sinus radiography is considered positive for acute sinusitis with the presence of air fluid level, complete opacification, or at least 6 mm of mucosal thickening; it has a reported sensitivity of 76% and specificity 79%.[8] There are considerable limitations to the sensitivity of plain films especially in diagnosing ethmoid and sphenoid disease.

- Nasal endoscopy, identifying purulent material within the drainage area of the sinuses, may be comparable to plain sinus radiography in diagnosing acute sinusitis.[8]

- In acute disease, computed tomography (CT) scanning is generally reserved for persistent or recurrent symptoms to confirm sinusitis, or to investigate infectious complications (**Figures 30-1** and **30-2**). It is unclear whether a full or limited scan is preferred. A recent study reported a sensitivity and specificity of 95.1% and 92.6%, respectively for a "three-slice" CT for identifying inflammatory sinus disease at one institution.[9]

DIFFERENTIAL DIAGNOSIS

- Upper respiratory tract infections-These are common infections, primarily viral (most commonly rhinovirus), that cause two to four infections per year in adults and six to eight infections per year in children. This frequency is tripled in children in day-care settings. Infections are self-limited (lasting approximately 7–10 days) and typical symptoms include rhinorrhea, nasal congestion, sore throat, and cough. Upper respiratory tract infections often precedes acute sinusitis.

Other causes of facial pain include:

- Migraine headache or cluster headache—moderate to severe head pain that is usually deep seated, persistent, and pulsatile. There is a history of multiple occurrences and head pain may be associated with nausea, vomiting, and photophobia, and scotomata. Attacks last 4 to 72 hours.

- Trigeminal neuralgia—painful condition characterized by excruciating, paroxysmal, shock-like pain lasting seconds to minutes along the distribution of the trigeminal nerve (ophthalmic, maxillary and/or mandibular branches). Pain may be triggered by face washing, air draft, and chewing.

- Dental pain—tooth pain may be secondary to caries or gingivitis. When caries extend into the tooth pulp, the tooth becomes sensitive to percussion and hot and cold food and beverages. If pulp necrosis occurs, pain becomes severe, sharp, throbbing and often worse when supine. Abscess formation results in pain, swelling and erythema of the gum and surrounding tissue, and possibly purulent drainage.

- Temporal arteritis—unilateral pounding headache that may be associated with visual changes and systemic symptoms (e.g., fever, weight loss, muscle aches). Onset is usually older adults (more than the age 50) and laboratory testing reveals an elevated erythrocyte sedimentation rate (i.e., more than 50 mm).

MANAGEMENT

Duration of illness assists in decision-making as most patients improve without specific treatment.

- Methods to improve sinus drainage include oral and topical (nasal) decongestants, nasal saline lavage. SOR **C**

- There have been no clinical trials of mucolytics reported in nonatopic children or adults with acute bacterial sinusitis. However, they may be useful in preventing crust formation and liquefying secretions. SOR **C**

- Patients who fail to improve or have severe symptoms may be offered oral antibiotics. SOR **A**
  - Adults (after 7 days)—Amoxicillin (875 mg twice daily) or trimethoprim-sulfamethoxazole (TMS-SMX) (1 DS twice daily) for 10 days.[3]
  - Children (after 10–14 days of symptoms)—Amoxicillin (40–90 mg/kg divided twice daily), Cefuroxime axetil (30 mg/kg divided twice daily) or Cefdinir (14 mg/kg daily) for 10 to 14 days.[3,4]

- In a Cochrane review of 49 trials evaluating antibiotic treatment for acute maxillary sinusitis, penicillin improved clinical cures compared with controls (relative risk 1.72; 95% CI 1.00–2.96).[10] SOR **A** Numbers needed to treat to benefit one patient ranged between three and six.[11] Treatment with amoxicillin did not significantly improve cure rates (relative risk 2.06; 95% CI 0.65–6.53) but there was significant variability between studies. Comparisons between classes of antibiotics showed no significant differences; therefore narrow-spectrum antibiotics should be first line therapy.[10]

- For those adults who fail initial treatment, consider Amoxicillin (1500 mg) plus clavulanate (125 mg) twice daily for 10 days, Amoxicillin (1500 mg) plus clindamycin (300 mg four times daily) for 10 days, or an antipneumococcal fluoroquinolone (e.g., levofloxacin, 500 mg daily) for 7 days.[3] SOR **C**

- With respect to alternative therapy, there is limited evidence that Sinupret and bromelain may be effective adjunctive treatments in acute rhinosinusitis.[12] SOR **B**

- Surgery and intravenous antibiotics are used for complications including abscess and cases with orbital involvement.[3]

- Patients with fungal sinusitis are treated with aggressive debridement and adjunctive antifungals (e.g., amphotericin).[3]

- It is clear that endoscopic sinus surgery does not confer benefit in all cases[13]. Patients should be selected based on the severity of disease (frequency of antibiotics/oral steroid use), comorbidities (asthma, aspirin sensitivity, etc.), and overall clinical picture (presence of polyps or fungal disease).

PATIENT EDUCATION

- Sinus pressure, nasal congestion, and purulent rhinitis are common symptoms accompanying many upper respiratory illnesses. These symptoms usually abate within 1 week.

- Methods to improve sinus drainage in the acute setting include oral and nasal decongestants and nasal saline lavage. Patients should be cautioned against using nasal decongestants for more than 3 days to avoid rebound symptoms. For longer-term management, topical nasal steroids and oral/topical antihistamines may prove useful.

- Patients should be encouraged to see their primary care provider if symptoms persist or worsen after 1 week, suggesting bacterial infection that may benefit from antibiotic treatment.

FOLLOW-UP

Based on a Cochrane review, relapse rates within 1 month of successful therapy were 7.7%.[10] Patients should be monitored for relapse and an alternate course of antibiotics prescribed (as above).

PATIENT RESOURCES

- **http://www.niaid.nih.gov/factsheets/sinusitis.htm.**
- **http://familydoctor.org/686.xml.**

PROVIDER RESOURCES

Clinical practice guideline: Management of sinusitis. *Pediatrics* 2001;108(3):798–808.

Snow V, Mottur-Pilson C, Hickner JM. Principles of appropriate antibiotic use for acute sinusitis in adults. *Ann Intern Med.* 2001; 134(6):495–497.

REFERENCES

1. Anand VK. Epidemiology and economic impact of rhinosinusitis. *Ann Otol Rhinol Laryngol Suppl.* 2004;193:3–5.

2. Holleman DR Jr, Williams JW Jr, Simel DL. Usual care and outcomes in patients with sinus complaints and normal results of sinus roentgenography. *Arch Fam Med.* 1995;4:246–251.

3. Rubin MA, Gonzales R, Sande MA. Infections of the upper respiratory tract. In: Kasper DL, Braunwald E, Fauci AS, Hauser SL, Longo DL, Jameson, JL eds. *Harrison's Principles of Internal Medicine*, 16th ed. New York, NY: McGraw-Hill Companies Inc., 2005: 185–188.

4. Ramadan HH. Pediatric sinusitis: Update. *J Otolaryngol.* 2005; 34(Suppl 1):S14–S17.

5. Bhattacharyya N. Clinical and symptom criteria for the accurate diagnosis of chronic rhinosinusitis. *Laryngoscope.* 2006;116(7 Pt 2 Suppl 110):1–22.

6. Gordts F, Clement PA, Destryker A, et al. prevalence of sinusitis signs on MRI in a non-ENT pediatric population. *Rhinology.* 1997;35:154–157.

7. Benninger MS, Payne SC, Ferguson BJ, et al. Endoscopically directed middle meatal cultures versus maxillary sinus taps in acute bacterial maxillary rhinosinusitis: A meta-analysis. *Otolaryngol Head Neck Surg.* 2006;134(1):3–9.

8. Berger G, Steinberg DM, Popoytzer A, Ophir D. Endoscopy versus radiography for the diagnosis of acute bacterial rhinosinusitis. *Eur Arch Otorhinolaryngol.* 2005;262(5):416–422.

9. Cagici CA, Cakmak O, Hurcan C, Tercan F. Three-slice computerized tomography for the diagnosis and follow-up of rhinosinusitis. *Eur Arch Otorhinolaryngol.* 2005;262(9):744–750.

10. Williams JW Jr, Aguilar C, Cornell J, et al. Antibiotics for acute maxillary sinusitis. *Cochrane Database Syst Rev.* 2003;(2): CD000243.

11. Arroll B. Antibiotics for upper respiratory tract infections: An overview of Cochrane reviews. *Respir Med.* 2005;99(3):255–261.

12. Guo R, Canter PH, Ernst E. Herbal medicines for the treatment of rhinosinusitis: A systematic review. *Otolaryngol Head Neck Surg.* 2006;135(4):496–506.

13. Khalil HS, Nunez DA. Functional endoscopic sinus surgery for chronic rhinosinusitis. *Cochrane Database Syst Rev.* 2006;3: CD004458.

SECTION 1   MOUTH AND THROAT

31 ANGULAR CHEILITIS

Linda French, MD
Richard P. Usatine, MD

PATIENT STORY

A middle-aged woman complains of soreness at the corners of her mouth for 4 months (**Figure 31-1**). On examination, she has cracking and fissures at the right corner of her mouth. She is diagnosed with angular cheilitis and treated with over-the-counter (OTC) miconazole cream twice daily. Within 2 weeks she was fully healed.

EPIDEMIOLOGY

- Most common in the elderly. In one study of institutionalized elderly patients in Scotland, angular cheilitis was present in 25% of patients.[1]

ETIOLOGY AND PATHOPHYSIOLOGY

- Maceration is the usual predisposing factor, which can be related to poor dentition or poorly fitting dentures in the elderly (**Figure 31-2**). Microorganisms, most often *Candida albicans*, can then invade the macerated area. It may also occur in infants and children related to drooling, thumb sucking, and lip licking.
- HIV or other types of immunodeficiency may lead to more severe case of angular cheilitis with overgrowth of Candida (**Figure 31-3**).
- Historically associated with vitamin B deficiency, which is rare in developed countries.

DIAGNOSIS

CLINICAL FEATURES
- Erythema and fissuring at the corners of the mouth, without exudates or ulceration (**Figures 31-1** and **31-2**).

TYPICAL DISTRIBUTION
Corners of the mouth (oral commissures)
  Biopsy not usually indicated.

DIFFERENTIAL DIAGNOSIS

- Impetigo—Yellowish crusts or exudates are characteristic of impetigo but not angular cheilitis (see Chapter 110, Impetigo).

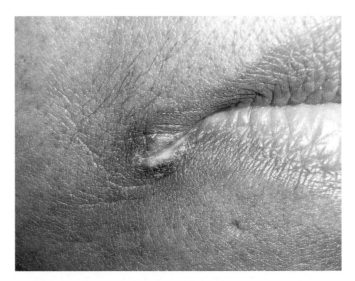

FIGURE 31-1 Angular cheilitis (perlèche). Note dry, erythematous, and fissured appearance. (*Courtesy of Richard P. Usatine, MD.*)

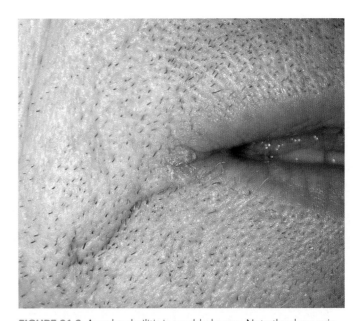

FIGURE 31-2 Angular cheilitis in an elderly man. Note the deep wrinkle line extending downward from the corner of his mouth indicating some change in his facial anatomy that can predispose to this condition. The perlèche started while he was waiting for his dentures to be repaired. (*Courtesy of Richard P. Usatine, MD.*)

- Herpes simplex (cold sores)—Initial blisters, followed by shallow ulcers are characteristic of herpes simplex, but not angular cheilitis (see Chapter 123, Herpes Simplex).

MANAGEMENT

- Attempt to relieve precipitating causes such as poorly fitting dentures.
- Prescribe nystatin ointment to be applied bid.[2] SOR **B**.
- OTC topical antifungal creams such as miconazole or clotrimazole should work equally well.
- Low potency topical corticosteroid such as 1% hydrocortisone cream bid may be added to treat the inflammatory component SOR **B**.
- Nystatin lozenges work well but their use is limited because of their unpleasant taste.[2] SOR **B**. If thrush is also present, prescribe clotrimazole troches for treatment of both conditions.
- One randomized controlled study showed that medicated chewing gum can decrease the risk of angular cheilitis in older occupants of nursing homes. Consider recommending xylitol-containing gum to elderly patients with angular cheilitis.[3] SOR **B**.
- Protective lip balm as needed.

PATIENT EDUCATION

Attempt to identify predisposing factors and correct if possible, such as:

- Edentulousness.
- Poorly fitting dentures.
- Drooling.
- Lip licking.

Protective lip balm may be helpful to prevent recurrences.

FOLLOW-UP

- As needed.

PATIENT AND PROVIDER RESOURCES

www.stevedds.com.

www.ncemi.org/cse/cse0409.htm.

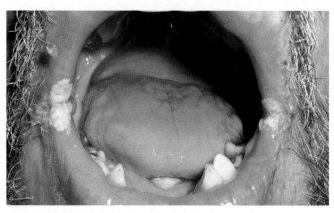

FIGURE 31-3 Severe angular cheilitis in an HIV positive man with thrush. Note the obvious white Candida growth on both corners of his mouth. (*Courtesy of Richard P. Usatine, MD.*)

REFERENCES

1. Samaranayake LP, Wilkieson CA, Lamey PJ, MacFarlane TW. Oral disease in the elderly in long-term hospital care. *Oral Dis.* 1995;1(3):147–151.

2. Skinner N, Junker JA, Flake D, Hoffman R. Clinical inquiries: What is angular cheilitis and how is it treated? *J Fam Pract.* 2005;54(5):470–471.

3. Simons D, Brailsford SR, Kidd EA, Beighton D. The effect of medicated chewing gums on oral health in frail older people: A 1-year clinical trial. *J Am Geriatr Soc.* 2002;50(8):1348–1353.

32 TORUS PALATINUS

Linda French, MD

PATIENT STORY

A 66-year-old woman is in the office for a physical examination. While looking in her mouth, a torus is seen at the midline on the hard palate (**Figure 32-1**). She states that she has had this for her whole adult life and it does not bother her. You explain to her that it is a torus palatinus and that nothing needs to be done. She is pleased to know the name of this lump and even happier to know that it is not harmful.

EPIDEMIOLOGY

- Most common bony maxillofacial exostosis.
- Usually in adults more than 30 years of age.
- More common in women than men.
- Some populations seem to be more predisposed (e.g., Middle-Eastern).[1]

ETIOLOGY AND PATHOPHYSIOLOGY

- Benign bony exostosis (bony growth) occurring in the midline of the hard palate.

DIAGNOSIS

CLINICAL FEATURES

- Hard lump protruding from the hard palate into the mouth covered with normal mucous membrane (**Figure 32-1**).

  Typical distribution—Hard palate in the midline

DIFFERENTIAL DIAGNOSIS

- Mandibular tori (torus mandibularis) are benign bony exostoses that occur from the mandible and under the tongue. These are usually bilateral and less common than torus palatinus (**Figure 32-2**).
- Squamous cell carcinoma on the palate is not as hard and the mucous membranes are usually ulcerated. Mucous membranes are normal in appearance with torus palatinus unless traumatized (see Chapter 42, Oral Cancer).

MANAGEMENT

- Excision can be considered if the lesion interferes with function such as the fit of dentures. This is performed as an outpatient procedure.[2,3]

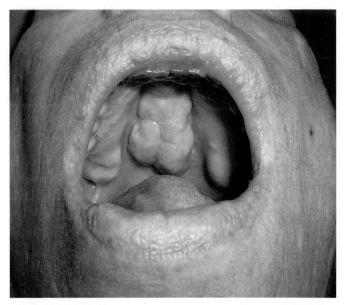

FIGURE 32-1 Torus palatinus in a 66-year-old woman. The patient was asymptomatic and this was an incidental finding. (*Courtesy of Richard P. Usatine, MD.*)

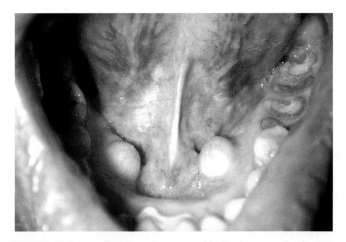

FIGURE 32-2 Mandibular tori (torus mandibularis) seen under the tongue caused by bony exostoses. Note these are bilateral and appear similar to a torus palatinus. While this patient had multiple untreated dental problems, the tori were asymptomatic and this was an incidental finding. (*Courtesy of Richard P. Usatine, MD.*)

PATIENT EDUCATION

- Patients should be informed about the benign nature of the lesion and that removal can be considered, if bothersome.

PATIENT RESOURCES

http://www.atlantadentist.com/torus_palatinus.htm.

PHYSICIAN RESOURCES

http://www.fpnotebook.com/DEN21.htm.

REFERENCES

1. Yildiz E, Deniz M, Ceyhan O. Prevalence of torus palatinus in Turkish school children. *Surg Radiol Anat.* 2005;27:368–371.

2. Al-Quran FA, Al-Dwairi ZN. Torus palatinus and torus mandibularis in edentulous patients. *J Contemp Dent Pract.* 2006;7:112–119.

3. Cagirankaya LB, Dansu O, Hatipoglu MG. Is torus palatinus a feature of a well-developed maxilla? *Clin Anat.* 2004;17:623–625.

33 SCARLET FEVER AND STRAWBERRY TONGUE

M. Jason Sanders, MD
Linda French, MD

PATIENT STORY

A 7-year-old boy is brought to the family physician's office with a rough red rash on his trunk (**Figures 33-1** and **33-2**) along with fever and a sore throat. The sandpaper rash and signs consistent with strep pharyngitis lead the physician to diagnose scarlet fever. The diagnosis is explained to the mother and oral Pen VK is prescribed. The boy feels markedly better by the next day, and the mother continues to give the penicillin for the full 10 days as directed.

EPIDEMIOLOGY

- Scarlet fever is predominately seen in school-aged children with no gender predilection.
  - Majority related to strep pharyngitis with 1 in 10 developing scarlet fever (**Figures 33-1, 33-2** and **33-3**).
  - Prevalent in late fall to early spring.
- Strawberry tongue (**Figure 33-4**) is most commonly seen in children in association with scarlet fever or Kawasaki disease.
  - Can be present with other group A streptococcus (strep) infection.
  - In cases of strep, a white membrane through which the papillae are seen can initially cover the tongue followed by desquamation of the membrane (with the appearance as in **Figure 33-4**).

ETIOLOGY AND PATHOPHYSIOLOGY

- Transmission of *streptococcus* occurs via respiratory secretions.
- Virulent *streptococcus pyogenes* (group A streptococcus or GAS) incubate more than 2 to 7 days. M protein serotypes of GAS are typically more invasive with greater potential for progression to rheumatic fever or acute glomerulonephritis if untreated.[2]
- Fever and rash are related to pyrogenic A–C and erythrogenic exotoxins produced by GAS.[1]
- Infection may originate from other sites like skin (e.g., cellulitis) and seed blood (bacteremia) or organ systems (e.g., pneumonia).
- Strawberry tongue results from a general inflammatory response during the early course of the disease.

DIAGNOSIS

CLINICAL FEATURES

- Headache, sore throat, lymphadenopathy, abdominal pain, nausea and vomiting, malaise, and fever may precede rash.

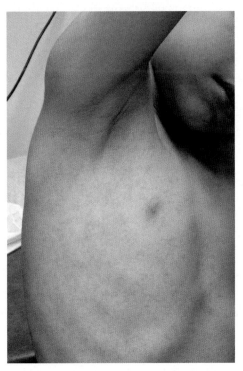

FIGURE 33-1 Sandpaper rash on the trunk and in the axilla of a 7 year-old boy with scarlet fever. (*Courtesy of Richard P. Usatine, MD.*)

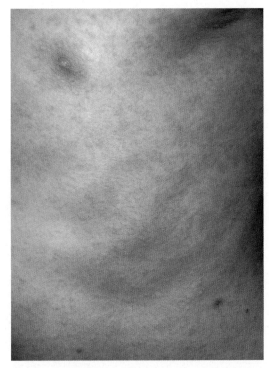

FIGURE 33-2 Scarlatiniform rash comprising small papules and erythema on the trunk of a febrile child with strep pharyngitis. (*Courtesy of Richard P. Usatine, MD.*)

- Oropharyngeal findings include:
  - Strawberry tongue—erythematous and sometimes edematous tongue with prominent papillae (**Figure 33-4**).
- May be covered by a white membrane/coat through which the papillae can be seen.
- Not typically painful.
  - Forchheimer spots—palatal and uvular petechiae and erythematous macules.
- Initial sandpaper rash, associated with blanching erythema and occasional pruritus, erupts in 1 to 2 days (**Figures 33-1 to 33-3**).[1]
- Pastia's lines are pink or red lines seen in the body folds (especially elbows and axilla) during scarlet fever. Linear hyperpigmentation may persist after the rash fades (**Figure 33-1**).
- Desquamation of the skin (especially of the hands and feet) ensues in 3 to 4 days as rash fades and can persist for 2 to 4 weeks.[2]

TYPICAL DISTRIBUTION

- Progresses centrally (torso) to peripherally (extremities) and can be prominent on the face, chest, palms, fingers, and toes.[2]

LABORATORY TESTS AND IMAGING

- Throat swab for rapid strep testing (screening) and/or culture (confirmation) is usually performed.
- CBC if indicated, to look for:
  - Elevation of white blood cell count with left shift.
  - Elevated platelet count—seen with Kawasaki disease (after 1 week).
- Antistreptolysin-O titer is obtained to confirm prior infection or support suspected poststreptococcal complication, such as rheumatic fever.[3]
- If Kawasaki disease is suspected, 2D echocardiography or angiography is obtained to detect coronary artery abnormalities. The initial echocardiogram should be performed as soon as the diagnosis is suspected to establish a baseline for longitudinal follow-up of coronary artery morphology, left ventricular and left valvular function, and the evolution and resolution of pericardial effusion when present.[4] SOR **G**

DIFFERENTIAL DIAGNOSIS

The rash of scarlet fever may be confused with the following:

- Allergic/contact dermatitis—often localized to areas of contact; prominent pruritus and skin vesicles often in linear streaks (see Chapter 139, Atopic Dermatitis and Chapter 140, Contact Dermatitis).
- Viral exanthem—many viral exanthems have prodromal phases with fever followed by skin rashes that can be macular or maculopapular including measles (see Chapter 119, Measles), rubella (tender retroauricular, cervical, and occipital lymphadenopathy and rash starts on face and spreads and fades quickly), and roseola (rash occurs at the end of a period of 3 to

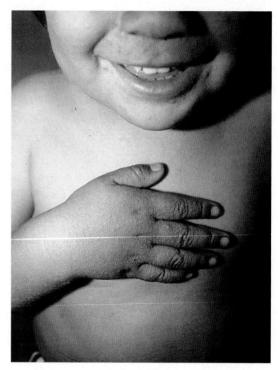

FIGURE 33-3 Sandpaper rash seen prominently on the hand of a child recovering from strep pharyngitis. (*Courtesy of Richard P. Usatine, MD.*)

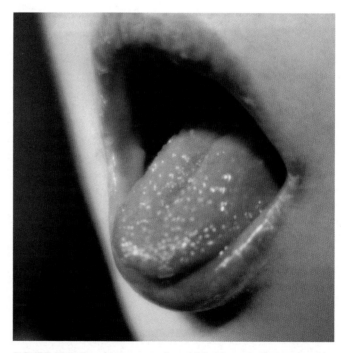

FIGURE 33-4 Strawberry tongue in a child with scarlet fever caused by strep pharyngitis; note marked erythema and prominent papillae. (*Courtesy of Richard P. Usatine, MD.*)

5 days of high fever). Lack of sand paper feel and oral findings help distinguish.

- Staphylococcal scalded skin syndrome—rash may also follow a prodrome of malaise and fever but is macular, brightly erythematous, and initially involves the face, neck axilla, and groin. Skin is markedly tender and large areas of the epidermis peel away.

- Erythema toxicum—rash of newborns; often blotchy, evanescent, macular erythema that can include pale yellow or white wheals or papules on an erythematous base (see Chapter 102, Normal Skin Changes).

The differential diagnosis for strawberry tongue includes

- Kawasaki disease—fever persists at least 5 days and there must be the presence of at least 4 principal features including the following:[4]
  - Changes in extremities—Acute: Erythema of palms, soles; edema of hands and feet or Subacute: Periungual peeling of fingers and toes in weeks 2 and 3.
  - Polymorphous exanthem.
  - Bilateral bulbar conjunctival injection without exudate.
  - Changes in lips and oral cavity—Erythema, lips cracking, strawberry tongue, diffuse injection of oral and pharyngeal mucosae.
  - Cervical lymphadenopathy (>1.5 cm diameter), usually unilateral.

- Viral stomatitis with eruptive lingual papillitis—Lack of other features for scarlet fever or Kawasaki's will assist in differentiating.

- Red-colored food dyes—History is helpful; edema and prominent papillae will be absent.

MANAGEMENT

- Supportive care with oral fluids and age-appropriate symptomatic measures such as salt-water gargles, and an antipyretic as needed are recommended.

- For scarlet fever and strawberry tongue caused by group A streptococcus:
  - Oral penicillin (penicillin VK 500 mg TID to QID for 10 days for adults or 25–50 mg/kg/d divided TID to QID for 10 days for children) or macrolide (erythromycin 250–500 mg QID for 10 days for adults or 30–50 mg/kg/d divided QID for 10 days for children) in penicillin-allergic patients for 10 days. Alternatively, a single intramuscular dose of penicillin (benzathine penicillin G 1.2 million U intramuscularly for adults and 300,000–600,000 U for children weighing less than 27 kg and 900,000–1.2 million U for children weighing over 27 kg) may be given.[3] SOR **A**
  - Cephalosporins are an efficacious alternative (e.g., cephalexin 250–500 mg QID for 10 days for adults or 25–50 mg/kg/d divided QID for 10 days for children); cephalosporins were better than penicillin in a meta-analysis.[5] SOR **A**
  - Symptoms typically resolve in 4 to 7 days.

- For strawberry tongue caused by Kawasaki disease:
  - Intravenous gamma globulin (IVIG), 2 g/kg in a single infusion, within 7 to 10 days of onset for Kawasaki disease to reduce subsequent coronary artery abnormalities.[6] SOR **A**

- In the acute phase, aspirin is also administered at 80 to 100 mg/kg per day in 4 doses with IVIG followed by low-dose aspirin (3–5 mg/kg per day) until the patient shows no evidence of coronary changes by 6 to 8 weeks after the onset of illness.[6] SOR **C**

PATIENT EDUCATION

- Contact physician for fever recurrence, atypical or persistent rash, and new symptoms or potential complications (meningitis, sinusitis, otitis media, oropharyngeal abscess, pneumonia, acute glomerulonephritis, or rheumatic fever). Completion of a prescribed antibiotic course is encouraged to decrease the incidence of recurrence and potential complications.[3]

FOLLOW-UP

- Routine follow-up is not required unless illness is protracted or complication is suspected.

- For patients with uncomplicated Kawasaki disease, echocardiographic evaluation should be performed at the time of diagnosis, at 2 weeks, and at 6 to 8 weeks after onset of the disease.[2] SOR **C** Recent studies have shown that repeat echocardiography performed 1 year after the onset of the illness is unlikely to reveal coronary artery enlargement in patients whose echocardiographic findings were normal at 4 to 8 weeks.[4]

PATIENT RESOURCES

http://www.kidshealth.org/parent/infections/bacterial_viral/scarlet_fever.html.

PROVIDER RESOURCES

http://www.emedicine.com/DERM/topic383.htm.

REFERENCES

1. Cherry JD. Contemporary infectious exanthems. *Clin Infect Dis.* 1993;16(2):199–205.

2. Cunningham MW. Pathogenesis of group A streptococcal infections. *Clin Microbiol Rev.* 2000;13(3):470–511.

3. Hahn RG, Knox LM, Forman TA. Evaluation of poststreptococcal illness. *Am Fam Physician.* 2005;71(10):1949–1954.

4. Cohen BA, Lehmann CU. http://www.dermatlas.com. Accessed August 16, 2006.

5. Casey JR, Pichichero ME. Meta-analysis of cephalosporin versus penicillin treatment of group A streptococcal tonsillopharyngitis in children. *Pediatrics.* 2004;113(4):866–882.

6. Newburger JW, Takahashi M, Gerber MA, et al. Diagnosis, treatment, and long-term management of Kawasaki disease: A statement for health professionals from the committee on rheumatic fever, endocarditis and Kawasaki disease, council on cardiovascular disease in the young, american heart association. *Circulation.* 2004;110(17):2747–2771.

34 PHARYNGITIS

Andreas Kuhn, MD
Richard P. Usatine, MD

PATIENT STORY

A 27-year-old woman complains of sore throat, fever, and chills for 2 days. She is unable to swallow anything other than fluids because of severe odynophagia. She denies any congestion or cough. On examination, she has bilateral tonsillar erythema and exudate (**Figure 34-1**). Her anterior cervical lymph nodes are tender. Based on the presence of fever, absence of cough, tender lymphadenopathy, and tonsillar exudate, she is diagnosed with a high probability of group A β-hemolytic streptococcus (GABHS) and placed on antibiotics.

EPIDEMIOLOGY

- Pharyngitis accounts for 1.1% of primary care visits.
  - An estimated 60% to 90% of cases of pharyngitis are from viral infections.
  - Between 5% and 30% are caused by bacterial infections depending upon the age of the population and the season.
  - The GABHS accounts for 5% to 10% of pharyngitis in adults and 15% to 30% in children. Up to 38% of cases of tonsillitis are because of GABHS.

- Highest prevalence in winter.

- Highest incidence in children between 4 and 7 years of age.

- Acute rheumatic fever is currently rare in the United States.

- Up to 14% of deep neck infections result from pharyngitis.[1]

ETIOLOGY AND PATHOPHYSIOLOGY

- Viruses and bacteria may cause inflammation of the pharyngeal mucosa by direct invasion of the mucosa or secondary to suprapharyngeal secretions.[2]

- The GABHS release exotoxins and proteases. Exotoxins are responsible for the development of the scarlatiniform exanthem (**Figure 34-2**). Secondary antibody formation may result in rheumatic fever and valvular heart disease. Antigen–antibody complexes may cause acute glomerulonephritis.

- Untreated GABHS pharyngitis can result in peritonsillar abscess formation (**Figure 34-3**).

DIAGNOSIS

CLINICAL FEATURES

- Rhinorrhea and cough are more consistent with viral etiology.

- Rapid onset odynophagia, tonsillar exudates, anterior cervical lymphadenopathy, and fever are consistent with streptococcal pharyngitis.

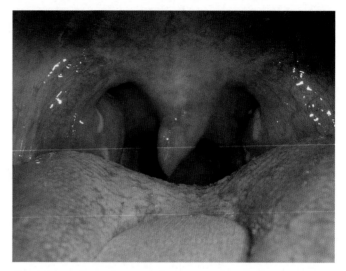

FIGURE 34-1 Strep pharyngitis showing tonsillar exudate and erythema. (*Courtesy of Michael Nguyen, MD.*)

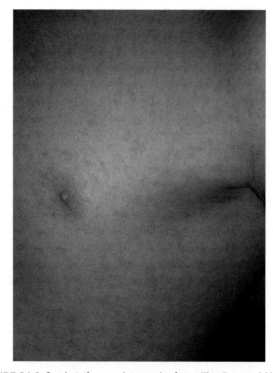

FIGURE 34-2 Scarlatiniform rash in scarlet fever. This 7-year-old boy has a typical sandpaper rash with his strep throat and fever. The erythema is particularly concentrated in the axillary area. (*Courtesy of Richard P. Usatine, MD.*)

- A sandpaper rash is suggestive of scarlet fever (**Figure 34-2**).

- Not all tonsillar exudates are caused by streptococcal pharyngitis. Mononucleosis and other viral pharyngitis can cause tonsillar exudates (**Figure 34-4** and **34-5**). The positive predictive value for tonsillar exudate and strep throat is only 31%. That is, 69% of patients with tonsillar exudate will have mononucleosis- or viral pharyngitis.

- Para- and supratonsillar edema with medial and/or anterior displacement of the involved tonsil and uvular displacement to the contralateral side suggest peritonsillar abscess (**Figure 34-3**). Anterior cervical and jugulodigastric lymphadenopathy with severe tenderness to palpation are additional findings.

- Palatal petechiae can be seen in all types of pharyngitis (**Figure 34-6**).

- Lymphoid hyperplasia can cause a cobblestone pattern on the posterior pharynx or palate from viral infections or allergies (**Figure 34-7**). While it usually is more suggestive of a viral infection or allergic rhinitis, lymphoid hyperplasia can be seen in strep pharyngitis (**Figure 34-8**).

- The following criteria are helpful in the diagnosis of GABHS pharyngitis:[3-7]
  ○ History of fever or temperature of 38°C (1 point).
  ○ Absence of cough (1 point).
  ○ Tender anterior cervical lymph nodes (1 point).
  ○ Tonsillar swelling or exudates (1 point).
  ○ Age:
    ▪ <15 years (1 point).
    ▪ 15 to 45 years (0 points).
    ▪ >15 years (−1 point).

  The probability of GABHS is approximately 1% with (−1 to 0 points) and approximately 51% with 4 to 5 points.[8]

LABORATORY TESTS AND IMAGING

- Rapid antigen detection is often used to diagnose GABHS. Test options include enzyme immunoassays, latex agglutination, liposomal method, and immunochromatographic assays; the latter has the highest reported sensitivity (0.97), specificity (0.97), positive (32.3), and negative (0.03) likelihood ratios.[9]

- The gold standard for the diagnosis of streptococcal infection is a positive throat culture. However, GABHS is part of the normal oropharyngeal flora in many patients and the diagnosis of acute streptococcal pharyngitis must include both the clinical signs of acute infection and a positive throat culture.

- False positive tests for streptococcal infection occur when the patient is colonized with GABHS but this is not the cause of the acute disease.

- False negative tests for streptococcal infection occur when poor sampling technique with the throat swab fails to recover the streptococcal organism when it is the cause of the acute infection.

- A positive mono spot (likelihood ratio in the first week of illness 5.7) and/or >40% atypical lymphocytes on the peripheral smear (likelihood ratio 39) indicate mononucleosis.[9]

- Viral cultures obtained from vesicles can be obtained in coxsackievirus and herpes infections but the diagnosis is usually based on clinical grounds.

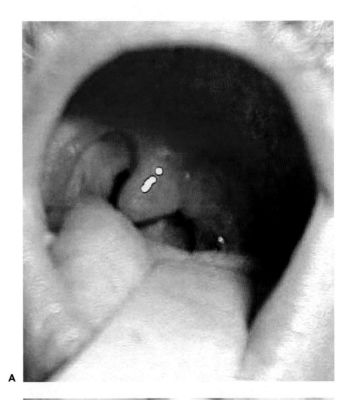

A

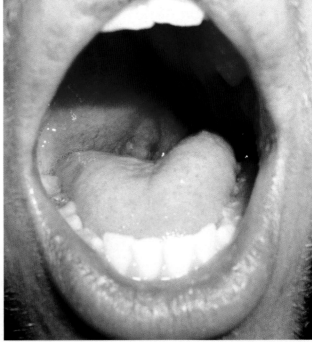

B

FIGURE 34-3 A. Peritonsillar abscess on the left showing uvular deviation away from the side with the abscess. B. Peritonsillar abscess with swelling and anatomic distortion of the right tonsillar region. (*Courtesy of Charlie Goldberg, MD, and The Regents of the University of California.*)

• Head-neck CT scan can assist in the diagnosis and localization of peritonsillar abscess and should be obtained if further extension into the deeper neck is suspected.

DIFFERENTIAL DIAGNOSIS

• Infectious mononucleosis—Nausea, anorexia without vomiting, uvular edema, and generalized symmetric lymphadenopathy, particularly in teenagers and young adults, is more suggestive of acute mononucleosis (Epstein–Barr virus [EBV]) although the pharyngeal examination has a similar appearance to GABHS (**Figure 34-4**). Hepatosplenomegaly is indicative of EBV in this group.

• Herpangina/coxsackievirus infection—Oropharyngeal vesicles and ulcers indicate herpangina, which is caused by coxsackievirus A16 in the majority of cases (**Figure 34-9**).

• Oral candida—Whitish plaques of the oropharyngeal mucosa indicate oral candida/thrush, which is mainly found in infants but can be found in adults with immunosuppression (see Chapter 130, Candida).

• Primary herpes gingivostomatitis causes oral ulcers and pain in the mouth. The wide distribution of ulcers with the first case of HSV-1 distinguishes this infection from other types of pharyngitis (see Chapter 122, Herpes Simplex).

• Cytomegalovirus (CMV)—Primary CMV infection in the immunocompetent host is usually asymptomatic. In the immunocompromised host, CMV may present with a mononucleosis-like syndrome clinically indistinguishable from EBV infection.

• Deep neck infections—Asymmetry of the neck, neck masses, and any displacement if the peripharyngeal wall should raise suspicion. Associated shortness of breath may be a warning sign of impending airway obstruction. Other complications include aspiration, thrombosis, mediastinitis, and septic shock.[10]

• Epiglottitis—Rapid onset fever, malaise, sore throat, and drooling in the absence of coughing characterize acute epiglottitis. Progression of the disease can lead to life-threatening airway obstruction. Fortunately, this is a rare condition because of the preventive effect of the Hib vaccine.

• Diphtheria—A rare condition since most patients today have been immunized. However, it needs to be considered, especially in immigrant populations. Pharyngeal diphtheria presents with sore throat, low-grade fever, and malaise. The pharynx is erythematous with a grayish pseudomembrane that cannot be scraped off. Complications include myocarditis resulting in acute and severe CHF, endocarditis, and neuropathies.

MANAGEMENT

• Hydration, with plenty of fluids.

• Acetaminophen (15–20 mg/kg every 4–6 hours for children and 1 g every 4 to 6 hours for adults) may be used for symptomatic relief of fever and pain. Ibuprofen is a powerful antipyretic and analgesic too.

• In severe cases of pharyngitis, viscous lidocaine 2%, one teaspoon in half glass of water to gargle with 20 to 30 minutes before meals helps the odynophagia. If patients use this for symptom relief, warn

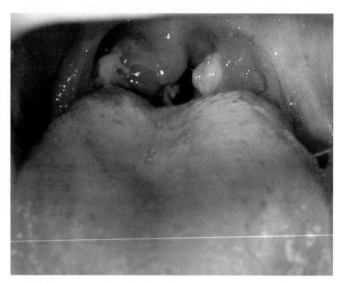

FIGURE 34-4 Mononucleosis in a young adult with considerable tonsillar exudate. (*Courtesy of Tracey Cawthorn, MD.*)

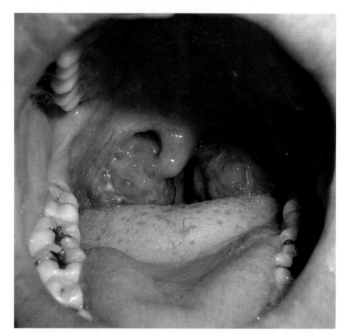

FIGURE 34-5 Viral pharyngitis in a young adult showing enlarged cryptic tonsils with some erythema and exudate. (*Courtesy of Richard P. Usatine, MD.*)

them to use caution with hot meals and beverages since they may not feel oral burns until the lidocaine wears off.

- Steroids (e.g., dexamethasone single 10 mg injection) are indicated in severe tonsillitis in patients without immunocompromise.[9] SOR **C** However, there is no good evidence to recommend steroids in EBV.[11]

- Use the clinical prediction rule (given above [Clinical Features]) for estimating the probability of GABHS:[3,6,7]
  ○ Low probability: (no test, no treat for GABHS) patients scoring (0 points should be treated symptomatically and not given antibiotics.
  ○ Intermediate probability: (test and treat based on result) patients with 1 to 3 points (probability of GABHS is approximately 18%) should undergo a rapid antigen test and be treated with antibiotics if positive.
  ○ High probability: (no test, treat for GABHS) patients with 4 to 5 points should be considered for empiric antibiotic treatment.

- For suspected or proven GABHS, penicillin V 500 mg orally bid to tid for 10 days is the treatment of choice for adults.[12] SOR **A** Erythromycin 500 mg orally qid may be used in penicillin allergic patients. Penicillin G 1.2 million U IM single dose may be used if unable to tolerate oral medication. Pediatric doses are Pen VK 25–50 mg/kg/d divided TID to QID and erythromycin 30–50 mg/kg/d divided QID for 10 days.

- Refer to ENT for patients with peritonsillar abscess. Incision and drainage is the treatment of choice in addition to using systemic antibiotics.

- If signs of airway impairment are present, the patient should be immediately transported to an emergency department. Intubation can be extremely difficult and risky.

- Penicillin G (600 mg IV q6h for 24–48 hours) in combination with metronidazole (15 mg/kg IV more than 1 hour followed by 7.5 mg/kg IV more than 1 hour every 6–8 hours) is recommended for peritonsillar abscess.

- Consider ENT referral for tonsillectomy in recurrent GABHS cases. SOR **C** However, there is no evidence to support tonsillectomy.[13]

PATIENT EDUCATION

- Explain to patients the difference between a viral and a bacterial infection so that they can understand why antibiotics were prescribed or not prescribed.

- Rest, fluids, and analgesics should not be minimized. It is inappropriate to give an antibiotic to the patient with an obvious viral infection even if they believe the antibiotic is what they need. Studies of patient satisfaction have demonstrated that spending time with the patient and explaining to them their disease process is associated with greater patient satisfaction than purely giving an antibiotic.[14]

- Patients with mononucleosis and splenomegaly should be warned to avoid contact sports that could result in splenic rupture.

FOLLOW-UP

- Follow-up if not improving within 72 hours or if deteriorating.

- Patients with mononucleosis may need more close follow-up if they have a severe case that lingers.

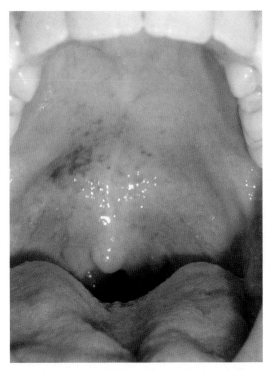

FIGURE 34-6 Viral pharyngitis with visible palatal petechiae. Palatal petechiae can be seen in all types of pharyngitis. (*Courtesy of Richard P. Usatine, MD.*)

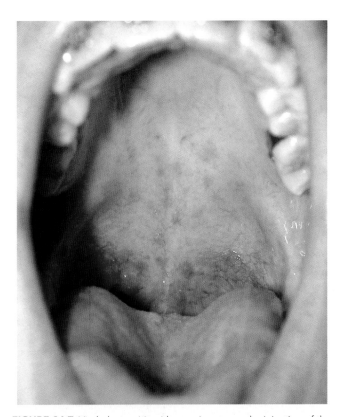

FIGURE 34-7 Viral pharyngitis with prominent vascular injection of the soft palate and lymphoid hyperplasia. (*Courtesy of Richard P. Usatine, MD.*)

PATIENT RESOURCES

Sore Throat: Easing the Pain of a Sore Throat

http://familydoctor.org/163.xml.

Strep Throat information for patients **http://familydoctor. org/670.xml.**

Mononucleosis information for patients **http://familydoctor.org/077.xml.**

PROVIDER RESOURCES

Del Mar CB, Glasziou PP, Spinks AB. Antibiotics for sore throat. Cochrane Database Syst Rev. 2006 Oct 18;(4): CD000023. Review.

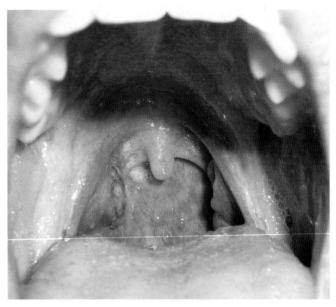

FIGURE 34-8 Strep pharyngitis with dark necrotic area on right tonsil and prominent lymphoid hyperplasia in a cobblestone pattern on the posterior pharynx. (*Courtesy of Richard P. Usatine, MD.*)

REFERENCES

1. Bottin R, Marioni G, Rinaldi R, Boninsegna M, Salvadori L, Staffieri A. Deep neck infection: A present-day complication. A retrospective review of 83 cases (1998–2001). *Eur Arch Otorhinolaryngol.* 2003;260(10):576–579.

2. Kazzi AA, Wills J. Pharyngitis. Emedicine. http://www.emedicine.com/EMERG/topic419.htm. Accessed November, 2006.

3. Ebell MH. Strep throat. *Am Fam Physician.* 2003;68(5):937–938.

4. Singh S, Dolan JG, Centor RM. Optimal management of adults with pharyngitis: A multi-criteria decision analysis. *BMC Med Inform Decis Making.* 2006;6:14.

5. Linder JA, Chan JC, Bates DW. Evaluation and treatment of pharyngitis in primary care practice: The difference between guidelines is largely academic. *Arch Intern Med.* 2006;166(13):1374–1379.

6. Vincent MT, Celestin N, Hussain AN. Pharyngitis. *Am Fam Physician.* 2004;69(6):1465–1470.

7. Merrill B, Kelsberg G, Jankowski TA, Danis P. Clinical inquiries. What is the most effective diagnostic evaluation of streptococcal pharyngitis? *J Fam Pract.* 2004;53(9):734, 737–738, 740.

8. McIsaac WJ, Goel V, to T, Low DE. The validity of a sore throat score in family practice. *CMAJ.* 2000;163:811–815.

9. Ebell MH. Sore throat. In: Sloane PD, Slatt LM, Ebell MH, Jacques LB eds. *Essentials of Family Medicine.* Baltimore, MD: Lippincott Williams & Wilkins, 2002:727–738.

10. Michelle C Marcincuk M, Alan D Murray, MD. Deep Neck Infections. Emedicine http://www.emedicine.com/ENT/topic669.htm. Accessed November, 2006.

11. Candy B, Hotopf M. Steroids for symptom control in infectious mononucleosis. *Cochrane Database Syst Rev.* 2006;3:CD004402.

12. Cooper RJ, Hoffman JR, Bartlett JG, et al. Principles of appropriate antibiotic use for acute pharyngitis in adults: background. *Ann Intern Med.* 2001;134(6):509–517.

13. Neill RA, Scoville C. Clinical inquiries. What are the indications for tonsillectomy in children? *J Fam Pract.* 2002;51(4):314.

14. Hamm RM, Hicks RJ, Bemben DA. Antibiotics and respiratory infections: Are patients more satisfied when expectations are met? *J Fam Pract.* 1996;43(1):56–62.

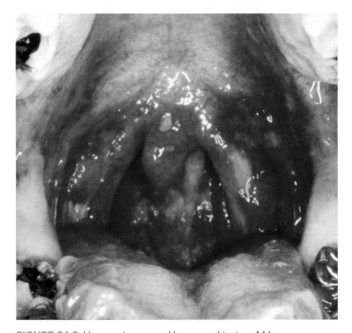

FIGURE 34-9 Herpangina caused by coxsackievirus A16.

35 THE LARYNX (HOARSENESS)

J. Michael King, MD
C. Blake Simpson, MD

PATIENT STORY

A 47-year-old man with a 40-pack-year history of smoking presents with worsening hoarseness that began approximately 6 weeks ago. He complains of globus sensation and difficulty swallowing solid foods. He denies odynophagia, otalgia, hemoptysis, and hematemesis. There is no associated cough, and he has not had any constitutional symptoms such as fevers, chills, or recent weight loss.

Hoarseness in a middle-aged man with the above symptoms is very common, and the differential diagnosis is long (all the diseases below are possibilities in this case scenario). The patient's smoking history and duration of symptoms should raise concern for a possible laryngeal malignancy. However, there is a higher incidence of laryngopharyngeal reflux (LPR) followed by benign vocal fold (cord) lesions.

EPIDEMIOLOGY

- The most common cause of hoarseness in adults and children overall is a viral infection causing laryngitis (**Figure 35-1**). It helps to know the anatomy of the normal larynx as a start (**Figure 35-2**).
- Laryngopharyngeal reflux may be present in up to 50% of patients presenting with voice and laryngeal disorders.[1]
- Squamous cell carcinoma (SCC) accounts for 95% of laryngeal cancer. Approximately 11,000 new cases are diagnosed in the United States each year. Peak incidence is in the sixth and seventh decades of life with a strong male predominance.[1]
- Recurrent respiratory papillomatosis (RRP) represents the most common benign neoplasm of the larynx among children and should be considered in children with chronic hoarseness. A known risk factor for juvenile onset is the triad of a first-born child (75%), teenage mother, and vaginal delivery. The incidence in children and adults is 4.3 and 1.8 per 100,000, respectively.[2] There is a known association between cervical human papillomavirus (HPV) infection in the mother and juvenile onset RRP, but the precise mode of transmission is unclear. The risk of a child contracting RRP after delivery from an actively infected mother with genital HPV ranges from 0.25% to 3%.[3] Since cesarean section does not prevent RRP in all cases, routine prophylactic cesarean section in mothers with active condyloma acuminata is currently *not* recommended.

ETIOLOGY AND PATHOPHYSIOLOGY

- Laryngitis is a nonspecific term to describe inflammation of the larynx from any cause. Most commonly this is caused by a viral upper respiratory infection. Laryngeal symptoms result from dry throat, mucous stasis, and recurrent trauma from coughing and throat clearing (**Figure 35-1**).

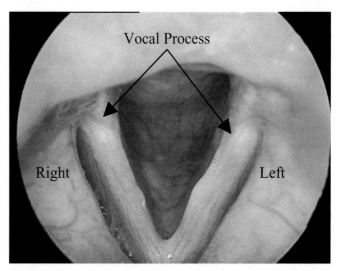

FIGURE 35-1 Laryngitis causing diffuse erythema and inflammation. Note how the vocal cords are not the normal white color that is seen in the following figure. (*Courtesy of C. Blake Simpson, MD.*)

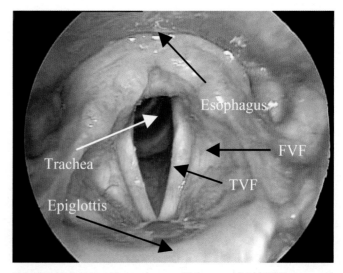

FIGURE 35-2 Normal larynx (true and false vocal folds). TVF, true vocal fold (cord); FVF, false vocal fold. (*Courtesy of C. Blake Simpson, MD.*)

- Vocal cord nodules, polyps, and cysts are benign lesions arising from mechanical trauma (vocal abuse or misuse). They are a common cause of dysphonia in singers, teachers, and other professional voice users (**Figures 35-3** and **35-4**).

- Recurrent respiratory papillomatosis (RRP) is caused by HPV. Onset is predominantly in young children although an adult-onset variant exists. Its course is unpredictable and highly variable. Tracheal and bronchopulmonary spread can occur. Malignant transformation to SCC is uniformly fatal and rare (**Figures 35-5** and **35-6**).

- Laryngopharyngeal reflux (LPR) is a distinct entity from GERD. Patients do *not* typically have heartburn, indigestion, and regurgitation as in GERD; patients do have a high incidence of hoarseness, globus, excessive throat clearing and chronic cough. The larynx is highly sensitive to even small amounts of acid/pepsin. Thus, patients who do not have severe enough reflux to cause esophagitis (GERD symptoms) may still develop symptomatic laryngeal mucosal injury secondary to LPR (**Figures 35-7** and **35-8**).[1,4,5]

- SCC has multifactorial etiology, but 90% of patients have a history of heavy tobacco and/or alcohol use. These risk factors have a synergistic effect. Other independent risk factors include professions like painters, metalworkers, persons exposed to diesel and gasoline fumes, and patients exposed to therapeutic doses of radiation (**Figure 35-9**).

- Causes of vocal cord paresis or paralysis are myriad:[1,6]
  - Iatrogenic surgical injury (25%) is most common (anterior spine fusion, carotid endarterectomy, thyroidectomy).
  - Nonlaryngeal malignancy (24%) (mediastinal, bronchopulmonary, and skull base).
  - No cause is identifiable (idiopathic) in 20% of cases.
  - Nonsurgical trauma (10%) (penetrating/blunt injury and intubation injury).
  - Neurologic (8%) causes include stroke, CNS tumors, MS, and ALS.
  - Inflammatory/infectious disease (2%–5%).

- Presbyphonia is a diagnosis of exclusion denoting vocal changes from aging of the larynx (gradually weakening voice, poor vocal projection, and vocal "roughness"). Hoarseness in elderly patients older than 60 years of age is most commonly caused by benign vocal cord lesions such as polyps followed by malignancy and vocal cord paralysis. Once a thorough evaluation has been done to rule out organic causes, presbyphonia is the cause of hoarseness in approximately 10% of elderly patients.[7]

DIAGNOSIS

CLINICAL FEATURES

- Key historical and physical examination findings can help differentiate benign pathology from potentially more serious problems:
  - Otalgia (ear pain)—often a source of referred pain from primary laryngeal and pharyngeal carcinomas.
  - Dysphagia and odynophagia (pain when swallowing)—nonspecific complaints, but potentially worrisome for obstructing lesions or reactive pharyngeal edema.

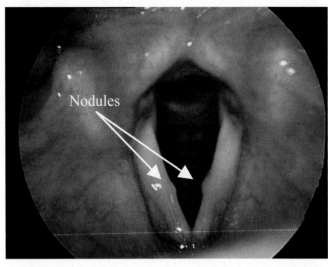

FIGURE 35-3 Vocal cord nodules. (*Courtesy of C. Blake Simpson, MD.*)

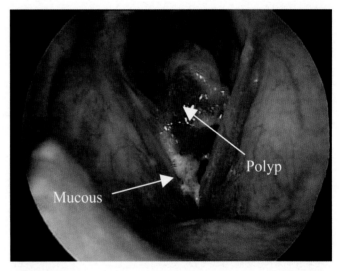

FIGURE 35-4 Large obstructing laryngeal polyp. (*Courtesy of C. Blake Simpson, MD.*)

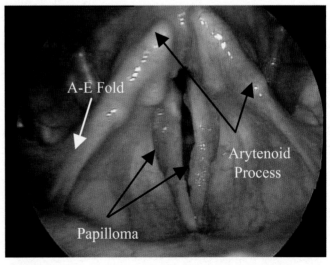

FIGURE 35-5 Adult recurrent respiratory papillomatosis (RRP). Aryepiglottic fold (A–E fold) (*Courtesy of C. Blake Simpson, MD.*)

- Stridor—"noisy breathing" with respiratory distress should be evaluated urgently to rule out impending airway obstruction.
- Globus—the persistent or intermittent nonpainful sensation of a lump or foreign body in the throat. This is commonly associated with LPR and GERD.
- Neck mass—associated unilateral or bilateral lymphadenopathy is suspicious for a laryngeal neoplasm until proven otherwise.
- Timing—onset, duration, and frequency of symptoms is important.

- "Red Flags" for laryngeal carcinoma include a history of smoking and/or alcohol abuse, hoarseness for more than 1 month, dysphagia/odynophagia, and otalgia.

- LPR symptoms include hoarseness, throat clearing, "postnasal drip," chronic cough, dysphagia, globus sensation, and sore throat. "Heartburn" is *not* a requisite symptom.

- Hallmark of diagnosis is direct visualization of the larynx with a flexible fiberoptic scope. Otolaryngology consultation may be necessary for office videostroboscopic evaluation and to biopsy suspicious lesions.

LABORATORY STUDIES AND IMAGING

- Laboratory studies are not usually helpful because the real diagnostic test is fiberoptic laryngoscopy.

- Plain films of the chest are useful to rule out bronchopulmonary or mediastinal masses as a cause of vocal cord paralysis, but are generally not helpful for primary laryngeal lesions.

- A contrasted CT of the neck is useful in cases of suspicion of carcinoma, especially if there is associated cervical lymphadenopathy.

- An MRI with and without gadolinium offers the best imaging for suspected primary CNS or skull base lesions.

- Referral to a gastroenterologist for dual-channel 24 hour pH probe monitoring (while on antireflux medications) is a useful diagnostic tool for patients with suspected LPR.

DIFFERENTIAL DIAGNOSIS OF A HOARSE VOICE

- Laryngitis (**Figure 35-1**).
- Vocal cord nodule (**Figure 35-2**).
- Vocal cord polyp (**Figure 35-3**).
- Vocal cord cyst.
- Laryngeal papillomatosis (**Figures 35-5** and **35-6**).
- LPR disease (**Figures 35-7** and **35-8**).
- SCC (**Figure 35-9**).
- Vocal cord paresis or paralysis.
- Neurological disorders (multiple sclerosis, Parkinson's disease, and essential tremor).
- Systemic diseases (Wegener granulomatosis, sarcoidosis, rheumatoid arthritis).
- Presbyphonia.

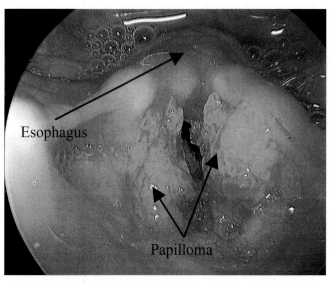

FIGURE 35-6 Recurrent respiratory papillomatosis in a 3-year-old child. The papillomas are nearly obstructing the airway and have required debridement. (*Courtesy of C. Blake Simpson, MD.*)

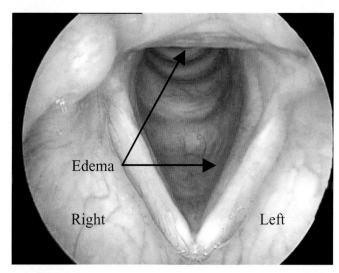

FIGURE 35-7 Laryngopharyngeal reflux disease (LPR). (*Courtesy of C. Blake Simpson, MD.*)

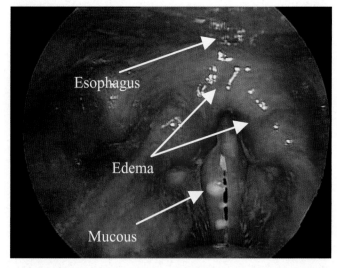

FIGURE 35-8 Laryngopharyngeal reflux during phonation with diffuse erythema, inflammation, and thick mucous. (*Courtesy of C. Blake Simpson, MD.*)

MANAGEMENT

- *Laryngitis*—Empiric treatment is aimed at alleviating symptoms such as cough and draining nasal/pharyngeal secretions. Hydration is critical for healing (steam showers, humidifiers, and saunas may help). Throat clearing should be discouraged and voice rest encouraged. Talking should be conserved, not prohibited. Inform patients that whispering causes more vocal strain and makes matters worse.

- *Vocal cord nodules, polyps, and cysts*—Initial management involves speech therapy accompanied by medical treatment of dehydration, allergies, sinonasal secretions (postnasal drip), and LPR. Refractory disease may require surgical excision.

- *Laryngeal papillomatosis*—Most children have a recalcitrant course that requires periodic surgical debridement by an otolaryngologist to prevent airway obstruction. Spontaneous remission may occur. Adjuvant therapy, such as cidofovir, is commonly utilized in more aggressive disease.

- *LPR*—Mainstay treatment involves patient education to modify diet and behavior (weight loss, tobacco cessation, limiting alcohol and caffeine, and avoiding meals shortly before lying down). Expert opinion suggests the use of *twice* daily proton pump inhibitors (PPIs) before meals. However, recommendations for empiric treatment of suspected LPR with PPIs are based on poor levels of evidence from uncontrolled studies. The few randomized, controlled trials have failed to demonstrate superiority of PPIs over placebo for treatment of suspected LPR.[8] SOR Ⓒ While there is no evidence to support adding an H2-blocker, such as ranitidine 300 mg, at bedtime, this is a commonly used treatment modality. SOR Ⓒ

- *SCC*—Multidisciplinary management is best. Depending on the staging and extent of disease, patients often receive one or more modalities of treatment including surgery, radiation, and chemotherapy.

- *Vocal cord paresis or paralysis*—Treatment is targeted at the underlying disorder. Some patients may be candidates for surgical intervention to reposition the paralyzed cord into the physiologic phonating position. These procedures restore voice quality and often alleviate chronic aspiration problems.

- *Neurologic diseases*—Laryngeal problems are associated with multiple sclerosis in young patients, and Parkinson's disease and essential tremor in the elderly. In addition to managing the underlying disorder, a trial of voice therapy is often useful.

- *Systemic diseases* such as Wegener granulomatosis, sarcoidosis, and rheumatoid arthritis may rarely involve the larynx. Voice and swallowing problems in these patients should be evaluated by an otolaryngologist to rule out associated laryngeal stenosis.

- *Presbyphonia* is first and foremost a diagnosis of exclusion. Once organic etiologies have been ruled out, a trial of voice therapy is recommended before considering surgical options (i.e., vocal cord augmentation).

PATIENT EDUCATION

- Efforts should focus on tobacco cessation and prevention of excessive alcohol use.

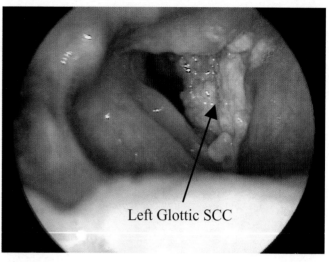

Left Glottic SCC

FIGURE 35-9 Squamous cell carcinoma (SCC), advanced stage with left true vocal cord paralysis. (*Courtesy of C. Blake Simpson, MD.*)

- Vocal cord nodules, polyps, and cysts typically occur in professional voice users (ministers, auctioneers, teachers, singers, etc.) Speech therapists can be integral in preventing and healing lesions by teaching patients how to avoid vocal misuse.

- Most benign laryngeal pathology will be improved by controlling both gastroesophageal and LPR disease. Patients should be educated about GERD/LPR risk factors:
  - Obesity.
  - Spicy or greasy foods.
  - Tobacco and alcohol abuse.
  - Caffeinated beverages (especially carbonated sodas).
  - Citric juices, chocolate, mints.
  - Eating meals within 2 to 3 hours of lying down.

FOLLOW-UP

- Close follow-up and/or urgent referral to an otolaryngologist for fiberoptic examination of the larynx is advisable when the history and physical are suspicious for carcinoma.

- Patients suspected of having LPR should be seen approximately 6 to 8 weeks after initiating empiric therapy. An otolaryngology and/or gastroenterology consultation is indicated when symptoms do not improve after optimized behavioral and medical management or who require long-term PPI therapy (longer than 12 months).

- When symptoms worsen or fail to resolve, referral to an otolaryngologist (or laryngologist) is indicated (see Provider Resources below to find a laryngologist in your area).

PATIENT RESOURCES

The American Academy of Otolaryngology—Head and Neck Surgery (AAO-HNS) health information for the public site—**http://www.entnet.org/healthinfo/index.cfm.**

Website designed to educate doctors and patients about Otolaryngology—**http://www.entusa.com.**

http://www.voiceproblem.org.

PROVIDER RESOURCES

http://www.voiceproblem.org.

Gallery of Laryngeal Pathology from UC Davis—**http://www.ucdvoice.org/gallery.html.**

Information about laryngeal pathology as well as an extensive list of laryngologists worldwide—**http://www.voicedoctor.net/links/physicians.html.**

REFERENCES

1. Ossoff R, Shapshay S, Woodson G, Netterville J. *The Larynx.* Philadelphia, PA: Lippincott Williams & Wilkins. 2003:270, 337, 499–500.

2. Derkay CS. Recurrent Respiratory Papillomatosis. *Laryngoscope.* 2001;111:57–69.

3. Rosen FS, Pou AM, Quinn FB, Ryan MW. Recurrent respiratory papillomatosis. Grand Rounds Presentation, UTMB, Dept. of Otolaryngology. June 25, 2003. http://www.utmb.edu/otoref/Grnds/Papillomatosis-2003–0625/Papillomatosis-2003-0625.htm. Accessed May 12, 2007.

4. Simpson CB. Patient of the Month Program. American Academy of Otolaryngology, Head and Neck Surgery Foundation. *Breathy Dysphonia (Diagnosis and Treatment of Vocal Fold Paralysis).* 2002;31(7): 19–28.

5. Koufmann JA, Amin MA, Panetti M. Prevalence of reflux in 113 consecutive patients with laryngeal and voice disorders. *Otolaryngol Head Neck Surg.* 2000;123:385–388.

6. Benninger MS, Gillen JB, Altman JS. Changing etiology of vocal fold immobility. *Laryngoscope.* 1998;108:1346–1349.

7. Kendall K. Presbyphonia: A review. *Curr Opin Otolaryngol Head Neck Surg.* 2007;15:137–140.

8. Karkos PD, Wilson JA. Empiric treatment of laryngopharyngeal reflux with proton pump inhibitors: A systematic review. *Laryngoscope.* 2006;116(1):144–148.

PART 6

ORAL HEALTH

36 BLACK HAIRY TONGUE

Wanda C. Gonsalves, MD

PATIENT STORY

A 60-year-old man who smokes presents to the physician's office smelling of alcohol. He complains of a black discoloration of his tongue and a gagging sensation without eating. The history determines that he brushes his teeth infrequently and goes to a dentist only if he has a toothache. He reports that he drinks >5 cups of coffee a day. **Figures 36-1** shows the man with poor dentition and a black hairy tongue (HT). The remaining teeth are horribly stained and his tongue shows elongated papillae with brown discoloration. The physician discuss his tobacco and alcohol addictions and offer him help to stop drinking and smoking. The physician also discuss how he needs to take care of his mouth and see a dentist.

EPIDEMIOLOGY

The prevalence of HT varies from 15% of the general population to 57% in persons incarcerated or addicted to drugs.[1] HT has been reported more commonly in males and increasing age.

ETIOLOGY AND PATHOPHYSIOLOGY

- HT (**Figure 36-1**), frequently called black hairy tongue (BHT) is an asymptomatic disorder characterized by elongation and hypertrophy of filiform papillae and defective desquamation of the papillae on the dorsal tongue resulting in a hair-like appearance.[2]

- These papillae, which are normally about 1 mm in length, may become as long as 12 mm.

- HT is found most frequently in heavy smokers, and it also has been associated with poor oral hygiene, use of oxidizing mouthwashes, *Candida albicans,* and certain medications (especially broad-spectrum antibiotics).[3]

DIAGNOSIS

CLINICAL FEATURES

The diagnosis is made by visual inspection:

- Most patients are asymptomatic.
- Rarely, patients may complain of burning (associated candidiases), gagging, or a metallic taste.
- Debris between elongated papillae can result in halitosis.
- HT may exhibit a thick coating of black, brown, or yellow discoloration depending on foods ingested, tobacco use, and amount of coffee or tea consumed.

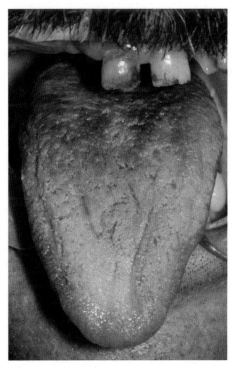

FIGURE 36-1 Black hairy tongue showing elongated filiform papillae with brown discoloration. (*Courtesy of Brad Neville, DDS.*)

Typical distribution: The lesion is restricted to the dorsum of the tongue, anterior to the circumvallate papillae, rarely involving the tip or sides of the tongue.

Laboratory tests: KOH preparation to rule out associated candidiasis.

DIFFERENTIAL DIAGNOSIS

- Leukoplakia—lesions begin as a white or red patch, progress to an ulceration, and later may become an endophytic or exophytic mass.

- Hairy leukoplakia—appears as faint white vertical keratotic streaks typically on the lateral side of the tongue (**Figure 36-2**). Do not confuse HT with oral hairy leukoplakia, an Epstein–Barr virus-related condition typically affecting the lateral tongue bilaterally in immunocompromised patients—especially those with human immunodeficiency virus infection.

- Pseudomembranous candidiasis—white plaques typically found on the buccal mucosa, tongue, and palate when removed has an erythematous base.

MANAGEMENT

Most patients improve with avoidance of predisposing factors (e.g., tobacco, mouthwashes, and antibiotics) and regular tongue brushing using a soft toothbrush or tongue scraper. If candidiasis is suspected, the use of an oral antifungal troche may be prescribed.

PATIENT EDUCATION

Tell patients to brush their tongue twice a day or to use a tongue scraper. Address addictions and offer help to quit. Suggest that patients eat firm foods like fresh apples that will help to clean the tongue.

PATIENT RESOURCES

Carr A. black hairy tongue. MayoClinic.com. **http://www.mayoclinic.com/health/black-hairy-tongue/HQ00325.** Accessed April 15, 2007.

PROVIDER RESOURCES

Hairy tongue. **http://www.usc.edu/hsc/dental/opath/Cards/HairyTongue.html.** Accessed April 15, 2007.

REFERENCES

1. Bouquot JE. Common oral lesions found during a mass screening examination. *J AM Dent Assoc.*1986;112(1):50–57.

2. Harada Y, Gaafar H. black hairy tongue. A scanning electron microscopic study. *J Laryngol Otol.* 1977;91:91–96.

3. Sarti GM, Haddy RI, Schaffer D, Kihm J. black hairy tongue. *Am Fam Physician.* 1990;41:1751–1755.

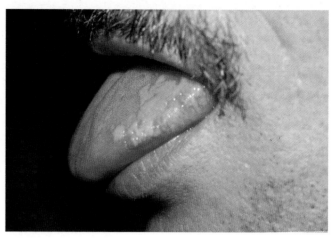

FIGURE 36-2 Oral hairy leukoplakia on the side of the tongue in a man with AIDS. (*Courtesy of Richard P. Usatine, MD.*)

37 GEOGRAPHIC TONGUE (BENIGN MIGRATORY GLOSSITIS)

Wanda C. Gonsalves, MD

PATIENT STORY

A 23-year-old male medical student presents to the physician's office complaining of his tongue's "strange appearance." He denies pain or discomfort and is unsure how long the lesions have been present. The lesions seem to change areas of distribution on the tongue. The examination reveals large, well-delineated, shiny and smooth, erythematous spots on the surface of the tongue (**Figure 37-1**). The diagnosis is geographic tongue (benign migratory glossitis). The physician explains that it is benign.

EPIDEMIOLOGY

Geographic tongue, also known as benign migratory glossitis, has an estimated prevalence of 1% to 3% of the population.[1] It may occur in either children or adults and exhibits a female predilection.

ETIOLOGY AND PATHOPHYSIOLOGY

- Geographic tongue is a common oral inflammatory condition of unknown etiology.
- Some studies have shown an increased frequency in patients with allergies, pustular psoriasis, stress, type 1 diabetes, fissured tongue, and hormonal disturbances.[2]
- Histopathologic appearances have resembled psoriasis.[3]

DIAGNOSIS

CLINICAL FEATURES

- The diagnosis is made by visual inspection and history of the lesion.
- Geographic tongue consists of large, well-delineated, shiny, and smooth, erythematous spots surrounded by a white halo, typically on the anterior two-thirds of the dorsal tongue mucosa.
- Suspect systemic intraoral manifestations of psoriasis or Reiter's syndrome if the patient has psoriatic skin lesions or has conjunctivitis, urethritis, arthritis, and skin involvement suggestive of Reiter's syndrome.
- Tongue lesions exhibit central erythema because of atrophy of the filiform papillae and are usually surrounded by slightly elevated, curving, white to yellow elevated borders (**Figures 37-1** and **37-2**).
- The condition typically waxes and wanes, and the lesions demonstrate a migrating pattern without scarring.
- Lesions may last days, months, or years.

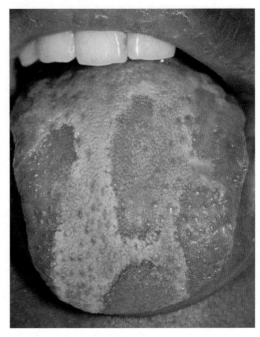

FIGURE 37-1 Geographic tongue (benign migratory glossitis). *(Reprinted with permission from Common Oral Lesions: Part II. Copyright © 2007 American Academy of Family Physicians. All right reserved. Gonsalves WC, Chi AC, Neville BW. Am Fam Phys 75(4): 501–508.)*

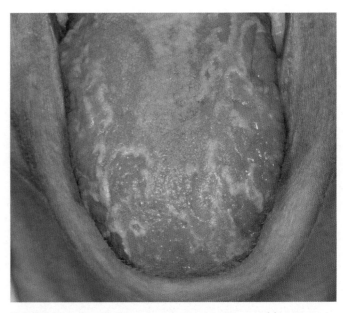

FIGURE 37-2 Geographic tongue lesions in a 71-year-old woman. *(Courtesy of Michael Huber, DMD.)*

- Most patients are asymptomatic, but some patients may complain of pain or burning, especially when eating spicy foods.

TYPICAL DISTRIBUTION

Geographic tongue usually affects the tongue, although other oral sites may be involved such as the buccal mucosa, the labial mucosa, and less frequently the soft palate.[2] This has sometimes been referred to as ectopic geographic tongue or erythema migrans.

DIFFERENTIAL DIAGNOSIS

- Erythroplakia or leukoplakia—may be suspected when lesions affect the soft palate (see Chapter 41, Leukoplakia).

- Lichen Planus—reticular forms are characterized by interlacing white lines commonly found on the buccal mucosa, or erosive forms, characterized by atrophic erythematous areas with central ulceration and surrounding radiating striae (**Figure 37-3**).

- Psoriasis—intraoral lesions have been described as red or white plaques associated with the activity of cutaneous lesions (see Chapter 145, Psoriasis) (**Figure 37-4**).

- Reiter's syndrome—a condition characterized by the triad of "urethritis, arthritis, and conjunctivitis," may have rare intraoral lesions described as painless ulcerative papules on the buccal mucosa and palate (see Chapter 148, Reiters).

MANAGEMENT

Most individuals are asymptomatic and do not require treatment. For symptomatic cases, several treatments have been proposed, including topical steroids, zinc supplements, and topical anesthetic rinses. No treatment has been proven to be uniformly effective.[3,4]

PATIENT EDUCATION

Patients should be reassured of the condition's benign nature. Tell patients with geographic tongue to avoid irritating spicy foods and liquids. Tell patients who use tobacco to stop.

FOLLOW-UP

Tell the patient to contact you if the symptoms continue past 10 days and to go to the emergency department immediately if:

- The tongue swells significantly,
- He/she has trouble breathing, or
- He/she has trouble talking or chewing/swallowing.[5]

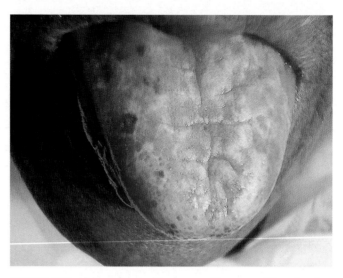

FIGURE 37-3 Lichen planus of the tongue. There are white striae; the surface is smooth because of the loss of papillae. (*Reproduced with permission from Photo Rounds: A sore and sensitive tongue. The Journal of Family Practice, January 2005; 54(1):33, Dowden Health Media.*)

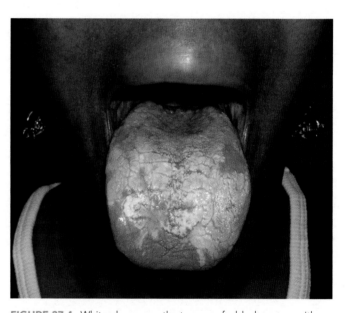

FIGURE 37-4 White plaques on the tongue of a black woman with severe cutaneous plaque psoriasis. (*Courtesy of E.J. Mayeaux, Jr., MD.*)

PROVIDER RESOURCES

Kelsch R. Geographic tongue. Updated January 24, 2007. eMedicine. **http://www.emedicine.com/derm/topic664.htm.** Accessed April 22, 2007.

MayoClinic.com. Geographic tongue. **http://www.mayoclinic. com/health/geographic-tongue/DS00819.** Accessed April 22, 2007.

REFERENCES

1. Redman RS. Prevalence of geographic tongue, fissured tongue, median rhomboid glossitis, and hairy tongue among 3,611 Minnesota schoolchildren. *Oral Surg Oral Med Oral Pathol.* 1970;30:390–395.

2. Assimakopoulos D, Patrikakos G, Fotika C, Elisaf M. Benign migratory glossitis or geographic tongue: An enigmatic oral lesion. *Am J Med.* 2002;113:751–755.

3. Espelid M, Bang G, Johannessen AC, Leira JI, Christensen O. Geographic stomatitis: Report of 6 cases. *J Oral Pathol Med.* 1991;20:425–428.

4. Gonsalves W, Chi A, Neville B. Common oral lesions: Part 1. Superficial mucosal lesions. *Am Fam Physician.* 2007;75:501–507.

5. Medline Plus. Geographic tongue. http://www.nlm.nih.gov/medlineplus/ency/article/001049.htm. Accessed April 22, 2007.

38 GINGIVITIS AND PERIODONTAL DISEASE

Wanda C. Gonsalves, MD
Richard P. Usatine, MD

PATIENT STORY

A 35-year-old woman presents to clinic for a routine physical examination. She says that for the last 6 months her gums bleed when she brushes her teeth. She reports smoking 1 pack of cigarettes per day. The oral examination finds generalized plaque and red swollen intradental papilla (**Figure 38-1**). The physician explains to her that she has gingivitis and that she should brush twice and use floss daily. The physician tells her that smoking is terrible for her health in all ways including her oral health. The physician offers her help to quit smoking and refers her to a dentist for a cleaning and full dental examination.

DEFINITIONS

- Gingivitis is the inflammation of the gingiva (gums). Gingivitis alone does not affect the underlying supporting structures of the teeth and is reversible (**Figure 38-1**).

- Periodontitis (periodontal disease) is a chronic inflammatory disease, which includes gingivitis along with loss of connective tissue and bone support for the teeth. It damages alveolar bone (the bone of the jaw in which the roots of the teeth are connected) and the periodontal ligaments that hold the roots in place. It is a major cause of tooth loss in adults (**Figures 38-2** to **38-4**).

EPIDEMIOLOGY

- Gingivitis and periodontal diseases are the most common oral diseases in adults.

- It is estimated that 35% of adults 30 years or older in the United States have periodontal disease: 22% have a severe form and 13% have a moderate to severe form.[1]

- Homeless persons are a very high-risk group for gingivitis, periodontitis, and all dental disease (**Figure 38-4**).

- Periodontal disease has been shown in some studies to be an associated factor in coronary artery disease and ischemic stroke. Periodontal disease in pregnancy has been associated with an increase in preterm birth.[2]

ETIOLOGY AND PATHOPHYSIOLOGY

- Periodontal diseases are caused by bacteria in dental plaque that create an inflammatory response in gingival tissues (gingivitis) or in the soft tissue and bone supporting the teeth (periodontitis).

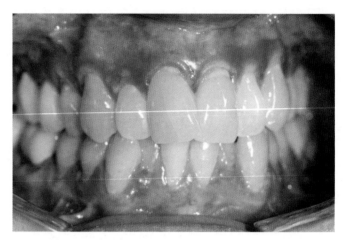

FIGURE 38-1 Chronic gingivitis in which the intradental papillae are edematous and blunted. There is some loss of gingival tissue. The gums bleed with brushing. (*Courtesy of Gerald Ferretti, DMD.*)

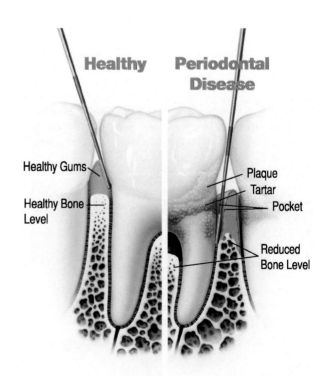

FIGURE 38-2 Healthy periodontal anatomy vs periodontal disease. (*Copyrighted by and reprinted with permission from the American Academy of Periodontology; http://www.perio.org/consumer/2a.html.*)

- The normal healthy gingival attachments form the gingival cuff around the tooth to help protect the underlying bone and teeth from the bacteria of the mouth.

- Gingivitis is caused by a reversible inflammatory process that occurs as the result of prolonged exposure of the gingival tissues to plaque and tartar (**Figure 38-2**).

- Gingivitis may be classified by appearance (e.g., ulcerative, hemorrhagic), etiology (e.g., drugs, hormones), duration (e.g., acute, chronic), or by quality (e.g., mild, moderate, or severe).

- A severe form, acute necrotizing ulcerative gingivitis (ANUG), (**Figure 38-5**) also known as Vincent's disease or trench mouth, is associated alpha-hemolytic streptococci, anaerobic fusiform bacteria, and nontreponemal oral spirochetes. The term trench mouth was coined in the World War I when ANUG was common among soldiers in the trenches. Predisposing factors now include diabetes, HIV, and chemotherapy.[2]

- Risk factors that contribute to the development of periodontal disease include poor oral hygiene, smoking, environmental factors (e.g., crowded teeth and mouth breathing), and comorbid conditions such as a weakened immune status (e.g., HIV, steroids, or diabetes) and low income.

- The most common form of gingivitis is chronic gingivitis induced by plaque (**Figure 38-1**). This type of gingivitis occurs in half of the population aged 4 years or older. The inflammation worsens as mineralized plaque forms calculus (tartar) at and below the gum surface (sulcus). The plaque that covers calculus causes destruction of bone (an irreversible condition) and loose teeth, which result in tooth mobility and tooth loss.

- Gingivitis may persist for months or years without progressing to periodontitis. This suggests that host susceptibility plays an important role in the development of periodontitis.[3]

- While common forms of periodontal disease have been associated with adverse pregnancy outcomes, cardiovascular disease, stroke, pulmonary disease, and diabetes, no causal relations have been established.[4]

DIAGNOSIS

CLINICAL FEATURES

- Simple or marginal gingivitis first cause swelling of the intradental papillae and later affect gingiva and dental interface (**Figures 38-1** to **38-4**).

- Mild gingivitis is painless and may bleed when brushing or eating hard foods.

- Acute necrotizing ulcerative gingivitis (ANUG) (**Figure 38-5**) is painful, ulcerative, and edematous and produces halitosis and bleeding gingival tissue. Patients with ANUG may have systemic symptoms such as myalgias and fever.

TYPICAL DISTRIBUTION

Gingivitis begins at the gingival and dental margins and may extend onto the alveolar ridges.

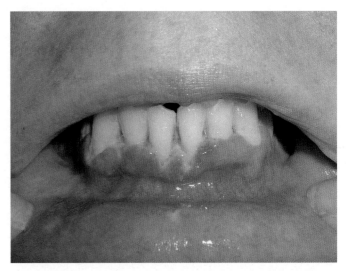

FIGURE 38-3 Severe periodontal disease in a woman who smokes and is addicted to cocaine. Note the blunting of the intradental papillae and the dramatic loss of gingival tissue. (*Courtesy of Richard P. Usatine, MD.*)

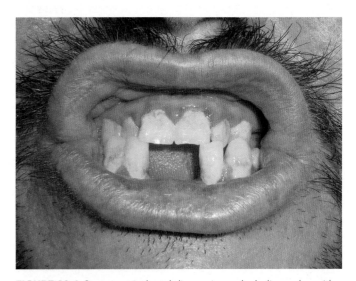

FIGURE 38-4 Severe periodontal disease in an alcoholic smoker with very edematous and blunted intradental papilla. This homeless man has already lost two teeth secondary to his severe periodontal disease. (*Courtesy of Richard P. Usatine, MD.*)

LABORATORY STUDIES AND IMAGING

The dentist will usually suggest radiographs of the mouth to evaluate for bone loss in periodontal disease.

DIFFERENTIAL DIAGNOSIS

- Gingivitis can be from poor dental hygiene only or secondary to conditions that affect the immune system such as diabetes, Addison disease, HIV, and pregnancy.
- Gingival hyperplasia is an overgrowth of the gingiva with various etiologies including medications such as calcium channel blockers, phenytoin, and cyclosporin. This can occur with or without coexisting gingivitis (see Chapter 39, Gingival Hyperplasia).

MANAGEMENT

- Recommend and teach good oral hygiene (i.e., tooth brushing at least twice a day and flossing daily). SOR **A**
- Some experts suggest that electric toothbrushes may have additional benefit over manual brushing.[2] SOR **C**
- Few poor quality studies suggest brushing followed by rinsing with chlorhexidine may be a reasonable alternative to brushing and flossing.[2] This alternative may be worth suggesting to patients who refuse to floss. SOR **C**
- Nonsteroidal anti-inflammatory drugs have been shown to speed the resolution of inflammation when teeth are being cleaned and scaled to remove plaque.[2] SOR **C**
- Avoid drugs that may precipitate gingival hyperplasia. SOR **C**
- In patients with ANUG, treatment involves antibiotics, nonsteroidal anti-inflammatory drugs, and topical 2% viscous lidocaine for pain relief. Saline rinses can help to speed resolution, and oral rinses with a hydrogen peroxide 3% solution also may be of benefit.[2] SOR **C**
- Antibiotics recommended for ANUG include Penicillin VK, erythromycin, doxycycline, and clindamycin.[2] SOR **C**
- Recommend smoking cessation for all patients who smoke. SOR **A**
- All patients should receive ongoing care from a dental professional.

PATIENT EDUCATION

- Advise the patient to use good oral hygiene (i.e., brushing twice a day and using floss daily for hard-to-reach areas).
- There is no safe level of smoking. Quitting is crucial to good health.
- Consult a dentist for regular check-ups and especially when the condition does not improve after using good oral hygiene.

FOLLOW-UP

Follow-up patients with ANUG closely. All patients need regular dental care and follow-up with their dentist.

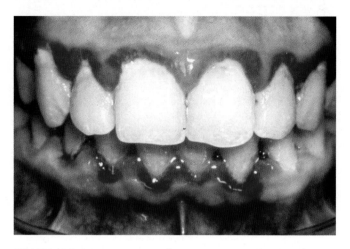

FIGURE 38-5 Acute necrotizing ulcerative gingivitis (ANUG) with intense erythema and ulcerations around the teeth. This is an acute infectious process. (*Courtesy of Gerald Ferretti, DMD.*)

PATIENT RESOURCES

MedlinePlus. Gingivitis. **http://www.nlm.nih.gov/ medlineplus/ency/article/001056.htm.** Accessed May 19, 2007.

The American Academy of Periodontology. **http://www. perio.org/consumer/2a.html.** Accessed May 19, 2007.

PROVIDER RESOURCES

Stephen J. Gingivitis. medicine. **http://www.emedicine.com/ emerg/topic217.htm.** Accessed May 19, 2007.

REFERENCES

1. Albandar JM, Brunelle JA, Kingman A. Destructive periodontal disease in adults 30 years of age and older in the united states, 1988–1994. *J Periodontol.* 1999;70:13–29.

2. Stephen J. Gingivitis. medicine. http://www.emedicine.com/ emerg/topic217.htm. Accessed May 19, 2007.

3. Kornman KS, Crane A, Wang HY, et al. The interleukin-1 genotype as a severity factor in adult periodontal disease. *J Clin Periodontol.* 1997;24:72–77.

4. Pihlstrom BL, Michalowicz BS, Johnson NW. Periodontal diseases. *Lancet.* 2005;366(9499):1809–1820.

39 GINGIVAL HYPERPLASIA

Wanda C. Gonsalves, MD
Richard P. Usatine, MD

PATIENT STORY

A 31-year-old woman with a history of seizure disorder notices increasing gum enlargement (**Figure 39-1**). She is unemployed and does not have dental insurance. She has not been to a dentist in at least 10 years. She brushes her teeth only once a day and does not floss at all. She has been on phenytoin (Dilantin) since early childhood and this does prevent her seizures. You talk to her about dental hygiene and refer her to a low-cost dental clinic that cares for persons with limited resources.

EPIDEMIOLOGY

- The prevalence of phenytoin-induced gingival hyperplasia is estimated at 15% to 50% in patients taking the medication.[1]

- The prevalence for cyclosporine transplant recipient patients is estimated at 27%.[1]

- The incidence of gingival hyperplasia has been reported as 10% to 20% in patients treated with calcium antagonists in the general population.[1]

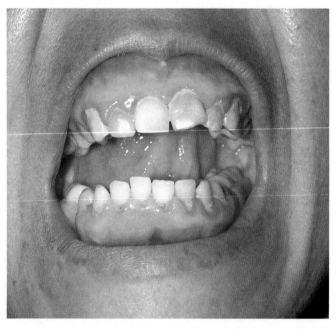

FIGURE 39-1 Gingival hyperplasia secondary to phenytoin (Dilantin) in a woman with epilepsy. (*Courtesy of Richard P. Usatine, MD.*)

ETIOLOGY AND PATHOPHYSIOLOGY

- The etiology of gingival hyperplasia or gingival overgrowth (GO) is not entirely known, however risk factors known to contribute to GO include the following: nonspecific chronic inflammation associated with poor hygiene, hormonal changes (pregnancy), medications (calcium channel blockers, phenytoin, and cyclosporin), and systemic diseases (leukemia, sarcoidosis, or Crohn's disease).

- More than 15 drugs have been shown to cause GO.

- The most common nonreversible drug-induced gingival enlargement is caused by phenytoin (**Figures 39-1** and **39-2**).[2] Severity relates to the serum concentration of phenytoin.

- Not all patients who take calcium channel blockers, phenytoin, or cyclosporine develop GO.

- Poor oral hygiene and the presence of periodontal disease are risk factors for development of GO.

- Histopathologically, tissue enlargement is the result of proliferation of fibroblasts, collagen fibers, and chronic inflammatory cells.

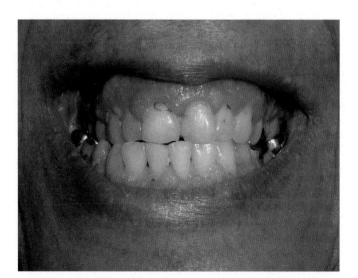

FIGURE 39-2 Multiple tiny hamartomas on the gums from Cowden's disease with gingival hyperplasia secondary to phenytoin. (*Courtesy of Richard P. Usatine, MD.*)

DIAGNOSIS

SIGNS/SYMPTOMS

- The diagnosis is made by visual inspection and obtaining a thorough history (**Figures 39-1** and **39-2**).

- The gingiva appears edematous and bulky with loss of its stippling. It may be soft or firm.

- Nonspecific chronic inflammation, hormonal and systemic causes such as leukemia appear red and inflamed and may bleed.

- Drug-induced hyperplasia looks more fibrous and noninflamed.

Typical distribution: Lobular gingiva enlargement occurs first at the interdental papillae and anterior facial gingiva approximately 2 to 3 months after starting the drug, and increases in maximum severity in 12 to 18 months.

Laboratory tests: Order a CBC to rule out anemia or leukemia.

Imaging: The periodontist or oral medicine specialist may order bitewing radiographs and periapical films to evaluate for the presence of periodontal disease.

Bite wing radiographs are the "gold standard" and are better than a Panorex film.

DIFFERENTIAL DIAGNOSIS

- Generalized gingivitis—gums around the teeth become inflamed. This condition often occurs with poor oral hygiene (see Chapter 38, Gingivitis and Periodontal Disease).

- Pregnancy gingivitis—Inflamed gums. More than half of pregnant women will develop gingivitis at some point bacause of hormonal changes.

- Pyogenic granuloma—A small red bump that may bleed and grow to approximately half an inch. These are most often found on the skin but can occur in the mouth secondary to trauma or pregnancy. When they occur in pregnancy they are sometimes called a pregnancy tumor. In reality, these are not pyogenic nor granulomatous but are a type of lobular capillary hemangioma (see Chapter 154, Pyogenic Granuloma) (**Figure 39-3**).

- Leukemia—leukemic cells may infiltrate the oral soft tissues producing a diffuse, boggy, nontender swelling that may or may not ulcerate.

MANAGEMENT

- Teach and emphasize good oral hygiene including cleanings at least every 3 months to control plaque.

- If possible, stop drugs that induce gingival hyperplasia since discontinuing the medications may reverse the condition in most cases except phenytoin.

- If drugs cannot be stopped, try reducing the dose, if possible, since gingival hyperplasia can be dose dependent.

- Try empiric antibiotic therapy with azithromycin.[1]

- Chlorhexidine 12% (Peridex) once before going to bed or Biotene mouthwash after meals is recommended for patients known to be at risk for gingivitis.[1] Warn patients that Chlorhexidine 12% will taste bad and can stain the teeth. This staining can be removed with a dental cleaning. This information should help improve adherence to the use of this mouthwash.

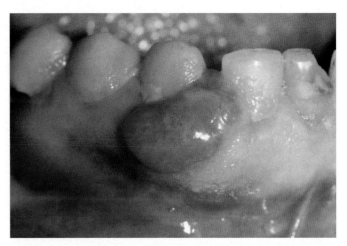

FIGURE 39-3 Pyogenic granuloma growing rapidly on the gums after minor trauma. (*Reprinted with permission from Common Oral Lesions: Part II. Copyright © 2007 American Academy of Family Physicians. All Rights Reserved. Gonsalves WC, Chi AC, Neville BW. Am Fam Phys 75(4):509–512.*)

- For patients who do not respond to the above measures, refer to dental health professional for possible gingivectomy. This can be done with a scalpel or with a laser.[1]

  All recommendations provided above are. SOR **C**

PREVENTION

Ensure healthy periodontal tissue prior to starting calcium channel blockers, phenytoin or before any organ transplantation in which cyclosporin will be prescribed.[1]

PATIENT EDUCATION

Advise patients to practice good oral hygiene (i.e., brush at least twice a day and floss at least once a day) and have regular follow-up with their dental health professional to monitor for worsening periodontal disease.

FOLLOW-UP

- Patients should be monitored by a periodontist or an oral medicine specialist as long as the patients are taking medicines that induce gingival hyperplasia.

PATIENT RESOURCES

The Merck Manual of Health and Aging. Periodontal Disease. **http://www.merck.com/pubs/mmanual_ha/sec3/ch39/ch39c.html.** Accessed April 21, 2007.

PROVIDER RESOURCES

Drug-induced Gingival Hyperplasia. **http://www.emedicine.com/derm/topic645.htm.** Accessed May 19, 2007.

REFERENCES

1. Vacharotayangul P. Drug-induced Gingival Hyperplasia. http://www.emedicine.com/derm/topic645.htm. Accessed May 19, 2007.

2. Silverstein, LH. Medication induced gingival enlargement: a clinical review. *Gen Dent*. 1997;45(4):371–376.

40 APHTHOUS ULCER

Wanda C. Gonsalves, MD

A 19-year-old woman presents with a painful sore in her mouth for almost 1 week (**Figure 40-1**). She denies fever or chills. She thinks she may have traumatized the area with a new firm toothbrush she got a few days ago. She is reassured that it is only a canker sore and some symptomatic treatments are suggested. She is also told about the benefits of using a soft bristled toothbrush and dental floss.

EPIDEMIOLOGY

- An oral ulcerative condition, also known as "canker sores."
- Reported prevalence range from 5% to 66% depending on the population studied.[1]
- Three clinical variations: Minor, major (1–3 cm), and herpetiform (<3 mm). The most common minor form appears as rounded, well-demarcated, single or multiple ulcers <1 cm in diameter that usually heal in 10 to 14 days without scarring.

ETIOLOGY/PATHOPHYSIOLOGY

- The precise etiopathogenesis of this condition remains unknown although a variety of host and environmental factors have been implicated.
- A variety of factors have been associated with recurrent aphthous stomatitis (RAS), including certain foods (milk sensitivity), medications (NSAIDs), vitamin deficiencies (zinc, iron, B_{12}, folate), environmental factors (trauma, stress), viruses (HSV, HIV), and systemic diseases (Celiac and Behçets) have been studied.[2,3]

DIAGNOSIS

CLINICAL FEATURES

- Recurring, painful, solitary or multiple ulcers, typically covered by a white to yellow pseudomembrane and surrounded by an erythematous halo (**Figure 40-2**).
- Symptoms may begin with a burning or pricking sensation. Lesions are never preceded by vesicles.
- The pain is exacerbated by moving the area affected by the ulcer.

Typical distribution: RAS usually involves nonkeratinizing mucosa (e.g., labial mucosa, buccal mucosa, ventral tongue).

Laboratory tests: Order CBC, ferritin, B_{12}, folate, ESR, viral culture, KOH, skin biopsy, or HIV testing if indicated.

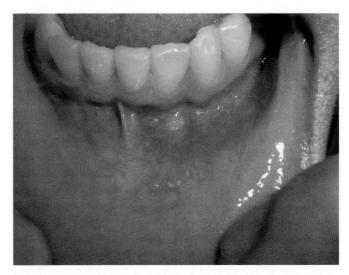

FIGURE 40-1 Small aphthous ulcer (canker sore) lingual mucosa. (*Courtesy of Richard P. Usatine, MD.*)

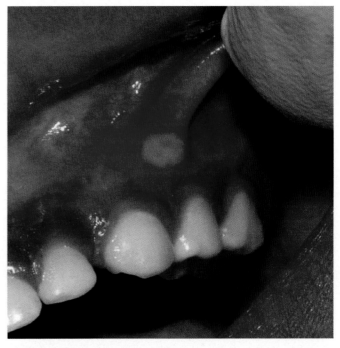

FIGURE 40-2 Aphthous ulcer located on *unkeratinized* (movable) mucosa in a 5 year-old girl. It is slightly raised, round, with a white-yellow necrotic center and an erythematous halo. (*Courtesy of Ellen Eisenberg, DMD.*)

DIFFERENTIAL DIAGNOSIS

- Herpes simplex virus (acute gingivostomatitis)—primary HSV infection that begins as vesicular yellow lesions, which quickly ulcerate accompanied by systemic manifestations such as fever, malaise, anorexia, and sore throat located on movable and nonmovable oral mucosa. Lesions may also appear on keratinized surfaces such as the lip (see Chapter 123, Herpes Simplex).

- Candidiasis—white plaque, when removed appear red with associated burning sensation (see Chapter 130, Mucocutaneous Candidiasis).

- Oral Cancer—ulcerative lesion that will not resolve by 2 weeks (see Chapter 42, Oral Cancer).

- Erythema multiforme—mucocutaneous lesion preceded by infection of HSV, mycoplasma pneumoniae, or exposure to certain drugs or medications. Oral lesions begin as patches and evolve into large shallow erosions and ulcerations with irregular borders. Common sites include the lip, tongue, buccal mucosa, floor of the mouth, and soft palate (see Chapter 170, Erythema Multiforme).

- Erosive lichen planus—erythematous ulcerative lesion with surrounding striae (see Chapter 147, Lichen Planus).

- Contact dermatitis—Acute or chronic forms that may resemble vesicular lesions that rapidly rupture. Lesions may appear white or erythematous and give a burning sensation.

- Behçet's syndrome—a condition with multiple ulcerative lesions that resemble aphthae involving the soft palate and oropharynx, infrequent sites for routine aphthae. Common cutaneous lesions include the genital and ocular mucosa (**Figure 40-3**).

- Hand, foot and mouth disease presents as mucocutaneous lesions involving the hand, foot, and mouth caused by enterovirus. Oral lesions resemble herpangina and may number up to 30. Any area of mucosa may be involved. Lesions resolve within 1 week (see Chapter 122, Hand, Foot and Mouth Disease).

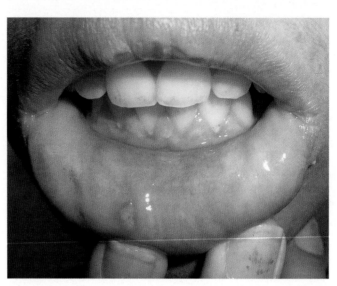

FIGURE 40-3 Behçet's disease characterized by recurrent oral and genital ulcers in a 17-year-old girl. (*Courtesy of Richard P. Usatine, MD.*)

MANAGEMENT

- Most require no treatment or only periodic topical therapy.

- Corticosteroids such as fluocinonide gel or dexamethasone elixir can promote healing and lessen the severity of RAS.[4] Patients should be instructed to dab the area of ulcer dry, apply the gel, paste, or cream after rinsing, and to avoid eating or drinking for at least 30 minutes. SOR **C**

- In severe cases, systemic therapy with thalidomide, colchicine, pentoxifylline, or azathioprine may be necessary.[5] SOR **C**

PATIENT EDUCATION

Recurrent lesions that do not respond to treatment, or severe cases should be seen by their oral health provider or primary care physician to look for an underlying cause. Foods that are spicy or acidic worsen pain and should be avoided.

PATIENT RESOURCES

MedicineNet.com. Canker sores (aphthous ulcers). **http://www.medicinenet.com/canker_sores/article.htm.** Accessed April 7, 2007.

PROVIDER RESOURCES

Dermnet NZ. Aphthous ulcers. **http://www.dermnetnz.org/site-age-specific/aphthae.html.**

Douglass A, Gonsalves W, Maier R, Silk H, Tysinger J, Wrightson S. Smiles for life: A national oral health curriculum for family medicine. **http://www.stfm.org/oralhealth/.** Accessed April 7, 2007.

National Center for Chronic Disease Prevention and Health Promotion. Oral health: Preventing cavities, gum disease, and tooth loss. **http://www.cdc.gov/nccdphp/publications/aag/oh.htm.** Accessed April 7, 2007.

World Health Organization. Oral Health. **http://www.who.int/oral_health/en/.** Accessed April 7, 2007.

REFERENCES

1. Neville BW, Damm DD, Allen CM, Bouqout JE. Recurrent aphthous stomatitis (Recurrent aphthous ulcerations, canker sores). In: *Oral & Maxillofacial Pathology*. Philadelphia: WB Saunders Company, 2002:285–290.

2. Natah S, Konttinen Y, Enattah N, et al. Recurrent aphthous ulcers today: A review of the growing knowledge. *Int J Oral Maxillofac Surg.* 2004;33:221–232.

3. Gonsalves W, Chi A, Neville B. Common Oral Lesions: Part 1. Superficial Mucosal Lesions. *AFP* 2007;75:501–507.

4. Casiglia JM. Recurrent aphthous stomatitis: Etiology, diagnosis and treatment. *Gen Dent.* 2002;50:157–166.

5. University of Texas at Austin, School of Nursing, Family Nurse Practitioner Program. Recommendations for the diagnosis and management of recurrent aphthous stomatitis. National Guideline Clearinghouse. http://www.guideline.gov. Accessed April 7, 2007.

41 LEUKOPLAKIA

Wanda C. Gonsalves, MD

PATIENT STORY

A 57-year-old male smoker presents at the physician's clinic with a 7-month history of a nonpainful white patch below his tongue. He admits to drinking two to three beers in the evening and smokes 1 pack per day. Your examination reveals a painless white, thick lesion with fissuring below the tongue (**Figure 41-1**). A biopsy shows this to be premalignant and the patient is told that he must stop smoking and drinking. He is also referred to an oral surgeon for further evaluation of the leukoplakia.

EPIDEMIOLOGY

- Leukoplakia occurs in 1% to 8% of adults and is most frequently seen in middle-aged and older men.[1,2]
- The World Health Organization defines leukoplakia as "a white patch or plaque that cannot be characterized clinically or pathologically as any other disease."[3]

ETIOLOGY AND PATHOPHYSIOLOGY

- Leukoplakia may be a premalignant change with an estimated malignant transformation potential of 4% lifetime risk.[2]
- Cause is unknown, however, it is frequently in smokers, but it may occur in nonsmokers. The lesions may be white (leukoplakia), red (erythroplakia), or combination of red and white (speckled leukoplakia) (**Figures 41-1 to 41-3**).[4]
- Alcohol has a strong synergistic effect with tobacco.[2]
- Biopsies have shown that erythroplakia and speckled leukoplakia are more likely than other types of leukoplakia to undergo malignant transformation with more severe epithelial dysplasia.[1]
- The determination of malignant transformation requires incisional biopsy.

DIAGNOSIS

CLINICAL FEATURES

- Precancer and early oral cancer can be subtle and asymptomatic.
- The lesions may be white, red, a combination of red and white (called speckled leukoplakia or erythroleukoplakia) depending on the degree of hyperkeratosis or epithelial atrophy, or warty (verrucous leukoplakia). The lesions cannot be removed with a gauze swab. Lesions first appear as a slightly elevated grayish-white plaque that later becomes thicker and whiter.[2] Lesions induced by smokeless tobacco are characterized by a wrinkled surface that ranges from opaque white to translucent and are located in the area where the tobacco (e.g., snuff) is held.

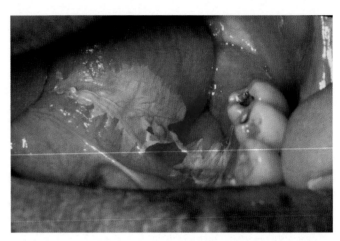

FIGURE 41-1 Leukoplakia showing white patch below tongue. (*Courtesy of Brad Neville, MD.*)

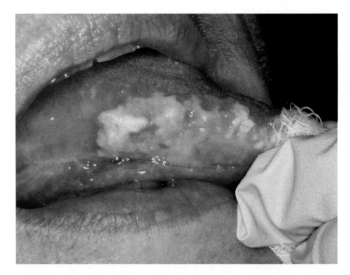

FIGURE 41-2 Leukoplakia with moderate dysplasia on the lateral border of the tongue of a 65 year-old woman with a long history of smoking. She presented with discomfort and a noticeable white plaque on her tongue and a biopsy proved this to be moderate dysplasia. This was the third white dysplastic lesion she had excised in this area. A new excision was performed and close follow-up is needed. Even though she quit smoking a few years ago, the damage done has led to a relentless dysplastic process. (*Courtesy of Ellen Eisenberg, DMD.*)

TYPICAL DISTRIBUTION

The lesions occur most often on the tongue, floor of mouth, and lower lip vermilion.

LABORATORY

Perform a biopsy to determine if a lesion is malignant.

DIFFERENTIAL DIAGNOSIS

- Frictional keratoses—hyperkeratotic lesions that result from chronic cheek chewing or occur when exposed edentulous sites are irritated during chewing.
- Nicotine stomatitis—hyperkeratotic epithelial changes on the hard palate that result from prolonged cigar smoking or cigarette smoking (**Figure 41-4**).
- Tobacco pouch keratoses—patches that appear wrinkled and grayish-white appearing patches that are usually located in the buccal or labial vestibule where tobacco is held.

MANAGEMENT

- Always biopsy leukoplakia in a patient with a history of tobacco use to determine the presence of epithelia dysplasia, carcinoma in situ, or squamous cell carcinoma.[5] SOR C
- Mild or moderate dysplasia may reverse if the patient stops using tobacco. However, lesions found to be severe dysplasia or carcinoma in situ have a low potential for reversal and should be managed by complete surgical excision.[6] SOR C
- If all physicians and dentists would do a thorough intraoral examination, more oral cancers would be found in the leukoplakia and dysplastic stages than in the more advanced stages in which they are typically found.

PATIENT EDUCATION

- Counsel patients who use tobacco (e.g., smoke or smokeless tobacco) to quit. Ask if they are ready to quit at each visit, and sign a contract with them that specifies the date and time they will quit. Provide tools (see "Patient Resources") they can use to quit.

FOLLOW-UP

Monitor patients who have lesions surgically removed for recurrence.

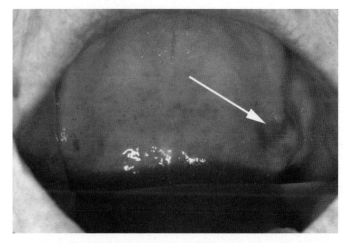

FIGURE 41-3 Erythroplakia with red patch on the upper alveolar ridge of an edentulous person. (*Courtesy of Gerald Ferritti, DMD.*)

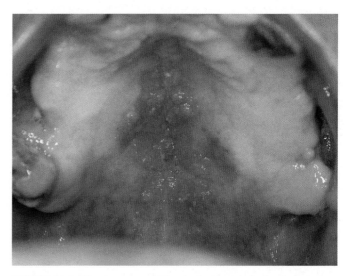

FIGURE 41-4 Nicotine stomatitis typically seen on the hard palate. (*From Rizzolo D, Chiodo TA. Photo Rounds: Lesion on the hard palate. J Fam Pract 2008;57(1):33–35, Dowden Health Media.*)

REFERENCES

1. Mashberg A, Samit A. Early diagnosis of asymptomatic oral and oropharyngeal squamous cancers. *CA Cancer J Clin.* 1995;45: 328–351.

2. Neville BW, Damm DD, Allen CM, et al. *Oral and Maxillofacial Pathology*, 2nd ed. Philadephia, PA: Saunders, 2002:337–369.

3. Kramer IR, Lucas RB, Pindborg JJ, Sobin LH. Definition of leuko- plakia and related lesions: An aid to studies on oral precancer. *Oral Surg Oral Med Oral Pathol.* 1978;46(4):518–539.

4. Salonen L, Axell T, Hellden L. Occurrence of oral mucosal lesions, the influence of tobacco habits and an estimate of treatment time in an adult Swedish population. *J Oral Pathol Med.* 1990;19:170–176.

5. Truman Bl, Gooch BF, Sulemana I, et al. Reviews of evidence on interventions to prevent dental caries, oral and pharyngeal cancers, and sport-related craniofacial injuries. *Am J Pre Med.* 2002;231 (1 suppl):21–54.

6. Mirbod S, Ahing S. Tobacco-associated lesions of the oral cavity: Part 1. Nonmalignant lesions. *J Can Dent Assoc.* 2000;66:252–256.

42 ORAL CANCER

Wanda C. Gonsalves, MD

PATIENT STORY

A 66-year-old man presents to the physician's office with a nonhealing painful lesion on the roof of his mouth (**Figure 42-1**). The lesion has increased in size recently and he is worried because his dad died from oral cancer. Your patient has smoked since he was 11 years old by getting cigarettes from his dad. He admits to being a heavy drinker. A biopsy shows squamous cell carcinoma and the patient is referred to a head and neck surgeon.

EPIDEMIOLOGY

- In the United States, cancers of the oral cavity and oropharynx are the ninth most common cancer, accounting for approximately 3% of malignancies among men and 2% of malignancies among women.[1,2]

- The prevalence of these cancers increases with age and approximately 90% of oral cancers are squamous cell carcinomas.[1] African American males have the highest incidence rate of oral cancer, 20.5 cases out of 100,000 versus 9.7 cases out of 100,000,[2] except for cancers of the lip vermilion that occur primarily in white men.[3]

ETIOLOGY AND PATHOPHYSIOLOGY

- Tobacco use and heavy alcohol consumption are the two principal risk factors for 75% of oral cancers. The other 25% results from nutrimental and genetic factors.[2]

- Other risk factors associated with oral cancer include: betel quid chewing, human papillomavirus, low intake of fruits and vegetables, lichen planus, and iron deficiency anemia in combination with dysphagia and esophageal webs (Plummer–Vinson syndrome).[4]

DIAGNOSIS

CLINICAL FEATURES

- Lesions begin as a thin white or red patch, progress to a superficial ulceration of the mucosal surface (**Figure 42-1**), and later become an endophytic or exophytic growth (**Figures 42-3** and **41-4**). Some lesions are solitary lumps.

- Early oral cancer and the more common precancerous lesions (leukoplakia) are subtle and asymptomatic. Larger, advanced cancers may be painful and may erode underlying tissue (**Figures 42-1 to 42-4**).

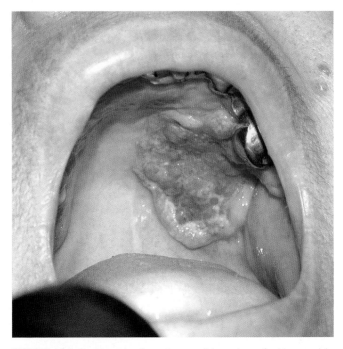

FIGURE 42-1 Squamous cell carcinoma of the palate of a 66-year-old man who smokes and drinks. (*Courtesy of Frank Miller, MD.*)

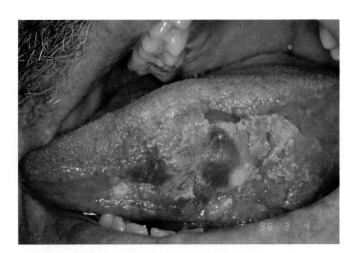

FIGURE 42-2 Squamous cell carcinoma on the lateral side of the tongue. This is a broad erythroleukoplakic mass with surface ulcerations. (*Courtesy of Ellen Eisenberg, DMD.*)

- Squamous cell carcinoma (SCC) is commonly found on the lower lip secondary to sun exposure. However, cigar smokers may get SCC on the inner lip (**Figure 42-5**).

- While melanoma is rare inside the mouth it can be seen in this location. In **Figure 42-6** it is found arising from the palate. Even a basal cell carcinoma can develop inside the mouth (**Figure 42-7**).

- Patients with lesions presenting on the lateral soft palate and tonsillar region may complain of dysphagia, odynophagia, and otalgia.

TYPICAL DISTRIBUTION

These cancers occur most commonly (in order of frequency) on the tongue, floor of mouth, and lower lip vermilion. The horseshoe-shaped region (lateral tongue extending to the lateral soft palate and tonsillar area) has the greatest risk of developing cancer.[4] Sixty percent of oral carcinomas are advanced by the time they are detected, and approximately 15% of patients will have another cancer in a nearby area as the larynx, esophagus, or lungs.[4]

LABORATORY AND IMAGING

CT scan with contrast and MRI have been used for staging.

DIFFERENTIAL DIAGNOSIS

- Tobacco-associated lesions (including frictional keratoses, nicotine stomatitis, tobacco pouch keratoses, and leukoplakia)—white hyperkeratotic lesions that result from chronic cheek chewing or occur when exposed edentulous sites are irritated during chewing.

- Hairy leukoplakia—may appear as a faint white vertical keratotic streak, typically on the lateral side of the tongue (see Chapter 36, black Hairy Tongue).

- Geographic tongue–well delineated, shiny and smooth, erythematous spots surrounded by a white halo, typically on the anterior two thirds of the dorsal tongue mucosa (see Chapter 37, Geographic Tongue).

- Candidiasis—white plaque typically found on the buccal mucosa, tongue, and palate when remove has an erythematous base (see Chapter 130, Mucocutaneous Candidiasis).

MANAGEMENT

- Evaluate any persistent red or white lesion in the mouth if it is present longer than 2 weeks.[5] SOR **C**

- A computer-assisted oral brush biopsy technique called Oral CDX has been shown to differentiate premalignant from malignant changes.[6,7] SOR **A** This method is not as definitive as a real biopsy. If you see a suspicious lesion, then it is best to do a shave or a punch biopsy and send it for histology. If this is out of your scope of practice, refer the patient to an oral surgeon.

PATIENT EDUCATION

Advise patients to discontinue smoking and/or drinking alcohol.

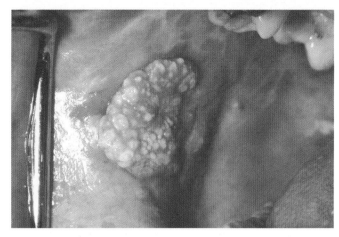

FIGURE 42-3 Squamous cell carcinoma arising on the buccal mucosa. (*Courtesy of Gerald Ferritti, DDS.*)

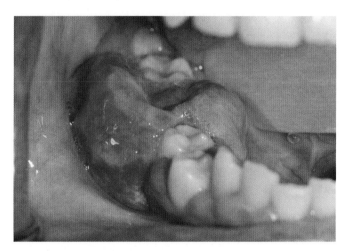

FIGURE 42-4 Exophytic cancer of the mouth. (*Courtesy of Gerald Ferritti, DDS.*)

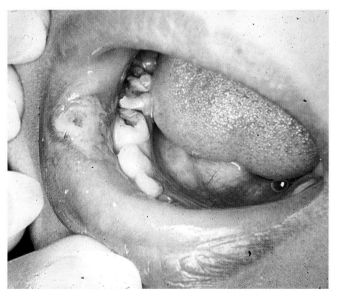

FIGURE 42-5 Squamous cell carcinoma of the lip inner lip in a cigar smoker. (*Courtesy of Gerald Ferritti, DDS.*)

FOLLOW-UP

Perform regular oral examinations and monitor patients for recurrent lesions.

PATIENT RESOURCES

The Oral Cancer Foundation. **http://www.oralcancer foundation.org/.** Accessed April 15, 2007.

Centers for Disease Control and Prevention, National Oral Health Surveillance System. **http://www.cdc.gov/nohss/ guideCP.htm.** Accessed April 15, 2007.

PROVIDER RESOURCES

The Oral Cancer Foundation. **http://www.oralcancer foundation.org/.** Accessed April 15, 2007.

National Cancer Institute. Lip and Oral Cavity Cancer (PDQ®): Treatment. **http://www.cancer.gov/cancertopics/pdq/ treatments/lip-and-oral-cavity/healthprofessional/** Accessed April 15, 2008.

http://www.emedicine.com/derm/topic565.htm# section~Clinical.

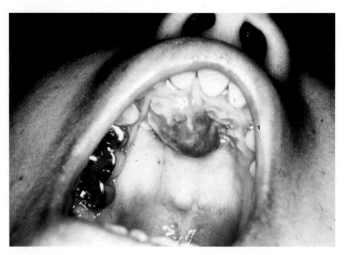

FIGURE 42-6 Malignant melanoma arising from the palate. (*Courtesy of Gerald Ferritti, DDS.*)

REFERENCES

1. Jemal A, Murray T, Ward E, et al. Cancer statistics. *CA Cancer J Clin.* 2005;55:10–30.

2. Silverman SJ. Demographics and occurrence of oral and pharyngeal cancers. The outcomes, the trends, the challenge. *J Am Dent Assoc.* 2001;132: 7S–11S.

3. Neville BW, Damm DD, Allen CM, Bouqout JE. *Oral and Maxillofacial Pathology.* Philadelphia: WB Saunders. 2002:337–369.

4. Weinberg MA, Estefan DJ. Assessing oral malignancies. *Am Fam Physician.* 2002;65:1379–1384.

5. Truman BL, Gooch Bf, Sulemana I, et al. Reviews of evidence on interventions to prevent dental caries, oral and pharyngeal cancers, and sports-related craniofacial injuries. *Am J Prev Med.* 2002;231 (1 supp l):21–54.

6. Neville B, Day T. Oral cancer and precancerous lesions. *CA Cancer J Clin.* 2002;52(4):195–215.

7. Sciubba JJ. Improving detection of precancerous and cancerous oral lesions. Computer-assisted analysis of the oral brush biopsy. U.S. collaborative oral CDX study group. *J Am Dent Assoc.* 1999; 130(10):1445–1457.

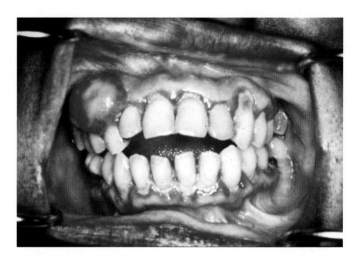

FIGURE 42-7 Basal cell carcinoma in the mouth. (*Courtesy of Gerald Ferritti, DDS.*)

43 EARLY CHILDHOOD CARIES

Wanda C. Gonsalves, MD

PATIENT STORY

A mother brings her 18-month-old son to the physician's clinic for his well-child examination. He is almost weaned from his bottle, but still drinks from a bottle to go to sleep. During the day, he uses a sippy cup to drink everything, from milk to soda. His mother has started giving him apple juice in the bottle instead of milk, since he tends to get constipated. On performing an oral examination, the physician notices that several of his teeth have "white spots" (**Figure 43-1**). The physician discusses dental hygiene and treats him with topical fluoride gel.

EPIDEMIOLOGY

- Early Childhood Caries [ECC] (tooth decay) is the single most common chronic childhood disease. It is five times more common than asthma and seven times more common than hay fever among children 5 to 7 years of age.[1]

- Tooth decay affects more than 25% of U.S. children from ages 2 to 5 years and about half of those aged 12 to 15.

- Disparities in oral health exist—32% of Mexican American and 27% of non-Hispanic black children aged 2 to 11 years had untreated decay in their primary teeth, compared to 18% of non-Hispanic white children.[3]

- ECC is defined as "the presence of one or more decayed (noncavitated or cavitated lesions), missing (due to caries), or filled tooth surfaces in any primary tooth in a child 71 months of age or younger (**Figures 43-2 to 43-4**)."[4]

- Consequences of ECC include the following: poor self-esteem, diminished physical development, decreased ability to learn, higher risk of new caries, and added cost.[4]

ETIOLOGY AND PATHOPHYSIOLOGY

- Dental caries is a multifactorial, infectious, communicable disease caused by the demineralization of tooth enamel (**Figure 43-1**) in the presence of a sugar substrate and acid-forming cariogenic bacteria, *Streptococcus mutans* (also known as *mutans streptococci*), which is considered to be the primary strain causing decay that are found in the soft gelatinous biofilm.

- Caries can develop at any time after tooth eruption. Early teeth are principally susceptible to caries caused by the transmission of *Streptococcus mutans* from the mouth of the caregiver or sibling(s) to the mouth of the infant or toddler. This type of tooth decay is called baby bottle tooth decay, nursing bottle caries, or ECC.

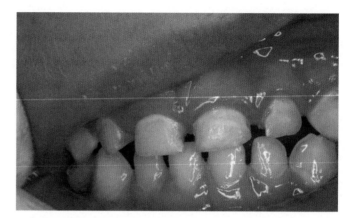

FIGURE 43-1 Demineralization at gingiva margins characterized by whitish discolorations. (*Courtesy of Gerald Ferretti, DMD.*)

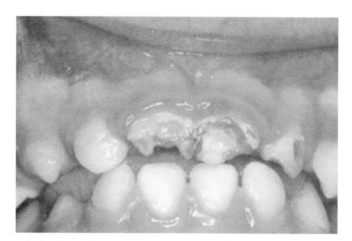

FIGURE 43-2 Central maxillary incisors with severe tooth decay, and bilateral maxillary lateral incisors with demineralized area near gingival line (yellow–brownish discolorations). The upper incisors are often the first teeth involved in nursing bottle caries. (*Courtesy of Gerald Ferretti, DMD.*)

- Risk factors for caries development include:
  - Frequent consumption of liquids.
  - Repetitive use of a "sippy cup" containing sugars (juice, milk, formula, soda).
  - Consumption of sticky foods.
  - Nursing ad lib or sleeping with a bottle, a caregiver with caries.
  - Drinking nonfluoridated community water or bottled water which is most often lacking in flouride.
  - Low socioeconomic status.
  - Taking medications that contain sugar or cause dryness and poor oral hygiene.

DIAGNOSIS

CLINICAL FEATURES

- Demineralized areas develop on the tooth surfaces, between teeth, and on pits and fissures. These areas are painless and appear clinically as opaque or brown spots (**Figure 43-1**).
- Infection allowed to progress forms a cavity that can spread to and through the dentin (the component of the tooth located below the enamel) and to the pulp (composed of nerves and blood vessels; an infection of the pulp is called pulpitis) causing pain, necrosis, and, perhaps, an abscess.

TYPICAL DISTRIBUTION

Demineralized (white or brown spots) and carious lesions generally occur at the margins of the gingiva upper incisors, and later first and second molars in pits and grooves of occlusal surfaces. Lower incisors are rarely affected.

LABORATORY AND IMAGING

Demineralized lesions may not be seen on radiographs, but advanced carious lesions between and on the occlusal surfaces are detected by x-ray.

DIFFERENTIAL DIAGNOSIS

- Developmental defects or pits—the tooth surface has defects (e.g., enamel that noticeably varies in thickness) or visible grooves.

MANAGEMENT

- Counsel patients about the importance of good oral hygiene practices and perform a caries risk assessment during well-child examination visits.[5,6] SOR **B**
- Refer to the dental health professional for the application of pit and fissure sealants.[5,6] SOR **B**
- Before prescribing supplemental fluoride, the primary care provider must determine the fluoride concentration in the child's primary source of drinking water. If fluoridated water is not available in the community, natural sources of fluoride are well water exposed to fluorite minerals and certain fruits and vegetables grown in soil irrigated with fluoridated water.[7] SOR **A**

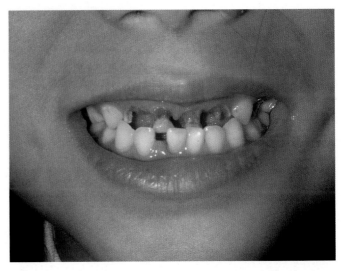

FIGURE 43-3 Severe early childhood caries in a 4-year-old with severe decay of all 4 maxillary incisors. (*Courtesy of Richard P. Usatine, MD.*)

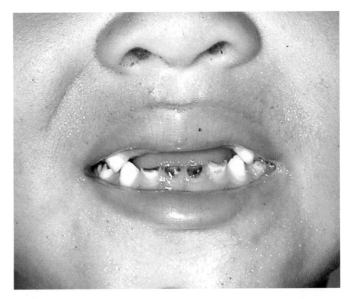

FIGURE 43-4 Severe Early Childhood Caries in a 3-year-old with multiple area of cavitary lesions involving the mandibular incisors and missing maxillary incisors secondary to decay. (*Courtesy of Richard P. Usatine, MD.*)

TABLE 43-1 Supplemental Fluoride Dosage Schedule

	Concentration of Fluoride in Water		
Age	<0.3 ppm F	0.3–0.6 ppm F	>0.6 ppm F
Birth to 6 mo	0	0	0
6 mo to 3 yr	0.25 mg	0	0
3–6 yr	0.50 mg	0.25 mg	0
6 yr to at least 16 yr	1.00 mg	0.50 mg	0

Source: The Guideline on Fluoride Therapy (2008 revision) is Copyright © 2007–08 by the American Academy of Pediatric Dentistry and is reproduced with their permission.

- Fluoride supplementation is not recommended for use by persons who live in communities whose water is optimally fluoridated (0.7–1.2 ppm or > 0.6 mg/L). See **Table 43-1** for fluoride supplementation.[7] SOR **A**

- Advice the caregiver to take the child to a dentist by age one.[6] SOR **C**

- Application of fluoride varnishes twice per year in moderate to high-risk children have been shown to prevent caries in demineralized enamel.[8] SOR **A**

PATIENT EDUCATION[6]

- Give the child's caregiver anticipatory guidance that is appropriate to the child's age and dental development. Before the teeth erupt, the caregiver should use a wash cloth or cotton gauze to clean a baby's mouth and to transition the child to tooth brushing.

- The caregiver should brush the child's teeth until the child is capable of doing an adequate job (usually around age 7 years) and should discourage children less than 3 years old from using fluoridated dentifrices because of the risk that the child may swallow toothpaste during brushing.

- A pea-sized amount of toothpaste is recommended for brushing. Educate caregivers about the benefits of fluoride and fluorosis, and the possible side effects of using too much fluoride.

- Advise caregivers to teach the child to drink from a "sippy cup" as soon as possible and to avoid giving the child milk, juice, or soda in either a bottle or sippy cup when putting the child to bed.

- Advise moms to avoid breastfeeding the child while going to sleep because it provides an excellent environment for caries-causing bacteria to grow and destroy the teeth.

FOLLOW-UP

Insure that any child whose teeth has "white spots" or visible caries taken to a dentist for evaluation and treatment so the teeth can be saved from decay or repaired.

PATIENT RESOURCES

American Academy of Pediatrics. Baby bottle tooth decay. **http://www.aap.org/pubed/ZZZKBW52R7C.htm? &sub_cat=11.** Accessed April 20, 2007.

Centers for Disease Control and Prevention. Brush up on healthy teeth. **http://www.cdc.gov/OralHealth/pdfs/Brush UpPoster.pdf.** Accessed April 20, 2007.

Douglass JM, Douglass AB, Silk HJ. Your baby's teeth. *Am Fam Physician.* 2004;70:2121. **http://www.aafp.org/afp/ 20041201/2121ph.html.** Accessed April 20, 2007.

PROVIDER RESOURCES

American Academy of Pediatric Dentistry. **http:// www.aapd.org/.** Accessed April 20, 2007.

Centers for Disease Control and Prevention. Oral Health: Preventing Cavities, Gum Disease, and Tooth Loss at a Glance 2007. **http://www.cdc.gov/nccdphp/publications/ AAG/oh.htm.** Accessed April 20, 2007.

Douglass A, Gonsalves W, Maier R, Silk H, Stevens N, Tysinger J, Wrightson AS (The Society of Teachers of Family Medicine Group on Oral Health Steering Committee). Smiles for Life: A National Oral Health Curriculum for Family Medicine. **http://www. stfm.org/oralhealth/ or http://www.fmdri.org/140.** Accessed April 20, 2007.

US Department of Health and Human Services, Oral health in America: A report of the Surgeon General-Executive Summary. Rockville, MD: US Department of Health and Human Services, National Institute of Dental and Craniofacial Research, National Institutes of Health, 2000. **http://www.nidr.nih.gov/sgr/ execsumm.htm.** Accessed March 16, 2007.

REFERENCES

1. US Department of Health and Human Services, Oral Health in America: A Report of the Surgeon General-Executive Summary. Rockville, MD: US Department of Health and Human Services, National Institute of Dental and Craniofacial Research, National Institutes of Health, 2000. http://www.nidr.nih.gov/sgr/ execsumm.htm. Accessed March 16, 2007.

2. Centers for Disease Control and Prevention. Oral health: Preventing cavities, gum disease, and tooth loss at a glance 2007. http://www.cdc.gov/nccdphp/publications/AAG/oh.htm. Accessed April 20, 2007.

3. Centers for Disease Control and Prevention. Oral health resources: New report finds improvements in oral health of Americans. http://www.cdc.gov/oralhealth/pressreleases/improvements.htm. Accessed June 2, 2007.

4. American Academy of Pediatric Dentistry, Council on Clinical Affairs. Definition of early childhood caries (ECC). 2006–07 *Definitions, Oral Health Policies, and Clinical Guidelines* (Revised 2003). http://www.aapd.org/media/Policies_Guidelines/D_ECC.pdf. Accessed April 19, 2007.

5. National Institutes of Health, Consensus Development Conference Statement, March 26–28, 2001. Diagnosis and Management of Dental Caries Throughout Life. Originally published as: Diagnosis and Management of Dental Caries Throughout Life. NIH Consensus Statement 2001 March 26–28; 18(1): 1–24. http://consensus. nih.gov/2001/2001DentalCaries115html.htm. Accessed April 20, 2007.

6. American Academy of Pediatric Dentistry, Clinical Affairs Committee – Infant Oral Health Subcommittee. Guideline on Infant Oral Health Care. http://www.aapd.org/media/Policies_ Guidelines/G_InfantOralHealthCare.pdf. Accessed April 20, 2007.

7. American Academy of Pediatric Dentistry, Liaison with Other Groups Committee, Council on Clinical Affairs. *Guideline on Fluoride Therapy*, p. 90. http://www.aapd.org/media/Policies_ Guidelines/G_FluorideTherapy.pdf. Accessed April 19, 2007.

8. Adair SM. Evidence base use of fluoride in contemporary pediatric dental medicine. *Ped Dent.* 2006;28(2):133–142 discussion 192–198.

44 ADULT DENTAL CARIES

Wanda C. Gonsalves, MD

PATIENT STORY

A 41-year-old homeless man presents to a clinic on "skid row" with a toothache (**Figure 44-1**). He has a history of alcoholism and smoking. Many of his teeth are loose and a number of his teeth have fallen out in the last year. He acknowledges that he does not floss or brush his teeth regularly. He has been sober for 60 days now and wants help to get his teeth fixed. He states that no one will hire him with his teeth as they are. He also has pain in a molar and wants something for the pain until he can see a dentist. On oral examination, you see missing teeth, generalized plaque, and teeth with multiple brown caries.

EPIDEMIOLOGY

- Many adults (e.g., 27% of those 20 to 39 years, 21% of those 40 to 59 years, and 19% of those 60 years and older) have untreated dental caries[1] (**Figure 44-1**) and two-thirds of adults aged 35 to 44 have lost at least one permanent tooth to dental caries.[2]

- In the older adult population, the percentage of teeth free of caries and restorations declined from 10.6% to 7.9% in those aged 55 to 64 years and from 9.6% to 6.5% in those aged 65 to 74 years.

- Many older adults suffer from root caries (decay on the roots of their teeth) (**Figure 44-2**). The percentage of adults with root caries increased with age: 9% of adults aged 20 to 39 years had root decay, compared with 18% of adults aged 40 to 59 years and 32% of adults 60 years and older.[1]

- Twice as many current smokers (28%) as nonsmokers (14%) had root caries.[1]

ETIOLOGY AND PATHOPHYSIOLOGY

- Dental caries result from the activity of dental bacterial plaque, a complex biofilm containing microorganisms that demineralize and proteolyse tooth enamel and dentin through their action on the fermentation of sucrose and other sugars. The main organism is *Streptococcus mutans*. When plaque is not removed regularly, it may calcify forming calculus (tartar).

- The risk factors for adult caries include the following[3]:
  - Physical and medical disabilities.
  - The presence of existing restorations or oral appliances.
  - Patients with Sjögren's syndrome.
  - Medications that decrease saliva flow (tricyclic antidepressants).
  - Illicit drugs such as methamphetamine and cocaine that also dry the mouth.
  - Radiation to the head and neck.
  - Gingival recession.
  - Low socioeconomic status with limited or no access to medical or dental care.

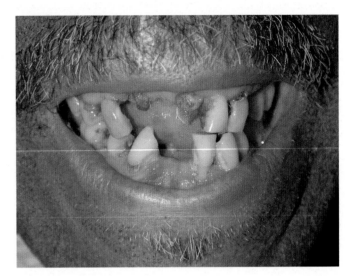

FIGURE 44-1 Severe caries in a homeless man. (*Courtesy of Richard P. Usatine, MD.*)

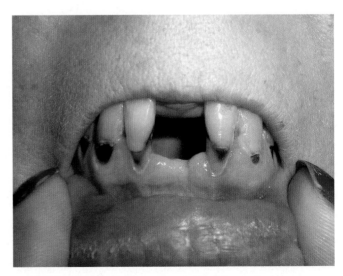

FIGURE 44-2 Root caries in a woman with a history of substance abuse. She has lost all of her upper teeth and is beginning to lose her lower teeth. Note the exposed and darkened roots. (*Courtesy of Richard P. Usatine, MD.*)

DIAGNOSIS

CLINICAL FEATURES

- Dental caries initially present as a painless white spot (demineralization of enamel) and progress to a brownish discoloration with cavitation through the dentin, where nonlocalized pain is produced upon exposure to heat, cold, or sweats. The pain subsides with removal of the stimulus. As the infection progresses to the pulp (pulpitis), the pain may be severe and persistent. If untreated, pulp necrosis and dental abscess may occur.

TYPICAL DISTRIBUTION

Any enamel or exposed dentin surface, including occlusal, interproximal, and root surfaces.

LABORATORY AND IMAGING

An x-ray will show cavities, but not demineralized areas.

DIFFERENTIAL DIAGNOSIS

- Trauma—usually involves maxillary incisors common in sports, accidents, violence, and epilepsy.
- Tooth erosion—results from consumption of carbonated beverages and fruit drinks, repeated vomiting associated with eating disorders, gastroesophageal reflux, and alcoholism.
- Tooth attrition—wearing down of teeth because of tooth grinding (bruxism) or an abrasive diet. Brushing with a hard brush and using abrasive toothpaste may also cause attrition.
- Bulimia can cause destruction of the teeth because of the gastric acids (**Figure 44-3**).

MANAGEMENT

- Demineralized lesions ("white spots") and caries—topical fluorides such as varnishes (2% NaF; 9040 ppm) that are applied by dental health providers or the primary care physician twice a year have been shown to decrease dental caries by 21%.[4] SOR Ⓐ
- Fluoride mouth rinses (0.2% NaF) are effective in controlling caries when used daily.[4] SOR Ⓐ
- Refer to a dental health professional for sealant treatment of pits and fissures.[5] SOR Ⓒ
- Refer patients with "white spots" and dental caries to a dental professional for treatment and/or restoration.[3] SOR Ⓒ
- Patients with xerostomia (dry mouth) may be treated with saliva substitutes such as oral balance in the biotene range.[3] SOR Ⓒ

PATIENT EDUCATION

- Advise patients to maintain good oral hygiene by brushing their teeth twice daily with small-headed, soft to medium hardness brush using a toothpaste that contains fluoride. Electric toothbrushes may

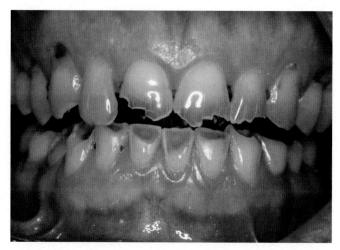

FIGURE 44-3 Destruction of the teeth in woman with bulimia. The gastric acids have dissolved the enamel. (*Courtesy of Gerald Ferretti, DMD.*)

be useful for those with poor manual dexterity. Counsel patients to floss once daily to remove plaque and food particles from between the teeth.

- Suggest that patients use antiplaque mouthwashes containing Chlorhexidine to inhibit *Streptococcus mutans*, but caution coffee, tea, or red wine drinkers that such mouthwashes may increase dental staining.[3]

- Those patients with xerostomia (dry mouth) should be advised to practice good oral hygiene and avoid sugary foods. Chewing sugar-free gum will induce salivation.[3]

- Advise patients that plaque formation may be reduced by chewing sugar-free gum or cheese after meals.

- Advise patients to visit a dental professional at least once a year for a cleaning and examination.

FOLLOW-UP

Remind adult patients who have "white spots" or active caries to go to a dentist for immediate treatment.

PATIENT RESOURCES

New York State Department of Health. Oral Health Resources and Links. **http://www.health.state.ny.us/prevention/dental/weblinks_oral_health.htm.** Accessed April 7, 2007.

PROVIDER RESOURCES

Douglass A, Gonsalves W, Maier R, Silk H, Tysinger J, Wrightson S. Smiles for life: A National Oral Health Curriculum for Family Medicine. **http://www.stfm.org/oralhealth/.** Accessed April 7, 2007.

National Center for Chronic Disease Prevention and Health Promotion. Oral Health: Preventing Cavities, Gum Disease, and Tooth Loss. **http://www.cdc.gov/nccdphp/publications/aag/oh.htm.** Accessed April 7, 2007.

World Health Organization. Oral Health. **http://www.who.int/oral_health/en/.** Accessed April 7, 2007.

REFERENCES

1. Centers for Disease Control and Prevention. Oral Health: Preventing Cavities, Gum Disease, and Tooth Loss At A Glance 2007. http://www.cdc.gov/nccdphp/publications/AAG/oh.htm. Accessed April 20, 2007.

2. US Department of Health and Human Services. Oral health in America: A Report of the Surgeon General-Executive Summary. Rockville, MD: US Department of Health and Human Services, National Institute of Dental and Craniofacial Research, National Institutes of Health, 2000. http://www.surgeongeneral.gov/library/oralhealth/. Accessed April 21, 2007.

3. Johnson, V, Chalmers, J. Oral hygiene care for functionally dependent and cognitively impaired older adults. National Guideline Clearinghouse, 2002. http://www.guideline.gov. Accessed June 2, 2007.

4. Ripa LW. A critique of topical fluoride methods (dentifrices, mouthrinses, operator, and self-applied gels) in an era of decreased caries and increased fluorosis prevalence. *J Public Health Dent*. 1991;51:23–41.

5. National Institutes of Health, Consensus Development Conference Statement, March 26–28, 2001. Diagnosis and Management of Dental Caries Throughout Life. Originally published as: Diagnosis and Management of Dental Caries Throughout Life. NIH Consensus Statement 2001;18(1):1–24.

PART 7

THE HEART AND CIRCULATION

45 CORONARY ARTERY DISEASE

Heidi Chumley, MD

PATIENT STORY

A 45-year-old man began having chest pressure with exertion that was relieved with rest. He did not have diabetes, high blood pressure, or high cholesterol and had never had a myocardial infarction. His examination and resting electrocardiogram were normal. On the basis of the testing modalities available, he was scheduled for exercise stress testing. After a positive test, he underwent coronary angiography that demonstrated a significant stenosis in the right coronary artery (**Figure 45-1**). He underwent a stenting procedure and was placed on aspirin and cholesterol-lowering medication.

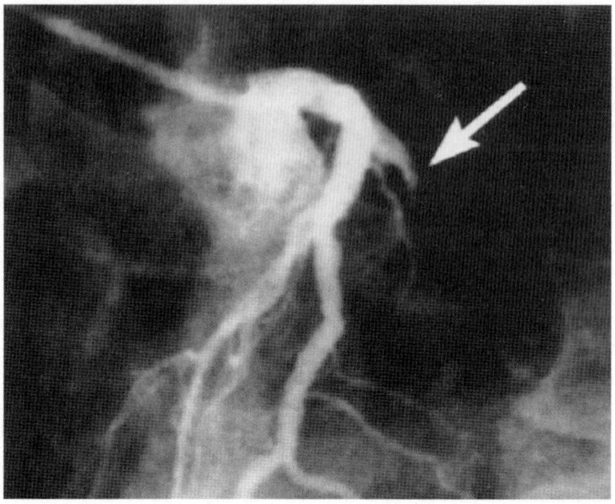

FIGURE 45-1 Coronary arteriogram demonstrating severe stenosis (white arrow) in the right coronary artery.

EPIDEMIOLOGY

* Coronary heart disease (CHD) is the leading cause of death in the United States, responsible for approximately 500,000 deaths in 2003.[1]

* 1.2 million myocardial infarctions occur per year (first and recurrent) with a 40% mortality rate.[1]

* An estimated 13 million people are living with CHD in the United States.[1]

* In 2002, the prevalence of CHD among U.S. adults older than 20 years of age was highest in white men and in blacks: 8.9% and 5.4% for white men and women, 7.4% and 7.5% in black men and women, and 5.6% and 4.3% for Hispanic men and women.[1]

ETIOLOGY AND PATHOPHYSIOLOGY

* CHD is one of several manifestations of atherosclerotic disease, which begins with endothelium dysfunction.[2]
  ○ Endothelium, when normal, balances vasoconstrictors and vasodilators, impedes platelet aggregation, and controls fibrin production.
  ○ Dysfunctional endothelium encourages macrophage adhesion, plaque growth, and vasoconstriction by recruiting inflammatory cells into the vessels walls, the initiating step of atherosclerosis.
  ○ The vessel wall lesions develop a cap of smooth muscle cells and collagen to become fibroadenomas.
  ○ The vessels with these lesions undergo enlargement, allowing progression of the plaque without compromising the lumen.

- Plaque disruption and thrombus formation, instead of progressive narrowing of the coronary artery lumen, is responsible for two-thirds of acute coronary events.[2]
  - Plaques most likely to rupture (high-risk plaques) have a large core of lipids, many macrophages, decreased vascular smooth muscle cells, and a thin fibrous cap.
  - After plaque rupture, the exposed lipid core triggers a superimposed thrombus that occludes the vessel.
  - Increased thrombosis is triggered by known cardiac risk factors including elevated low-density lipoprotein (LDL) cholesterol, cigarette smoking, and hyperglycemia.

- The other one-third of acute coronary events occurs at the site of very stenotic lesions (**Figure 45-2**).[2]

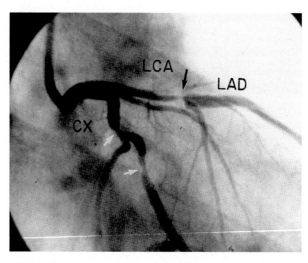

FIGURE 45-2 Coronary angiogram of a left coronary artery (LCA) with a tight stenosis in the proximal left anterior descending (LAD) artery (black arrow). The circumflex artery (CX) has two moderately severe stenoses (white arrows).

DIAGNOSIS

CLINICAL FEATURES

- Typical angina is chest pain or pressure, brought on by exertion or stress, and relieved with rest or nitroglycerine.

- Atypical angina has 2 of the 3 features of typical angina; however, women with coronary artery disease report more neck, throat, or jaw pain.[3]

- Noncardiac chest pain has 0 to 1 of the 3 features of typical angina.

LABORATORY STUDIES

- Risk factor assessment: lipid profile and fasting blood glucose.

- Acute coronary syndrome: cardiac specific troponin is now preferred; when troponin cutoff is 0.1 −g/L, sensitivity is 93%, specificity is 91%, LR+ 10.33, and LR− 0.08.

COMMON NONINVASIVE TESTING[4]

- Exercise treadmill testing: sensitivity 52% and specificity 71%, LR+ 1.79, LR− 0.68.

- Stress echocardiogram: sensitivity 85% and specificity 77%, LR+ 3.70, LR− 0.19.

- Stress thallium: sensitivity 87% and specificity 64%, LR+ 2.42, LR− 0.20.

  Newer methods being tested: CT for diagnosis:[5]

- 4- or 16-slice study: sensitivity 95% and specificity 84%, LR+ 5.94, LR− 0.06, with 78% and 91% of segments evaluable.

- 64-slice study: sensitivity 100% and specificity 100% with 100% of segments evaluable.

DIFFERENTIAL DIAGNOSIS

Chest pain can be caused by several conditions including:

- Cardiac: pericarditis—slower onset of pain, pain aggravated by movement or inspiration, characteristic EKG changes.

- Respiratory: pneumothorax—acute onset with shortness of breath and characteristic radiographic findings; pneumonia—often accompanied by fever, cough, shortness of breath/hypoxia, and/or radiographic findings; pulmonary embolism—acute onset of shortness of breath, positive ventilation/perfusion scan or spiral CT.

- Gastrointestinal: gastroesophageal reflux—related to eating, responds to H2 blockers or PPI.

- Musculoskeletal: costochondritis—chest muscles tender to palpation.

MANAGEMENT

- In general, send patients with typical angina and high-risk patients with a typical angina for further evaluation.

- Refer patients with positive noninvasive testing to be evaluated for cardiac catheterization.

- Consult with cardiologists and cardiothoracic surgeons to determine optimal management.
  - Traditionally, patients with >50% stenosis of left main, proximal stenosis of three major arteries, or significant stenosis of the proximal left anterior descending and one other major artery have been treated with coronary bypass surgery.[6] SOR **A**
  - Advancements with drug-eluding stents may increase in the patients who benefit from stenting.[6]
  - Medical management (managing risk factors and treating symptoms) can be used for nonsignificant stenoses.

- Managing risk factors
  - Advise patients who smoke to stop to lower risk for a subsequent cardiac event by at least 33%.[7] SOR **A**
  - Recommend 30 minutes of physical activity 5 to 7 days per week.[8] SOR **B**
  - Advise patients in weight management with a goal BMI of 18.5 to 24.9.[8] SOR **B**
  - Lower LDL cholesterol using lifestyle modification and HMG-CoA reductase inhibitors to decrease major coronary events and coronary mortality by approximately 25%. In one trial, number needed to treat (NNT) was 22 for 6 years to prevent 1 event.[9] SOR **A**
  - Lower blood pressure to 140/90 or 130/80 (with diabetes or chronic renal disease); treat patients who are post MI with a beta-blocker, thiazide diuretic, or aldosterone antagonist.[10] SOR **A**
  - Prescribe aspirin in patients with prior ST elevation or non-ST elevation acute coronary event or chronic stable angina. Prescribe clopidogrel alone in chronic stable angina or with aspirin in non-ST elevation acute coronary syndrome.[11] SOR **A**
  - Prescribe a beta antagonist—several trials demonstrate mortality decreases of 25% to 40% with various beta-blockers used in the acute MI or post-MI period.[12]

- Treat symptoms
  - Nitroglycerin sublingual or spray for immediate relief of angina.[13] SOR **B**
  - Long-acting nitrates or calcium antagonists if beta-blockers are contraindicated, do not control symptoms, or have unacceptable side effects.[13] SOR **B**

PATIENT EDUCATION

Advise patients in the importance of lifestyle modification and medications in the long-term management of CHD.

FOLLOW-UP

Follow-up frequency is based on the extent of illness and symptoms and may include primary care and subspecialty care. Patients should have ongoing evaluation of risk factors and symptoms every 4 to 12 months. Expert guidelines recommend annual exercise stress testing for patients with chronic stable angina.[13] SOR **C**

PATIENT RESOURCES

Patient educational materials for reducing risk of coronary artery disease can be found at **www.aafp.org.**

The American Heart Association has information about the warning signs of heart attacks and living a healthy lifestyle at **www.americanheart.org.**

PROVIDER RESOURCES

Online calculator for pre- and posttest probability of CAD based on history and physical located at **http://www.sgim.org/tools.cfm.**

The National Heart, Blood, and Lung Institute has information for health professionals including PDA downloads and health assessment tools at **http://www.nhlbi.nih.gov/index.htm.**

REFERENCES

1. The American Heart Association. http://www.americanheart.org. Accessed January 7, 2007.

2. Viles-Gonzalez JF, Fuster V, Badimon JJ. Atherothrombosis: A widespread disease with unpredictable and life-threatening consequences. *Euro Heart J.* 2004;25(14):1197–1207.

3. Philpott S. Boynton PM. Feder G. Hemingway H. Gender differences in descriptions of angina symptoms and health problems immediately prior to angiography: The ACRE study. Appropriateness of Coronary Revascularisation study. *Soc Sci Med.* 2001;52(10):1565–1575.

4. Pryor DB, Shaw L, McCants CB, et al. Value of the history and physical in identifying patients at increased risk for coronary artery disease. *Ann Intern Med.* 1993;118(2):81–90.

5. Stein PD, Stein PD, Beemath A, et al. Multidetector computed tomography for the diagnosis of coronary artery disease: A systematic review. *Am J Med.* 2006;119(3):203–216.

6. Schofield PM. Indications for percutaneous and surgical revascularisation: How far does the evidence base guide us? *Heart.* 2003;89(5):565–570.

7. Critchley J, Capewell S. Smoking Cessation for the secondary prevention of Coronary Heart Disease. Last update Aug 1, 2003. www.cochrane.org. Accessed January 1, 2007.

8. Smith SC, et al. AHA/ACC Guidelines for Secondary Prevention for Patients With Coronary and Other Atherosclerotic Vascular Disease: 2006 Update. *Circulation.* 2006;113:2363–2372.

9. Colquhoun D, Keech A, Hunt D, et al. LIPID Study Investigators. Effects of pravastatin on coronary events in 2073 patients with low levels of both low-density lipoprotein cholesterol and

high-density lipoprotein cholesterol: Results from the LIPID study. *Euro Heart J.* 2004;25(9):771–777.

10. The seventh report of the joint national committee on prevention, detection, evaluation and treatment of hypertension. http://www.nhlbi.nih.gov/guidelines/hypertension/index.htm. Accessed January 1, 2007.

11. Tran H, Anand SS. Oral antiplatelet therapy in cerebrovascular disease, coronary artery disease, and peripheral arterial disease. *JAMA.* 2004;292(15):1867–1874.

12. Ellison KE, Gandhi G. Optimising the use of beta-adrenoceptor antagonists in coronary artery disease. *Drugs.* 2005;65(6): 787–797.

13. Gibbons RJ, Abrahms J, Chatterjee K, et al. ACC/AHA 2002 guideline update for the management of patients with chronic stable angina. http://www.americanheart.org. Accessed January 7, 2007.

46 CONGESTIVE HEART FAILURE

Heidi Chumley, MD

PATIENT STORY

A 60-year-old man presents to the emergency department with shortness of breath increasing in severity over the past several days, along with paroxysmal nocturnal dyspnea and orthopnea. He does not have a history of heart failure or previous myocardial infarction. On examination it was found that he had a third heart sound and an elevated jugular venous pressure. His chest radiograph showed cardiomegaly (**Figure 46-1**) and his B-type natriuretic peptide (BNP) was elevated at 600 pg/mL. He was diagnosed with congestive heart failure, evaluated for underlying causes including coronary artery disease, and treated initially with an ACE inhibitor and a diuretic. Later, he will be started on a beta-blocker and an aldosterone inhibitor.

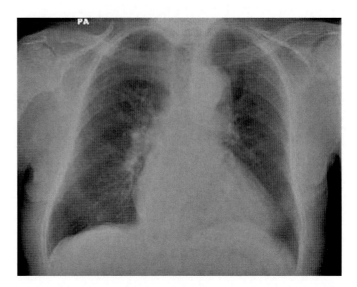

FIGURE 46-1 Cardiomegaly demonstrated in a posteroanterior (PA) view. The widest part of the heart is greater than 50% of the diameter of the chest. (*Courtesy of Kansas University Medical Center.*)

EPIDEMIOLOGY

- The prevalence of CHF in the community increases with age: 0.7% (45–54 years); 1.3% (55–64 years); 1.5% (65–74 years); and 8.4% (75 years or older).[1]

- More than 40% of patients in the community with CHF have an ejection fraction greater than 50%.[1]

- At age 40 years, the lifetime risk for CHF is 21.0% (95% CI 18.7% to 23.2%) for men and 20.3% (95% CI 18.2% to 22.5%) for women.[2]

ETIOLOGY AND PATHOPHYSIOLOGY

- Heart pumping capacity declines from any cause (i.e., myocardial infarction or ischemia, hypertension, valvular dysfunction, cardiomyopathy, or infections such as endocarditis or myocarditis).

- Cardiac dysfunction activates the adrenergic and renin-angiotensin-aldosterone systems.

- These systems provide short-term compensation, but chronic activation leads to myocardial remodeling and eventually worsening cardiac function.

- Norepinephrine, angiotensin II, aldosterone, and tissue necrosis factor each contribute to disease progression.

- Angiotensin II directly causes cell death through necrosis and apoptosis, as well as cardiac hypertrophy.

DIAGNOSIS

Many history, examination, radiographic, electrocardiogram, and laboratory features are helpful in making the diagnosis of congestive heart failure for patients presenting with dyspnea in the emergency department:[3]

- History of heart failure (LR+ = 5.8), myocardial infarction (LR+ = 3.1).[3]
- Symptoms of paroxysmal nocturnal dyspnea (LR+ = 2.6), orthopnea (LR+ = 2.2), edema (LR+ = 2.1).[3]
- Examination finding of third heart sound (LR+ = 11), hepatojugular reflex (LR+ = 6.4), jugular venous distention (LR+ = 5.1).[3]
- Radiographic finding of pulmonary venous congestion (**Figure 46-2**) (LR+ = 12.0), interstitial edema (LR+ = 12.0), alveolar edema (LR+ = 6.0), cardiomegaly (**Figures 46-1 to 46-3**) (LR+ = 3.3).[3]
- Electrocardiogram finding of atrial fibrillation (LR+ = 3.8), T wave changes (LR+ = 3.0), any abnormality (LR+ = 2.2). A normal EKG lowers likelihood (LR− = 0.640).[3]
- Laboratory value of BNP ≥250 (LR+ = 4.6); BNP <100 decreases likelihood of heart failure.[3]

DIFFERENTIAL DIAGNOSIS

Gradually increasing shortness of breath can also be caused by:

- Chronic obstructive pulmonary disease may have dyspnea with exertion but does not have orthopnea; chest radiograph shows a normal size heart, hyperinflated lungs, and flattened diaphragms; pulmonary function tests may be abnormal.
- Deconditioning has a normal chest radiograph.
- Metabolic acidosis from any cause can be differentiated with an arterial blood gas.
- Anxiety has episodic shortness of breath, not associated with exertion and a normal chest radiograph.
- Neuromuscular weakness may have abnormal pulmonary function tests and a normal chest radiograph.
- Pneumonia may have fever and an infiltrate on chest radiograph.

MANAGEMENT

Individually, ACE inhibitors (ACE-I), beta-blockers (BB), and aldosterone antagonists (AA) lower mortality and should be considered for all patients without contraindications.

- Prescribe an ACE-I. SOR **A** ACE-Is lower mortality rates by 23% overall. Use in patients with asymptomatic left ventricular dysfunction and all other stages of heart failure.[4]
- Prescribe a BB. SOR **A** BBs reduce mortality by 32%.[5] Begin at a small dose and double the dose every 2 to 4 weeks until the target dose is reached or the patient cannot tolerate the increased dose. One study demonstrating a decrease in mortality had a large percentage of patients in the control and intervention groups already on an ACE-I, indicating that the 2 together may decrease mortality more than an ACE-I alone.[4] SOR **B**
- Prescribe an AA when the creatinine is less than 2.0; monitor renal function and potassium.[4] SOR **A** AAs lowered mortality in patients already on ACE-I.[5] SOR **B**

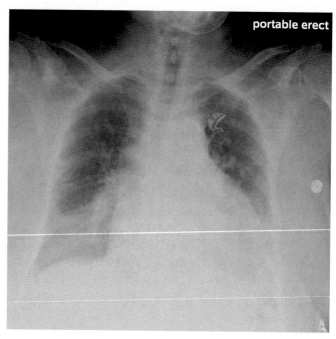

FIGURE 46-2 Cardiomegaly with pulmonary venous congestion and bilateral pleural effusions. (*Courtesy of Kansas University Medical Center.*)

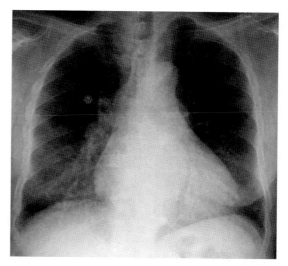

FIGURE 46-3 Cardiomegaly with increased pulmonary vasculature and Kerley B lines (2–3 cm horizontal lines in the lower lung fields). (*Courtesy of Kansas University Medical Center.*)

- Consider an angiotensin II receptor blocker (ARB) for patients who cannot tolerate an ACE-I.[4] Patients with moderate, severe, or advanced heart failure may benefit from an ACE-I plus an ARB or AA SOR **Ⓑ**, but the safety of all three is unknown.[4]

- After a myocardial infarction, an ARB has shown equivalent reductions in mortality to an ACE-I, but the combination does not improve outcomes.

- Refer for evaluation for implantable cardiac-defibrillator (ICD) placement in patients with NYHA class II-IV and LVEF<35% SOR **Ⓒ**. ICDs have been shown to reduce mortality up to 30% and may offer greater risk reduction than anti-arrhythmic medical therapy for some patients.[6]

Non-potassium sparing diuretics, calcium channel blockers, and digoxin may improve symptoms but do not lower mortality.

- Non-potassium sparing diuretics (i.e., furosemide) have been associated with worse outcomes, including higher mortality when used alone. Use for volume overload with ACE-I, BB, AA $+/-$ ARB as above.[5]

- Calcium channel blockers (verapamil and nifedipine) are avoided in systolic heart failure. CCBs improve symptoms in diastolic heart failure, but do not lower mortality.[7] SOR **Ⓐ**

- Digoxin reduces hospitalizations and improves clinical symptoms, but does not lower mortality.[5] Consider adding digoxin when patients have symptoms despite adequate therapy with ACE-I, BB, AA $+/-$ ARB.

PATIENT EDUCATION

Fluid and sodium restriction are often advised, but there is little evidence to support their use. One small trial (fluid restriction $=$ 1.5 L/d; sodium restriction $=$ 2 to 2.4 g/d) demonstrated small improvements in quality-of-life measures.[8]

PATIENT RESOURCES

The American Heart Association has patient information about heart failure and a caregiver's guide under diseases and conditions—**http://www.americanheart.org.**

MedlinePlus has an interactive online patient education program in English or Spanish—**http://www.nlm.nih.gov/medlineplus/heartfailure.html.**

PROVIDER RESOURCES

The American Heart Association professionals page has statistics, presentations, and publications—**http://www.americanheart.org.**

REFERENCES

1. Redfield MM, Jacobsen SJ, Burnett JC, Jr., Mahoney DW, Bailey KR, Rodeheffer RJ. Burden of systolic and diastolic ventricular dysfunction in the community: Appreciating the scope of the heart failure epidemic. [see comment]. *JAMA.* 2003;289(2):194–202.

2. Lloyd-Jones DM, Larson MG, Leip EP et al. Lifetime risk for developing congestive heart failure: The Framingham Heart Study. [see comment]. *Circulation.* 2002;106(24):3068–3072.

3. Wang CS, FitzGerald JM, Schulzer M, Mak E, Ayas NT. Does this dyspneic patient in the emergency department have congestive heart failure? [Review]. *JAMA.* 2005;294(15):1944–1956.

4. Mielniczuk L, Stevenson LW. Angiotensin-converting enzyme inhibitors and angiotensin II type I receptor blockers in the management of congestive heart failure patients: What have we learned from recent clinical trials? [Review]. *Curr Opin Cardiol.* 1920;250–255.

5. Yan AT, Yan RT, Liu PP. Narrative review: Pharmacotherapy for chronic heart failure: Evidence from recent clinical trials.[summary for patients in Ann Intern Med. 2005;142(2):I53;PMID: 15657154]. [Review]. *Ann Intern Med.* 2005;142(2):132–145.

6. Kadish A, Mehra M. Heart failure devices: Implantable cardioverter-defibrillators and biventricular pacing therapy. [Review]. *Circulation.* 2005;111(24):3327–3335.

7. Haney S, Sur D, Xu Z. Diastolic heart failure: A review and primary care perspective. [Review]. *J Am Board Fam Pract.* 2005;18(3):189–198.

8. Colin RE, Castillo ML, Orea TA, Rebollar GV, Narvaez DR, Asensio LE. Effects of a nutritional intervention on body composition, clinical status, and quality of life in patients with heart failure. *Nutrition.* 1920;890–895.

47 PERICARDIAL EFFUSION

Heidi Chumley, MD

PATIENT STORY

A 30-year-old woman presented to her family physician with increasing shortness of breath over the past 2 weeks. Prior to this, she had a flu-like illness and felt like she never recovered. She denied chest pain and edema, did not take any medications, and had not had any recent trauma or surgery. She had a normal examination. Her chest radiograph showed a classic globular heart as demonstrated in **Figure 47-1.** She had nonspecific ST changes on her EKG. An echocardiogram confirmed pericardial effusion (**Figure 47-2**). The underlying etiology was not elucidated and she recovered spontaneously over the next several months.

EPIDEMIOLOGY

- Six and a half percent of adults (<1% age 20–30; 15% >80 years of age) had echocardiogram findings consistent with pericardial effusion in a population-based study of 5652 adults and adult family members of participants in the Framingham Heart Study.[1]
- Seventy-seven percent of patients after cardiac surgery for valves or bypass have pericardial effusions, which rarely (<1%) require therapy.[2]
- Forty percent of healthy pregnant women have small, asymptomatic pericardial effusions in the third trimester.[3]

ETIOLOGY AND PATHOPHYSIOLOGY

Pericardial effusion, acute or chronic, occurs when there is increased production or decreased drainage of pericardial fluid allowing accumulation in the pericardial space. The underlying etiology is apparent clinically approximately 25% of the time and can be determined with testing in another 25% of cases, leaving 50% of cases idiopathic.[4] Underlying causes include:

- Congestive heart failure of other cardiac disease such as rheumatic heart disease, cor pulmonale, or cardiomyopathy.[5]
- Postop cardiac surgery or postmyocardial infarction.[2]
- Connective tissue disorders (scleroderma, lupus erythematous, rheumatoid arthritis).[5]
- Neoplasms: benign (atrial myxoma); primary malignant (mesothelioma); secondary malignant (i.e., lung or breast cancer).[5]
- Chronic renal disease (uremia or hemodialysis) or other causes of hypoalbuminemia.
- Infections: acute (enterovirus, adenovirus, influenza virus, streptococcus pneumonia, *Coxiella burnetii*—responsible for Q fever or chronic (tuberculosis, fungus, parasites).[4]
- Medications (procainamide, hydralazine) or after radiation.[5]
- Severe hypothyroidism with myxedema.[5]

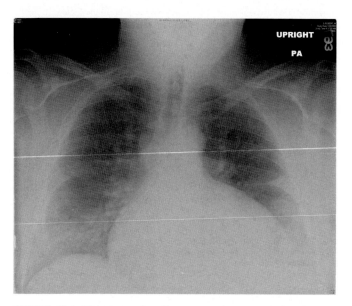

FIGURE 47-1 Globular cardiac silhouette or classic "water-bottle heart" seen with a pericardial effusion can be difficult to distinguish from cardiomegaly on plain radiographs. (*Courtesy of Kansas University Medical Center.*)

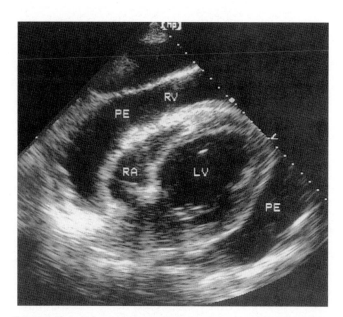

FIGURE 47-2 Echocardiogram showing right ventricular (RV) compression from a pericardial effusion (PE). RA, right atrium; LV, left ventricle. (*Courtesy of Kansas University Medical Center.*)

DIAGNOSIS

Clinical features, chest radiograph, and electrocardiogram suggest pericardial effusion, which is confirmed by echocardiogram. The underlying etiology is identifiable in approximately 50% of cases.

CLINICAL FEATURES

Signs and symptoms occur when the volume of fluid is large enough to affect hemodynamics. This occurs at 150 to 200 mL in acute pericardial effusion. Chronic pericardial effusion allows stretching overtime and may require up to 2 liters to cause significant symptoms[5]:

- Hypotension, increased jugular venous pressure, and soft heart sounds form the classic triad of acute cardiac tamponade, but all three are present only in approximately 30% of cases.[5]

- Common symptoms include anorexia (90%), dyspnea (78%), cough (47%), and chest pain (27%).[5]

- Common physical examination findings include pulsus paradoxus (77% with acute tamponade, 30% with chronic effusions), sinus tachycardia (50%), jugular venous distension (45%), hepatomegaly and peripheral edema (35%).[5]

- Electrocardiogram is abnormal in 90%. Findings include low QRS voltage and nonspecific ST-T changes (59% to 63%) and electrical alternans (0% to 10%).[5]

- Chest radiograph shows a globular enlarged cardiac silhouette (see **Figure 47-1**) (sensitivity 78%, specificity 34% with moderate or severe effusions); and pericardial fat stripe (**Figure 47-3**) (sensitivity 22%, specificity 92%).[5]

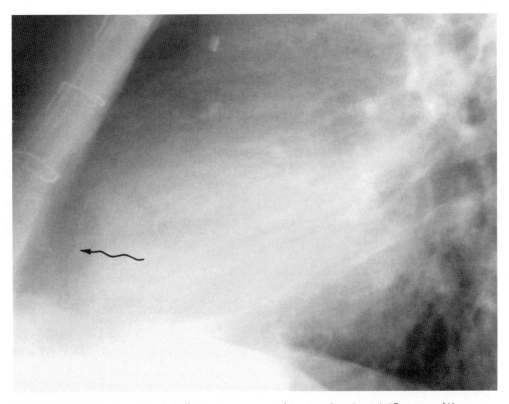

FIGURE 47-3 Moderate pericardial effusion is seen as a wide pericardium (arrow). (*Courtesy of Kansas University Medical Center.*)

LABORATORY STUDIES

When the diagnosis remains unclear, pericardial fluid can be sent for cell count and differential, protein, lactate dehydrogenase, glucose, gram stain, bacterial cultures, fungal cultures, mycobacterial acid fast stain and culture, and tumor cytology. Measure rheumatoid factor, antinuclear antibody, and complement levels when collagen vascular disease is suspected.[5] Check HIV status in at-risk patients.

When there is no obvious cause, ordering this set of specific tests determined the underlying etiology more often than seen in historic controls (27.3% vs. 3.9%; $p < 0.001$).[6]

- Aerobic and anaerobic blood cultures.
- Throat swab cultures for influenza, adenovirus, and enterovirus.
- Serological tests for cytomegalovirus, influenza, *C. burnetii*, mycoplasma pneumonia, and toxoplasma.
- Blood tests for ANA and TSH.

DIFFERENTIAL DIAGNOSIS

- Congestive heart failure has many similar signs and symptoms (dyspnea, jugular venous distention, hepatomegaly, and edema) but may have pulmonary rales, which are unusual in pericardial effusions. A lateral radiograph in a patient with congestive heart failure (without pleural effusion) should have a normal thin pericardium (**Figure 47-4**).
- Pleural effusions may also present with dyspnea, but have different physical examination and radiographic findings.

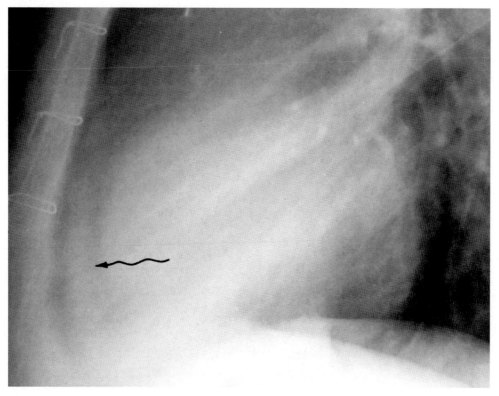

FIGURE 47-4 The lateral view demonstrates the normal thin pericardium (arrow), which should be less than 2 mm. (*Courtesy of Kansas University Medical Center.*)

- Acute pericarditis (without pericardial effusion) can present with chest pain and nonspecific EKG changes also seen with pericardial effusion. In contrast, acute pericarditis often has elevated inflammatory markers and a normal chest radiograph.

MANAGEMENT

In addition to treating any identified underlying cause, pericardial effusion may require removal of fluid when there is hemodynamic compromise.

- Pericardiocentesis is performed by a specialist under local anesthesia as follows: elevate the patient to a 45-degree angle. Insert a needle in the angle between the left costal arch and the xiphoid process, directed 15-degree posterior, and angled toward the head or either shoulder. Complications are reduced when this procedure is guided by echocardiography. Fluid often reaccumulates. An indwelling catheter can be placed for up to 72 hours without increasing the risk of infection, until a more permanent procedure can be performed to decrease the likelihood of reaccumulation.

- Sclerosing therapy reduces the recurrence of symptoms from reaccumulation or the need for a repeat procedure for 30 days in more than 70% of patients. A caustic substance such as bleomycin or tetracycline is instilled into the pericardial space and held there for up to 4 hours.

- Other options to reduce recurrence include balloon pericardiotomy performed in a cardiac catheterization laboratory, radiation therapy, and surgery (i.e., pericardial window).

PATIENT EDUCATION

- The underlying cause of a pericardial effusion is identified only 50% of the time; however, specific tests should be done to find treatable causes.

- In patients without an obvious underlying illness, infections (like the flu, Q fever, or tuberculosis) and cancer are the two most common identified causes of pericardial effusions.

FOLLOW-UP

Follow-up is based on the underlying cause. Pericardial effusions often disappear when the underlying illness resolves, and reappear when the underlying illness does not resolve (metastatic cancer).

PATIENT RESOURCES

Patient information about pericardial effusions can be found at Your-Heart, a United Kingdom-based website—**www.yourheart.org.uk.**

REFERENCES

1. Savage DD, Garrison RJ, Brand F, et al. Prevalence and correlates of posterior extra echocardiographic spaces in a free-living population based sample (the Framingham study). *Am J Cardiol.* 1983; 51(7):1207–1212.

2. Ikaheimo MJ, Huikuri HV, Airaksinen KE, et al. Pericardial effusion after cardiac surgery: Incidence, relation to the type of surgery, antithrombotic therapy, and early coronary bypass graft patency. *Am Heart J.* 1988;116(1 Pt 1):97–102.

3. Ristic AD, Seferovic PM, Ljubic A, et al. Pericardial disease in pregnancy. *Herz* 2003;28(3):209–215.

4. Levy PY, Corey R, Berger P, et al. Etiologic diagnosis of 204 pericardial effusions. *Medicine.* 2003;82(6):385–391.

5. Karam N, Patel P, deFilippi C. Diagnosis and management of chronic pericardial effusions. *Am J Med Sci.* 2002;322(2):79–87.

6. Levy PY, Moatti JP, Gauduchon V, Vandenesch F, Habib G, Raoult D. Comparison of intuitive versus systematic strategies for aetiological diagnosis of pericardial effusion. *Scand J Infect Dis.* 2005;37(3): 216–120.

48 BACTERIAL ENDOCARDITIS

Heidi Chumley, MD

PATIENT STORY

A 25-year-old man, addicted to injecting cocaine, came to the office because he had been feeling tired and feverish for several weeks. On examination, he was febrile and had a heart murmur of which he was previously unaware. His fingernails showed splinter hemorrhages (**Figure 48-1**). His funduscopic examination revealed Roth spots (**Figure 48-2** and **48-3**). An echocardiogram demonstrated vegetation on the tricuspid valve. He was hospitalized and treated empirically for bacterial endocarditis. After his blood cultures returned *Staphylococcus aureus*, his regimen was adjusted based on sensitivities and continued for 6 weeks.

EPIDEMIOLOGY

- 1.7 to 6.2 cases per 100,000 patient-years with an in-hospital mortality of 16%.[1]
  - Incidence in intravenous drug users is 3 per 1000 person-years or 1% to 5% per year.[2]
  - Incidence in HIV-positive intravenous drug users 13.8 per 1000 person-years.[2]
- Male-to-female ratio of 2:1.
- Nosocomial infections make up 22% of endocarditis cases.[1]
  - Seen in immunosuppressed with central venous catheters or hemodialysis patients.
  - Mortality is approximately 50%.
- Prosthetic valve endocarditis makes up 10% to 15% of endocarditis cases.[1]
  - Incidence of 0.1% to 2.3% person-year.[1]
  - Can occur early (2 months after surgery) or late.
- Common organisms include *S. aureus* (IV drug users, nosocomial infections, prosthetic valve patients), *Streptococcus bovis* (elderly patients), enterococci (nosocomial infections), and *Staphylococcus epidermis* (early infection in prosthetic valve patients).

ETIOLOGY AND PATHOPHYSIOLOGY

- Endothelium is injured by mechanical or inflammatory processes.
- Microbes adhere to compromised endothelium during transient bacteremia.
- Blood contacts subendothelial factors, which promotes coagulation.
- Pathogens bind and activate monocyte, cytokine, and tissue factor production enlarging the vegetations on the heart valves.
- The vegetations enlarge and damage the heart valves (**Figure 48-4**). This process can lead to death if not treated adequately in time.

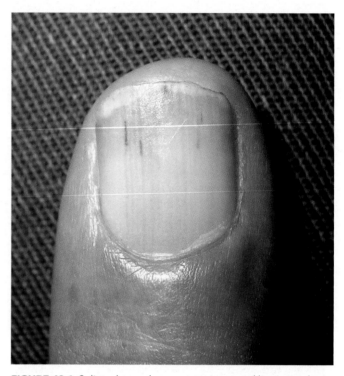

FIGURE 48-1 Splinter hemorrhages appearing as red linear streaks under the nail plate and within the nail bed. While endocarditis can cause this, splinter hemorrhages are more commonly seen in psoriasis and trauma. (*Courtesy of Richard P. Usatine, MD.*)

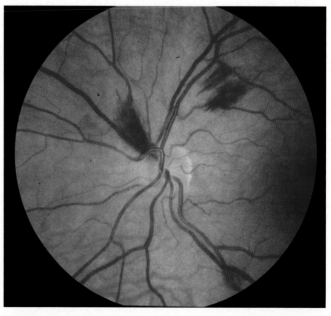

FIGURE 48-2 Roth spots that are retinal hemorrhages with white centers seen in bacterial endocarditis. These can also be seen in leukemia and diabetes. (*Courtesy of Paul D. Comeau.*)

- Septic emboli can occur, most commonly in the brain, spleen, or kidney.[1]

DIAGNOSIS

- Duke criteria use a combination of history, physical examination, laboratory, and echocardiogram findings and have a sensitivity of approximately 80% across several studies.[3]
- Diagnosis is considered definite when patients have two major, one major and three minor, or five minor criteria.[3]
- Diagnosis is considered possible with one major and one minor or three minor criteria.[3]
- Major criteria include:[3]
  - Positive blood culture with:
    - *Viridans streptococcus*, *S. bovis*, *S. aureus*, *Haemophilus*, *Actinobacillus*, *Cardiobacterium*, *Eikenella*, *Kingella*.
    - *Enterococcus* (community acquired) without a primary focus.
    - Microorganisms consistent with prior positive blood cultures.
    - *Coxiella burnetii* or IgG antibody titer for *Coxiella* >1:800.
  - Endocardial involvement as evidenced by echocardiogram evidence of vegetation, abscess, or new partial dehiscence of a prosthetic valve.
  - New valvular regurgitation.
- Minor criteria include:[3]
  - Predisposition (e.g., heart condition such as a congenital or acquired valvular defect, injection drug use, prior history of endocarditis).
  - Temperature >38°C.
  - Clinical signs: arterial emboli, septic pulmonary infarcts, mycotic aneurysms, intracranial hemorrhages, Janeway lesions (**Figures 48-5** and **48-6**).
  - Glomerulonephritis, Osler nodes, Roth spots, or positive rheumatoid factor (**Figures 48-2, 48-3** and **48-6**).
  - Positive blood culture not meeting major criteria.

CLINICAL FEATURES

- Fever—seen in 85% to 99% of patients, typically low-grade, approximately 39°C.
- New or changing heart murmur—seen in 20% to 80% of patients.
- Septic emboli—seen in up to 60%, largely dependent on the size (over 10 mm) and mobility of the vegetation.
- Intracranial hemorrhages—in 30% to 40% of patients, bleeding from septic emboli or cerebral mycotic aneurysms.
- Mycotic aneurysms—aneurysms resulting from infectious process in the arterial wall, most commonly in the thoracic aorta, also found in the cerebral arteries.
- Janeway lesions—very rare, flat, painless, red to bluish-red spots on the palms and soles (**Figures 48-5** and **48-6**).
- Splinter hemorrhages—red, linear streaks in the nail beds of the fingers or toes (**Figure 48-1**).
- Glomerulonephritis—immune mediated that can result in hematuria and renal insufficiency, occurs in approximately 15% of patients with endocarditis.

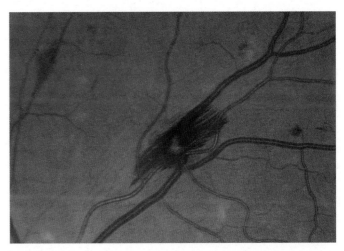

FIGURE 48-3 Close-up of a Roth spot, which is actually a cotton wool spot surrounded by hemorrhage. The cotton wool comes from ischemic bursting of axons and the hemorrhage comes from ischemic bursting of an arteriole. (*Courtesy of Paul D. Comeau.*)

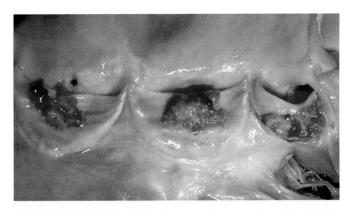

FIGURE 48-4 Pathology specimen of a patient who died of bacterial endocarditis. Bacterial growth can be seen on the three cusps of this heart valve. (*Courtesy of Larry Fowler, MD.*)

- Osler nodes—tender, subcutaneous nodules in the pulp of the digits: (**Figure 48-6**).
- Roth spots—retinal hemorrhages from microemboli, seen in approximately 5% of endocarditis (**Figures 48-2** and **48-3**).
- Positive rheumatoid factor—seen in up to 50% of patients.

TYPICAL DISTRIBUTION

- Native endocarditis: mitral valve (prior rheumatic fever or mitral valve prolapse), followed by aortic (prior rheumatic fever, calcific aortic stenosis of bicuspid valve).
- Prosthetic valve endocarditis: site of any prosthetic valve.
- In intravenous drug users: tricuspid valve, followed by aortic.

LABORATORY AND IMAGING STUDIES

In addition to blood cultures, consider a complete blood count for anemia and leukocytosis, ESR (elevated in approximately 90%), and urinalysis for proteinuria or microscopic hematuria (seen in approximately 50%).

- Positive blood culture—first two sets of cultures are positive in 90%.[1]
- Abnormal echocardiogram in 85%.[3]
- If trans-thoracic echocardiogram is normal and endocarditis is still suspected, order a trans-esophageal echo.[4] SOR **A**

DIFFERENTIAL DIAGNOSIS

Fever without a clear cause may be seen with:

- Connective tissue disorders—typically with other signs depending on the disorder, negative blood cultures, normal echocardiogram.
- Fever of unknown origin—negative blood cultures or positive cultures with atypical organisms, normal echocardiogram in noncardiac causes.
- Intra-abdominal infections—fever and positive blood cultures, normal echocardiogram.

Echocardiogram findings similar to bacterial endocarditis may be seen with:

- Noninfective vegetations—no fever and negative blood cultures.
- Cardiac tumors—embolic complications, right or left heart failure, often located off valves in cardiac chambers, negative blood cultures.
- Cusp prolapse—no fever and negative blood cultures.
- Myxomatous changes—extra connective tissue in the valve leaflets.
- Lambl's excrescences—stranding from wear and tear on the valve, most commonly aortic, no fever and negative blood cultures.

MANAGEMENT

- Draw blood cultures (2–3 sets) and admit suspected cases to the hospital for IV antibiotics.

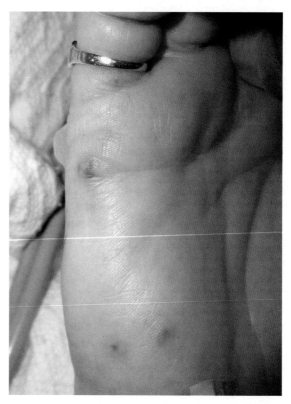

FIGURE 48-5 Janeway lesions on the palm of a woman hospitalized with acute bacterial endocarditis. These were not painful. (*Courtesy of David A. Kasper DO, MBA.*)

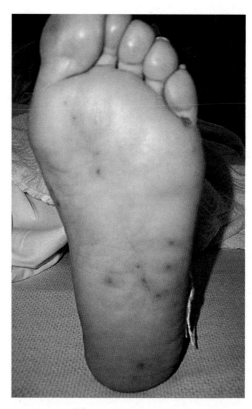

FIGURE 48-6 Osler's node causing pain within pulp of the big toe in the same woman hospitalized with acute bacterial endocarditis. (Osler's nodes are painful – remember "O" for Ouch and Osler.) Note the multiple painless flat Janeway lesions over the sole of the foot. (*Courtesy of David A. Kasper DO, MBA.*)

- Start antibiotics empirically—(SOR **C** for specific regiments).
  - Cover streptococcus in native valve endocarditis: penicillin G 12 to 18 million units divided every 4 hours and gentamicin 1.5 mg/kg loading dose, then 1 mg/kg every 8 hours.
  - Cover staphylococcus in intravenous drug abusers: nafcillin 2 g every 4 hours and gentamicin; use vancomycin instead of nafcillin when concerned about MRSA (prior history of MRSA infection).
  - Cover MRSA in prosthetic valve endocarditis: vancomycin 30 mg/kg per day divided every 8 hours and gentamicin.
- Alter antibiotics based on culture results. SOR **A**
- Treat gram positive with a beta-lactam; current evidence does not support adding an aminoglycaside.[5] SOR **A**
- Consider consultation for surgical excision of infected tissue, particularly when:
  - Congestive heart failure is severe with mitral or aortic regurgitation.
  - Fever and/or bacteremia persist for 7 to 10 days despite adequate antibiotic therapy, abscesses or perivalvular involvement occurs, or fungal organisms are identified.
  - Embolic events recur on adequate antibiotic therapy or the risk of embolic events is high because of vegetations larger than 10 mm. SOR **C**
- Anticoagulation and aspirin are not indicated for infective endocarditis and are contraindicated with cerebral complications or aneurysms.

PATIENT EDUCATION

- Bacterial endocarditis is a serious life-threatening disease requiring long-term antibiotics and close follow-up.
- Educate patients with high risk for endocarditis of the importance of prophylactic antibiotics before certain procedures. Following are the 2007 American Heart Association recommendations:[6]
  - Prescribe prophylactic antibiotics only to patients at the highest risk: SOR **B**
    - Patients with prosthetic cardiac valves.
    - Patients with previous bacterial endocarditis.
    - Cardiac transplant recipients with cardiac valvuloplasty.
    - Patients with these congenital heart defects (CHD): unrepaired cyanotic CHD, CHD repaired with prosthetic material within the last 6 months, repaired CHD with a residual defect at or adjacent to the site of a prosthetic device.
    - Prophylactic antibiotics are *no longer recommended* for patients with mitral valve prolapse.
  - Prescribe prophylactic antibiotics only to patients undergoing one of the following:
    - Any dental procedure that involves manipulation of gingival tissue or the periapical region of teeth or perforation of the oral mucosa. SOR **C**
    - Respiratory procedures involving incision or biopsy of the respiratory mucosa such as a tonsillectomy or adenoidectomy. SOR **C**
    - Procedures on infected skin or musculoskeletal tissue.
  - Endocarditis prophylaxis is *no longer recommended* for patients undergoing gastrointestinal or genitourinary procedures. SOR **B**

- Prescribe a one dose regimen to be taken 30 minutes to 1 hour before the procedure:[6]
  - Amoxicillin 2.0 g orally for adults, 50 mg/kg for children.
  - Unable to take oral medications: ampicillin 2.0 g IM or IV for adults, 50 mg/kg for children 30 minutes before the procedure; *or* cefazolin or ceftriaxone 1 g IM or IV for adults, 50 mg/kg for children.
  - Penicillin allergic: clindamycin 600 mg po, IM, or IV for adults; 20 mg/kg po, IM, or IV for children; *or* azithromycin or clarithromycin 500 mg po for adults, 15 mg/kg po for children. If allergy to penicillin is *not* anaphylaxis, angioedema, or urticaria, may also use cephalexin 2.0 g po for adults, 50 mg/kg po for children; *or* cefazolin or ceftriaxone 1 g IM or IV for adults, 50 mg/kg for children.

FOLLOW-UP

- Most patients with bacterial endocarditis will require 4 to 6 weeks of IV antibiotics.
- Depending on the antibiotics, some patients will need to have medication levels monitored.
- Repeat blood cultures to ensure response to therapy.
- An echocardiogram at the end of treatment provides baseline imaging, as patients with endocarditis are at risk for another episode.[4] SOR **C**

PATIENT RESOURCES

General information on bacterial endocarditis can be found on the American Academy of Family Physicians website—
http://www.aafp.org.

The American Heart Association has information about who is at risk for bacterial endocarditis and a printable wallet card for at risk patient, available in English or Spanish—
http://www.americanheart.org.

PROVIDER RESOURCES

The American Heart Association has complete information about who should receive endocarditis prophylaxis and medication regiments—**http://www.americanheart.org.**

REFERENCES

1. Prendergast BD. The changing face of infective endocarditis. *Heart.* 2006;92(7):879–885.

2. Wilson LE, Thomas DL, Astemborski J, Freedman TL, Vlahov D. Prospective study of infective endocarditis among injection drug users. *J Infect Dis.* 2002;185(12):1761–1766.

3. Habib G. Management of infective endocarditis. *Heart.* 2006;92(1):124–130.

4. Baddour LM, Wilson WR, Bayer AS, Fowler BG, Bolger AF, Levison ME. American Heart Association Scientific Statement on Infective Endocarditis. *Circulation.* 2005;111:e394–e434.

5. Falagas ME, Matthaiou DK, Bliziotis IA. The role of aminoglycosides in combination with a beta-lactam for the treatment of bacterial endocarditis: A meta-analysis of comparative trials. *J Antimicrob Chemother*. 2006;57(4):639–647.

6. Wilson W, Taubert KA, Gewitz M, et al. Prevention of infective endocarditis: A guideline from the American Heart Association. *Circulation*. 2007;116: 1736–1754.

SECTION 2 PERIPHERAL

49 CLUBBING

Heidi Chumley, MD

PATIENT STORY

A 31-year-old man with congenital heart disease has had these clubbed fingers since his childhood (**Figures 49-1** and **49-2**). A close view of the fingers shows a widened club-like distal phalanx. He has learned to live with the limitations from his congenital heart disease and his fingers do not bother him at all.

EPIDEMIOLOGY

Prevalence in the general population is unknown:

- 2% of adult patients admitted to a Welsh general medicine or surgery service.[1]
- 38% and 15% of patients with Crohn's disease and ulcerative colitis, respectively.[2]
- 33% and 11% of patients with lung cancer and COPD, respectively.[3]

ETIOLOGY AND PATHOPHYSIOLOGY

- The etiology of clubbing is poorly understood.
- Megakaryocytes and platelet clumps leak into systemic circulation; platelets release platelet-derived growth factor, which may cause thickening at the nail bed.[4]

DIAGNOSIS

CLINICAL FEATURES

- Typically painless.
- Abnormal nail fold angles[5] (**Figure 49-3**).
  - Profile angle (ABC) ≥180 degrees.
  - Hyponychial (ABD) ≥192 degrees.
- Phalangeal depth ratio (BE:GF) ≥1[5] (**Figure 49-3**).

TYPICAL DISTRIBUTION

- Bilateral, involves all fingers and often toes.
- Rarely unilateral or involves one or some digits.

DIFFERENTIAL DIAGNOSIS

PRIMARY CLUBBING

- Pachydermoperiostosis.
- Familial clubbing.
- Hypertrophic osteoarthropathy.

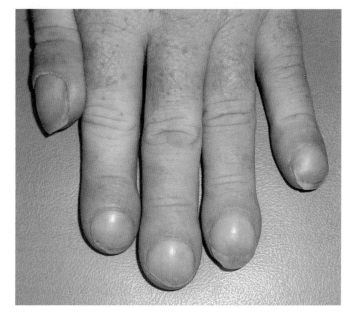

FIGURE 49-1 Clubbing of all the fingers in a 31-year-old man with congenital heart disease. Note thethickening around the proximal nail folds. (*Courtesy of Richard P. Usatine, MD.*)

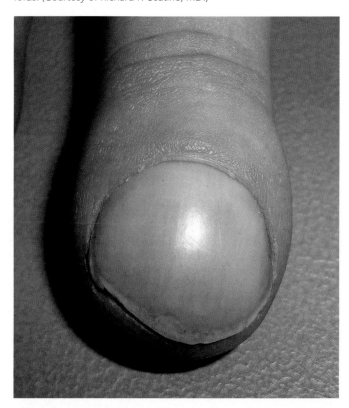

FIGURE 49-2 Close-up view of a clubbed finger. (*Courtesy of Richard P. Usatine, MD.*)

SECONDARY CLUBBING

Secondary clubbing can be caused by many conditions including the following ones:[4]

- Gastrointestinal—Inflammatory bowel disease, cirrhosis, and celiac disease.
- Pulmonary—Malignancy, asbestosis, chronic obstructive pulmonary disease, and cystic fibrosis.
- Cardiac—Congenital heart disease, endocarditis, atrioventricular malformations, or fistulas.

MANAGEMENT

- Clubbing improves with the management of the underlying disease.[2]
- Evaluate patients without an obvious associated disease for lung cancer.[4] SOR **C**
- Evaluate patients with COPD and a phalangeal depth ratio >1 for lung cancer.[3] (LR 3.9, SOR **B**)

REFERENCES

1. White HA, Alcolado R, Alcolado JC. Examination of the hands: An insight into the health of a Welsh population. *Postgrad Med J.* 2003; 79(936):588–589.

2. Kitis G, Thompson H, Allan RN. Finger clubbing in inflammatory bowel disease: Its prevalence and pathogenesis. *BMJl.* 1979; 2(6194):825–828.

3. Baughman RP, Gunther KL, Buchsbaum JA, Lower EE. Prevalence of digital clubbing in bronchogenic carcinoma by a new digital index. *Clin Exp Rheumatol.* 1998;16(1):21–26.

4. Fawcett RS, Linford S, Stulberg DL. Nail abnormalities: Clues to systemic disease. *Am Fam Physician.* 2004;69(6):1417–1424.

5. Myers KA, Farquhar DR. The rational clinical examination. Does this patient have clubbing?[Comment]. *JAMA.* 2001;286(3): 341–347.

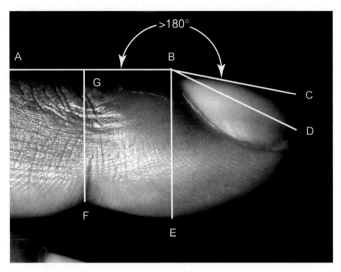

FIGURE 49-3 Clubbing of fingers in a 55-year-old man with COPD. Abnormal profile angle (ABC) and hyponychial angle (ABD); distal phalangeal depth (BE) greater than interphalangeal depth (GF). (*Courtesy of Richard P. Usatine, MD.*)

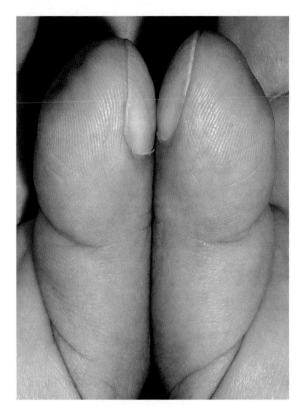

FIGURE 49-4 Schamroth sign: Loss of the normal diamond shape formed when right and left thumbs are opposed in a person with clubbing of the fingers. (*Courtesy of Richard P. Usatine, MD.*)

50 VENOUS INSUFFICIENCY

Maureen K. Sheehan, MD

PATIENT STORY

A 45-year-old woman presents to her physician's office with complaints of heaviness and fatigue in her legs (**Figure 50-1**). She does not experience the symptoms in the morning but they become more noticeable as the day progresses and with prolonged standing. When she stands for many hours, she develops swelling in both of her legs. The symptoms are concentrated over her medial calf where she has prominent tortuous veins. She first noted the veins about 20 years ago when she was pregnant. Initially, they did not cause her any discomfort but have progressively enlarged now and over the past 10 years have become increasingly painful. She recalls that her mother had similar veins in her legs.

EPIDEMIOLOGY

- Varies by definition and region, but generally venous insufficiency affects 27% of population.[1]
- Prevalence estimates vary by some reports, indicating a prevalence of 10.4% to 23% in men and 29.5% to 39% in women.[2,3]
- More frequent in women as compared to men.
- Symptomatic in more than two-third of those affected.
- Varicose veins are notable only in half of patients with venous insufficiency.[4]

ETIOLOGY AND PATHOPHYSIOLOGY

- Most frequently it is a result of valvular dysfunction.
- Valvular dysfunction may be primary or secondary (result of trauma, DVT, or May-Thurner syndrome).
- It may affect deep system (i.e., femoral veins), superficial system (i.e., saphenous vein), or both.
- The superficial system is involved in 88% of cases either alone or in conjunction with the deep system.
- Dysfunction leads to loss of compartmentalization of veins, leading to distension and increased pressure (**Figures 50-1** and **50-2**).
- Increased pressure in veins is transmitted to microvasculature leading to basement membrane thickening, increased capillary elongation, and visual skin changes (**Figures 50-3** and **50-4**).

DIAGNOSIS

- Symptoms: Heaviness, fatigue, and edema; not present immediately in the morning; get worse with prolonged standing or walking; relieved with elevation.

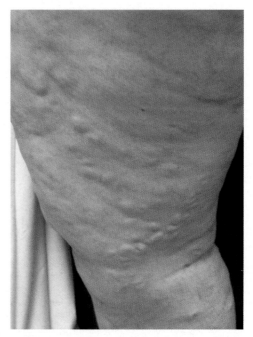

FIGURE 50-1 Uncomplicated varicose veins of thigh. (*Courtesy of Maureen K. Sheehan, MD.*)

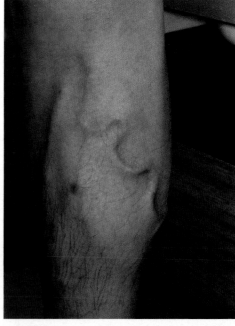

FIGURE 50-2 Varicose veins of posterior calf *without* hemosiderin deposition, lipodermatosclerosis, or ulceration. (*Courtesy of Maureen K. Sheehan, MD.*)

- Typical distribution: Varicose veins can be present anywhere on the leg depending upon affected segments or branches; ulcers from venous disease tend to be near the medial malleoli (**Figure 50-5**).

- Tests: Duplex scanning to assess valve closure; normal valve closure takes 0.5 to 1.0 seconds.

DIFFERENTIAL DIAGNOSIS

- Arterial ulcers—Tend to be at toes, shin, and pressure points (heels or sides of feet).

- Diabetic ulcers—Occur at ambulatory pressure points, mostly at first metatarsal head.

- Malignancy (basal cell or squamous cell carcinoma).

- Chronic infectious diseases (osteomyelitis, leprosy).

- Vasculitides—Irregular border, black necrosis, erythema, or bluish or purplish discoloration of adjacent tissue.

MANAGEMENT

- Graduated compression hose for superficial or deep system insufficiency: SOR **C**
  - 15 to 20 mm Hg—Minor reflux and minimal symptoms.
  - 20 to 30 mm Hg—Moderate to severe reflux and symptoms; moderate edema; postsurgical.
  - 30 to 40 mm Hg—Severe reflux and symptoms; severe edema.

- Compression for open ulcer.[5] SOR **B**

- Compression hose treat symptoms, not underlying pathophysiology. Effective only when being worn.

- Surgical intervention is available either with endovenous ablation or with stripping and ligation if superficial system involved.

- If only deep system involvement, then compression hose is the mainstay of therapy. SOR **C**

- When superficial and deep systems are affected, treatment of superficial system leads to improvement of deep system reflux in one-third of the patients.

- A study randomizing patients to stripping and ligation versus compression therapy demonstrated an improved quality of life in the surgical arm.[7] SOR **A**

- Endovenous therapy uses radiofrequency or laser energy to ablate vein. Since the vein is usually accessed with a needle under ultrasound guidance, an incision is avoided in most all instances.

- Decreased postoperative pain and analgesic use in patients undergoing endovenous ablation compared to those undergoing stripping and ligation.[8] SOR **A**

- Adjunctive phlebectomies for branch varicosities may be necessary with either operative approach.

PATIENT EDUCATION

Venous insufficiency is not merely a cosmetic concern. Long-standing disease can give rise to skin changes (**Figures 50-3** and **50-4**) and

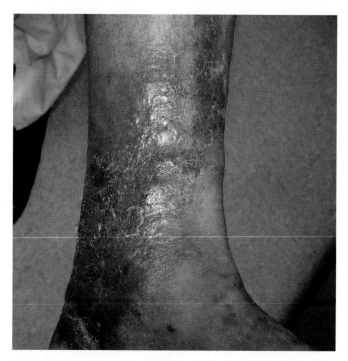

FIGURE 50-3 Lipodermatosclerosis with hemosiderin deposition. (*Courtesy of Maureen K. Sheehan, MD.*)

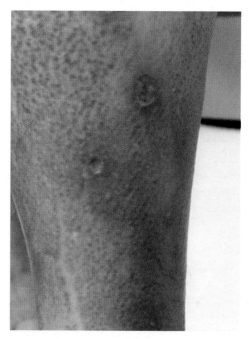

FIGURE 50-4 Healed ulcers with hemosiderin deposition. (*Courtesy of Maureen K. Sheehan, MD.*)

ulcers (**Figure 50-5**). Compliance with compression hose is necessary. Compression hose only treats symptoms, not the underlying disease process. Even after surgical intervention, new varicose veins may appear as the process is chronic.

FOLLOW-UP

• It depends on the treatment and severity of disease.

• Unna boots for ulceration need to be changed at least weekly.

• Compression hose needs to be replaced every 6 months.

• Following surgical intervention, follow-up depends upon intervention. Stripping and ligation requires wound checks, whereas endovenous ablations require ultrasound monitoring.

PATIENT RESOURCES

• American Venous Forum—**http://www.venous-info.com/welcome/patients.html**.

• American College of Phlebology patient care information—**http://www.phlebology.org/index.cfm?sector=patients&page=brochure&b=ip**.

PROVIDER RESOURCES

American College of Phlebology—**http://www.phlebology.org/**.

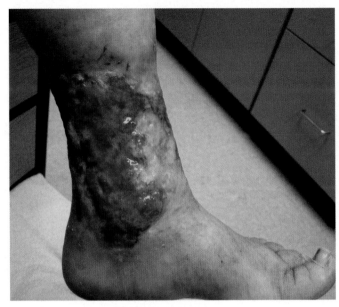

FIGURE 50-5 Venous stasis ulcer in the typical location around the medial malleolus. (*Courtesy of Maureen K. Sheehan, MD.*)

REFERENCES

1. White JV, Ryjewski C. Chronic Venous Insufficiency. *Perspect Vasc Surg Endovasc Ther.* 2005;17:319–327.

2. Beebe-Dimmer JL, Pfeifer JR, Engle JS, Schottenfeld D. The epidemiology of chronic venous insufficiency and varicose veins. *Ann Epidemiol.* 2005;15:175–184.

3. Mundy L, Merlin TL, Fitridge RA, Hiller JE. Systematic review of endovenous laser treatment for varicose veins. *Brit J Surg.* 2005;92:1189–1194.

4. Reichenberg J, Davis M. Venous Ulcers. *Semin Cutan Med Surg.* 2005;24:216–226.

5. Cullum N, Nelson EA, Fletcher AW, Sheldon TA. Compression for venous leg ulcers. *Coch. Data. Syst. Rev.* 2000; Issue 3, Art No.: CD000265.

6. Puggioni A, Lurie F, Kistner RL, et al. How often is deep venous reflux eliminated after saphenous vein ablation? *J Vasc Surg.* 2003; 38:517–521.

7. Michaels JA, Brazier JE, Campbell WB, et al. Randomized clinical trial comparing surgery with conservative treatment for uncomplicated varicose veins. *Brit J Surg.* 2006;93:175–181.

8. Rautio T, Ohinmaa A, Perala J, et al. Endovenous obliteration versus conventional stripping operation in the treatment of primary varicose veins: A randomized controlled trial with the comparison of the costs. *J Vasc Surg.* 2002;35:958–965.

PART 8

THE LUNGS

51 COMMUNITY-ACQUIRED PNEUMONIA

Mindy A. Smith, MD, MS

PATIENT STORY

A 55-year-old man complains of a terrible cough and fever for several days' duration. His cough is productive with rusty colored sputum. He is otherwise healthy. His chest x-ray is similar to the one shown in **Figure 51-1**. He is diagnosed with probable bacterial pneumonia and is placed on antibiotics.

EPIDEMIOLOGY

- Four million adults per year in United States with community-acquired pneumonia (CAP) (8–15/1000 persons/year).

- Twenty percent patients are admitted to hospital; half with *S. pneumoniae.*

- Increased incidence in men and blacks versus whites.

- Other risk factors include smoking, alcohol (relative risk (RR, 9), asthma (RR, 4.2), immune suppression (RR, 1.9), and age >70 (RR 1.5 vs. 60–69 year olds).[1]

ETIOLOGY AND PATHOPHYSIOLOGY

Pneumonia refers to an infection in the lower respiratory tract (distal airways, alveoli, and interstitium of the lung).

- Most common route of infection is microaspiration of oropharyngeal secretions colonized by pathogens. In this setting, *S. pneumoniae* and *Haemophilus influenza* are the most common pathogens.

- Pneumonia secondary to gross aspiration occurs postoperatively or in those with central nervous system disorders; anaerobes and gram-negative bacilli are common pathogens.

- Hematogenous spread, most often from the urinary tract, results in *Escherichia coli* pneumonia, and hematogenous spread from intravenous catheters or in the setting of endocarditis may cause *Staphyloccocus aureus* pneumonia.

- *Mycobacterium tuberculosis* (TB), fungi, *legionella,* and many respiratory viruses are spread by aerosolization.

- Etiology is unknown in up to 70% of cases of CAP.

DIAGNOSIS

The history can provide clues to the likely pathogen:[1]

- Alcoholism—Consider *Strep. pneumoniae, Kleibsiella, S. aureus,* and anaerobes.

- Chronic obstructive pulmonary disease: Consider *S. pneumoniae, Haemophilus influenza,* and *Moraxella.*

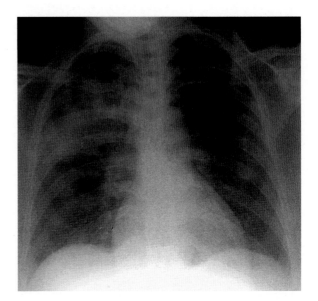

FIGURE 51-1 Chest x-ray (CXR) showing right upper lobe consolidation. (*From Miller WT, Jr. Diagnostic Thoracic Imaging, p. 218, Figure 5-1 B, Copyright 2006, McGraw-Hill.*)

- Uncontrolled diabetes mellitus—Consider *S. pneumoniae* and *S. aureus*.

- Sickle-cell disease—Consider *S. pneumoniae*.

- HIV with low CD4 count—*S. pneumoniae*, *Pneumocystis carinii*, *Haemophilus influenza*, *cryptococcus*, and TB.

CLINICAL FEATURES

- Constellation of symptoms include cough, fever, chills, pleuritic chest pain, and sputum production.

- Signs include increased respiratory rate, dullness to percussion, bronchial breathing, egophony, crackles, wheezes, and pleural-friction rub.

LABORATORY STUDIES

- Sputum gram stain may be helpful in determining etiology in hospitalized patients. An adequate specimen has >25 WBC and <10 epithelial cells per high powered field. Testing of induced sputum has established merit only for detection of TB and *Pneumocystis carinii*.[2] SOR **A**

- Special stains are needed for detecting TB, *Pneumocystis carinii*, and fungi.

- Blood cultures should be considered in ambulatory patients with a temperature >38.5°C or <36°C or in those who are homeless or abusing alcohol.[1] SOR **C**

- Blood cultures (two sets prior to administration of antibiotics) are suggested for hospitalized patients SOR **C** and are positive in 6% to 20%. Investigators in a Canadian study found that blood cultures had limited usefulness in the routine management of patients admitted to the hospital with uncomplicated CAP; only 1.97% (15 of 760 patients) had a change of therapy directed by blood culture results.[3]

- Urinary antigens may be useful in diagnosing legionnaires disease (*L. pneumophila*) and *S. pneumoniae*.[2] SOR **B**

- Serology (IgM titer) may be useful in diagnosing *Mycoplasma pneumoniae*, *Chlamydia pneumoniae*, legionnaires, and viral pneumonia such as influenza.[2] SOR **C**

IMAGING

The diagnosis of pneumonia based on clinical history and examination is only 47% to 69% sensitive and 58% to 75% specific and therefore chest x-ray (CXR) is considered a standard part of evaluation. If the initial CXR is negative in a patient with clinical features of pneumonia, the CXR should be repeated in 24 to 48 hours or a chest CT be considered. SOR **C**

There are four general patterns of pneumonia seen on CXR:

- Lobar—Consolidation involves the entire lobe (**Figures 51-1** to **51-5**). A cavity with an air-fluid level is sometimes seen within the area of consolidation representing abscess formation (**Figure 51-5**).

- Bronchopneumonia—Patchy involvement of one or several lobes that may be extensive (**Figures 51-6** and **51-7**), usually in the dependent lower and posterior lungs (**Figure 51-3**).

- Interstitial pneumonia—Inflammatory process involves the interstitium; usually patchy and diffuse (**Figure 51-8**). A nodular interstitial pattern is seen in patients with histoplasmosis (**Figure 51-9**), miliary TB, pneumoconiosis, and sarcoidosis.

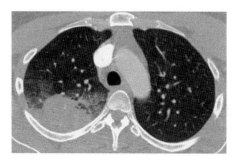

FIGURE 51-2 CT scan in the patient in **Figure 51-1**, demonstrating a confluent region of lung consolidation with ground-glass opacification on the margins of the consolidated lung commonly seen in bacterial pneumonia. (*From Miller WT, Jr. Diagnostic Thoracic Imaging, p. 218, Figure 5-1 C, Copyright 2006, McGraw-Hill.*)

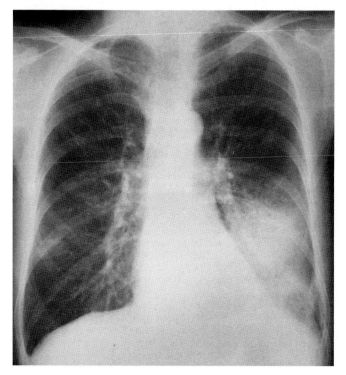

FIGURE 51-3 Posteroanterior chest x-ray consolidation in the left lower lobe occupying all three basilar segments. There is blunting of the left costophrenic angle indicating a parapneumonic effusion. (*From Miller WT, Jr. Diagnostic Thoracic Imaging, p. 219, Figure 5-2 C, Copyright 2006, McGraw-Hill.*)

• Miliary pneumonia—Numerous discrete lesions from hematogenous spread (see tuberculosis) (see Chapter 52, Tuberculosis).

DIFFERENTIAL DIAGNOSIS

• Upper respiratory illnesses, including bronchitis, can cause cough, fever, chills, and sputum production with a negative chest x-ray (CXR).

• Pulmonary embolus should be considered in patients with pleuritic chest pain or hypoxia and a negative CXR (see Chapter 53, Pulmonary Embolus).

• Asthma can cause cough, wheezing, dyspnea, and hypoxia, whereas CXR tests negative unless mucous plugging causes collapse of airways.

MANAGEMENT

• Initial determination of severity of illness:
  ◦ Respiratory rate (RR) >30 breaths/minute without underlying disease is single best predictor.
  ◦ British Thoracic Society (BTS) rule—The presence of one or more of the following four: confusion; blood urea nitrogen >7 mmol/L; RR > 30/min; systolic blood pressure <90 mm Hg or diastolic blood pressure <60 mm Hg. If none are present, mortality is 2.4%; one present 8%; two present 23%; three present 33%; and all four present 80%.
  ◦ A number of other severity scores are available, but a recent study found that the modified BTS performed best, although they recommend validation in each clinical setting.[4]

• Assessment of oxygen consumption/hypoxia.

• Consider hospitalization if severe (BTS score >0), hypoxic, worsening symptoms, preexisting conditions are present that compromise safety of home care or fail to improve in more than 72 hours.

• Empiric antibiotic treatment: [1]
  ◦ Outpatient, uncomplicated—Macrolide (erythromycin, azithromycin, or clarithromycin) or doxycycline. SOR Ⓐ
  ◦ Outpatient with cardiac disease or high risk for drug resistant *S. pneumoniae*—Quinolone with enhanced activity against *S. pneumoniae* (i.e., levofloxacin, moxifloxacin, and gatifloxacin) or beta-lactam plus macrolide or doxycycline or telithromycin. Telithromycin was recently reported to be associated with serious liver toxicity in three patients following administration.[5] Hospitalized patient—beta-lactam plus macrolide combination or quinolone with enhanced activity (as above).[2] SOR Ⓐ
  ◦ Nursing home—Amoxicillin/clavulanic acid plus macrolide or quinolone with enhanced activity against *S. pneumoniae* or ceftriaxone or cefotaxime plus macrolide.
  ◦ Aspiration pneumonia—No antibiotics for 24 hours; if poor dental hygiene or alcoholic treat with metronidazole or piperacillin/tazobactam or imipenem plus quinolone (as above) or ceftriaxone or cefotaxime.

• Duration 10 to 14 days SOR Ⓒ; 5 days if long-acting antibiotic (i.e., azithromycin), possibly 5 days with a quinolone if uncomplicated CAP[6] and 21 days if treating legionnaires disease.

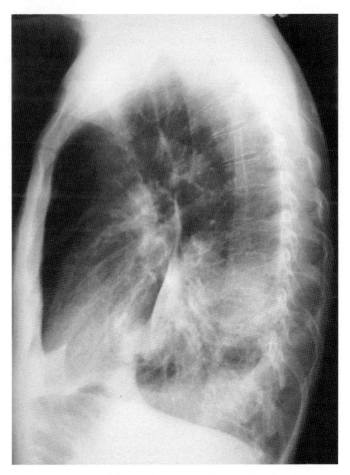

FIGURE 51-4 Lateral CXR in the patient in **Figure 51-3** showing posterior displacement of the major fissure indicating some atelectasis of the left lower lobe. (*From Miller WT, Jr. Diagnostic Thoracic Imaging, p. 219, Figure 5-2 D, Copyright 2006, McGraw-Hill.*)

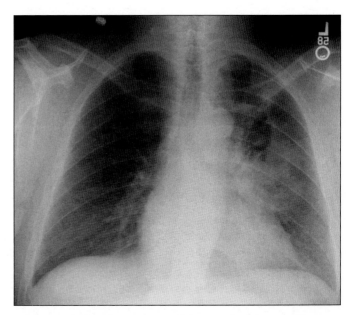

FIGURE 51-5 CXR showing a consolidation in the left upper lobe; note oval lucency that represents cavitation within the infiltrate. This patient had *Klebsiella* pneumonia. (*From Miller WT, Jr. Diagnostic Thoracic Imaging, p. 223, Figure 5-6 A, Copyright 2006, McGraw-Hill.*)

PATIENT EDUCATION

- Patients who smoke should be offered cessation assistance.

- Improvement is expected in healthy outpatients younger than 65 years in 48 to 72 hours with their returning to work in approximately 4 to 5 days and complete improvement within 2 weeks.

- In hospitalized patients, clinical stability is expected in 3 to 7 days; mortality is 8% with 70% developing a complication such as respiratory failure, congestive heart failure, shock, dysrhythmia, myocardial infarction, gastrointestinal bleeding, or renal insufficiency.

FOLLOW-UP SOR Ⓒ

- Assess need and provide pneumococcal and influenza vaccination.

- Monitor improvement and treat comorbid illness (which may worsen).

- Repeat CXR until clear, if patient is older than 40 years or smokes —2% of them may have underlying cancer.[1]

PATIENT RESOURCES

Sites where patients may obtain additional information:

- National Institutes of Health: **www.nlm.nih.gov/ medlineplus/pneumonia.html.**

- Mayo clinics patient education site: **www.mayoclinic.com/ health/pneumonia.**

PROVIDER RESOURCES

Several evidence-based guidelines are available at **www.guideline.gov.** (Includes Ref. 2 and Institute for Clinical Systems Improvement (ICSI). Community-acquired pneumonia in adults. Bloomington, MN: ICSI; 2005.)

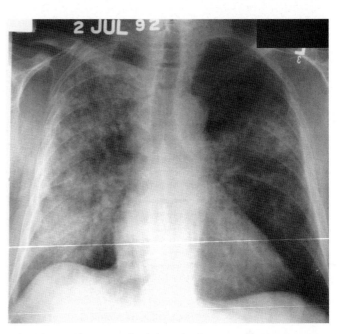

FIGURE 51-6 This patient has bilateral pulmonary infiltrates worsening despite antibiotics characteristic of severe bronchopneumonia. Note air bronchograms on the right side. He was diagnosed with *Legionella* pneumonia. (*From Miller WT, Jr. Diagnostic Thoracic Imaging, p. 221, Figure 5-4 B, Copyright 2006, McGraw-Hill.*)

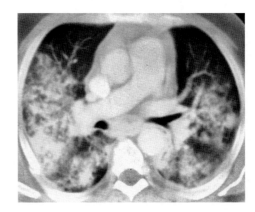

FIGURE 51-7 CT scan in the patient in **Figure 51-6** at the level of the main pulmonary arteries showing extensive pulmonary consolidation in both lungs. (*From Miller WT, Jr. Diagnostic Thoracic Imaging, p. 221, Figure 5-4 D, Copyright 2006, McGraw-Hill.*)

REFERENCES

1. Marrie TJ, Campbell GD, Walker DH, Low DE. Pneumonia. In: Kasper DL, Braunwald E, Fauci AS, Hauser SL, Longo DL, Jameson JL eds. *Harrison's Principles of Internal Medicine*, 16th ed. New York: McGraw-Hill, 2005:1528–1541.

2. Mandell LA, Bartlett JG, Dowell SF, File TM Jr, Musher DM, Whitney C. Update of practice guidelines for the management of community-acquired pneumonia in immunocompetent adults. *Clin Infect Dis*. 2003;37(11):1405–1433.

3. Campbell SG, Marrie TJ, Anstey R, et al. The contribution of blood cultures to the clinical management of adult patients admitted to the hospital with community-acquired pneumonia: A prospective observational study. *Chest*. 2003;123(4):1142–1150.

4. Buising KL, Thursky KA, Black JF, et al. Reconsidering what is meant by severe pneumonia: A prospective comparison of severity scores for community-acquired pneumonia. *Thorax*. 2006;61(5): 419–424.

5. Clay KD, Hanson JS, Pope SD, et al. Brief communication: Severe hepatotoxicity of telithromycin: Three case reports and literature review. *Ann Intern Med*. 2006;144(6):415–420.

6. Shorr AF, Zadeikis N, Xiang JX, et al. A multicenter, randomized, double-blind, retrospective comparison of 5- and 10-day regimens of levofloxacin in a subgroup of patients aged >/=65 years with community-acquired pneumonia. *Clin Ther*. 2005;27(8): 1251–1259.

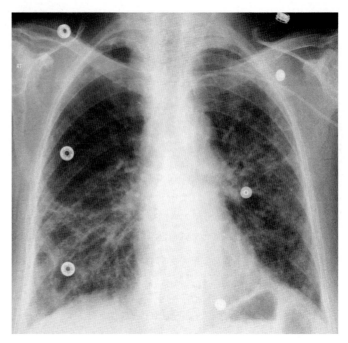

FIGURE 51-8 Chest x-ray showing basilar predominant interstitial lung disease in this 70-year old woman; given her age, idiopathic pulmonary fibrosis is the most likely diagnosis. (*From Miller WT, Jr. Diagnostic Thoracic Imaging, p. 81, Figure 3-10 A, Copyright 2006, McGraw-Hill.*)

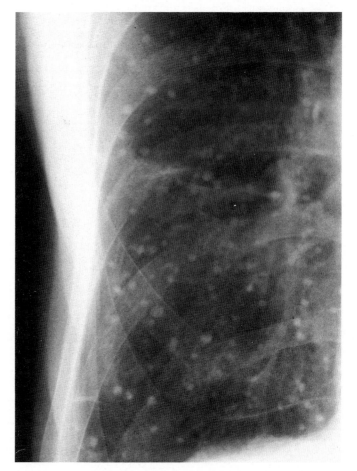

FIGURE 51-9 Nodular interstitial pattern with many calcified granulomas in a patient with histoplasmosis. (*From Schwartz DT and Reisdorff EJ. Emergency Radiology, p. 460, Figure 17-15, Copyright 2000, McGraw-Hill.*)

52 TUBERCULOSIS

Mindy A. Smith, MD, MS

PATIENT STORY

A 57-year-old emergency department nurse presents with a persistent cough for the last 3 weeks with low-grade fever and night sweats. She had an episode of hemoptysis last night and fears that she may have lung cancer. She smokes an occasional cigarette and her only medical problem is diabetes, which is fairly well controlled on oral medication. Her chest x-ray (CXR) is similar to the radiograph in **Figure 52-1**. She is initially treated for pneumonia, but fails to respond to antibiotic treatment. At follow-up, sputum cultures became positive for tuberculosis (TB) and she is started on a 2-month initial treatment phase with anti-TB medications.

EPIDEMIOLOGY[1]

- Primarily involves the lungs although other organs are involved in one-third of cases.

- Estimated 8.5 million cases worldwide in 2001, 90% of cases occurring in developing countries.

- About 15,000 cases reported in the United States in 2002.

- Most cases in the United States are reported in the elderly, HIV-infected young adults, and in immigrant and disadvantaged populations subject to overcrowding. In a study of hospital personnel, only the percentage of low-income persons within the employee's residential postal zone was independently associated with conversion (odds ratio 1.39, 95% CI, 1.09–1.78).[2]

- Without treatment, approximately one-third will die within 1 year and half within 5 years. Of those who survive 5 years, 60% will have undergone spontaneous remission and the remaining will continue to be infectious.

- Treatment of those with latent TB (infection without active disease—usually diagnosed by skin test conversion from negative to positive) will reduce the risk of active TB by ≥ 90%. SOR Ⓐ

ETIOLOGY AND PATHOPHYSIOLOGY

- Most human cases caused by *Mycobacterium tuberculosis (M.TB)*.

- Infection is transmitted by aerosolized respiratory droplet nuclei.

- About 10% of those infected develop active TB, usually within 1–2 years of exposure; risk factors for the development of active TB include recent infection (<1 year) (relative risk [RR] 12.9 versus old infection), fibrotic lesions (spontaneously healed) (RR 2–20), HIV infection (RR 100), jejunoileal bypass (RR 30–60), silicosis (RR 30), chronic renal failure/hemodialysis (RR 10–25), intravenous drug use (RR 10–30), immunosuppressive treatment (RR 10), and malnutrition (RR 2).[1]

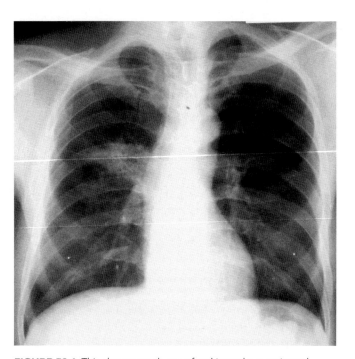

FIGURE 52-1 This chest x-ray shows a focal irregular marginated opacity in the right upper lobe. Initially treated for pneumonia, the patient failed to respond to antibiotic treatment for pneumonia; sputum cultures became positive for TB. (*From Miller WT, Jr. Diagnostic Thoracic Imaging, p. 289, Figure 6-5 A, Copyright 2006, McGraw-Hill.*)

- There are 3 host responses to infection: Immediate non specific macrophage ingestion of those bacilli reaching the alveoli, later tissue-damaging response (delayed-type hypersensitivity reaction), and specific macrophage activating response—the latter, if effective, walling off infection into granulomas.

- In areas of high prevalence, TB is often seen in children. The disease process usually localizes to the middle and upper lung zones accompanied by hilar and paratracheal lymphadenopathy (as the tubercle bacilli spread from lung to lymphatic vessels). The primary focus usually heals spontaneously and may disappear entirely or, if encapsulated by fibroblasts and collagen fibers, be visible as a calcified lung nodule (Ghon [primary] lesion) (**Figure 52-2**).

DIAGNOSIS

The diagnosis of TB requires a high index of suspicion. Manifestations of active TB can be classified as pulmonary or extrapulmonary.

CLINICAL FEATURES

- Pulmonary:
  - Early nonspecific signs and symptoms: fever, night sweats, fatigue, anorexia, weight loss.
  - Later nonproductive cough or cough with purulent sputum.
  - Patients with extensive disease may develop dyspnea or acute respiratory distress syndrome.
  - Physical examination findings also nonspecific with crackles or rhonchi.

- Extrapulmonary TB, caused by hematogenous spread, occurs in the following order of frequency:
  - Lymph nodes: painless swelling of cervical and supraclavicular nodes (scrofula).
  - Pleura: pleural effusion with exudates.
  - Genitourinary tract: may cause urethral stricture, kidney damage or infertility (in women, affects the fallopian tubes and endometrium).
  - Bones and joints: pain in the spine (Pott's disease), hips, or knees.
  - Other less common sites are meninges, peritoneum, and pericardium.

SKIN TESTING

Skin testing with purified protein derivative is not useful in diagnosing active TB but is used to detect latent infection in exposed or high-risk individuals. A positive test is 10 mm induration at the inoculation site or 5 mm induration in a patient who is immune-compromised.

A new in vitro test, QuantiFERON-TB Gold (QFT-G, Cellestis Limited, Carnegie, Victoria, Australia), received approval from the U.S. Food and Drug Administration as an aid for diagnosing *M. TB* infection.[3] This test detects the release of interferon-gamma in fresh heparinized whole blood from sensitized persons when it is incubated with mixtures of synthetic peptides representing two proteins present in M. TB; the test may be more sensitive than testing with purified protein derivative.

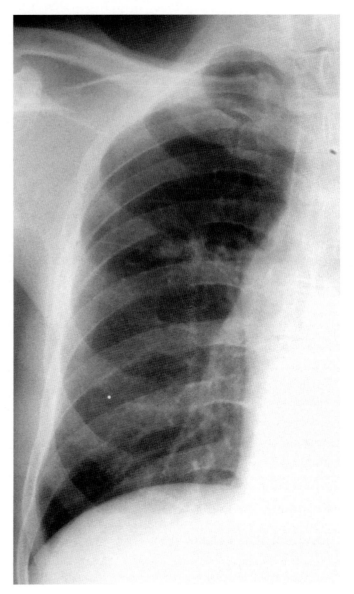

FIGURE 52-2 One year later, a chest x-ray of the patient in **Figure 52-1** shows the primary TB has coalesced into a small granuloma. (*From Miller WT, Jr. Diagnostic Thoracic Imaging, p. 289, Figure 6-5 E, Copyright 2006, McGraw-Hill.*)

LABORATORY STUDIES

- Nonspecific findings include mild anemia and leukocytosis.

- Urinalysis may show pyuria and hematuria with urinary tract involvement.

- Acid-fast bacilli may be seen on gram stain from sputum or pleural or peritoneal fluid. They may also be seen upon staining tissue from fine needle aspiration or biopsy of lymph nodes or other tissues as above.

- Definitive diagnosis is based on culture of sputum, urine (3 morning specimens—positive in 90% with urinary tract infection), or from tissue or bone biopsy. *M. TB* is slow growing and may take 4 to 8 weeks to identify. Once identified, testing for drug sensitivity should be performed.

- Obtaining baseline liver enzymes is suggested for monitoring drug toxicity.

IMAGING

- CXR classically shows upper lobe infiltrate with cavitation (**Figure 52-3**) but any pattern may be seen ranging from a solitary nodule (**Figure 52-2**) to diffuse infiltrates that may represent bronchogenic spread (**Figures 52-4** and **52-5**).
  - CXR pattern in children often shows an infiltrate with hilar and paratracheal lymphadenopathy (**Figure 52-6**).
  - In disseminated TB, innumerable tiny nodules are seen throughout both lungs (**Figure 52-7**).

- X-ray, CT, or MRI of bone may show destructive lesions.

BIOPSY

Histology reveals granulomatous lesions.

DIFFERENTIAL DIAGNOSIS

Because any pattern on CXR may be seen with active TB, the differential diagnosis includes:

- Bacterial or viral pneumonia—No TB contacts, sputum or serum culture may reveal the infecting organism, and the patient will usually respond to antibacterial drugs and/or time.

- Fungal respiratory infections:
  - Acute histoplasmosis is usually asymptomatic or causes only mild symptoms and CXR typically shows hilar adenopathy with or without pneumonitis (**Figure 52-8**); patients with chronic pulmonary histoplasmosis have gradually increasing cough, weight loss and night sweats and CXR shows uni- or bilateral fibronodular, apical infiltrates.
  - Coccidiomycosis has similar clinical features to TB and CXR may show infiltrate, hilar adenopathy, and pleural effusion; serologic tests are useful in the diagnosis.

MANAGEMENT

Patients may be managed by their primary care provider, by public health departments, or jointly, but in all cases the health department is ultimately responsible for ensuring availability of appropriate diagnostic and treatment services and for monitoring the results of therapy.

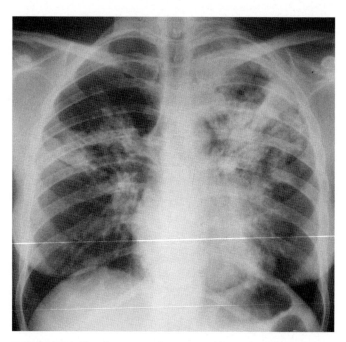

FIGURE 52-3 This chest x-ray of a 29-year-old patient with cough and fever demonstrates a focal area of consolidation in the left upper lobe with several areas of cavitation. (*From Miller WT, Jr. Diagnostic Thoracic Imaging, p. 393, Figure 8-2 A, Copyright 2006, McGraw-Hill.*)

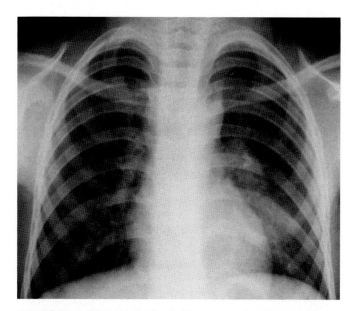

FIGURE 52-4 CT scan at the level of the aortic arch shows multiple cavities and consolidation in the left lung and multiple tree-in-bud opacities in the right lung typical of bronchogenic spread. (*From Miller WT, Jr. Diagnostic Thoracic Imaging, p. 394, Figure 8-2 E, Copyright 2006, McGraw-Hill.*)

For adult patients with *active-TB* there are four major drugs used for treatment. The first-line anti-TB medications should be administered together; split dosing should be avoided. A few combination medications are available but are more costly. The following regimen is suggested by the American Thoracic Society, Infectious Diseases Society of America and the Center for Disease Control and Prevention[1]: SOR **C**

- Two-month initial-treatment phase with all four medications (isoniazid 5 mg/kg daily (maximum 300 mg) or 15 mg/kg thrice weekly (maximum 900 mg); rifampin (10 mg/kg daily or thrice weekly (maximum 600 mg); pyrazinamide (20–25 mg/kg daily (maximum 2 gm) or 30–40 mg/kg thrice weekly (maximum 3 g); and ethambutol (15–20 mg/kg daily or 25–30 mg/kg thrice weekly).[1]

- Four-month continuation phase with isoniazid and rifampin; treatment is extended to 7 months for patients with cavitary pulmonary TB who remain sputum positive after initial treatment or if pregnant.

- To prevent isoniazid-related neuropathy, pyridoxine 10–25 mg/d may be given, especially to those at risk for vitamin B6 deficiency (i.e., alcoholic, malnourished, pregnant or lactating women, HIV-positive, and those with chronic disease).

- Drug-resistant TB is treated with a variety of injectable drugs including streptomycin, kanamycin, and amikacin or oral drugs including fluoroquinolones, ethionamide, cycloserine, and *p*-aminosalicylic acid.[1] In a Cochrane review of 10 small trials on the use of fluoroquinolones in TB regimens, investigators found no difference in trials substituting ciprofloxacin or ofloxacin for first-line drugs in relation to cure (89 participants, 2 trials), treatment failure (388 participants, 3 trials), or clinical or radiologic improvement (216 participants, 2 trials).[4] Substituting ciprofloxacin into first-line regimens in drug-sensitive TB led to a higher incidence of relapse in HIV-positive patients.

- Research into adjuvant immunotherapy (e.g., antitumor necrosis factor therapies) is underway to determine whether this treatment will accelerate the response to treatment.

Treatment may be given daily or intermittently (3 times a week throughout or twice weekly after the initial phase). For patients who are HIV-seronegative with noncavitary pulmonary TB and negative cultures at 2-months, treatment may be given once weekly.

For adult patients with *latent TB*, the following options are used:

- Isoniazid 5 mg/kg daily (maximum 300 mg) for 9 months; SOR **A** twice weekly regimens (15 mg/kg (maximum 900 mg)) may be considered if the patients is under direct observation therapy and 6 month therapy may be considered for adults who are not HIV-infected and have no fibrotic lesions on CXR. SOR **B**

- Rifampin (10 mg/kg daily; maximum 600 mg) for 4 months if isoniazid-resistant TB or allergy.

PATIENT EDUCATION

Identifying and testing household and other intimate contacts and maintaining follow-up are extremely important for preventing

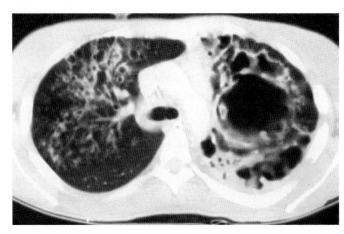

FIGURE 52-5 One month later, the patient in **Figure 52-4** has had progression of disease with confluent nodular areas of consolidation in the lower zones of the left lung consistent with bronchogenic spread and additional areas of consolidation in the right upper lobe indicating spread. He had not been able to adhere to medication regimen. (*From Miller WT, Jr. Diagnostic Thoracic Imaging, p. 393, Figure 8-2 B, Copyright 2006, McGraw-Hill.*)

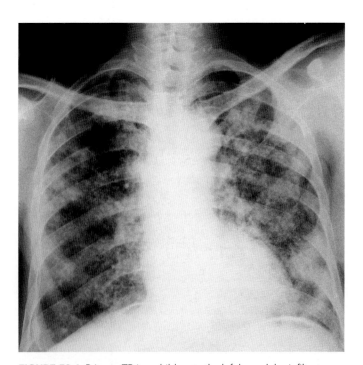

FIGURE 52-6 Primary TB in a child; note the left lower lobe infiltrate and the left hilar lymphadenopathy and right paratracheal adenopathy. (*From Schwartz DT and Reisdorff EJ. Emergency Radiology, p. 469, Figure 17-28, Copyright 2000, McGraw-Hill.*)

spread, insuring cure, and monitoring for drug toxicity (as below). The potential severity of TB should be emphasized.

If available, patients should consider receiving treatment through a Directly Observed Therapy Short course program. Directly Observed Therapy Short course is composed of five distinct elements: Political commitment; microscopy services; drug supplies; surveillance and monitoring systems and use of highly efficacious regimens; and direct observation of treatment.[5] Although data are conflicting about the benefits of such programs, they may be better equipped to provide the intense services needed, especially in resource poor communities.

FOLLOW-UP[1] SOR Ⓒ

- Monitor compliance with treatment; risk factors for non-compliance include lack of motivation, lack of perceived vulnerability, and poverty.

- Monitor response to treatment—monthly sputum cultures should be obtained until culture negative (80% expected by 2 months); If culture positive at ≥3 months, consider drug resistance or treatment failure. For those with extra-pulmonary TB, monitor clinically.

- CXR is not used for monitoring treatment as clearing lags behind clinical improvement. A CXR should be completed at the end of treatment for later comparison if reactivation is suspected.

- Monitor drug toxicity:
  - Gastrointestinal side effects and pruritus are common and can generally be managed without suspending treatment.
  - Hepatitis is the most common serious adverse event (symptoms include dark urine and decreased appetite); elevation of liver enzymes up to 3 times normal occurs in 20% and is of no clinical importance. Treatment (isoniazid, pyrazinamide, or rifampin) should be discontinued for elevations of 5 times or more or with symptoms and drugs re-introduced one at a time after liver function has normalized.
  - Hypersensitivity reactions usually require discontinuing treatment.
  - Hyperuricemia and arthralgias may occur with pyrazinamide and can be managed with aspirin; the drug should be discontinued if the patient develops gouty arthritis.
  - Autoimmune thrombocytopenia may be caused by rifampin and requires discontinuing the drug.
  - Optic neuritis may occur with ethambutol and the drug should be discontinued.

- Routine measurements of hepatic and renal function and platelet count are not necessary during treatment unless patients have baseline abnormalities or are at increased risk of hepatotoxicity (e.g., hepatitis B or C virus infection, alcohol abuse).

PATIENT RESOURCES

Patient education materials can be found at—
www.cdc.gov/nchstp/tb/faqs/qa.htm;
www.nlm.nih.gov/medlineplus/tuberculosis.html.

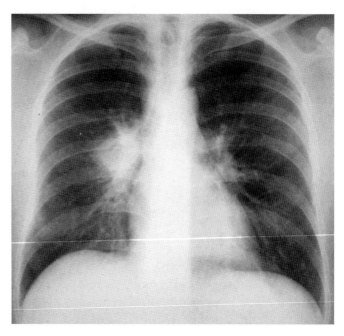

FIGURE 52-7 Disseminated (miliary) TB with tiny innumerable nodules throughout both lungs. (*From Schwartz DT and Reisdoff EJ. Emergency Radiology, p. 470, Figure 17-30 (upper block only), Copyright 2000, McGraw-Hill.*)

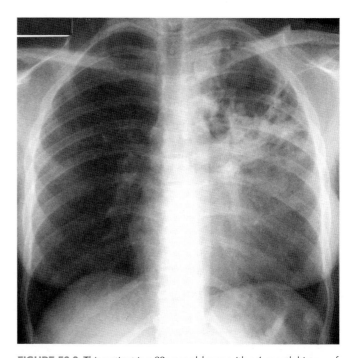

FIGURE 52-8 This patient is a 33-year-old man with a 6-month history of fatigue; chest x-ray shows a 4 cm mass overlying the right hilum and a lumpy contour of the left hilum that indicates lymphadenopathy. Histoplasmosis was diagnosed on bronchoscopy. (*From Miller WT, Jr. Diagnostic Thoracic Imaging, p. 357, Figure 7-52 A, Copyright 2006, McGraw-Hill.*)

PROVIDER RESOURCES

Evidence-based guidelines are available at—**www.guideline.gov.**

Neff M. ATS, CDC, and IDSA update recommendations on the treatment of tuberculosis *Am Fam Physician* 2003;68(9):1854, 1857–1858, 1861–1862; Treatment of tuberculosis. *MMWR Recomm Rep.* 2003 Jun 20;52(RR-11):1–77.

Information about occupational exposure and TB can be found at—**www.osha.gov/SLTC/tuberculosis/index.html.**

REFERENCES

1. Raviglione MC, O'Brien RJ. Tuberculosis. In: Kasper DL, Braunwald E, Fauci AS, Hauser SL, Longo DL, Jameson, JL eds. *Harrison's Principles of Internal Medicine*, 16th ed. New York: McGraw-Hill, 2005:953–966.

2. Bailey TC, Fraser VJ, Spitznagel EL, Dunagan WC. Risk factors for a positive tuberculin skin test among employees of an urban, midwestern teaching hospital. *Ann Intern Med.* 1995;122(8):580–585.

3. Mazurek GH, Jereb J, Lobue P, et al. Guidelines for using the QuantiFERON-TB Gold test for detecting Mycobacterium tuberculosis infection, United States. *MMWR Recomm Rep.* 2005; 54(RR–15):49–55.

4. Ziganshina LE, Vizel AA, Squire SB. Fluoroquinolones for treating tuberculosis. *Cochrane Database Syst Rev.* 2005;20(3):CD004795.

5. Davies PD. The role of DOTS in tuberculosis treatment and control. *Am J Respir Med.* 2003;2(3):203–209.

53 PULMONARY EMBOLISM

Mindy A. Smith, MD, MS

PATIENT STORY

A 52-year-old woman developed acute shortness of breath 3 weeks after a hysterectomy. She denied leg pain or swelling. She has no chronic medical problems and takes no medications. Her pulse is 105 beats per minute, respiratory rate is 20 breaths per minute, and the rest of her examination is unremarkable. She had an elevated hemidiaphragm on chest x-ray (CXR). These findings placed her at moderate risk for pulmonary embolism (PE) based on the Geneva score. Chest computed tomography (CT) demonstrated a moderate-sized PE similar to the one shown in **Figure 53-1**. She was treated with anticoagulation without complications.

EPIDEMIOLOGY

Population estimate of the age- and sex-adjusted annual incidence of deep vein thrombosis (DVT) is 48 per 100,000 and 69 per 100,000 for PE; the incidence increases with age.[1]

ETIOLOGY AND PATHOPHYSIOLOGY

- Most commonly caused by embolization of a thrombus from a proximal leg or pelvic vein that enters the pulmonary artery circulation and obstructs a vessel. Pulmonary emboli may also be caused by:
  - An upper extremity thrombus (from indwelling catheters or pacemakers) (**Figure 53-1**).
  - Fat embolus (following surgery or trauma).
  - Hair/talc/cotton embolus (from intravenous drug use).
  - Amniotic fluid embolus (from a tear at the placental margin in a pregnant woman).

- In a population study, independent risk factors for DVT included[2]:
  - Surgery (OR, 21.7; 95% CI, 9.4–49.9).
  - Trauma (OR, 12.7; 95% CI, 4.1–39.7).
  - Hospital or nursing home confinement (OR, 8.0; 95% CI, 4.5–14.2).
  - Malignant neoplasm with (OR, 6.5; 95% CI, 2.1–20.2) or without (OR, 4.1; 95% CI, 1.9–8.5) chemotherapy.
  - Central venous catheter or pacemaker (OR, 5.6; 95% CI, 1.6–19.6).
  - Superficial vein thrombosis (OR, 4.3; 95% CI, 1.8–10.6).
  - Neurologic disease with extremity paresis (OR, 3.0; 95% CI, 1.3–7.4).

- Other risk factors for PE include hormonal treatment (i.e., oral contraceptives or menopausal hormone therapy), pregnancy, obesity, smoking, chronic obstructive pulmonary disease, and clotting disorders.

- Genetic predisposition includes factor V Leiden and prothrombin gene mutations.

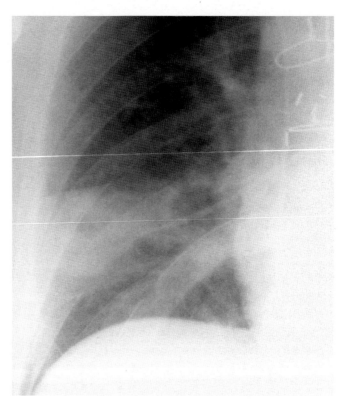

FIGURE 53-1 Chest x-ray showing a wedge-shaped pulmonary infarction with the base on the pleural surface and the apex at the tip of a pulmonary artery catheter; the catheter caused the occlusion of a peripheral artery. (*From Miller WT, Jr. Diagnostic Thoracic Imaging, p. 272, Figure 5-61, Copyright 2006, McGraw-Hill.*)

- Although most PE are asymptomatic and do not alter physiology, PE can cause:
  - Increased pulmonary, vascular, and airway resistance (from obstruction of vessels or distal airways).
  - Impaired gas exchange (from increased dead space and right to left shunting).
  - Alveolar hyperventilation (from stimulation of irritant receptors).
  - Decreased pulmonary compliance (from lung edema, hemorrhage, or loss of surfactant).
  - Right ventricular (RV) dysfunction (from increased pulmonary vascular resistance, increased RV wall tension, and reduced right coronary artery flow).

DIAGNOSIS

CLINICAL FEATURES

- Dyspnea—the most common symptom and tachycardia the most common sign.
- Chest pain—may be caused by a small, peripheral PE with pulmonary infarction.
- Other signs—include fever, neck vein distention, and accentuated pulmonic component of the second heart sound.
- Massive PE—may present with shock, syncope, and cyanosis.
- Clinical scoring systems—useful for determining the clinical (pretest) probability of PE; the two most frequently used are the Geneva and the Wells score.[3,4] The Geneva score appears to be the most consistent across experience of examiner.[5] Scores <5 indicate a low probability of PE; 5–8 indicates a moderate probability of PE; >8 indicates a high probability of PE. The Geneva score is derived by summing the following points:
  - Age (+1 for 60–79 years and +2 for ≥80 years).
  - Previous DVT or PE (+2).
  - Recent surgery (<4 weeks ago, +3).
  - Heart rate >100 bpm (+1).
  - $PaCO_2$ (<35 mm Hg +2 or 35–39 mm Hg +1).
  - PaO_2 (<49 mm Hg +4, 49–59 mm Hg +3, 60–71 mm Hg +2, 72–82 mm Hg +1).
  - CXR with band atelectasis (+1) and/or elevated hemidiaphragm (+1).

LABORATORY STUDIES AND ECG

- Plasma D-dimer immunosorbent assay may be useful to rule out a PE (sensitive but not specific).[6] SOR **B** The test is suggested for patients with low clinical probability of a PE—if negative, there is only approximately a 0.4% chance that the patient has a PE. 90% of patients with a PE will have a value greater than 500 ng/mL.
- The most frequent, sensitive, and specific ECG finding is T wave inversion in leads V_{1-4} indicative of RV strain. Other findings include tachycardia, new onset atrial fibrillation or flutter, S in Lead I, Q and inverted T in lead III, and a QRS axis >90 degrees.

IMAGING

- CXR is often nonspecific and dyspnea with a near normal CXR should suggest PE. Findings that may be seen on CXR include:

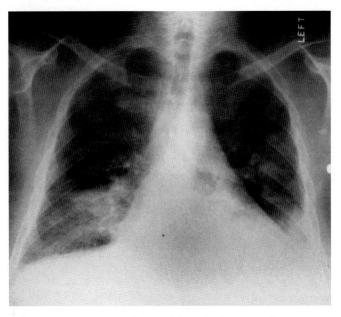

FIGURE 53-2 Chest x-ray showing bilateral pulmonary infiltrates thought to represent pneumonia. (*From Miller WT, Jr. Diagnostic Thoracic Imaging, p. 273, Figure 5-63 A, Copyright 2006, McGraw-Hill.*)

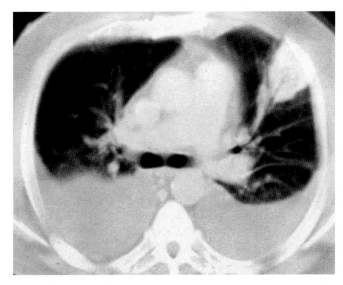

FIGURE 53-3 CT scan from the patient in **Figure 53-2** demonstrates several large wedge-shaped pulmonary opacities with air bronchograms characteristic of pulmonary infarcts. (*From Miller WT, Jr. Diagnostic Thoracic Imaging, p. 273, Figure 5-63 B, Copyright 2006, McGraw-Hill.*)

○ Triad of basal infiltrate, blunted costophrenic angle, and elevated hemi-diaphragm.

○ Infiltrates similar to pneumonia (**Figure 53-2**) that may be diagnosed using CT (**Figure 53-3**).

○ A peripheral wedge-shaped density (**Figure 53-1**).

○ Decreased vascular markings (**Figure 53-4**).

• Chest CT scan with contrast is suggested as the initial test for patients with high probability of PE who have normal kidney function and no allergy to dye. CT is effective in diagnosing large central PE (**Figure 53-3**) and providing evidence of alternate diagnoses.

• A lung scan is considered the initial test for patients with high probability of PE who have renal insufficiency or dye allergy. A high probability scan for PE (positive predictive value of 90%) has 2 or more segmental perfusion defects with normal ventilation.

• If the CT scan or lung scan is nondiagnostic, a leg ultrasound may be performed. If positive for a DVT, proceed with treatment as below. If normal or nondiagnostic, a pulmonary angiogram is suggested.

• Pulmonary angiography is generally reserved for patients with inadequate CT, lung scans, or nondiagnostic leg ultrasound and for patients who will undergo embolectomy or catheter-directed thrombolysis. An intraluminal filling defect may be seen along with truncated arteries associated with regions of diminished perfusion (**Figure 53-5**).

DIFFERENTIAL DIAGNOSIS

The differential diagnosis of a symptomatic PE includes:

• Pneumonia—symptoms include chills, fever, and pleuritic chest pain (the latter two can occur with PE); physical findings include dullness to percussion, bronchial breathing, egophony (E to A change), and crackles with area of infiltrate/pneumonia usually confirmed on CXR (see Chapter 51, Pneumonia).

• Congestive heart failure—history of previous heart failure or myocardial infarction; symptoms of paroxysmal nocturnal dyspnea, orthopnea or the presence of bilateral lower extremity edema, third heart sound, hepatojugular reflex, and jugular venous distention. CXR may show pulmonary venous congestion, interstitial or alveolar edema, and cardiomegaly (see Chapter 46, Congestive Heart Failure).

• Pneumothorax—history of previous pneumothorax or chronic obstructive pulmonary disease, or current rib fracture; physical findings include absence of breath sounds and CXR may show free air, an elevated hemi diaphragm or a shift of the mediastinum to the contralateral side with a tension pneumothorax.

MANAGEMENT[7]

• Primary treatment of PE is considered for patients with hemodynamic instability, RV dysfunction, or infarct.

• In selected patients with massive PE, systemic administration of thrombolytic therapy is suggested.[7] SOR **B** Highly compromised patients who are unable to receive thrombolytic therapy or whose

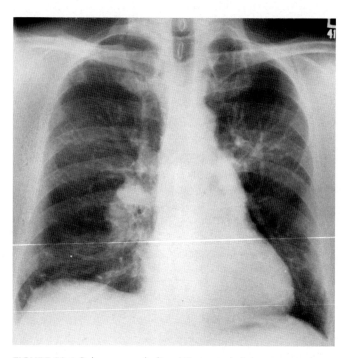

FIGURE 53-4 Pulmonary embolism: Westermark sign—an avascular zone because of obstructed vessel from a blood clot. In this patient, both lung apices and the mid to lower thorax have decreased vascular markings. Note the fusiform enlargement of both hila and the prominent pulmonary artery mediastinal shadow characteristic of pulmonary hypertension. (*From Miller WT, Jr. Diagnostic Thoracic Imaging, p. 748, Figure 14-19A, Copyright 2006, McGraw-Hill.*)

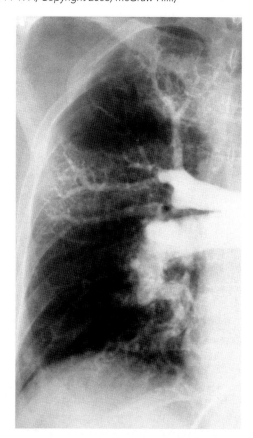

FIGURE 53-5 Pulmonary angiogram in the patient in **Figure 53-4** showing abruptly truncated pulmonary arteries associated with regions of diminished perfusion typical of chronic pulmonary emboli. (*From Miller WT, Jr. Diagnostic Thoracic Imaging, p. 748, Figure 14-19B, Copyright 2006, McGraw-Hill.*)

critical status does not allow sufficient time to infuse thrombolytic therapy may be treated with pulmonary embolectomy.[7] SOR **C**

- Moderate to large PE may be treated similarly or with anticoagulation only. In a recent Cochrane review, authors found no trials comparing thrombolytic therapy to surgical intervention and were unable to determine whether thrombolytic therapy was better than heparin for PE.[8]

- Smaller PEs or proximal DVT are treated with oral anticoagulation to prevent future PE. In addition to beginning oral anticoagulation (e.g., warfarin 5 mg daily, adjusted based on INR), options include unfractionated intravenous heparin using a weight-based nomogram or low-molecular-weight heparin (1 mg/kg twice daily) for a minimum of 5 days.[7] SOR **A** Once the international normalized ratio is therapeutic (range 2–3), oral anticoagulation is continued for a minimum of 6 to –12 months or indefinitely unless there is a known reversible or time-limited risk factor (e.g., recent surgery) when oral anticoagulation may be discontinued after 3 months.[7] SOR **A**

- Selective factor Xa (e.g., fondaparinux sodium) and direct thrombin inhibitors (e.g., ximelagatran) appear to be as effective as low-molecular-weight heparin in prevention of venous thromboembolism and treatment of pulmonary embolism, may have fewer side effects, and will not need routine monitoring. They are not considered initial therapy using current guidelines.

- Inferior vena cava filter placement is reserved for patients with contraindications to anticoagulation or for failure of anticoagulation (i.e., recurrence).[7] SOR **C** While decreasing recurrent PE, they do not appear to improve long-term survival.

- Adjunctive therapy, if needed, includes pain relief, supplemental oxygen, and psychological support. RV failure/shock may be treated with dobutamine.

- Knee-high compression stockings (30–40 mm Hg) are recommended to reduce recurrence.[7] SOR **A**

PATIENT EDUCATION

- Patients should be instructed about the importance of remaining on an extended course of oral anticoagulation and use of compression stockings to decrease the likelihood of recurrence.

- Use of an anticoagulation service or home self-monitoring[9] may be considered to improve adherence and reduce complications.

- Avoidance of periods of prolonged immobilization is suggested.

FOLLOW-UP

- Patients should be monitored based using a standard protocol.

- For patients with serious bleeding complications, management includes holding warfarin, giving vitamin K1 10 mg slow IV plus fresh frozen plasma or prothrombin complex concentrate, and repeating vitamin K1 every 12 hours as needed. SOR **C**

REFERENCES

1. Silverstein MD, Heit JA, Mohr DN, et al. Trends in the incidence of deep vein thrombosis and pulmonary embolism. A 25-year population-based study. *Arch Intern Med.* 1998;158:585–593.

2. Heit JA, Silverstein MD, Mohr DN, et al. Risk factors for deep vein thrombosis and pulmonary embolism: A population-based case-control study. *Arch Intern Med.* 2000;160(6):809–815.

3. Wicki J, Perneger TV, Junod AF, et al. Assessing clinical probability of pulmonary embolism in the emergency ward: A simple score. *Arch Intern Med,* 2001;161:92–97.

4. Wells PS, Anderson DR, Rodger M, et al. Derivation of a simple model to categorize patients probability of pulmonary embolism: Increasing the model's utility with the SimpliRED D-dimer. *Thromb Haemost.* 2000;83:416–420.

5. Iles S, Hodges AM, Darley JR, et al. Clinical experience and pre-test probability scores in the diagnosis of pulmonary embolism. *Q J Med.* 2003;96:211–215.

6. Clinical policy: Critical issues in the evaluation and management of adult patients presenting with suspected pulmonary embolism. *Ann Emerg Med.* 2003;41(2):257–270.

7. Buller HR, Agnelli G, Hull RD, Hyers TM, Prins MH, Raskob GE. Antithrombotic therapy for venous thromboembolic disease: The Seventh ACCP Conference on Antithrombotic and Thrombolytic Therapy. *Chest.* 2004;126(3 Suppl):401S-428S.

8. Dong B, Jirong Y, Liu G, et al. Thrombolytic therapy for pulmonary embolism. *Cochrane Database Syst Rev.* 2006;19:CD004437.

9. Menendez-Jandula, et al. Comparing self-management of oral anti-coagulant therapy with clinic management. *Ann Intern Med.* 2005;142(1):1.

54 CHRONIC OBSTRUCTIVE PULMONARY DISEASE (COPD)

Mindy A. Smith, MD, MS

PATIENT STORY

A 74-year-old woman and longtime smoker presents with fatigue and shortness of breath. She has not seen a physician for many years and says she has basically been healthy. On physical examination, she is found to be pale, mildly cachectic, and her lips are cyanotic. Her breath sounds are distant, although crackles can be heard in both lung bases. Her heart sounds are best heard in the epigastrium; a third heart sound is present. She has mild peripheral edema. Her resting pulse oximetry is 74%. Her chest x-ray (CXR) shows emphysema (**Figure 54-1**) and her echocardiogram confirms heart failure.

EPIDEMIOLOGY

- Prevalence of chronic obstructive pulmonary disease (COPD) in the United States of more than 16 million cases.[1]

- Fourth leading cause of death both in United States and worldwide.

- Risk factors include smoking (direct and passive), airway hypersensitivity, and occupational exposures (e.g., gold and coal mining, cotton textile dust).[1]

ETIOLOGY AND PATHOPHYSIOLOGY

- Standard definition (Global Initiative for Chronic Obstructive Lung Disease): "a disease state characterized by airflow limitation that is not fully reversible."[2]

- Mediated by chronic inflammatory responses to environmental factors, especially cigarette smoke, that results in recruitment of inflammatory cells in terminal airspaces and release of elastolytic proteinases that damage the extracellular lung matrix and cause ineffective repair of elastin and other matrix components.

- The inflammatory process leads to obstruction and later fibrosis of small airways and the destruction of lung parenchyma.

- Genetic mutations (α_1-antitrypsin deficiency [1%–2% of cases]) are present in some patients and likely others. Suspect a genetic mutation when emphysema is found in a patient ≤ age 50, a positive family history, primarily basilar disease, or a minimal smoking history.[1]

DIAGNOSIS

CLINICAL FEATURES

- COPD's three most common symptoms are cough, sputum production, and exertional dyspnea.

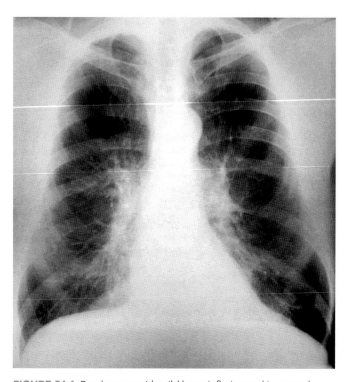

FIGURE 54-1 Emphysema with mild hyperinflation and increased interstitial markings. (*From Miller WT, Jr. Diagnostic Thoracic Imaging, p. 106, Figure 3-37 A. Copyright 2006, McGraw-Hill.*)

- Physical findings may include:
  - Tobacco odor and nicotine staining of fingernails.
  - Increased expiratory phase or expiratory wheezing.
  - Signs of hyperinflation—barrel chest, poor diaphragmatic excursion.
  - Use of accessory muscles of respiration—intercostals, sternocleidomastoid, and scalene muscles.
  - Late in illness: cyanosis of the lips and nail beds, wasting, and *cor pulmonale* (right-sided heart failure—signs include increased jugular-venous distention, right ventricular heave, third heart sound, ascites, and peripheral edema).

LABORATORY STUDIES

Postbronchodilator spirometry secures the diagnosis and provides the severity classification[2]:

- At risk: Chronic cough and sputum production with normal spirometry.
- Mild COPD: FEV1/FVC (forced expiratory volume in 1 second divided by forced vital capacity) < 0.7 and FEV 1 $\geq 80\%$ predicted.
- Moderate COPD: FEV1/FVC < 0.7 and $50\% \leq$ FEV 1 $< 80\%$ predicted.
- Severe COPD: FEV1/FVC < 0.7 and $30\% \leq$ FEV 1 $< 50\%$ predicted.
- Very severe COPD: FEV1/FVC < 0.7 and FEV 1 $< 30\%$ predicted or FEV1 $< 50\%$ with respiratory failure or signs of right-sided heart failure.

Additional tests that may be useful in management are sputum culture (in acute exacerbations to assist in confirming pneumonia) and blood gases (confirms hypoxia or respiratory failure $PCO_2 > 45$). A serum level of α_1-antitrypsin should be measured if you suspect a genetic mutation.

IMAGING

Findings on CXR include[3]:

- Hyperinflation manifested by the following (**Figures 54-1** to **54-3**):
  - Dark lung fields.
  - Increased AP diameter.
  - Increased retrosternal air space.
  - Infracardiac air.
  - Low-set flattened diaphragms (best assessed in lateral chest).
  - Vertical heart.
- Bullae are difficult to recognize in CXR but are easily seen on CT (**Figures 54-4** to **54-6**).
- Paucity of vascular markings in periphery (**Figure 54-2**).
- Pulmonary hypertension (CXR shows enlarged central pulmonary arteries).
- The emphysematous changes in both bases and the upper lobes may be normal in patients with α_1-antitryptin deficiency. The vascular markings are prominent in the upper lobes "cephalization."

The chest CT scan is the current definitive test for emphysema, but the findings do not influence treatment.[1] Cystic and bullous lesions are better delineated with CT scan (**Figures 54-4, 54-5,** and **54-7**)

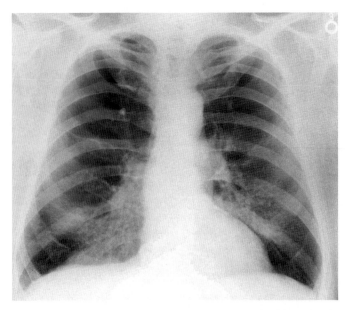

FIGURE 54-2 PA radiograph showing flattened hemidiaphragms and decreased vascular markings. (*From Miller WT, Jr. Diagnostic Thoracic Imaging, p. 108, Figure 3-40 A and B, Copyright 2006, McGraw-Hill.*)

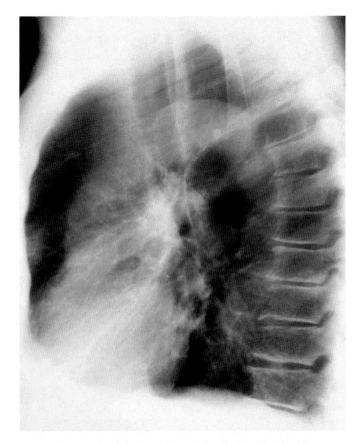

FIGURE 54-3 Lateral view in the patient in **Figure 54-2** showing increased AP diameter. (*From Miller WT, Jr. Diagnostic Thoracic Imaging, p. 108, Figure 3-40 A and B, Copyright 2006, McGraw-Hill.*)

and collapsing airways with inspiration and expiration can also be demonstrated with CT.

DIFFERENTIAL DIAGNOSIS

The differential diagnosis of an individual with persistent productive cough and dyspnea includes:

- Asthma—begins before age 40 in most, usually episodic and characterized by increased responsiveness to many stimuli (e.g., allergens, occupational exposures). Nocturnal awakenings with symptoms are common. This condition is reversible with bronchodilators.

- Lung cancer—symptoms may occur with central or endobronchial growth of the tumor (e.g., cough, hempotysis, wheeze, stridor, dyspnea), collapse of airways from tumor obstruction (e.g., postobstructive pneumonitis), involvement of the pleura or chest wall (e.g., pleuritic chest pain), or from regional spread of the tumor (e.g., dysphagia, hoarseness from recurrent laryngeal nerve paralysis, dyspnea, and elevated hemidiaphragm from phrenic nerve paralysis). Findings on CXR or chest CT may be focal or unilateral and tissue confirms diagnosis.

- Pneumonia—symptoms include fever, chills, and pleuritic chest pain; physical findings include dullness to percussion, bronchial breathing, egophony (E to A change), and crackles with area of infiltrate/pneumonia usually confirmed on chest x-ray.

Any of these processes/illnesses may occur in conjunction with emphysema.

MANAGEMENT

For patients with *stable COPD*, only smoking cessation and oxygen therapy have been shown to improve outcome.[1] SOR **A**

- To assist with smoking cessation, consider nicotine replacement therapy, bupropion (150 mg, twice daily) and supportive counseling and follow-up; using these interventions improves rates of smoking cessation by approximately two-fold. SOR **B**

- Oxygen therapy is initiated with a resting O_2 saturation < 88% or < 90% in a patient with pulmonary hypertension or right-sided heart failure; chronic administration (<15 h/d) in patients with chronic respiratory failure is associated with greater survival.[2] SOR **A**

Nonpharmacologic therapies that should be considered for all patients are[1,2]:

- Vaccination against influenza and pneumococcal vaccination. SOR **C**

- Patient education (multidisciplinary and self-management training) has been shown to improve patient outcomes and reduce costs and hospitalizations.[2,4] SOR **A**

- Pulmonary rehabilitation programs have been shown to decrease hospitalization at 6–12 months, increase quality of life, and improve dyspnea and exercise capacity.[5] SOR **A**

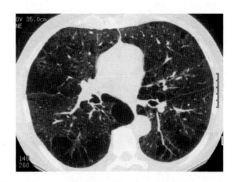

FIGURE 54-4 CT scan showing multiple cystlike lesions (darker round areas) representing emphysema of the entire secondary pulmonary lobule—the most severe form of centrilobular emphysema. (*From Miller WT, Jr. Diagnostic Thoracic Imaging, p. 109, Figure 3-40 E, Copyright 2006, McGraw-Hill.*)

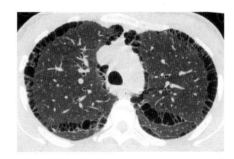

FIGURE 54-5 CT at the level of the aortic arch showing a pattern of cysts in the subpleural lung with an upper-lung zone predominance characteristic of mild paraseptal emphysema. (*From Miller WT, Jr. Diagnostic Thoracic Imaging, p. 110, Figure 3-41 D, Copyright 2006, McGraw-Hill.*)

The following are recommended for symptomatic relief:

- Inhaled bronchodilators: β-agonists (e.g., albuterol) or anticholinergic agents (e.g., ipratropium bromide)—intermittent use, SOR Ⓐ these agents are comparable in efficacy and the choice of agent should be based on patient preference.[2]

- Inhaled long-acting β-agonists (e.g., salmeterol)—regular treatment is more effective, but more costly and may be associated with tachycardia and tremor. SOR Ⓐ On November 18, 2005, the U.S. Food and Drug Administration notified manufacturers of Advair Diskus®, Foradil Aerolizer®, and Serevent Diskus® to update their existing product labels with warnings that these medicines may increase the chance of severe asthma episodes and death when those episodes occur. Long-acting β-agonists can be combined with inhaled anticholinergic agents to provide incremental benefit for symptoms.[2] SOR Ⓑ

- Inhaled glucocorticoids—Data are conflicting, but there may be a small decrease in the frequency of exacerbations (approximately half-a-day per month), but an increase in oral candidiasis, easy bruising, and bone loss.[1] SOR Ⓐ These agents are recommended for patients with moderate to severe COPD or for frequent exacerbations. Parenteral steroids do not benefit patients with stable COPD.

- Theophylline—mildly effective, but associated with nausea.[6] SOR Ⓐ

- Mucolytic agents (e.g., guafenesin, potassium iodide)—produce a small decrease in the frequency of exacerbations (2.7 exacerbations/year [control group] versus 0.79 per year [intervention group]) and in disability days.[7] SOR Ⓐ Global Initiative for Chronic Obstructive Lung Disease does not recommend these medications for routine use.[2]

Two surgical therapies may be considered for patients with severe disease despite optimal medical therapy:

- Lung volume reduction surgery—patients with upper lobe predominant disease and low postrehabilitation exercise capacity appear to gain the most symptom benefit.[2]

- Lung transplant—considered for patients who are ≤ age 65 with no comorbid disease. However, investigators from Norway found no obvious survival benefit from lung transplantation in a cohort of 219 patients accepted onto the lung transplant waiting list.[8]

Acute exacerbations occur approximately 1 to 3 times a year in patients with moderate or severe COPD. For acute exacerbations (defined as an increase in symptoms and change in the amount and character of the sputum), the following interventions should be considered:

- Assess severity[1]: SOR Ⓒ
  - Consider CXR for those with moderate to severe symptoms and focal lung findings.
  - Consider blood gas for those with moderate to severe symptoms, advanced COPD, history of hypercarbia, or mental status changes.

- Hospitalize—base on clinical judgment, the presence of respiratory acidosis, hypercarbia, hypoxemia, severe underlying disease, or poor home situation.[1] SOR Ⓒ

- Inhaled bronchodilators—both β-agonist and anticholinergics can be used alone or in combination; metered dose inhalers with

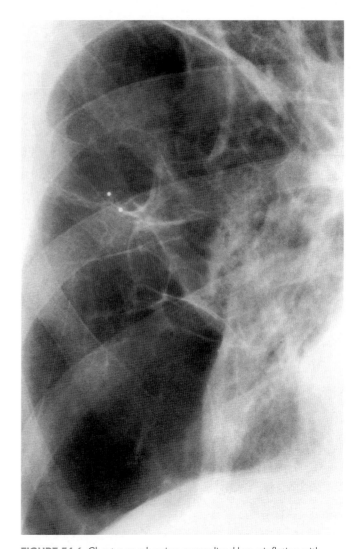

FIGURE 54-6 Chest x-ray showing generalized hyperinflation with large regions of hyperlucency particularly at the lung bases suggesting multiple large bullae. (*From Miller WT, Jr. Diagnostic Thoracic Imaging, p. 111, Figure 3-42 and C, Copyright 2006, McGraw-Hill.*)

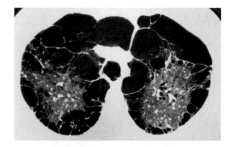

FIGURE 54-7 CT scan in the patient in **Figure 54-6** (at the level of the pulmonary veins) showing multiple large peripheral bullae; the patient was diagnosed with severe paraseptal emphysema. (*From Miller WT, Jr. Diagnostic Thoracic Imaging, p. 111, Figure 3-42 and C, Copyright 2006, McGraw-Hill.*)

proper patient instruction perform as well as nebulized treatments and are less expensive.[2] SOR **A**

- Antibiotics—treating COPD with antibiotics is controversial. In a systematic review, investigators found four placebo-controlled clinical trials and a meta-analysis that demonstrated significant improvements in outcome for patients treated with an antibiotic versus placebo.[9] In contrast, six studies failed to demonstrate statistical differences. Global Initiative for Chronic Obstructive Lung Disease recommends the use of antibiotics in the presence of purulent sputum during an exacerbation of symptoms.[2] SOR **B** The choice of antibiotic does not appear to influence outcome.

- Glucocorticoid—use oral (30–40 mg/d for 10–14 days) or intravenous glucocorticoids if the patient is unable to tolerate oral medication. Steroids have been shown to decrease hospital length of stay and relapse rates.[1] SOR **A**

- Oxygen therapy—use to maintain O_2 saturation above 89%.[2] SOR **C**

- Mechanical ventilatory support—may be needed for patients with respiratory failure.
  - Noninvasive positive pressure ventilation has been shown to decrease mortality, decrease the need for intubation, and reduce hospital length of stay.[2] SOR **A** However, patients may find it difficult to tolerate. It should be considered for patients with moderate to severe dyspnea, moderate to severe acidosis (pH $<$ 7.35), hypercapnea ($PaCO_2$ $>$ 6.0 kPa, 45 mm Hg), and respiratory rate $>$ 25 per minute.[2]
  - Mechanical ventilation support should be considered for patients with severe dyspnea, life threatening hypoxemia (PaO_2 $<$ 5.3 kPa, 40 mm Hg or PaO2/FiO2 $<$ 200 mm Hg), severe acidosis (pH $<$ 7.25) and hypercapnia ($PaCO_2$ $>$ 8.0 kPa, 60 mm Hg) and respiratory arrest.[2] SOR **C**

PATIENT EDUCATION

Smoking cessation should be strongly and repeatedly encouraged. Progressive exercise should also be encouraged, activities that brace the arms and allow use of accessory muscles of respiration are better tolerated—these include, pushing a cart, walker or wheelchair, and use of a treadmill.

PATIENT RESOURCES

For general information, these sites are helpful:

- American Lung Association—**http://www.lungusa.org/** Click on Diseases A to Z to find COPD Fact Sheet. Accessed May 11, 2008.
- Journal of the American Medical Association, Chronic Obstructive Pulmonary Disease, Patient Page with good diagram.— **http://jama.ama-assn.org/cgi/content/full/290/17/2362.** Accessed May 11, 2008.
- The Family of COPD Support Programs, COPD Support, Inc. This website provides information and links to support groups—**www.copd-support.com.** Accessed August 9, 2006.

PROVIDER RESOURCES

Several evidence-based guidelines are available at— www.guideline.gov; **http://www.guideline.gov/** and search on COPD.

Evidence-based guidelines are also available on Global Initiative for Chronic Obstructive Lung Disease (GOLD) at— **http://www.goldcopd.com/.**

World Health Organization (WHO), National Heart, Lung, and Blood Institute (NHLBI). Global strategy for the diagnosis, management, and prevention of chronic obstructive pulmonary disease. Bethesda, MD: Global Initiative for Chronic Obstructive Lung Disease, World Health Organization, National Heart, Lung, and Blood Institute. 2005.

Another website which has links to National Heart, Lung, and Blood Institute, American Academy of Family Physicians, and others, patient education materials and an interactive tutorial is— **www.nlm.nih.gov/medlineplus/copdchronicobstructiv epulmonarydisease.html.**

REFERENCES

1. Reilly JJ, Silverman EK, Shapiro SD. Chronic Obstructive Pulmonary Disease. In: Kasper DL, Braunwald E, Fauci AS, Hauser SL, Longo DL, Jameson, JL eds. *Harrison's Principles of Internal Medicine*. New York: McGraw-Hill, 2005:1547–1554.

2. The Global Initiative for Chronic Obstructive Lung Disease (GOLD). http://www.goldcopd.com. Accessed August 10, 2006.

3. Atlas of Radiologic Images. Loyola University Chicago, Stritch School of Medicine. http://www.meddean.luc.edu/lumen/MedEd/Radio/curriculum/Harrisons/Harrisons_f.htm. Accessed April 5, 2006.

4. Gadoury MA, Schwartzman K, Rouleau M, et al. Chronic obstructive pulmonary disease axis of the respiratory health network, fonds de la recherche en sante du quebec (FRSQ). Self-management reduces both short- and long-term hospitalisation in COPD. *Eur Respir J*. 2005;26(5):853–857.

5. Ries AL, Make BJ, Lee SM, et al. National emphysema treatment trial research group. The effects of pulmonary rehabilitation in the national emphysema treatment trial. *Chest*. 2005;128(6):3799–3809.

6. Ram FS. Use of theophylline in chronic obstructive pulmonary disease: Examining the evidence. *Curr Opin Pulm Med*. 2006;12(2):132–139.

7. Poole PJ, Black PN. Mucolytic agents for chronic bronchitis or chronic obstructive pulmonary disease. *Cochrane Database Syst Rev*. 2003;(2):CD001287.

8. Stavem K, Bjortuft O, Borgan O, et al. Lung transplantation in patients with chronic obstructive pulmonary disease in a national cohort is without obvious survival benefit. *J Heart Lung Transplant*. 2006;25(1):75–84.

9. Russo RL, D'Aprile M. Role of antimicrobial therapy in acute exacerbations of chronic obstructive pulmonary disease. *Ann Pharmacother*. 2001;35(5):576–581.

55 LUNG CANCER

Mindy A. Smith, MD, MS

PATIENT STORY

A 60-year-old woman comes in to the clinic for a solid, nontender, movable mass on her upper chest that's been there for 6 months. When she first noticed the mass it was the size of a dime. It began growing more rapidly over the past month (**Figure 55-1A**). She has lost 10 pounds over the last year without dieting. She admits to smoking one pack of cigarettes per day since age 18. She started smoking at age 13 and gets short of breath easily. She drinks 1 to 2 glasses of wine per night and has no history of using illegal drugs. Her "smoker's cough" has gotten worse in the last few months and occasionally she coughs up some blood-tinged sputum. Her family physician excised the mass in the office and sent it to pathology (**Figure 55-1B**). When the result demonstrated squamous cell carcinoma of the lung, a CXR was ordered (**Figure 55-2A**). The lung cancer was easily visible on the CXR, but the radiologist suggested a CT to confirm the diagnosis (**Figure 55-2B**). The patient chose to have no treatment and passed away in 10 months of her lung cancer.

EPIDEMIOLOGY[1]

- Lung cancer affects 93,000 men and 80,000 women each year in the United States. Although the rate is decreasing in men, it continues to increase in women.

- It is the No. 1 cause of cancer deaths with a 5-year survival rate of 14%.

- Smoking is the major risk factor; a smoking history (current or former) is present in 90% with a relative risk ratio of 13 (passive smoke exposure has a risk ratio of 1.5). Currently 28% of men, 25% of women, and 38% of high school seniors smoke in the United States.

- Women have a higher susceptibility to the carcinogens in tobacco.

- Occupations and exposures that increase risk of lung cancer include asbestos mining and processing, welding, pesticide manufacturing (arsenic), metallurgy (chromium), polycyclic hydrocarbons (through coke oven emissions), iron oxide, vinyl chloride, and uranium.

ETIOLOGY AND PATHOPHYSIOLOGY

- Lung cancer arises from respiratory epithelium (bronchi, bronchioles/alveoli).

- Likely caused by a multistep process involving both carcinogens and tumor promoters; a number of genetic mutations are present in lung cancer cells including activation of dominant oncogenes and inactivation of tumor suppressor oncogenes.[1]

- There are four major cell types responsible for 88% of cases[1]:
  ○ Adenocarcinoma (including bronchoalveolar)—32% of cases (5-year survival: 17%).

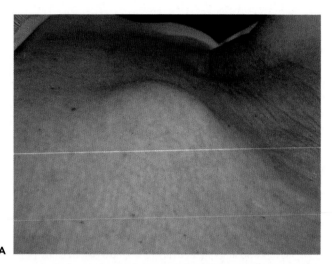

A

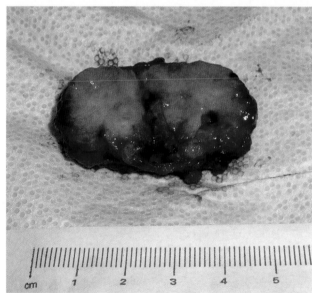

B

FIGURE 55-1 (A) Growing chest nodule in a 60-year-old woman who smoked tobacco her whole adult life. The pathology demonstrated metastatic squamous cell carcinoma from the lung. (B) The resected nodule was surgically removed by the family physician in the office. (*Courtesy of Leonard Chow, MD and Ross Lawrer, MD.*)

○ Squamous or epidermoid carcinoma—29% of cases (5-year survival: 15%).

○ Small cell (or oat cell) carcinoma—18% of cases (5-year survival: 5%).

○ Large cell (or large cell anaplastic)—9% of cases (5-year survival: 11%).

• Ten to twenty percent of squamous and large cell carcinomas cavitate.

DIAGNOSIS

Signs and symptoms depend on location, tumor size, and the presence of local or distant spread.

• Five to fifteen percent of patients are asymptomatic—the cancer is found on chest imaging performed for another reason.

• Systemic symptoms (e.g., anorexia, cachexia, weight loss [seen in 30% of patients]) may be seen but the cause is unknown.

The diagnosis of lung cancer requires tissue confirmation through sputum cytology, bronchoscopy, lymph node biopsy, operative specimen, needle aspiration, biopsy under CT guidance, or cell block from pleural effusion.[2]

• For suspicious central lung lesions, sputum cytology (at least three specimens) is a reasonable first step followed by bronchoscopy if needed. SOR Ⓑ

• In patients with a suspicious peripheral lung lesion (especially < 2 cm), if sputum cytology fails to confirm the diagnosis, transthoracic needle aspiration has a higher sensitivity than bronchoscopy. SOR Ⓐ

• In patients with a lesion that is moderately suspicious for lung cancer who appear to have limited disease, excisional biopsy and subsequent lobectomy if a lung cancer is confirmed is recommended. SOR Ⓑ

CLINICAL FEATURES

• Symptoms may occur in the following situations:
  ○ Central or endobronchial growth of the tumor may produce cough, hemoptysis, wheezing, stridor, and dyspnea.
  ○ Collapse of airways from tumor obstruction may cause postobstructive pneumonitis.
  ○ Involvement of the pleura or chest wall may cause pleuritic chest pain, dyspnea on a restrictive bases, or lung abscess from tumor cavitation.
  ○ Regional spread of the tumor may cause tracheal obstruction; dysphagia from esophageal spread; hoarseness from recurrent laryngeal nerve paralysis; dyspnea, and elevated hemidiaphragm from phrenic nerve paralysis; and Horner's syndrome (enophthalmos, ptosis, miosis, ipsilateral loss of sweating from sympathetic nerve paralysis).
  ○ Spread to lymph nodes may be detected as firm masses in the supraclavicular area, axilla, or groin.
  ○ Extrathoracic metastases are common (found at autopsy in 50%–95%) and may cause neurologic symptoms with brain metastases; pain and fracture with bone metastases; cytopenias or leukoerythroblastosis from bone marrow involvement; and liver dysfunction from metastases to the liver.
  ○ Paraneoplastic syndromes are common and include endocrine syndromes (seen in 12%) such as hypercalcemia and

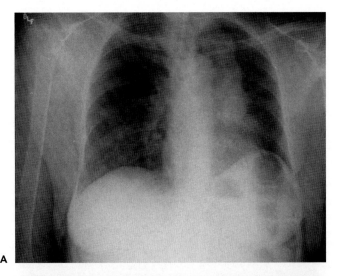

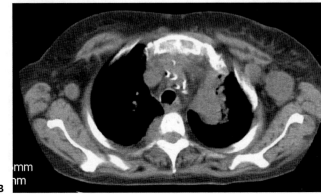

FIGURE 55-2 (A) Chest x-ray showing squamous cell carcinoma of the lung. (B) CT scan demonstrating the architecture of the squamous cell carcinoma of the lung. (*Courtesy of David A. Kasper DO, MBA.*)

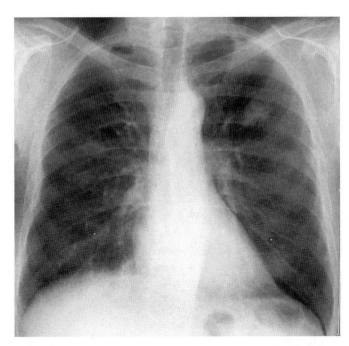

FIGURE 55-3 Chest x-ray demonstrating a 2.5-cm irregular nodule in the left upper lobe.

hypophosphatemia from elevated parathyroid hormone or parathyroid-hormone related peptide; hyponatremia from secretion of antidiuretic hormone; and electrolyte disturbances seen with secretion of adrenocorticotropic hormone.

○ Skeletal and connective tissue syndromes including clubbing (seen in 30%, especially with non-small cell carcinoma) and hypertrophic pulmonary osteoarthropathy with pain and swelling from periostitis (1%–10%, especially with adenocarcinoma).

○ Skin nodules from lung cancer metastases may not be painful but are a poor prognostic sign (**Figures 55-1** and **55-2**).

IMAGING

• CXR and CT scans are both recommended for staging purposes (see below).
  ○ CXR and/or CT scan may show a nodule (**Figures 55-3** and **55-4**) or diffuse lung abnormalities often confused with pneumonia (**Figures 55-5** to **55-7**).
• Although the US Preventive Services Task Force found that that screening with low dose CT, CXR, or sputum cytology could detect lung cancer at an earlier stage, there was poor evidence that any screening strategy for lung cancer decreased mortality. They concluded that there is insufficient evidence to recommend for or against screening for lung cancer.[3]

TYPICAL DISTRIBUTION

• Squamous and small cell carcinoma tend to present as central masses with endobronchial growth.
• Adeno and large cell carcinoma tend to present as peripheral masses, frequently with pleural involvement.

BIOPSY: HISTOLOGY[1]

• Small cell tumors have scant cytoplasm, hyperchromatic nuclei with fine chromatin pattern, nucleoli that are indistinct, and diffuse sheets of cells.
• Non-small cell tumors have abundant cytoplasm, pleomorphic nuclei with coarse chromatin pattern, prominent nucleoli, and glandular or squamous architecture.

DIFFERENTIAL DIAGNOSIS

The differential diagnosis of an individual with lung findings (e.g., productive cough, and dyspnea) includes:

• Emphysema—most common symptoms are cough, sputum production and exertional dyspnea. Although hemoptysis may occur, imaging (chest CT is most definitive) will not show a tumor. There is an increased risk of lung cancer in these patients (see Chapter 54, Chronic Obstructive Pulmonary Disease).

• Pneumonia—symptoms include fever, chills, and pleuritic chest pain; physical findings include dullness to percussion, bronchial breathing, egophony (E to A change), and crackles with area of infiltrate(pneumonia usually confirmed on chest x-ray (CXR) (see Chapter 51, Pneumonia).

Both these processes may occur in conjunction with lung cancer.

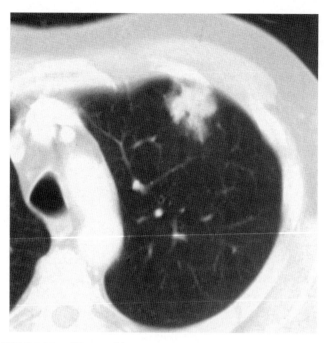

FIGURE 55-4 CT scan of the patient in **Figure 55-3** shows a spiculated mass confirmed at surgery to be an adenocarcinoma.

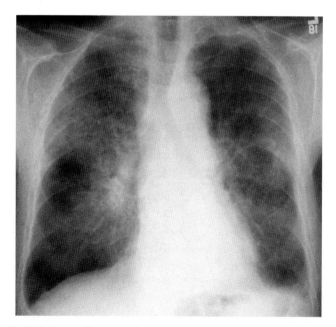

FIGURE 55-5 Diffuse lung abnormality seen on chest x-ray best characterized as ground-glass opacity, slightly worse in the right upper lobe. Open biopsy demonstrated bronchoalveolar carcinoma.

MANAGEMENT

Treatment is based on staging—both anatomic (physical location of tumor) and physiologic (patient's ability to withstand treatment). All patients should undergo the following[1]: SOR **C**

- Complete history and physical.

- Laboratory tests: Complete blood count with platelets, electrolytes, glucose, calcium, phosphorus, and renal and liver function tests.

- Electrocardiogram.

- CXR, CT scans of chest and abdomen (or chest CT extending inferiorly to include the liver and adrenal glands). If symptoms are suggestive of disease, also obtain CT scan of brain, radionuclide scan of bones, barium-swallow (e.g., esophageal symptoms), or pulmonary function studies.

- Fiberoptic bronchoscopy (unless contraindicated or late stage) or biopsy of accessible lesions if more appropriate.

- For patients with non-small cell tumors who may be candidates for curative surgery or radiotherapy, obtain PET scan to evaluate the mediastinum and detect metastases, pulmonary function tests, coagulation tests, and possible cardiopulmonary exercise testing.

- For patients with small cell or advanced tumors, CT of the brain and bone marrow aspiration/biopsy are suggested.

Staging for patients with non-small cell tumors is based on the TNM classification system where T describes the size of the tumor, N describes any regional lymph node involvement, and M notes the presence or absence of distant metastases. At diagnosis, approximately one-third have localized disease (stage I [no node involvement or metastatic disease], II, and IIIA [no metastatic disease]) and one-third have distant metastases (stage IV).

Staging for patients with small cell tumors is divided into two groups, limited disease (confined to one hemithorax and regional lymph node system) or extensive disease. Limited disease is present in one-third at diagnosis.

Management of patients with non-small cell tumors includes the following:

- Localized stage I and II: Pulmonary resection.[4] SOR **C** For patients with early superficial squamous cell carcinoma who are not surgical candidates, photodynamic therapy should be considered as a treatment option.[5] SOR **B** The role of photodynamic therapy for patients undergoing surgery is under investigation. Investigators in a recent systematic review found postoperative adjuvant platinum-based chemotherapy improved survival compared with surgery alone in completely resected non-small cell lung cancer.[6]

- Stage IIIA and favorable age, cardiovascular function, and anatomy: Possible surgery with adjuvant platinum-based chemotherapy with or without radiation.

- Stage IIIB: Consider pneumonectomy. For patients with unresectable, locally advanced stage III non-small cell lung cancer, chemotherapy in association with definitive thoracic irradiation is appropriate for selected patients.[7]

- Stage IV: Options include radiation therapy to symptomatic local sites, chemotherapy, chest tube for malignant effusion, and consider resection of primary or isolated brain or adrenal metastases.

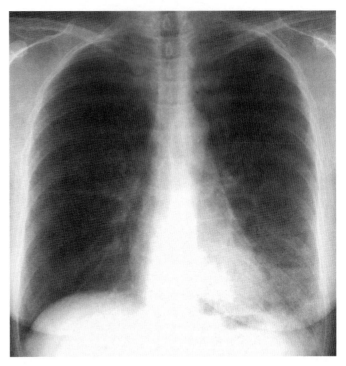

FIGURE 55-6 Chest x-ray showing local area of consolidation in the left lower lobe. Worsening consolidation for the subsequent 2 months despite antibiotic treatment lead to a surgical biopsy, which confirmed bronchoalveolar carcinoma.

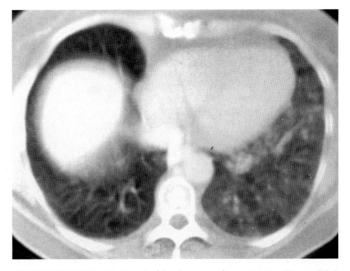

FIGURE 55-7 CT at the level of the bases in the patient in **Figure 55-6** showing areas of ground-glass opacification in the left lower lobe and lingula.

Management of patients with small cell limited disease includes combination, platinum-based chemotherapy, and chest radiation therapy.[4] SOR Ⓐ

- Patients with limited-stage small cell lung cancer should be offered thoracic irradiation concurrently with the first or second cycle of chemotherapy or following completion of chemotherapy if there has been at least a good partial response within the thorax.

- For patients with extensive disease, thoracic irradiation should be considered following chemotherapy if there has been a complete response at distant sites and at least a good partial response within the thorax.[4]

Supportive care for the patient and family and palliative care of the patient should be provided, including adequate pain relief.

- Opioids, such as codeine or morphine, may also reduce cough.

- External beam radiotherapy could be considered for the relief of breathlessness, cough, hemoptysis, or chest pain.

PATIENT EDUCATION

- Smoking cessation, never initiating smoking, and avoidance of occupational and environmental exposure to carcinogenic substances are recommended to reduce the risk of a second primary in curatively treated patients. In patients with metastatic disease, although smoking cessation has little effect on overall prognosis, it may improve respiratory symptoms.

- Information about local hospice services and support groups should be provided. A Web site that can be used to find support groups is listed below.

FOLLOW-UP

Surveillance for the recognition of a recurrence of the original lung cancer and/or the development of a metachronous tumor should be coordinated through a multidisciplinary team approach.

- This team should develop a lifelong surveillance plan appropriate for the individual circumstances of each patient immediately following initial curative-intent therapy. SOR Ⓒ

- In lung cancer patients following curative-intent therapy, the use of blood tests, positron emission tomography scanning, sputum cytology, tumor markers, and fluorescence bronchoscopy is not currently recommended for surveillance.[2]

PATIENT RESOURCES

Information for patients can be accessed at the website of National Cancer Institute—**www.cancer.gov/cancertopics/wyntk/lung.**

More information for patients can be accessed from—**www.mayoclinic.com/health/lung-cancer/DS00038.**

American Lung Association—**www.lungusa.org.**

Support groups for patients and families can be found at the following website—**www.lungcanceralliance.org/facing/support_groups.html.**

REFERENCES

1. Minna JD. Neoplasms of the lung. In: Kasper DL, Braunwald E, Fauci AS, Hauser SL, Longo DL, Jameson, JL eds. *Harrison's Principles of Internal Medicine,* 16th ed. New York: McGraw-Hill, 2005: 506–516.

2. Rivera MP, Detterbeck F, Mehta AC. Diagnosis of lung cancer: The guidelines. *Chest.* 2003;123(1 Suppl):129S–136S.

3. U.S. Preventive Services Task Force. Lung cancer screening: Recommendation statement. *Ann Intern Med.* 2004;140(9):738–739.

4. National Collaborating Centre for Acute Care. The Diagnosis and Treatment of Lung Cancer. London (UK): National Institute for Clinical Excellence (NICE); 2005 Feb. 350 p. www.guideline.gov. Accessed May 19, 2006.

5. Mathur PN, Edell E, Sutedja T, Vergnon JM. Treatment of early stage non-small cell lung cancer. *Chest.* 2003;123(1 Suppl): 176S–180S.

6. Alam N, Darling G, Evans WK, et al. Adjuvant chemotherapy for completely resected non-small cell lung cancer: A systematic review. *Crit Rev Oncol Hematol.* 2006; 58(2):146–155.

7. Pfister DG, Johnson DH, Azzoli CG, et al. American society of clinical oncology treatment of unresectable non-small-cell lung cancer guideline: Update 2003. *J Clin Oncol.* 2004;22(2):330–353.

PART 9

THE GUT

56 PEPTIC ULCER DISEASE

Hend Azhary, MD

PATIENT STORY

A 41-year-old man presents with a 4-month history of epigastric pain. The pain is dull, achy, and intermittent; there is no radiation of the pain and it has not changed in character since it began. Coffee intake seems to exacerbate the symptoms while eating or drinking milk helps. Infrequently, he is awakened at night from the pain. He reports no weight loss, vomiting, melena, or hematochezia. On examination, there is mild epigastric tenderness with no rebound or guarding. The reminder of the examination is unremarkable. A stool antigen test is positive for *H. pylori*, and the patient is treated for peptic ulcer disease with eradication therapy.

EPIDEMIOLOGY

- Peptic ulcer disease (PUD) is a common disorder affecting approximately 4.5 million people annually in the United States. It encompasses both gastric and duodenal ulcers (**Figures 56-1** and **56-2**).[1]

- One-year point prevalence is 1.8%, and the lifetime prevalence is 10% in the United States.[1]

- Prevalence is similar in both sexes with increase incidence with age.[2]

- Duodenal ulcers most commonly occur in patients between the age of 30 and 55 years.[1]

- Gastric ulcers are more common in patients between the ages of 55 and 70 years.[1]

- PUD incidence in *Helicobacter (H) pylori*-infected individuals is about 1% per year (6–10-fold higher than uninfected subjects).[2]

- Physician office visit and hospitalization for PUD have decreased in the last few decades.[2]

- Hospitalization rate is approximately 30 per 100,000 cases.[3]

- Mortality rate is approximately 1 per 100,000 cases.[3]

ETIOLOGY AND PATHOPHYSIOLOGY

- Ulcers are breaks in the mucosal surface >5 mm in size, with depth reaching submucosal layer.[2]

- Causes of PUD include:
  - Major causes are nonsteroidal anti-inflammatory drugs (NSAIDs), chronic *H. pylori* infection, and acid hypersecretory states such as Zollinger–Ellison syndrome.[1]
  - Uncommon causes include cytomegalovirus (especially in transplant recipients), systemic mastocytosis, Crohn's disease, lymphoma, and medications (e.g., alendronate).[1]
  - Up to 10% of ulcers are idiopathic.[1]

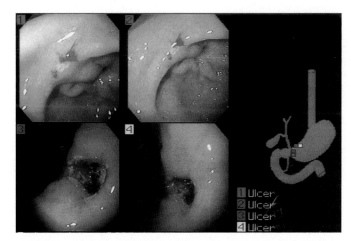

FIGURE 56-1 Endoscopic pictures of a gastric ulcer. Plates 1 and 2 show erosions. Note that the bleeding is from biopsy. Plates 3 and 4 show a large crater with evidence of recent bleeding. Both are consistent with severe ulcer disease. (*Courtesy of Michael Harper, MD.*)

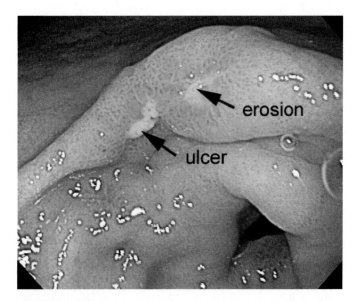

FIGURE 56-2 Endoscopic view of a pyloric ulcer and an erosion of the mucosa. The ulcer and erosion are benign PUD and not malignant. (*Courtesy of Marvin Derezin, MD.*)

- Infection with *H. pylori*, a short, spiral-shaped, microaerophilic gram-negative bacillus, is the leading cause of PUD. It is associated with up to 70% to 80% of duodenal ulcers.[1]
  - *H. pylori* colonize the deep layers of the gel that coats the mucosa and disrupt its protective properties causing release of certain enzymes and toxins. These make the underlying tissues more vulnerable to damage by digestive juices thus cause injury to the stomach (**Figures 56-1** to **56-3**) and duodenum cells.[2]
- NSAIDs are the second most common cause of PUD and account for many *H. pylori*-negative cases.
  - NSAIDs and aspirin inhibit mucosal cyclooxygenase activity reducing the level of mucosal prostaglandin causing defects in the protective mucus layer.
  - There is a 10% to 20% prevalence of gastric ulcers and a 2% to 5% prevalence of duodenal ulcers in long-term NSAID users.[1]

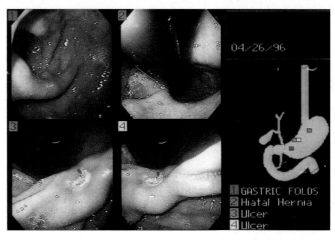

FIGURE 56-3 Stomach ulcer in a patient with a hiatal hernia. (*Courtesy of Michael Harper, MD.*)

DIAGNOSIS

CLINICAL FEATURES

- Epigastric pain (dyspepsia), the hallmark of PUD, is present in 80% to 90% of patients; however, this symptom is not sensitive or specific enough to serve as a reliable diagnostic criterion for PUD. Pain is typically described as a gnawing or burning, occurring 1 to 3 hours after meals and relieved by food or antacids. It can occur at night, and sometimes radiates to the back.[1]
- Other dyspeptic symptoms including belching, bloating, and distention are common but also not specific features of PUD since they are commonly encountered in many other conditions.
- Additional symptoms include fatty food intolerance, heartburn, and chest discomfort.
- Less than 25% of patients with dyspepsia have ulcer disease at endoscopy.
- Nausea and anorexia may occur with gastric ulcers.
- Significant vomiting and weight loss are unusual with uncomplicated ulcer disease and suggest gastric outlet obstruction or gastric malignancy.[1]
- Twenty percent of patients with ulcer complications such as bleeding and nearly 61% of patients with NSAID-related ulcer complications have no antecedent symptoms.
- Rare and nonspecific physical findings include:
  - Epigastric tenderness.
  - Heme-positive stool.
  - Hematemesis or melena in cases of gastrointestinal bleeding.

TYPICAL DISTRIBUTION

- Duodenal ulcers occur most often in the first portion of the duodenum (>95%), with approximately 90% of ulcers located within 3 cm of the pylorus.[2]
- Benign gastric ulcers are located most commonly in the antrum (60%) and at the junction of the antrum and body on the lesser curvature (25%) (**Figure 56-3**).[2]

LABORATORY STUDIES

- In most patients with uncomplicated PUD, routine laboratory tests are not helpful.[3]
- Noninvasive tests include serum *H. pylori* antibody detection, fecal antigen tests, and urea breath tests; the latter two, if positive, indicate active disease.
- Obtaining a serum gastrin is useful in patients with recurrent, refractory, or complicated PUD and is useful in patients with a family history of PUD to screen for Zollinger-Ellison syndrome.[4]

IMAGING

- Upper endoscopy is the procedure of choice for the diagnosis of duodenal and gastric ulcers (**Figures 56-1** to **56-3**).[1]
  - Endoscopy provides better diagnostic accuracy than barium radiography and affords the ability to biopsy for the presence of malignancy and *H. pylori* infection. Endoscopy is usually reserved for the following situations:
    - Patients with red flag signs (e.g., bleeding, dysphagia, severe pain, abdominal mass, recurrent vomiting, weight loss).
    - Patients who fail initial therapy.
    - Patients whose symptoms recur after appropriate therapy.
- Duodenal ulcers are virtually never malignant and do not require biopsy.[1]
- Gastric ulcers should be biopsied because 3% to 5% of benign-appearing gastric ulcers prove to be malignant.[1]
- Barium upper gastrointestinal series is an acceptable alternative to endoscopy but is not as sensitive for the diagnosis of small ulcers (<0.5 cm).[3]
  - Patient's testing positive for PUD should undergo noninvasive testing for *H. pylori*.
  - Upper gastrointestinal series has limited accuracy in distinguishing benign from malignant gastric ulcers, therefore all patients diagnosed this way should be reevaluated with endoscopy after 8 to 12 weeks of therapy.

DIFFERENTIAL DIAGNOSIS

Disease processes that may present with "ulcer-like" symptoms include:

- Nonulcer or functional dyspepsia (FD)—The most common diagnosis among patients seen for upper abdominal discomfort, it is a diagnosis of exclusion. Dyspepsia has been reported to occur in up to 30% of the US population and up to 60% of patients seeking medical care for dyspepsia have a negative diagnostic evaluation.[4]
- Gastroesophageal reflux—Classic symptoms are heartburn (i.e., substernal pain that may be associated with acid regurgitation or a sour taste) aggravated by bending forward or lying down, especially after a large meal. Endoscopy is considered if symptoms fail to respond to treatment (e.g., histamine-2-receptor agonist, proton pump inhibitor [PPI]) or red flag signs and symptoms occur.
- Gastric cancer—Most patients do not become symptomatic until late in the disease; symptoms include upper abdominal pain, postprandial fullness, anorexia and mild nausea, vomiting (especially with pyloric tumors), weight loss and a palpable mass. Endoscopic biopsy is used to make this diagnosis (see Chapter 57, Gastric Cancer).

- Biliary colic is characterized by discrete, intermittent episodes of pain that should not be confused with other causes of dyspepsia.
- Gastroduodenal Crohn's disease—symptoms include epigastric pain, nausea, and vomiting. On endoscopy, patients often have *H. pylori*-negative gastritis and may develop gastric outlet obstruction. Extra-intestinal manifestations include erythema nodosum, peripheral arthritis, conjunctivitis, uveitis, and episcleritis. Endoscopy shows an inflammatory process with skip lesions, fistulas, aphthous ulcerations, and rectal sparing. Small bowel involvement is seen on imaging with longitudinal and transverse ulceration (cobblestoning) in addition to segmental colitis and frequent stricture.

MANAGEMENT

- Given current understanding of the pathogenesis of PUD, the majority of patients with PUD are treated successfully medically with cure of *H. pylori* infection and/or avoidance of NSAIDs, along with appropriate use of antisecretory therapy.
- The goals of treatment of active *H. pylori*-associated ulcers are to relieve dyspeptic symptoms, to promote ulcer healing, and to eradicate *H. pylori* infection.
  - Triple therapy for 14 days is considered the treatment of choice for *H. pylori* infection, which result in a cure rate of infection and healing in approximately 85% to 90% of cases. SOR Ⓐ Two forms of triple therapy are available, including PPI-based triple therapy and bismuth-based triple therapy.
    - PPI–based triple therapy consists of a proton-pump inhibitor (PPI) (e.g., omeprazole 20 mg, lansoprazole 30 mg, rabeprazole 20 mg, esomeprazole 40 mg) and 2 antibiotics (clarithromycin 500 mg and amoxicillin 1 g or clarithromycin 500 mg and metronidazole 500 mg in penicillin-allergic patients), each given twice daily for 2 weeks. A once-daily PPI must be administered for an additional 2 to 4 weeks for duodenal ulcer or 4 to 6 weeks for gastric ulcer after completion of the antibiotic regimen to ensure complete ulcer healing.[3]
    - Bismuth-based triple therapy consists of bismuth 525 mg and 2 antibiotics (tetracycline 500 mg, metronidazole 250 mg), each given four times daily for 2 weeks. In the setting of an active ulcer, addition of an antisecretory agent, such as an H2-receptor antagonist (e.g., ranitidine 150 mg twice daily), is recommended to optimize ulcer healing.[3]
    - Treat NSAID-induced ulcers with cessation of NSAIDs, if possible, and an appropriate course of standard ulcer therapy with a histamine 2–receptor antagonist or a PPI. If NSAIDs are continued, prescribe a PPI. SOR Ⓐ
    - *H. pylori*-negative ulcers that are not caused by NSAIDs can be treated with appropriate antisecretory therapy, either H2-receptor antagonist or PPI. SOR Ⓐ

PATIENT EDUCATION

- Patients with PUD should be encouraged to eat balanced meals at regular intervals, avoid heavy alcohol use, and avoid smoking (which has been shown to retard the rate of ulcer healing and increase the frequency of recurrences); stress reduction counseling might be helpful in individual cases.

FOLLOW-UP

- Endoscopy is required to document healing of gastric ulcers and to rule out gastric cancer, this is performed 6–8 weeks after the initial diagnosis.

- Confirmation of *H. pylori* eradication in patients with uncomplicated ulcers is not necessary.

- Confirmation of healing with endoscopy is required in all patients with ulcer complicated by bleeding, perforation, or obstruction.

PATIENT RESOURCES

National Digestive Diseases Information Clearing House—**http://digestive.niddk.nih.gov/ddiseases/pubs/pepticulcers_ez/index.htm.**

Centers for Disease Control and Prevention—**http://www.cdc.gov/ulcer/.**

PROVIDER RESOURCES

www.emedicine.com/med/topic1776.htm.

REFERENCES

1. McPhee SJ, Papadakis MA, Tierney LW, Jr. *Current Medical Diagnosis and Treatment*. New York: McGraw-Hill, 2007:518–526.

2. Del Valle J. Peptic ulcer disease and related disorders. In: Kasper DL, Braunwald E, Fauci AS, Hauser SL, Longo DL, Jameson, JL eds. *Harrison's Principles of Internal Medicine,* 16th ed. New York: McGraw-Hill, 2005:1746–1762.

3. Le TH, Fantry GT. Peptic Ulcer Disease. eMedicine. 10 15, 2007 and the URL is http://www.emedicine.com/med/TOPIC1776.HTM

4. Andrew SH. Diagnosis of peptic ulcer disease. UptoDate. 2001. http://patients.uptodate.com/topic.asp?file=acidpep/7766

57 GASTRIC CANCER

Mindy A. Smith, MD

PATIENT STORY

A 72-year-old Japanese immigrant was brought in by his family with complaints of difficulty in eating, vague abdominal pain, and weight loss. Endoscopy and biopsy confirmed gastric adenocarcinoma (**Figure 57-1**). Liver metastases were found on abdominal CT. The family and the patient chose only comfort measures and the patient passed away in 6 months.

EPIDEMIOLOGY

- Despite a marked decrease in the incidence and mortality rate from stomach cancer in the past 6 decades, stomach cancer occurs in 5 per 100,000 men and 2.3 per 100,000 women in a year.[1]
- The incidence of stomach cancer in the United States in 2004 was 22,710 individuals with 11,780 deaths reported.[1]
- The median age at diagnosis is 65 years (range 40–70 years). Gastric cancers that occur in younger patients may represent a more aggressive variant.[2]
- High rates of stomach cancer still occur in Japan, China, Chile, and Ireland. A rigorous early screening program developed in Japan has resulted in earlier stage at diagnosis and better survival rates; some speculate, however, that there is a biologic difference between the disease as it manifests in Asia vs Western countries leading to the improved survival.[2]

ETIOLOGY AND PATHOPHYSIOLOGY

- The vast majority (85%) of stomach cancers are adenocarcinomas with 15% lymphomas and gastrointestinal stromal tumors.[1] Adenocarcinoma is further divided into two types:
  - Diffuse type—characterized by absent cell cohesion, these tumors affect younger individuals infiltrating and thickening the stomach wall; the prognosis is poor.
  - Intestinal type—characterized by adhesive cells forming tubular structures, these tumors frequently ulcerate.
- Most tumors are thought to arise from ingestion of nitrates that are converted by bacteria to carcinogens. Two broad categories of factors contribute to this process[1]:
  - Exogenous sources of nitrates—includes foods that are dried, smoked, and salted. *H. pylori* infection may contribute to carcinogenicity by creating gastritis, loss of acidity, and bacterial growth. It is not known whether *H. pylori* eradication will prevent cancer. Similarly, previous gastric surgery has been implicated as a risk factor as a result of alteration of the normal pH.
  - Endogenous factors—Atrophic gastritis (including postsurgical vagotomized patients) and pernicious anemia are conditions that favor the growth of nitrate-converting bacteria. In addition,

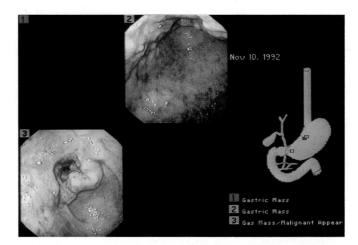

FIGURE 57-1 Endoscopy showing a raised and irregular mass in the antrum of the stomach deforming the pylorus. It fills the distal one-half of the antrum. The lesion was hard when probed with biopsy forceps. Biopsy indicated adenocarcinoma. (*Courtesy of Michael Harper, MD.*)

intestinal-type cells that develop metaplasia and possibly atypia can replace the gastric mucosa in these patients. Genetic polymorphisms (e.g., interleukin-1B-511, interleukin-1RN, and tumor necrosis factor-alpha) also appear to play a role.

- Additional risk factors for gastric carcinoma are smoking, low socioeconomic class, lower educational level, exposure to certain pesticides (e.g., those who work in the citrus fruit industry in fields treated with 2,4-D, chlordane, propargite, and trifluin[3]), and blood type A.

- Gastric tumors are classified for staging using the T (tumor) N (nodal involvement) M (metastases) system. Two important prognostic factors are depth of invasion through the gastric wall (less than T2 [tumor invades muscularis propria or subserosa]) and presence or absence of regional lymph node involvement (N0).[2]

- Gastric cancer spreads in multiple ways[2]:
  - Local extension to omenta, pancreas, diaphragm, transverse colon, and duodenum is common.
  - Lymphatic drainage through numerous pathways leads to multiple nodal group involvement (i.e., gastric, gastroepiploic, celiac, porta hepatic, splenic, suprapancreatic, pancreaticoduodenal, paraesophageal, and paraaortic lymph nodes).
  - Hematogenous spread is also common with liver metastases.

DIAGNOSIS

CLINICAL FEATURES

- Asymptomatic, if superficial and/or early.
- Upper abdominal pain that ranges from vague to severe, especially if onset after age 45.
- Postprandial fullness.
- Anorexia and mild nausea are common.
- Nausea and vomiting occur with pyloric tumors.
- Late symptoms include weight loss and a palpable mass (regional extension).
- Late complications include peritoneal and pleural effusions; obstruction of the gastric outlet; bleeding from esophageal varices or postsurgical site; and jaundice.[2]
- Physical signs are also late features and include[2]:
  - Palpable enlarged stomach with succussion splash (splashing sound on shaking, indicative of the presence of fluid and air in a body cavity).
  - Primary mass (rare).
  - Enlarged liver.
  - Enlarged, firm to hard, lymph nodes (i.e., left supraclavicular (Virchow), periumbilical region (Sister Mary Joseph node), and peritoneal cul-de-sac (Blumer shelf; palpable on vaginal or rectal examination).

TYPICAL DISTRIBUTION

Tumors occur in the proximal third (cardia; 37%), distal stomach (pylorus; 30%), mid-portion of the stomach (body; 20%), and entire stomach (13%).[1] Metastases spread to adjacent liver, colon, and pancreas, and regional lymph nodes affected include intraabdominal and supraclavicular areas.

IMAGING AND ENDOSCOPY

- Diagnosis can be made on endoscopy (**Figures 57-1** and **57-2**) with biopsy of suspicious lesions.

- Double-contrast radiography is an alternative to endoscopy and can detect large primary tumors but only occasionally detects their spread to the esophagus and duodenum.[2]

- Although endoscopy is not necessary when radiography demonstrates a benign appearing ulcer with evidence of complete healing at 6 weeks, some authors recommend routine endoscopy, biopsy, and brush cytology when any gastric ulcer is identified.[1]

- Work-up for metastases includes[4]: SOR **C**
  - Chest radiograph.
  - CT scan or MRI of the abdomen and pelvis.

- Endoscopic sonography is useful as a staging tool when the CT scan fails to find evidence of locally advanced or metastatic disease.[2]

LABORATORY STUDIES

- A hemoglobin or hematocrit can identify anemia, present in approximately 30% of patients.[2]

- Electrolyte panels and liver function tests can assist in assessing the patient's clinical state and any liver involvement.[2]

DIFFERENTIAL DIAGNOSIS

- Peptic ulcer—typical symptoms include epigastric pain (described as a gnawing or burning), occurring 1–3 hours after meals and relieved by food or antacids. Patients may also have nausea and vomiting, bloating, abdominal distention, and anorexia. Endoscopy confirms diagnosis (see Chapter 56, Peptic Ulcer Disease).

- Nonulcer dyspepsia—includes gastroesophageal reflux disease and functional dyspepsia. Classic symptoms of gastroesophageal reflux disease are heartburn (i.e., substernal pain that may be associated with acid regurgitation or a sour taste) aggravated by bending forward or lying down, especially after a large meal; individual symptoms, however, do not help to distinguish these patients from those with peptic ulcer disease. Endoscopy is considered if symptoms fail to respond to treatment (e.g., histamine-2 receptor agonist, proton pump inhibitor) or red flag signs/symptoms occur (e.g., bleeding, dysphagia, severe pain, weight loss).

- Chronic gastritis—includes autoimmune (body-predominant) and *H. pylori* related (antral-predominant) types; mucosal inflammation (primarily lymphocytes) may progress to atrophy and metaplasia. Abdominal pain and dyspepsia are common symptoms and patients may have pernicious anemia.

- Esophagitis—may be mechanical or infectious (primarily viral and fungal). Symptoms include heartburn (retrosternal wave-like pain that may radiate to the neck or jaw) and painful swallowing (odynophagia); regurgitation of sour or bitter tasting material may occur with obstruction. Barium swallow or esophagoscopy can be used to establish the diagnosis.

- Esophageal cancer—relatively uncommon malignancy of two cell types—squamous cell cancers (largely related to smoking, excessive alcohol consumption, and other agents causing mucosal

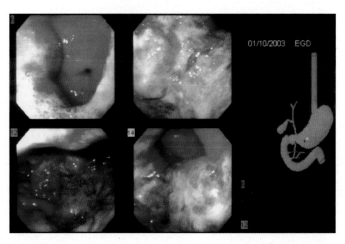

FIGURE 57-2 Endoscopy showing a deep ulcer with yellow/brown exudate in center of mass, consistent with cancer. Pathology confirmed a high-grade diffuse large B-cell lymphoma of the stomach. (*Courtesy of Michael Harper, MD.*)

trauma) and adenocarcinomas (usually arising in the distal esophagus related to reflux disease). Symptoms include progressive dysphagia and weight loss; the diagnosis is confirmed on esophagoscopy and biopsy.

MANAGEMENT

- Complete resection including adjacent lymph nodes.[1]
  - Proximal tumors—total gastrectomy; 5-year survival: less than 10%.
  - Distal tumors—subtotal gastrectomy; 5-year survival: 20%.
  - In a meta-analysis, laparoscopy-assisted distal gastrectomy compared to conventional distal gastrectomy was associated with a lower morbidity, less pain, faster bowel function recovery, and shorter hospital stay; anastomotic and wound complications and mortality rates were similar.[5]
- Radiation is useful for palliation for pain.
- Chemotherapy using 5-flurouricil and doxorubicin with or without cisplatin or mitomycin C is somewhat helpful (partial response in 30% to 50%).[1]
  - In one randomized clinical trial, perioperative epirubicin, cisplatin, and infused fluorouracil decreased tumor size and stage and significantly improved progression-free and overall survival for patients with operable gastric or lower esophageal adenocarcinomas.[6]
  - In a meta-analysis, three-drug regimens containing FU, an anthracycline, and cisplatin administered as adjunct therapy appeared to have the best survival rates.[7]
  - Following surgical resection, adjuvant chemotherapy is recommended for patients whose tumors penetrated the muscularis propria or involved regional lymph nodes.[8] SOR Ⓒ When combined with radiation, there is some decrease in recurrence and increased survival. However, the guideline developers note that there is insufficient evidence from randomized trials to recommend neoadjuvant chemotherapy, or neoadjuvant or adjuvant radiation therapy or immunotherapy, either alone or in combination, outside of a clinical trial.[8]
- A study is currently underway to determine whether eradication of *H. pylori* infection will reduce recurrence of gastric cancer.[9]
- Limited data are available regarding prevention of gastric cancer, but in a population of poorly nourished Chinese subjects, combined supplementation with beta-carotene, alpha-tocopherol, and selenium reduced the incidence of and mortality rate from gastric cancer and the overall mortality rate from cancer by 13% to 21%.[10]

PATIENT EDUCATION

- Postoperative mortality is approximately 1% to 2%.[2]
- Early postoperative complications include anastomotic failure, bleeding, ileus, cholecystitis, pancreatitis, pulmonary infections, and thromboembolism. Further surgery may be required for anastomotic leaks.[2]

- Late mechanical and physiologic complications include dumping syndrome, vitamin B-12 deficiency, reflux esophagitis, and bone disorders, especially osteoporosis.
- Postgastrectomy patients often are immunologically deficient.

FOLLOW-UP

- Recurrences occur in the first 8 years.
- Follow-up varies from evaluation based on clinical suspicion of relapse to intensive investigations to detect early recurrences; unfortunately there are no data to show that early detection of local recurrence by endoscopy or CT improves survival or quality of life because these recurrences are invariably incurable.[11]
  - Isolated liver metastasis identified on CT, however, may be resectable.
  - Tumor markers have been used with some success to detect subclinical recurrences and could be used to target more invasive or expensive procedures.[11]

PATIENT RESOURCES

National Cancer Institute—**http://www.cancer.gov/cancertopics/types/stomach/.**

Medline Plus—**http://www.nlm.nih.gov/medlineplus/stomachcancer.html.**

PROVIDER RESOURCES

National Cancer Institute—**http://www.cancer.gov/cancertopics/types/stomach/.**

REFERENCES

1. Mayer R. Gastrointestinal tract cancer. In: Kasper DL, Braunwald E, Fauci AS, Hauser SL, Longo DL, Jameson, JL eds. *Harrison's Principles of Internal Medicine*, 16th ed. New York: McGraw-Hill, 2005:523–533.

2. Mehta VK, Fisher G. Gastric Cancer. www.emedicine.com. Accessed January 27, 2007.

3. Mills PK, Yang RC. Agricultural exposures and gastric cancer risk in Hispanic farm workers in California. *Environ Res.* 2007;104(2): 282–289.

4. Society for Surgery of the Alimentary Tract (SSAT). Surgical treatment of gastric cancer. Manchester, MA: Society for Surgery of the Alimentary Tract (SSAT); 2004;15:4.

5. Hosono S, Arimoto Y, Ohtani H, Kanamiya Y. Meta-analysis of short-term outcomes after laparoscopy-assisted distal gastrectomy. *World J Gastroenterol.* 2006;12(47):7676–7683.

6. Cunningham D, Allum WH, Stenning SP, et al. Perioperative chemotherapy versus surgery alone for resectable gastroesophageal cancer. *N Engl J Med.* 2006;355(1):11–20.

7. Wagner AD, Grothe W, Haerting J, et al. Chemotherapy in advanced gastric cancer: A systematic review and meta-analysis based on aggregate data. *J Clin Oncol.* 2006;24(18):2903–2909.

8. Gastrointestinal Cancer Disease Site Group. Earle CC, Maroun J, Zuraw L. Neoadjuvant or adjuvant therapy for resectable gastric cancer [full report]. Toronto (ON): Cancer Care Ontario (CCO); 2003 May 21 [online update]. 21 p. (Practice guideline; no. 2–14).

9. Kato M, Asaka M, Ono S, et al. Eradication of Helicobacter pylori for primary gastric cancer and secondary gastric cancer after endoscopic mucosal resection. *J Gastroenterol.* 2007;42(Suppl 17): 16–20.

10. Huang HY, Caballero B, Chang S, et al. The efficacy and safety of multivitamin and mineral supplement use to prevent cancer and chronic disease in adults: A systematic review for a National Institutes of Health state-of-the-science conference. *Ann Intern Med.* 2006;145(5):372–385.

11. Whiting J, Sano T, Saka M, et al. Follow-up of gastric cancer: A review. *Gastric Cancer.* 2006;9(2):74–81.

58 LIVER DISEASE

Mindy A. Smith, MD, MS

PATIENT STORY

A 64-year-old woman presents with complaints of itchy skin and fatigue. She is noted on physical examination to have scleral icterus and jaundice (**Figure 58-1**). Laboratory testing revealed elevated liver enzymes, particularly the serum alkaline phosphatase and gamma-glutamyltranspeptidase, and positive antinuclear and antimitochondrial antibodies. A liver biopsy confirmed primary biliary cirrhosis. Two months later, she vomits up some blood and on endoscopy is found to have esophageal varices from her portal hypertension (**Figure 58-2**).

EPIDEMIOLOGY

- Common causes of liver disease include:
  - Alcohol, excessive use—approximately 5% of the population are at risk; this includes women who drink >2 drinks per day and men who drink >3 drinks per day.[1]
  - Drug-induced liver disease[2]:
    - Drugs causing hepatitis include phenytoin, captopril, enalapril, isoniazid, amitriptyline, and ibuprofen.
    - Drugs causing cholestasis include oral contraceptives, erythromycin, and nitrofurantoin.
    - Drugs causing both of the above include azathioprine, carbamazepine, statins, nifedipine, verapamil, amoxicillin-clavulanic acid, and trimethoprim-sulfamethoxazole.
  - Infectious disease—viral hepatitis, infectious mononucleosis, cytomegalovirus, and coxsackievirus are most common. Viral hepatitis infections include:
    - Hepatitis A—In the 1970s, 40% of urban populations in the United States had serologic evidence of prior hepatitis A infection; rates in recent years have been decreasing.[3]
    - Hepatitis B—Five to ten percent of volunteer blood donors in the United States have evidence of prior infection with 1%–10% of those infected progressing to chronic infection.[3]
    - Hepatitis C—In the United States, 1.8% of the general population have had hepatitis C with 50%–70% developing chronic hepatitis and 80%–90% chronic infection.[3]
- Less common disorders include:
  - Genetic inheritance—Wilson disease (defective copper transport with copper toxicity; autosomal recessive with 1 per 40,000 affected), hemochromatosis (disorder of iron storage; autosomal recessive—among individuals of northern European heritage, one in 10 individuals is a heterozygous carrier and 0.3%–0.5% have the disease), alpha1 antitrypsin deficiency (autosomal recessive with 1%–2% of patients with chronic obstructive pulmonary disease affected).
  - Autoimmune liver disease—Eleven to twenty-three percent of patients with chronic liver disease and accounts for approximately 6% of liver transplantations in the United States.[4]

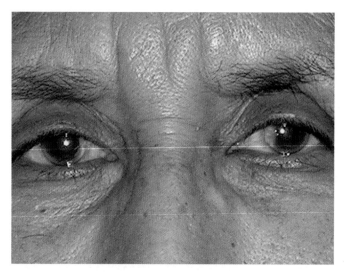

FIGURE 58-1 Scleral icterus in a 64-year-old Hispanic woman with primary biliary cirrhosis. (*Courtesy of Javid Ghandehari, MD.*)

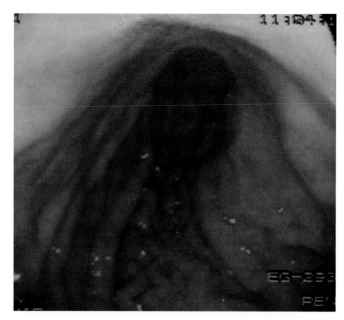

FIGURE 58-2 Esophageal varices in the patient in **Figure 58-1** secondary to her cirrhosis and portal hypertension. (*Courtesy of Javid Ghandehari, MD.*)

◦ Primary biliary cirrhosis (approximately 5 per 100,000 worldwide)—a disease of unknown etiology characterized by inflammatory destruction of the small bile ducts and gradual liver cirrhosis (**Figures 58-1** and **58-2**).

ETIOLOGY AND PATHOPHYSIOLOGY

To understand liver disease, the anatomy and key functions are briefly described here.

• The hepatic artery (20%) and the portal vein (80%) provide the vascular supply of the liver.[1] The liver is organized functionally into acini which are divided into three zones[1]:
  ◦ Zone 1—the portal areas where blood enters from both sources.
  ◦ Zone 2—the hepatocytes and sinusoids where blood flows.
  ◦ Zone 3—the terminal hepatic veins.

• Hepatocytes, the predominant cells in the liver, perform several vital functions including the synthesis of essential serum proteins (e.g., albumin, coagulation factors); production of bile and its carriers (e.g., bile acids, cholesterol); regulation of nutrients (e.g., glucose, lipids, amino acids); and metabolism and conjugation of lipophilic compounds (e.g., bilirubin, various drugs) for excretion into the bile or urine.[1]

• There are two basic patterns of liver disease and one mixed pattern[1]:
  ◦ Hepatocellular—features of this type are direct liver injury, inflammation, and necrosis. Examples are alcoholic and viral hepatitis.
  ◦ Cholestatic (obstructive)—involves inhibition of bile flow. Examples are gallstone disease, malignancy, primary biliary cirrhosis, and some drug-induced disease.
  ◦ Both patterns—evidence of direct damage and obstruction. Examples are cholestatic form of viral hepatitis and some drug-induced diseases.

• Cirrhosis occurs following irreversible hepatic injury with hepatocyte necrosis resulting in fibrosis and distortion of the vascular bed. This in turn can cause portal hypertension.

• Risk factors for liver disease include[1]:
  ◦ Alcohol and intravenous drug use.
  ◦ Drugs (e.g., oral contraceptives).
  ◦ Personal and sexual habits.
  ◦ Travel to underdeveloped countries.
  ◦ Exposure to contaminant in food (e.g., shellfish) or individuals with liver disease (includes needle stick injuries).
  ◦ Family history.
  ◦ Blood transfusion prior to 1992.

DIAGNOSIS

The goals of diagnosis are to determine the etiology and severity of the liver disease and, where appropriate, the stage of the disease including whether it is acute or chronic, early or late in the course of the disease, and whether there is cirrhosis present and to what degree.

CLINICAL FEATURES

- Constitutional symptoms including fatigue (most common; especially following activity), weakness, anorexia, and nausea.
- Skin alterations[1]:
  ○ Jaundice (hallmark of obstructive pattern)—best seen in the sclera or below the tongue, the latter is particularly useful in dark-skinned individuals. Not detected until serum bilirubin levels reach 2.5 mg/dL (43 micromol/L). Early, jaundice may manifest as dark (tea colored) urine and later with light colored stools. Jaundice without dark urine is usually from indirect hyperbilirubinemia as seen in patients with hemolytic anemia or Gilberts Syndrome.
  ○ Palmar erythema—can be seen in both acute and chronic disease but also seen in normal individuals and during pregnancy (**Figure 58-3**).
  ○ Spider angiomas (superficial, tortuous arterioles that flow outward from the center)—also seen in both acute and chronic disease, in normal individuals, and during pregnancy (**Figure 58-4**).
  ○ Excoriations—pruritus is prominent in acute obstructive disease and in chronic cholestatic diseases such as primary biliary cirrhosis.
  ○ Palpable purpura—seen with hepatitis C and chronic hepatitis B.
- Abdominal distention/bloating—secondary to ascites (accumulation of excess fluid within the peritoneal cavity) (**Figure 58-5**).
  ○ Ascites may be detected on examination by shifting dullness on percussion (ascitic fluid will flow to the most dependent portions of the abdomen and the air-filled intestines will float on top of this fluid. The fluid/air interface is detected with the patient supine and then turned onto the side where the "line" shifts upward) (**Figures 58-6** and **58-7**).
- Pain in the right upper quadrant (caused by stretching or irritation of Glisson's capsule surrounding the liver) with tenderness on examination in the liver area. Pain and fever in a patient with ascites should suggest the diagnosis of spontaneous bacterial peritonitis (SBP).
- Hepatomegaly and splenomegaly (congestive splenomegaly from portal hypertension)—seen in patients with cirrhosis, venoocclusive disease, malignancy, and alcoholic hepatitis.[1]
- Features of hyperestrogenemia in men including gynecomastia (**Figure 58-8**) and testicular atrophy.
- Physical signs of specific liver disease include:
  ○ Kayser-Fleischer rings—brown copper pigment deposits around the periphery of the cornea seen in Wilson's disease (**Figure 58-9**).
  ○ Excessive skin pigmentation (slate gray hue/bronzing), diabetes mellitus, polyarticular arthropathy, congestive heart failure, and hypogonadism (hemochromatosis).
  ○ Cachexia, wasting, and firm hepatomegaly (primary hepatocellular carcinoma [HCC] or metastatic liver disease).
- Features of patients with advanced disease include muscle wasting, ascites, edema, dilated abdominal veins (e.g., caput medusa—collateral veins seen radiating from the umbilicus, bruising, hepatic fetor (i.e., sweet, ammonia odor), asterixis (i.e., flapping of the hands when extended), and mental confusion, stupor, or coma.[1]

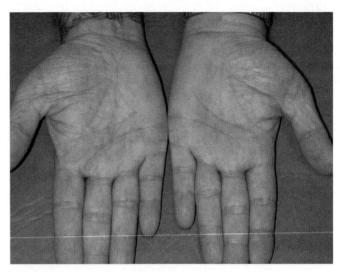

FIGURE 58-3 Palmar erythema in a man with cirrhosis secondary to alcoholism. (*Courtesy of Richard P. Usatine, MD.*)

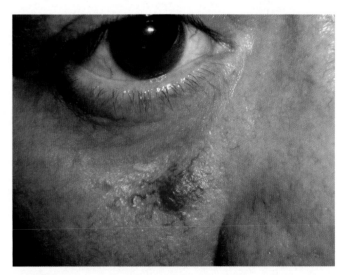

FIGURE 58-4 Spider angioma on the face of a woman with cirrhosis secondary to chronic hepatitis C. (*Courtesy of Richard P. Usatine, MD.*)

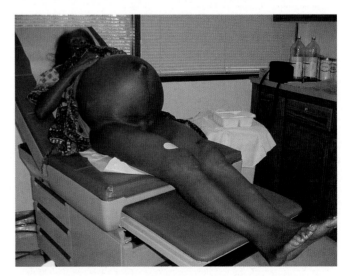

FIGURE 58-5 Tense ascites in a woman with cirrhosis from her alcoholism. An umbilical hernia is also seen from the increased intra-abdominal pressure. (*Courtesy of Richard P. Usatine, MD.*)

- Hepatic failure, defined as the occurrence of signs and symptoms of hepatic encephalopathy, may begin with sleep disturbance, personality changes, irritability, and mental slowness.[1] Mental confusion, disorientation, or coma may occur later along with physical signs as above.

LABORATORY STUDIES AND IMAGING

- Initial evaluation with bilirubin, albumin, alanine aminotransferase (ALT), aspartate aminotransferase (AST), gamma-glutamyl transpeptidase (GGT), and alkaline phosphatase (AlkP).[1]
  - Acute disease (less than 6 months) with hepatocellular pattern (↑↑ ALT) or mixed (↑ ALT, ↑ AlkP)—Consider hepatitis panel (hepatitis A, B, and C), antinuclear antibodies and smooth muscle antibody (autoimmune hepatitis), monospot (hepatitis associated with mononucleosis), and ceruloplasmin (decreased in Wilson's disease). Also look for a history of alcohol or drug use. Additional tests that may be considered, based on history and clinical picture, include a toxicology screen, acetaminophen level, and ammonia level.
  - Acute disease with cholestatic pattern (↑↑ AlkP, ↑↑ GGT, ↑ bilirubin, ↑ ALT)—Consider antimitochondrial antibody (primary biliary cirrhosis), ultrasound and/or magnetic resonance imaging (gallstone, biliary duct dilation, fatty liver, masses), magnetic resonance cholangiopancreatography (visualize biliary tree) and/or endoscopic retrograde cholangiopancreatography (good for detecting ampullary lesions, primary sclerosing cholangitis, and to obtain biopsy).
  - Chronic disease (more than 6 months duration) with hepatocellular pattern (↑↑ ALT) or mixed (↑ ALT, ↑ AlkP)—Consider hepatitis panel (hepatitis B and C); iron saturation and ferritin (hemochromatosis), ceruloplasmin (Wilson's disease), alpha1 antitrypsin; antinuclear antibodies and smooth muscle antibody (autoimmune hepatitis); and ultrasound. Look for alcohol history.
  - Chronic disease with cholestatic pattern (↑↑ AlkP, ↑↑ GGT, ↑ bilirubin, ↑ ALT)—Consider AMA; peripheral antineutrophil cytoplasmic antibody (primary sclerosing cholangitis); ultrasound and magnetic resonance cholangiopancreatography or endoscopic retrograde cholangiopancreatography.
  - Bilirubin, albumin, and prothrombin time along with the presence or absence of ascites and hepatic encephalopathy are part of the Child-Pugh classification of cirrhosis that has been used to estimate the likelihood of survival and complications of cirrhosis; it is also used to determine candidacy for liver transplant.[5] Another scoring system, the model for end-stage liver disease, that uses the international normalized ratio, serum bilirubin, and serum creatinine provides a more objective measure of disease severity and is currently used to establish priority for liver transplant.[6]
- Suspected SBP can be confirmed following paracentesis of the ascitic fluid showing a polymorphonuclear leukocyte count greater than or equal to 250 cells/mm³.

Biopsy: Liver biopsy is the gold standard for diagnosing those with acute disease where the etiology is unclear or for those with chronic disease (e.g., chronic hepatitis B, hepatitis C) to assist in staging the disease and for prognosis.

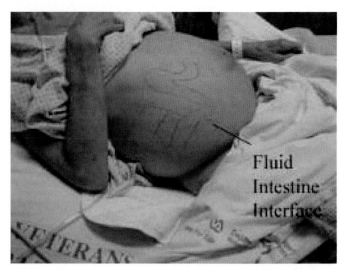

FIGURE 58-6 Patient with ascites and jaundice; lines drawn demonstrate the position of the fluid dullness to percussion (solid stripes), intestines (tubular structure), and the fluid intestine interface (dotted line). (*Courtesy of Charlie Goldberg, MD, copyrighted by the University of California, San Diego.*)

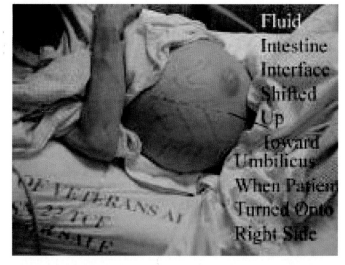

FIGURE 58-7 When patient is turned to the right side, the fluid intestine interface is shifted upward as shown—this is the sign called shifting dullness. (*Courtesy of Charlie Goldberg, MD, copyrighted by the University of California, San Diego.*)

- It may be possible to predict significant fibrosis and inflammation among patients with chronic hepatitis B using noninvasive markers, thereby limiting the number of biopsies needed.
  - In one study, significant liver fibrosis was predicted in patients who were hepatitis B e-antigen (HBeAg) negative using the HBV DNA levels, AlkP, albumin, and platelet counts with an area under Receiver Operating Characteristic curve of 0.91 for the training group and 0.85 for the validation group.[7]
  - The best model for predicting significant inflammation included the variables age, HBV DNA levels, AST, and albumin with an area under the curve of 0.93 in the training and 0.82 in the validation group. In HBeAg positive patients, no factor could accurately predict stages of liver fibrosis, but the best factor for predicting significant inflammation was AST with an area under the curve of 0.87.

MANAGEMENT

Management decisions are based on the etiology, acuity, and severity of the disease.

- Alcoholic cirrhosis—Discontinue alcohol and provide supportive therapy. Alcoholic hepatitis is treated with either glucocorticoids or pentoxifylline.[8]
- Drug-induced disease—withdrawal of agent.
- Viral hepatitis—Hepatitis A and acute hepatitis B are treated supportively; virtually all patients recover without specific treatment. Chronic hepatitis B may be treated with antiviral therapy (interferon) and the nucleoside analogue lamivudine or the acyclic nucleotide analogue adefovir.[3,9] Hepatitis C is currently treated with pegylated interferon and ribavirin.[3] All persons with chronic hepatitis B who are not immune to hepatitis A should receive 2 doses of hepatitis A vaccine 6 to 18 months apart.[9] Patients with hepatitis C should be vaccinated against Hepatitis A and B if they are seronegative for these other forms of hepatitis. SOR **B** Newborns of hepatitis B virus-infected mothers should receive hepatitis B immunoglobulin and hepatitis B vaccine at delivery and complete the recommended vaccination series.[9] SOR **A**
- Wilson's disease is treated with zinc acetate (50 mg three times daily) with or without trientine, a chelating agent (500 mg twice daily).[10]
- Hemochromocytosis is treated with weekly or twice weekly phlebotomy.
- Primary biliary cirrhosis is managed with ursodiol (13–15 mg/kg/d) single dose and eventual liver transplant.[11] SOR **A** In a meta-analysis of seven trials, ursodeoxycholic acid treatment resulted in a significant reduction of the incidence of liver transplantation (OR 0.65, $p = 0.01$) and a marginally significant reduction of the rate of death or liver transplantation.[12]
- Autoimmune hepatitis is treated with glucocorticoid therapy with or without azathioprine.
- Management of the complications of cirrhosis include:
  - Control ascites with salt restriction (2g/d of NaCl), fluid restriction if hyponatremic (1000 mL/d), gentle diuresis to avoid electrolyte disturbance (spironolactone 100–400 mg/d) with or without furosemide (40–160 mg/d).[11] SOR **A**

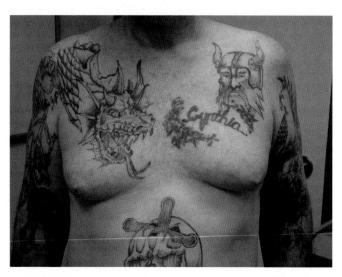

FIGURE 58-8 Gynecomastia in a man with cirrhosis secondary to alcoholism. (*Courtesy of Richard P. Usatine, MD.*)

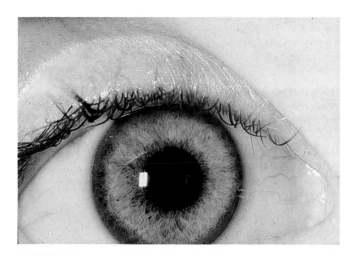

FIGURE 58-9 Kayser-Fleischer ring around the cornea in a patient with Wilson's disease. (*Courtesy of Marc Solioz, University of Berne.*)

○ SBP is treated with empiric antibiotic therapy (e.g., intravenous cefotaxime 2 g every 8 hours).[13] SOR **A**

○ Portal hypertension may be managed with shunting.

PATIENT EDUCATION

• Patients with liver disease should be counseled about avoidance of alcohol and medications that may cause liver injury. They should avoid aspirin use (coagulation impaired) and use acetaminophen at lower doses (2g/d).

• For those with infectious causes of liver disease, prevention of the spread of disease should be emphasized including limiting alcohol, safe-sex practices, and avoiding needle sharing. Screening for sexual contacts and household members should be offered along with vaccination for hepatitis B, if nonimmune and noninfected.[9] SOR **A**

FOLLOW-UP

• Hepatitis B virus carriers with high risk for HCC (e.g., men above 45 years of age, those with cirrhosis, and individuals with a family history of HCC, should be screened periodically with both alpha-fetoprotein and ultrasonography.[9] SOR **C**

• Patients who have survived an episode of SBP should receive long-term prophylaxis with daily norfloxacin or trimethoprim/sulfamethoxazole.[13] SOR **A**

PATIENT RESOURCES

Patients may select among specific topics as desired from the website—**http://www.nlm.nih.gov/medlineplus/ency/article/000205.htm.**

For information on autoimmune hepatitis—**http://www.cumc.columbia.edu/dept/gi/autoimmune.html.**

For information on primary biliary cirrhosis—**http://www.cumc.columbia.edu/dept/gi/PBC.html.**

PROVIDER RESOURCES

A number of disease-specific evidence-based guidelines can be found through the National Guideline Clearinghouse—**http://www.guideline.gov.**

Lok AS, McMahon BJ. Chronic hepatitis B. Alexandria, VA: American Association for the Study of Liver Diseases; 2004, p. 25.

Czaja AJ, Freese DK. Diagnosis and treatment of autoimmune hepatitis. *Hepatology* 2002;36(2):479–497.

Polson J, Lee WM. AASLD position paper: The management of acute liver failure. *Hepatology* 2005;41(5):1179–1197.

Runyon BA. Management of adult patients with ascites due to cirrhosis. *Hepatology* 2004;39(3):841–856.

REFERENCES

1. Ghany M, Hoofnagle JH. Approach to the patient with liver disease. In: Kasper DL, Braunwald E, Fauci AS, Hauser SL, Longo DL, Jameson, JL eds. *Harrison's Principles of Internal Medicine*, 16th ed. New York: McGraw-Hill, 2005:1808–1813.

2. Dientag JL, Isselbacher KJ. Toxic and drug-induced hepatitis. In: Kasper DL, Braunwald E, Fauci AS, Hauser SL, Longo DL, Jameson, JL eds. *Harrison's Principles of Internal Medicine*, 16th ed. New York: McGraw-Hill, 2005:1840.

3. Dienstag JL, Isselbacher KJ. Acute viral hepatitis. In: Kasper DL, Braunwald E, Fauci AS, Hauser SL, Longo DL, Jameson, JL eds. *Harrison's Principles of Internal Medicine*, 16th ed. New York: McGraw-Hill, 2005:1822–1838.

4. Wolf DC, Raghuraman UV. Autoimmune Hepatitis. http://www.emedicine.com. Accessed November 15, 2006.

5. Kamath PS, Wiesner RH, McDiarmid SV, et al. A model to predict survival in patients with end-stage liver disease. *Hepatology.* 2001;33(2):464–470.

6. www.mayo.edu/int-med/gi/model/. Accessed November 5, 2006.

7. Mohamadnejad M, Montazeri G, Fazlollahi A, et al. Noninvasive markers of liver fibrosis and inflammation in chronic hepatitis B-virus related liver disease. *Am J Gastroenterol.* 2006;101(11):2537–2545.

8. Mailliard ME, Sorrell NF. Alcoholic liver disease. In: Kasper DL, Braunwald E, Fauci AS, Hauser SL, Longo DL, Jameson, JL eds. *Harrison's Principles of Internal Medicine*, 16th ed. New York: McGraw-Hill, 2005:1855–1857.

9. Lok AS, McMahon BJ. Chronic hepatitis B. Alexandria, VA: American Association for the study of liver diseases; 2004. 25 p. http://www.guideline.gov; http://www.aasld.org. Accessed November 5, 2006.

10. Brewer GJ. Wilson disease. In: Kasper DL, Braunwald E, Fauci AS, Hauser SL, Longo DL, Jameson, JL eds. *Harrison's Principles of Internal Medicine*, 16th ed. New York: McGraw-Hill, 2005:2313–2315.

11. Chung RT, Podolsky DK. Cirrhosis and its complications. In: Kasper DL, Braunwald E, Fauci AS, Hauser SL, Longo DL, Jameson, JL eds. *Harrison's Principles of Internal Medicine*, 16th. New York: McGraw-Hill, 2005:1808–1813.

12. Shi J, Wu C, Lin Y, et al. Long-term effects of mid-dose ursodeoxycholic acid in primary biliary cirrhosis: A meta-analysis of randomized controlled trials. *Am J Gastroenterol.* 2006;101(7):1529–1538.

13. Runyon BA. Management of adult patients with ascites due to cirrhosis. *Hepatology.* 2004;39(3):841–856.

59 GALLSTONES

Mindy A. Smith, MD, MS

PATIENT STORY

A 44-year-old woman reports frequent episodes of severe pain that usually occur shortly after her evening meal and sometimes at night in the mid and upper-right-side of her abdomen. She is obese, but otherwise healthy. The pain lasts for several hours and is steady and often causes vomiting. On physical examination she complains of slight tenderness in the right upper quadrant (RUQ). An ultrasound confirms the presence of a gallstone (**Figure 59-1**).

EPIDEMIOLOGY

- Based on autopsy data, 20% of women and 8% of men have gallstones.[1]

- Approximately 20 million people in the United States are affected, with 1 million new cases each year.[1]

- Among pregnant women, 5% to 12% have gallstones and 20% to 30% have gallbladder sludge (thick mucous material containing cholesterol crystals and mucin thread or mucous gels). Gallbladder sludge is a possible precursor form of gallstone disease.[1]

- First-degree relatives of patients with gallstones have a higher risk of gallstones: In a case control study, the prevalence of gallstones was 28.6% in first-degree relatives of subjects with gallstones versus 12.4% in first-degree relatives of subjects without gallstones (relative risk (RR) 1.80, 95% confidence interval (CI) 1.29–2.63).[2]

- Patients with asymptomatic gallstones have a 1% to 2% risk per year of developing symptoms or complications of gallstones. Based on data primarily for men, this will occur in 10% by 5 years, 15% by 10 years, and 18% by 15 years following diagnosis.[1]

- Gallstone disease is responsible for approximately 10,000 deaths per year in the United States. Most (7,000) of these deaths are attributable to acute gallstone complications (e.g., cholecystitis, pancreatitis, cholangitis).[2]

- Approximately 2000–3000 deaths per year are caused by gallbladder cancers, 80% of which occur in the setting of gallstone disease with chronic cholecystitis.[3]

ETIOLOGY AND PATHOPHYSIOLOGY

- There are two types of gallstones: Cholesterol stones (80%) and pigmented stones (primarily calcium bilirubinate, 20%).

- The solute components of bile include bile acids (80%), lecithin and other phospholipids (16%), and unesterified cholesterol (4%).[1] Cholesterol gallstones form when there is excess cholesterol or an abnormal ratio of cholesterol, bile acids, and lecithin.

- Excess biliary cholesterol can occur from a secondary increase in secretion of cholesterol caused by obesity, high cholesterol diet,

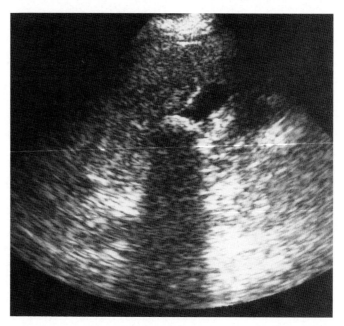

FIGURE 59-1 Ultrasound showing echogenic gallstone (arrow) in the gallbladder (asterisk). Note the absence of echoes posterior to the gallstone called "shadowing" (arrowheads). (*From Schwartz DT and Reisdorff EJ. Emergency Radiology p. 537, Fig. 19-39. Copyright 2000, McGraw-Hill.*)

clofibrate therapy, or a genetic predisposition to increased hydroxymethylglutaryl-coenzyme A reductase.

- The excess cholesterol becomes supersaturated and can precipitate out of solution in a process called nucleation, forming solid cholesterol monohydrate crystals that can become trapped in gallbladder mucus, producing sludge, and/or grow and aggregate to form cholesterol gallstones.

- Genetic mutations can result in reduction of bile acids and lecithin that predispose some patients to stone formation. A high prevalence of gallstones is found in first-degree relatives of patients with gallstones and among Native Americans, Chilean Indians, and Chilean Hispanics.[1]

- Gallbladder hypomotility is a predisposing and possibly necessary factor in stone formation because of the failure to completely empty supersaturated or crystal-containing bile.[1] Situations associated with hypomotility include pregnancy, prolonged parenteral nutrition, surgery, burns, and use of oral contraceptives or estrogen therapy.

- Pigmented stones occur when increasing amounts of unconjugated bilirubin in bile precipitate to form stones. Bilirubin, a yellow pigment derived from the breakdown of heme, is actively secreted into bile by liver cells. In situations of high heme turnover, such as chronic hemolytic states (e.g., sickle cell anemia), calcium bilirubinate can crystallize from solution and form stones.

- Other risk factors for gallstones include rapid weight loss (20–30% form stones within 4 months),[3] increasing age, liver or ileal disease, and cystic fibrosis.

- Chronic gallstones may cause progressive fibrosis of the gallbladder wall and loss of function.[3]

- Gallbladder adenocarcinoma is uncommon, but usually develops in the setting of gallstones and chronic cholecystitis.[3]

DIAGNOSIS

CLINICAL FEATURES

- Symptoms of gallstones are caused from inflammation or obstruction as stones migrate into the cystic or common bile duct (CBD).
  - Biliary colic is a steady, severe pain or ache, usually of sudden onset, located in the epigastrium or RUQ. Pain episodes last between 30 minutes and 5 hours and may radiate to the interscapular area, right scapula, or right shoulder.
  - Gallstone-related pain may be precipitated by a fatty meal, a regular meal or a large meal followed by a prolonged fast.
  - Pain is recurrent and often nocturnal.
- RUQ tenderness may be elicited on physical examination.
- Nausea and vomiting are common.
- Accompanying fever and chills suggests a complication of gallstones. Complications are more common in patients with a calcified gallbladder or in those who have had a previous episode of acute cholecystitis.[1]

LABORATORY STUDIES

- No laboratory testing is usually indicated since the results are usually normal. However, an elevated gamma-glutamyl transpeptidase suggests a CBD stone. In a study of patients with acute calculous gallbladder disease, investigators found a one in three chance of CBD stones when the gamma-glutamyl transpeptidase level was above 90 units/L and a one in 30 chance when the level was less than 90 units/L.[4]

IMAGING

- Ultrasound is the diagnostic test of choice and is 95% accurate for stones as small as 2 mm in diameter (**Figure 59-1**).[1] Shadowing, a discrete acoustic shadow caused by the absorption and reflection of sound by the stone that changes with patient positioning, is an important diagnostic feature that is shown in **Figures 59-1** and **59-2**.

- Gallstones may be seen on plain film, but only calcified stones are seen (**Figures 59-3** and **59-4**). This includes only 10% to 15% of cholesterol stones and 50% of pigmented stones.[1] Stones may be single or multiple and the gallbladder wall may be calcified (referred to as a "Porcelain gallbladder") indicating severe chronic cholecystitis or adenocarcinoma.

- Computed tomography (CT) is less sensitive and more expensive than ultrasound for the detection of gallstones (**Figures 59-5** and **59-6**). However, CT can detect both radio-opaque stones and radiolucent stones and is superior to ultrasound in visualizing gallstones in the distal CBD.[3]

- An oral cholecystogram can be used to assess cystic duct patency and emptying function. This test has largely been replaced by gallbladder ultrasound.

- Radioisotope scans (e.g., Technetium Tc-99m hepatoiminodiacetic acid) can be used to confirm acute cholecystitis (nonvisualizing gallbladder) and can be useful in evaluating functional abnormalities.

- Endoscopic retrograde cholangiopancreatography is used for imaging bile ducts. Stones in bile appear as filling defects in the opacified ducts. Endoscopic retrograde cholangiopancreatography is usually performed in conjunction with endoscopic retrograde sphincterotomy and gallstone extraction.[3]

DIFFERENTIAL DIAGNOSIS

Severe epigastric and RUQ pain can be seen in the following conditions[5]:

- Acute cholecystitis—pain may radiate to the back, and fever is usually present. Physical examination can reveal RUQ rigidity and guarding with a positive Murphy's sign (RUQ pain worsening with deep inspiration while the examiner maintains steady pressure below the right costal margin). White blood count, serum amylase, aspartate transaminase and alanine transaminase may all be elevated.

- Pancreatitis—pain is located in the mid-epigastrium and left upper quadrant, but may radiate to the RUQ. Abdominal distention and diminished bowel sounds may be present. Elevations in lipase and amylase are found and pancreatic pseudocysts or abscess may be present on ultrasound.

- Peptic ulcer disease—Pain may be described as burning and is usually epigastric and often relieved by antacids. Onset is 1 to 3 hours after meals or following nonsteroidal antiinflammatory drugs usage. Stool hemoccult testing may be positive. An ulcer may be visualized on upper gastrointestinal barium swallow or endoscopy.

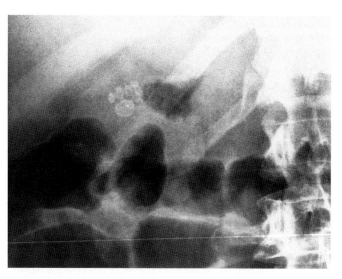

FIGURE 59-2 Plain film showing multiple gallstones (white arrow). (*From Schwartz DT and Reisdorff EJ. Emergency Radiology p. 536, Fig. 19-37. Copyright 2000, McGraw-Hill.*)

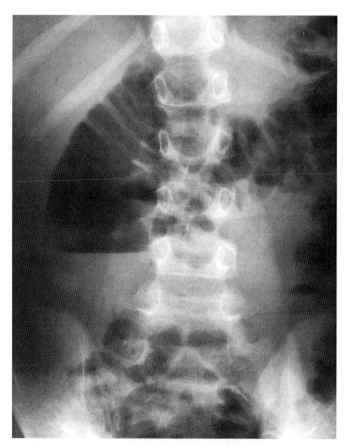

FIGURE 59-3 Gallstone ileus in an elderly patient with diabetes; note dilated loops of small bowel and an ectopic gallstone (arrow). (*From Schwartz DT and Reisdorff EJ. Emergency Radiology p. 527, Fig. 19-21. Copyright 2000, McGraw-Hill.*)

- Hepatitis—Other symptoms and signs include malaise, anorexia, pruritus, tender liver and low-grade fever. Jaundice may be present and urine may be dark (i.e., bilirubinuria). Aspartate transaminase and alanine transaminase are elevated.

MANAGEMENT

- Silent gallstones may be managed expectantly; prophylactic cholecystectomy is unwarranted based on the few who develop symptoms over time and the very low rate of complications (3%).[6] SOR Ⓐ

- Cholecystectomy should be considered for patients with[1]:
  - Frequent symptoms that interfere with daily life.
  - A prior complication of gallstone disease.
  - The presence of an underlying condition (e.g., calcified gallbladder) that predisposes the patient to increased risk of complications.

- Laparoscopic cholecystectomy is the surgical treatment of choice because of the low rate of complications (4%) and mortality (<0.1%), shortened hospital stay, and reduced cost.[1] Conversion to an open laparotomy is infrequent (5%).[1]

- Medical therapy with ursodeoxycholic acid may be considered for patients with functioning gallbladders and small stones (<10 mm).[1] Approximately 50% of these patients will have complete dissolution of stones in 6–24 months, but recurrences are common (30–50% at 3–5 year follow-up).[1]

- Medical therapy can also be used to prevent gallstone formation in patients with expected rapid weight loss caused by very low-calorie diets or bariatric surgery. Administration of ursodeoxycholic acid at a dose of 600 mg daily for 16 weeks reduces incidence of gallstones by 80% in this setting.[3]

- Extracorporeal shock wave lithotripsy combined with medical therapy may be considered for patients with radiolucent, solitary stones less than 2 cm, and a functional gallbladder.[1]

PATIENT EDUCATION

- Patients with asymptomatic gallstones may be managed expectantly—the rates of developing symptoms and complications should be reviewed. They should be encouraged to report symptoms of biliary colic and acute cholecystitis or pancreatitis (described above).

- Laparoscopic cholecystectomy appears to be very successful for symptom resolution, although chronic diarrhea may occur (see "Follow-up" below) and abdominal pain may persist in approximately 30% of patients.[7]

FOLLOW-UP

- Approximately 5% to 10% of patients develop chronic diarrhea, attributed to increased bile salts reaching the colon, following cholecystectomy.[3] Diarrhea is usually mild and can be managed with over-the-counter antidiarrheal agents (e.g., loperamide).

- Some patients may experience recurrent pain resembling biliary colic (called postcholecystectomy syndrome). Some of these

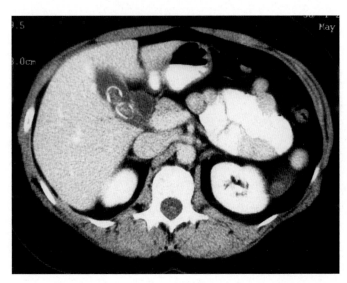

FIGURE 59-4 CT scan showing two large gallstones that have a rim of calcification (large arrows). (*From Schwartz DT and Reisdorff EJ. Emergency Radiology p. 538, Fig. 19-41A. Copyright 2000, McGraw-Hill.*)

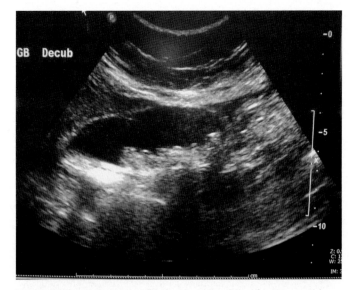

FIGURE 59-5 Gallstones visible in the gallbladder of a 43-year-old woman with RUQ pain and a positive Murphy's sign. Note the shadowing effect behind the gallstones as they reflect the sound back to the transducer. (*Courtesy of Jeff Russell, MD.*)

patients have an underlying motility disorder of the sphincter of Oddi that can be treated with endoscopic retrograde sphincterotomy.[3]

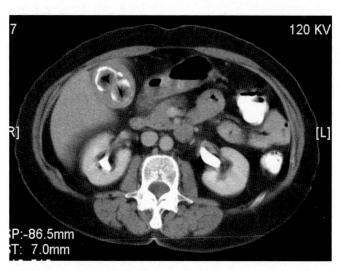

FIGURE 59-6 Radiographic sign seen on a CT cut through the gallbladder (the gallstones produce a pattern that resembles Mercedes-Benz logo). (*Courtesy of Mike Freckleton, MD.*)

REFERENCES

1. Greenberger NJ, Paumgartner G. Diseases of the gallbladder and bile ducts. In: Kasper DL, Braunwald E, Fauci AS, Hauser SL, Longo DL, Jameson, JL eds. *Harrison's Principles of Internal Medicine*, 16th ed. New York: McGraw-Hill, 2005: 1880–1884.

2. Attili AF, De Santis A, Attili F, et al. Prevalence of gallstone disease in first-degree relatives of patients with cholelithiasis. *World J Gastroenterol.* 2005;11(41):6508–6511.

3. Heuman DM, Mihas A, Allen J, Cuschieri A. http://www. emedicine.com. Accessed October 10, 2006.

4. Peng WK, Sheikh Z, Paterson-Brown S, Nixon SJ. Role of liver function tests in predicting common bile duct stones in acute calculous cholecystitis. *Br J Surg.* 2005;92(10):1241–1247.

5. Curran D. Gallbladder disease. In: Smith MA, Shimp LA eds. *20 Common Problems in Women's Health Care*. New York: McGraw-Hill, 2000:616.

6. Gracie WA, Ransohoff DF. The natural history of asymptomatic gallstones: The innocent gallstone is not a myth. *N Engl J Med.* 1982;307:798–800.

7. Gui GP, Cheruvu CV, West N, et al. Is cholecystectomy effective treatment for symptomatic gallstones? Clinical outcomes after long-term follow-up. *Ann R Coll Surg.* 1998;80:25–32.

60 COLON POLYP

Cathy Abbott, MD
Mindy A. Smith, MD, MS

PATIENT STORY

A 62-year-old woman presents to her physician for routine annual examination. She has no known family history of colon disease and is asymptomatic. Stool cards and flexible sigmoidoscopy were recommended and on flexible sigmoidoscopy a 2.4-cm polyp was noted at 35 cm. A colonoscopy was performed and additional polyps were identified in the descending colon and cecum (**Figure 60-1**).

EPIDEMIOLOGY

- More than 30% of middle-aged or elderly patients are found to have adenomatous polyps on screening and based on autopsy surveys less than 1% will become malignant.[1]

- Patients with an adenomatous polyp have a 30% to 50% risk for developing another adenoma and are at higher risk for colon cancer. This risk is greatest in the first 4 years after diagnosis of the first polyp, and greater if a villous adenoma or more than 3 polyps were found.

- Familial adenomatous polyposis of the colon is a rare autosomal dominant disorder. Thousands of adenomatous polyps appear in the large colon, generally by age 25, and colorectal cancer develops in almost all of these patients by age 40.[1] Other hereditary polyposis syndromes include Gardner syndrome, Turcot syndrome, Peutz-Jeghers syndrome, Cowden disease, familial juvenile polyposis, and hyperplastic polyposis.[2]

ETIOLOGY AND PATHOPHYSIOLOGY

- Polyps are growths that arise from the epithelial cells lining the colon. There are several types including:
  - Hyperplastic polyps—contain increased numbers of glandular cells with decreased cytoplasmic mucous and an absence of nuclear hyperchromatism, stratification, or atypia. Traditionally thought to be benign, recent evidence suggests malignant potential particularly for right-sided polyps, especially proximal hyperplastic serrated polyps[1] and those associated with hyperplastic polyposis syndrome (a familial disorder with multiple (>30) hyperplastic polyps proximal to the sigmoid colon with 2 or more >10 mm).[2] The percentage of polyps reported to be in this category ranges from 12% to 90%.[2,3]
  - Adenomatous polyps—may be tubular, villous (papillary), or tubulovillous. In a case series of 582 patients who had a polyp removed, 81% were adenomatous including 65.0% that were tubular, 25.8% tubulovillous, 7.2% villous adenomas, and 0.5% mixed adenomatous hyperplastic polyps; 12 (1.4%) were invasive carcinomas.[3]

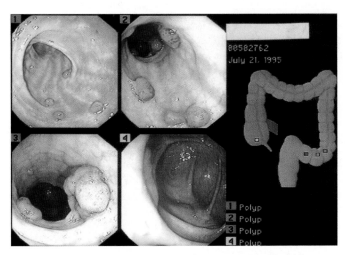

FIGURE 60-1 Colon polyps seen on colonoscopy. (*Courtesy of Michael Harper, MD.*)

- Adenomatous polyps may be pedunculated or sessile; cancers more frequently develop in sessile polyps.[1]
  - Villous polyps can cause hypersecretory syndromes characterized by hypokalemia and profuse mucous discharge; these more frequently harbor carcinoma in situ or invasive carcinoma than other adenomas.[2] Villous polyps are 3 times more likely to develop into cancers.[1]
  - Non-neoplastic hamartoma (juvenile polyp)—benign cystic polyps with mucus filled glands, most commonly found in male children, aged 2 to 5 years; often as singular lesions but additional polyps are found on panendoscopy in 40% to 50% of children. Juvenile polyps in adolescence may be associated with hereditary syndromes that carry malignant potential.[4]
- A series of genetic/molecular changes have been found that are thought to represent a multi-step process from normal colon mucosa to malignant tumor.[2] These include:
  - Point mutations in the K'ras protooncogene leading to gene activation and deletion of DNA at the site of tumor suppressor gene.
  - This results in an altered proliferative pattern and polyp formation.
  - Mutational activation of an oncogene, coupled with loss of tumor suppressor genes, leads to malignant transformation.
- Patients with familial polyposis inherit a germline alteration that leads into the above pathway.
- Diet appears to be associated with colon polyps and colon cancer. Animal fats may alter anaerobes in the gut microflora increasing conversion of normal bile acids to carcinogens. Also, increased cholesterol is associated with an enhanced risk of development of adenomas.
- Insulin resistance, with increased concentrations of insulin-like growth factor type I, may also stimulate proliferation of the intestinal mucosa.
- There is an association between *Helicobacter* exposure and colonic polyps.[5]

DIAGNOSIS

CLINICAL FEATURES

- Usually asymptomatic.
- Patients may experience overt or occult rectal bleeding.
- Diarrhea or constipation can occur, often with decreased stool caliber.
- Secretory villous adenomas can occasionally manifest as a syndrome of severe diarrhea with massive fluid and electrolyte loss.[2]

TYPICAL DISTRIBUTION

In the past, 60% of polyps were found in the rectosigmoid colon, but the distribution has moved more proximal for unknown reasons so that cancer distribution is approximately equal between the right and left colon. Juvenile polyps are usually found in the rectosigmoid region.

IMAGING AND ENDOSCOPIC FEATURES

Polyps may be identified on barium enema, flexible sigmoidoscopy, or colonoscopy (including virtual computer tomography colonoscopy) (**Figures 60-1** to **60-3**).

- A polyp is defined as grossly visible protrusion from the mucosal surface.

- Colonoscopy must be subsequently performed to identify additional lesions and remove all lesions.

- Synchronous lesions occur in one third of cases (**Figure 60-1**).

LABORATORY STUDIES

- Occult blood in the stool is found in <5% of patients with polyps.[1] Of the 2% to 4% of asymptomatic patients who have heme positive stool on screening, 20% to 30% will have polyps.[1]

- For patients with a family history of familial adenomatous polyposis, DNA testing may be performed to detect the *adenomatous polyposis coli (APC)* gene mutation; this can lead to a definitive diagnosis before the development of polyps. SOR Ⓒ[1] A positive test finding only indicates susceptibility, not the actual presence of a polyp.[2]

- Genetic testing can also be considered for patients with a family history of hereditary nonpolyposis colorectal cancer (HNPCC) which is caused by germline mutation of the DNA mismatch repair genes (*hMLH1, hMSH2, hPMS1, hPMS2, hMSH6*).[6] SOR Ⓒ

BIOPSY

Upon removal polyps are sent for histology to determine type and whether dysplasia or carcinoma in situ are present (**Figure 60-3**).

DIFFERENTIAL DIAGNOSIS

Other causes of rectal bleeding include:

- Infectious agents—*Salmonella, shigella,* certain *Campylobacter* species, enteroinvasive *E. coli, C. difficile,* and *entamoeba histolytica* can cause bloody, watery diarrhea and are identified by culture. Bacterial toxins may be identified with *C. difficile*. Additional symptoms include fever and abdominal pain and the disease is often self-limited.

- Hemorrhoids and fissures—bleeding is usually bright red blood and seen in the toilet or with wiping after bowel movements. Hemorrhoids can sometimes be visible as a protruding mass often associated with pruritus and fissures are identified as a cut or tear occurring in the anus. Hemorrhoidal pain is described as a dull ache but may be severe if thrombosed (see Chapter 63, Hemorrhoids).

- Diverticula—bleeding is usually abrupt in onset, painless, and may be massive but often stops spontaneously. These may be seen on endoscopy or on radiographic study.

- Vascular colonic ectasias—bleeding tends to be chronic resulting in anemia. Bleeding source may be identified during colonoscopy but a radionuclide scan or angiography may be needed.

- Colon cancer—other symptoms include abdominal cramping, tenesmus (i.e., urgency with a feeling of incomplete evacuation), narrow caliber stool, occasional obstruction, and rarely perforation. Imaging studies often can distinguish and biopsy confirms malignancy (see Chapter 61, Colon Cancer).

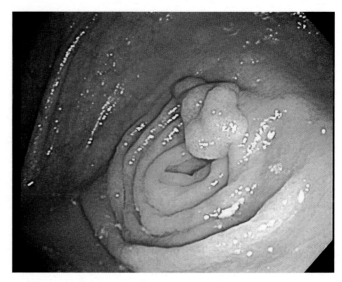

FIGURE 60-2 Polyp in the cecum seen on colonoscopy. (*Courtesy of Marvin Derezin, MD.*)

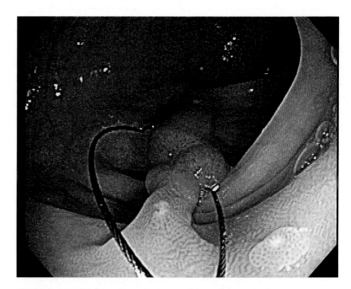

FIGURE 60-3 Polypectomy being performed through the colonoscope. (*Courtesy of Marvin Derezin, MD.*)

• Inflammatory bowel disease—includes ulcerative colitis and Crohn's disease; symptoms include diarrhea, tenesmus, passage of mucus, and cramping abdominal pain. Extra-intestinal manifestations are more common in Crohn's disease and include skin involvement (e.g., erythema nodosum), rheumatologic symptoms (e.g., peripheral arthritis, symmetric sacroiliitis), and ocular problems (e.g., uveitis, iritis). Diagnosis may be made on endoscopy.

MANAGEMENT

• Removal of a solitary polyp may be completed during sigmoidoscopy or colonoscopy (**Figure 60-3**).
• Colonic resection is advocated for patients with familial polyposis and patients with long-standing ulcerative colitis who have developed high-grade dysplasia or a dysplasia-associated lesion or mass.[2]

PATIENT EDUCATION

• Primary prevention of colon cancer should be encouraged:
  ◦ Dietary alterations may be useful; decreasing animal fats as diets high in animal fats are thought to be a major factor based on epidemiologic studies. However, in the Women's Health Initiative study, a low-fat dietary intervention did not reduce the risk of colorectal cancer in postmenopausal women during 8.1 years of follow-up.[7] Additional dietary fiber has not been shown to be helpful in controlled studies. Increasing water consumption to eight glasses per day may also be helpful.
  ◦ Calcium supplements, hormone therapy in women, and folic acid have all been shown to reduce the risk of colon cancer.[1] SOR Ⓐ
  ◦ Low dose aspirin (81 mg/d) was found to decrease recurrent adenomas, including those containing advanced neoplasms.[8] In patients with familial adenomatous polyposis, once-daily treatment with 25 mg rofecoxib significantly decreased the number and size of rectal polyps in one randomized trial.[9]
  ◦ Smoking cessation.
  ◦ Increasing physical activity to decrease insulin resistance may be helpful.
  ◦ Screening options for colon cancer include use of Hemoccult cards, flexible sigmoidoscopy, colonoscopy, and air contrast barium enema.
• Patients should be encouraged to engage in continued surveillance for polyps and colon cancer. Those at increased risk for a subsequent advanced neoplasia (see below) should have a follow-up colonoscopy at 3 years. SOR Ⓑ For other patients, follow-up is recommended at 5–10 years.[10] SOR Ⓒ

FOLLOW-UP

There is some debate regarding the frequency of screening. Guidelines developed by the U.S. Multi-Society Task Force on Colorectal Cancer and the American Cancer Society were recently published based on available evidence.[10] They recommend that:

- People at increased risk for a subsequent advanced neoplasia (i.e., patients who have either three or more adenomas, high-grade dysplasia, villous features, or an adenoma ≥1 cm in size) have a 3-year follow-up colonoscopy.

- People at lower risk (e.g., those with one or two small (<1 cm) tubular adenomas with no high-grade dysplasia) have a follow-up in 5 to 10 years.

- People with hyperplastic polyps only should have a 10-year follow-up similar to average-risk people.

PATIENT RESOURCES

http://digestive.niddk.nih.gov/ddiseases/pubs/colonpolyps_ez/index.htm.

http://www.mayoclinic.com/health/colonpolyps/DS00511/DSECTION=4.

PROVIDER RESOURCES

http://www.emedicine.com/med/topic414.htm.

REFERENCES

1. Mayer R. Gastrointestinal tract cancer. In: Kasper DL, Braunwald E, Fauci AS, Hauser SL, Longo DL, Jameson, JL eds. *Harrison's Principles of Internal Medicine*, 16th ed. New York: McGraw-Hill, 2005:523–533.

2. Enders GH, El-Deiry WS. http://www.emedicine.com. Accessed December 22, 2006.

3. Khan A, Shrier I, Gordon PH. The changed histologic paradigm of colorectal polyps. *Surg Endosc.* 2002;16(3):436–440.

4. Barnard J. Gastrointestinal polyps and polyp syndromes in adolescents. *Adolesc Med Clin.* 2004;15(1):119–129.

5. El-Deiry WS. http://www.emedicine.com/med/topic413.htm. Accessed December 22, 2006.

6. American Gastroenterological Association medical position statement: Hereditary colorectal cancer and genetic testing. *Gastroenterology.* 2001;121(1):195–197.

7. Beresford SA, Johnson KC, Ritenbaugh C, et al. Low-fat dietary pattern and risk of colorectal cancer: The women's health initiative randomized controlled dietary modification trial. *JAMA.* 2006;295(6):643–654.

8. Baron JA, Cole BF, Sandler RS, et al. A randomized trial of aspirin to prevent colorectal adenomas. *N Engl J Med.* 2003;348(10):891–899.

9. Higuchi T, Iwama T, Yoshinaga, K, et al. A randomized, double-blind, placebo-controlled trial of the effects of rofecoxib, a selective cyclooxygenase-2 inhibitor, on rectal polyps in familial adenomatous polyposis patients. *Clin Cancer Res.* 2003;9(13):4756–4760.

10. Winawer SJ, Zauber AG, Fletcher RH, et al. Guidelines for colonoscopy surveillance after polypectomy: A consensus update by the US multi-society task force on colorectal cancer and the american cancer society. *CA Cancer J Clin.* 2006;56(3):143–159.

61 COLON CANCER

Mindy A. Smith, MD, MS

PATIENT STORY

A 72-year-old man reports rectal bleeding with bowel movements over the past several months and the stool seems narrower with occasional diarrhea. He has a history of hemorrhoids but at this time is not experiencing rectal irritation or itching, as with previous episodes. His medical history is significant for controlled hypertension and a remote history of smoking. On digital rectal examination, his stool sample tests positive for blood but anoscopy fails to identify the source of bleeding. On colonoscopy, a mass is seen at 25 cm (**Figure 61-1**). A biopsy was obtained and pathology confirmed adenocarcinoma.

EPIDEMIOLOGY

Colon cancer is the third most common cancer in both men and women in the United States.

• It is second only to lung cancer, as a cause of death in the United States, although the mortality rate has been decreasing, especially for women.[1]

• The incidence has been unchanged for the past 30 years with 146,940 new cases and 56,730 deaths reported in 2004.[1]

• Onset is after age 50.

• Proximal colon carcinoma rates in blacks are higher than in whites.[2]

ETIOLOGY AND PATHOPHYSIOLOGY

• Most cases are adenocarcinomas arising from adenomatous polyps; mutational events occur within the polyp including activation of oncogenes and loss of tumor suppressor genes.

• The probability of a polyp undergoing malignant transformation increases for the following cases:[1]
  ○ The polyp is sessile, especially if villous histology.
  ○ Larger size—Malignant transformation is rare if <1.5 cm, 2% to 10% if 1.5 to 2.5 cm, and 10% if >2.5 cm.

• Risk factors:[1]
  ○ Ingestion of animal fats.
  ○ Hereditary syndromes—Polyposis coli and nonpolyposis syndromes.
  ○ Inflammatory bowel disease.
  ○ Bacteremia with *Streptococcus bovis*—Increased incidence of occult tumors.
  ○ Following ureterosigmoidostomy procedures (5%–10% incidence over 30 years).
  ○ Smoking.
  ○ Alcohol consumption.[2]
  ○ Family history of colon cancer in a first-degree relative.

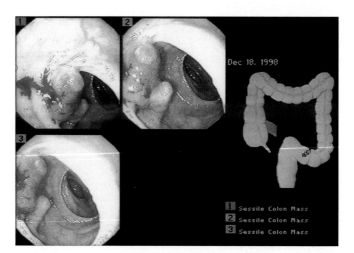

FIGURE 61-1 A sessile colon mass seen at 35 cm. At surgery, this was found to be a Duke's stage A adenocarcinoma. (*Courtesy of Michael Harper, MD.*)

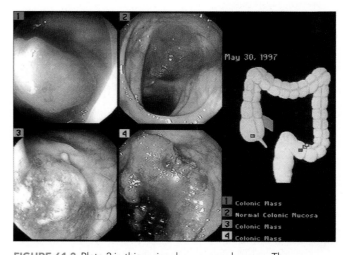

FIGURE 61-2 Plate 2 in this series shows normal cecum. The remaining frames show a large friable mass. Biopsy confirmed adenocarcinoma. The tumor was resected and determined to be Duke's stage B adenocarcinoma. Colonoscopy 3 years later was negative. (*Courtesy of Michael Harper, MD.*)

DIAGNOSIS

The diagnosis is sometimes made following a positive screening test (i.e., digital rectal examination, fecal occult blood testing (FOBT), sigmoidoscopy, colonoscopy, or barium enema). The U.S. Preventive Services Task Force (USPSTF) strongly recommends that clinicians screen men and women 50 years of age or older for colorectal cancer.[2] SOR **A**

- FOBT—This test will be positive in 2% to 4% of asymptomatic patients; less than 10% will have colon cancer.[1] There is a good evidence that periodic FOBT reduces mortality from colorectal cancer.[2,3]

- Flexible sigmoidoscopy (FSG)—There is fair evidence that sigmoidoscopy alone or in combination with FOBT reduces mortality from colon cancer.[2] The ideal interval for surveillance is unknown. Although 5-year interval has been recommended,[3] in a study of 1292 patients returning 3 years after an initial negative flexible sigmoidoscopy, 13.9% had a polyp or mass detected and 3.1% (292/9317) were found to have an adenoma or cancer.[4]

- Colonoscopy—Although there is no direct evidence that screening colonoscopy is effective in reducing colorectal cancer mortality, efficacy is supported by extrapolation from sigmoidoscopy studies, limited case–control evidence, and the ability of colonoscopy to inspect the proximal colon.[2] Examples of colonoscopy pictures are shown in **Figures 61-1** to **61-3**.

- Double-contrast barium enema—This test offers an alternative means of whole-bowel examination, but is less sensitive than colonoscopy, and there is no direct evidence that it is effective in reducing mortality rates.[2] **Figure 61-4** shows a sessile tumor of the cecum and **Figure 61-5** displays a classic "apple-core deformity" of the descending colon.

CLINICAL FEATURES

Symptoms vary, primarily based on anatomic location, as follows:[1]

- Right-sided colon tumors commonly ulcerate occasionally causing anemia without change in stool or bowel habits. Approximately 30% of patients diagnosed with colon cancer present with occult bleeding.[2]

- Tumors in the transverse and descending colon often impede stool passage causing abdominal cramping, occasional obstruction, and rarely perforation (**Figure 61-5**). Approximately 50% of patients diagnosed with colon cancer present with abdominal cramping and 15% with obstruction.[2]

- Tumors in the rectosigmoid region are associated more often with hematochezia, tenesmus (i.e., urgency with a feeling of incomplete evacuation), narrow caliber stool, and uncommonly, anemia. Approximately 35% of patients are diagnosed with colon cancer present with altered bowel habits.[2]

PHYSICAL SIGNS[2]

- Weight loss and cachexia.
- Abdominal distention, discomfort, or tenderness.
- Abdominal or rectal mass.

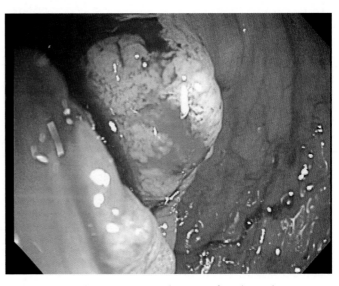

FIGURE 61-3 Adenocarcinoma in the cecum found on colonoscopy. (*Courtesy of Marvin Derezin, MD.*)

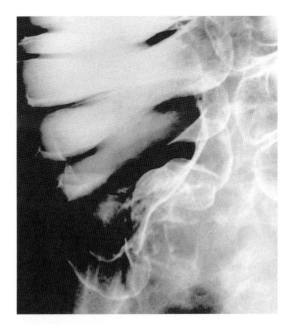

FIGURE 61-4 Sessile tumor of the cecum seen on double-contrast air-barium enema in a patient with iron-deficiency anemia and guaiac-positive stool. The lesion at surgery was a stage B adenocarcinoma. (*From Kasper DL, Braunwald E, Fauci AS, Hauser SL, Longo DL, Jameson JL. Harrison's Internal Medicine, 16th ed, Figure 77-1. Copyright 2005, McGraw-Hill.*)

- Ascites.
- Rectal bleeding, or occult blood on rectal examination.

TYPICAL DISTRIBUTION

Colon cancers are approximately equally distributed between the right and left colon.[5]

IMAGING, ENDOSCOPY, AND WORK-UP

- Colonoscopy of the entire colon is recommended to identify additional neoplasms or polyps (**Figures 61-1** and **61-2**).
- Evaluation for metastatic disease includes:
  - Chest x-ray.
  - Abdominal/pelvic CT scans.
  - Liver function test.
  - Preoperative carcinoembryonic antigen (CEA)—An elevated CEA level can be used to monitor for recurrence. CEA may be elevated for reasons other than colon cancer, such as pancreatic or hepatobiliary disease; elevation does not always reflect cancer or disease recurrence.[2]
- At surgery, surgeons perform an examination of the liver, pelvis, hemi-diaphragm, and full length of the colon for evidence of tumor spread.[1]

BIOPSY

Colonic adenocarcinomas may be microscopically well-differentiated or poorly differentiated glandular structures. Normal topologic architecture of colonic epithelium is lost. Anorectal lesions have a squamous morphology.[2] The addition of cytology brushings to forceps biopsies may increase the diagnostic yield, especially in the setting of obstructing tumors that cannot be traversed.[6]

DIFFERENTIAL DIAGNOSIS

Other causes of abdominal pain in patients in this age group:

- Inflammatory bowel disease includes ulcerative colitis and Crohn's disease; symptoms include bloody diarrhea, tenesmus, passage of mucus, and cramping abdominal pain. Extraintestinal manifestations, more common in Crohn's disease, include skin involvement (e.g., erythema nodosum), rheumatologic symptoms (e.g., peripheral arthritis, symmetric sacroiliitis), and ocular problems (e.g., uveitis, iritis). Diagnosis may be made on basis of endoscopy.

- Diverticulitis—Patients present with fever, anorexia, lower left-sided abdominal pain, and diarrhea. Abdominal distention and peritonitis may be found on physical examination. Diagnosis is usually made on the basis of abdominal CT scan.

- Appendicitis—Initial symptoms include periumbilical or epigastric abdominal pain with time becoming more severe and localized to the right lower quadrant. Additional symptoms include fever, nausea, vomiting, and anorexia.

Other causes of rectal bleeding:

- Infectious agents—Salmonella, shigella, certain campylobacter species, enteroinvasive *Escherichia coli*, *Clostridium difficile*, and

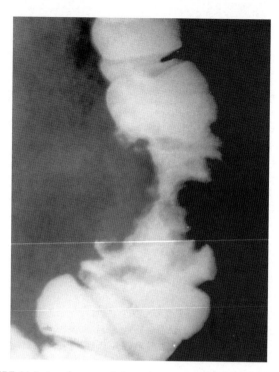

FIGURE 61-5 Annular, constricting adenocarcinoma of the descending colon. This radiographic appearance is referred to as an "apple-core" lesion and is highly suggestive of malignancy. (*From Kasper DL, Braunwald E, Fauci AS, Hauser SL, Longo DL, Jameson JL. Harrison's Internal Medicine, 16th ed, Figure 77-2. Copyright 2005, McGraw-Hill.*)

Entamoeba histolytica can cause bloody, watery diarrhea, and are identified by culture test. Bacterial toxins may be identified with *C. difficile*. Additional symptoms include fever and abdominal pain and the disease is often self-limited.

- Hemorrhoids and fissures—Bleeding is usually bright red blood and seen in the toilet or with wiping after bowel movements. Hemorrhoids can sometimes be visible as a protruding mass often associated with pruritus and fissures are identified as a cut or tear occurring in the anus. Hemorrhoidal pain is described as a dull ache but may be severe if thrombosed.

- Diverticula—Bleeding is usually abrupt in onset, painless, and may be massive, but often stops spontaneously. These may be seen in endoscopy or in radiographic study.

- Vascular colonic ectasias—Bleeding tends to be chronic resulting in anemia. Bleeding source may be identified during colonoscopy, but a radionuclide scan or angiography may be needed.

- Colon polyp—Usually asymptomatic, although abdominal pain, diarrhea, or constipation can occur often with decreased stool caliber. Imaging studies often can distinguish and biopsy confirms absence of malignancy.

Other causes of intestinal obstruction include adhesions, peritonitis, inflammatory bowel disease, fecal impaction, strangulated bowels, and ileus.[2]

MANAGEMENT

- Total resection of the tumor is completed for attempted cure or for symptoms; laparoscopic techniques may be used. Sphincter replacement by electrically stimulated skeletal muscle neosphincter and artificial anal sphincter can be used to provide a continence option for patients with end-stage fecal incontinence and those requiring abdominoperineal resection.[2]

- Total colonic resection is performed for patients with familial polyposis and multiple colonic polyps.

- For rectal carcinoma, sharp dissection is recommended (vs. blunt) for rectal tumors to reduce recurrence to ~10%.[1] In addition, radiation therapy of the pelvis also decreases regional recurrence.[1] Postoperative treatment with 5-Flurouracil (FU) and radiation decreases recurrence for stage B2 and C tumors.[1]

- Preoperative radiation therapy can be used to shrink large tumors prior to resection.

- Solitary metastases to the liver can be treated with partial liver resection.

- Chemotherapy with 5-FU, irinotecan, with or without leucovorin (LV) is of marginal benefit with overall responses in approximately 15% to 20% of patients.[1] Six months of postoperative treatment with 5-FU and LV decreased recurrence for Duke's C tumors by 40% and increased survival by 30%.[1] A reduction in relapse rate and a modest increase in 3-year disease-free survival was also seen in patients with Dukes B and C colon cancer by adding oxaliplatin to 5-FU/leucovorin.[2]

- Antivascular endothelial growth factor (VEGF) therapy with bevacizumab prolongs survival in advanced colorectal cancer when combined with irinotecan, 5-FU, and leucovorin.[2]

PATIENT EDUCATION

- Most recurrences occur within the first 4 years, so survival at 5-years is a good indication of cure.[1]

- Surveillance for recurrence should be conducted over the first 5 years following treatment as noted below. In addition to identifying recurrence, a second tumor is found in 3% to 5% and adenomatous polyps will be found in >15% over that period.[1]

- Secondary prevention—Low-dose aspirin (81 mg) has been shown to prevent adenomas in patients with previous colon cancer.[7]

FOLLOW-UP

- Staging is based on tumor depth and spread and predicts survival as follows:[1]
  ○ Duke's A (T1N0M0)—Cancer limited to mucosa and submucosa; 90%; 5-year survival.
  ○ Duke's B1 (T2N0M0)—Cancer extends into muscularis; 85%; 5-year survival.
  ○ Duke's B2 (T3N0M0)—Cancer extends into or through serosa; 70% to 80%; 5-year survival.
  ○ Duke's C (TxN1M0)—Cancer involves regional lymph nodes; 35% to 65%; 5-year survival.
  ○ Duke's D (TxNxM1)—Distant metastases (i.e., lung, liver); 5%; 5-year survival.

- In addition to node involvement and metastases, poor outcome is associated with[1]:
  ○ Number of regional lymph nodes involved.
  ○ Tumor penetration or perforation through the bowel wall.
  ○ Histology of poor differentiation.
  ○ Tumor adherence to adjacent organs.
  ○ Venous invasion.
  ○ Elevated preoperative CEA (i.e., >5 ng/mL).
  ○ Aneuploidy.
  ○ Specific chromosomal deletion (e.g., allelic loss on chromosome 18q).

- Surveillance should be conducted as follows: [8]
  ○ Office visits and CEA evaluations should be performed at a minimum of three times per year for the first 2 years of follow-up. SOR **A**
  ○ There is insufficient data to recommend for or against chest x-ray (CXR) as a part of routine colorectal cancer follow-up. SOR **C**
  ○ Posttreatment colonoscopy should be performed at 3-year intervals. SOR **A**
  ○ Periodic anastomotic evaluation is recommended for patients who have undergone resection/anastomosis or local excision of rectal cancer. SOR **B**
  ○ Serum hemoglobin, Hemoccult II (FOBT), and liver function tests (hepatic enzymes tests) should not be routine components of a follow-up program. SOR **A**

- For patients with progressive disease, options for further therapy must be discussed including discontinuing therapy, intrahepatic chemotherapy (if appropriate), and experimental (i.e., phase I) therapy.[2]

PATIENT RESOURCES

- www.nlm.nih.gov/medlineplus/ency/article/ 000262.htm.
- www.cancer.gov/cancertopics/pdq/treatment/colon.

PROVIDER RESOURCES

- http://www.emedicine.com/med/topic413.htm.
- U.S. Preventive Services Task Force. Screening for colorectal cancer: Recommendations and rationale. *Ann Intern Med.* 2002 Jul 16;137(2):129–131.

REFERENCES

1. Mayer R. Gastrointestinal tract cancer. In: Kasper DL, Braunwald E, Fauci AS, Hauser SL, Longo DL, Jameson JL eds. *Harrison's Principles of Internal Medicine.* 16th ed. New York: McGraw-Hill, 2005: 523–533.

2. El-Deiry WS. http://www.emedicine.com/med/topic413.htm. Accessed December 22, 2006.

3. U.S. Preventive Services Task Force. Screening for colorectal cancer: Recommendations and rationale. *Ann Intern Med.* 2002;137(2): 129–131.

4. Schoen RE, Pinsky PF, Weissfeld JL, et al. Results of repeat sigmoidoscopy 3 years after a negative examination. *JAMA.* 2003;290(1): 41–48.

5. Topazian M. Gastrointestinal endoscopy. In: Kasper DL, Braunwald E, Fauci AS, Hauser SL, Longo DL, Jameson JL eds. *Harrison's Principles of Internal Medicine.* 16th ed. New York: McGraw-Hill, 2005: 1730–1739.

6. Davila RE, Rajan E, Adler D, et al. ASGE guideline: The role of endoscopy in the diagnosis, staging, and management of colorectal cancer. *Gastrointest Endosc.* 2005;61(1):1–7.

7. Sandler RS, Halabi S, Baron JA, et al. A randomized trial of aspirin to prevent colorectal adenomas in patients with previous colorectal cancer. *N Engl J Med.* 2003;348(10):883–890.

8. Anthony T, Simmang C, Hyman N, et al. Practice parameters for the surveillance and follow-up of patients with colon and rectal cancer. *Dis Colon Rectum.*2004;47(6):807–817.

62 ULCERATIVE COLITIS

Mindy A. Smith, MD, MS

PATIENT STORY

A 20-year-old man presents with several days of diarrhea with a small amount of rectal bleeding with each bowel movement. This is his second episode of bloody diarrhea; the first seemed to resolve after several days and occurred several weeks ago. He has cramps that occur with each bowel movement, but feels fine between bouts of diarrhea. He has no travel history outside of the United States. He is of Jewish descent and has a cousin with Crohn's disease. Colonoscopy shows mucosal friability with superficial ulceration and exudates confined to the rectosigmoid colon, and he is diagnosed with ulcerative colitis (**Figure 62-1**).

EPIDEMIOLOGY

- Incidence of ulcerative colitis (UC) in the United States is 11/1000,000; higher than the incidence in Europe or Asia.[1]

- Age of onset is bimodal with peaks at 15 to 30 years and 60 to 80 years.[1]

- Predilection for those of Jewish ancestry (especially Ashkenazi Jews) followed in order by non-Jewish Caucasians, African Americans, Hispanic, and Asians.[1]

- Inheritance (polygenic) plays a role with a concordance of 20% in monozygous twins and a risk of 10% in first-degree relatives of an incidence case.[1]

ETIOLOGY AND PATHOPHYSIOLOGY

- Unknown etiology—Current theory is that the colitis is an inappropriate response to microbial gut flora or a lack of regulation of intestinal immune cells with failure of the normal suppression of the immune response and tissue repair.[1]

- Multiple bowel pathogens (e.g., *salmonella, Shigella* species, and *campylobacter*) may trigger UC. This is supported by a large cohort study where the hazard ratio of developing inflammatory bowel disease (IBD) was 2.4 (95% confidence interval [CI], 1.7–3.3) in the group who experienced a bout of infectious gastroenteritis compared with the control group; the excess risk was greatest during the first year after the infective episode.[2]

- Psychological factors (e.g., major life change, daily stressors) are associated with worsening symptoms.

- Patients with long-standing UC are at higher risk of developing colon dysplasia and cancer. For patients with pancolitis, the risk is 0.5% to 1% per year after 8 to 10 years of disease.[1] A cohort study confirmed a higher risk of colon cancer, but only for those patients with UC who had extensive colitis.[3]

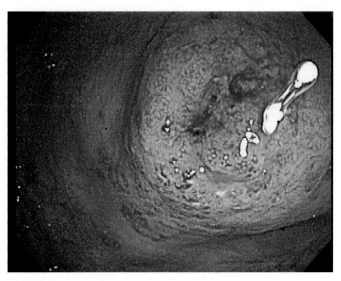

FIGURE 62-1 Ulcerative colitis in the rectosigmoid colon as viewed through the colonoscope. (*Courtesy of Marvin Derezin, MD.*)

DIAGNOSIS

The diagnosis depends on the clinical evaluation; sigmoid appearance; histology; and a negative stool for bacteria, *Clostridium difficile* toxin, and ova and parasites.[1]

CLINICAL FEATURES

- Major symptoms—Diarrhea, rectal bleeding, tenesmus (i.e., urgency with a feeling of incomplete evacuation), passage of mucus, and cramping abdominal pain.

- For patients with active disease, a sigmoidoscopy is performed to evaluate the mucosa.

- The disease is classified by severity based on the clinical picture and results of endoscopy[1]; treatment is based on disease classification.
  - Mild: Less than four bowel movements (BM) per day, small amount of stool blood, no or mild anemia, sedimentation (sed) rate <30 mm, and mucosal erythema with fine granularity and decreased vascular pattern.
  - Moderate: Four to six BM per day, moderate stool blood, low-grade fever, anemia (75%), mucosa with marked erythema, course granularity, absent vascular markings, and contact bleeding, but no ulcers.
  - Severe: More than six BM per day, severe stool blood, fever, tachycardia, variable anemia, sed rate >30 mm, and mucosa with spontaneous bleeding and ulcers.

- Extraintestinal manifestations are more common in Crohn's disease[1]:
  - Dermatologic—Erythema nodosum (10%) that correlates with disease activity and pyogenic gangrenosum (pustule that spreads concentrically and ulcerates surrounded by violaceous borders) in 1% to 12% of patients.
  - Rheumatologic—Peripheral arthritis, ankylosing spondylitis, and symmetric sacroiliitis (<10%).
  - Ocular—Conjunctivitis, uveitis, iritis, and episcleritis (1%–10%).
  - Hepatobiliary—Hepatic steatosis (fatty liver).
  - Cardiovascular—Increased risk of deep venous thrombosis, pulmonary embolus, and stroke (because of a hypercoagulable state from thrombocytosis and gut losses of antithrombin III among other factors); endocarditis; myocarditis; and pleuropericarditis.
  - Bone—Osteoporosis and osteomalacia from vitamin D deficiency and calcium malabsorption.

- Severe complications include toxic colitis (15% initially present with catastrophic illness), massive hemorrhage (1% of those with severe attacks), toxic megacolon (i.e., transverse colon diameter >5–6 cm) (5% of attacks; may be triggered by electrolyte abnormalities and narcotics), and bowel obstruction (caused by strictures and occurring in 10% of patients).[1]

TYPICAL DISTRIBUTION

- With respect to mucosal involvement, half of the patients have disease limited to the rectum or rectosigmoid, 30% to 40% have disease extending beyond the rectum, but not involving the entire colon, 20% of them have total colon involvement (**Figure 62-1**).

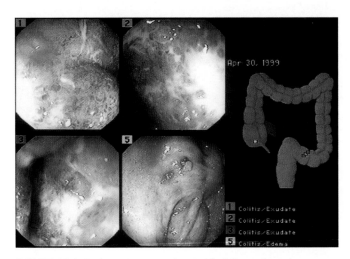

FIGURE 62-2 Endoscopic image showing friability and exudates over superficial ulceration in the sigmoid colon. There is edema in the cecum that, all together, indicates pan colitis. Biopsy confirmed ulcerative colitis. (*Courtesy of Michael Harper, MD.*)

LABORATORY TESTS

- Acute disease can result in a rise of acute phase reactants (e.g., C-reactive protein) and elevated sed rate (rare in patients with just proctitis).

- Obtain hemoglobin (to assess for anemia) and platelets (to assess for reactive thrombocytosis).

- Serologic markers may be available in the future to assist in distinguishing UC from Crohn disease and other diarrheal illnesses.[4]

ENDOSCOPY AND IMAGING

- Colonoscopy with ileoscopy and mucosal biopsy should be performed in the evaluation of IBD and for differentiating UC from Crohn's disease[5] (**Figure 62-1** to **62-5**). SOR **B**

- Colonoscopy can show pseudopolyps in both active UC (**Figure 62-3**) and inactive UC (**Figure 62-4**).

- In patients with severe disease, a plain supine film may show edematous, irregular colon margins, mucosal thickening, and toxic dilation.[1]

- Single contrast barium enema—Fine mucosal granularity in early disease to thickened mucosa with shallow ulcers; edematous Haustral folds with loss of folds in long-standing disease along with colon shortening and narrowing. With deep ulcers, ulceration through the mucosa appears as "collar-button" ulcers.[1]

- Computed tomography (CT) is of limited usefulness but can show mural thickening, absence of small bowel thickening, increased perirectal and presacral fat, and adenopathy.[1]

DIFFERENTIAL DIAGNOSIS

- Crohn's disease—Similar features may be seen but gross blood and mucus in the stool are less frequent and systemic symptoms, extra-colonic features, pain, perineal disease, and obstruction are more common.[1] On endoscopy, rectal sparing is frequent and cobble-stoning of the mucosa is seen. Small bowel involvement is seen on imaging in addition to segmental colitis and frequent strictures (**Figure 62-5**).

- Infections of the colon—*Salmonella, Shigella* species, and *Campylobacter* have a similar appearance with bloody diarrhea and abdominal pain but disease is usually self-limited and stool culture can confirm the presence of these bacteria. *C. difficile* and *Escherichia coli* can also mimic inflammatory bowel disease.

- Numerous infectious agents including mycobacterium, cytomegalovirus and protozoan parasites can mimic UC in immunocompromised patients.

- Ischemic colitis—May present with sudden onset of left lower quadrant pain, urgency to defecate, and bright red blood per rectum. It can be chronic and diffuse and should be considered in elderly patients following abdominal aorta repair or when a patient has a hypercoagulable state. Endoscopic examination often demonstrates normal rectal mucosa with a sharp transition to an area of inflammation in the descending colon or splenic flexure (**Figure 62-6**).

- Colitis associated with nonsteroidal anti-inflammatory drugs (NSAIDs)—Clinical features of diarrhea and pain, but may be

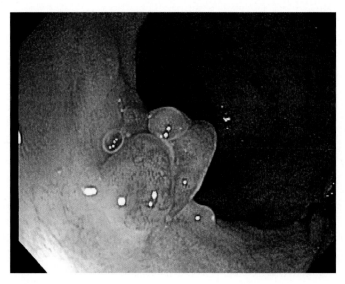

FIGURE 62-3 Pseudopolyps in active UC viewed through colonoscope. (*Courtesy of Marvin Derezin, MD.*)

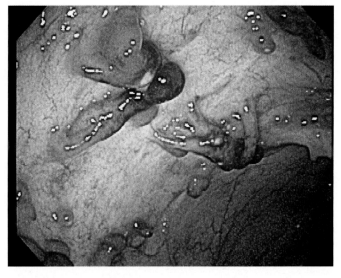

FIGURE 62-4 Pseudopolyps in inactive UC viewed through colonoscope. (*Courtesy of Marvin Derezin, MD.*)

complicated by bleeding, stricture, obstruction, and perforation. History is helpful and symptoms improve with withdrawal of the agent.

MANAGEMENT

Treatment of acute disease is based on disease activity as follows:

- Mild disease—Oral 5-aminosalicylic acid (ASA) agent (e.g., sulfasalazine (4–8 g/d), Asacol (2.4–4.8 g/d), and Pentasa (2–4 g/d); topical enemas of mesalamine are also effective. SOR Ⓐ Fifty to seventy-five percent of patients will show clinical improvement with 2 g/d of 5-ASA and a similar percentage will maintain remission will doses of 1.5 to 4 g/d.[1]

- Moderate disease—5-ASA (oral or enema), plus glucocorticoid enema or oral form (40–60 mg/d or 1 mg/kg/d of prednisone or equivalent).[6] SOR Ⓐ Following a positive response (average 7–14 days), steroids may be tapered by 5 mg/week of prednisone to a dose of 20 mg and then 2.5 to 5 mg/week below 20 mg.[6] SOR Ⓑ

- Severe—Same as for moderate disease but glucocorticoids may be delivered intravenously (IV) (methylprednisolone 40–60 mg/d or hydrocortisone 200–300 mg/d) following hospitalization.[6] SOR Ⓐ

- Fulminant—IV glucocorticoid plus IV cyclosporine (2–4 mg/kg/d). Intravenous cyclosporine is effective as a means of avoiding surgery in patients with severe corticosteroid-refractory UC.[6] SOR Ⓐ

- Immunomodulators (e.g., azathioprine, 6-mercaptopurine) should be considered for patients with chronic active corticosteroid-dependent disease (AZA 2.0–3.0 mg/kg/d or 6-MP 1.0–1.5 mg/kg/d) in an effort to lower or preferably eliminate corticosteroid use. Infliximab is another option in this situation, as is combination infliximab/antimetabolite therapy.[6] SOR Ⓐ

- Biological therapy (e.g., antitumor necrosis factor antibodies) is being used increasingly in patients with IBD, but side effects include serious infections, induction of autoimmune phenomena, and neurotoxicity.[7]

- For patients with refractory UC, oral tacrolimus may be an option.[8] SOR Ⓒ

Surgery (total proctocolectomy with ileostomy or continence-preserving operation (i.e., IPAA) is performed in approximately half of patients with UC within 10 years of disease onset. Indications for surgery include the following:[1]

- Intractable or fulminant disease
- Toxic megacolon
- Massive hemorrhage
- Colonic obstruction
- Colon cancer, dysplasia, or for cancer prophylaxis

PATIENT EDUCATION

- Patients should be informed about the unpredictable course of this disease and the need for frequent contact with an experienced provider for medical management, support, and surveillance.

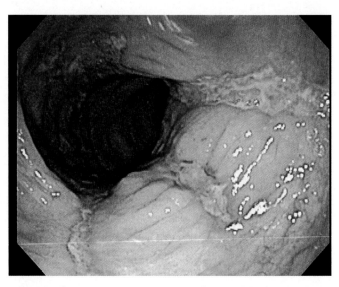

FIGURE 62-5 Crohn's colitis with deep longitudinal ulcers and normal appearing tissue in between. The biopsies that showed normal tissue between the ulcers clinched the diagnosis for Crohn's disease. Ulcerative colitis is diffuse whereas Crohn's disease often skips areas as seen in this patients colon. (*Courtesy of Marvin Derezin, MD.*)

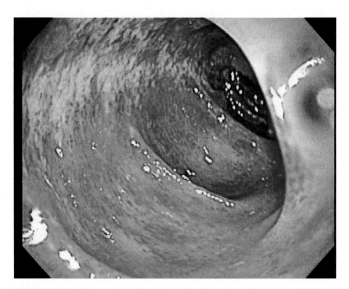

FIGURE 62-6 Ischemic colitis in an elderly patient. (*Courtesy of Marvin Derezin, MD.*)

- Should surgery be necessary, options should be reviewed and women with UC should be informed that IPAA increases the risk of infertility by approximately threefold.[9]

FOLLOW-UP

- Support and patient education should be provided to address medication side effects, the uncertain nature of the disease, and potential complications.
- Periodic bone mineral density assessment is recommended for patients on long-term corticosteroid therapy (>3 months).[6] SOR **A**
- Annual ophthalmologic examinations are recommended for patients on long-term corticosteroid therapy.[6] SOR **C**
- Patients with longstanding UC are at higher risk of developing colon dysplasia and cancer. For patients with pancolitis, the risk is 0.5% to 1% per year after 8 to 10 years of disease.[1] Options include prophylactic surgery or annual or biennial colonoscopy with biopsy for surveillance. There is no clear evidence, however, that surveillance colonoscopy prolongs survival in patients with extensive colitis. There is evidence that cancers tend to be detected at an earlier stage in patients who are undergoing surveillance.[10]

PATIENT RESOURCES

- **digestive.niddk.nih.gov/ddiseases/pubs/colitis/.**
- **www.ccfa.org** (Crohn's and Colitis Foundation of America).

PROVIDER RESOURCES

Lichtenstein GR, Abreu MT, Cohen R, Tremaine W. American Gastroenterological Association Institute medical position statement on corticosteroids, immunomodulators, and infliximab in inflammatory bowel disease. *Gastroenterology.* 2006;130(3):935–939.

REFERENCES

1. Friedman S, Blumberg RS. Inflammatory bowel disease. In: Kasper DL, Braunwald E, Fauci AS, Hauser SL, Longo DL, Jameson JL eds. *Harrison's Principles of Internal Medicine.* 16th ed. New York: McGraw-Hill, 2005:1776–1789.

2. Garcia Rodriguez LA, Ruigomez A, Panes J. Acute gastroenteritis is followed by an increased risk of inflammatory bowel disease. *Gastroenterology.* 2006;130(6):1588–1594.

3. Jess T, Loftus EV, Jr., Velayos FS, et al. Risk of intestinal cancer in inflammatory bowel disease: A population-based study from olmsted county, Minnesota. *Gastroenterology.* 2006;130(4): 1039–1046.

4. Buckland MS, Mylonaki M, Rampton D, Longhurst HJ. Serological markers (anti-Saccharomyces cerevisiae mannan antibodies and antineutrophil cytoplasmic antibodies) in inflammatory bowel disease: Diagnostic utility and phenotypic correlation. *Clin Diagn Lab Immunol.* 2005;12(11):1328–1330.

5. Leighton JA, Shen B, Baron TH, et al. Standards of practice committee, American society for gastrointestinal endoscopy. ASGE guideline: Endoscopy in the diagnosis and treatment of inflammatory bowel disease. *Gastrointest Endosc.* 2006;63(4):558–565.

6. Lichtenstein GR, Abreu MT, Cohen R, Tremaine W. American gastroenterological association institute medical position statement on corticosteroids, immunomodulators, and infliximab in inflammatory bowel disease. *Gastroenterology.* 2006;130(3): 935–939.

7. Van Assche G, Vermeire S, Rutgeerts P. Safety issues with biological therapies for inflammatory bowel disease. *Curr Opin Gastroenterol.* 2006;22(4):370–376.

8. Ogata H, Matsui T, Nakamura M, et al. A randomised dose finding study of oral tacrolimus (FK506) therapy in refractory ulcerative colitis. *Gut.* 2006;55(9):1255–1262.

9. Waljee A, Waljee J, Morris A, Higgins PD. Three-fold increased risk of infertility: A meta-analysis of infertility after pouch surgery in ulcerative colitis. *Gut.* 2006;55(11):1575–1580.

10. Collins PD, Mpofu C, Watson AJ, Rhodes JM. Strategies for detecting colon cancer and/or dysplasia in patients with inflammatory bowel disease. *Cochrane Database Syst Rev.* 2006;(2): CD000279.

63 HEMORRHOIDS

Mindy A. Smith, MD, MS

PATIENT STORY

A 42-year-old woman complains of rectal pressure and occasional bright red blood on the toilet paper when wiping after bowel movements. She has had difficulty with constipation off and on for many years and had bad hemorrhoids during her last pregnancy. Physical examination confirms the diagnonis of external hemorrhoids (**Figure 63-1**).

EPIDEMIOLOGY

- More than 1 million people in western civilization suffer from hemorrhoids each year.[1]
- Estimated at 4.4% prevalence in the general population.[2]
- Increases with age; peaks at 45 to 65 years of age.[2]
- More frequent in whites, especially in those from higher socioeconomic status and from rural areas.[2]

ETIOLOGY AND PATHOPHYSIOLOGY

- Hemorrhoidal cushions (subepithelial connective tissues and smooth muscle) surround and support distal anastomoses between the superior rectal arteries and the superior, middle, and inferior rectal veins.[2] The hemorrhoidal cushions form three hemorrhoidal complexes that cross the anal canal and aid in fecal continence by contributing to resting anal pressure and preventing anal sphincter muscle damage.
- Hemorrhoidal tissue provides important sensory information, enabling the differentiation between solid, liquid, and gas.[2]
- Abnormal swelling of the anal cushions, often from straining during bowel movements, causes dilatation and engorgement of the arteriovenous plexuses, which can lead to stretching of the suspensory muscles and eventual prolapse of rectal tissue through the anal canal.[2] The engorged anal mucosa is easily traumatized, leading to rectal bleeding. Prolapse predisposes to incarceration and strangulation.
- Hemorrhoids are classified with respect to their position relative to the dentate line.
  - Internal hemorrhoids develop above the dentate line and are covered by columnar epithelium of anal mucosa. Internal hemorrhoids lack somatic sensory innervation (**Figure 63-2**).
  - External hemorrhoids arise distal to the dentate line. They are covered by stratified squamous epithelium and receive somatic sensory innervation from the inferior rectal nerve (**Figure 63-1**).
- Hemorrhoids are further classified in four stages of disease severity[1,2]:
  - Stage I—Enlargement and bleeding.
  - Stage II—Protrusion of hemorrhoids with spontaneous reduction.

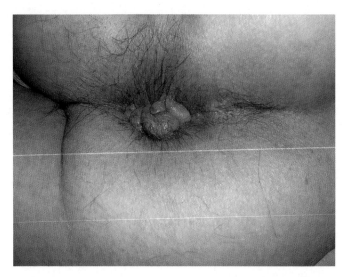

FIGURE 63-1 External hemorrhoid that is symptomatic. The patient had some bleeding with bowel movements. (*Courtesy of Richard P. Usatine, MD.*)

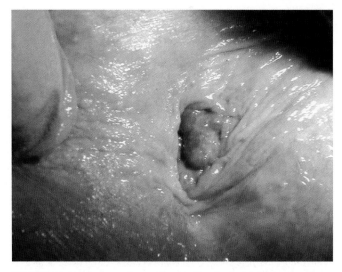

FIGURE 63-2 A large prolapsed internal hemorrhoid. (*Courtesy of Charlie Goldberg, MD and the Regents of the University of California.*)

○ Stage III—Protrusion of hemorrhoids with manual reduction possible.

○ Stage IV—Irreducible protrusion of hemorrhoids usually containing both internal and external components with or without acute thrombosis or strangulation (**Figure 63-1**).

• Risk factors include family history, personal history of constipation or diarrhea, pregnancy, and history of prolonged sitting or heavy lifting.[2]

DIAGNOSIS

CLINICAL FEATURES

• Bleeding described as bright red blood (because of the high blood oxygen content within the arteriovenous anastomoses) seen in the toilet or with wiping after bowel movements.

• Protrusion/mass (**Figure 63-1**).

• Pain described as a dull ache or severe, if thrombosed.

• Inability to maintain personal hygiene/staining/soiling secondary to prolapse.

• Pruritus, also secondary to prolapse.

Diagnosis is made on visual inspection and anoscopy, with and without straining:

○ Physical findings of swollen blood vessels protruding from the anus suggest external hemorrhoids. These are generally soft and compressible unless they become thrombosed.

○ A thrombosed hemorrhoid will be tender and firm, and appear as a circular purplish bulge adjacent to the anal opening. There may be a black discoloration, if there is accompanying necrosis.

○ Internal hemorrhoids may be visualized on anoscopy as swollen purple blood vessels arising above the dentate line. Internal hemorrhoids may prolapse and then become visible on anal inspection (**Figure 63-2**).

○ Excoriations may also be seen on the skin surrounding the anus.

• Other physical findings that may accompany hemorrhoids are redundant tissue and skin tags from old thrombosed external hemorrhoids.

DIFFERENTIAL DIAGNOSIS

• Rectal prolapse—Full-thickness circumferential protrusion appearing as a bluish, tender perianal mass. More common in women (sixfold higher incidence) and associated with other pelvic floor disorders (e.g., cystocele, urinary incontinence). It can present as an anal mass with bleeding.[1]

• Condyloma acuminata—Appears as flesh-colored, exophytic lesions on perianal skin. They may be flat, verrucous, or pedunculated (see Chapter 127, Genital Warts).

• Signs of infection or abscess formation—Tender mass, sometimes feeling fluctuant, with overlying skin erythema (**Figure 63-3**). If cellulitis is also present, then skin may have a woody hard feel. Fistulas may also form and an opening may be seen on the buttock.

• Fissures—A cut or tear occurring in the anus that extends upwards into the anal canal. Common and occurring at all ages; fissures cause pain during bowel movements in addition to bleeding (**Figure 63-4**).

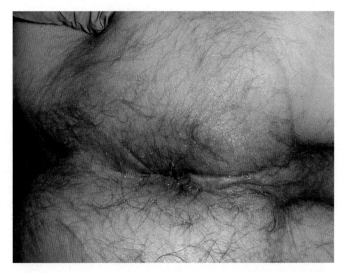

FIGURE 63-3 Perirectal abscess: Note surrounding erythema that extends onto the right buttock. (*Courtesy of Charlie Goldberg, MD, copyrighted by the University of California, San Diego.*)

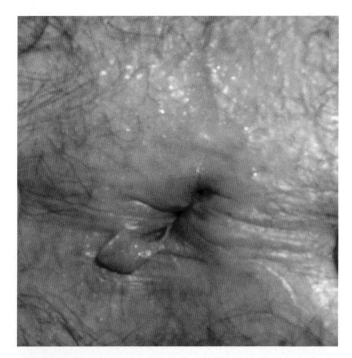

FIGURE 63-4 Rectal fissure with prominent skin tag. (*Courtesy of Charlie Goldberg, MD, copyrighted by the University of California, San Diego.*)

MANAGEMENT

- All patients with hemorrhoids should increase dietary fiber and/or add a fiber supplement to reduce severity and duration of symptoms. SOR Ⓐ

- Short course of a topical steroid cream or suppositories, twice daily.

- Stool softener and encourage adequate fluid intake if constipation is a factor.

- Stage I hemorrhoids can also be treated with sclerotherapy (1–2 mL of sclerosing agent such as sodium tetradechol sulfate injected via a 25-guage needle into the submucosa of the hemorrhoidal complex).[1] Sclerotherapy, however, has a higher rate of postprocedure pain; impotence, urinary retention, and abscess formation have also been reported.[2] Recurrence rates are as high as 30%.[2]

- Stage II and III hemorrhoids, above the dentate line, can be treated with banding (i.e., rubber band ligation). Two bands are placed around the engorged tissue producing ischemia and fibrosis of the hemorrhoid.

- Lower stage hemorrhoids can also be treated with infrared coagulation, bipolar electrocautery, laser therapy, or low-voltage direct current (the latter works for higher grade hemorrhoids).

- Stage IV hemorrhoids can be treated with surgery using stapling or traditional excision. In a recent small randomized clinical trial comparing the two, investigators found less postoperative pain, earlier discharge, and less time off work with similar complications for stapled hemorrhoidectomy.[3]

- Complications of surgery include infection, bleeding, fecal incontinence (if sphincter muscle damage), anal stenosis, and rectal prolapse. Indications for surgery include the following:[2]
  - Failure of nonsurgical treatment (persistent bleeding or chronic symptoms).
  - Grade III and IV hemorrhoids with severe symptoms.
  - Presence of other anorectal conditions (e.g., anal fissure or fistula) requiring surgery.
  - Patient preference.

- In a Cochrane review comparing excisional hemorrhoidectomy with banding for grade III hemorrhoids, only three methodologically poor trials were identified.[4] Results with surgery were better resolution of symptoms but increased postprocedural pain, higher complications, and more time off work.

- Acutely thrombosed external hemorrhoids may be safely excised in the office or emergency department for patients who present within 48 to 72 hours of symptom onset. A local anesthetic containing epinephrine is used followed by elliptical incision (not extending beyond the anal verge or deeper than the cutaneous layer) and excision of the thrombosed hemorrhoid and overlying skin.[2] Simple incision and clot evacuation is inadequate therapy for complete resolution,[2] although it may relieve pain. A pressure dressing is applied for several hours after which the wound is left to heal by secondary intention.

PATIENT EDUCATION

- Most hemorrhoids resolve spontaneously or with medical therapy alone. However, the recurrence rate with nonsurgical therapy is

10% to 50% (over a 5-year period) and, for surgical treatment, recurrence is approximately 26%.[2]

- Patients should be counseled to avoid aggravating factors including constipation and prolonged sitting.

- Advise patients who elect rubber band ligation, that complications, based on one follow-up study, include pain (at 1 week, 75% of patients were pain-free and 7% were still experiencing moderate-to-severe pain), rectal bleeding (in 65% on the day after banding, persisting in 24% at 1 week), and relatively low satisfaction (only 59% were satisfied with their experience and would undergo the procedure again).[5]

- Advice patients who elect or are recommended for surgery about potential complications of infection, thrombosis, ulceration, and incontinence.

FOLLOW-UP

- Necrotizing pelvic sepsis is a rare, but serious complication of rubber band ligation. The diagnosis should be suspected by the triad of severe pain, fever, and urinary retention.[2] It occurs 1 to 2 weeks after ligation, frequently in immune compromised patients, and requires prompt surgical debridement.[2]

- After excision of a thrombosed hemorrhoid, patient instructions should include initial bed rest for several hours, sitz baths three times daily, stool softeners, and topical or systemic analgesia.[2] The patient should return in 48 to 72 hours for a wound check.[2]

PATIENT RESOURCES

http://digestive.niddk.nih.gov/ddiseases/pubs/hemorrhoids/index.htm.

PROVIDER RESOURCES

http://www.nlm.nih.gov/medlineplus/hemorrhoids.html.

REFERENCES

1. Hemorrhoidal Disease. In: Kasper DL, Braunwald E, Fauci AS, Hauser SL, Longo DL, Jameson JL eds. *Harrison's Principles of Internal Medicine*. 16th ed. New York,: McGraw-Hill, 2005:1801–1802.

2. Gurley DR, Sinert R, Pilar Guerrero, MD. http://www.emedicine.com/emerg/topic242.htm. Accessed October 10, 2006.

3. Bikhchandani J, Agarwal PN, Kant R, Malik VK. Randomized controlled trial to compare the early and mid-term results of stapled versus open hemorrhoidectomy. *Am J Surg*. 2005;189(1):56–60.

4. Shanmugam V, Thaha MA, Rabindranath KS, et al. Rubber band ligation versus excisional haemorrhoidectomy for haemorrhoids. *Cochrane Database Syst Rev*. 2005;3:CD005034.

5. Watson NF, Liptrott S, Maxwell-Armstrong CA. A prospective audit of early pain and patient satisfaction following out-patient band ligation of haemorrhoids. *Ann R Coll Surg Engl*. 2006;88(3):275–279.

PART 10

THE URINARY TRACT

64 URINARY SEDIMENT—HEMATURIA, PYURIA, AND CASTS

Mindy A. Smith, MD, MS
Richard P. Usatine, MD

PATIENT STORY

A 47-year-old woman presents to the office with severe right flank pain that does not radiate. Dipstick urinalysis shows hematuria and microscopic examination confirms the presence of many red blood cells per high power field (**Figure 64-1**). There is no pyuria or bacteriuria. The physician gives her some pain medication and sends her to get a CT urogram. The CT urogram shows a stone in the right ureter and some mild hydronephrosis. Fortunately for the patient, she passes the stone when urinating after the imaging study is complete.

EPIDEMIOLOGY

- A finding of hematuria (2–5 RBC/HPF) on a single urinalysis in an asymptomatic person is common and most often due to menses, allergy, exercise, viral illness, or mild trauma.[1]

- One study of servicemen, conducted for a period of 10 years, found an incidence of 38%.[1]

- Persistent (>3 RBC/HPF over three specimens) and significant hematuria (>100 RBC/HPF or gross hematuria) was associated with significant lesions in 9.1% of more than 1000 patients.[1]

- Isolated pyuria (>2–10 white blood cells per high power field (WBC/HPF) is uncommon, since inflammatory processes in the urinary tract are usually associated with hematuria.[1]

ETIOLOGY AND PATHOPHYSIOLOGY

- Hematuria (**Figure 64-1**) has many causes including[1]:
  - Idiopathic (increasing incidence in the young).
  - Stones.
  - Neoplasms (increasing incidence with increase in age).
  - Trauma.
  - Infection/inflammation including acute cystitis, urethritis, pyelonephritis, and prostatitis.
  - Metabolic abnormalities including hypercalcemia and hyperuricemia.
  - Glomerular diseases such as IGA nephropathy, hereditary nephritis, and thin basement membrane disease.

- Hematuria with dysmorphic RBC or RBC casts (**Figure 64-2**) and excess protein excretion (>500 mg/dL) indicates glomerulonephritis.

- Gross hematuria suggests a postrenal source in the collecting system.

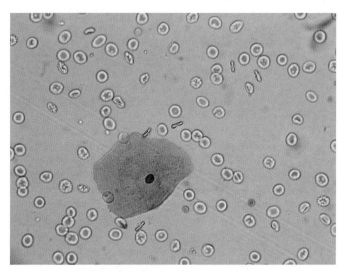

FIGURE 64-1 Red blood cells seen in the urine of a woman passing a kidney stone. Some of the RBCs are crenated and there is one epithelial cell visible. (*Courtesy of Richard P. Usatine, MD.*)

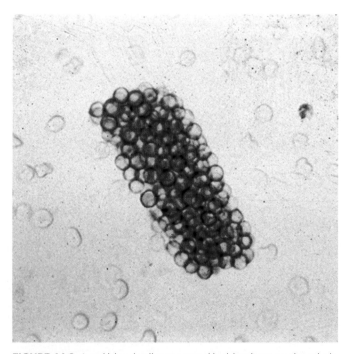

FIGURE 64-2 A red blood cell cast caused by bleeding into the tubule from the glomerulus. These casts are seen in glomerulonephritis, IgA nephropathy, lupus nephritis, Goodpasture's syndrome, and Wegener's granulomatosis. RBC casts are always pathologic. (*Courtesy of ABF/Vanderbilt Collection.*)

- Pyuria (**Figure 64-3**) is often the result of urinary tract infection.
  - The presence of bacteria ($>10^2$ organisms per mL or $>10^5$ using a midstream urine specimen) suggests infection.
  - The presence of WBC casts (**Figure 64-4**) with bacteria indicates pyelonephritis.
- WBCs and/or WBC casts can be seen in tubulointerstitial processes like interstitial nephritis, systemic lupus erythematosus, or transplant rejection.
- Urinary casts are formed only in the distal convoluted tubule (DCT) or in the collecting duct (distal nephron).
- Hyaline casts are formed from mucoprotein secreted by the tubular epithelial cells within the nephrons. These translucent casts are the most common type of cast and can be seen in normal persons after vigorous exercise or with dehydration. Low urine flow and concentrated urine from dehydration can contribute to the formation of hyaline casts (**Figure 64-5**).
- Granular casts are the second most common type of cast seen (**Figure 64-6**). These casts can result from the breakdown of cellular casts or the inclusion of aggregates of albumin or immunoglobulin light chains. They can be classified as fine or coarse based on the size of the inclusions. There is no diagnostic significance to the classification of fine or coarse.

DIAGNOSIS

CLINICAL FEATURES

- Other signs and symptoms of glomerular disease include various degrees of renal failure, edema, oliguria, and hypertension.
- Hematuria is often asymptomatic in patients with glomerular disease or metabolic abnormalities. Renal stones can cause pain in the ipsilateral flank and/or abdomen with radiation to the ipsilateral groin, testicle or vulva or irritative symptoms of frequency, urgency and dysuria, if located in the bladder.
- Symptoms of urinary tract infection include dysuria, nocturia, urgency, offensive odor of urine, or a combination of these; positive likelihood ratios, however, are low (1–2).[2]
- Symptoms of pyelonephritis include chills and rigor, fever, nausea and vomiting, and flank pain; positive likelihood ratios are 1.5 to 2.5.
- Family history of renal failure or microscopic hematuria or history of trauma, weight loss, and changes in urine volume may be useful.

LABORATORY AND IMAGING

The work-up for persistent or significant hematuria includes the following:[1]

- Urinary sediment looking for dysmorphic cells or RBC casts (**Figure 64-2**) and a 24-hour urine sample for proteinuria.
  - If positive, suspect glomerular disease and consider blood cultures, anti-glomerular basement membrane (GBM) antibody, antineutrophil cytoplasmic (ANCA) antibody, complement, cryoglobulins, hepatitis serologies, venereal disease research laboratory (VDRL), HIV and antistreptolysin O; a renal biopsy may be indicated.

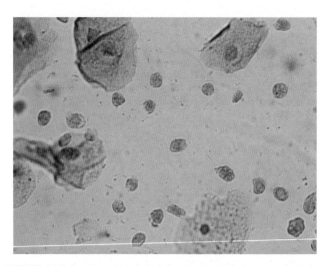

FIGURE 64-3 Pyuria and bacteriuria in a woman with a urinary tract infection. A simple stain was added to the wet mount of spun urine. Although there are epithelial cells present, the culture demonstrated a true UTI and not merely a contaminated urine. (*Courtesy of Richard P. Usatine, MD.*)

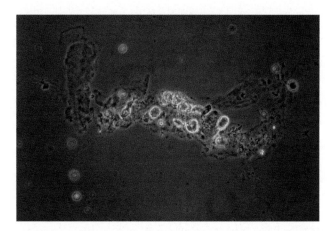

FIGURE 64-4 White blood cell casts seen in pyelonephritis. These can be differentiated from a clump of WBCs by their cylindrical shape and the presence of a hyaline matrix. (*Courtesy of ABF/Vanderbilt Collection.*)

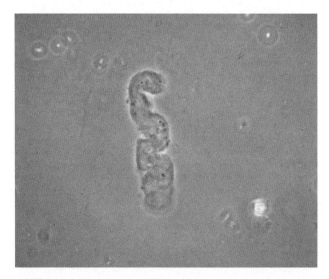

FIGURE 64-5 Hyaline casts are translucent and proteinaceous. These are the most common casts found in the urine and can be seen in normal individuals. Concentrated urine with low flow usually caused by dehydration, exercise, and/or diuretics can lead to hyaline cast formation. (*Courtesy of ABF/Vanderbilt Collection.*)

- If negative and the sediment contains WBCs (**Figure 64-3**) or WBC casts (**Figure 64-4**), suspect infection and obtain a urine culture; *E. coli* is the most common organism (80%) in uncomplicated cystitis. WBCs seen in conjunction with many epithelial cells, particularly in women, can indicate a contaminated specimen and a repeat of specimen should be considered.

- If negative and no WBCs, obtain a hemoglobin electrophoresis, urine cytology, UA from family members looking for hematuria or signs of glomerular disease, and a 24-hour urine for calcium and uric acid.

- If the above is negative, obtain an intravenous pyelography (IVP) and/or renal ultrasound.

- If the above is negative, perform cystoscopy.

- If the above is negative, perform a renal CT scan; if positive, an open renal biopsy may be indicated.

- If the above is negative, consider periodic follow-up.

- If RBC casts (**Figure 64-2**) are seen on urinalysis in addition to proteinuria, also consider nephrotic syndrome caused by diabetes or amyloidosis.

- Note that RBC casts are fragile and are best seen in a fresh urine specimen (**Figure 64-2**).

MANAGEMENT

Treatment will depend on the underlying etiology:

- Cystitis is treated with appropriate antibiotics based on knowledge of the sensitivities of *E. coli* in your practice location (e.g., nitrofurantoin is usually a good choice).

- Uncomplicated pyelonephritis is treated with appropriate antibiotics as an outpatient (e.g., an oral quinolone for 7–14 days or intravenous single dose ceftriaxone (1 g) or gentamicin (3–5 mg/kg) followed by an oral quinolone for 7–14 days). The urine should always be cultured in pyelonephritis to help guide therapy. Pregnant women may need hospitalization.

- See Chapter 65 for management of patients with kidney stones.

PROVIDER RESOURCES

http://library.med.utah.edu/WebPath/TUTORIAL/URINE/URINE.html.

REFERENCES

1. Denker BM, Brenner BM. Azotemia and urinary abnormalities. In: Kasper DL, Braunwald E, Fauci AS, Hauser SL, Longo DL, Jameson JL eds. *Harrison's Principles of Internal Medicine*. 16th ed. New York,: McGraw-Hill, 2005:250–251.

2. Bergus GR. Dysuria. In: Sloane PD, Slatt LM, Ebell MH, Jaques LB eds. *Essentials of Family Medicine*. 4th ed. Lippencott Williams & Wilkins, 2002:495–510.

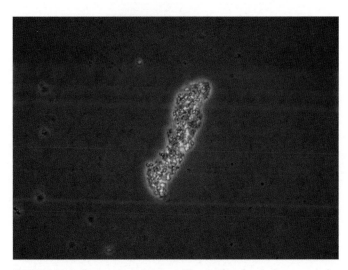

FIGURE 64-6 Coarse granular cast. All granular casts indicate underlying renal disease. These are nonspecific and may be seen in diverse renal conditions. (*Courtesy of ABF/Vanderbilt Collection.*)

65 KIDNEY STONES

Mindy A. Smith, MD, MS

PATIENT STORY

A 47-year-old man is seen in the emergency department with severe pain in the right flank. The pain began suddenly after supper and increased dramatically over the next hour. He is given pain medication and a plain film revealed a stone in the right midureter (**Figure 65-1A** and **B**). A retrograde pyelogram was performed to better define the anatomy of the urinary collecting system (**Figure 65-1C**). This is his first episode of kidney stone but he reports that his father and brother had stones in the past.

EPIDEMIOLOGY

- Prevalence: 2% to 3% in the general population with a lifetime risk for men of 12%.

- African Americans have a lower rate of kidney stones than whites; this may be due to differences in renal handling of dietary calcium and oxalate.[1]

There are four major types of kidney stones[2]:

- Calcium containing stones (calcium oxalate and calcium phosphate) are most common (75%–85%) with an average onset in the third or fourth decade; more common in men (ratio 2:1).

- Struvite stones occur in 10% to 15% of cases as a result of infection. They are more common in women (ratio 5:1) and in patients with chronic indwelling catheters. These stones can grow large, filling the renal pelvis, and extending into the calyces (staghorn calculi, **Figure 65-2**).

- Uric acid stones occur in 5% to 8% of patients. Among those with gout (50%), there is a male predilection (3 to 4:1), but the ratio is 1:1 for patients with idiopathic hyperuricemia.

- Cystine stones are rare and there is no difference in rates by gender.

ETIOLOGY AND PATHOPHYSIOLOGY

Most stones form when there is supersaturation of insoluble materials usually from increased excretion of these compounds or extreme dehydration. Urine pH is also a factor—Alkaline urine contains more phosphate while uric acid predominates in acidic urine (pH <5.5).
  Risk factors vary, with type of stone as follows:

- Calcium stones may be increased by supplemental calcium and animal protein; elevated body mass index and weight gain;[3] and medications including triamterene, indinavir, and acetazolamide.

- Struvite stones are most often caused by urease-producing bacteria like Proteus.

- Uric acid stones are associated with gout and other conditions that cause hyperuricemia and subsequent hyperuricosuria from myeloproliferative disorders or chemotherapy.

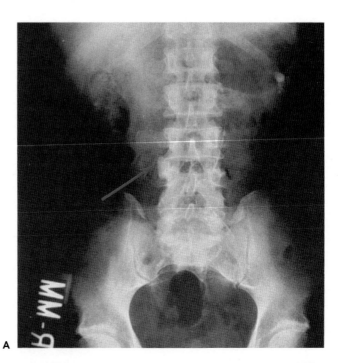

A

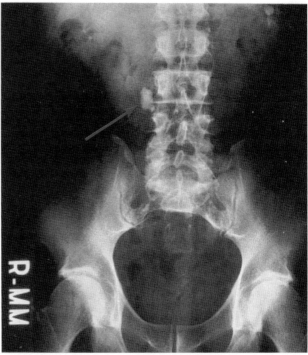

B

FIGURE 65-1 Plate A is a plain x-ray showing a large, right ureteral stone (red arrow) somewhat obscured by the spinal column. Plate B is a slightly oblique view of the same patient that reveals the large stone (red arrow) in the right midureter. (*continued*)

- Cystine stones are primarily due to an autosomal recessive disorder of cystine transport.

DIAGNOSIS

CLINICAL FEATURES

- Stone passage causes pain and bleeding (hematuria). The pain generally begins suddenly in the ipsilateral flank and/or abdomen in waves (renal colic), gradually increasing in intensity in the next 20 to 60 minutes. As the stone moves downward, pain occurs in the ipsilateral groin, testicle, or vulva.
- Stones within the bladder cause frequency, urgency, and dysuria.

LABORATORY

- Urinalysis usually reveals microscopic hematuria and limited pyuria.
- Laboratory work-up is recommended for adults with recurrent stones and for children with a first stone.[2] SOR **C**
- Two 24-hour urine collections (weekday and weekend due to the importance of diet) for pH, volume, oxalate, and citrate.
- Simultaneous serum tests for calcium, uric acid, electrolytes, and creatinine.
- In patients with elevated serum calcium, parathyroid hormone (PTH) should be measured.

IMAGING

- Plain film will demonstrate calcium, struvite, and cystine stones and is recommended for patients with a prior radiopaque stone (**Figures 65-1** to **65-3**).
- Unenhanced helical CT (**Figure 65-4**) has largely replaced intravenous urography because it can detect uric acid stones, involves no radiocontrast agent, and may provide clues on diagnoses outside the urinary system.
- Ultrasound is recommended for pregnant women, women with suspected gynecologic processes, and for patients with suspected cholelithiasis.

DIFFERENTIAL DIAGNOSIS

Other causes of flank and lower pelvic/groin pain:

- Gynecologic conditions in women (ovarian torsion, cyst, or ectopic pregnancy)—These can often be distinguished on ultrasound.
- In men, epididymitis, prostatitis, or testicular tumor may be confused with kidney stones. Physical examination can help differentiate these conditions.
- Cholelithiasis—Biliary colic is usually described as a steady, severe pain or ache, usually of sudden onset, located in the epigastrium or RUQ (see Chapter 59). RUQ tenderness may be elicited on physical examination and ultrasound usually shows stones in the gallbladder.
- Urologic disorders including ureteropelvic junction obstruction, renal subcapsular hematoma, and renal cell carcinoma. Imaging assists in differentiating these from kidney stones.

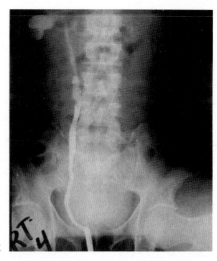

FIGURE 65-1 (*Continued*) Plate C is a retrograde pyelogram performed to better define the anatomy of the urinary collecting system in this patient. Note that we are only viewing the right-sided collecting system and the stone has already passed. (*From Brunicardi CF, Andersen K, BIlliar TR, Hunter JG, Pollock RE. Schwartz's Principles of Surgery; 8/e, Figure 39-28, p. 1547. Copyright 2005, McGraw-Hill.*)

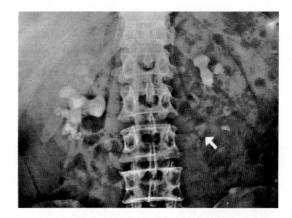

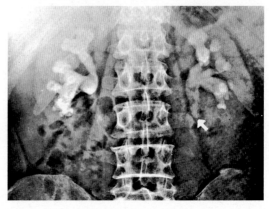

FIGURE 65-2 Bilateral staghorn calculi and left upper ureteral stone (arrow). (*From Doherty GM. Current Surgical Diagnosis and Treatment; Figure 40-17, p. 1023. Copyright 2006, McGraw-Hill.*)

Abdominal pain from renal stones may be confused with:

- Colitis, appendicitis, and diverticulitis—Systemic symptoms such as fever are often seen. Symptoms of colitis include diarrhea, rectal bleeding, tenesmus (i.e., urgency with a feeling of incomplete evacuation), passage of mucus, and cramping abdominal pain (see Chapter 62). Gastrointestinal symptoms with kidney stones are limited to nausea and vomiting from stimulation of the celiac plexus.

- Aortic aneurysm—Peak incidence is later, usually in the sixth and seventh decades. Pain is described as severe and tearing localized to the front or back of the chest and associated with diaphoresis. Syncope and weakness may also occur.

Stones within the bladder mimic urinary tract infection (UTI). Helpful indictors of UTI are a urine dipstick positive for nitrates (LR+ 26.5) and urinary sediment showing 10 or more bacteria/ high power field (LR+ 85).

MANAGEMENT

Acute management of kidney stones depends on the size and type of stone.[4]

- Urgent urologic consultation is recommended for patients with urosepsis, anuria, or renal failure.[5] SOR ⓒ Urologic consultation is also recommended for patients with refractory pain and nausea, extremes of age, major comorbidities, and stones >5 mm. SOR ⓒ

- Effective pain control should be provided using a combination of narcotics and nonsteroidal anti-inflammatory drugs (NSAIDs). NSAIDs should be avoided if planning lithotripsy because of increased risk of perinephric bleeding.

- Stones <0.5 cm are likely to pass spontaneously. The probability of passage is greater with stones in the distal (approximately three-fourth of the stones will pass) vs proximal (approximately half of them) ureter.

Indications for operative intervention:

- Infection.

- Persistent symptoms of flank pain, nausea, and vomiting.

- Failure to pass a ureteral stone after an appropriate trial of observation (2–4 weeks).

Alternative treatment: Several types of juice may be protective against renal stones including black current (increases urinary pH) and cranberry juice (decreases urinary pH), but data are conflicting about their effects on other urine components and there are no data available from clinical trials.

PATIENT EDUCATION

- Half of the patients with a first calcium-containing stone have a recurrence within 10 years. Twenty-five percent of patients with struvite stones recur if there was incomplete removal of the stone.

- Long-term complications are uncommon. The proportion of nephrolithiasis-related ESRD appears small (3.2%).[5]

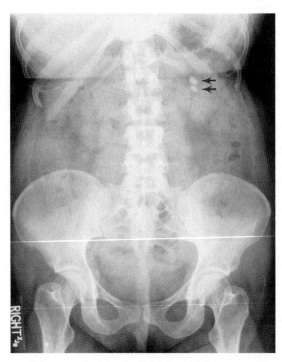

FIGURE 65-3 X-ray shows two dense 1-cm calcifications (arrows) projecting over the mid-portion of the left kidney consistent with kidney stones. (*From Chen MY, Pope TL, Jr, Ott DJ. Basic Radiology; Figure 9-33, p. 243. Copyright 2004, McGraw-Hill.*)

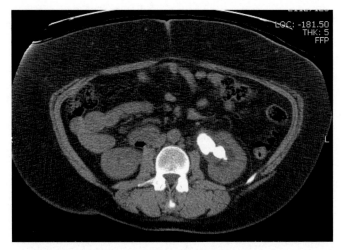

FIGURE 65-4 An unenhanced CT performed on a 49-year-old woman with known renal stones reveals a large left staghorn calculus. The striated appearance of the left renal cortex is seen in obstruction, infection, and ischemia. (*Courtesy of Michael Freckleton, MD.*)

• For long-term management, increased fluid intake to at least 2.5 L/d (specific gravity of 1.005) is recommended for most patients as this fluid level has been shown to reduce recurrences by half.[2]

FOLLOW-UP

Additional treatments may be warranted based on the type of stone[2]:

• Patients with recurrent calcium-containing stones caused by idiopathic hypercalcuria are treated with a thiazide diuretic (reduces recurrence by 50% over 3 years). Hypokalemia should be avoided; low potassium reduces urinary citrate. Hyperoxaluria (present in 10%–30%) is treated with a low-oxalate diet (decreasing spinach, nuts, and chocolate) and possibly an oxalate-binding resin cholestyramine (8–16 g/d).

• Low-calcium diets should not be used (increases stone formation and lowers bone mineral density).

• Idiopathic stone disease is treated with oral phosphate, fluids, and potassium citrate (2 g/d).

• Struvite stones can be treated with percutaneous nephrolithotomy (PCNL), lithotripsy, or open surgery.

• Uric acid stones associated with gout are treated with allopurinol and a low-purine diet.

• For cystine stones, nighttime fluids, alkalinizing the urine to a pH ≥7.5, and a low sodium diet are recommended. D-penicillamine has also been used.

REFERENCES

1. Rodgers AL, Lewandowski S. Effects of five different diets on urinary risk factors for calcium oxalate kidney stone formation: Evidence of different renal handling mechanisms in different race groups. *J Urol.* 2002;168(3):931–936.

2. Asplin JR, Coe FL, Ravus, MJ. Nephrolithiasis. In: Kasper DL, Braunwald E, Fauci AS, Hauser SL, Longo DL, Jameson JL eds. *Harrison's Principles of Internal Medicine*, 16th ed. New York,: McGraw-Hill, 2005:1710–1714.

3. Taylor EN, Stampfer MJ, Curhan GC. Obesity, weight gain, and the risk of kidney stones. *JAMA.* 2005;293(4):455–462.

4. Portis AJ, Sundaram CP. Diagnosis and initial management of kidney stones. *Am Fam Physician.* 2001;63(7):1329–1338.

5. Jungers P, Joly D, Barbey F, et al. ESRD caused by nephrolithiasis: Prevalence, mechanisms, and prevention. *Am J Kidney Dis.* 2004;44(5):799–805.

66 HYDRONEPHROSIS

Mindy A. Smith, MD, MS

PATIENT STORY

A 74-year-old man presented with a 2-day history of severe, steady pain radiating down to the lower abdomen and left testicle. He has had urinary frequency, nocturia, hesitancy, and urinary dribbling for several years with slight worsening with time. CT scan revealed left-sided hydronephrosis (**Figure 66-1**). In this patient, an irregular mass was seen at the left ureterovesical junction compressing the bladder. Prostate cancer was found on biopsy.

EPIDEMIOLOGY

- The most common cause of congenital bilateral hydronephrosis is posterior urethral valves (in males). Other causes include narrowing of the ureteropelvic or ureterovesicular junction.

- Among acquired causes in adults, pelvic tumors, renal calculi, and urethral stricture predominate.[1] If renal colic is present, renal stone is likely present (90% in one study).[2]

- Hydronephrosis is common in pregnancy because of the compression from the enlarging uterus and functional effects of progesterone.

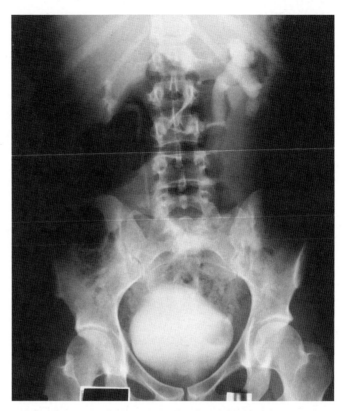

FIGURE 66-1 Intravenous urogram showing left hydronephrosis and hydroureter. (*From Schwartz DT and Reisdorff EJ. Emergency Radiology p. 540, Fig. 19-45, Copyright 2000, McGraw-Hill.*)

ETIOLOGY AND PATHOPHYSIOLOGY

- Bilateral hydronephrosis is caused by a blockage to urine flow occurring at or below the level of the bladder.

- Unilateral hydronephrosis is caused by a blockage to urine flow occurring above the level of the bladder.

- Multiple causes result in this condition including congenital, acquired intrinsic (e.g., calculi, inflammation, and trauma) and acquired extrinsic (e.g., pregnancy or uterine leiomyoma, retroperitoneal fibrosis). Within these groupings, obstruction may be due to mechanical or functional (e.g., neurogenic bladder) defects.

DIAGNOSIS

In children, the diagnosis of hydronephrosis or megaureter is often made by a routine ultrasound. A workup for hydronephrosis in adults is often triggered by the discovery of azotemia (due to impaired excretory function of sodium, urea, and water). Sudden or new onset of hypertension (because of the increased renin release with unilateral obstruction) may also trigger an investigation. A first step in the evaluation is to perform bladder catheterization. If diuresis occurs, the obstruction is below the bladder neck.

CLINICAL FEATURES

- Pain is the symptom that most commonly leads an adult patient to seek medical attention. This is caused by distention of the collecting system or renal capsule. The pain is often described as severe, steady, and radiating down to the lower abdomen, testicles, or labia. Flank pain with urination is pathognomonic for vesicoureteral reflux.

- Disturbed excretory function or difficulty in voiding: Oliguria and anuria are symptoms of complete obstruction whereas polyuria and nocturia occur with partial obstruction (impaired concentrating ability causes osmotic diuresis).

- The physical examination may reveal distention of the kidney or bladder. Rectal exam may show an enlarged prostate or rectal/pelvic mass and pelvic examination may reveal an enlarged uterus or pelvic mass.

LABORATORY STUDIES

Urinalysis may show hematuria, pyuria, or bacteruria but the sediment is often normal.[1]

IMAGING

- Ultrasound imaging has a sensitivity and specificity of 90% for identifying the presence of hydronephrosis, if no diuresis occurs following bladder catheterization.[1]

- If a source remains unidentified, an IV urogram and/or CT scan should be obtained to diagnose intraabdominal or retroperitoneal causes (**Figures 66-1** and **66-2**).

- One study of MR pyelography (vs. ultrasound and urography) reported a sensitivity in detecting stones, strictures, and congenital ureteropelvic junction obstructions of 68.9%, 98.5%, and 100%, respectively, with a specificity of 98%.[3] Accuracy regarding the level of obstruction was high (100%).

- Antegrade urography (percutaneous placement of ureteral catheter) or retrograde urography (cystoscopic placement of ureteral catheter) may be needed in patients with azotemia and poor excretory function or in those at high risk or acute renal failure from IV contrast (i.e., diabetes, multiple myeloma).

- A voiding cystourethrogram is useful in the diagnosis of vesicoureteral reflux and bladder neck and urethral obstructions.

DIFFERENTIAL DIAGNOSIS

Hydronephrosis is usually found during an investigation for symptoms such as flank pain or renal failure. Following are the other causes of flank pain:

- Pyelonephritis—Fever, chills, nausea, vomiting, and diarrhea often occurring with or without symptoms of cystitis.

- Cholelithiasis—Pain is more typically in the epigastrium and right upper quadrant (biliary colic) and often nausea and vomiting occurs (see Chapter 59, Gallbladder Disease).

- Other urologic disorders include ureteropelvic junction obstruction, renal subcapsular hematoma, and renal cell carcinoma.

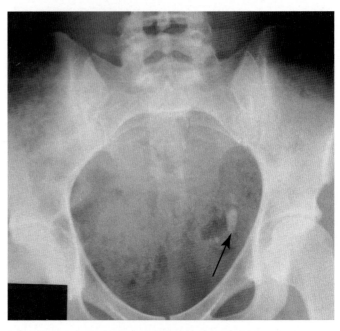

FIGURE 66-2 Large irregular calcification (arrow) representing ureterolithiasis in the left side of the pelvis in the patient in **Figure 66-1**. (*From Schwartz DT and Reisdorff EJ. Emergency Radiology p. 539, Fig. 19-43, Copright 2000, McGraw-Hill.*)

Causes of unexplained renal failure in adults:

- Hypoperfusion (prerenal failure).
- Acute tubular necrosis (ATN), interstitial, glomerular, or small vessel disease (intrarenal failure).
- Hypoperfusion and acute tubular necrosis account for the majority of cases of acute renal failure.

MANAGEMENT

- Spontaneous resolution or decrease in urinary tract dilatation is expected for most cases of neonatal hydronephrosis and primary megaureter diagnosed prenatally.[4,5]
- Patients with hydronephrosis, complicated by infection, should be treated with appropriate antibiotics for 3 to 4 weeks. Chronic or recurrent unilateral infections may require nephrectomy. SOR **A**
- Patients with renal failure can be treated with dialysis. SOR **A**
- Elective surgery for drainage is performed for persistent pain or progressive loss of renal function. SOR **C**
- Functional causes may be treated by frequent voiding or catheterization and/or anticholinergic drugs.

FOLLOW-UP

- Neonates and children with unresolved hydronephrosis or megaureter should be followed periodically with ultrasonography and possibly renal scan.
- Prognosis for an adult patient depends on the duration and completeness of the obstruction and associated complications like infection; complete obstruction for 1 to 2 weeks may be followed by partial return of renal function, but after 8 weeks, recovery is unlikely.[1]
- Postobstructive diuresis can cause loss of sodium, potassium, and magnesium that may require replacement in the setting of hypovolemia, hypotension, or electrolyte imbalance.

PATIENT RESOURCES

- National Kidney Foundation (800-622-9010) or **www.kidney.org.**
- National Institutes of Health **www.nlm.nih.gov/medlineplus.**

PROVIDER RESOURCES

Guideline: American College of Radiology (ACR), Expert Panel on Urologic Imaging. Radiologic investigation of causes of renal failure. Reston (VA): American College of Radiology (ACR); 2001. 8 p (ACR appropriateness criteria).

REFERENCES

1. Seifter JL, Brenner BM. Urinary tract obstruction. In: Kasper DL, Braunwald E, Fauci AS, Hauser SL, Longo DL, Jameson JL eds. *Harrison's Principles of Internal Medicine.* 16th ed. New York,: McGraw-Hill, 2005:1722–1724.

2. Pepe P, Motta L, Pennisi M, Aragona F. Functional evaluation of the urinary tract by color-Doppler ultrasonography (CDU) in 100 patients with renal colic. *Eur J Radiol*. 2005;53(1):131–135.

3. Blandino A, Gaeta M, Minutoli F, et al. MR pyelography in 115 patients with a dilated renal collecting system. *Acta Radiol*. 2001; 42(5):532–536.

4. Shukla AR, Cooper J, Patel RP, et al. Prenatally detected primary megaureter: A role for extended followup. *J Urol*. 2005;173(4): 1353–1356.

5. Upadhyay J, McLorie GA, Bolduc S, et al. Natural history of neonatal reflux associated with prenatal hydronephrosis: Long-term results of a prospective study. *J Urol*. 2003;169(5):1837–1841.

67 POLYCYSTIC KIDNEY DISEASE

Mindy A. Smith, MD, MS

PATIENT STORY

A 43-year-old woman with newly diagnosed hypertension reports persistent bilateral flank pain. She has a family history of "kidney problems." On urinalysis, she is noted to have microscopic hematuria. An ultrasound and abdominal CT scan show bilateral polycystic kidneys (**Figure 67-1**).

EPIDEMIOLOGY

- Most common tubular disorder of the kidney, affecting 1 in 300 individuals.
- Autosomal dominant in 90% of cases, rarely as an autosomal recessive trait.[1]
- Sporadic mutation in approximately 1:1000 individuals.
- Accounts for 40% of end-stage renal disease (ESRD) in the United States.
- Most frequently seen in the third and fourth decades, but can be diagnosed at any age.

ETIOLOGY AND PATHOPHYSIOLOGY

- Autosomal dominant polycystic kidney disease (PKD) results from abnormal regulation of cell-cell or cell-matrix interactions and up-regulation of keratinocyte growth factor and receptors, which may stimulate proliferation of cyst-lining epithelial cells.[2]
- Few (1%–5%) nephrons actually develop cysts.
- Remaining renal parenchyma shows varying degrees of tubular atrophy, interstitial fibrosis, and nephrosclerosis.
- Cysts are also found in other organs such as liver (**Figure 67-2**), spleen, pancreas, and ovaries.

DIAGNOSIS

Family history is a useful tool for diagnosing early autosomal dominant PKD.

CLINICAL FEATURES

- Chronic flank pain as a result of the mass effect of enlarged kidneys.
- Acute pain with infection, obstruction, or hemorrhage into a cyst.
- Hypertension is common in adults (75%) and may be present in 20% to 30% of children.

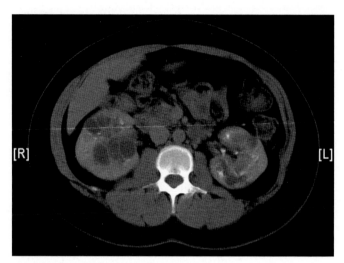

FIGURE 67-1 Polycystic kidneys in a 43-year-old woman with hematuria. (*Courtesy of Michael Freckleton, MD.*)

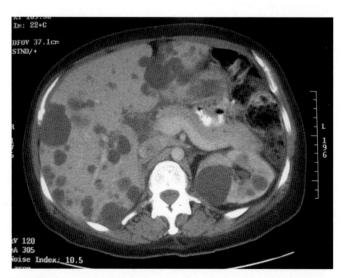

FIGURE 67-2 CT scan showing multiple liver cysts and multiple cysts in both kidneys in a patient with PKD. (*Courtesy of Vesselin Dimov, MD, Cleveland Clinic, ClinicalCases.org.*)

- Kidney stones (calcium oxalate and uric acid) develop in 15% to 20% because of urinary stasis from distortion of the collecting system, low urine pH, and low urinary citrate.

- Nocturia may also be present from impaired renal concentrating ability.

LABORATORY STUDIES AND IMAGING

- Gross or microscopic hematuria.

- Diagnosis often made with ultrasound. More than 80% of patients have cysts present by age 20 and 100% by age 30. In one study, the sensitivity of ultrasound in individuals younger than 30 years, who were at risk, was 67% to 95% based on the type of PKD present.[3] For younger patients or those with small cysts, CT scan (**Figures 67-1** and **67-2**) or MRI may be preferred.

- Cysts are commonly found in the liver (50%–70%) (**Figure 67-2**), spleen, pancreas, and ovaries.

- Increased incidence of intracranial aneurysms (5%–10%).

MANAGEMENT

The role of therapy in PKD is to slow the rate of progression of renal disease and minimize symptoms. The following therapies have been suggested, although little benefit has been demonstrated:

- Neither protein restriction nor tight blood pressure control decreased the decline in glomerular filtration rate (GFR) in clinical trials.[4,5]

- Treat infection as early as possible. If pyocyst is suspected, agents that penetrate cysts such as trimethoprim-sulfamethoxazole, chloramphenicol, and ciprofloxacin are used. SOR **C**

- Cyst puncture and a sclerosing agent (i.e., ethanol) can be used in painful cysts. SOR **C**

- For patients with ESRD as a result of PKD, transplant and dialysis are options.

- Genetic linkage analysis can be offered, particularly if an ultrasound is negative or for family members who are being screened for kidney donation.

PATIENT EDUCATION

Explain the genetics and prognosis to patients. Referral to a genetic counselor may be useful for patients considering childbearing.

FOLLOW-UP

Approximately 50% progress slowly to ESRD. Following are the characteristics that predict a faster rate of decline in GFR in persons with ADPKD:[4]

- Greater serum creatinine (independent of GFR).

- Greater urinary protein excretion.

- Higher mean arterial pressure (MAP).

- Young age.

The prognosis for patients following renal transplant is fairly good. In a follow-up study of patients with autosomal dominant PKD, adult cadaveric renal transplant survival at 5 years was found to be 79%.[6]

PATIENT AND PROVIDER RESOURCES

National Kidney Foundation (800-622-9010)—**www.kidney.org.**

National Institutes of Health—**www.nlm.nih.gov/ medlineplus.**

REFERENCES

1. Asplin JR, Coe FL. Tubular disorders. In: Kasper DL, Braunwald E, Fauci AS, Hauser SL, Longo DL, Jameson, JL eds. *Harrison's Principles of Internal Medicine.* 16th ed. New York, NY: McGraw-Hill, 2005:1694–1696.

2. Mei C, Mao Z, Shen X, et al. Role of keratinocyte growth factor in the pathogenesis of autosomal dominant polycystic kidney disease. *Nephrol Dial Transplant.* 2005;20(11):2368–2375.

3. Nicolau C, Torra R, Bandenas C, et al. Autosomal dominant polycystic kidney disease types 1 and 2: Assessment of US sensitivity for diagnosis. *Radiology.* 1999;213(1):273–276.

4. Klahr S, Breyer JA, Beck GJ, et al. Dietary protein restriction, blood pressure control, and the progression of polycystic kidney disease. Modification of Diet in Renal Disease Study Group. *J Am Soc Nephrol* 1995;6(4):1318.

5. Schrier R, McFann K, Johnson A, et al. Cardiac and renal effects of standard versus rigorous blood pressure control in autosomal-dominant polycystic kidney disease: Results of a seven-year prospective randomized study. *J Am Soc Nephrol.* 2002;13(7):1733–1739.

6. Johnston O, O'Kelly P, Donohue J, et al. Favorable graft survival in renal transplant recipients with polycystic kidney disease. *Ren Fail.* 2005;27(3):309–314.

68 RENAL CELL CARCINOMA

Mindy A. Smith, MD, MS

PATIENT STORY

A 56-year old man with hypertension presents with a 2-week history of left-sided flank pain. Urinalysis shows microscopic hematuria and a CT scan (**Figures 68-1** and **68-2**) demonstrates a solid left renal mass. Work-up for metastatic disease was negative. A biopsy confirmed renal cell carcinoma and a radical nephrectomy was performed.

EPIDEMIOLOGY

- Ninety to ninety-five percent of kidney neoplasms are renal cell carcinomas (RCC).
- There are 36,000 cases per year and about 12,300 deaths per year from RCC.[1]
- Peak incidence is between age 50 and 70 with a male-to-female ratio of 2:1.
- Metastatic disease at presentation occurs in 23% to 33%; the most common sites of distant metastases (in descending order) are lung, bone, skin, liver, and brain.

ETIOLOGY AND PATHOPHYSIOLOGY

RCCs are a heterogeneous group of tumors depending on their morphology and histology that range from benign to high-grade malignancy. Risk factors include smoking, obesity, and acquired cystic disease associated with ESRD. The majority of tumors fall into the following categories:

- Clear cell carcinoma (60%).
- Papillary carcinoma (5%–15%).
- Chromophobic tumors (5%–10%).
- Oncocytomas (5%–10%).[1]

DIAGNOSIS

CLINICAL FEATURES

- Hematuria (40%) and flank pain (40%).
- Weight loss and anemia (about 33%).
- Flank mass (about 25%).

The classic triad of hematuria, flank pain, and flank mass occurs in 5% to 10%.[1] Other reported symptoms include night sweats, bone pain, fatigue, and sudden onset of left varicocele.

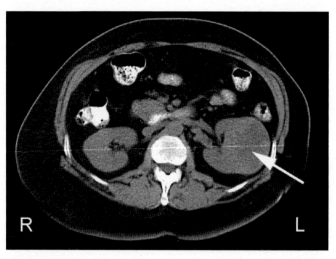

FIGURE 68-1 Renal cell carcinoma: CT shows solid mass in the left kidney (arrow). (*Courtesy of Michael Freckleton, MD.*)

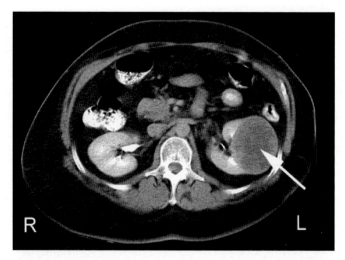

FIGURE 68-2 CT with contrast in the same patient shows the solid hypodense renal cell carcinoma mass (arrow) in the left kidney and contrasting normal parenchyma. The contrast is taken up better by the remaining normal kidney tissue and the tumor becomes more visible. (*Courtesy of Michael Freckleton, MD.*)

LABORATORY AND IMAGING

Potentially useful studies: SOR Ⓒ

- Hemoglobin (anemia).
- Liver chemistries (metastatic disease or paraneoplastic syndrome).
- Urine analysis (hematuria—gross or microscopic).
- Urine cytology (neoplastic cells).

The standard work-up for a suspected RCC, based on consensus opinion of the American College of Radiology,[2] includes:

- Chest x-ray (tumor may extend into the hilar lymph nodes—Stage IIIB).
- Dynamic-enhanced computed tomography (CT) scan of the abdomen (**Figures 68-1** and **68-2**) (solid renal mass; signs suggestive of renal vein or caval thrombus include filling defects, enlargement of the vessel, and rim enhancement) or abdominal MRI (slightly more sensitive for thrombus detection).
- Bone scans and brain MRI should be reserved for patients with abnormal blood chemistries, symptoms, or large and locally aggressive or metastatic primary renal cancers.

DIFFERENTIAL DIAGNOSIS

The differential diagnosis of a renal mass includes:

- Simple cysts.
- Renal calculi/nephrolithiasis (see Chapter 65, Kidney Stones).
- Benign neoplasms (infrarenal hematoma, adenoma, angiomyolipoma, and oncocytoma).
- Inflammatory lesions (focal bacterial nephritis, abcess, pyelonephritis, and renal tuberculosis); patients often present with systemic signs and symptoms of infection such as fever and chills.
- Other primary or metastatic tumors (neoplastic tumors involving the kidney include squamous cell carcinoma of the collecting system, transitional cell carcinomas of the renal pelvis or collecting system, sarcoma, lymphoma, nephroblastoma, and melanoma).

These can frequently be differentiated from RCC on CT scan, but biopsy may be necessary.

MANAGEMENT

- Surgery (radical nephrectomy—complete removal of the kidney and Gerota's fascia) for local disease and potentially solitary metastases. SOR Ⓒ

- Regional lymphadenectomy is controversial.
- Investigational therapy for advanced disease because chemotherapy and immunotherapy are ineffective. The clinical course is highly variable and spontaneous remissions have occurred.

PATIENT EDUCATION

Several prognostic algorithms, or nomograms, for RCC survival are available that may be useful in counseling patients about their probable clinical course and facilitating treatment planning.[3]

FOLLOW-UP

Prognosis of renal cell carcinoma is based on stage at diagnosis with 5-year survival as follows:

- Stage I (confined to kidney) 66% to 100%; greater survival is seen with tumors smaller than 2.5 cm.
- Stage II disease (extending through the capsule but within Gerota's fascia) or stage IIIA 60% to 64%.
- Stage IIIB (as above) 20%.
- Stage IV (distant metastases) 11%.

PATIENT RESOURCES

- National Kidney Foundation (800-622-9010): **www.kidney.org.**
- National Institutes of Health **www.nlm.nih.gov/medlineplus.**

PROVIDER RESOURCES

Kidney Cancer Trial Search Tool (800) 850-9132; **http://kidneycancercare.org.**

REFERENCES

1. Scher HI, Motzer RJ. Bladder and Renal Cell Carcinomas. In: Kasper DL, Braunwald E, Fauci AS, Hauser SL, Longo DL, Jameson JL eds. *Harrison's Principles of Internal Medicine.* 16th ed. New York,: McGraw-Hill, 2005:541–543.

2. American College of Radiology (ACR), Expert Panel on Urologic Imaging. Renal cell carcinoma staging. Reston (VA): *American College of Radiology.* (ACR); 2001.

3. Lane BR, Kattan MW. Predicting outcomes in renal cell carcinoma. *Curr Opin Urol.* 2005;15(5):289–297.

69 BLADDER CANCER

Mindy A. Smith, MD, MS

PATIENT STORY

A 68-year-old man, who is a retired painter and in good health, comes to the office at the insistence of his wife. He reports that his urinary stream is smaller and he has occasional dysuria. He has no major medical problems, although he continues to smoke one pack of cigarettes per day. His urinalysis in the office shows microscopic hematuria and an irregular mass is seen in the bladder on CT (**Figure 69-1**). Cystoscopy shows a bladder tumor (**Figure 69-2**). Complete endoscopic resection is performed and confirms transitional cell carcinoma.

EPIDEMIOLOGY

- Fourth most common cause of cancer in men and tenth in women.

- More than 60,000 new cases and more than 12,700 deaths in 2004.[1]

- Male-to-female ratio of 4:1 and more prevalent in whites vs. blacks (ratio of 2:1).[1]

- Risk factors include smoking (odds ratio increased by three- to fourfold; 50% attributable risk), aniline dyes (e.g., workers in chemical plants exposed to benzidine or *o*-toluidine), the drugs phenacetin and chlornaphazine, external beam radiation, and exposure to Schistosoma haematobium.

- There is an increased risk in certain occupations, particularly those involving exposure to metals, including aluminum, paint and solvents, polycyclic aromatic hydrocarbons, diesel engine emissions, and textiles.[2] An increased risk was also seen with drinking tap water (OR for > 2L/d vs. ≤ 0.5 L/d was 1.46 (1.20–1.78)), with a higher risk among men (OR = 1.50, 1.21–1.88).[3]

ETIOLOGY AND PATHOPHYSIOLOGY

- Ninety-five percent are transitional cell cancers (3% squamous cell, 2% adenocarcinoma)[1] (**Figures 69-1 to 69-4**). Transitional cells line the urinary tract from the renal pelvis to the proximal two-third of the urethra.

- Ninety percent of transitional cell tumors develop in the bladder and the others develop in the renal pelvis, ureters or urethra.[1]

- Most are superficial (75%) with 20% invading the muscle of the bladder wall and 5% presenting with distant metastases.[1]

- The most common sites of hematogenous spread are lung, bone, liver, and brain. Superficial lesions do not metastasize until they invade deeply and may remain indolent for years.[1]

DIAGNOSIS

CLINICAL FEATURES

- Hematuria in 80% to 90%.

- Irritative symptoms (i.e., dysuria, frequency) are the most common presentation.

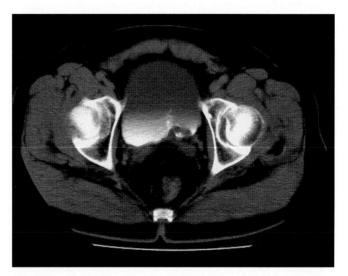

FIGURE 69-1 CT with contrast reveals a bladder cancer in a 68-year-old man with hematuria. (*Courtesy of Michael Freckleton, MD.*)

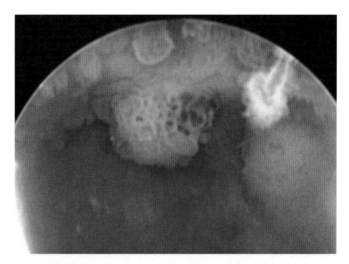

FIGURE 69-2 Cystoscopic view of the transitional cell carcinoma in the man in **Figure 69-2**. (*Courtesy of Carlos Enrique Bermejo, MD.*)

LABORATORY AND IMAGING

- Urine cytology (high specificity [90% to 95%] but low sensitivity [23% to 60%]), CT scan of the pelvis (**Figures 69-1, 69-3** and **69-4**) or IVP, and cystoscopy (**Figure 69-2**) comprise the basic work-up.[1]

- For pretreatment staging of invasive bladder cancer, the American College of Radiology recommends an IVP, chest x-ray (with chest CT if equivocal), and possibly MRI of the pelvis.[4] SOR **C**

- CT or MRI of the chest or abdomen and a bone scan may be needed for suspected metastatic disease. Bone scanning may be limited to patients with bone pain and/or elevated levels of serum alkaline phosphatase.[4]

DIFFERENTIAL DIAGNOSIS

- Among adult patients with microscopic hematuria, most patients have benign pathology with 25% having prostate cancer and only 2% have bladder cancer.[1]

- Among adult patients with gross hematuria, 22% have benign cystitis and 15% have bladder cancer.[1]

MANAGEMENT

Depends on the extent or spread of the disease as given below:

- Superficial disease—Complete endoscopic resection with or without intravesical treatment (bacillus Calmette-Guérin [BCG] weekly for 6 weeks or interferon or mitomycin C). In a meta-analysis of 3 trials, tumor recurrence was significantly lower with intravesical BCG but there was no difference in disease progression or survival.[5] SOR **B** BCG treatment causes dysuria, urinary frequency, and rarely systemic granulomatous infection requiring antituberculosis treatment.

- Persistent or recurrent superficial disease—Second course of BCG or intravesical chemotherapy (valrubicin or gemcitabine).[1]

- Invasive disease (extends to muscle or lymph nodes)—Radical cystectomy with or without systemic chemotherapy. SOR **C** In men, radical cystectomy includes removal of the prostate, seminal vesicles, and proximal urethra resulting in impotence. In women, the uterus, ovaries, and anterior vaginal wall are removed. Most patients receive cutaneous reservoirs (bowel or orthotopic neobladder) drained by intermittent self-catheterization. In a recent meta-analysis of adjuvant chemotherapy for patients with invasive disease it was found that there is a 25% relative reduction in risk of death but the authors concluded that there was insufficient evidence on which to reliably base treatment decisions.[6] SOR **B**

- Metastatic disease—Systemic chemotherapy with or without surgery. SOR **C**

PATIENT EDUCATION

Based on a simple scoring system derived from six clinical and pathologic factors (number of tumors, tumor size, prior recurrence rate, T category, carcinoma in situ, and grade), tables have been created that provide probabilities of recurrence and disease progression.[7] This information can be useful in discussions with patients to determine the most appropriate treatment and frequency of follow-up.

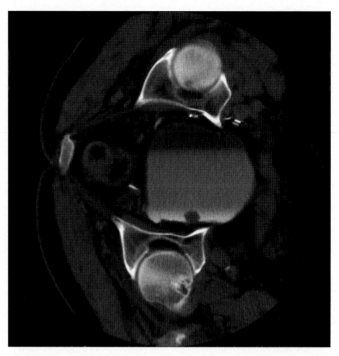

FIGURE 69-3 CT with contrast of a small transitional cell carcinoma of the bladder that was barely visible until the patient was scanned on side. A small bladder diverticulum is visible as well. (*Courtesy of Michael Freckleton, MD.*)

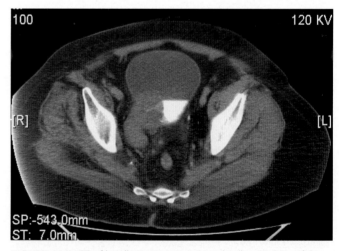

FIGURE 69-4 CT of locally-invasive transitional cell carcinoma of the bladder extending outside of the bladder in a 71-year-old man. The contrast on the left is adjacent to the tumor on the right. (*Courtesy of Michael Freckleton, MD.*)

FOLLOW-UP

- Recurrence rates overall are 50% with a median recurrence at 1 year (0.4–11 years). Patients should be seen every 3 months for the first year. SOR **C**
- Bladder tumor markers from voided urine will likely improve detection of recurrence in the future, but they are not widely accepted.[8]
- Five to twenty percent progress to a more advanced stage.
- Five-year survival rates for superficial disease are 90%; infiltrating (stage II or III) 35% to 70%; metastatic disease (stage IV) 10% to 20%.[1]

PATIENT AND PROVIDER RESOURCES

- Information for both patients and providers can be found at: **www.nlm.nih.gov/medlineplus/bladdercancer.html.**
- **http://www.cancerbacup.org.uk/Cancertype/Bladder.**

REFERENCES

1. Scher HI, Motzer RJ. Bladder and Renal Cell Carcinomas. In: Kasper DL, Braunwald E, Fauci AS, Hauser SL, Longo DL, Jameson JL eds. *Harrison's Principles of Internal Medicine.* 16th ed. New York: McGraw-Hill, 2005:539–540.

2. Band PR Le ND MacArthur AC, et al. Identification of occupational cancer risks in British Columbia: A population-based case-control study of 1129 cases of bladder cancer. *J Occup Environ Med.* 2005; 47(8):854–858.

3. Villanueva CM, Cantor KP, King WD, et al. Total and specific fluid consumption as determinants of bladder cancer risk. *Int J Cancer.* 2006;118(8):2040–2047.

4. American College of Radiology (ACR), Expert Panel on Urologic Imaging. Pretreatment staging of invasive transitional cell carcinoma of the bladder. Reston (VA): American College of Radiology (ACR); 2001. (ACR appropriateness criteria).

5. Shelley MD, Wilt TJ, Court J, et al. Intravesical bacillus Calmette-Guerin is superior to mitomycin C in reducing tumour recurrence in high-risk superficial bladder cancer: a meta-analysis of randomized trials. *BJU Int.* 2004;93(4):485–490.

6. Advanced Bladder Cancer (ABC) Meta-analysis Collaboration. Adjuvant chemotherapy in invasive bladder cancer: A systematic review and meta-analysis of individual patient data Advanced Bladder Cancer (ABC) Meta-analysis Collaboration. *Eur Urol.* 2005;48(2):189–199.

7. Sylvester RJ, van der Meijden AP, Oosterlinck W, et al. Predicting recurrence and progression in individual patients with stage ta t1 bladder cancer using eortc risk tables: a combined analysis of 2596 patients from seven eortc trials. *Eur Urol.* 2006;49(3):466–475.

8. Lokeshwar VB, Habuchi T, Grossman HB, et al. Bladder tumor markers beyond cytology: International consensus panel on bladder tumor markers. *Urology.* 2005;66:35–63.

PART 11

WOMEN'S HEALTH

SECTION 1 PREGNANCY

70 SKIN FINDINGS IN PREGNANCY

E.J. Mayeaux, Jr., MD

PATIENT STORY

A 32-year-old G3P2 woman presents with persistent itching in her 31st week of pregnancy. The itching is constant and worse at night. Her pregnancy had been uncomplicated and she has no past history of medical problems. Many excoriations are noted and there are no blisters (**Figure 70-1**). She has no jaundice or scleral icterus. Her transaminases were over 300 and her total bilirubin was elevated at 2.1. Her bile salts were elevated and her hepatitis panel was negative. The ultrasound showed gallstones but no obstruction was seen. A diagnosis of "intrahepatic cholestasis of pregnancy" was made and the patient was treated with oral ursodiol (a bile salt binding agent) and topical 1% hydrocortisone cream. The bile salts and transaminases were decreased and the patient's pruritus improved but did not resolve until after delivery.[1]

EPIDEMIOLOGY

- Maternal skin and skin structures undergo numerous changes during pregnancy.

- Almost all pregnant women develop some increase in skin pigmentation. This usually occurs in discrete areas, probably because of differences in melanocyte density.

- Another common finding is prurigo of pregnancy (now called atopic eruption of pregnancy), with an incidence of approximately 1 in 300 to 1 in 450 pregnancies.[2,3]

ETIOLOGY

- The most common skin pigmentary change is darkening of the linea alba (**Figure 70-2**), which is then called the linea nigra.[4] It may span from the pubic symphysis to the umbilicus or all the way to the xiphoid process.

- The skin around the areola may also darken and develop a reticular type pattern. Other anatomic areas that develop hyperpigmentation are the nipples, axillae, vulva, perineum, anus, inner thighs, and neck.[5] Darkening may also occur in nevi during pregnancy.

- Atopic eruption of pregnancy is most common in the second or third trimester, but has been reported in all trimesters. It presents with erythematous, excoriated papules on the extensor surfaces of the limbs and trunk.[2,3] Lesions are grouped and may appear eczematous. The eruption usually resolves in the immediate postpartum

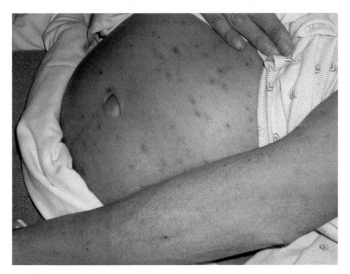

FIGURE 70-1 Pruritus and excoriations in a patient with intrahepatic cholecystasis of pregnancy. All the lesions are secondary to patient scratching. (*Courtesy of Richard P. Usatine, MD.*)

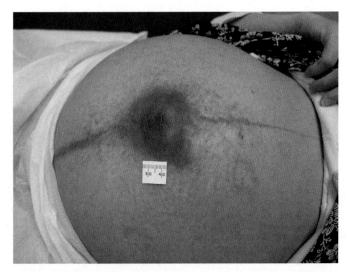

FIGURE 70-2 Darkened linea alba (linea nigra) in a pregnant patient. (*Courtesy of Dan Stulberg, MD.*)

period, although it can persist for months. This should not be confused with intrahepatic cholestasis of pregnancy, which is most common in the third trimester and has no primary skin lesions (**Figure 70-1**).

- As pregnancy progresses, increased eccrine activity may result in hyperhidrosis (increased sweating) and/or miliaria ("prickly heat").[6] Apocrine activity decreases during pregnancy but increases postpartum, so hidradenitis suppurativa improves during pregnancy but may rebound later.[6]

- Hypertrophy of sebaceous glands produces small, brown papules on the areolae (Montgomery's tubercles, **Figure 70-3**) in up to half of pregnant women. They usually regress postpartum.[6]

- Spider angiomas, arterial spiders, or spider nevi may develop, especially in Caucasians. They occur mostly on the neck, face, upper chest, arms, and hands.[4] Almost all regress postpartum.

- Palmar erythema may develop and may be limited to the thenar or hypothenar eminence, or may be diffuse and mottled.[6]

- Saphenous, vulvar, and hemorrhoidal varicosities may increase in number and/or size (see Chapter 63, Hemorrhoids). This may be because of increased blood volume, increased venous pressure, or genetic predisposition. Jacquemier sign refers to venous distention in the vestibule and vagina and is associated with vulvar varicosities, which are particularly difficult to treat.[6] Varicosities regress, at least partially, postpartum.

- Vascular type tumors may develop or enlarge during pregnancy. Pyogenic granulomas (**Figure 70-4**) (granuloma gravidarum, pregnancy tumor, pregnancy epulis) are reddish purple papules that are made up of granulation tissue (see Chapter 154, Pyogenic Granuloma). They usually begin in the first half of pregnancy and then partially regress postpartum. They most commonly appear on the gingiva, but are also common on fingers. Hemangiomas, subcutaneous hemangioendotheliomas, and glomangiomas (glomus tumors) may also occur.

- Stretch marks (striae distensae, striae graviduram) begin as pink/violaceous linear patches in the sixth to seventh month of gestation and are a common cosmetic concern among pregnant women. They evolve into hypopigmented linear depressions. They are most common on the abdomen, breasts, and thighs, but may also arise on the lower back, buttocks, and upper arms.[6] There is a familial predisposition to striae gravidarum, and women with preexisting breast or thigh striae are also more prone to this condition.[7] Although striae fade postpartum, they do not completely disappear.

- Acrochordons (skin tags) may develop, enlarge, or increase on the face, neck, axillae, chest, groin, and inframammary area during the second half of pregnancy. Some may regress postpartum.[8]

- Keloids, leiomyomas, dermatofibromas, and neurofibromas may enlarge during pregnancy.[8]

- Scalp hair appears thicker during pregnancy as a result of slowing of the normal progression of hairs to the telogen ("resting") stage, thereby creating a relative increase in anagen hair. Hair loss (telogen effluvium) is common 1 to 5 months postpartum as the percentage of telogen hairs in the scalp normalizes or increases (**Figure 70-5**).[8] Telogen effluvium resolves within 15 months postpartum, but the scalp hair may never return to prepregnancy thickness.[8]

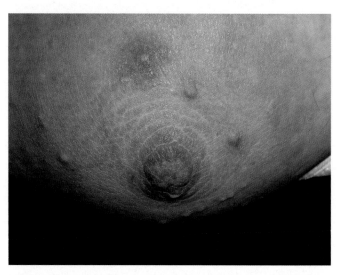

FIGURE 70-3 Montgomery's tubercles in a pregnant woman. The brown papules on the areola are caused by hypertrophy of the normal sebaceous glands. (*Courtesy of Richard P. Usatine, MD.*)

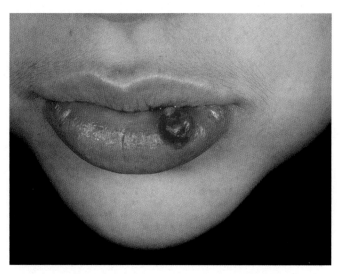

FIGURE 70-4 Pyogenic granuloma in a pregnant woman. (*Courtesy of Richard P. Usatine, MD.*)

- Hirsutism may occur on the face, arms, legs, back, and suprapubic region.[8] Hirsutism appears to be a result of increased levels of ovarian and placental androgens. Frontoparietal hair loss (androgenic alopecia) may develop late in pregnancy but usually resolves postpartum.

MANAGEMENT

- Changes such as hypertrophy of sebaceous glands, spider angiomas, palmar erythema, and varicosities that regress postpartum often require only symptomatic or no therapy. SOR ⓒ

- The primary treatment for pruritus in pregnancy is symptomatic. SOR ⓒ Topical low to mid-potency corticosteroids are safe and can give symptomatic relief of itching. Oral antihistamines such as diphenhydramine may be used to relieve itching. SOR ⓒ see Chapters 71 and 72 for specific treatment of various pruritic diseases in pregnancy.

- Persistent, bothersome pyogenic granulomas can be excised and should be sent to pathology to rule out amelanotic melanoma (see Chapter 154, Pyogenic Granuloma). SOR ⓒ

- Varicosities may be treated with leg elevation, compression with support hose, sleeping on the left side to ease uterine pressure on the great veins, exercise, and avoidance of long periods of standing or sitting. SOR ⓒ (see Chapter 50, Venous Stasis).

- Physical lesions such as skin tags, fibromas, and angiomas may be treated by local surgical or destructive therapies. SOR ⓒ

- Treatment of stretch marks after pregnancy with 0.1% tretinoin was reported to be beneficial but should not be used during pregnancy because of the risk of birth defects with any retinoid.[9] SOR ⓑ

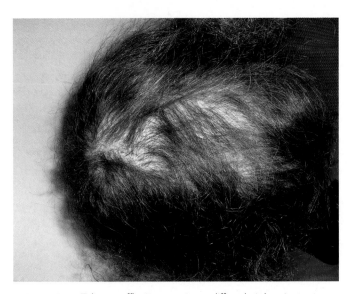

FIGURE 70-5 Telogen effluvium causing a diffuse hair loss in a woman 5 months postpartum. There was no scalp inflammation or scarring. A gentle hair pull test showed that over 25% of her hairs were in the telogen phase. Her hair returned to normal within 1 year of this visit. (*Courtesy of Richard P. Usatine, MD.*)

PATIENT EDUCATION

- The primary aim of treatment for most skin conditions in pregnancy is to relieve symptoms, since many conditions improve or resolve postpartum. Those conditions which do not resolve can usually be safely treated postpartum when there is no risk to the pregnancy.

FOLLOW-UP

- Conditions should be monitored during pregnancy and the patient regularly reassured. Postpartum, the patient may be followed or treated as needed.

REFERENCES

1. Orr B, Usatine RP, Pruritus in pregnancy. *J Fam Pract.* 2007; 56(11):913–916.

2. Roger D, Vaillant L, Fignon A, et al. Specific pruritic diseases of pregnancy: A prospective study of 3192 pregnant women. *Arch Dermatol.* 1994;130:734–739.

3. Holmes, RC, Black, MM. The specific dermatoses of pregnancy. *J Am Acad Dermatol.* 1983;1405–1412.

4. Esteve E, Saudeau L, Pierre F, et al. Physiological cutaneous signs in normal pregnancy: A study of 60 pregnant women. *Ann Dermatol Venereol.* 1994;121:227–231.

5. Muzaffar F, Hussain I, Haroon TS. Physiologic skin changes during pregnancy: A study of 140 cases. *Int J Dermatol.* 1998; 37(6): 429–431.

6. Martin AG, Leal-Khouri S. Physiologic skin changes associated with pregnancy. *Int J Dermatol.* 1992;31(6):375–378.

7. Chang AL, Agredano YZ, Kimball AB. Risk factors associated with striae gravidarum. *J Am Acad Dermatol.* 2004;51(6):881–885.

8. Winton GB, Lewis CW. Dermatoses of pregnancy. *J Am Acad Dermatol.* 1982;6(6):977–998.

9. Kang S, Kim KJ, Griffiths CE, et al. Topical tretinoin (retinoic acid) improves early stretch marks. *Arch Dermatol.* 1996;132(5): 519–526.

71 PRURITIC URTICARIAL PAPULES AND PLAQUES OF PREGNANCY (PUPPP)

E.J. Mayeaux, Jr., MD

PATIENT STORY

A 26-year-old pregnant woman presents at 36 weeks of gestation with a progressive itchy rash. The rash started within the abdominal striae (**Figure 71-1**) and spread to her proximal extremities. This is her first pregnancy and she has never had any rashes like this before. The itching "is maddening." The patient is diagnosed with pruritic urticarial papules and plaques of pregnancy (PUPPP) and treated with topical steroids and oral antihistamines.

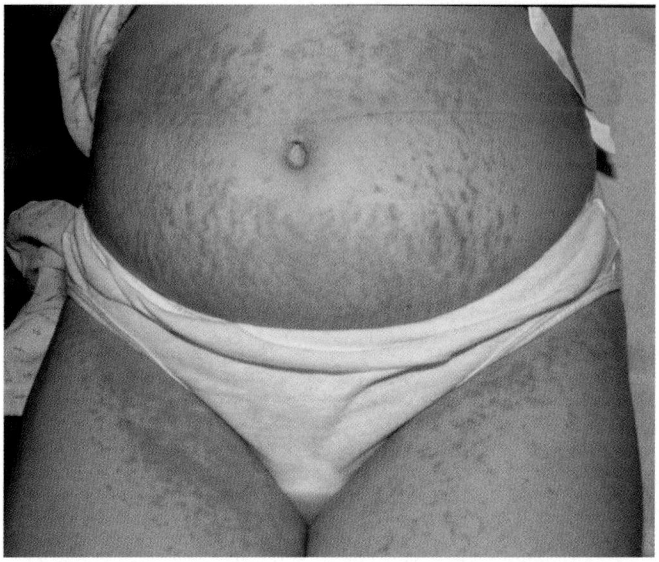

EPIDEMIOLOGY

- The incidence of pruritic urticarial papules and plaques of pregnancy (PUPPP) is 1/160 to 1/300 pregnancies, making it the most common defined dermatosis of pregnancy.[1]

- Nulliparous patients account for more than 75% of patients with classic PUPPP.[2]

- PUPPP is also more common with multiple gestations, possibly because of increased abdominal distension or higher hormone levels.[3]

ETIOLOGY AND PATHOPHYSIOLOGY

- PUPPP is a dermatosis of pregnancy characterized by a papulovesicular or urticarial eruption on the trunk and limbs.

- PUPPP is also known as polymorphic eruption of pregnancy (in the United Kingdom), toxic erythema of pregnancy, and linear IgM dermatosis of pregnancy.[1]

- The etiology of PUPPP is unknown. PUPPP is more common with excessive stretching of the skin, possibly because of damage to connective tissue, which could result in exposure of antigens that trigger an inflammatory response.[1,4] The disease may also represent an immunologic reaction to circulating fetal antigens.

- Onset of PUPPP is usually late in the third trimester, but may develop postpartum.[2,5] There are case reports of first and second trimester disease.[2] Pruritus may worsen after delivery, but generally resolves by 15 days postpartum. The PUPPP may resolve prior to delivery.

DIAGNOSIS

CLINICAL FEATURES

PUPPP typically presents with erythematous papules and plaques within striae (**Figures 71-1** and **71-2**). Pruritus is a hallmark of the disease and is present in all patients.[5]

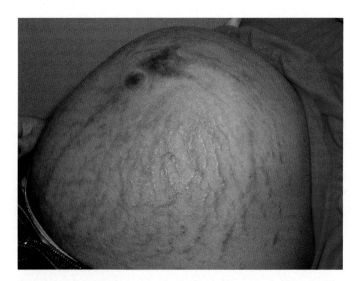

FIGURE 71-1 Pruritic urticarial papules and plaques of pregnancy (PUPPP) presenting as pruritic stria on the abdomen. (*Courtesy of University of Texas Health Sciences Center, Division of Dermatology.*)

FIGURE 71-2 PUPPP occurring in the first pregnancy of a 20-year-old woman during her third trimester. Note how it involves the stria of her abdomen. She also has darkening of her linea alba and umbilicus. (*Courtesy of Rachel Giese.*)

TYPICAL DISTRIBUTION

Abdominal striae are the most common initial site.[2] The lesions usually spread to the extremities and coalesce to form urticarial plaques (**Figure 71-3**). The face, palms, soles, and periumbilical region are usually spared. White halos often surround the erythematous papules, and are target-like, exhibiting three distinct rings or color.[2]

BIOPSY

Biopsy is not necessary when the clinical picture is classic. When the diagnosis is uncertain, perform a punch biopsy and consider immunofluorescent studies. It is preferable to biopsy a lesion off the abdomen to avoid wound-healing problems on a distended abdomen.

DIFFERENTIAL DIAGNOSIS

- Pemphigoid gestationis can be differentiated from PUPPP by its bullous lesions (see Chapter 72, Pemphigoid Gestationis).

- Erythema multiforme produces target lesions that may affect the palms and soles (see Chapter 170, Erythema Multiforme).

- Drug reactions produce various types of erythematous eruptions on the trunk and extremities. History of a new drug exposure helps to distinguish this from PUPPP (see Chapter 196, Cutaneous Drug Reactions).

- Scabies infestations produce severe itching from the mite burrows that are common between the fingers and in areas of skin folds (see Chapter 137, Scabies).

- Viral exanthems may produce all types of erythematous eruptions that can be pruritic at times. The history of a fever along with upper respiratory symptoms should help to differentiate these eruptions from PUPPP (see Chapters 120 and 121, Measles and Fifth Disease).

MANAGEMENT

- First-line therapy consists of topical steroids and antihistamines to alleviate symptoms. Systemic corticosteroids are occasionally required in cases of extreme pruritus. SOR Ⓒ
  - Start with a mid-potency topical corticosteroid such as 0.1% triamcinolone bid to tid. Pregnancy class B. SOR Ⓒ High-potency, topical, corticosteroids such as fluocinonide may be applied sparingly bid to tid as severity warrants. Pregnancy class B. SOR Ⓒ
  - For more severe symptoms, prednisone at a dose of 0.5 to 1 mg/kg/d PO may be used and tapered after symptoms improve. Pregnancy class C. SOR Ⓒ
  - Diphenhydramine 25 to 50 mg PO bid to qid or similar antihistamines may be used for symptomatic relief of pruritus. Pregnancy class B. SOR Ⓒ

- Symptom control is the main goal. Aggressive therapy is not recommended since the condition is self-limiting. SOR Ⓒ

- Early delivery to relieve symptoms is rarely required. Other than maternal itching, PUPPP poses no increased risk to fetal or maternal morbidity.[5] The rate of recurrence with subsequent pregnancies is unknown.

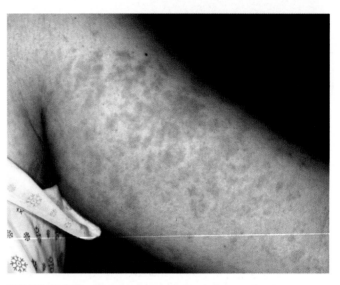

FIGURE 71-3 Pruritic urticarial papules and plaques of pregnancy (PUPPP) on the arm. (*Courtesy of Richard P. Usatine, MD.*)

PATIENT EDUCATION

- When discussing treatment options, inform the patient that the condition is self-limited, so therapy is based on making the patient comfortable while the minimizing the potential risks involved in the use of medications.

- Symptom control with topical steroids and antihistamines is the main goal.

FOLLOW-UP

Routine prenatal and postpartum care should be continued.

PATIENT RESOURCES

About.com: PUPPP **http://dermatology.about.com/cs/ pregnancy/a/puppp.htm.**

DermNet NZ:PUPPP **http://dermnetnz.org/reactions/ puppp.html.**

PROVIDER RESOURCES

EMedicine: Pruritic Urticarial Papules and Plaques of Pregnancy—**http://www.emedicine.com/derm/ topic351.htm.**

REFERENCES

1. Vaughan Jones SA, Black MM. Pregnancy dermatoses. *J Am Acad Dermatol*. 1999;40:233.

2. Aronson IK, Bond S, Fiedler VC, et al. Pruritic urticarial papules and plaques of pregnancy: Clinical and immunopathologic observations in 57 patients. *J Am Acad Dermatol*. 1998;39:933.

3. Kroumpouzos G, Cohen LM. Specific dermatoses of pregnancy: An evidence-based systematic review. *Am J Obstet Gynecol*. 2003;188: 1083.

4. Beckett MA, Goldberg NS. Pruritic urticarial plaques and papules of pregnancy and skin distention. *Arch Dermatol*. 1991;127:125.

5. Yancey KB, Hall RP, Lawley TJ. Pruritic urticarial papules and plaques of pregnancy. Clinical experience in twenty-five patients. *J Am Acad Dermatol*. 1984;10:473.

72 PEMPHIGOID GESTATIONIS

E.J. Mayeaux, Jr., MD

PATIENT STORY

A 37-year-old pregnant woman presented to the hospital with severe preeclampsia. After all medical methods were tried and failed to control her severe preeclampsia, a joint decision was made to induce labor to save the life of the mother. The pregnancy was too early for the fetus to survive. The following day she began to develop the lesions seen in **Figures 72-1** through **72-4**. A diagnosis of pemphigoid gestationis was made. Her past history includes antiphospholipid syndrome with multiple pregnancy losses but two live children. This was her third episode of pemphigoid gestationis. A photograph of her previous episode is included to see how similar the periumbilical bulla was to her current episode of pemphigoid gestationis. A new biopsy was not performed given that her previous biopsy was on file and the clinical picture was consistent with a recurrence of this disease. She was treated with oral prednisone and began to improve rapidly (**Figure 72-5**).

EPIDEMIOLOGY

- Pemphigoid gestationis is a rare disease that occurs in 1/1700 to 1/50,000 pregnancies.[1,2]

ETIOLOGY AND PATHOPHYSIOLOGY

- Pemphigoid gestationis, which has classically been called herpes gestationis, is defined as a bullous or blistering disease that is associated with pregnancy or with trophoblastic tumors.

- As there is no connection with a herpes virus, the preferred name is now pemphigoid gestationis. It is associated with an increased risk of fetal morbidity and mortality (see "Follow-Up").

- The pathophysiology of the disease involves IgG antibodies that attack cells in the skin.

- The IgG attacks the same antigen (bullous pemphigoid antigen) as in bullous pemphigoid.[2] This antigen is a transmembrane protein that is part of the hemidesmosome, which connects the basal cells of the epidermis to the basement membrane.

- When the inflammatory response is activated, the hemidesmosomes are destroyed and the epidermis separates from the dermis.[2]

- It is unknown why some patients form these antibodies.

- Rarely, pemphigoid gestationis persists for years postpartum.[1,2]

- There is no scarring from the lesions.

DIAGNOSIS

CLINICAL FEATURES

- Pemphigoid gestationis typically erupts during the second or third trimester, and rarely postpartum and first trimester.

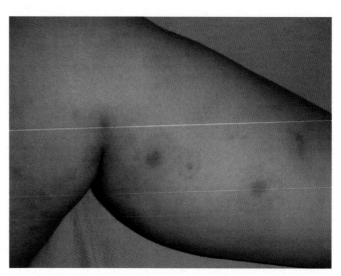

FIGURE 72-1 Pemphigoid gestationis in the pruritic papular stage. The lesions resemble the target lesions of erythema multiforme. (*Courtesy of Richard P. Usatine, MD.*)

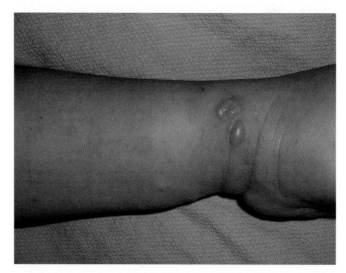

FIGURE 72-2 Pemphigoid gestationis with bullous lesions on the wrist. (*Courtesy of Richard P. Usatine, MD.*)

- Pruritus sometimes precedes the rash and vesicles may develop early.
- The eruption spreads rapidly and forms bullae (**Figures 72-1** to **72-5**).

LABORATORY STUDIES

There are no diagnostic laboratory tests.

TYPICAL DISTRIBUTION

The rash begins on the trunk around the umbilicus as pruritic papules or plaque and may progress to bullae (**Figures 72-4** to **72-5**).[1,2] Lesions may occasionally be seen on the palms and soles, and rarely on the face or mucous membranes.

BIOPSY

Skin biopsy including the edge of a blistering lesion reveals a subepidermal vesicle with a perivascular lymphocytic and eosinophilic infiltrate.

- Eosinophils may appear at the dermoepidermal junction and inside the vesicle; the degree of eosinophilia correlates with disease severity.
- Basal cell necrosis and papillae edema are usually present.

A skin biopsy of perilesional skin for indirect immunofluorescent staining shows complement 3 in a homogeneous linear band at the basement membrane, which is pathognomonic for pemphigoid gestationis in a pregnant patient.

DIFFERENTIAL DIAGNOSIS

- Papular urticarial papules and plaques of pregnancy (PUPPP) may mimic pemphigoid gestationis, especially early in the disease. However, PUPPP usually begin in the striae, while pemphigoid gestationis is usually periumbilical. Most importantly, PUPPP does not develop large bullae as does pemphigoid gestations (see Chapter 71, PUPPP).
- Dermatitis herpetiformis is a very pruritic, vesicular skin eruption. It is a chronic recurrent symmetric vesicular eruption that is usually associated with gluten-induced enteropathy. Men are more often affected than women (see Chapter 179, Bullous Other).
- Erythema multiforme secondary to pregnancy, infection, or drug exposure can mimic pemphigoid gestationis. Biopsy with routine histology can usually distinguish between these disorders (see Chapter 170, Erythema Multiforme).
- Contact dermatitis and drug reactions may have a similar appearance and history of exposure to a contact allergen or medication can help to distinguish between these reactions and pemphigoid gestationis (see Chapters 140, Contact Dermatitis and 196, Cutaneous Drug Reactions).

MANAGEMENT

- Topical steroids and antihistamines should be administered in early or mild cases, but are usually ineffective in more severe cases. SOR **C**
- Systemic steroids, such as prednisone (0.5 mg/kg per day), are effective to control most cases.[3] SOR **C** The dose may be tapered and eventually discontinued in many pregnancies.

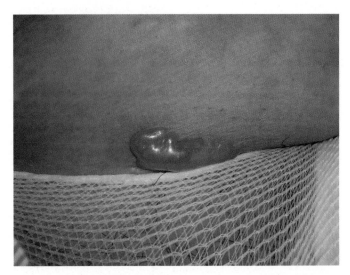

FIGURE 72-3 Pemphigoid gestationis—close up of a bullous lesion on the abdomen. (*Courtesy of Richard P. Usatine, MD.*)

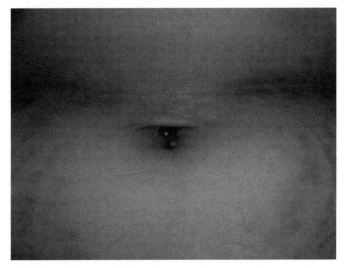

FIGURE 72-4 Pemphigoid gestationis with a bulla in the umbilicus. Lesions typically begin in the periumbilical region. (*Courtesy of Richard P. Usatine, MD.*)

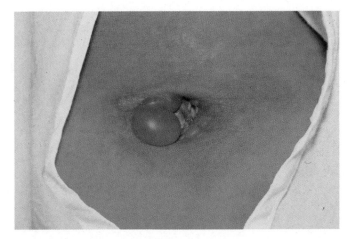

FIGURE 72-5 Close-up of a large bulla in the umbilicus in a previous case of pemphigoid gestationis in the same patient 5 years before. (*Courtesy of University of Texas Health Sciences Center, Division of Dermatology.*)

PATIENT EDUCATION

- Pemphigoid gestationis may abate prior to delivery, but 75% of patients flare postpartum requiring reinstatement of treatment.
- At least 25% of patients will flare with oral contraceptive pill use or during menses.
- Most cases spontaneously resolve in the weeks to months following delivery.
- The disease usually recurs with future pregnancies and often worsens with repeated episodes, but may also skip some pregnancies.[2,4]

FOLLOW-UP

- Follow-up of the mother and child are essential because of the following issues: The fetus during a pregnancy in which the mom has pemphigoid gestationis is at risk for growth restriction and prematurity. Mild placental insufficiency may result from an immune response between placental antigens and the disease-related antibodies.[5]
- Occasionally newborns present with the eruption. They typically have a mild course that resolves within weeks. The newborn has minimal risk of adrenal suppression, regardless of the mother's dose of steroids.
- The mother is at high risk of recurrent pemphigoid gestationis with subsequent pregnancies and at an increased lifetime risk of Grave's disease.[2,4]

PATIENT RESOURCES

About.com. Pemphigoid gestationis—**http://dermatology. about.com/cs/pregnancy/a/pemphgest.htm.**

DermNet NZ—**http://www.dermnetnz.org/immune/ pemphigoid-gestationis.html.**

PROVIDER RESOURCES

EMedicine. Pemphigoid Gestationis—**http://www.emedicine. com/derm/topic178.htm.**

The Merck Manual Online—**http://www.merck.com/ mrkshared/mmanual/section18/chapter252/252h.jsp.**

REFERENCES

1. Roger D, Vaillant L, Fignon A, et al. Specific pruritic diseases of pregnancy. A prospective study of 3192 pregnant women. *Arch Dermatol.* 1994;130:734.

2. Shornick JK. Dermatoses of pregnancy. *Semin Cutan Med Surg.* 1998; 17:172.

3. Jenkins RE, Hern S, Black MM. Clinical features and management of 87 patients with pemphigoid gestationis. *Clin Exp Dermatol.* 1999;24(4):255-259.

4. Jenkins RE, Hern S, Black MM. Clinical features and management of 87 patients with pemphigoid gestationis. *Clin Exp Dermatol.* 1999;24:255.

5. Jenkins, RE, Shornick, JK, Black, BL. Pemphigoid gestationis. *J Eur Acad Dermatol Venereol.* 1993;2:163.

73 FIRST TRIMESTER ULTRASOUND

E.J. Mayeaux, Jr., MD

PATIENT STORY

A 22-year-old woman presents with no menstrual period for approximately 2 months (she has irregular menses.) She is complaining of morning sickness but is otherwise feeling well. A urine pregnancy test confirms she is pregnant. **Figure 73-1** shows a fetus of 9 weeks estimated gestational age (EGA).

EPIDEMIOLOGY

- Women who receive antenatal care have lower maternal and perinatal mortality and better pregnancy outcomes.[1] However, the optimal components of prenatal care have not been rigorously examined in well-designed studies.

- In the United States in 2003, 84.1% of pregnant women obtained prenatal care in the first trimester, and only 3.5% received no care or initiated prenatal care in the third trimester.

- Ultrasonography (US) allows for a relatively detailed assessment of fetal gestational age, development, and anatomy in utero. Most pregnancies in the United States undergo ultrasound imaging for various indications.

ETIOLOGY AND PATHOPHYSIOLOGY

- Ultrasound is used to estimate gestational age and to calculate the expected date of delivery (EDD). Ultrasound is especially helpful when menses are irregular, the last menstrual period (LMP) is unknown, or in patients who conceived while using hormonal contraceptives.

- The routine antenatal diagnostic imaging with ultrasound (RADIUS) trial was a randomized trial of routine obstetrical ultrasound screening.[2] It included over 15,000 women in the United States. The trial showed that routine ultrasound screening was associated with a significantly increased detection of fetal anomalies, but no improvement in any perinatal outcome, including mortality, preterm birth, birth weight, and neonatal morbidity.

- First trimester vaginal bleeding is found in 20% to 40% of pregnancies. The differential diagnoses include possible spontaneous abortion, ectopic pregnancy, and gestational trophoblastic disease.

- Ectopic pregnancy causes a significant degree of morbidity and mortality if untreated, often through tubal rupture with potentially life-threatening hemorrhage. Identification of an intrauterine pregnancy effectively excludes the possibility of an ectopic in almost all cases, unless conception involved assisted reproductive technology.

- Threatened, incomplete, or complete spontaneous abortion may cause first trimester bleeding. Up to one-third of recognized pregnancies end

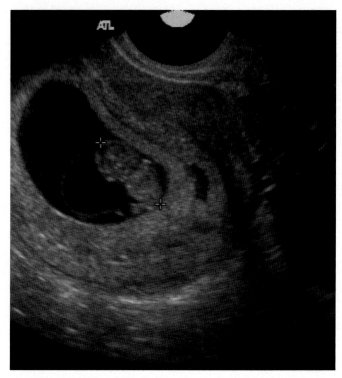

FIGURE 73-1 Ultrasound examination of a fetus of 9 weeks estimated gestational age. The ultrasound was performed with a vaginal probe and the membranes are visible. (*Courtesy of E.J. Mayeaux, Jr., MD.*)

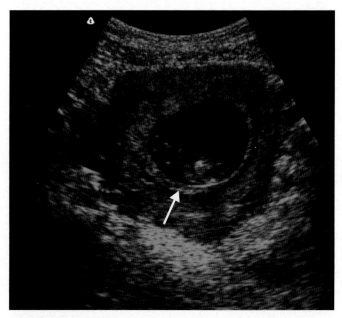

FIGURE 73-2 Ultrasound examination of a 9-week EGA twin with abdominal probe. The arrow is pointing to the yolk sac. Only one of the twins is visible. (*Courtesy of E.J. Mayeaux, Jr., MD.*)

in early pregnancy loss. Ectopic pregnancy may also be a concern. US may be used to determine if a gestational sac is present in the uterus.

- Ultrasound used in conjunction with serum screening is the most sensitive way to detect aneuploidy. When performed in the first trimester, the two modalities can detect over 90% of fetuses with Down's syndrome or with other aneuploidies. The majority of abnormal serum tests recalculated based on US corrected expected date of delivery.

DIAGNOSIS

- The goals of a basic first trimester ultrasound examination include:[3]
  - Confirm the presence of an intrauterine (or evaluate suspected extrauterine) pregnancy.
  - Assess gestational age.
  - Determine fetal viability.
  - Determine whether a multiple gestation is present.
  - Evaluate maternal pelvic organs for congenital or acquired abnormalities.
- Fetal biometric measurements are used to calculate gestational age and weight and may be performed via the transvaginal ultrasonography and/or the transabdominal ultrasonography route. Since the variation in size from fetus to fetus is minimal in the first trimester, this is the optimal time to obtain an estimate of gestational age. Transvaginal ultrasonography is typically used early for evaluation of the gestational sac, yolk sac, and developing embryo, while transabdominal ultrasonography usually provides better visualization later in the first trimester.
- During the first 5 weeks of pregnancy, the endometrium has a "triaminar" appearance, and usually does not show distinct evidence of an intrauterine pregnancy. The gestational sac is the first detectable sign on ultrasound. Initial gestational age measurements are based on diameter of the sac. The yolk sac (**Figure 73-2**) is the first anatomic structure to appear within the gestational sac around the fifth week of gestation. A gestational sac diameter of 8 mm or greater with an empty or no fetal pole yolk sac indicates an abnormal gestation.[4]
- The embryonic disc becomes visible at about a gestational age of 5 to 6 weeks.[5] If the embryo is visible, but too small to measure, detection of cardiac activity establishes a gestational age of approximately 6 weeks. Direct measurement of the crown-rump length of the embryo provides the most accurate estimate of gestational age once the fetal pole is evident (**Figure 73-3**). The crown-rump length is the mean of three measurements of the longest straight-line length of the embryo from the outer margin of the cephalic pole to the rump.
- The biparietal diameter may be used later in the first trimester (**Figure 73-4**). It is highly reproducible and can predict gestational age within 7 days when measured between 14 and 20 weeks of gestation. The biparietal diameter should be measured on a plane of section that intersects both the third ventricle and thalami. The falx cerebri should be visible. The cursors are placed on the outer edge of the proximal skull and the inner edge of the distal skull to take the measurement. The femur length can be assessed by 10 weeks gestational age, but is more accurate after 20 weeks gestation.

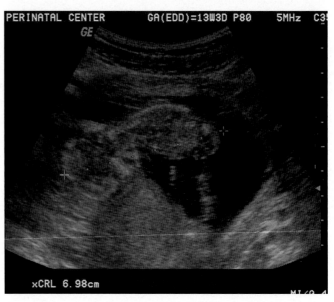

FIGURE 73-3 Ultrasound examination of a 13-week 3-day fetus by dates showing the head and spine with crown-to-rump length measurement of 6.98 cm. This represents an EGA of 13-week 3-day by ultrasound estimation. (essentially equal to dates.) (*Courtesy of E.J. Mayeaux, Jr., MD.*)

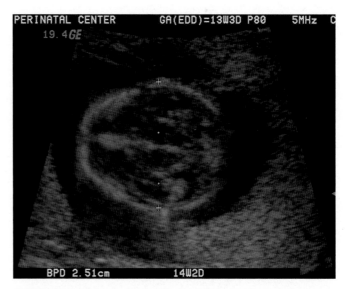

FIGURE 73-4 Ultrasound examination of the same 13-week 3-day fetus showing the biparietal diameter of 2.51 cm producing an EGA of 14 week and 2 days. A 1-week disparity is within the measurement error of ultrasound at this stage of the pregnancy. (*Courtesy of E.J. Mayeaux, Jr., MD.*)

REFERENCES

1. Villar J, Bergsjo P. Scientific basis for the content of routine antenatal care. Philosophy, recent studies, and power to eliminate or alleviate adverse maternal outcomes. *Acta Obstet Gynecol Scand.* 1997;76:1.

2. Ewigman BG, et al. Effect of prenatal ultrasound screening on perinatal outcome. RADIUS Study Group. *N Engl J Med.* 1993;329:821.

3. American Institute of Ultrasound in Medicine. AIUM Standards and Guidelines. http://www.aium.org/publications/clinical/obstetrical.pdf. Accessed July 4, 2006.

4. Levi CS, Lyons EA, Lindsay DJ. Early diagnosis of nonviable pregnancy with endovaginal US. *Radiology.* 1988;167:383.

5. Goldstein SR, Wolfson R. Endovaginal ultrasonographic measurement of early embryonic size as a means of assessing gestational age. *J Ultrasound Med.* 1994; 13:27.

74 SECOND TRIMESTER ULTRASOUND

E.J. Mayeaux, Jr., MD

PATIENT STORY

A 23-year-old pregnant G2P1 woman is being seen for ultrasound because of her uncertain dates. Her best recollection of her last period gave her an estimated gestational age (EGA) of 19 weeks. Her vital signs are normal and her fundal height is 20 cm. **Figures 74-1** to **74-3** are still images taken from her ultrasound examination demonstrating a EGA of 21 weeks and 6 days by measurement of the baby's biparietal diameter (BPD), head circumference (HC), abdominal circumference (AC), and femur length (FL). All four measurements allow the computer to calculate an estimated fetal weight of 431 g. The pregnancy proceeded without complications and the patient delivered a healthy boy at 40⅓ weeks based on the ultrasound calculated estimated date of delivery. No interventions were needed for postdates because of the ultrasound calculations earlier in the pregnancy.

INDICATIONS FOR ULTRASOUND

- Second and third trimester ultrasound examination can be used to determine fetal number and presentation, and for documentation of fetal cardiac activity, placental location, and amniotic fluid volume.

- Second trimester is a good time to perform ultrasound for fetal assessment for gestational age and weight, and it is also an integral part of performing amniocentesis.

- Fetal anatomy evaluation is best performed now. If fetal abnormalities are detected, a more detailed examination (level 2 ultrasound) by a specialized sonogropher is indicated.

- Ultrasound examination is indicated to establish the number of fetuses when multiple gestation is suspected. Risk factors for multiple gestation pregnancy include assisted reproductive technology, family history of twins (or higher multiples), and uterine size larger than that expected by menstrual dating. The number of fetuses can be best established by obtaining an image that includes a cross-section of all fetal poles that have distinct cardiac activity within a single frame.

- The cervix and lower uterine segment may be imaged in the second trimester to look for funneling (membranes protruding into the cervical canal), a short cervix or placenta previa.[1]

PATHOPHYSIOLOGY

- Fetal abnormalities that may be reliably diagnosed by ultrasound include achondroplasia, anencephaly, cleft lip, clubfoot, duodenal

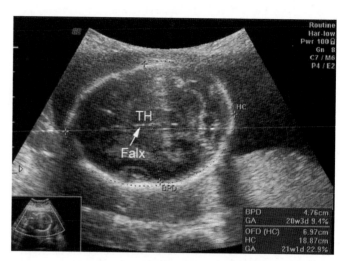

FIGURE 74-1 Ultrasound examination of a 21-week EGA fetus showing measurement of the baby's biparietal diameter (BPD) and head circumference (HC). Note the presence of the falx cerebri and the thalamus (TH) to ensure the measurement is at the right anatomic level. (see arrows). (*Courtesy of E.J. Mayeaux, Jr., MD.*)

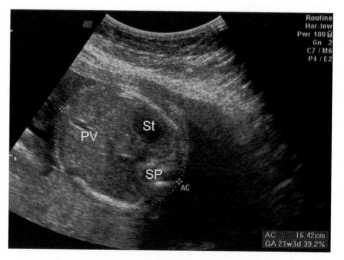

FIGURE 74-2 Ultrasound examination of a 21-week EGA fetus showing measurement of the baby's abdominal circumference (AC). Note how the stomach, spine, and portal vein are all visible to ensure that the measurement is at the right anatomic level. (*Courtesy of E.J. Mayeaux, Jr., MD.*)

atresia, fetal hydrops, gastroschisis, hydrocephalus, myelomeningo-
cele, omphalocele, renal abnormalities, and spina bifida. If anomalies are suspected, a level 3 ultrasound with an experienced sonog-
rapher is indicated.

- Up to 5% of pregnancies will have placentas that partially or completely cover the internal cervical os at 16 to 18 weeks of gestation.
Only one in ten of these will continue to cover the internal os in
the late third trimester.[2] Placentas that are clear of the cervix in
early pregnancy will not encroach upon it later.

INDICATIONS FOR OB ULTRASOUNDS IN SECOND TRIMESTER

- Evaluating the possibility of a fetal anomaly is best done by
ultrasound examination after 16 weeks of gestation since earlier
examination may be limited by fetal size and development.

- The sensitivity and specificity of the procedure for detecting
congenital abnormalities varies depending upon the specific defect,
the gestational age, the quality of the ultrasound unit, and the skill
of the ultrasonographer.

- Ultrasound examination is the main diagnostic modality used to
evaluate second and third trimester bleeding. The major placental
causes of vaginal bleeding at this time are placenta previa and
abruptio placentae. A transvaginal obstetric ultrasound examination
can identify placental location, and is safe even when placenta previa is present. The images should be obtained after the mother has
emptied her bladder to avoid displacement of the anterior lower
uterine segment thus producing a false positive test.[3]

- Fetal intrauterine growth limiting disorders are more likely when
the uterine size is less than appropriate for gestational age, a prior
pregnancy has been affected by growth restriction, with maternal
hypertension, and in multiple gestations. Ultrasound cannot distinguish between a constitutionally small fetus and a pathologically
small fetus. Decreased amniotic fluid volume and below normal interval growth make placental insufficiency more likely.

PERFORMING THE PROCEDURE

- The four standard biometric parameters commonly used to
estimate gestational age and/or fetal weight in the second are: BPD,
HC (**Figure 74-1**), AC (**Figure 74-2**), and FL (**Figure 74-3**).[4]
They are usually obtained by transabdominal ultrasound examination, and the fetal weight is calculated.

- The BPD (**Figure 74-1**) is a highly reproducible measurement and
can predict gestational age within ±7 days when the ultrasound is
performed between 14 and 20 weeks gestation, although the best
time to get an accurate date is in the first trimester. The BPD
should be measured on a plane that includes both the third ventricle
and the thalamus. The cursors are placed on the outer edge of the
proximal skull and the inner edge of the distal skull and the BPD
measured.

- The cephalic index is ratio of the BPD and the occipitofrontal diameter multiplied by 100. It should be used where the BPD may be

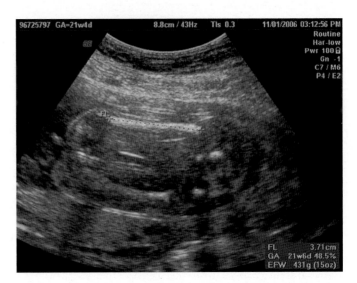

FIGURE 74-3 Ultrasound measurement of the same baby's femur
length giving an EGA of 21 weeks and 6 days. Note the buttocks and
penis are visible. All four measurements from Figures 74-1 to 74-3 allow
the computer to calculate an estimated fetal weight (EFW) of 431
grams. (*Courtesy of E.J. Mayeaux, Jr., MD.*)

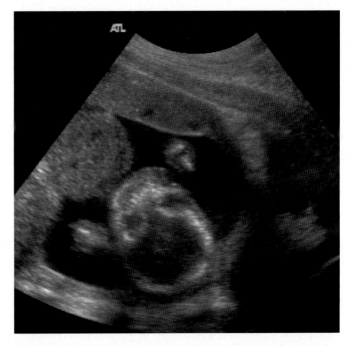

FIGURE 74-4 Ultrasound examination of a 15-week EGA fetus showing the baby's face. (*Courtesy of E.J. Mayeaux, Jr., MD.*)

inaccurate, such as with breech presentations, oligohydramnios, premature rupture of the membranes, and neural tube abnormalities.

- The measurement of fetal HC also accurately estimates gestational age, and is especially useful in the setting of growth disorders (**Figure 74-1**). The accuracy decreases in the second half of pregnancy. The HC should be measured on a plane that includes the third ventricle, the thalamus, the cavum septum pellucidum anteriorly, and the tentorial hiatus posteriorly. Unlike the BPD measurements, the HC measurement is obtained by placing the cursors on the outer margins of the calvarium bilaterally.

- The AC (**Figure 74-2**) is the least accurate in predicting gestational age, being accurate within 2 weeks in the second trimester. It is most often used for estimations of fetal weight and interval growth evaluations rather than fetal dating. The measurement should be taken at the level of the largest diameter of the fetal liver where the right and left portal veins join. The four calipers are placed around the abdomen on the skin edge to draw a circular line for AC measurement.

- Femur length (**Figure 74-3**) can be measured and is accurate to within 1 week before 20 weeks gestation. Align the transducer along the long axis of the femoral bone and visualize either the femoral head or the greater trochanter proximally, and the end of the femur or the femoral condyle distally. Make sure you are measuring the femur and not another long bone in the arm or leg. Place the calipers at the bone and cartilage junction and measure only ossified bone, not including the femoral head.

- Many providers will often show expectant parents images of the baby's face (**Figures 74-4** and **74-5**), hands (**Figure 74-6**), and sex (**Figures 74-7** and **74-8**).

- The cervix and placenta should be examined for signs of placenta previa.

PATIENT RESOURCES

OB Ultrasound A Comprehensive Guide—**http://www.ob-ultrasound.net/**.

RadiologyInfo—**http://www.radiologyinfo.org/en/info.cfm?pg=obstetricus&bhcp=1**.

PROVIDER RESOURCES

The Society of Obstetricians and Gynaecologists of Canada (SOGC) recommends a single "routine" ultrasound evaluation at 16 to 20 weeks in all pregnancies and suggests that 8 markers be evaluated based on an EBM review of the literature—**http://www.sogc.org/guidelines/pdf/JOGC-june05-Fetalmarkers-revised-ENG-CPG.pdf**.

Perinatology.com, Level 2 Ultrasound—**http://www.perinatology.com/ultrasound.htm**.

FP Notebook has a number of chapters—**http://www.fpnotebook.com/OB167.htm**.

The Fetus.net—**http://www.thefetus.net/page.php?id=593**.

Obstetric Ultrasound by Dr. Joseph Woo—**http://www.ob-ultrasound.net/**.

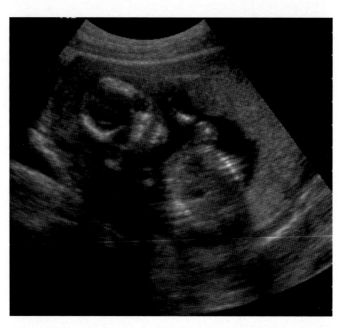

FIGURE 74-5 Ultrasound examination of a 15-week EGA fetus showing another view of the baby's face. (*Courtesy of E.J. Mayeaux, Jr., MD.*)

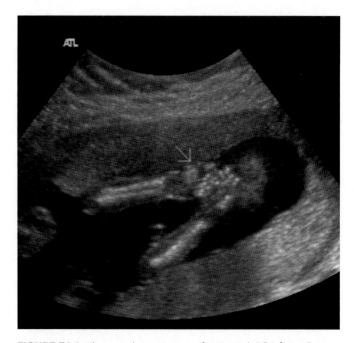

FIGURE 74-6 Ultrasound examination of a 19-week EGA fetus showing the baby's hands and forearms. Arrow is pointing at the right hand. (*Courtesy of E.J. Mayeaux, Jr., MD.*)

REFERENCES

1. Expert Panel on Women's Imaging. Premature cervical dilatation. American College of Radiology, Reston, Virginia 1999. http://www.acr.org/s_acr/sec.asp?CID=1845&DID=16050. Accessed July 4, 2006.

2. Townsend, RR, Laing, FC, Nyberg, DA, et al. Technical factors responsible for "placental migration": sonographic assessment. *Radiology* 1986;160:105.

3. American Institute of Ultrasound in Medicine. AIUM Standards and Guidelines. http://www.aium.org/publications/clinical/obstetrical.pdf. Accessed July 4, 2006.

4. Hadlock, FP. Sonographic estimation of fetal age and weight. *Radiol Clin North Am* 1990;28:39.

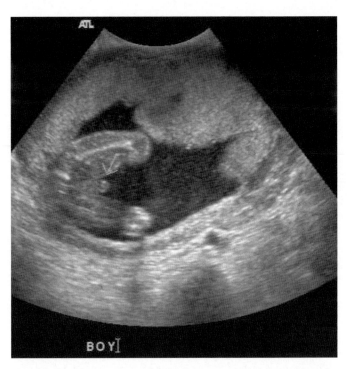

FIGURE 74-7 Ultrasound examination of a 19-week EGA fetus showing the baby is a boy (arrow). (*Courtesy of E.J. Mayeaux, Jr., MD.*)

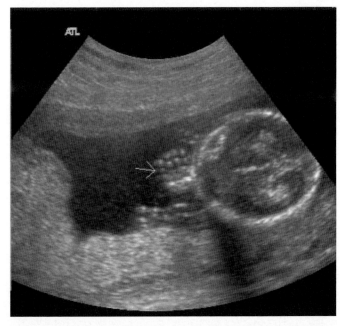

FIGURE 74-8 Ultrasound examination of a 19-week EGA fetus sucking his thumb (arrow). The two hemispheres of the brain are visible with the falx cerebri in between. (*Courtesy of E.J. Mayeaux, Jr., MD.*)

75 OBSTETRICS—THIRD TRIMESTER ULTRASOUND

E.J. Mayeaux, Jr., MD

PATIENT STORY

A 26-year-old woman gravida 3, para 2-0-0-2 with a singleton pregnancy at 27 weeks gestation is concerned because her sister had a fetal demise and she thinks her baby is moving less. An ultrasound demonstrating normal anatomy (**Figures 75-1** to **75-3**) and strong fetal heart motion is very reassuring (**Figure 75-4**).

INDICATIONS FOR USE

- Third trimester ultrasound examination can be used to determine fetal number and presentation, and for documentation of fetal cardiac activity, placental location, and amniotic fluid volume.

- A Cochrane review of seven studies showed no difference in obstetric, antenatal, or neonatal interventions between women undergoing routine late ultrasound examination after 24 weeks and those who did not.[1] In addition, there was no difference in perinatal outcome measures, such as admission to a neonatal intensive care unit, birthweight <10th percentile, or perinatal mortality.

- Hydrops fetalis is the accumulation of fluid in fetal tissues and body cavities usually due to immune pathologic conditions (**Figure 75-5**). Serial ultrasound examinations are useful for following pregnancies at risk for developing hydrops or to evaluate treatment.

- Ultrasound may also be used to evaluate third trimester bleeding. The major placental causes of vaginal bleeding at this time are placenta previa (**Figure 75-6**) and abruptio placentae.

- Ultrasound can safely image maternal abdominal organs during pregnancy. Ovarian cysts, uterine leiomyoma, renal obstruction, and gallbladder or liver disease can be evaluated without using ionizing radiation.

VALUE OF ULTRASOUND IN THIRD TRIMESTER

- Ultrasound-based determination of EDD has been shown to improve dating and thus reduce intervention for postterm pregnancy. One randomized controlled trial evaluated the effect of routine ultrasound examinations at 18 and 32 weeks of gestation on the accuracy of dating and pregnancy outcome in a low-risk population.[2] They found that ultrasound screening reduced the incidence of induced labor for postterm pregnancy by 70%, and also reduced the incidence of induction for all causes. They also found that the proportion of 5 minute Apgar scores <8 and the need for positive pressure ventilation were both lower in the screened group.

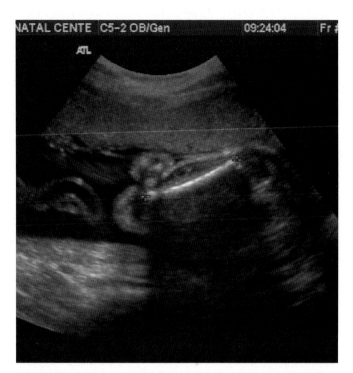

FIGURE 75-1 Ultrasound examination of a 27-week estimated gestational age (EGA) fetus showing measurement of the baby's humerus. (*Courtesy of E.J. Mayeaux, Jr., MD.*)

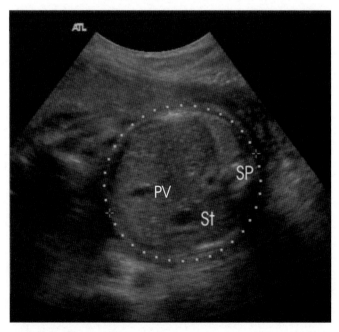

FIGURE 75-2 Ultrasound examination of a 27-week EGA fetus showing the baby's stomach (ST), abdomen, spine (SP), and left portal vein (LPV). (*Courtesy of E.J. Mayeaux, Jr., MD.*)

- Although ultrasound EDD determination as late as 34 weeks can reduce the number of pregnancies diagnosed as postterm, first trimester ultrasound in a low-risk population is more effective than later ultrasound in decreasing postterm pregnancy.

- Accurate assessment of gestational age is important so as not to inappropriately initiate tocolysis for near-term labor.

- Signs suggestive of fetal maturity may also be found on ultrasound. The femoral epiphyseal ossification center can be visualized by 32 weeks gestational age, and proximal tibial center can be visualized by 35 weeks. The proximal humeral epiphysis also appears in the late third trimester and correlates well with fetal lung maturity.

- Twin pregnancies are at increased risk of complications, such as fetal heart rate abnormalities and complications as a result of malpresentation. When both twins are found on ultrasound to be vertex (42% of twins) a trial of labor with the goal of a vaginal delivery is appropriate. When one twin is nonvertex (38% of twins) options include cesarean delivery of both twins, or attempted vaginal delivery of one or both twins.[3,4]

- Parents are now paying for 3D ultrasounds so that they can see and get pictures of their developing child. The 3D ultrasound is not a standard medical device (**Figure 75-7**).

FOLLOW-UP

- When a patient has placenta previa diagnosed on ultrasound, advise patient to avoid coitus, digital cervical examination, and exercise. Counsel her to seek immediate medical attention if there is any vaginal bleeding or uterine contractions. Advise her that cesarean delivery is the delivery route of choice.[5]

PATIENT RESOURCES

Ob Ultrasound A Comprehensive Guide—**http://www.ob-ultrasound.net/**.

March of Dimes pregnancy education center—**http://www.marchofdimes.com/pnhec/159_523.asp**.

PROVIDER RESOURCES

FP Notebook has a number of chapters—**http://www.fpnotebook.com/OB167.htm**.

The Fetus.net—**http://www.thefetus.net/page.php?id =593**.

Obstetric Ultrasound by Dr. Joseph Woo—**http://www.ob-ultrasound.net/**.

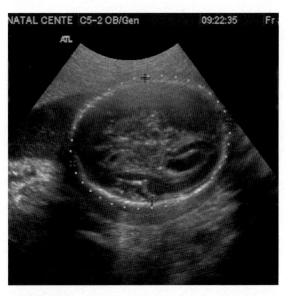

FIGURE 75-3 Ultrasound examination of a 27-week EGA fetus showing measurement of the baby's biparietal diameter (BPD). (*Courtesy of E.J. Mayeaux, Jr., MD.*)

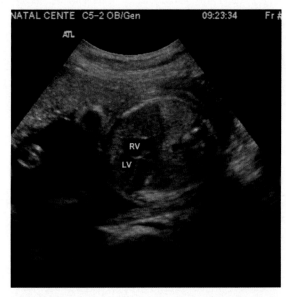

FIGURE 75-4 Ultrasound examination of a 27-week EGA fetus showing all four chambers of the baby's heart. (*Courtesy of E.J. Mayeaux, Jr., MD.*)

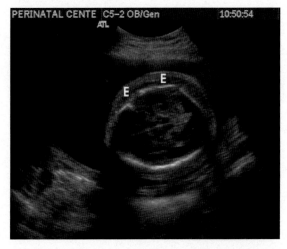

FIGURE 75-5 Ultrasound examination showing scalp edema (E) associated with hydrops fetalis. (*Courtesy of E.J. Mayeaux, Jr., MD.*)

REFERENCES

1. Bricker L, Neilson, JP. Routine ultrasound in late pregnancy (after 24 weeks gestation). *Cochrane Database Syst Rev.* 2000; CD001451.

2. Eik-Nes SH, Salvesen KA, Okland O, Vatten LJ. Routine ultrasound fetal examination in pregnancy: The 'Alesund' random-ized controlled trial. *Ultrasound Obstet Gynecol.* 2000;15:473.

3. Chasen ST, Spiro SJ, Kalish RB, Chervenak FA. Changes in fetal presentation in twin pregnancies. *J Matern Fetal Neonatal Med.* 2005;17:45.

4. Dodd JM, Crowther CA. Evidence-based care of women with a multiple pregnancy. *Best Pract Res Clin Obstet Gynaecol.* 2005;19:131.

5. Bhide A, Prefumo F, Moore J, et al. Placental edge to internal os distance in the late third trimester and mode of delivery in placenta praevia. *BJOG.* 2003;110:860.

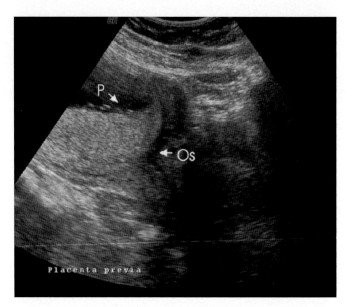

FIGURE 75-6 Ultrasound examination showing the placenta (P) cover-ing the cervical os (Os) in placenta previa. (*Courtesy of E.J. Mayeaux, Jr., MD.*)

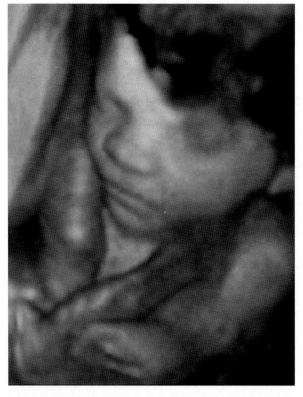

FIGURE 75-7 3D ultrasound showing a 25-week fetus. (*Courtesy of E.J. Mayeaux, Jr., MD.*)

SECTION 2   VAGINITIS AND CERVICITIS

76 VAGINITIS

E.J. Mayeaux, Jr., MD

EPIDEMIOLOGY

- Vaginal discharge is a frequent presenting complaint in primary care. The three most common causes are bacterial vaginosis, candidiasis and trichomoniasis. However, a significant number of patients with vaginal discharge will have some other condition such as atrophic vaginitis.

- The reported rates of chlamydia and gonorrhea are highest among females aged 15 to 19 years. Adolescents are at greater risk for STDs because they frequently have unprotected intercourse, are biologically more susceptible to infection, are often engaged in partnerships of limited duration, and face multiple obstacles to utilization of health care.[1]

ETIOLOGY AND PATHOPHYSIOLOGY

- Physicians must refrain from "diagnosing" a vaginitis based solely on the color and consistency of the discharge, since this may lead to misdiagnosis and may miss concomitant infections.[1]

- Before starting an examination, determined whether the patient douched recently, because this can lower the yield of diagnostic tests and increase the risk of pelvic inflammatory disease.[2] Patients who have been told not to douche will sometimes start wiping the vagina with soapy washcloths, which also irritates the vagina and cervix and may cause a discharge.

- There are many causes of vaginitis in humans. Infectious causes include bacterial vaginosis (40% to 50% of cases) (**Figures 76-1** and **76-2**), vulvovaginal candidiasis (20% to 25%), and trichomonas (15% to 20%) (**Figure 76-3**).[3] Less common causes include atrophic vaginitis, foreign body (especially in children), cytolytic or desquamative inflammatory vaginitis, streptococcal vaginitis, ulcerative vaginitis, and idiopathic vulvovaginal ulceration associated with HIV infection.

- Rarer noninfectious causes include chemicals, allergies, hypersensitivity, contact dermatitis, trauma, postpuerperal atrophic vaginitis, erosive lichen planus, collagen vascular disease, Behçet's syndrome, and pemphigus syndromes.

DIAGNOSIS (Table 76-1)

- Examine the external genitalia for irritation or discharge (**Figure 76-2**). Speculum examination is done to determine the amount and character of the discharge (**Figure 76-4**). A chlamydia and gonorrhea test should always be done in sexually active females. Look

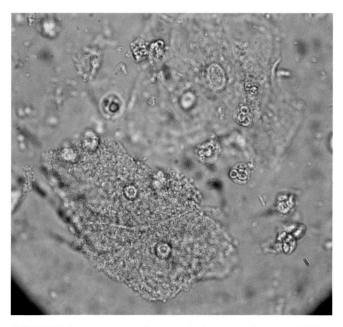

FIGURE 76-1 A wet mount of vaginal discharge in saline under high power light microscopy. Note the presence of vaginal epithelial cells, smaller white blood cells (polymorphonucleocytes) and bacteria. The bacteria are the coccobacilli of *Gardnerella vaginalis* covering the cell membranes of the two vaginal epithelial cells near the lower end of the field. These are clue cells seen in patients with bacterial vaginosis. (*Courtesy of Richard P. Usatine, MD.*)

closely at the cervix for discharge and signs of infection, dysplasia or cancer (**Figure 76-3**). Bimanual examination may show evidence of cervical, uterine, or adnexal tenderness. **Table 76-1** shows diagnostic values for examination of vaginitis.

- Vaginal pH testing can be helpful in the diagnosis of vaginitis. The pH can be checked by applying pH paper to the vaginal sidewall. Do not place the pH paper in contact with the cervical mucus. A pH above 4.5 is seen with menopausal patients, trichomonas infection, or bacterial vaginosis.

- Wet preps are obtained by applying a cotton-tipped applicator to the vaginal sidewall and placing the sample into normal saline. A drop of the suspension is then placed on a slide and examined for the presence and number of white blood cells (WBCs), trichomonads, candidal hyphae, or clue cells (**Figure 76-1**).

- A KOH prep is made by adding a drop of KOH solution to a drop of saline suspension of the discharge. The KOH lyses epithelial cells in 5 to15 minutes (faster if the slide is warmed briefly over a flame) and allows easier visualization of candidal hyphae. The use of KOH with DMSO allows for quicker lyses of the epithelial cells and immediate examination of the smear.

- Another diagnostic procedure is the "whiff" test, which is performed by placing a drop of KOH on a slide of the wet prep and smelling for a foul, fishy odor. The odor is indicative of anaerobic overgrowth or infection. The "whiff" test is positive if the fishy amine odor is detected during the exam and it is then not necessary to add KOH and "whiff" again.

- Nucleic acid amplification tests are highly sensitive tests for *N. gonorrhoeae*, *Chlamydia*, and *C. trachomatis* that can be performed on genital specimens or urine. Urine screening for gonorrhea, chlamydia, or both using nucleic acid amplification test can be used successfully in difficult-to-reach adolescents.[4]

MANAGEMENT

- Management is based on the identification of the causative agent.
- Health food store lactobacilli are the wrong strain and not adhere well to the vaginal epithelium. Ingestion of live-culture, nonpasteurized yogurt does not significantly change the incidence of candidal vulvovaginitis or bacterial vaginosis.[5]

PATIENT RESOURCES

Centers for Disease Control and Prevention. 2006 Guidelines for Treatment of Sexually Transmitted Diseases—**http://www.cdc.gov/std/treatment/default.htm#tg2006.**

Indiana University Health Center—**http://www.indiana.edu/~health/vaginiti.html.**

Planned parenthood—**http://www.plannedparenthood.org/pp2/portal/files/portal/medicalinfo/femalesexualhealth/pubvaginitis.xml.**

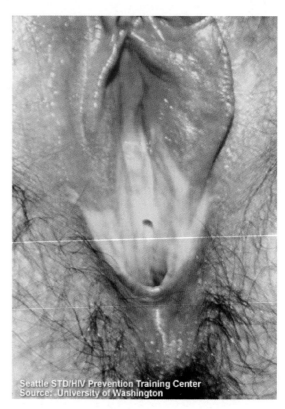

FIGURE 76-2 Thin white discharge from bacterial vaginosis seen covering the introitus prior to speculum exam. (*Courtesy of University of Washington STD/HIV Prevention Training Center.*)

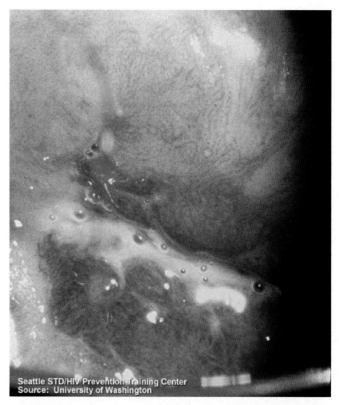

FIGURE 76-3 Colposcopic view of the cervix in a patient infected with trichomonas vaginalis. Note the frothy discharge with visible bubbles and the cervical erythema. (*Courtesy of University of Washington STD/HIV Prevention Training Center.*)

TABLE 76-1 Diagnostic Values for Vaginal Infections

Diagnostic Criteria	Normal	Bacterial Vaginosis	Trichomonas Vaginitis	Candida Vulvovaginitis
Vaginal pH	3.8–4.2	>4.5	4.5	<4.5 (usually)
Discharge	White, thin, flocculent	Thin, white, gray	Yellow, green, or gray, frothy	White, curdy, "cottage cheese"
Amine odor "whiff" test	Absent	Fishy	Fishy	Absent
Microscopic	Lactobacilli, epithelial cells	Clue cells, adherent cocci, no WBCs	Trichomonads, WBCs >10/hpf	Budding yeast, hyphae, pseudohyphae

(Courtesy of E.J. Mayeaux, Jr., MD.)

PROVIDER RESOURCES

Centers for Disease Control and Prevention. 2006 Guidelines for Treatment of Sexually Transmitted Diseases— **http://www.cdc.gov/std/treatment/default.htm#tg2006.**

CDC STD Page—**http://www.cdc.gov/std/.**

EMedicine—**http://www.emedicine.com/med/topic 2358.htm.**

American Family Physician—**http://www.aafp.org/afp/ 20000901/1095.html.**

REFERENCES

1. CDC. Sexually transmitted disease surveillance 2001. Atlanta, Georgia: U.S. Department of Health and Human Services, CDC, 2002.

2. Zhang J, Thomas AG, Leybovich E. Vaginal douching and adverse health effects: A meta-analysis. *Am J Public Health.* 1997;87: 1207–1211.

3. Sobel JD. Vaginitis. *N Engl J Med.* 1997;337:1896–1903.

4. Monroe KW, Weiss HL, Jones M, Hook EW, 3rd. Acceptability of urine screening for Neisseria gonorrheae and Chlamydia trachomatis in adolescents at an urban emergency department. *Sex Transm Dis.* 2003;30:850–853.

5. Pirotta M, Gunn J, Chondros P, et al. Effect of lactobacillus in preventing post-antibiotic vulvovaginal candidiasis: A randomised controlled trial. *BMJ.* 2004;329:548.

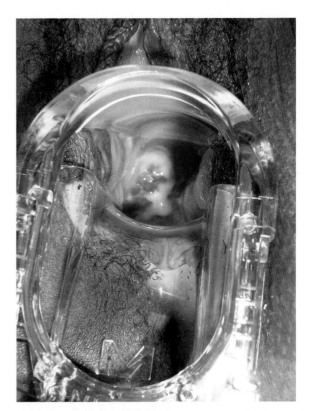

FIGURE 76-4 Speculum exam showing mucopurulent discharge with a friable appearing cervix. (*Courtesy of Richard P. Usatine, MD.*)

77 ATROPHIC VAGINITIS

E.J. Mayeaux, Jr., MD

PATIENT STORY

A 60-year-old woman with vaginal dryness and irritation is seen to
follow-up on an inflammatory pap smear. She denies discharge, odor,
douching, and STD exposure. She does admit to some postcoital
bleeding. Her cervix has atrophic changes and an endocervical polyp
(**Figure 77-1**). The polyp was removed easily with a ring forceps and
no dysplasia was found on pathology. She also had thinning of the hair
and thinning and erythema of vulvar skin associated with atrophic vulvitis (**Figure 77-2**).

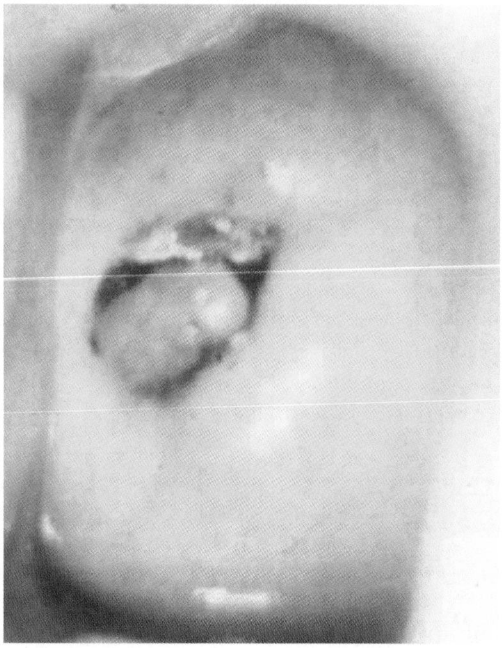

EPIDEMIOLOGY

- The average age of menopause is 51 years in the United States.

- Approximately 5% of women experience menopause after age 55
  (late menopause), and another 5% experience the transition
  between the ages 40 to 45 years (early menopause). This means that
  in the United States, most women will live a significant portion of
  their lives during menopause. Women who in menopause have surgical menopause or have ovarian suppression without estrogen supplementation (progestin only contraceptives) are susceptible to atrophic changes in their lower genital tract.

ETIOLOGY AND PATHOPHYSIOLOGY

- After menopause, circulating estrogen levels dramatically decrease
  to a level at least one-sixth their premenopausal levels.[1] Changes
  that occur in the vaginal and cervical epithelium include proliferation
  of connective tissue, loss of elastin, and hyalinization of collagen.

- A long-term decrease in estrogen is generally necessary before
  symptoms become apparent. Genital symptoms include decreased
  vaginal lubrication, dryness, burning, dyspareunia, leukorrhea, itching, and yellow malodorous discharge.

- Urinary symptoms such as frequency, hematuria, urinary tract infection, dysuria, and stress incontinence are usually late symptoms. Over
  time, the lack of vaginal lubrication often results in sexual dysfunction.

- Cervical polyps (**Figure 77-1**) are pedunculated tumors that usually arise from the endocervical canal mucosa, and are common in
  patients with atrophic vaginitis. Many will show squamous metaplasia, and they may develop squamous dysplasia. Polyps are most
  commonly asymptomatic unless they bleed.

- Menopause is the most common cause of atrophic vaginitis. In premenopausal women, radiation therapy, chemotherapy, immunologic
  disorders, and oophorectomy may greatly decrease production of
  ovarian estrogen and lead to atrophic vaginitis. Antiestrogen medications may also result in atrophic vaginitis. Women who are naturally premenopausally estrogen deficient, smoke cigarettes, or have
  not given vaginal birth tend to have more severe symptoms.[1]

FIGURE 77-1 Colposcopic photograph (scanning objective with 10X
eyepiece) demonstrating atrophic vaginitis. Note thinned white epithelium, friable epithelium with bleeding, and a cervical polyp. (*Courtesy
of E.J. Mayeaux, Jr., MD.*)

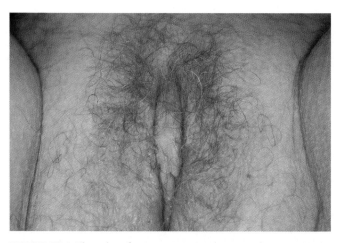

FIGURE 77-2 The vulva of a postmenopausal women demonstrating
thinning of the hair and thinning and erythema of vulvar skin associated
with atrophic vulvitis. (*Courtesy of Gordon Davis, MD., Arizona Vulva
Clinic, Inc.*)

DIAGNOSIS

CLINICAL FEATURES

Atrophic vaginal and cervical epithelium appears pale, smooth, relatively dry, and shiny. Inflammation with patchy erythema, petechiae, and friability are common in more advanced cases. The external genitalia may demonstrate diminished elasticity, turgor of skin, sparsity of pubic hair, dryness of labia, erythema (**Figure 77-2**), and fusion of the labia minora.

LABORATORY STUDIES

A serum follicle stimulating hormone (FSH) level greater than 40 ImU/mL is diagnostic of menopause. A Papanicolaou smear can confirm the presence of urogenital atrophy. Cytologic examination of smears from the upper one-third of the vagina shows an increased proportion of parabasal cells and a decreased percentage of superficial cells. An elevated vaginal pH level (>5), monitored by a pH strip in the vaginal vault, and may also be a sign of vaginal atrophy.[1]

DIFFERENTIAL DIAGNOSIS

- Atrophic vaginitis symptoms can be exacerbated by coinfection of candidiasis, trichomoniasis, or bacterial vaginosis. These can be identified by wet-prep, pH, and whiff test.

- Sexually transmitted diseases including gonorrhea, trichomonas, and chlamydia also may coexist with or mimic atrophic vaginitis. Cultures or nucleic acid amplification tests can identify these infections. It is important not to assume a diagnosis of solely atrophic vaginitis in the postmenopausal patient who presents with urogenital complaints.

MANAGEMENT

- Estrogen replacement therapy relieves menopausal symptoms including atrophic vaginitis.[2] SOR **A** Routes of administration include oral, transdermal, and intravaginal. Risks associated with estrogen use including breast cancer, coronary heart disease, stroke, and venous thromboembolism.

- A Cochrane review found that estrogen creams, pessaries, vaginal tablets and the estradiol vaginal ring appeared to be equally effective for the symptoms of vaginal atrophy.[2] SOR **A** One trial found significant side effects following conjugated equine estrogen cream administration when compared to tablets causing uterine bleeding, breast pain, and perineal pain. Another trial found significant endometrial overstimulation following use of the conjugated equine estrogen cream when compared to the ring. Women appeared to favor the estradiol-releasing vaginal ring for ease of use, comfort of product, and overall satisfaction.[2] SOR **A**

- The amount of estrogen and the duration of time required to eliminate symptoms depend on the degree of vaginal atrophy, and will vary among patients. Progestin therapy should be considered in any women with an intact uterus to avoid causing endometrial cancer. When oral estrogen is used at typical doses atrophic symptoms will persist in 10% to 25% of patients.[3]

- Topical administration of estrogen is an excellent treatment for genitourinary symptoms of atrophy, because exposure of other organs can be minimized if low doses of topical estrogens are used. Absorption rates with topical therapy increase with treatment duration because of the enhanced vascularity of the epithelium.

- Moisturizers and lubricants may be used to help maintain natural secretions and comfort during intercourse. Sexual activity has been shown to encourage vaginal elasticity and pliability, and the lubricative response to sexual stimulation.

- Nonhormonal local vaginal moisturizers may be used regularly to help treat symptoms of atrophic vaginitis. These can be especially helpful during sexual intercourse. One open-label study indicated that (Replens) a bioadhesive vaginal moisturizer was a safe and effective alternative to estrogen vaginal cream, with both therapies exhibiting statistically significant increases in vaginal moisture, vaginal fluid volume, and vaginal elasticity.[4] SOR **B**

PATIENT EDUCATION

Encourage patients to discuss the risks and benefits of estrogen replacement therapy. Water-soluble vaginal lubricants (OTC) may safely help prevent pain during intercourse.

FOLLOW-UP

Follow-up is needed for all patients placed on estrogen therapy to monitor for estrogen-related side effects. Otherwise, follow-up can be as needed.

PATIENT RESOURCES

University of Iowa—**http://obgyn.uihc.uiowa.edu/patinfo/Vulvar/vaginitis.htm.**

Medline Plus—**http://www.nlm.nih.gov/medlineplus/ency/article/000892.htm.**

PROVIDER RESOURCES

American Family Physician—**http://www.aafp.org/afp/20000515/3090.html.**
http://www.aafp.org/afp/20040501/cochrane.html.

REFERENCES

1. Pandit L, Ouslander JG. Postmenopausal vaginal atrophy and atrophic vaginitis. *Am J Med Sci.* 1997;314:228–231.

2. Suckling J, Lethaby A, Kennedy R. Local oestrogen for vaginal atrophy in postmenopausal women. *Cochrane Database Syst Rev.* 2006;4:CD001500. Doi: 10.1002/14651858.Cd001500.Pub2.

3. Smith P, Heimer G, Lindskog M, Ulmsten U. Oestradiol-releasing vaginal ring for treatment of postmenopausal urogenital atrophy. *Maturitas.* 1993;16:145–154.

4. Nachtigall Le. Comparative study: Replens versus local estrogen in menopausal women. *Fertil Steril.* 1994;61:178.

78 BACTERIAL VAGINOSIS

E.J. Mayeaux, Jr., MD
Richard P. Usatine, MD

PATIENT STORY

A 31-year-old woman presents with a malodorous vaginal discharge for 3 weeks. There is no associated vaginal itching or pain. She is married and monogamous. She admits to douching about once per month to prevent any odor but it is not working this time. On examination, her discharge is visible (**Figure 78-1**). It is thin and off-white. Wet prep examination shows that more than 50% of the epithelial cells are clue cells (**Figure 78-2**). The patient is treated with oral metronidazole 500 mg bid for 7 days with good results.

EPIDEMIOLOGY

- Bacterial vaginosis (BV) is a clinical syndrome resulting from alteration of the vaginal ecosystem. It is estimated to be the most prevalent cause of vaginal discharge or malodor. However, more than 50% of women with BV are asymptomatic.[1] It accounts for more than 10 million outpatient visits per year.[2]

ETIOLOGY AND PATHOPHYSIOLOGY

- Hydrogen peroxide-producing Lactobacillus is the most common organism composing normal vaginal flora.[1] In BV, normal vaginal lactobacilli are replaced by high concentrations of anaerobic bacteria such as *Mobiluncus, Prevotella, Gardnerella, Bacteroides,* and *Mycoplasma* species.[1,2]

- This is called a vaginosis, not a vaginitis, because of the fact that the tissues themselves are not actually infected, but only have superficial involvement. More than half of women with the disorder are asymptomatic.[1]

- BV has been associated with adverse pregnancy outcomes, including premature rupture of membranes, preterm labor, and preterm birth.[2] It has also been linked to an increased risk of miscarriage in the first trimester.[3] The presence of normal *Lactobacillus* species has been shown to be inversely associated with preterm delivery.[2]

- Hydrogen peroxide-producing *Lactobacillus* is the most common organism comprising normal vaginal flora. The hydrogen peroxide produced by the *Lactobacillus* may help in inhibiting the growth of atypical flora.

- In BV, normal vaginal lactobacilli are replaced by high concentrations of anaerobic bacteria such as *Mobiluncus, Prevotella, Gardnerella, Bacteroides,* and *Mycoplasma* species.

- The odor of BV is caused by the aromatic amines produced by the altered bacterial flora in the vagina. These aromatic amines include putrescine and cadaverine—aptly named to describe their foul odor.

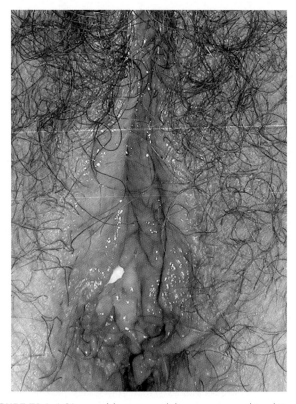

FIGURE 78-1 A 31-year-old woman with homogeneous, thin white malodorous vaginal discharge. (*Courtesy of Richard P. Usatine, MD.*)

DIAGNOSIS

- The physical examination should include inspection of the external genitalia for irritation or discharge. Speculum examination is done to determine the amount and character of the discharge. A nucleic acid amplification test for *Neisseria gonorrhoeae, Chlamydia*, and/or *C. trachomatis* (or similar test) should be performed on genital specimens (urethral or cervical) or urine.

- Vaginal pH testing can be very helpful in the diagnosis of vaginitis. The normal vaginal pH is usually 3.5 to 4.5. A pH above 4.5 is seen with menopausal patients, trichomonas infection, or BV.

- Wet preps are obtained using a cotton-tipped applicator applied to the vaginal sidewall, placing the sample of discharge into normal saline (not water). Observe for clue cells, number of white blood cells, trichomonads, and candidal hyphae. Clue cells are squamous epithelial cells whose borders are obscured by attached bacteria. More than 20% to 25% of epithelial cells seen in BV should be clue cells (**Figure 78-2**).

- BV can be clinically diagnosed by finding three of the following four signs and symptoms:
  - Homogeneous, thin, white discharge that smoothly coats the vaginal walls (**Figure 78-3**).
  - Presence of clue cells on microscopic examination (**Figure 78-2**).
  - pH of vaginal fluid >4.5.
  - A fishy odor of vaginal discharge before or after addition of 10% KOH (i.e., the whiff test).[1]

DIFFERENTIAL DIAGNOSIS

- Trichomonas also may have the odor of aromatic amines and, therefore, easily confused with BV at first glance. Look for the strawberry cervix on examination and moving trichomonads on the wet prep (see Chapter 80, Trichomonas Vaginitis).

- Candida vaginitis tends to present with a cottage-cheese-like discharge and vaginal itching (see Chapter 79, Candida Vaginitis).

- Gonorrhea and chlamydia should not be missed in patients with vaginal discharge. Consider testing for these STDs based on patients' risk factors and the presence of purulence clinically and white blood cells on the wet prep (see Chapter 81, Chlamydia Cervicitis).

MANAGEMENT

CDC Recommended Regimens[1]SOR Ⓐ

Metronidazole 500 mg orally twice a day for 7 days

OR

Metronidazole gel 0.75%, one full applicator (5 g) intravaginally, once a day for 5 days

OR

Clindamycin cream 2%, one full applicator (5 g) intravaginally at bedtime for 7 days

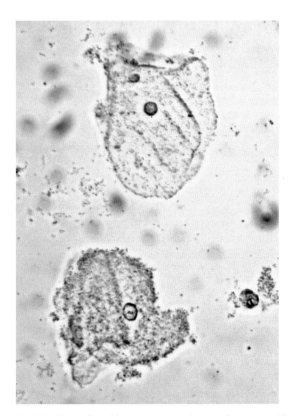

FIGURE 78-2 Clue cell and bacteria seen in bacterial vaginosis. The lower cell is a clue cell covered in bacteria while the upper cell is a normal epithelial cell. Light microscope under high power. (*Courtesy of E.J. Mayeaux, Jr., MD.*)

CDC Alternative Regimens[1] SOR **A**

Clindamycin 300 mg orally twice a day for 7 days

OR

Clindamycin ovules 100 mg intravaginally once at bedtime for 3 days

CDC Recommended Regimens for Pregnant Women[1] SOR **A**

Metronidazole 500 mg orally twice a day for 7 days

OR

Metronidazole 250 mg orally three times a day for 7 days

OR

Clindamycin 300 mg orally twice a day for 7 days

Metronidazole 2 g single-dose therapy has the lowest efficacy for BV and is no longer a recommended or alternative regimen. Clindamycin cream is oil-based and might weaken latex condoms and diaphragms for 5 days after use. Topical clindamycin preparations should not be used in the second half of pregnancy.[1] Multiple studies and meta-analyses have *not* demonstrated an association between metronidazole use during pregnancy and teratogenic or mutagenic effects in newborns.[1] SOR **A**

- The established benefits of therapy for BV in nonpregnant women are to (1) relieve vaginal symptoms and signs of infection and (2) reduce the risk for infectious complications after abortion or hysterectomy.[1] SOR **A** Other potential benefits might include a reduction in risk for other infections (e.g., HIV and other STDs).[1] SOR **B**

- Pregnancy: BV during pregnancy is associated with adverse pregnancy outcomes, including premature rupture of the membranes, preterm labor, preterm birth, intra-amniotic infection, and postpartum endometritis. The established benefit of therapy for BV in pregnant women is to relieve vaginal symptoms and signs of infection.[1] SOR **A**

- Additional potential benefits of therapy include (1) reducing the risk for infectious complications associated with BV during pregnancy and (2) reducing the risk for other infections (e.g., other STDs or HIV). The results of several investigations indicate that treatment of pregnant women with BV who are at high risk for preterm delivery (i.e., those who previously delivered a premature infant) might reduce the risk for prematurity.[1] SOR **B** Therefore, clinicians should consider evaluation and treatment of high-risk pregnant women with asymptomatic BV.[1] SOR **B**

- Routine treatment of sex partners is not recommended based on the results of clinical trials that indicate that a woman's response to therapy and the likelihood of relapse or recurrence are not affected by treatment of her sex partner(s).[1] SOR **A**

- Tinidazole, which is now indicated in the United States to treat trichomonas, also may be a useful option in women with recurrent BV.[4] SOR **C**

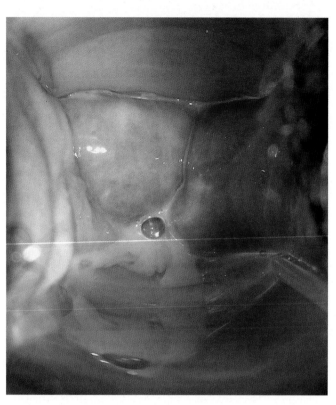

FIGURE 78-3 A homogeneous, off-white creamy malodorous discharge that adheres to the vaginal walls and pools in the vaginal vault in a women with bacterial vaginosis. (*Courtesy of Richard P. Usatine, MD.*)

- Extended ingestion of live culture, nonpasteurized yogurt may theoretically increase colonization by the bacteria and decrease the episodes of BV.[5] SOR Ⓒ However, health food store lactobacilli are the wrong strain and are not well-retained by the vagina.

- One randomized trial for persistent BV indicated that metronidazole gel 0.75% twice per week for 6 months after completion of a recommended regimen was effective in maintaining a clinical cure for 6 months.[6] SOR Ⓑ

PATIENT EDUCATION

Avoid consuming alcohol during treatment with metronidazole and for 24 hours thereafter. Women should be advised to return for additional therapy if symptoms recur because recurrence of BV is not unusual.

FOLLOW-UP

- Follow-up visits are unnecessary in nonpregnant women if symptoms resolve.[1]

- Treatment of BV in asymptomatic pregnant women who are at high risk for preterm delivery might prevent adverse pregnancy outcomes. Therefore, a follow-up evaluation 1 month after completion of treatment should be considered to evaluate whether therapy was effective.[1] SOR Ⓒ

- If symptoms do recur, consider a treatment regimen different from the original regimen to treat recurrent disease.[1] SOR Ⓒ

PATIENT RESOURCES

CDC Bacterial Vaginosis Fact Sheet—**http://www.cdc.gov/ std/BV/STDFact-Bacterial-Vaginosis.htm.**

Family Doctor.org from the AAFP—**http://familydoctor.org/ 234.xml.**

MedicineNet.com—**http://www.medicinenet.com/ bacterial_vaginosis/article.htm.**

ASCCP—**http://asccp.org/pdfs/patient_edu/bacterial_ vaginosis.pdf.**

PROVIDER RESOURCES

Centers for Disease Control and Prevention. 2006 Guidelines for Treatment of Sexually Transmitted Diseases—**http://www.cdc. gov/std/treatment/default.htm#tg2006.**

REFERENCES

1. Centers for Disease Control and Prevention. 2006 Guidelines for Treatment of Sexually Transmitted Diseases. http://www.cdc.gov/ std/treatment/default.htm#tg2006. Accessed February 9, 2008.

2. Martius J, Krohn MA, Hillier SL, Stamm WE, Holmes KK, Eschenbach DA. Relationships of vaginal lactobacillus species, cervical chlamydia trachomatis, and bacterial vaginosis to preterm birth. *Obstet Gynecol*. 1988;71:89–95.

3. Ralph SG, Rutherford AJ, Wilson JD. Influence of bacterial vaginosis on conception and miscarriage in the first trimester: Cohort Study. *BMJ*. 1999;319:220–223.

4. Shalev E, Battino S, Weiner E, Colodner R, Keness Y. Ingestion of yogurt containing acidophilus compared with pasteurized yogurt as prophylaxis for recurrent candidal vaginitis and bacterial vaginosis. *Arch Fam Med*. 1996;5:593–596.

5. Baylson FA, Nyirjesy P, Weitz MV. Treatment of recurrent bacterial vaginosis with tinidazole. *Obstet Gynecol*. 2004;104 (5 Pt 1):931–932.

6. Sobel JD, Ferris D, Schwebke J, et al. Suppressive antibacterial therapy with 0.75% metronidazole vaginal gel to prevent recurrent bacterial vaginosis. *Am J Obstet Gynecol*. 2006;194:1283–1289.

79 CANDIDA VULVOVAGINITIS

E.J. Mayeaux, Jr., MD
Richard P. Usatine, MD

PATIENT STORY

A 35-year-old woman presents with severe vaginal and vulvar itching. She also complains of a thick white discharge. **Figure 79-1** demonstrates the appearance of her vagina and cervix and **Figure 79-2** shows her vulva. **Figure 79-3** shows her wet-prep. Treatment with an over-the-counter intravaginal preparation was successful.

EPIDEMIOLOGY

- 75% of all women in the United States will experience at least one episode of vulvovaginal candidiasis. The most common organism involved is *Candida albicans*.[1] The incidence of the disease appears to be rising.

- It is a frequent iatrogenic complication of antibiotic treatment, secondary to altered vaginal flora. Nearly half of all women experience multiple episodes, and up to 5% experience recurrent disease.[1]

- Recurrent yeast vaginitis is usually caused by relapse, and less often by reinfection. Recurrent infection may be caused by *Candida* recolonization of the vagina from the rectum.[2] It is defined as four or more episodes of symptomatic disease annually and affects <5% of women.[1]

ETIOLOGY AND PATHOPHYSIOLOGY

- Most vulvovaginal Candidiasis is caused by *C. albicans* (**Figure 79-3**).[3] Two new species, *Candida glabrata* and *Candida tropicalis*, now cause one-quarter of all candida vulvovaginal infections. Those organisms are resistant to the over-the counter imidazole creams. *Glabrata* and *Tropicalis* species mutate out of the activity of treatment drugs much faster than *Albicans* species.

- The disease is suggested by pruritus in the vulvar area, together with erythema of the vagina and vulva (**Figures 79-1** and **79-2**). The familiar reddening of the vulvar tissues is caused by an ethanol by-product of the *Candida* infection. This ethanol compound also produces pruritic symptoms. A scalloped edge with satellite lesions is characteristic of the erythema on the vulva.

DIAGNOSIS

- The diagnosis is usually suspected by characteristic findings (**Figure 79-1**). A white discharge may or may not be present. Vaginitis solely caused by *Candida* generally has a vaginal pH <4.5.

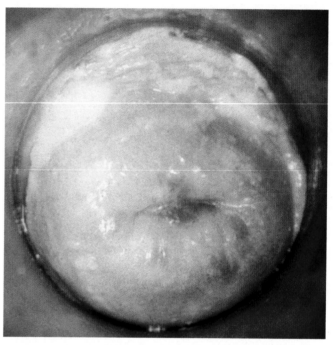

FIGURE 79-1 Candida vaginitis. Note the thick white adherent "cottage-cheese like" discharge. (*Courtesy of the CDC and Stuart Brown, MD.*)

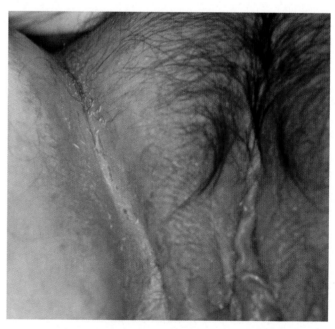

FIGURE 79-2 *Candida* on the vulva showing whitish patches with erythema. (*Courtesy of Gordon Davis, MD.*)

- The wet prep or KOH smear may demonstrate yeast or pseudohyphae (**Figure 79-3**). Wet preps may also demonstrate white blood cells, trichomonads, candidal hyphae, or clue cells.

- The KOH prep is made by adding a drop of KOH solution to a drop of saline suspension of the discharge. The KOH lyses epithelial cells in 5 to 15 minutes (faster if the slide is warmed briefly over a flame) and allows easier visualization of candidal hyphae.[1]

- Rapid antigen testing is also available for *Candida*. The detection of vaginal yeast by rapid antigen testing is feasible for office practice and more sensitive than wet mount. A negative test result, however, was not found to be sensitive enough to rule out yeast and avoid a culture.[3] SOR **A**

- Fungal culture is advised for persistent symptoms despite negative KOH.

DIFFERENTIAL DIAGNOSIS

- Trichomoniasis can be confused with candidiasis because patients may report itching and a discharge in both diagnoses. Look for the strawberry cervix on examination and moving trichomonads on the wet prep (see Chapter 80, Trichomonas Vaginitis).

- Bacterial vaginosis can be confused with Candidiasis because patients may report a discharge and an odor in both diagnoses. The odor is usually much worse in bacterial vaginosis and the quality of the discharge can be different. The wet prep should allow for differentiation between these two infections (see Chapter 78, Bacterial Vaginosis).

- Gonorrhea and chlamydia should not be missed in patients with vaginal discharge. Consider testing for these STDs based on patients' risk factors and the presence of purulence clinically and white blood cells on the wet prep (see Chapter 81, Chlamydia Cervicitis).

- Cytolytic vaginosis, or Döderlein's cytolysis, can be confused with candidiasis. Cytolytic vaginosis is produced by a massive desquamation of epithelial cells related to excess lactobacilli in the vagina. The signs and symptoms are similar to candida vaginitis except no yeast are found on wet prep. The wet prep will show an overgrowth of lactobacilli. The treatment is to discontinue all antifungals and other agents or procedures that alter the vaginal flora.

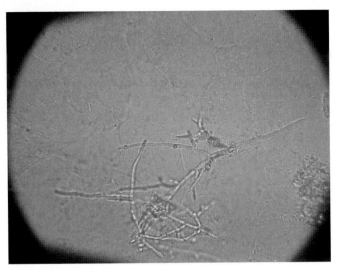

FIGURE 79-3 Wet mount with KOH of Candida albicans in a woman with candida vaginitis. Seen under high power demonstrating branching pseudohyphae and budding yeast. (*Courtesy of Dan Stulberg, MD.*)

MANAGEMENT

CDC Recommended Regimens[1]

Intravaginal Agents:

Butoconazole 2% cream 5 g intravaginally for 3 days*

Butoconazole 2% cream 5 g (Butaconazole1-sustained release), single intravaginal application

OR

Clotrimazole 1% cream 5 g intravaginally for 7 to 14 days*

Clotrimazole 100 mg vaginal tablet for 7 days

Clotrimazole 100 mg vaginal tablet, two tablets for 3 days

OR

Miconazole 2% cream 5 g intravaginally for 7 days*

Miconazole 100 mg vaginal suppository, one suppository for 7 days*

Miconazole 200 mg vaginal suppository, one suppository for 3 days*

Miconazole 1200 mg vaginal suppository, one suppository for 1 day*

OR

Nystatin 100,000-unit vaginal tablet, one tablet for 14 days

OR

Tioconazole 6.5% ointment 5 g intravaginally in a single application*

OR

Terconazole 0.4% cream 5 g intravaginally for 7 days

Terconazole 0.8% cream 5 g intravaginally for 3 days

Terconazole 80 mg vaginal suppository, one suppository for 3 days

Oral Agent:

Fluconazole 150 mg oral tablet, one tablet in single dose

*Over-the-counter preparations.

MANAGEMENT OF SEX PARTNERS

- Vulvovaginal candidiasis (VVC) is not usually acquired through sexual intercourse; treatment of sex partners is not recommended but may be considered in women who have recurrent infection. Some male sex partners might have balanitis (see Chapter 130, Mucocutaneous Candidiasis).

RECURRENT VULVOVAGINAL CANDIDIASIS

- Recurrent vulvovaginal candidiasis (RVVC) is defined as four or more episodes of symptomatic VVC in 1 year. It affects a small percentage of women (<5%). The pathogenesis of RVVC is poorly understood, and the majority of women with RVVC have no apparent predisposing or underlying conditions. Vaginal cultures should be obtained from patients with RVVC to confirm the clinical diagnosis and to identify unusual species, including nonalbicans species, particularly *C. glabrata* (*C. glabrata* does not form pseudohyphae or hyphae and is not easily recognized on microscopy).[1] SOR Ⓑ
C. glabrata and other nonalbicans *Candida* species are observed in 10% to 20% of patients with RVVC.[1] See below for therapy of nonalbicans *Candida*.

- Given the frequency at which RVVC occurs in the immunocompetent healthy population, the occurrence of RVVC <u>alone</u> should not be considered an indication for HIV testing.[1] SOR Ⓒ

- Each individual episode of RVVC caused by *C. albicans* usually responds well to short duration oral or topical azole therapy. To maintain clinical and mycologic control, some specialists recommend a longer duration of initial therapy (e.g., 7–14 days of topical therapy or a 100 mg, 150 mg, or 200 mg oral dose of fluconazole every third day for a total of 3 doses (day 1, 4, and 7) to attempt mycologic remission before initiating a maintenance antifungal regimen.[1] SOR **C**

MAINTENANCE REGIMENS

- Oral fluconazole (i.e., 100-mg, 150-mg, or 200-mg dose) weekly for 6 months is the first line of treatment. If this regimen is not feasible, some specialists recommend topical clotrimazole 200 mg twice a week, clotrimazole (500-mg dose vaginal suppositories once weekly), or other topical treatments used intermittently.[1] SOR **C**

- Suppressive maintenance antifungal therapies are effective in reducing RVVC.[1] SOR **A** However, 30% to 50% of women will have recurrent disease after maintenance therapy is discontinued. Routine treatment of sex partners is controversial. *C. albicans* azole resistance is rare in vaginal isolates, and susceptibility testing is usually not warranted for individual treatment guidance.

SEVERE VULVOVAGINITIS CANDIDIASIS

- Severe VVC (i.e., extensive vulvar erythema, edema, excoriation, and fissure formation) is associated with lower clinical response rates in patients treated with short courses of topical or oral therapy. Either 7 to 14 days of topical azole or 150 mg of fluconazole in two sequential doses (second dose 72 hours after initial dose) is recommended.[1] SOR **C**

NONALBICANS VULVOVAGINITIS CANDIDIASIS

- The optimal treatment of nonalbicans VVC remains unknown. Options include longer duration of therapy (7 to 14 days) with a nonfluconazole azole drug (oral or topical) as first-line therapy.[1] SOR **C** If recurrence occurs, 600 mg of boric acid in a gelatin capsule is recommended, administered vaginally once daily for 2 weeks. This regimen has clinical and mycologic eradication rates of approximately 70%.[1] SOR **B**

COMPROMISED HOST

- Women with underlying debilitating medical conditions (e.g., those with uncontrolled diabetes or those receiving corticosteroid treatment) do not respond as well to short-term therapies. Efforts to correct modifiable conditions should be made, and more prolonged (i.e., 7–14 days) conventional antimycotic treatment is necessary.[1] SOR **C**

PREGNANCY

- VVC frequently occurs during pregnancy. Only topical azole therapies, applied for 7 days, are recommended for use among pregnant women.[1] SOR **C**

HIV INFECTION

- Symptomatic VVC is more frequent in seropositive women and correlates with severity of immunodeficiency. In addition, among HIV-infected women, systemic azole exposure is associated with the isolation of nonalbicans *Candida* species from the vagina.

- According to the available data, therapy for VVC in HIV-infected women should not differ from that for seronegative women.[1] SOR **B**

OTHER

- *Lactobacillus acidophilus* does not adhere well to the vaginal epithelium, and it does not significantly change the incidence of candidal vulvovaginitis.[2,5]

- The cure rates with single-dose oral fluconazole and all the intravaginal treatments are equal.[6] Fluconazole (Diflucan) 150 mg single dose has become very popular, but may have clinical cure rates of approximately only 70%. SOR **A** Systemic allergic reactions are possible with the oral agents.

- Oral agents fluconazole, ketoconazole, and itraconazole also appear to be effective.[1] SOR **B**

PATIENT EDUCATION

Studies have shown that women whose condition has previously been diagnosed with VVC are not necessarily more likely to be able to diagnose themselves.[1] Any woman whose symptoms persist after using an OTC preparation, or who has a recurrence of symptoms within 2 months, should be evaluated with office-based testing. Explain that unnecessary or inappropriate use of OTC preparations can lead to a delay in the treatment of other vulvovaginitis etiologies, which can result in adverse clinical outcomes.[1]

FOLLOW-UP

Patients should be instructed to return for follow-up visits only if symptoms persist or recur within 2 months of onset of initial symptoms.[1]

PATIENT RESOURCES

FamilyDoctor.org from AAFP-**http://familydoctor.org/ online/famdocen/home/women/reproductive/ vaginal/206.html.**

PROVIDER RESOURCES

Centers for Disease Control and Prevention. 2006 Guidelines for Treatment of Sexually Transmitted Diseases—**http://www.cdc.gov/std/treatment/default.htm#tg2006.**

American Family Physician Management of Vaginitis—**http://www.aafp.org/afp/20041201/2125.html.**

REFERENCES

1. Centers for Disease Control and Prevention. 2006 Guidelines for Treatment of Sexually Transmitted Diseases. http://www.cdc.gov/std/treatment/default.htm#tg2006. Accessed February 9, 2008.

2. Shalev E, Battino S, Weiner E, Colodner R, Keness Y. Ingestion of yogurt containing acidophilus compared with pasteurized yogurt as prophylaxis for recurrent candidal vaginitis and bacterial vaginosis. *Arch Fam Med.* 1996;5:593–596.

3. Cohen DA, Nsuami M, Etame RB, et al. A school-based chlamydia control program using DNA amplification technology. *Pediatrics.* 1998;(1):101.

4. Chatwani AJ, Mehta R, Hassan S, Rahimi S, Jeronis S, Dandolu V. Rapid testing for vaginal yeast detection: A prospective study. *Am J Obstet Gynecol.* 2007;196:309.e1–e4.

5. Pirotta M, Gunn J, Chondros P, et al. Effect of lactobacillus in preventing post-antibiotic vulvovaginal candidiasis: A randomised controlled trial. *BMJ.* 2004;329:548.

6. Sobel JD, Brooker D, Stein GE, et al. Single oral dose fluconazole compared with conventional clotrimazole topical therapy of candida vaginitis. *Am J Obstet Gynecol.* 1995;172:1263–1238.

80 TRICHOMONAS VAGINITIS

E.J. Mayeaux Jr., MD
Richard P. Usatine, MD

PATIENT STORY

A 27-year-old woman presents with a vaginal itching, odor, and discharge for 1 week. She has one partner who is asymptomatic. Speculum examination shows a strawberry cervix seen with trichomonas infections (**Figure 80-1**). This strawberry pattern is caused by inflammation and punctate hemorrhages on the cervix. There is a scant white discharge with a fishy odor. Wet mount shows trichomonads swimming in saline under high power (**Figure 80-2**). The trichomonads are larger than WBCs and have visible flagella and movement. She is diagnosed with *Trichomoniasis* and treated with 2 g of metronidazole in a single dose. The patient is tested for other STDs and her partner is treated with the same regimen.

EPIDEMIOLOGY

• In the United States, there are an estimated 7.4 million new cases of trichomoniasis annually.[1]

• There has been a decline in incidence of trichomonas since the 1970s because of increased knowledge of the disease, effectiveness of metronidazole treatment, treatment of sexual partners, improved diagnosis, and correctly identifying patients.

ETIOLOGY AND PATHOPHYSIOLOGY

• Trichomonas infection is caused by the unicellular protozoan *Trichomonas vaginalis*.[2]

• The majority of men (90%) infected with *T. vaginalis* are asymptomatic, but many women (50%) report symptoms.[3]

• The infection is predominantly transmitted via sexual contact. The organism can survive up to 48 hours at 10°C (50°F) outside the body, making transmission from shared undergarments or from infected hot spas possible.

• Trichomonas infection is associated with low-birth-weight infants, premature rupture of membranes, and preterm delivery in pregnant patients.[4]

• In a person coinfected with HIV, the pathology induced by *T. vaginalis* infection can increase HIV shedding. Trichomonas infection may also act to expand the portal of entry for HIV in an HIV-negative person. Studies from Africa have suggested that *T. vaginalis* infection may increase the rate of HIV transmission by approximately twofold.[5]

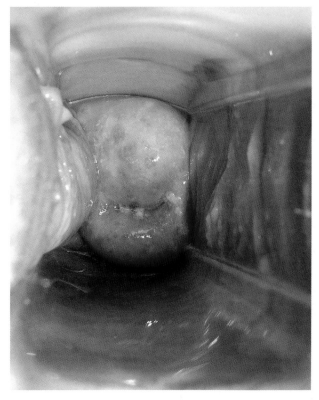

FIGURE 80-1 Speculum examination showing the strawberry cervix pattern seen with trichomonas infections. This strawberry pattern is caused by inflammation and punctate hemorrhages on the cervix. There is a scant white discharge. (*Courtesy of Richard P. Usatine, MD.*)

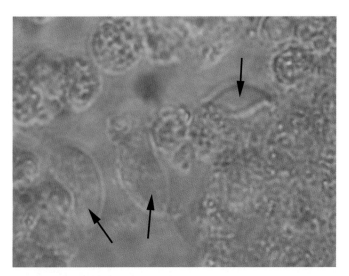

FIGURE 80-2 Wet mount showing trichomonas (arrows) in saline under high power. The smaller more granular cells are white blood cells. (*Courtesy of Richard P. Usatine, MD.*)

DIAGNOSIS

- Trichomoniasis is a common disease associated with vaginal discharge. A complete examination—including assays or cultures, wet preps, pH evaluation, and examination—should be performed if reasonably possible.

- The physical examination should include inspection of the external genitalia for irritation or discharge. Speculum examination is done to determine the amount and character of the discharge and to look for the characteristic strawberry cervix (**Figure 80-3**).

- Typically, women with trichomoniasis have a diffuse, malodorous, yellow-green discharge with vulvar irritation.[2] Vaginal and vulvar itching and irritation are common.

- It should be determined whether the patient douched recently, because this can lower the yield of diagnostic tests. Patients who have been told not to douche will sometimes start wiping the vagina with soapy washcloths to "keep clean" as an alternative. This greatly irritates the vagina and cervix, lowers test sensitivity, and may cause a discharge.

LABORATORY TESTS

- Wet preps are obtained using a cotton-tipped applicator applied to the vaginal side-wall, placing the sample of discharge into normal saline (not water). A drop of the suspension is then placed on a slide, covered with a cover-slip, and carefully examined with the low-power and high-dry objective lenses. Under the microscope, observe for motile trichomonads, which are often easy to visualize because of their lashing flagella (**Figure 80-2**).

- A vaginal pH above 4.5 is seen with menopausal patients, trichomonas infection, or bacterial vaginosis.[3]

- Wet prep has a sensitivity of only approximately 60%–70% and requires immediate evaluation of wet preparation slide for optimal results. Other FDA-cleared tests for trichomoniasis in women include OSOM Trichomonas Rapid Test and the Affirm™ VP III. Both tests are performed on vaginal secretions at the point-of-care and have a sensitivity greater than 83% and a specificity greater than 97%. The results of the OSOM Trichomonas Rapid Test are available in approximately 10 minutes, and results of the Affirm™ VP III are available within 45 minutes.[2]

- Culture is the most sensitive and specific method of diagnosis. In women in whom trichomoniasis is suspected but not confirmed by microscopy, vaginal secretions should be cultured for *T. vaginalis*.[2]

DIFFERENTIAL DIAGNOSIS

- Bacterial vaginosis and trichomonas may have the odor of aromatic amines and therefore easily confused with each other. Look for clue cells and trichomonads on the wet prep to differentiate between the two (see Chapter 78, Bacterial Vaginosis).

- Candida vaginitis tends to present with a cottage-cheese like discharge and vaginal itching (see Chapter 79, Candida Vaginitis).

- Gonorrhea and chlamydia and should not be missed in patients with vaginal discharge. Consider testing for these STDs based on

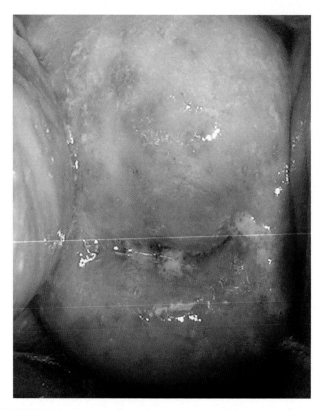

FIGURE 80-3 Close-up of strawberry cervix in a trichomonas infection demonstrating inflammation and punctate hemorrhages. (*Courtesy of Richard P. Usatine, MD.*)

patients' risk factors and the presence of purulence clinically and WBCs on the wet prep (see Chapter 81, Chlamydia Cervicitis).

MANAGEMENT

CDC Recommended Regimens[2] SOR Ⓐ
Metronidazole 2 g orally in a single dose

OR

Tinidazole 2 g orally in a single dose

CDC Alternative Regimen[2] SOR Ⓐ
Metronidazole 500 mg orally twice a day for 7 days

- Metronidazole 2 g orally as a single dose, or 500 mg bid for 7 days (including pregnant patients) are the best treatments by Cochrane analysis.[6] SOR Ⓐ

- Tinidazole (Tindamax), a second-generation nitroimidazole, is indicated as a one-time dose of 2 g for the treatment of trichomoniasis (including metronidazole-resistant trichomoniasis).[2] SOR Ⓐ It has been shown to be an effective therapy in nonresistant and resistant *T. vaginalis*.[7,8] The contraindications (including ETOH) to the use of tinidazole are similar to those for metronidazole.

- A nucleic acid amplification test for *Neisseria gonorrhoeae*, and/or *Chlamydia trachomatis* should be performed on all patients with trichomonas.

- Pregnant women may be treated with 2 g of metronidazole in a single dose. Metronidazole is pregnancy category B. Vaginal trichomoniasis has been associated with adverse pregnancy outcomes, particularly premature rupture of membranes, preterm delivery, and low birthweight. Unfortunately, data do not suggest that metronidazole treatment results in a reduction in perinatal morbidity and treatment may even increase prematurity or low birth weight.[2] Treatment of *T. vaginalis* might relieve symptoms of vaginal discharge in pregnant women and might prevent respiratory or genital infection of the newborn and further sexual transmission. The CDC recommends that clinicians counsel patients regarding the potential risks and benefits of treatment during pregnancy.[2]

- Some strains of *T. vaginalis* can have diminished susceptibility to metronidazole. Low-level metronidazole resistance has been identified in 2%–5% of cases of vaginal trichomoniasis. These infections should respond to tinidazole or higher doses of metronidazole. High-level resistance is rare.

PATIENT EDUCATION

- Sexual partners of patients with trichomonas should be treated. Patients can be sent home with a dose for a partner when it is believed that the partner will not come in on his own. Patients

should be instructed to avoid sex until they and their sex partners are cured (i.e., when therapy has been completed and patient and partner(s) are asymptomatic).[2]

FOLLOW-UP

- Follow-up is unnecessary for men and women who become asymptomatic after treatment or who are initially asymptomatic.[2]

PATIENT RESOURCES

CDC information—**http://www.cdc.gov/ncidod/dpd/ parasites/trichomonas/factsht_trichomonas.htm**; **http://www.dpd.cdc.gov/dpdx/HTML/ Trichomoniasis.htm.**

Medline-plus—**http://www.nlm.nih.gov/medlineplus/ ency/article/001331.htm.**

PROVIDER RESOURCES

CDC information—**http://www.dpd.cdc.gov/dpdx/ HTML/Trichomoniasis.htm**; **http://www.cdc.gov/ncidod/dpd/parasites/ trichomonas/moreinfo_trichomonas.htm.**

E-Medicine—**http://www.emedicine.com/med/ topic2308.htm.**

REFERENCES

1. Centers for Disease Control and Prevention. Trichomoniasis. http://www.cdc.gov/std/trichomonas/default.htm.

2. Centers for Disease Control and Prevention. 2006 Guidelines for Treatment of Sexually Transmitted Diseases. http://www.cdc.gov/std/treatment/default.htm#tg2006.

3. Gjerdngen D, Fontaine P, Bixby M, Santilli J, Welsh J. The impact of regular vaginal pH screening on the diagnosis of bacterial vaginosis in pregnancy. *J Fam Pract*. 2000;49:3–43.

4. Cotch MF, Pastorek JG 2nd, Nugent RP, et al. Trichomonas vaginalis associated with low birth weight and preterm delivery: The Vaginal Infections and Prematurity Study Group. *Sex Transm Dis*. 1997;24:353–360.

5. Sorvillo F, Smith L, Kerndt P, Ash L. Trichomonas vaginalis, HIV, and African-Americans. *Emerg Infect Dis*. 2001;7(6):927–932.

6. Epling J. What is the best way to treat trichomoniasis in women? (Cochrane review) *Am Fam Physician*. 2001;64:1241–1243.

7. Mammen-Tobin A, Wilson JD. Management of metronidazole-resistant trichomonas vaginalis—A new approach. *Int J STD AIDS*. 2005;16(7):488–490.

8. Hager WD. Treatment of metronidazole-resistant trichomonas vaginalis with tinidazole: Case reports of three patients. *Sex Transm Dis*. 2004;31(6):343–345.

81 CHLAMYDIA CERVICITIS

E.J. Mayeaux, Jr., MD
Richard P. Usatine, MD

THE PATIENT'S STORY

A 17-year-old girl presents to the STD clinic because her boyfriend was diagnosed with a Chlamydia urethritis. Both she and her boyfriend admit to having had sexual partners in the past before starting to be sexually active with each other. On physical examination, there is ectopy and some mucoid discharge (**Figure 81-1**). The cervix bled easily while obtaining discharge and cells for a wet mount and genetic probe test. The wet mount showed many WBCs but no visible pathogens. The patient was treated with 1 g of azithromycin taken in front of a clinic nurse. She was sent to the laboratory for a Rapid plasma reagin (RPR) and HIV test and given a follow-up appointment in one week. The genetic probe test was positive for chlamydia and all the other examinations were negative. This information was given to the patient on her return visit and safe sex was discussed.

EPIDEMIOLOGY

- A very common sexually transmitted disease, chlamydia is the most frequently reported infectious disease in the United States (excluding HPV).[1] An estimated three million cases occur annually in the United States at a cost of more than $2 billion. The CDC estimates screening and treatment programs can be conducted at an annual cost of $175 million. Every dollar spent on screening and treatment saves $12 in complications that result from untreated chlamydia.[2]

- It is common among sexually active adolescents and young adults.[1] As many as 1 in 10 adolescent girls tested for chlamydia is infected. Based on reports to Centers for Disease Control and Prevention (CDC) provided by states that collect age-specific data, teenage girls have the highest rates of chlamydial infection. In these states, 15 to 19-year-old girls represent 46% of infections and 20 to 24-year-old women represent another 33%.[2]

ETIOLOGY AND PATHOPHYSIOLOGY

- *C. trachomatis* is a small gram-negative bacterium with unique biologic properties among living organisms. Chlamydia is an obligate intracellular parasite that has a distinct life-cycle consisting of two major phases: The small elementary bodies that attach and penetrate into cells, and the metabolically active reticulate bodies that form large inclusions within cells.

- It has a long growth cycle, which explains why extended courses of treatment are often necessary. Immunity to infection is not long-lived, so reinfection or persistent infection is common.

- The infection may be asymptomatic and the onset often indolent. It can cause cervicitis, endometritis, pelvic inflammatory disease (PID),

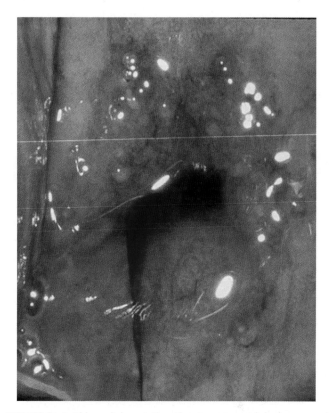

FIGURE 81-1 Chlamydial cervicitis with ectopy, mucoid discharge, and bleeding. The cervix is inflamed and friable. (*Courtesy of Connie Celum and Walter Stamm, Seattle STD/HIV Prevention Training Center.*)

urethritis, epididymitis, neonatal conjunctivitis, and pediatric pneumonia. Of exposed babies, 50% develop conjunctivitis and 10–16% develop pneumonia.

- Chlamydia infections may lead to Reiter's syndrome which presents with arthritis, conjunctivitis, and urethritis (see Chapter 149, Reiter's Disease). Past or ongoing *Chlamydia trachomatis* infection may be a risk factor for ovarian cancer.[3,4]

- Up to 40% of women with untreated chlamydia will develop PID. Undiagnosed PID caused by chlamydia is common. Of those with PID, 20% will become infertile; 18% will experience debilitating, chronic pelvic pain; and 9% will have a life-threatening tubal pregnancy. Tubal pregnancy is the leading cause of first-trimester, pregnancy-related deaths in American women.[2]

DIAGNOSIS

PHYSICAL EXAMINATION

- The cervix is inflamed, friable, and may bleed easily with manipulation. The cervix may show ectopy (columnar cells on the ectocervix). The discharge is usually mucoid or mucopurulent (**Figure 81-1**).

- Swab test—a white cotton-tip applicator is placed in the endocervical canal and removed to view. A visible mucopurulent discharge constitutes a positive swab test for chlamydia (**Figure 81-2**). This is not specific for Chlamydia as other genital infections can cause a mucopurulent discharge.

LABORATORY STUDIES

- A significant proportion of patients with Chlamydia are asymptomatic, providing a reservoir for infection. All pregnant women and sexually active women <25 years of age should be screened with routine examinations. A wet prep is usually negative for other organisms. Only WBCs and normal flora are seen.

- Chlamydia cannot be cultured on artificial media because it is an obligate intracellular organism. Tissue culture is required to grow the live organism. When testing for chlamydia, a wood-handled swab must not be used, since substances in wood may inhibit chlamydia organism. Culture has sensitivity of 70% to 100% and a specificity of almost 100%, which makes it the gold standard.

- The ELISA technique (Chlamydiazyme) has a sensitivity of 70% to 100% and a specificity of 97% to 99%.[1] Fluorescein-conjugated monoclonal antibodies test (MicroTrak) has a sensitivity of 70% to 100% and a specificity of 97% to 99%.[1]

- *C. trachomatis* can be detected using nucleic acid amplification techniques on voided urine specimens. These tests are used for urine screening to detect gonorrhea and chlamydia. Nucleic acid amplification tests have been used successfully in difficult-to-reach adolescents ("street kids") as well as in pediatric emergency departments and school-based settings.[5,6] Screening in school-based settings was associated with significant reduction in chlamydia rates during a one-year period.

- Specimens collected for liquid-based Pap smears can be used for nucleic acid amplification testing as well.

- Consider culture confirmation of positive test results in low-risk patients, since false positives do occur.[1]

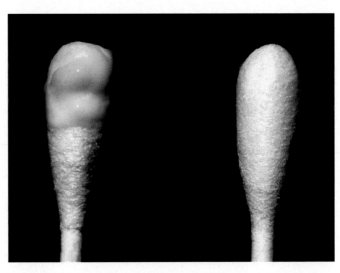

FIGURE 81-2 Mucopurulent discharge on the left swab from a cervix infected with chlamydia (positive swab test). (*Courtesy of Claire Stevens and Ronald Roddy, Seattle STD/HIV Prevention Training Center.*)

DIFFERENTIAL DIAGNOSIS

- Gonorrhea frequently coexists with chlamydia and should be tested for when patient is thought to have chlamydia. The discharge of gonorrhea may be more purulent but this is not always the case.
- Bacterial vaginosis—the aromatic amine odor and clue cells help to distinguish between these infections (see Chapter 208, Gonococcal Urethritis).
- Trichomoniasis—look for the strawberry cervix and trichomonas on the wet prep. There may also be a positive whiff test (see Chapter 80, Trichomonas Vaginitis).

MANAGEMENT

CDC Recommended Regimens[7]

Azithromycin 1 g orally in a single dose

OR

Doxycycline 100 mg orally twice a day for 7 days

CDC Alternative Regimens

Erythromycin base 500 mg orally four times a day for 7 days

OR

Erythromycin ethylsuccinate 800 mg orally four times a day for 7 days

OR

Ofloxacin 300 mg orally twice a day for 7 days

OR

Levofloxacin 500 mg orally once daily for 7 days

CDC Recommended Regimens in Pregnancy

Azithromycin 1 g orally in a single dose

OR

Amoxicillin 500 mg orally three times a day for 7 days

Alternative Regimens in Pregnancy

Erythromycin base 500 mg orally four times a day for 7 days

OR

Erythromycin base 250 mg orally four times a day for 14 days

OR

Erythromycin ethylsuccinate 800 mg orally four times a day for 7 days

OR

Erythromycin ethylsuccinate 400 mg orally four times a day for 14 days

- Patients' diagnosed with chlamydia cervicitis should be tested for other STDs.[7]

- Azithromycin (Zithromax) 1000 mg one-time dose is easy and may be directly observed in the clinic.[7] SOR Ⓐ It is the first-line therapy for chlamydia during pregnancy.

- Other treatments include doxycycline 100 mg po bid × 7 days or tetracycline 500 mg bid × 7 days.[7] SOR Ⓐ Avoid dairy products around time of dosing.

- Ofloxacin (Floxin) 300 mg po bid × 7 days is an alternative that should be taken on an empty stomach.[7] SOR Ⓐ It is contraindicated in children or pregnant and lactating women, but may also cover *N. gonorrhea* infection. Levofloxacin 500 mg orally for 7 days is another fluoroquinolone alternative.[7] SOR Ⓐ

- A meta-analysis of 12 randomized clinical trials of azithromycin versus doxycycline for the treatment of genital chlamydial infection demonstrated that the treatments were equally efficacious, with microbial cure rates of 97% and 98%, respectively.[8]

- Partners need treatment. If concerns exist that sex partners will not seek evaluation and treatment then delivery of antibiotic therapy (either a prescription or medication) to their partners is an option.[7]

PATIENT EDUCATION

- To minimize transmission, persons treated for chlamydia should be instructed to abstain from sexual intercourse for 7 days after single-dose therapy or until completion of a 7-day regimen.

- To minimize the risk for reinfection, patients also should be instructed to abstain from sexual intercourse until all of their sex partners are treated.[7]

FOLLOW-UP

- Test-of-cure (repeat testing 3 to 4 weeks after completing therapy) is not recommended for persons treated with the recommended or alterative regimens, unless therapeutic compliance is in question, symptoms persist, or reinfection is suspected. However, test-of-cure is recommended in pregnant women.[7]

PATIENT RESOURCES

- National Institute of Allergy and Infectious Diseases (NIAID) fact sheet—**http://www3.niaid.nih.gov/healthscience/healthtopics/chlamydia/index.htm.**
- CDC patient information—**http://www.cdc.gov/std/Chlamydia/STDFact-Chlamydia.htm.**

PROVIDER RESOURCES

- CDC Sexually Transmitted Diseases Treatment Guidelines 2006 for chlamydia—**http://www.cdc.gov/std/treatment/2006/urethritis-and-cervicitis.htm#uc4.**
- Emedicine.com—**http://www.emedicine.com/emerg/topic925.htm.**

REFERENCES

1. Skolnik NS. Screening for Chlamydia trachomatis infection. *Am Fam Physician*. 1995;51:821–826.

2. Centers for Disease Control and Prevention. http://www.cdc.gov/std/Chlamydia/STDFact-Chlamydia.htm. Accessed February 9, 2008.

3. Martius J, Krohn MA, Hillier SL, Stamm WE, Holmes KK, Eschenbach DA. Relationships of vaginal lactobacillus species, cervical chlamydia trachomatis, and bacterial vaginosis to preterm birth. *Obstet Gynecol*. 1988;71:89–95.

4. Ness RB, Goodman MT, Shen C, Brunham RC. Serologic evidence of past infection with Chlamydia trachomatis, in relation to ovarian cancer. *J Infect Dis*. 2003;187:1147–1152.

5. Monroe KW, Weiss HL, Jones M, Hook EW, 3rd. Acceptability of urine screening for Neisseria gonorrheae and chlamydia trachomatis in adolescents at an urban emergency department. *Sex Transm Dis*. 2003;30:850.

6. Rietmeijer CA, Bull SS, Ortiz CG, et al. Patterns of general health care and STD services use among high-risk youth in denver participating in community-based urine chlamydia screening. *Sex Transm Dis*. 1998;25:457.

7. Centers for Disease Control and Prevention. 2006 Guidelines for Treatment of Sexually Transmitted Diseases. http://www.cdc.gov/std/treatment/default.htm#tg2006. Accessed February 9, 2008.

8. Lau C-Y, Qureshi AK. Azithromycin versus doxycycline for genital chlamydial infections: A meta-analysis of randomized clinical trials. *Sex Transm Dis* 2002;29:497–502.

SECTION 3   VULVA

82 PAGET'S DISEASE OF THE VULVA

E.J. Mayeaux, Jr., MD

PATIENT'S STORY

A 60-year-old woman presented with vulvar pruritis for 1 year that is now constant. On physical examination, there is one large red lesion surrounded by white epithelium (**Figure 82-1**). A 3-mm punch biopsy was done of the white island within the red lesion using local anesthesia. The pathology showed Paget's disease of the vulva. The patient underwent a wide local excision of the involved area and no malignancy was found.

EPIDEMIOLOGY

- The frequency of malignancy in extramammary Paget's disease is approximately 20%, which is less than that of Paget's disease of the nipple.

- It accounts for less than 1% of all vulvar malignancies.[1]

- Most patients are white and in their 6th or 7th decade of life.

- Approximately 4% to 17% of patients with genital Paget's disease have an underlying neoplasm.[1,2] Associated malignancies include carcinomas of the Bartholin glands, urethra, bladder, vagina, cervix, endometrium, or adnexal apocrine tissue.

- Perianal Paget's disease (**Figure 82-2**) is associated with underlying colorectal carcinoma in 25% to 35% of cases.

ETIOLOGY AND PATHOPHYSIOLOGY

- Extramammary Paget's disease is an intraepithelial adenocarcinoma.

- It arises from apocrine gland tissue, usually as a primary cutaneous adenocarcinoma. The epidermis becomes infiltrated with neoplastic cells showing glandular differentiation.

DIAGNOSIS

CLINICAL FEATURES

- Lesions present on the vulva as geographic red macules that often appear excoriated or have an eczematoid appearance (**Figures 82-1** to **82-3**). The lesions are often dotted with small, white patches (islands of tissue).

- The patient may have no symptoms or feel an itching and/or burning sensation.

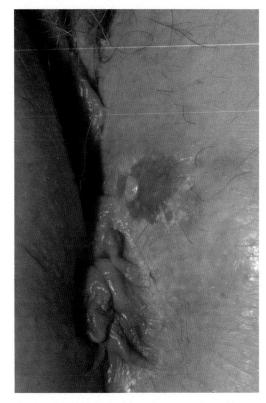

FIGURE 82-1 Paget's disease of the vulva. Note the red lesion with the "white island." (*Courtesy of Hope Haefner, MD.*)

- Pruritus is the most common symptom, present in 70% of patients.

- The lesions are well-demarcated and have slightly raised edges.

- Vulvar Paget's disease is similar in gross appearance to Paget's disease of the breast.

   Typical distribution: It is usually multifocal and may occur anywhere on the vulva, mons, perineum, perianal area, inner thigh, nipple, or bladder. It rarely occurs in males (**Figure 82-3**).

   Biopsy: Biopsy of gross lesions must be performed to determine the diagnosis and the depth and nature of stromal invasion. A punch biopsy should be taken from the center of the lesion and include underlying dermis and connective tissue so the depth of stromal invasion can be determined. If multiple abnormal areas are present, then multiple biopsies should be taken.

- The diagnosis is made by identification of "pagetoid" cells in the epidermis.
  ○ These cells are round in shape and considerably larger than the surrounding keratinocytes or melanocytes.
  ○ The cytoplasm is pink and the nuclei are large, round, and have prominent nucleoli.
  ○ The pagetoid cells cluster and form small nests in the rete pegs, but single cells spread into the superficial epidermis.
  ○ The appearance is similar to superficial melanoma, and sometimes special stains using markers that separate malignant melanocytes from Pagetoid cells may be necessary to identify the correct neoplasm.

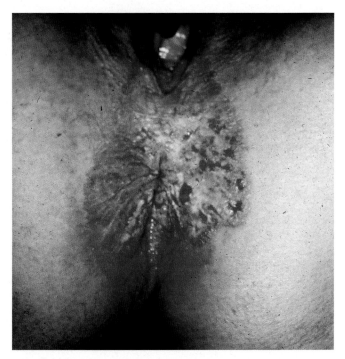

FIGURE 82-2 Perianal Paget's disease. Note the appearance is very similar to vulvar Paget's. (*Courtesy of University of Texas Health Sciences Center, Division of Dermatology.*)

DIFFERENTIAL DIAGNOSIS[3]

- Leukoplakia is an elevated white plaque seen before applying of acetic acid (see Chapter 83, Vulvar Intraepithelial Neoplasia).

- Squamous cell carcinoma of the vulva which can appear as expanding ulcerative lesions but without the "white islands" (see Chapter 164, Squamous Cell Carcinoma).

- Hidradenitis suppurativa also tends to form in apocrine areas but usually presents as chronic recurring abscesses (see Chapter 109, Hidradenitis Suppurativa).

- Amelanotic melanoma of the vulva can occur although vulvar melanoma is usually a pigmented lesion with irregular borders. Vulvar melanoma accounts for 5% of primary vulvar neoplasms, and occurs predominantly in postmenopausal white women (see Chapter 165, Melanoma).

- Condylomata accuminata (genital condylomas) are common and, when flat or excoriated, may be confused with vulvar Pagets disease. More than one-third of women have associated cervical intraepithelial neoplasia. Exophytic condylomas are typically verrucous, and usually occur in clusters along the vulvar surface (see Chapter 127, Genital Warts).

- Herpes simplex virus 1 and 2 are associated with ulcerative genital lesions and characteristic systemic symptoms (see Chapter 123, Herpes Simplex).

- Funfal infections commonly affect the vulva and are usually caused by Candida albicans. Patients present with vulvar itching and

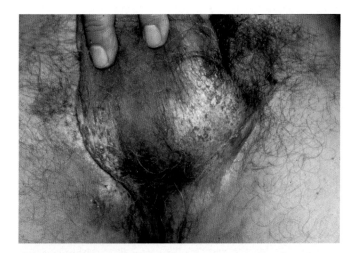

FIGURE 82-3 Paget's disease of the scrotum. (*Courtesy of University of Texas Health Sciences Center, Division of Dermatology.*)

burning. On inspection, the skin surface is red and may demonstrate small satellite lesions. A white "cottage cheese" discharge may also be present. Tinea cruris presents as a reddened area with raised sharp borders that occurs along the inner aspect of the thigh and often extends into the perianal and perineal region (see Chapter 130, Mucocutaneous Candidiasis).

- Lichen sclerosus is grossly and histologically similar to morphea (circumferential or localized scleroderma) which appears as white sclerotic or atrophic areas (**Figure 82-4**).

- Other dermatoses including seborrheic or contact dermatitis, psoriasis, lichen planus, and lichen simplex chronicus can resemble Paget's disease when these conditions occur in the vulva or perineum.

MANAGEMENT

- Treatment usually consists either of wide local excision or vulvectomy, if the disease is more extensive.[2] SOR **B** Local recurrence is common even in the face of negative surgical margins, presumably because the disease tends to be multicentric or from microscopic extension of disease beyond the margins.[2]

- Treatment with Moh's micrographic surgery may have a lower recurrence rate.[3] SOR **B**

- The role of radiation therapy and chemotherapy (topical and systemic) in the treatment of vulvar Paget's disease is not well-defined, but may be an option for some patients. SOR **C**

FOLLOW-UP

- Long-term follow-up is indicated because of the high risk of recurrence (even years after initial therapy) and the increased risk of noncontiguous carcinoma.

- The patient's vulva should be inspected annually and biopsy performed with any suggestion of abnormality.

- Screening and surveillance for tumors at other sites (breast, lung, colorectum, gastric, pancreas, and ovary) following national guidelines and U.S. Preventive Services Task Force guidelines should be considered.

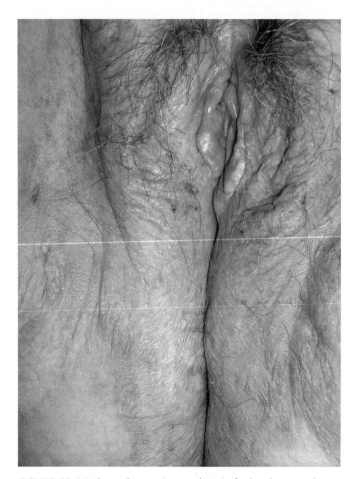

FIGURE 82-4 Lichen sclerosus (et atrophicus) of vulva showing white sclerotic plaques and epidermal atrophy. This was biopsy proven to rule out Paget's disease of the vulva and other possible malignancies. (*Courtesy of Richard P. Usatine, MD.*)

REFERENCE

1. Parker LP, Parker JR, Bodurka-Bevers D, et al. Paget's disease of the vulva: Pathology, pattern of involvement, and prognosis. *Gynecol Oncol.* 2000;77:183.

2. Fanning J, Lambert HC, Hale TM, et al. Paget's disease of the vulva: Prevalence of associated vulvar adenocarcinoma, invasive Paget's disease, and recurrence after surgical excision. *Am J Obstet Gynecol.* 1999;180:24.

3. Hendi A, Brodland DG, Zitelli JA. Extramammary Paget's disease: Surgical treatment with Mohs micrographic surgery. *J Am Acad Dermatol.* 2004;51:767.

83 VULVAR INTRAEPITHELIAL NEOPLASIA

E.J. Mayeaux, Jr., MD

PATIENT STORY

A 63-year-old black woman presents with a "knot" on her labia majora (**Figures 83-1** and **83-2**). She is a smoker but is otherwise healthy. The lesion is occasionally pruritic but is generally asymptomatic. She found it approximately 6 months ago, and it has been slowly increasing in size. There is no significant family history of cancer. On physical exam she is found to have exophytic condyloma acuminata around the introitus and a growth labelled VIN that the patient called a "knot." A 3-mm punch biopsy is performed and demonstrates vulvar intraepithelial neoplasia (VIN) III. The patient is referred to GYN oncology.

EPIDEMIOLOGY

- Vulvar cancer is the fourth most common gynecologic cancer (following cancer of the endometrium, ovary, and cervix) and accounts for 5% of lower female genital tract malignancies.[1] There are about 3900 new cases and 870 deaths each year in the United States from this disease.[1]

- Seventy-five percent of vulvar intraepithelial neoplasia (VIN) cases occur in premenopausal women, with no racial predisposition.

- Although the rate of invasive vulvar carcinoma has remained stable in the past two decades, the incidence of in situ disease (VIN) has more than doubled. This may be the result of improved surveillance and treatment of VIN, or the apparent increase in cases of VIN in younger women.[2]

ETIOLOGY AND PATHOPHYSIOLOGY

- VIN is the associated preneoplastic condition that is associated with the loss of epithelial cell maturation and nuclear abnormalities.

- Risk factors are similar to those for vulvar and cervical dysplasia, and include human papillomavirus infection, cigarette smoking, and altered immune status.[3]

- The cervix, vagina, vulva, anus, and lower three centimeters of rectal mucosa is derived from the embryonic cloaca. Most squamous intraepithelial lesions in this area affect multiple anatomic sites.

- The risk of neoplastic progression appears to be lower with VIN than with cervical intraepithelial neoplasia. VIN I probably has minimal malignant potential, but VIN III often progresses to invasive cancer if left untreated (see Biopsy).[4]

DIAGNOSIS

The vulva is best examined using a good source of white light and magnification from a handheld magnifying lens or a colposcope. The

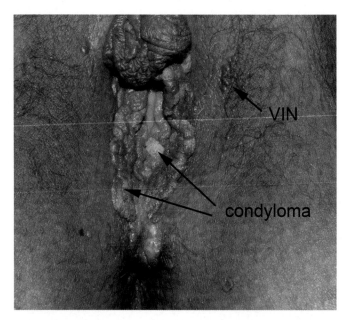

FIGURE 83-1 Patient with multiple exophytic condyloma and VIN III. The large clitoral hood is an incidental finding unrelated to the VIN. (*Courtesy of Hope Haefner, MD.*)

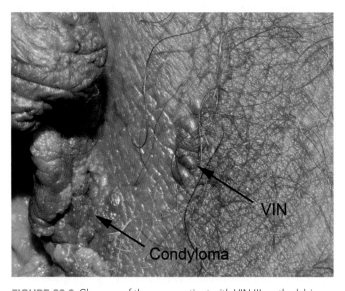

FIGURE 83-2 Close-up of the same patient with VIN III on the labia majora. (*Courtesy of Hope Haefner, MD.*)

examination should be systematic and incorporate all aspects of the vulvar surface. Vulvar examination may be aided by dilute acetic acid solution, which acts on the vulva much the same way as it does on the cervix and vagina. More acetic acid solution and a longer soaking time are required to achieve the aceto-white effect.

CLINICAL FEATURES

- VIN often appears as raised plaques and papules on the surface of the vulva and perineum (**Figures 83-1** and **83-2**).

- Approximately one-quarter of these lesions are pigmented (usually brown).

- Fifty percent of VINs are white (leukoplakia) or become aceto-white after soaking with dilute acetic acid (**Figure 83-3**).

- Lesions may occasionally be red and ulcerate (**Figure 83-4**). white areas may also indicate malignant changes (**Figures 83-5** and **83-6**).

- VIN can appear warty, so lesions that are diagnosed as condyloma but do not respond to conservative therapy should be biopsied to rule out VIN.

- More than 50% of patients presenting with vulvar dysplasia are without symptoms. Of patients with symptoms, pruritis is the most common.

- Lesions may become confluent, involving the labia majora, minora, and perianal skin.

TYPICAL DISTRIBUTION

Unlike cervical intraepithelial neoplasia, VIN is usually multifocal and can be located throughout the vulva, anus, and perineum. The inter-labial grooves, posterior fourchette, and perineum are the most frequent locations (**Figures 83-1 to 83-6**).

BIOPSY

Tissue biopsy is necessary for a definitive diagnosis of abnormal or ambiguous areas. After infiltration with lidocaine and epinephrine, 3 mm punch biopsies are performed in all suspicious areas. Bleeding can be stopped with a chemical hemostatic agent or electrosurgery. The biopsy sites usually do not need to be sutured and will heal well by secondary intention. Areas of ulceration should be sampled along the edge (**Figure 83-4**).

- On histology, VIN may be graded as VIN I (mild dysplasia), VIN II (moderate dysplasia), or VIN III (severe dysplasia, carcinoma in situ) based upon the depth of epithelial involvement.

- VIN III lesions are subdivided into three morphologic types; the basaloid type which shows a thickened epithelium with a relatively flat, smooth surface, the warty type which is characterized by a surface that has a condylomatous appearance, and the differentiated type in which the epithelium is thickened and parakeratotic with elongated and anastomosing rete ridges.

DIFFERENTIAL DIAGNOSIS

- Micropapillae of the inner labia minora have commonly been misinterpreted as being secondary to human papillomavirus. Micropapillomatosis is a condition in which the vestibular papillae are atypically prominent. It is a benign normal variant.

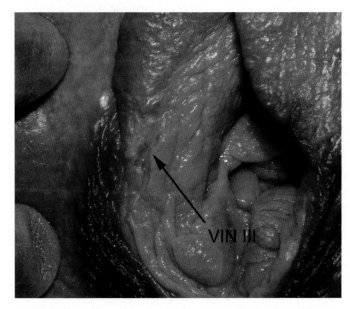

FIGURE 83-3 Diffuse white VIN III with ulceration. (*Courtesy of Hope Haefner, MD.*)

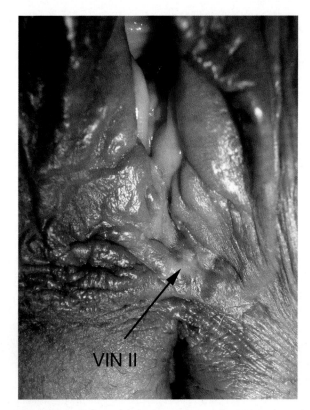

FIGURE 83-4 A small painful ulcer turned out to be VIN II on punch biopsy. A 3-mm punch biopsy was performed on the edge of the ulcer. (*Courtesy of Richard P. Usatine, MD.*)

- Sebaceous hyperplasia may be found as multiple small yellowish papules from Hart's line (junction of the keratinized skin and mucosa) to the junction of the hairbearing skin. This is a benign condition.

- Human papillomavirus causes condylomata accuminata (genital condylomas). More than one-third of women have associated cervical intraepithelial neoplasia. Exophytic condylomas are typically verrucous, and usually occur in clusters. They can be found at any site along the vulvar surface, and diagnosis is usually made by their characteristic appearance (see Chapter 127, Genital Warts).

- Herpes simplex virus 1 and 2 produce grouped vesicles and ulcers, and are associated with genital lesions (see Chapter 123, Herpes Simplex).

- Molluscum contagiosum lesions appear as small papules with central umbilicated cores that contain a cheesy material (see Chapter 124, Molluscum Contagiosum).

- Secondary syphilis usually appears as a gray, plaque-like lesion (condyloma lata) (see Chapter 209, Syphilis).

- Granuloma inguinale produces small red lesions appear from 3 weeks to three months after inoculation. These evolve into erosive ulcerations resulting in fibrosis and loss of superficial labial structures.

- Fungal infections commonly affect the vulva and are usually caused by Candida albicans. Patients present with vulvar itching and burning. On inspection, the skin surface is red and may demonstrate small satellite lesions. A white "cottage cheese" discharge may also be present (see Chapter 79, Candida Vaginitis).

- Tinea cruris presents as a reddened area with raised sharp borders that occurs along the inner aspect of the thigh and often extends into the perianal and perineal region (see Chapter 133, Tinea Cruris).

- Lichen sclerosus is grossly and histologically similar to morphea (circumferential or localized scleroderma) and appears as white atrophic patches with erythema and loss of hair. Areas suspicious for VIN should be biopsied (**Figure 83-7**).

- Other dermatoses including psoriasis, lichen planus, and lichen simplex chronicus may present on the vulva and be confused with VIN.

- Nevi are benign melanocytic skin tumors that may occur in any area of the body, including the vulva.

MANAGEMENT

- Patients with VIN 1 can be followed by close observation. SOR Ⓑ

- Patients with VIN grade 2 and 3 should have their lesions removed. Basaloid and warty VINs may be treated with ablation on non-hair bearing epithelium. Differentiated VINs and any lesions in hair bearing areas are generally treated with a wide local excision. Resected VIN specimens should be examined for residual disease in the margin.[5] SOR Ⓑ

- The 5-FU cream has been a traditional treatment for VIN that causes a chemical desquamation of the lesion.[6] It may result in significant burning, pain, inflammation, edema, and occasional painful

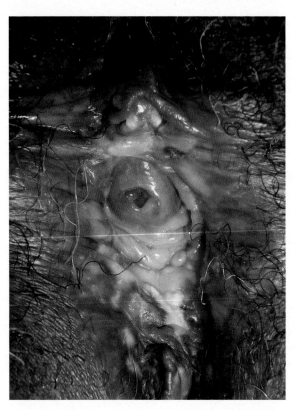

FIGURE 83-5 A 59-year-old woman with long history of condyloma and CIN presents with a vaginal irritation. In addition to her cystocele after her hysterectomy, she is found to have Trichomonas and evidence of atrophic changes. However, the most concerning areas are the leukoplakia at 6-, 11-, and 12- o'clock positions. These are most suspicious for VIN. (*Courtesy of Richard P. Usatine, MD.*)

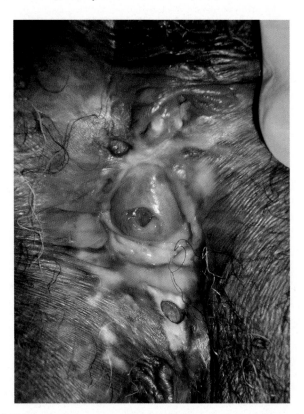

FIGURE 83-6 The woman in **Figure 83-5** after punch biopsies are performed of the most suspicious areas. Both biopsies show moderate epithelial dysplasia, VIN II along with associated human papilloma virus changes. (*Courtesy of Richard P. Usatine, MD.*)

ulcerations. Biopsy to exclude invasive disease is mandatory prior to 5-FU treatment.[6] SOR **B**

- Imiquimod cream is a topical immune response modifier that is FDA-approved for the treatment of anogenital warts, actinic keratosis, and certain basal cell carcinomas.[7] It has been used to treat multifocal VIN II or III in a few small pilot studies. The cream is self-administered three times per week for periods of 6 to 34 weeks.[7] SOR **B**

PATIENT RESOURCES

- Oncolink—Cervical, Vaginal, Vulvar Cancers—**http://oncolink.upenn.edu/types/types.cfm?c/=6.**

- Information on patient education is available with the International Society for the Study of Vulvovaginal Disease—**http://www.issvd.org/patient_education/patient_education.htm.**

- Vulvar Self Examination—**http://www.ivf.com/vse.html.**

- Vulva Self-examination—**http://wso.williams.edu/orgs/peerh/women/wsexam.html.**

PROVIDER RESOURCE

- Practice Management Materials from the American Society for Colposcopy and Cervical Pathology—**http://asccp.org/edu/practice/vulva.shtml** for the vulva.

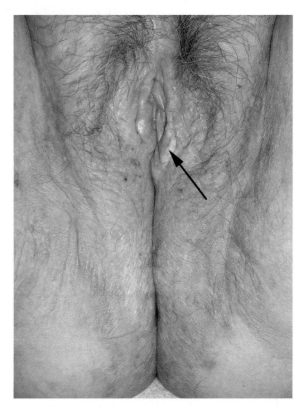

FIGURE 83-7 A 55-year-old woman with lichen sclerosus (et atrophicus). A biopsy was taken at the site indicated by the arrow to confirm the diagnosis and make sure that there was no VIN arising in that area. (*Courtesy of Richard P. Usatine, MD.*)

REFERENCE

1. Jemal A, Murray T, Ward W, et al. Cancer statistics. 2005. *CA Cancer J Clin.* 2005;55:10.

2. Sturgeon SR, Brinton LA, Devesa SS, Kurman RJ. In situ and invasive vulvar cancer incidence trends (1973–87). *Am J Obstet Gynecol.* 1992;166:1482.

3. Modesitt SC, Waters AB, Walton L, et al. Vulvar intraepithelial neoplasia III: Occult cancer and the impact of margin status on recurrence. *Obstet Gynecol.* 1998;92:962.

4. Jones RW, Rowan DM. Vulvar intraepithelial neoplasia III: A clinical study of the outcome in 113 cases with relation to the later development of invasive vulvar carcinoma. *Obstet Gynecol.* 1994;84:741.

5. Di Saia PJ, Rich WM. Surgical approach to multifocal carcinoma in situ of the vulva. *Am J Obstet Gynecol.* 1981;140:136.

6. Krupp PJ. 5-fluorouracil topical treatment of in situ vulvar cancer. *Obstet Gynecol.* 1978;51:702.

7. Le T, Menard C, Hicks-Boucher W, et al. Final results of a phase 2 study using continuous 5% Imiquimod cream application in the primary treatment of high-grade vulva intraepithelial neoplasia. *Gynecol Oncol.* 2007;106:579.

84 COLPOSCOPY—NORMAL AND NONCANCEROUS FINDINGS

E.J. Mayeaux, Jr., MD

PATIENT STORY

A 21-year-old woman presents for her well-woman examination. She has been followed by her physician for many years and has no complaints. She has been sexually active for a little more than 2 years with one mutually monogamous partner. She does not smoke, has never had a sexually transmitted disease (STD), and uses oral contraceptive pills for contraception. On speculum exam, her cervix appears normal (**Figure 84-1**) and a Pap smear is performed.

EPIDEMIOLOGY

- The Papanicolaou smear (Pap smear) is a commonly employed screening test for dysplasia and cancer of the uterine cervix. More than 50 million Pap smears are performed each year in the United States.[1] Colposcopy is the diagnostic test to evaluate patients with an abnormal cervical cytological smear or abnormal-appearing cervix.

ETIOLOGY AND PATHOPHYSIOLOGY

- Colposcopy entails the use of a field microscope to examine the cervix. The cervix and vagina are examined under magnification, and all abnormal areas are identified.

- If the colposcopy is satisfactory (the entire transformation zone (TZ) is examined and the extent of all lesions is seen) (**Figure 84-2**). Directed biopsies of the most abnormal areas are performed to obtain a tissue diagnosis.

- Colposcopy begins after visualization of the cervix prior to application of acetic acid to look for leukoplakia and abnormal vessels. 3–5% acetic acid is applied with a cotton ball held in a ring forceps or with a rectal swab. Scan the cervix with low power (typically 5x) and determine if the entire TZ, including the entire squamocolumnar junction (SCJ) can be seen. The borders of all lesions must be entirely visible (not disappearing into the canal) for the examination to be adequate.

- Most of the normal cervical findings are derived from the physiologic transformation of the exposed columnar epithelium to squamous epithelium (**Figures 84-1** and **84-2**). Noncancerous findings may include epithelial thinning and whitening as a result of

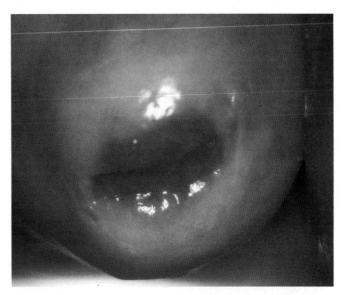

FIGURE 84-1 Normal cervix as seen through a colposcope without the application of vinegar. The red color around the os is produced by columnar cells and the lighter pink on the remainder of the cervix result from normal squamous cells. The presence of visible columnar cells outside the internal os is called ectropian and is a normal finding in young women and women on estrogen-containing contraception. The junction between the two cell types and colors is the squamocolumnar junction. (*Courtesy of E.J. Mayeaux, Jr., MD.*)

lack of estrogen, and polyp formations. The damage to the cervical epithelium from various infections often produces inflammation, friability, discharge, and bleeding.

DIAGNOSIS

- Normal colposcopic findings include[2]:
  - *Original Squamous Epithelium*, which is a featureless, smooth, pink epithelium without gland openings or Nabothian cysts (**Figure 84-3**).
  - *Columnar Epithelium* is a single-cell layer, mucous producing, epithelium that extends between the endometrium and the squamous epithelium. Columnar epithelium appears red and irregular with stromal papillae and clefts (**Figure 84-3**). With acetic acid application and magnification, columnar epithelium has a grape-like or "sea-anemone" appearance.
  - *SCJ* is a clinically visible line seen on the ectocervix or within the distal canal, which demarcates endocervical tissue from squamous (or squamous metaplastic) tissue (**Figure 84-3**).
  - *Squamous Metaplasia* is the physiologic, normal process whereby columnar epithelium transforms into squamous epithelium. At the SCJ, it appears as a "ghostly white" or white-blue film with the application of acetic acid. It is usually sharply demarcated toward the cervical os and has very diffuse borders peripherally (**Figure 84-3**).
  - *TZ* is the geographic area between the original squamous epithelium (before puberty) and the current SCJ. It may contain gland openings, Nabothian cysts, and islands of columnar epithelium surrounded by metaplastic squamous epithelium (**Figures 84-2** and **84-3**).
- Other nondysplastic colposcopic findings:
  - *Cervicitis* from an infection may make colposcopic assessment for dysplasia and cervical cancer difficult. *Cervicitis* appears as friable, inflamed epithelium, often in the presence of a vaginal discharge Trichomonas may cause an inflamed cervix that has a strawberry appearance (**Figure 84-4**) (see Chapter 80, Trichomonas Vaginitis).
  - *Atrophic vaginal or cervical epithelium* is frequently white and easily traumatized (**Figure 84-5**) (see Chapter 77, Atrophic Vaginitis).
  - *Nabothian cysts* are normal areas of mucus-producing epithelium that are "roofed over" with squamous epithelium (**Figure 84-3**). They do not require any treatment.

DIFFERENTIAL DIAGNOSIS

- Friability from infections must be differentiated from dysplastic changes by a history of possible exposure to STDs, presence of discharge, wet prep, and STD testing.

MANAGEMENT

- *Atrophic vaginal or cervical epithelium* can be treated with intravaginal estrogen for 2 to 4 weeks before colposcopy in order to "normalize"

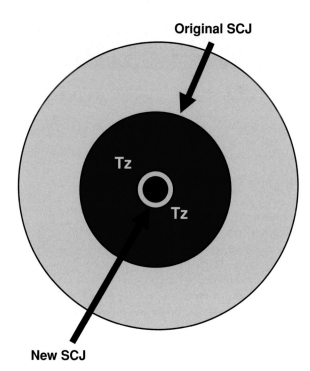

FIGURE 84-2 Schematic demonstration of the development of the transformation zone (TZ). The TZ extends from the original (prepubertal) squamocolumnar junction (SCJ) to the new (current) SCJ. This transformation zone in the area at highest risk for cervical cancer. (*Courtesy of E.J. Mayeaux, Jr., MD.*)

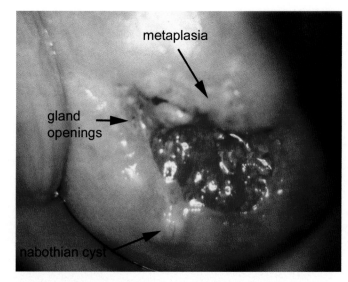

FIGURE 84-3 Normal transformation zone (TZ) viewed with colposcopy. Note the squamocolumnar junction separating the red columnar epithelium from the pink squamous epithelium. Gland openings, nabothian cysts and metaplasia are all part of this normal TZ. There is a white area of normal metaplasia on the anterior lip and a yellowish nabothian cyst on the posterior lip. (*Courtesy of E.J. Mayeaux, Jr., MD.*)

the epithelium. SOR ⊙ This is generally safe, even if dysplasia or cancer is present, because the duration of therapy is short, and these lesions do not express any more estrogen receptors than a normal cervix.[3]

- *Vaginocervicitis* is treated once the source is diagnosed

- *Nabothian cysts* do not require any treatment. If you tell patients that they have a Nabothian cyst, please tell them that this is a normal finding.

- *Cervical dysplastic changes* should be handled according to national evidence-based guidelines (see Chapters 85–87).[4]

PATIENT EDUCATION

- Patients should be discouraged from douching since it irritates the mucus membranes, disrupts normal flora, and makes acquisition of an STD more likely if exposed. Safer-sex education should be give to all patients at risk of acquiring an STD.

FOLLOW-UP

- If an infection coexists with an abnormal Pap smear or grossly abnormal appearing cervix, the infection should be treated and the colposcopic assessment should be performed 1 month later.

PATIENT RESOURCE

- National Cancer Institute, Cervical Cancer Screening— **http://lib-sh.lsuhsc.edu/fammed/atlases/colpo.html.**

PROVIDER RESOURCE

- American Society for Colposcopy and Cervical Pathology (includes colposcopy and treatment algorithms)— **http://www.asccp.org.**

REFERENCES

1. Sirovich BE, Welch HG. The frequency of Pap smear screening in the united States. *J Gen Intern Med.* 2004;19:243–250.

2. Stafl A, Wilbanks GD. An international terminology of colposcopy: Report of the nomenclature committee of the International federation of cervical pathology and colposcopy. *Obstet Gynecol.* 1991;77: 313–314.

3. Sadan O, Frohlich RP, Driscoll JA, Apostoleris A, Savage N, Zakust H. Is it safe to prescribe hormonal contraception and replacement therapy to patients with premalignant and malignant uterine cervices? *Gynecol Oncol.* 1986;34:159–163.

4. Wright TC Jr., Cox JT, Massad LS, Twiggs LB, Wilkinson EJ. For the 2001 ASCCP-sponsored consensus conference. Consensus guidelines for the management of women with cervical cytological abnormalities and cervical cancer precursors. part I: Cytological abnormalities. *JAMA.* 2002;287(18):2120–2129.

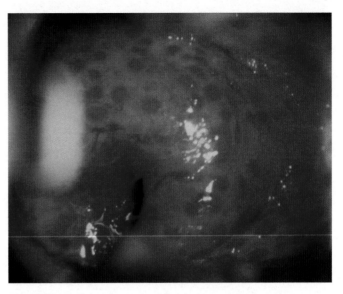

FIGURE 84-4 Colposcopic view of trichomonas infection. Note disruption of the epithelium with petechiae and pinpoint bleeding producing the "strawberry" cervix. (*Courtesy of E.J. Mayeaux, Jr., MD.*)

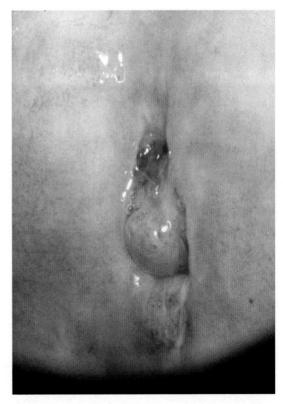

FIGURE 84-5 Colposcopic view of cervical atrophy and a benign endocervical polyp in a postmenopausal woman. Note the pale epithelium and the polyp extending from the cervical os. (*Courtesy of E.J. Mayeaux, Jr., MD.*)

85 COLPOSCOPY OF LOW-GRADE DISEASE

E.J. Mayeaux, Jr., MD

PATIENT STORY

A 23-year-old woman has a low-grade squamous intraepithelial lesion on her Pap smear. One colposcopic view of her cervix shows acetowhite changes consistent with a cervical intraepithelial neoplasia grade I lesion (CIN I) (**Figure 85-1**). She has no other suspicious findings and biopsy of the acetowhite area confirms CIN I. The endo-cervical curettage is negative for disease. During the follow-up visit the doctor and patient together decide to proceed with watchful waiting and repeat Pap smears at 6 and 12 months.

EPIDEMIOLOGY

- In low-grade squamous intraepithelial lesion (LGSIL) smears, the abnormalities are typically associated with human papillomavirus (HPV) infection or cervical intraepithelial neoplasia (CIN) grade I lesions.[1] Overall rates of Pap smear abnormalities are often estimated from regional studies. For example, in an observational cohort study of routine cervical smears in the Northwest United States, in women of all ages ($n = 150,052$), atypical squamous cells was diagnosed at a rate of 9.8 per 1000, low-grade squamous intraepithelial lesion was diagnosed at a rate of 3.5 per 1000, and negative routine smears occured at a rate of 278.5 per 1000.[2]

ETIOLOGY AND PATHOPHYSIOLOGY

- Essentially all CIN is caused by HPV. Ten to 15% of CIN I lesions progress to CIN II–III, and that 0.3% progress to cervical cancer.[3]
- There is no way to determine which CIN I lesions (**Figures 85-1** to **85-3**) or simple HPV lesions (**Figures 85-4** and **85-5**) will regress or progress.
- Colposcopy is the standard of care for assessing cervical dysplasia. It entails the use of a field microscope to examine the cervix after acetic acid (**Figures 85-1** to **85-4**) and Lugol's iodine (**Figure 85-5**) are applied to temporarily stain the cervix. The cervix and vagina are examined under magnification, and all abnormal areas are identified. If the colposcopy is satisfactory (the entire transformation zone is examined and the extent of all lesions is seen), directed biopsies of all lesions and especially the most severe lesions are performed.
- An atypical transformation zone is defined as a transformation zone with findings suggesting cervical dysplasia or neoplasia. Differences in thickness, density of the cells, degree of differentiation, and keratin production determine the color and opacity of the epithelium, and may produce the abnormal findings of leukoplakia and acetowhite (AW) epithelium.

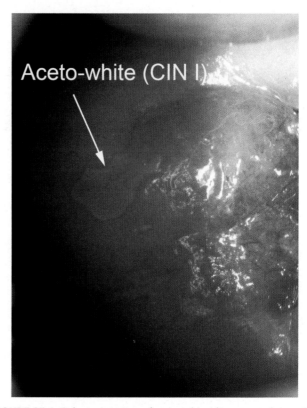

FIGURE 85-1 Colposcopic view of aceto-white changes on the cervix of CIN I lesions after the application of acetic acid. Note the irregular geographic borders. (*Courtesy of E.J. Mayeaux, Jr., MD.*)

DIAGNOSIS

- The diagnosis of low-grade cervical abnormalities is made on colposcopic examination. Findings consistent with this diagnosis include[1]:
  - **Acetowhite** changes (**Figures 85-1** to **85-4**). A transient, white-appearing epithelium following the application of acetic acid may be abnormal and correlates with higher nuclear density. The more sharp and angular the margin is, the likelier it is to be dysplastic. The margins of low-grade disease are usually feathery or geographic borders. Most low-grade lesions are snowy white with a shiny surface. A uniformly papillary surface is often indicative of HPV disease.
  - **Punctation** is a stippled appearance of small looped capillaries seen end-on, often found within AW area, appearing as fine-to-coarse red dots. Fine punctuation has fine caliber vessels that are regularly spaced, and is usually associated with benign conditions or low-grade disease (**Figures 86-3** and **86-4**).
  - **Lack of iodine** staining (Schiller's test) may be used when further clarification of potential biopsy sites is necessary (**Figure 85-5**). It need not be used in all cases. The sharp outlining afforded by Lugol's solution can be dramatic and very helpful.
- Biopsy is usually indicated to establish the histological grade of the abnormalities present.

DIFFERENTIAL DIAGNOSIS

- CIN I and HPV lesions must be differentiated from nonmalignant inflammatory lesions such as yeast vaginitis and sexually transmitted diseases, which usually present with vaginal itching, odor, and/or discharge (see Chapter 79, Candida Vulvovaginitis).
- High-grade dysplasia (CIN II/III) and cancer must also be ruled out, usually by colposcopic examination and biopsy (see Chapter 86, High-Grade Lesions).

MANAGEMENT

- According to the 2006 consensus guideline, the preferred treatment for women with CIN I and satisfactory colposcopy is repeat cytology at six and 12 months or DNA testing for HPV types at 12 months.[3,4] SOR **B** Most cases of CIN I spontaneously regress.
- Observation without treatment is acceptable in pregnant women and adolescents with CIN I and unsatisfactory colposcopy.[3,4] SOR **B**
- Treatment options for CIN can be grouped into chemically destructive, surgical ablative, and surgical excisional methods. Cryotherapy, laser, and loop electrosurgical methods are commonly employed when treatment is selected.
- Candidates for outpatient cervical cryotherapy are patients with smaller lesions that do not enter the cervical os. Endocervical sampling is recommended before applying any ablative treatment.[3,4] SOR **B**

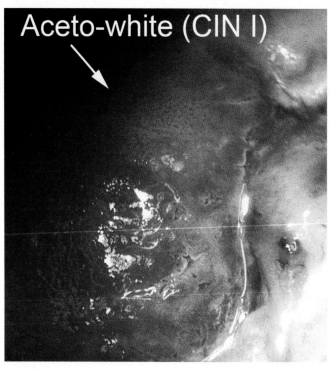

FIGURE 85-2 Another colposcopy view of acetowhite changes on the cervix of CIN I lesions. (*Courtesy of E.J. Mayeaux, Jr., MD.*)

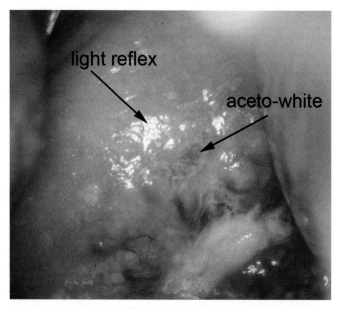

FIGURE 85-3 Colposcopy view of an indistinct AW lesion on the anterior lip. Note the light reflex just above the lesion that may be confused with an actual lesion. (*Courtesy of E.J. Mayeaux, Jr., MD.*)

- Large lesions (more than 1″ in diameter, more than 0.5″ from the os, or involving more than two cervical quadrants) may be more appropriate loop or laser therapy.[3,4] SOR Ⓑ

PATIENT EDUCATION

- Smoking cessation counseling is an important part of therapy for women who continue to smoke.
- The patient should also be counseled that an HPV vaccine may still be of benefit if indicated. The Advisory Committee on Immunization Practices (ACIP) recommends giving the vaccine to women in the indicated age group even if they have had an abnormal Pap smear since although it will not change the course of the current infection, it will protect from any HPV types the patient has not been exposed to yet.[5]

FOLLOW-UP

- Follow-up is in 4- to 6-month intervals until the patient has 2 serial normal examinations, with colposcopy or colposcopy interspersed with Pap smears. Recurrence is most common in the first 2 years after therapy. Recurrences are most common in the os and on the outside margins.
- After two consecutive negative Pap smears or one negative high risk-HPV DNA test, patients should continue to be screened at annual intervals.

PATIENT RESOURCES

- American Social Health Association-HPV—**http://www. ashastd.org/hpv/hpv_learn.cfm.**
- Oncolink: Cervical, Vaginal, Vulvar Cancers—**http:// oncolink.upenn.edu/types/types.cfm?c=6.**

PROVIDER RESOURCE

- Treatment algorithms based on the American Society for Colposcopy and Cervical Pathology 2006 Consensus guidelines for the management of women with abnormal Cervical Cancer Screening Tests available at **http://www.asccp.org/ consensus/cytological.shtml.**

REFERENCES

1. Stafl A, Wilbanks GD. An international terminology of colposcopy: Report of the nomenclature committee of the International federation of cervical pathology and colposcopy. *Obstet Gynecol.* 1991;77:313–314.

2. Insinga RP, Glass AG, Rush BB. Diagnoses and outcomes in cervical cancer screening: A population-based study. *Am J Obstet Gynecol.* 2004;191:105–113.

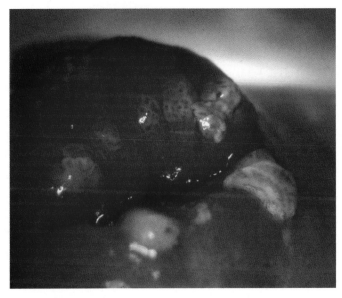

FIGURE 85-4 Colposcopy view of condyloma of the cervix. Note the bright AW effect that is common on condyloma. (*Courtesy of E.J. Mayeaux, Jr., MD.*)

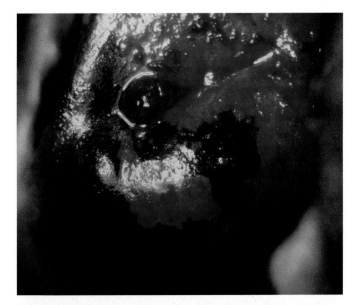

FIGURE 85-5 Colposcopic view of a cervix after Lugol's solution is applied. The abnormal CIN I lesion is the area on the cervix that does not stain brown with the iodine in the Lugol's solution. The areas that do not stain can then be biopsied. This is called Schiller's test. (*Courtesy of E.J. Mayeaux, Jr., MD.*)

3. Spitzer M, Apgar BS, Brotzman GL. Management of histologic abnormalities of the cervix. *Am Fam Physician*. 2006;73:105–112.

4. Wright TC, Jr., Massad LS, Dunton CJ, Spitzer M, Wilkinson EJ, Solomon D; 2006. American Society for Colposcopy and Cervical Pathology-sponsored Consensus Conference. 2006 consensus guidelines for the management of women with cervical intraepithelial neoplasia or adenocarcinoma in situ. *Am J Obstet Gynecol*. 2007;197(4):340–5. Available at http://www.asccp.org/consensus/histological.shtml

5. Advisory Committee on Immunization Practices (ACIP). ACIP recommendations for the use of quadrivalent HPV vaccine. Available at: http://www.cdc.gov/nip/recs/provisional_recs/hpv.pdf. Accessed February 18, 2008.

86 COLPOSCOPY OF HIGH-GRADE DISEASE

E.J. Mayeaux, Jr., MD

PATIENT STORY

A 36-year-old woman presented for follow-up of a persistently abnormal Pap smear. She is a smoker and has had multiple new sexual partners in the last few years. Although she has had several "abnormal Pap smears" in the past, she states she has never needed treatment. She was found to have a dense acetowhite (AW) lesion on colposcopy that was biopsied (**Figure 86-1**). The pathology returned cervical intraepithelial neoplasia (CIN) III and the patient was treated with loop electrosurgery. She had negative margins on the loop electrosurgical excision procedure specimen and remained recurrence free at 3 years.

EPIDEMIOLOGY AND PATHOPHYSIOLOGY

- Overall rates of Pap smear abnormalities are usually estimated from local or regional studies. For example, in an observational cohort study of routine cervical smears in the Northwest United States, in women of all ages ($n = 150,052$), high-grade squamous intraepitheliel lesion was diagnosed at a rate of 0.8 per 1000 compared to negative routine smears was diagnosed at a rate of 278.5 per 1000.[1]

ETIOLOGY AND PATHOPHYSIOLOGY

- In high-grade squamous intraepitheliel lesion smears, the abnormalities are in immature parabasilar cell types. They have increased nuclear to cytoplasmic ratio, enlarged hyperchromatic nucleoli, few nucleoli, and a reticular or granular appearance.

- On histology, abnormal maturation and nuclear atypia defines CIN. Koilocytosis (perinuclear cytoplasmic vacuolization) is indicative of human papillomavirus (HPV) infection and may be found with high-grade CIN. High-grade CIN is diagnosed when immature basaloid cells with nuclear atypia occupy greater than the lower one-third of the epithelium. With increasing lesion severity, there is also increased nuclear crowding, pleomorphism, normal and abnormal mitosis, and loss of polarity.

- For untreated CIN II, approximately 43% will spontaneously regress, 35% will persist, and 22% will progress to carcinoma in situ or invasive cancer.[2] The regression rate of CIN II is higher in adolescents.

- For untreated CIN III, approximately 32% will regress; 56% will persist, and 14% of CIN III will progress to carcinoma in situ or invasive cancer.[2]

- Traditionally, high-grade CIN is thought to arise as a small focus within a larger area of low-grade CIN that expands and eventually replaces much of the low-grade lesion.

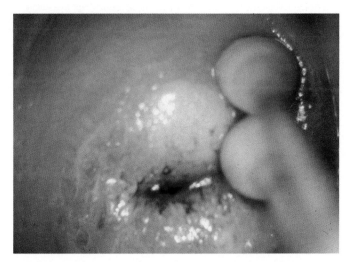

FIGURE 86-1 Dense acetowhite (white after application of vinegar) lesions with "rolled" edges in a patient with high-grade disease. Her colposcopically directed biopsies showed CIN III. (*Courtesy of E.J. Mayeaux, Jr., MD.*)

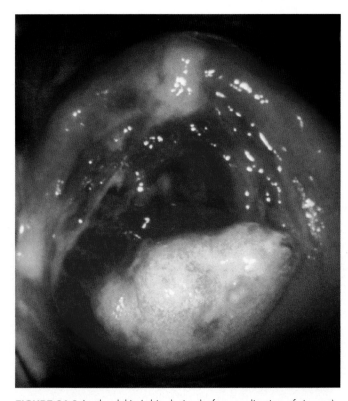

FIGURE 86-2 Leukoplakia (white lesion before application of vinegar) of the cervix seen with colposcopy in a patient with high-grade SIL. (*Courtesy of E.J. Mayeaux, Jr., MD.*)

- This "monoclonal" theory is supported by the fact that there is a 5-year difference between the peak prevalence of CIN I and CIN II/III, and detection of a low-grade squamous intraepitheliel lesion Pap greatly increases the risk that a high-grade CIN will be found on subsequent smears.
  - It has been difficult to document the rate of progression because most studies use cervical biopsy to establish an accurate diagnosis, which influences the rate of disease progression.
- With the discovery that most CIN I lesions regress or persist, the question has been raised as to whether high-grade CIN might be a process that develops concurrently and somewhat independently from low-grade CIN.
  - This theory is supported by the fact that CIN III can develop without a detectable preceding low-grade CIN lesion, and high-grade CIN is almost always found closer to the squamo-columnar junction than concomitant low-grade lesions. It has also been found that women who turned HPV 16/18 positive had a 39% rate of high-grade CIN at 2 years compared to HPV negative women.
  - Schiffman, et al. reported that both CIN I and CIN II/III lesions developed within the same time frame in a large group of women who turned HPV positive and were followed for 4 years.[3]
- Which theory is most correct is a matter of debate. Many practitioners still treat CIN I level lesions on the basis of the monoclonal theory or on the theory that if both lesions arise concomitantly, then treating CIN I lesions may be the best way of eliminating high-grade CIN. Others promote the idea of observing CIN I lesions and treating only high-grade CIN lesions.

DIAGNOSIS

- Leukoplakia, as shown in **Figure 86-2**, is typically an elevated, white plaque seen prior to the application of acetic acid. It is caused by a thick keratin layer that obscures the underlying epithelium, and may signal severe dysplasia or cancer. Although it may be associated with benign findings, it always warrants a biopsy.
- AW epithelium following the application of acetic acid is typical for CIN II/III lesions (**Figure 86-1**). The AW effect tends to develop more slowly than in lower-grade lesions and to persist longer. The margins of high-grade CIN are straighter and sharper compared to the vague, feathery, geographic borders of CIN I or HPV disease.
- When high-grade CIN coexists in the same lesion with a lower-grade lesion, the higher-grade lesion often presents with a sharply defined internal border (also known as a border-within-a-border).
- With increasing levels of CIN, desmosomes (intracellular bridges) that attach the epithelium to the basement membrane are often lost, producing an edge that easily peels. This loss of tissue integrity should raise the suspicion of high-grade dysplasia. The extreme expression of this effect is the ulceration that sometimes forms with invasive disease.
- High-grade CIN lesions are usually proximal to or touch the squamo-columnar junction, even when contained in larger lesions (**Figures 86-1 to 86-5**).

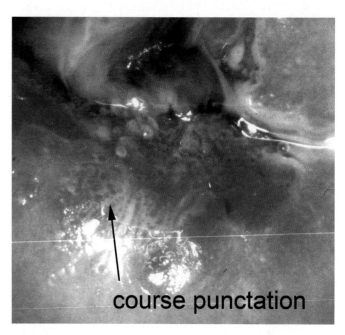

FIGURE 86-3 Course punctuation of the cervix seen through the colposcope in a patient with high-grade disease. (*Courtesy of E.J. Mayeaux, Jr., MD.*)

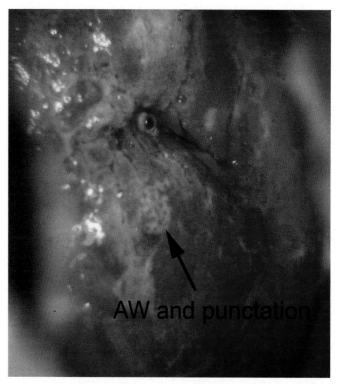

FIGURE 86-4 AW epithelium and course punctuation on the same cervix (arrow). The biopsies of this area showed CIN 3. (*Courtesy of E.J. Mayeaux, Jr., MD.*)

- Nodular elevations on the surface of lesions and ulceration are suspicious for high-grade or invasive cancer.

- Increases in local factors such as tumor angiogenesis factor or vascular endothelial growth factor, which are much more commonly produced by CIN III lesions, cause growth of abnormal surface vasculature, producing punctuation (**Figures 86-3** and **86-4**), mosaicism (**Figure 86-5**), and frankly abnormal vessels. However, most high-grade lesions do not develop any abnormal vessels.

- Punctation is a stippled appearance of small looped capillaries seen end-on, often found within AW area, appearing as fine-to-coarse red dots (**Figures 86-3** and **86-4**). Course punctation represents increased caliber vessels that are spaced at irregular intervals, and is more highly associated with increasing levels of dysplasia.

- Mosaicism is an abnormal pattern of small blood vessels suggesting a confluence of "tiles" or a "chicken-wire pattern" with reddish borders. Mosaicism represents capillaries that grow on or near the surface of the lesion that forms partitions between blocks of proliferating epithelium (**Figure 86-5**). It develops in a manner very similar to punctation and is often found in the same lesions. Course mosaic forms a consistently irregular cobblestone effect with dilated coarse vessels which is highly associated with CIN II/III.

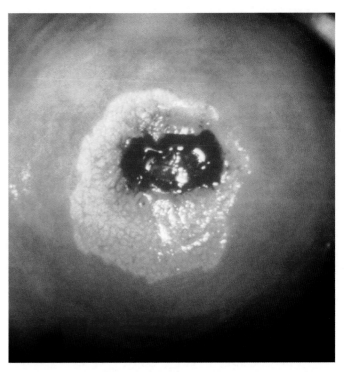

FIGURE 86-5 Colposcopy with findings of mosaicism in a patient with CIN 3. (*Courtesy of E.J. Mayeaux, Jr., MD.*)

DIFFERENTIAL DIAGNOSIS

- CIN II/III lesions must be differentiated from nonmalignant inflammatory lesions, especially Trichomoniasis and Chlamydia infections, which usually present with vaginal itching, odor, and/or discharge (see Chapter 80, Trichomonas Vaginitis, and Chapter 81, Chlamydia Cervicitis).

- Flat HPV lesions may mimic the dense AW lesions of CIN II/III.

- CIN II/III lesions must be differentiated from both CIN I and cancer (see Chapter 85, Colposcopy of Low-Grade Disease, and Chapter 87, Colposcopy of Cervical Cancer).

MANAGEMENT

- Except in special circumstances, women with biopsy-confirmed CIN II/III should be treated. CIN II may be followed with colposcopy and Pap smears in patients who have not attained their 21st birthday.[4,5]

- Effective treatment of CIN II/III requires the removal of the entire transformation zone rather than just the removal of the lesion. When colposcopy is satisfactory, any ablative or excisional modality will treat CIN effectively.[4] SOR **A** However, because excisional modalities allow for the pathologic identification of unanticipated microinvasive or occult invasive cancer, some physicians prefer these methods to treat biopsy-confirmed CIN II/III.[2] SOR **C**

- Both excision and ablation are acceptable treatment choices for nonpregnant adult women with a histological diagnosis of CIN II/III and satisfactory colposcopy. For adolescents and young women with a histological diagnosis of CIN II, observation with colposcopy and cytology at 6 month intervals is preferred but treatment is acceptable.

- Observation is unacceptable in women with CIN II except during pregnancy and in very compliant adolescents with satisfactory colposcopy and negative results on endocervical curettage.[5] SOR **C**

- A randomized clinical trial demonstrated that condom use promotes regression of CIN and clearance of HPV.[6] SOR **B**

- Because a small number of women with biopsy-confirmed CIN II/III and unsatisfactory colposcopy have occult invasive cancer, excisional procedures should be performed. Cold knife and loop electrosurgical excision procedure conizations effectively diagnose and treat these women.[5] SOR **B**

PATIENT EDUCATION

- Tobacco smoking has been linked to the development and recurrence of CIN. Part of any treatment program should include smoking cessation.

FOLLOW-UP

- After treatment for CIN II/III, acceptable management methods include cytology with or without colposcopy at 4- to 6-month intervals until three negative evaluations have been obtained, or HPV DNA testing no sooner than six months after treatment.[4,5] SOR **C**

- The preferred management for CIN identified at the margin of a diagnostic excisional procedure or in postprocedure endocervical sampling is colposcopy and endocervical sampling at the 4- to 6-month follow-up evaluation.[4,5] SOR **C**

PATIENT RESOURCES

- For information on Cervical Cancer Screening: National Cancer Institute—**http://www.cancer.gov/cancertopics/ types/cervical.**

- Oncolink—Cervical, Vaginal, Vulvar Cancers—**http:// oncolink.upenn.edu/types/types.cfm?c=6.**

- For more information on Patient Education: The International Society for the Study of Vulvovaginal Disease—**http://www. issvd.org/patient_education/patient_education.htm.**

PROVIDER RESOURCES

- Shreveport Colposcopy Atlas, Louisiana State University Health Sciences Center—**http://lib-sh.lsuhsc.edu/fammed/ atlases/colpo.html.**

- Treatment algorithms based on the American Society for Colposcopy and Cervical Pathology 2001 Consensus guidelines for the management of women with CIN are available at— **http://www.asccp.org/.**

REFERENCES

1. Insinga RP, Glass AG, Rush BB. Diagnoses and outcomes in cervical cancer screening: A population-based study. *Am J Obstet Gynecol.* 2004;191:105–113.

2. Spitzer M, Apgar BS, Brotzman GL. Management of histologic abnormalities of the cervix. *Am Fam Physician*. 2006;73:105–112.

3. Schiffman MH, Bauer HM, Hoover RN, et al. Epidemiological evidence showing that human papillomavirus infection causes most cervical intraepithelial neoplasia. *J Natl Cancer Inst*. 1994;85: 958–964.

4. Wright Jr., TC, Massad LS, Dunton CJ, et al. 2006 consensus guidelines for the management of women with cervical intraepithelial neoplasia or adenocarcinoma in situ. *Am J Obstet Gynecol*. 2007;197(4):340–345.

5. Wright Jr., TC, Massad LS, Dunton CJ, et al. 2006 consensus guidelines for the management of women with abnormal cervical cancer screening tests. *Am J Obstet Gynecol*. 2007;197(4):346–355.

6. Hogewoning CJ, Bleeker MC, van den Brule AJ, et al. Condom use promotes regression of cervical intraepithelial neoplasia and clearance of human papillomavirus: A randomized clinical trial. *Int J Cancer*. 2003;107:811–816.

87 COLPOSCOPY OF CERVICAL CANCER

E.J. Mayeaux, Jr., MD

PATIENT STORY

A 51-year-old woman presents with postcoital bleeding. She has not had a period in 3 years, but has started spotting after intercourse. Her last Pap smear was after the birth of her last child 25 years ago and was normal. Other than an occasional mild hot-flash, she has no other complaints. On colposcopy she was found to have a densely acetowhite lesion with abnormal vessel near the cervical os. Biopsy demonstrated invasive squamous cell carcinoma. The patient then had a radical hysterectomy with pelvic/paraaortic lymphadenectomy. Fortunately her lymph nodes were all negative.

EPIDEMIOLOGY

- Carcinoma of the cervix is one of the second most common cancers in women worldwide with an estimated 400,000 to 500,000 cases of cervical cancer diagnosed each year.[1,2]

- In the United States, an estimated 11,150 new cases and approximately 3670 deaths annually, even though more than 50 million Pap smears are performed each year.[3]

- Half of the cases will occur in women never screened and an additional 10% in women not screened within the past 5 years.[4]

- Ninety-three percent of invasive cervical cancer are squamous cell cancers (**Figures 87-1 to 87-4**). They almost all contain Human Papillomavirus (HPV) DNA, and 90% are subtypes 16/18 which are most virulent.[5]

- Approximately 7% of cases are adenocarcinomas but these are on the rise[5] (**Figure 87-5**).

- It is rare to find invasive cancer of the uterine cervix in pregnancy. The incidence varies from 1 to 15 cases per 10,000 pregnancies, and the prognosis is similar to that of nonpregnant patients.[6]

ETIOLOGY AND PATHOPHYSIOLOGY

- Oncogenic HPV serve as initiators, and other factors relating to immune status such as cigarette smoking, nutrition, or other genital infections may be promoters.[7]

- Cervical cancer is unique in that no other human cancer has been shown to have such a clearly identified cause, which is oncogenic strains of HPV.

DIAGNOSIS

- Leukoplakia is typically an elevated, white plaque seen prior to the application of acetic acid. It is caused by a thick keratin layer that obscures the underlying epithelium (**Figure 87-1**). It always warrants a biopsy.

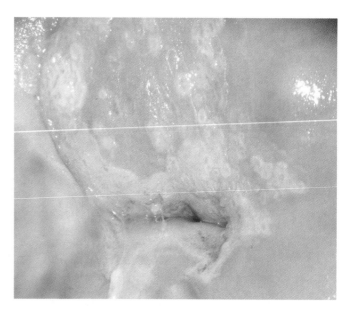

FIGURE 87-1 Colposcopic view of invasive squamous cell carcinoma. The lesion is densely acetowhite with abnormal vessels on the anterior lip just above the cervical os. (*Courtesy of E.J. Mayeaux, Jr., MD.*)

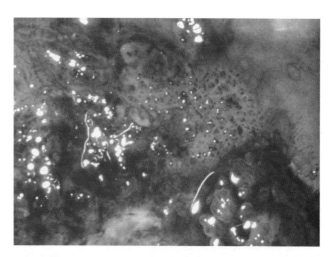

FIGURE 87-2 Colposcopic view of invasive squamous cell carcinoma with abnormal vessels. (*Courtesy of E.J. Mayeaux, Jr., MD.*)

- Early invasion often is associated with a decline in the acetowhite reaction. Yellow hued color change is also a marker for early or frank invasive lesions (**Figure 87-4**).

- With increasing levels of CIN, desmosomes (intracellular bridges) that attach the epithelium to the basement membrane are often lost, producing an edge that easily peels. This loss of tissue integrity should raise the suspicion of high-grade dysplasia. The extreme expression of this effect is the ulceration that sometimes forms with invasive disease. The ulcer can have a rolled edge around the ulcer without vessels visible in the ulcer cavity.

- Nodular elevations and ulceration are suspicious for high-grade or invasive cancer.

- Course punctation and course mosaic patterns may be associated with high-grade dysplasia or cancer (see Chapter 86, Colposcopy of High-Grade Lesions).

- Abnormal blood vessels are atypical irregular surface vessels that have lost their normal arborization or branching pattern (**Figures 87-1** and **87-2**). This represents an exaggeration of the abnormalities of punctation and mosaicism, and it usually represents increasing severity of the lesion. They can be indicative of invasive cancer, but can occasionally be seen with high-grade CIN. These vessels are often best seen before application of acetic acid. They are usually nonbranching, appear with abrupt courses and patterns, and often appear as commas, corkscrews, hairpins, or spaghetti. They may also appear as coarse parallel vessels. There is no definite repetitive pattern as with punctation or mosaic.

- A thin watery vaginal discharge is the most common early complaint of a woman with cervical cancer. As the lesions progress or enlarge, complaints occur of post coital bleeding or painless intermenstrual bleeding.

- More advanced lesions present with heavier and frequent bleeding until it may become continuous. Pain, hematuria, obstipation, and rectal bleeding are symptoms of late disease because of local direct invasion of surrounding para cervical structures. Lower extremity edema may occur with pelvic side-wall involvement of tumor. Hemorrhage and uremia are preterminal events.

- Findings on speculum examination include an exophytic mass (**Figures 87-3** and **87-5**), cervical ulcer, or barrel shaped cervix.

- Colposcopy and biopsy are needed to make the diagnosis. A histologic biopsy that is suspicious, but not confirmatory, of invasion requires cervical conization for definitive diagnosis. A biopsy of microinvasive carcinoma requires conization for definitive diagnosis and to rule out a more invasive lesion. A biopsy with definitive invasion greater than 5 mm does not require conization to plan therapy. Any frank lesion of the cervix requires biopsy for diagnosis.

- The staging of cervical cancer remains clinical. Physical examination with cystoscopy and proctoscopy usually starts the process. Routine x-ray studies are also used, including chest x-ray, intravenous pyelogram, and barium enema.

DIFFERENTIAL DIAGNOSIS

- Since some cancers of the cervix ulcerate, it must be differentiated from nonmalignant ulcerative diseases such as herpes virus infections (see Chapter 123, Herpes Simplex).

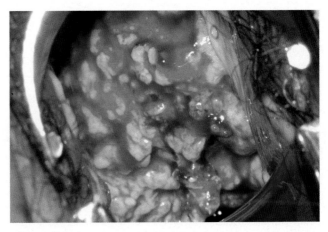

FIGURE 87-3 Colposcopic view of invasive squamous cell carcinoma. Note how the cancer has replaced the entire surface of the cervix with friable epithelium. (*Courtesy of Daron Ferris, MD.*)

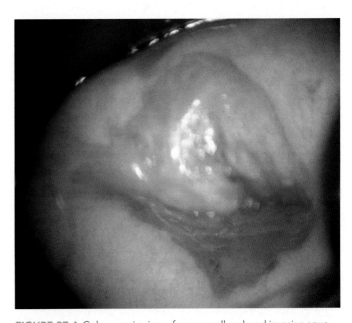

FIGURE 87-4 Colposcopic view of a rarer yellow-hued invasive squamous cell carcinoma of the cervix. (*Courtesy of E.J. Mayeaux, Jr., MD.*)

- Cervical cancer must be differentiated from CIN II/III lesions (see Chapter 86, Colposcopy of High-Grade Disease).

- Flat HPV lesions may mimic dense acetowhite lesions or leukoplakia. A colposcopically directed biopsy can distinguish between these conditions.

MANAGEMENT

- **Table 87-1** shows the staging and treatment methods for cervical cancer.

PATIENT EDUCATION

- Fertility sparing surgery is available for very early stage cervical cancer. Menopausal symptoms are a common side-effect of chemotherapy.

FOLLOW-UP

- Early stage (International Federation of Gynecology and Obstetrics stage IA–IIA) squamous cell carcinoma is treated with radical hysterectomy and pelvic/paraaortic lymphadenectomy or radiation therapy. In patients with positive resection margins or positive lymph nodes, postoperative chemotherapy and/or radiotherapy is often used.

- Stage IB2 and IIA disease is treated with either chemoradiotherapy alone, surgery followed by chemoradiotherapy, or chemotherapy and radiotherapy followed by hysterectomy.

- For patients with stages IIB, III, and IVA cervical squamous cell carcinoma, chemotherapy plus radiotherapy is usually recommended over radiation therapy alone.

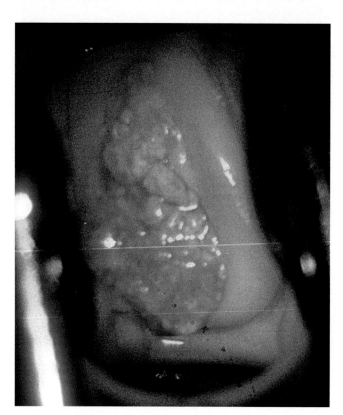

FIGURE 87-5 Adenocarcinoma of the cervix. (*Courtesy of E.J. Mayeaux, Jr., MD.*)

PATIENT RESOURCES

- Oncolink—Cervical, Vaginal, Vulvar Cancers— **http://oncolink.upenn.edu/types/types.cfm?c=6.**

- Womenshealth.gov—**http://womenshealth.gov/faq/ ccervix.htm.**

- National Cervical Cancer Coalition—**http://www. nccconline.org/.**

PROVIDER RESOURCES

- Wright TC Jr., Massad LS, Dunton CJ, Spitzer M, Wilkinson EJ, Solomon D; 2006 American Society for Colposcopy and Cervical Pathology-sponsored Consensus Conference. 2006 consensus guidelines for the management of women with cervical intraepithelial neoplasia or adenocarcinoma in situ. *Am J Obstet Gynecol.* 2007;197(4):340–5. Available at: **http://www. asccp.org/consensus/histological.shtml.**

- National Cancer Institute, NIH—**http://www.cancer.gov/ cancerinfo/types/cervical.**

TABLE 87-1 Staging and Treatment of Cervical Cancer[1,2]

Stage	Description	Treatment	5-Year Survival (%)
0	Carcinoma in situ		
I	Tumor is confined to the cervix		91.3
IA	Microinvasive disease with the lesion not grossly visible. No deeper than 5 mm and no wider than 7 mm	Simple hysterectomy or careful observation after cone biopsy (with clear margins)	98.1
IB	Larger tumor than in IA or grossly visible, confined to cervix	Radical hysterectomy with pelvic node dissection or external beam and intracavitary radiotherapy (equally effective)	88.2
II	Extends beyond the cervix, but does not involve the pelvic side wall or lowest third of the vagina		60.7
IIA	Involvement of the upper two-thirds of vagina, without lateral extension into the parametrium		67.2
IIB	Lateral extension into parametrial tissue	Pelvic radiotherapy	57.9
III	Involves the lowest third of the vagina or pelvic side wall or causes hydronephrosis		46.8
IIIA	Involvement of the lowest third of the vagina		38.6
IIIB	Involvement of pelvic side wall or hydronephrosis or nonfunctioning kidney		47.7
IV	Extensive local infiltration or has spread to a dissent site		
IVA	Spread of the tumor onto adjacent pelvic organs		15.5
IVB	Distant metastases	Chemotherapy with or without pelvic radiotherapy	14.6

[1]Staging system based on the Federation of International Gynecologists and Obstetricians: http://www.cancer.gov/cancertopics/pdq/treatment/cervical/HealthProfessional/page4#Section_61
[2]Survival data based on the SEER Survival Monograph: Cancer Survival Among Adults: US SEER Program, 1988–2001, Patient and Tumor Characteristics. Chapter 14: Cancer of the Cervix Uteri. http://seer.cancer.gov/publications/survival/surv_cervix_uteri.pdf

REFERENCES

1. Schiffman M, Herrero R, Hildesheim A, et al. HPV DNA testing in cervical cancer screening: results from women in a high-risk province of Costa Rica. *JAMA* 2000;283(1):87–93.

2. Parkin DM, Bray F. The burden of HPV-related cancers. *Vaccine* 2006;24(suppl3):511–525.

3. Jemal A, Siegel R, Ward E, Murray T, Xu J, Thun MJ. Cancer statistics, 2007. CA *Cancer J Clin* 2007;57:43.

4. NIH Consensus Statement Online 1996 April 1–3. Accessed October 28, 2003. 1–38.

5. Schiffman MH, Bauer HM, Hoover RN, et al. Epidemiological evidence showing that human papillomavirus infection causes most cervical intraepithelial neoplasia. *J Natl Cancer Inst.* 1994;85: 958–964.

6. Campion MJ, Sedlacek TV. Colposcopy in pregnancy. *Obstet Gynecol Clin North Am.* 1993;20(1):153–63.

7. Berrington DE, Gonzalez A, Green J. Comparison of risk factors for invasive squamous cell carcinoma and adenocarcinoma of the cervix: collaborative reanalysis of individual data on 8,097 women with squamous cell carcinoma and 1,374 women with adenocarcinoma from 12 epidemiological studies. *Int J Cancer* 2007;120:885.

88 MASTITIS AND BREAST ABSCESS

E.J. Mayeaux, Jr., MD

PATIENT STORY

A 23-year-old woman, who is currently breast feeding and 6 weeks postpartum presents with a hard, red, tender, indurated area medial to her right nipple (**Figure 88-1**). She also has a low-grade fever. There is a local area of fluctuance and so incision and drainage is recommended. The area is anesthetized with 1% lidocaine and epinephrine and drained with a No. 11 scalpel. A lot of purulence is expressed and the wound is packed. The patient is started on cephalexin 500 mg qid for 10 days to treat the surrounding cellulitis and seen in follow-up the next day. The patient was already feeling better the next day and went on to full resolution in the following weeks.

EPIDEMIOLOGY

- The prevalence of mastitis is estimated to be at least 1% to 3% of lactating women. Risk factors include a history of mastitis with a previous child, cracks and nipple sores, use of an antifungal nipple cream in the same month, and use of a manual breast pump.[1]

- Breast abscess is an uncommon problem in breast-feeding women with a incidence of approximately 0.1%.[3] Risk factors include maternal age more than 30 years of age, primiparity, gestational age of 41 weeks, and mastitis.[2,3] Breast abscess develops in 5% to 11% of women with mastitis, often caused by inadequate therapy.[2]

ETIOLOGY AND PATHOPHYSIOLOGY

- Mastitis, defined as an infection of the breast, and breast abscesses are typically found in breast-feeding women (**Figure 88-1**). A breast abscess can occur in older women unrelated to pregnancy and breast feeding (**Figure 88-2**).

- Mastitis is most commonly caused by *Staphylococcus aureus*, streptococcus species, and *Escherichia coli*.

- Recurrent mastitis can result from poor selection or incomplete use of antibiotic therapy, or failure to resolve underlying lactation management problems. Mastitis that repeatedly recurs in the same location, or does not respond to appropriate therapy, may indicate the presence of breast cancer.[2]

DIAGNOSIS

CLINICAL FEATURES

- Mastitis causes a hard, red, tender, swollen area on the breast (**Figures 88-1** and **88-2**).

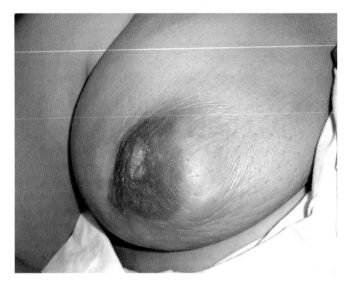

FIGURE 88-1 Localized cellulitis and breast abscess in a breast-feeding mother. Note the Peau d' orange appearance of the edematous breast tissue. (*Courtesy of Nicolette Deveneau, MD.*)

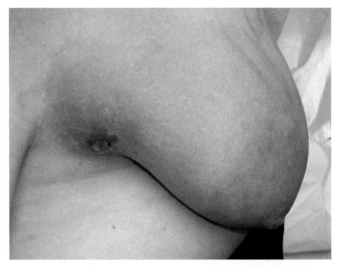

FIGURE 88-2 Breast abscess and cellulitis in a 40-year-old woman. Pus was already draining at the time of presentation, but a further incision and drainage through the openings yielded another 30 cc of pus. The patient was treated with oral antibiotics and scheduled to get a momentum when the infection is cleared. (*Courtesy of Richard P. Usatine, MD.*)

- Fever is common.

- Pain usually extends beyond the indurated area.

- It is often associated with other systemic complaints including myalgia, chills, malaise, and flu-like symptoms.

- Breast abscess can occur with mastitis, except a fluctuant mass is palpable. (In **Figure 88-3**, the fluctuant mass is close to the midline with two openings of spontaneous drainage. The remainder of the erythema is cellulitis.)

- Typical distribution is usually unilateral.

- Biopsy is unnecessary, but in persistent cases, a mid-stream milk sample may be cultured and antibiotics prescribed based upon the identification and sensitivity of the specific pathogen.

DIFFERENTIAL DIAGNOSIS

- Mastitis should be distinguished from plugged lacrimal ducts, which present as hard, locally tender, red areas without associated regional pain or fever.

- Tinea corporis can cause erythema and scaling on any part of the body including breast. It is often annular and pruritic (see Chapter 132, Tinea Corporis).

MANAGEMENT

- Management of mastitis includes supportive measures such as continued breast-feeding and bed rest. SOR **C** If the infant cannot relieve breast fullness during nursing, breast massage during nursing or pumping afterwards may help reduce discomfort.

- Acetaminophen or an anti-inflammatory agent such as ibuprofen may be used for pain control.

- Antibiotic treatment should be initiated with dicloxacillin or cephalexin (500 mg po 4 times daily) for 10 to 14 days.[4] SOR **A** Consider clindamycin if the patient is allergic to penicillin and/or cephalosporins.[4] Clindamycin may be a good choice if methicillin-resistant S. aureus (MRSA) is suspected. All of the antibiotics recommended are safe for the baby during pregnancy and lactation. Trimethoprim/sulfamethoxazole is an alternative for MRSA and/or penicillin allergic patients but it should be avoided near term pregnancy and in the first 2 months of breast-feeding because of a risk to the baby of kernicterus. Shorter courses of antibiotic therapy may be associated with higher relapse rates. SOR **C**

- The management of a breast abscess consists of drainage of the abscess.[4] SOR **A** Antibiotic therapy should be considered and is especially important if there is surrounding cellulitis (**Figures 88-2** and **88-3**).
  - Drainage can usually be performed by needle aspiration, with the addition of ultrasound guidance if necessary.
  - If needle aspiration is not effective, incision and drainage should be performed. Incision and drainage is often preferred because it allows for continued drainage through the opening. In many cases a cotton wick is placed to keep the abscess open while the purulence drains in the following days.
  - Breast-feeding may continue on both breasts if the incision isn't too painful and it does not interfere with the baby latching on. Otherwise a breast pump may be used on the affected breast for 3 to 4 days until nursing can resume.

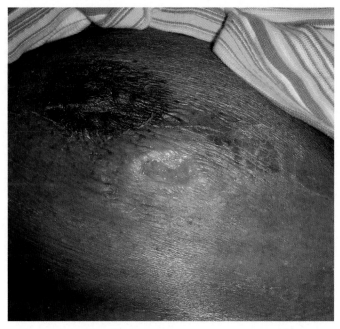

FIGURE 88-3 Healing after drainage of an abscess and antibiotics for cellulitis. (*Courtesy of E.J. Mayeaux, Jr., MD.*)

PATIENT EDUCATION

- The patient may take acetaminophen or ibuprofen for pain since these medications are safe while breast-feeding and are indicated for use in children.

- Warm compresses applied before and after feedings can provide some pain relief. A warm bath may also help.

- Instruct the patient to finish the antibiotic prescription, even if they feel better in a few days, to lower the risk of bacterial resistance or relapse.

- Continue feedings and use a breast pump to completely empty the breast if necessary.

- Educate the parents that the mastitis or the antibiotics will not harm the baby, and that the source of the infection was probably the baby's own mouth.

- Continue to drink plenty of water and eat well-balanced meals.

FOLLOW-UP

- If no response is seen within 48 hours or if MRSA is a possibility, antibiotic therapy should be switched to trimethoprim-sulfamethoxazole 1 double strength po twice a day, or Clindamycin 300 mg orally q6h. Avoid trimethoprim/sulfamethoxazole near term pregnancy and in the first 2 months of breast-feeding.

- Hospitalization and intravenous antibiotics are rarely needed but should be considered if the patient is systemically ill and not able to tolerate oral antibiotics.

PATIENT RESOURCES

- Medline plus—**http://www.nlm.nih.gov/medlineplus/ency/article/001490.htm.**

- National Health Service (Brittan) Direct Online Health Encyclopaedia—**http://www.nhsdirect.nhs.uk/articles/article.aspx?articleId=62.**

- University of Michigan info—**http://www.med.umich.edu/1libr/pa/pa_mastitis_hhg.htm.**

PROVIDER RESOURCES

- Emedicine—**http://www.emedicine.com/EMERG/topic68.htm.**

- Andolsek KM and Copeland JA. Benign breast conditions and disease: Mastitis. In: Tayor RB ed. *Family Medicine Principles and Practice*. 6th ed. New York, NY: Springer, 2003:898.

REFERENCES

1. Foxman B, D'Arcy H, Gillespie B, et al. Lactation mastitis: Occurrence and medical management among 946 breastfeeding women in the united states. *Am J Epidemiol.* 2002;155:103.

2. Berens PD. Prenatal, intrapartum, and postpartum support of the lactating mother. *Pediatr Clin North Am.* 2001;48:365.

3. Kvist LJ, Rydhstroem H. Factors related to breast abscess after delivery: A population-based study. *BJOG.* 2005;112:1070.

4. Stevens DL, Bisno AL, Chambers HF, et al. Practice guidelines for the diagnosis and management of skin and soft-tissue infections. *Clin Infect Dis.* 2005;41:1373–1406.

89 BREAST CANCER

E.J. Mayeaux, Jr., MD

A 55-year-old woman presents for routine screening mammogram. The patient does not have any complaints but has a family history of breast cancer in a sister at age of 40 years. Her mammogram demonstrates an irregular mass with possible local spread (**Figures 89-1** and **89-2**). She is referred to a breast surgeon and the biopsy confirms the diagnosis of breast cancer.

EPIDEMIOLOGY

- In 2007, approximately 178,000 women in the United States were diagnosed with breast cancer.[1] Breast cancer incidence in the United States has doubled over the past 60 years. Since the early 1980s, most of the increase has been in early stage and in situ cancers because of mammogram screening (**Figures 89-1 to 89-4**).

- In the 1990s, the mortality rate began declining annually. However, it is estimated that over 40,000 women died from breast cancer in the US in 2007.[1]

- Locally advanced breast cancer (LABC) has been decreasing in frequency over the past several decades, at least partially as a result of earlier diagnosis because of better screening (**Figures 89-5 to 89-7**). It represents 30 to 50% of newly diagnosed breast cancers in medically underserved populations.[2]

- Primary inflammatory breast cancer (IBC) is relatively rare, accounting for 0.5 to 2% invasive breast cancers.[3] However, it accounts for a greater proportion of cases presenting with more advanced disease. IBC is a clinical diagnosis. At presentation, almost all women with primary IBC have lymph node involvement and approximately one-third have distant metastases.[4]

ETIOLOGY AND PATHOPHYSIOLOGY

- The incidence of breast cancer increases with age. White women are more likely to develop breast cancer than black women. 1% of breast cancers occur in men.

- Primary risk factors for the development of breast cancer include age greater than 50 years, female sex, increased exposure to estrogen (including early menarche and late menopause), and a family history in a first-degree maternal relative (especially if diagnosed premenopausally.)

- Approximately one-half of the 8% of hereditary breast cancers are associated with mutations in genes BRCA1 and BRCA2. It is more common in premenopausal women, multiple family generations, and bilateral breasts.[5] Typically, several family members are affected over at least three generations and can include women from the paternal side of the family.

- A history of a proliferative breast abnormality such as atypical hyperplasia may increase a woman's risk for developing breast cancer.

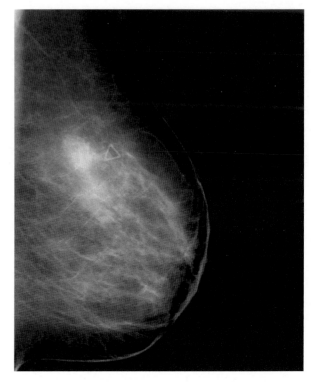

FIGURE 89-1 A mammogram that demonstrates an irregular mass with possible local spread. (*Courtesy of John Braud, MD.*)

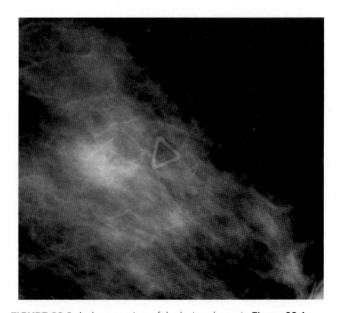

FIGURE 89-2 A close-up view of the lesion shown in **Figure 89-1**. (*Courtesy of John Braud, MD.*)

- The selective estrogen receptor modulator tamoxifen (and possibly raloxifene) reduces the risk of developing breast cancer.

- The American Cancer Society, American College of Radiology, American Medical Association, and American College of Obstetrics and Gynecology all recommend starting routine screening at age 40.[6]

- The United States Preventive Services Task Force and the 2002 statement by the American Academy of Family Physicians recommend screening mammography every 1 to 2 years for women ages 40 and older.[7]

- Women who have a family history of BRCA mutation should begin annual mammography between 25 and 35 years of age.[8] SOR Ⓐ

- MRI screening is more sensitive for detecting breast cancers than mammography and is being used to screen women with BRCA mutations.[9] It is not proven that surveillance regimens that include MRI will reduce mortality from breast cancer in high-risk women.[9]

- While the sensitivity of MRI is higher than that of conventional imaging. MRI has a lower specificity. One study suggests that unnecessary biopsies can be avoided with second-look ultrasound when MRI is positive and mammography is not. Second-look ultrasound can be used to recognize false positive MRI results and guide biopsies.[10]

DIAGNOSIS

CLINICAL FEATURES

- Detection of a breast mass is the most common presenting breast complaint. However, 90% of all breast masses are caused by benign lesions. Breast pain is also a common presenting problem. Physical examination of the breast should be performed in the upright (sitting) and supine positions. Inspect for differences in size, retraction of the skin or nipple (**Figures 89-5** and **89-6**), prominent venous patterns and signs of inflammation (**Figures 89-5** and **89-6**). Palpate the breast tissue, axillary area, and supraclavicular areas for masses or adenopathy. Gently squeeze the nipple to check for discharge.

- Most LABC are both palpable and visible (**Figure 89-7**). Careful palpation of the skin, breasts, and regional lymph nodes is the initial step in diagnosis.

- IBC usually presents clinically as a diffuse brawny induration of the skin of the breast with an erythematous edge, and usually without an underlying palpable mass. Patients with de novo IBC typically present with pain and a rapidly enlarging breast. The skin over the breast is warm, and thickened, with a "peau d'orange" (skin of an orange) appearance (**Figures 89-5** and **89-6**). The skin color can range from a pink flushed discoloration to a purplish hue.

TYPICAL DISTRIBUTION

A mass that is suspicious for breast cancer is usually solitary, discrete, hard, unilateral, and nontender. It may be fixed to the skin or the chest wall.

BIOPSY

- Fine-needle aspiration biopsy generally uses a 20 to 23 gauge needle to obtain samples from a solid mass for cytology. Ultrasound or

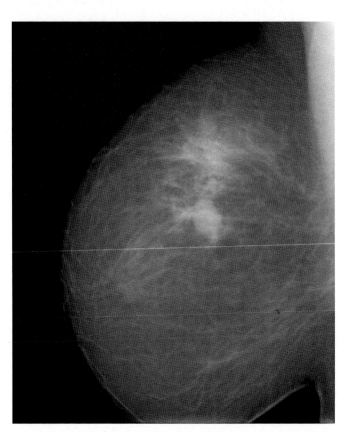

FIGURE 89-3 A screening mammogram of a 55-year-old woman who is without breast complaints. The mammogram demonstrates a significant mass with spiculations. (*Courtesy of John Braud, MD.*)

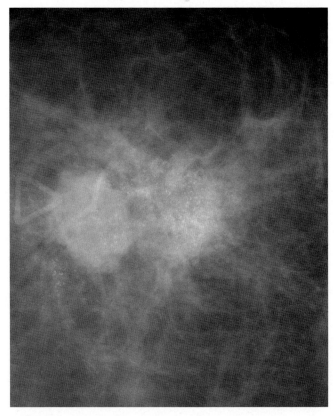

FIGURE 89-4 Close-up view of the mass (given in **Figure 89-3**) demonstrating clear spiculations and microcalcifications. (*Courtesy of John Braud, MD.*)

stereotactic guidance is used to assist in collecting a fine-needle aspiration from a nonpalpable lump. Core biopsy uses a 14-gauge or similar needle to remove cores of tissue from a mass. Excisional biopsy is done as the initial procedure or when needle biopsies are negative when the clinical suspicion is high. Guided biopsy and nonguided biopsy are also commonly used to make a definitive diagnosis.

TESTING

- Screening tests are available that detect BRCA mutations. Genetic testing is controversial and raises issues about test reliability and what use may be made of the test results. Diagnostic mammography is done to evaluate suspected cancer. Digital mammography is similar to standard mammography, but images are stored digitally and can be enhanced by modifying the brightness or contrast. Computer-aided diagnosis is being applied to the digital images and may enhance their accuracy.

DIFFERENTIAL DIAGNOSIS

- Fibroadenoma usually present as smooth, rounded, rubbery masses in women in their 20s and 30s. A clinically suspicious mass should be biopsied even if mammography findings are normal.

- Benign cysts are rubbery and hollow feeling in women in their 30s and 40s. A cyst can be diagnosed by ultrasound imaging. A simple cyst can be aspirated, but a residual mass requires further evaluation. Ultrasound is useful to differentiate between solid and cystic breast masses, especially in young women with dense breast tissue.

- Bilateral mastalgia is rarely associated with breast cancer, but it does not eliminate the possibility. It is usually related to fibrocystic changes in premenopausal women that are associated with diffuse lumpy breasts. A unilateral breast lump with pain must be evaluated for breast cancer.

- Nipple discharge may be from infection which is usually purulent, and from pregnancy, stimulation, or prolactinoma which produces a thin, milky, often bilateral discharge. A pregnancy test may be helpful. A suspicious discharge from a single duct can be evaluated with a ductogram.

- Infectious mastitis and breast abscess, which typically occur in lactating women, appear similar to IBC but are generally associated with fever and leukocytosis (see Chapter 88, Breast Abscess and Mastitis).

- Ductal ectasia with inflammation appears similar but is usually localized.

- Leukemic involvement of the breast may mimic IBC, but the peripheral blood smear is typically diagnostic.

MANAGEMENT

- Surgical resection is required in all patients with invasive breast cancer. Oncologic outcomes are similar with mastectomy and breast conserving therapy (lumpectomy plus breast radiation

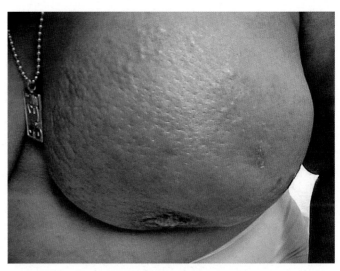

FIGURE 89-5 Woman with advanced breast cancer and Peau d' orange sign. The skin looks like the skin of an orange due to lymphedema. (*Courtesy of Richard P. Usatine, MD.*)

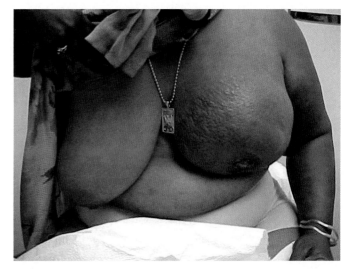

FIGURE 89-6 The patient in **Figure 89-5** showing breast retraction and brawny edema of the breast and arm. (*Courtesy of Richard P. Usatine, MD.*)

therapy) in appropriately selected patients. For women undergoing mastectomy, breast reconstruction may be performed at the same time as the initial breast cancer surgery, or deferred to a later date.[11] SOR **A**

- Adjuvant systemic therapy consists of administration of hormone therapy, chemotherapy, and/or trastuzumab (a humanized monoclonal antibody directed against HER-2/neu) after definitive local therapy for breast cancer. It benefits most women with early stage breast cancer, but the magnitude of benefit is greatest for those with node-positive disease.[12] SOR **A**

- The most common approach for advanced breast cancer is preoperative chemotherapy followed by surgery and radiotherapy. Questions regarding sequencing and choice of specific chemotherapy regimens and extent of surgery (including the utility of the sentinel node biopsy) persist. SOR **B**

- Preoperative (as opposed to postoperative) chemotherapy has several advantages for advanced breast cancer (**Figure 89-7**) treatment. It can reduce the size of the primary tumor, thus allowing for breast conserving surgery, permits assessing an identified mass to determine the sensitivity of the tumor cells to drugs with discontinuation of ineffective therapy (thus avoiding unnecessary toxicity), and enables drug delivery through an intact tumor vasculature.[13] SOR **B**

- Tamoxifen and aromatase inhibitors may be used in selective patients as neoadjuvant hormone therapy of decrease overall tumor volume. SOR **C**

- Long-term survival can be obtained in approximately 50% of women with LABC who are treated with a multimodality approach.[14] Prognostic factors include age, menopausal status, tumor stage and histologic grade, clinical response to neoadjuvant therapy, and ER status.

- In general, women with IBC are approached similarly to those with noninflammatory LABC except that breast conservation therapy is generally considered inappropriate for these women.[15] SOR **B**

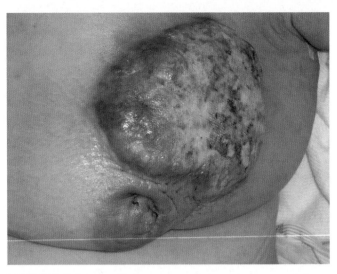

FIGURE 89-7 Advanced breast cancer with fungating mass and distortion of the normal breast anatomy. (*Courtesy of Kristen Sorenson, MD.*)

PATIENT EDUCATION

The contralateral breast is at increased risk of breast cancer and should be monitored. Patients on tamoxifen should be monitored for endometrial hyperplasia or cancer.

FOLLOW-UP

Regular follow-up will usually be maintained during treatment. After treatment, life-long regular follow-up for surveillance should be maintained.

PATIENT RESOURCES

- Breast cancer support group for survivors— **http://bcsupport.org/.**
- Breastcancer.org—**http://www.breastcancer.org/.**

REFERENCES

1. American Cancer Society. *Cancer Facts and Figures* 2007. Atlanta: American Cancer Society, 2007.

2. Hortobagyi GN, Sinigletary SE, Strom EA. Treatment of locally advanced and inflammatory breast cancer. In: Harris JR, Lippman ME, Morrow M, Osborne CK eds. *Diseases of the Breast*. 2nd ed. Philadelphia: Lippincott Williams and Wilkins, 2000;645–660.

3. Hance KW, Anderson WF, Devesa SS, et al. Trends in inflammatory breast carcinoma incidence and survival: The surveillance, epidemiology, and end results program at the national cancer institute. *J Natl Cancer Inst*. 2005;97:966.

4. Kleer CG, van Golen KL, Merajver SD. Molecular biology of breast cancer metastasis: Inflammatory breast cancer: Clinical syndrome and molecular determinants. *Breast Cancer Res*. 2000;2:423.

5. Krainer M, Silva-Arrieta S, FitzGerald MG, et al. Differential contributions of BRCA1 and BRCA2 to early-onset breast cancer. *N Engl J Med*. 1997;336:1416–1421.

6. Smith RA, Saslow D, Sawyer KA, et al. American cancer society guidelines for breast cancer screening: Update 2003. *CA Cancer J Clin*. 2003;53:141.

7. U.S. Preventive Services Task Force. Guide to Clinical Preventive Services, 3rd ed. www.ahrq.gov/clinic/uspstfix.htm. Accessed March 7, 2005.

8. Burke W, Daly M, Garber J, et al. Recommendations for follow-up care of individuals with an inherited predisposition to cancer. II. BRCA1 and BRCA2. *JAMA*. 1997;277:997–1003.

9. Warner E, Plewes DB, Hill KA, et al. Surveillance of BRCA1 and BRCA2 mutation carriers with magnetic resonance imaging, ultrasound, mammography, and clinical breast examination. *JAMA*. 2004;292(11):1317–1325.

10. Trecate G, Vergnaghi D, Manoukian S, et al. MRI in the early detection of breast cancer in women with high genetic risk. *Tumori*. 2006;92(6):517–523.

11. Vandeweyer E, Hertens D, Nogaret JM, Deraemaecker R. Immediate breast reconstruction with saline-filled implants: No interference with the oncologic outcome? *Plast Reconstr Surg*. 2001; 107:1409.

12. Goldhirsch A, Glick JH, Gelber RD, Coates AS, Thurlimann B, Senn HJ. Meeting highlights: International expert consensus on the primary therapy of early breast cancer 2005. *Ann Oncol*. 2005;16:1569.

13. Fisher B, Gunduz N, Saffer EA. Influence of the interval between primary tumor removal and chemotherapy on kinetics and growth of metastases. *Cancer Res*. 1983;43:1488.

14. Brito RA, Valero V, Buzdar AU, et al. Long-term results of combined-modality therapy for locally advanced breast cancer with ipsilateral supraclavicular metastases: The University of Texas M.D. Anderson Cancer Center experience. *J Clin Oncol*. 2001;19: 628.

15. Lyman GH, Giuliano AE, Somerfield MR, et al. American society of clinical oncology guideline recommendations for sentinel lymph node biopsy in early-stage breast cancer. *J Clin Oncol*. 2005;23:7703.

90 PAGET'S DISEASE OF THE BREAST

E.J. Mayeaux, Jr., MD

PATIENT STORY

A 62-year-old woman presents with a 6-month history of an eczematous, scaly, rash near her nipple. It is mildly pruritic. On physical examination, you find a hard mass in the lateral lower quadrant of the same breast (**Figure 90-1**).

EPIDEMIOLOGY

- The incidence of Paget's disease of the breast is approximately 1.1% in women in the United States, according to National Cancer Institute SEER data.[1] Paget's disease is rare in men as are all breast cancers.

- It is associated with underlying in situ and/or invasive breast cancer 97% of the time. Paget's disease and breast cancer should be in the differential diagnosis of any persistent nipple abnormality or one that doesn't respond to appropriate therapy.

ETIOLOGY AND PATHOPHYSIOLOGY

- Most patients delay presentation, assuming the abnormality is a benign condition of some sort. The median duration of signs and symptoms prior to diagnosis is 6 to 8 months.[2]

- Presenting symptoms are sometimes limited to persistent pain, burning, and/or pruritus of the nipple (**Figures 90-1** and **90-2**).

- A palpable breast mass is present in 50% of cases, but is often located more than 2 cm from the nipple-areolar complex.[3]

- Twenty percent of cases will have a mammographic abnormality without a palpable mass, and 25% of cases will have neither a mass nor abnormal mammogram, but will have an occult ductal carcinoma.

- In less than 5% of cases, Paget's disease of the breast is an isolated finding.[3]

- There are two theories regarding the pathogenesis of Paget's disease of the breast, the choice of which affects treatment choices.
  - The more widely accepted epidermotropic theory proposes that the Paget cells arise from an underlying mammary adenocarcinoma that migrates through the ductal system of the breast to the skin of the nipple. It is supported by the fact that Paget's disease is usually associated with an underlying ductal carcinoma, and both Paget's cells and mammary ductal cells usually express similar immunochemical staining patterns and molecular markers. This could mean that there is a common genetic alteration and/or a common progenitor cell for both Paget's cells and the underlying ductal carcinoma.
  - The much less widely accepted transformation theory proposes that epidermal cells in the nipple transform into malignant

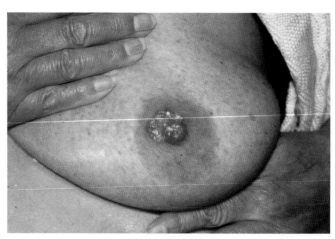

FIGURE 90-1 Paget's disease of the breast that presented as a persistent eczematous lesion. (*Courtesy of the University of Texas Health Sciences Center, Division of Dermatology.*)

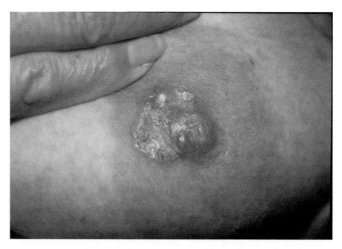

FIGURE 90-2 Close up of Paget's disease of the breast. Note the erythematous, eczematous, scaly appearance of the lesion. (*Courtesy of the University of Texas Health Sciences Center, Division of Dermatology.*)

Paget's cells, and that Paget's disease of the breast represents an independent epidermal carcinoma in situ. It is supported by the fact that there is no parenchymal cancer identified in a small percentage of cases, and underlying breast carcinomas are often located at some distance to the nipple. Most pathologists disagree with the transformation theory.

DIAGNOSIS

CLINICAL FEATURES

Paget's disease of the breast presents clinically in the nipple/areolar complex as a dermatitis that may be erythematous, eczematous, scaly, raw, vesicular, or ulcerated (**Figures 90-1** and **90-2**). The nipple is usually initially involved, and the lesion then spreads to the areola. Spontaneous improvement or healing of the nipple dermatitis can occur and should not be taken as an indication that Paget's disease is not present. The diagnosis is made by finding malignant, intraepithelial adenocarcinoma cells on pathology.

TYPICAL DISTRIBUTION

Paget's disease of the breast is almost always unilateral, although bilateral cases have been reported.

BIOPSY

The diagnosis is made by full-thickness punch or wedge biopsy which show Paget's cells. Nipple scrape cytology can diagnose Paget's disease and may be considered for screening eczematous lesion of the nipple.

DIFFERENTIAL DIAGNOSIS

- Eczema of the areola is the most common cause of scaling of the breast (**Figures 90-3** and **90-4**). If the patient (**Figure 90-3**) had new nipple inversion with the onset of skin changes, this would be more suspicious for Paget's disease.

- Bowen's disease is squamous cell carcinoma-in-situ and can differentiate from Paget's disease by histology. Also, Bowen's expresses high molecular weight keratins, whereas Paget's expresses low molecular weight keratins (see Chapter 159, Actinic Keratosis/Bowen's Disease and Chapter 164, Squamous Cell Carcinoma).

- Superficial spreading malignant melanoma may be confused with Paget's but histological study and immunohistochemical staining can separate the two (**Figure 90-5**) (see Chapter 165, Melanoma).

- Seborrheic keratoses and benign lichenoid keratoses can occur on and around the areola and be suspicious for Paget's disease (**Figure 90-6**). A biopsy is the best way to make the diagnosis (see Chapter 151, Seborrheic Keratosis).

- Nipple adenoma which usually presents as an isolated mass with redness can be diagnosed with biopsy.

MANAGEMENT

- The treatment and prognosis of Paget's disease of the breast is first based on the stage of any underlying breast cancer. Simple mastectomy

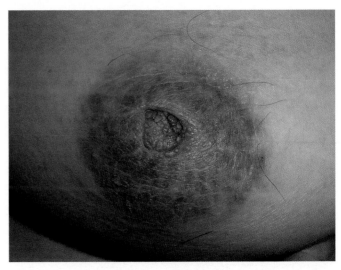

FIGURE 90-3 Eczema of the areola in a 43-year-old woman who has had an inverted nipple her whole adult life. She remembers having difficulty breast-feeding her children. The current eczema has been present on the areola on and off for more than 10 years and always responds to topical corticosteroids. Breast examination and mammography are negative. (*Courtesy of Richard P. Usatine, MD.*)

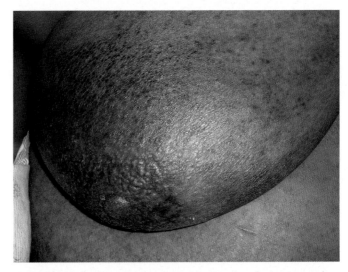

FIGURE 90-4 Widespread eczema on the breast and other parts of the body. (*Courtesy of Richard P. Usatine, MD.*)

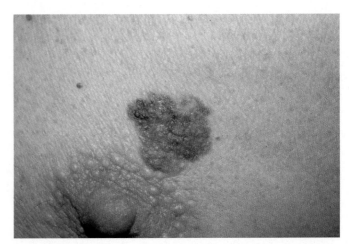

FIGURE 90-5 Superficial spreading melanoma adjacent to the areola. (*Courtesy of the University of Texas Health Sciences Center, Division of Dermatology.*)

has traditionally been the standard treatment for isolated Paget's disease of the breast, but breast conserving treatment is being used more often. Breast conserving surgery combined with breast irradiation is gaining wider acceptance. The surgically conservative approaches includes excision of the complete nipple-areolar complex with margin evaluation. Sentinel lymph node biopsy should be performed to evaluate axillary lymph node status.[4] SOR **B**

- Patients with non invasive Paget's disease of the nipple have excellent cancer outcome with conservative surgery with survival rates similar to those achieved with mastectomy.[5,6] SOR **B**

PATIENT EDUCATION

- All lesions of the breast that do not heal should be checked for cancer.

- The patient's prognosis is based on the underlying cancer, if present, not the Paget's disease itself.

PATIENT RESOURCES

- Imaginis.com—**http://imaginis.com/breasthealth/ pagets_disease.asp.**

- American Cancer Society—**http://www.cancer.org/ docroot/CRI/content/CRI_2_4_1X_What_is_breast_ cancer_5.asp.**

PROVIDER RESOURCES

- New South Wales Breast Cancer Institute—**http://www.bci. org.au/medical/protocol_pdfs/pagets.pdf.**

- National Cancer Institute (NCI)—**http://www.cancer.gov/ cancertopics/factsheet/Sites-Types/pagets-breast.**

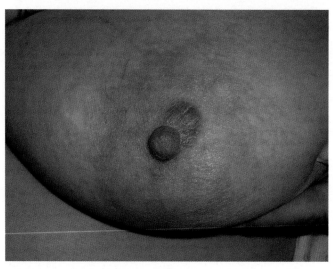

FIGURE 90-6 Benign lichenoid keratosis on the areola proven by biopsy. (*Courtesy of Richard P. Usatine, MD.*)

REFERENCES

1. Berg JW, Hutter RV. Breast cancer. *Cancer*. 1995;75:257.

2. Chaudary MA, Millis RR, Lane EB, Miller NA. Paget's disease of the nipple: A ten year review including clinical, pathological, and immunohistochemical findings. *Breast Cancer Res Treat*. 1986;8:139.

3. Ashikari R, Park K, Huvos AG, Urban JA. Paget's disease of the breast. *Cancer*. 1970;26:680.

4. Caliskan M, Gatti G, Sosnovskikh I, et al. Paget's disease of the breast: the experience of the European institute of oncology and review of the literature. *Breast Cancer Res Treat*. 2008 Feb 1 [Epublication ahead of print] http://www.springerlink.com/content/6270v27346461v08/. Accessed February 25, 2008.

5. Marshall JK, Griffith KA, Haffty BG, et al. Conservative management of Paget disease of the breast with radiotheraphy: 10- and 15-year results. *Cancer*. 2003;97(9):2142–2149.

6. Pezzi CM, Kukora JS, Audet IM, Herbet SH, Horvick D, Richter MP. Breast conservation surgery using nipple-areolar resection for central breast cancers. *Arch Surg*. 2004;139(1):32–37.

PART 12

MUSCULOSKELETAL PROBLEMS

91 OSTEOARTHRITIS

Heidi Chumley, MD

PATIENT STORY

A 70-year-old woman presents with pain and swelling in the joints of both hands, which impedes her normal activities. Her pain is better in the morning after resting and worse after she has been working with her hands. She denies stiffness. On examination, you find bony enlargement of most distal interphalangeal (DIP) and proximal interphalangeal (PIP) joints on both hands (**Figure 91-1**). Radiographs confirm the presence of Heberden's and Bouchard's nodes. She begins taking 1 g of acetaminophen twice a day and has significant improvement in her pain and function.

EPIDEMIOLOGY

- Osteoarthritis is the most common type of arthritis, affecting more than 40 million Americans, approximately 15% of the population.[1]

- The incidence and prevalence of osteoarthritis increases with age.[1]

- The incidence of knee osteoarthritis ranges from 164 to 240 per 100,000 person-years.[1]

- In the Framingham cohort (mean age 71 at baseline) women and men developed symptomatic knee osteoarthritis at the rate of 1% and 0.7% per year, respectively.[1]

- Risk of developing osteoarthritis increases with knee injury in adolescence or adulthood (RR = 2.95) and obesity (RR = 1.51–2.07).[1]

- Occupational physical activity and abnormal joint loading also increase the risk.[1,2]

ETIOLOGY AND PATHOPHYSIOLOGY

- Biomechanical factors and inflammation upset the balance of articular cartilage biosynthesis and degradation.

- Chondrocytes attempt to repair the damage; however, eventually enzymes produced by the chondrocytes digest the matrix and accelerate cartilage erosion.

DIAGNOSIS

The American College of Rheumatology uses the following criteria for the most common joints involved in osteoarthritis.

- Knee: knee pain, osteophytes on radiograph, and one of three: age > 50, stiffness < 30 minutes, or crepitus on physical examination (sensitivity = 91%, specificity = 86%).[3]

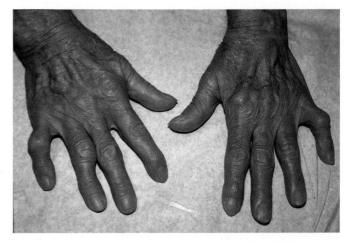

FIGURE 91-1 Bony enlargement of most distal interphalangeal (DIP) and proximal interphalangeal (PIP) joints consistent with Heberden's and Bouchard's nodes. (*Courtesy of Richard P. Usatine, MD.*)

- Hip: hip pain and two of three: ESR $<$ 20 mm/h; femoral or acetabular osteophytes by radiograph; superior, axial, or medial joint space narrowing by radiograph (sensitivity = 89%, specificity = 91%).[3]

- Hand: hand pain, aching, or stiffness and three of four: Hard tissue enlargement of $\geq$2 DIP joints, $<$3 swollen MCP joints, hand tissue enlargement of $\geq$2 selected joints, deformity of $\geq$1 selected joint. Selected joints include second and third DIP, second and third PIP, first CMC on either hand (sensitivity = 94%, specificity = 87%).[3]

CLINICAL FEATURES

- Typically, joint pain worsened with movement and relieved by rest; however, a small subset may demonstrate inflammatory symptoms including prolonged stiffness.

- Loss of function (i.e., impaired gait with knee or hip osteoarthritis, impaired manual dexterity with hand osteoarthritis).

- Radicular pain when vertebral column osteophytes impinge nerve roots.

- Bony enlargement of the DIP joints (Heberden's nodes) or PIP joints (Bouchard's nodes) (**Figure 91-1**).

- Normal ESR and synovial fluid WBC $<$ 2000 per mm.[3]

- Loss of joint space or osteophytes on radiographs (**Figures 91-2** to **91-5**).

DIFFERENTIAL DIAGNOSIS

Musculoskeletal pain can also be caused by

- Connective tissue diseases (scleroderma and lupus) which have other specific systemic signs.

- Fibromyalgia—pain at trigger points instead of joints.

- Polyarticular gout—erythematous joints and crystals in joint aspirate (see Chapter 94, Gout).

- Polymyalgia rheumatica—proximal joint pain without deformity, elevated ESR.

- Seronegative spondyloarthropathies—asymmetric joint involvement, spine often involved (see Chapter 93, Ankylosing Spondylitis).

- Reactive arthritis—history of infection, sexually transmitted disease, or bowel complaints. Reiter's disease is one example of a reactive arthritis (see Chapter 148, Reiter's Disease).

- Rheumatoid arthritis—symmetric soft tissue swelling in distal joints, stiffness after inactivity, positive rheumatoid factor. Ulnar deviation of the fingers at the MCP joints is a distinct finding in rheumatoid arthritis (**Figure 91-6**) (see Chapter 92, Rheumatoid Arthritis).

- Bursitis—pain at one site, often increased with direct pressure.

MANAGEMENT

- Recommend therapeutic low-impact exercises to maintain range of motion and strengthen muscles surrounding affected joints.[4] SOR Ⓐ

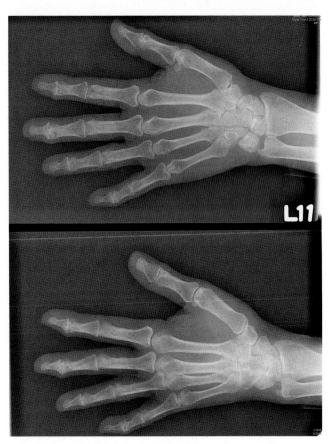

FIGURE 91-2 Joint space narrowing, marginal osteophytes, and Heberden's nodes at the distal interphalangeal (DIP) joints of the second through fifth fingers. (*Courtesy of Kansas University Medical Center.*)

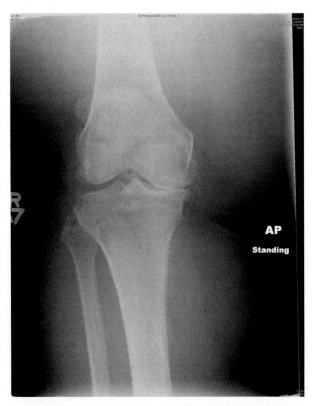

FIGURE 91-3 Osteoarthritis of the knee causing joint space narrowing, sclerosis, and bony spurring in all three compartments of the right knee, most pronounced in the medial compartment. (*Courtesy of Kansas University Medical Center.*)

- Recommend weight loss for knee osteoarthritis. Weight loss may not improve current pain, but may slow progression and can be recommended for numerous other health reasons.[2] SOR **C**

- Recommend glucosamine, which has been demonstrated to reduce pain and increase function in patients with knee or hip arthritis.[5] SOR **B**

- Prescribe an NSAID for moderate to severe hip or knee osteoarthritis in patients at low risk for GI complications. A 2006 Cochrane review found NSAIDS were slightly more effective than acetaminophen, although more likely to produce adverse GI events.[6] SOR **A**

- Prescribe acetaminophen (2–4 g/d) for pain relief in patients at higher risk for GI complications, including patients older than 65 years. In a pooled analysis, acetaminophen improved pain by 5%, NNT 4 to 14.[6] SOR **A**

- Consider topical capsaicin 0.025% cream 4 times a day over the affected joint.[2] SOR **B**

- Consider an intra-articular corticosteroid injection for knee osteoarthritis.[2] SOR **B**

- Consider a knee brace that alters knee mechanics (i.e., CounterForce brace).[7] SOR **B**

- Consider an injection of sodium hyaluronate or hylan G-F 20. Current studies demonstrate none to small improvements in pain and function.[2] SOR **C**

- Refer patients who do not respond to conservative therapy to a specialist for evaluation for newer disease modifying therapies or a surgeon for evaluation for arthroplasty or joint replacement.

PATIENT EDUCATION

Osteoarthritis is a chronic, progressive disease. Nonpharmacologic and pharmacologic therapies can reduce pain and preserve function.

FOLLOW-UP

There are no recommended intervals for follow-up; however, it is reasonable to see patients periodically to assess pain management and function.

PATIENT RESOURCES

- Patient information handouts on hyaluronate injections, knee bracing, and staying active are available on **www.familydoctor.org.**
- Patient information about osteoarthritis is also available through the American College of Rheumatology at **www.rheumatology.org.**

PROVIDER RESOURCES

- Current diagnostic criteria for many rheumatologic disorders including osteoarthritis are available at **www.rheumatology. org.**

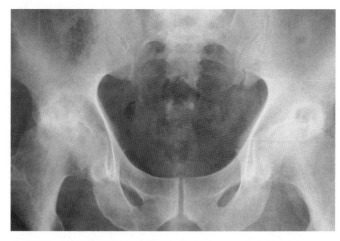

FIGURE 91-4 Articular space narrowing, sclerosis, and subchondral cyst formation of both hips due to osteoarthritis. (*From Chen MYM, Pope TL, Jr., Ott DJ. Basic Radiology, p. 189, Fig. 7-34, New York: McGraw-Hill, Copyright 2004.*)

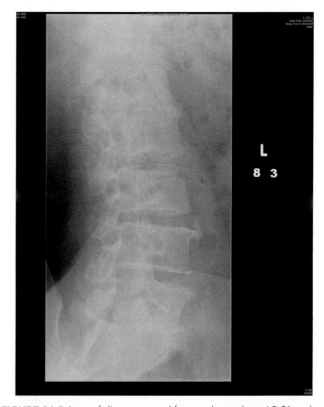

FIGURE 91-5 Loss of disc space and facet arthropathy at L5-S1 and small osteophytes, best seen on L4 and L5. These changes are due to osteoarthritis. (*Courtesy of Kansas University Medical Center.*)

REFERENCES

1. Sharma L, Kapoor D, Issa S. Epidemiology of osteoarthritis: An update. [Review]. *Curr Opin Rheumatol.* 2006;18(2):147–156.

2. Manek NJ, Lane NE. Osteoarthritis: Current concepts in diagnosis and management. *Am Fam Physician.* 2000;61:1795–1804.

3. American College of Rheumatology. http://www.rheumatology. org. Accessed August 30, 2006.

4. Ottawa panel evidence-based clinical practice guidelines for therapeutic exercises and manual therapy in the management of osteoarthritis. [Review] [178 refs]. *Phys Ther.* 2005;85:907–971.

5. Fox BA, Schmitz ED, Wallace R. FPIN's clinical inquiries. Glucosamine and chondroitin for osteoarthritis. [Review] [12 refs]. *Am Fam Physician.* 2006;73:1245–1246.

6. Towheed TE, Maxwell L, Judd MG, Catton M, Hochberg MC, Wells G. Acetaminophen for osteoarthritis. Update in *Cochrane Database Syst Rev.* 2003;(2):CD004257; PMID: 12804508. [Review] [81 refs]. *Cochrane Database Syst Rev.* 2006;(1): CD004257.

7. Barnes CL, Cawley PW, Hederman B. Effect of counterForce brace on symptomatic relief in a group of patients with symptomatic unicompartmental osteoarthritis: A prospective 2-year investigation. *Am J Orthop.* 2002;31:396–401.

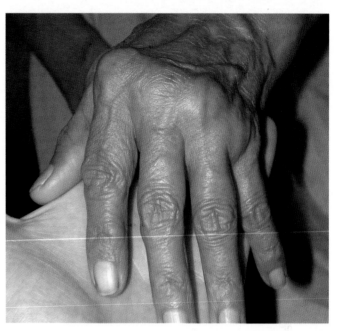

FIGURE 91-6 Rheumatoid arthritis showing ulnar deviation at the MCP joints. (*Courtesy of Richard P. Usatine, MD.*)

92 RHEUMATOID ARTHRITIS

Heidi Chumley, MD

PATIENT STORY

A 79-year-old woman with late-stage rheumatoid arthritis comes for routine follow-up (**Figures 92-1** to **92-4**). She began having hand pain and stiffness approximately 40 years ago. She took over-the-counter medications for pain for approximately 10 years before seeing a physician. She was diagnosed with rheumatoid arthritis on the basis of combination of clinical, laboratory, and radiograph findings. She was treated with prednisone and tried most of the disease-modifying agents as they became available; however, her disease progression continued. Approximately 10 years ago, she began having increased foot pain and difficulty walking. Today, she works with a multidisciplinary team to control pain and preserve hand function and independence.

EPIDEMIOLOGY

- 0.8% of the adult population worldwide.[1]
- Twice as common in women as compared to men (54 per 100,000 vs. 25 per 100,000).[1]
- Typical age of onset is 30 to 50 years.[1]

ETIOLOGY AND PATHOPHYSIOLOGY

- Genetic predisposition coupled with an autoimmune or infection-triggering incident.
- Synovial macrophages and fibroblasts proliferate, leading to increased lymphocytes and endothelial cells.
- Increased cellular material occludes small blood vessels, causing ischemia, neovascularization, and inflammatory reactions.
- Inflamed tissue grows irregularly causing joint damage.
- Damage causes further release of cytokines, interleukins, proteases, growth factors, resulting in more joint destruction and systemic complications.

DIAGNOSIS

American Rheumatism Association criteria (with positive likelihood ratio abbreviated as LR+):[2]

- Stiffness around joint for 1 hour after inactivity (LR+1.9).
- Three or more of these have soft tissue swelling: Wrist, PIP, MCP, elbow, knee, ankle, MTP (LR+1.4).
- Hand joints involved (LR+1.5) (**Figures 92-1, 92-4,** and **92-5**).
- Symmetrical involvement of one of these: Wrist, PIP, MCP, elbow, knee, ankle, MTP (LR+1.2).

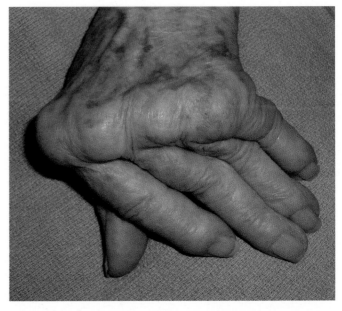

FIGURE 92-1 Ulnar deviation at metacarpophalangeal joints in advanced rheumatoid arthritis. Also note the swelling at the distal interphalangeal joints, seen best on the first finger. (*Courtesy of Richard P. Usatine, MD.*)

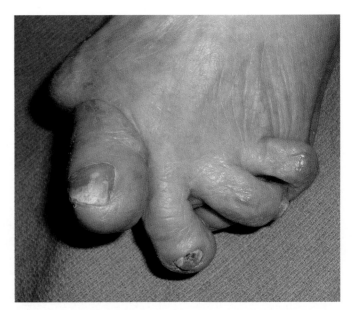

FIGURE 92-2 Rheumatoid arthritis in the foot of a 79 year-old woman with subluxation of the first MTP joint. (*Courtesy of Richard P. Usatine, MD.*)

- Subcutaneous nodules (3.0) (**Figures 92-5** and **92-6**).

- Positive serum rheumatoid factor (8.4).

- Osteopenia or erosion of surrounding joints on hand or wrist films (11) (**Figures 92-7** and **92-8**).

LABORATORY TESTS HELPFUL IN MAKING THE DIAGNOSIS[3]

- C-reactive protein (>0.7 picog/mL) or erythrocyte sedimentation rate (>30 mm/h).

- Rheumatoid factor (negative in 30% of patients; positive in many connective tissue, neoplastic, and infectious diseases).

- Complete blood count (normocytic or microcytic anemia, thrombocytosis).

RADIOGRAPHS

- Hand or wrist radiographs may show soft tissue swelling, osteopenia, erosions, subluxations, and deformities.

DIFFERENTIAL DIAGNOSIS

Rheumatoid arthritis can mimic many systemic diseases and should be differentiate from the following:[1]

- Connective tissue diseases (scleroderma and lupus), which have other specific systemic signs.

- Fibromyalgia—pain at trigger points instead of joints.

- Hemochromatosis—abnormal iron studies and skin changes.

- Infectious endocarditis—heart murmurs, high fever, risk factors, such as IV drug use.

- Polyarticular gout—erythematous joints and crystals in joint aspirate.

- Polymyalgia rheumatica—proximal joint pain without deformity.

- Seronegative, spondyloarthropathies—asymmetric joint involvement, spine often involved.

- Reactive arthritis—history of infection, sexually transmitted disease, or bowel complaints.

MANAGEMENT

The American College of Rheumatology Subcommittee on Rheumatoid Arthritis makes the following recommendations:[3]

- Disease-modifying agents reduce disease progression. Consider for all patient early in the disease (within 3 months of onset of symptoms).[3] SOR **A**
  - If erosions are not present, treat with hydroxychloroquine, sulfasalazine, or minocycline.
  - If erosions are present, consider methotrexate (10–15 mg/wk) with or without hydroxychloroquine or sulfasalazine.
  - If ineffective, increase methotrexate dose to 20 mg/wk orally or 25 mg/wk SC or IM.
  - Consider leflunomide or azathioprine.

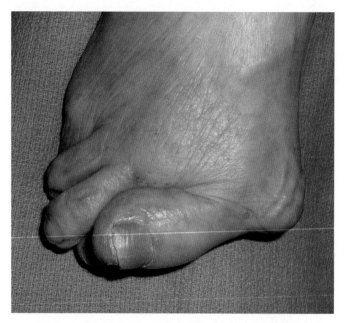

FIGURE 92-3 Deviation at the metatarsalphalangeal joints from bony destruction in advanced rheumatoid arthritis. (*Courtesy of Richard P. Usatine, MD.*)

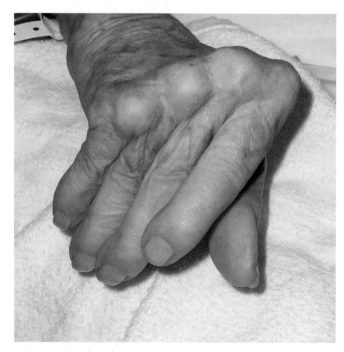

FIGURE 92-4 Ulnar deviation at metacarpophalangeal joints seen in a 79-year-old woman with advanced rheumatoid arthritis. (*Courtesy of Kelly Foster, MD.*)

- Nonsteroidal anti-inflammatory medications for pain control.[3] SOR **A**
  - Do not alter disease progression and should not be used alone.
  - Patients with rheumatoid arthritis are twice as likely to have serious GI complications, monitor carefully.
- Systemic corticosteroids relieve pain and slow progression,[3] SOR **A** but have serious side effects and should be used at lowest dose possible with added bone protection (e.g., calcium and vitamin D or a bisphosphonate).
- Monitor for complications:
  - Anemia—25% will respond to iron therapy.
  - Cancer—twofold increase risk of lymphomas and leukemias.
  - Cardiac complications such as pericarditis or pericardial effusion (30% at diagnosis).
  - Cervical spine disease—atlas instability; careful with intubation and avoid flexion films after trauma until atlas visualized.
- Use of multidisciplinary team improves outcomes.[4] SOR **B**
- Alternative therapies:
  - Diet modifications—omega 3 polyunsaturated fatty acids may decrease anti-inflammatory medication use.[1] SOR **B**
  - Exercise improves aerobic capacity and strength without increases in pain or disease activity.[3] SOR **B**

PATIENT EDUCATION

Rheumatoid arthritis is a chronic illness. Twenty to forty percent of patients will have remission with therapy. Early treatment can prevent complications and allow the person to maintain function. It is best to stay active and exercise to the best of your ability.

FOLLOW-UP

Multidisciplinary follow-up with primary care, rheumatologist, occupational and physical therapists, and patient educators improves outcomes.

PATIENT RESOURCES

American College of Rheumatology has a patient and public page accessible through **http://www.rheumatology.org.**

PROVIDER RESOURCES

American College of Rheumatology keeps an updated list of classification and treatment guidelines on the members and professionals page accessible through **http://www.rheumatology.org.**

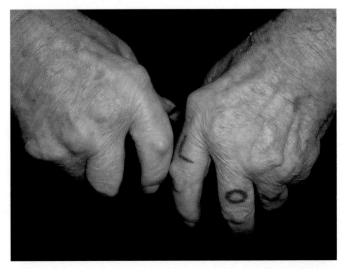

FIGURE 92-5 Rheumatoid nodules in the hands. (*Courtesy of Richard P. Usatine, MD.*)

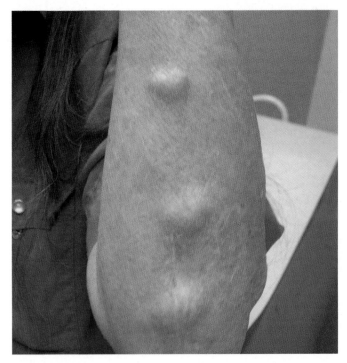

FIGURE 92-6 Rheumatoid nodules in the arms. (*Courtesy of Richard P. Usatine, MD.*)

REFERENCES

1. Rindfleisch JA and Muller D. Diagnosis and Management of Rheumatoid Arthritis. *Am Fam Physician.* 2005;72(6):1037–1047, 1049–1050.

2. Saraux A, Berthelot JM, Chales G, et al. Ability of the American college of rheumatology 1987 criteria to predict rheumatoid arthritis in patients with early arthritis and classification of these patients two years later. *Arthritis Rheum.* 2001;44(11):2485–2491.

3. American College of Rheumatology Subcommittee on Rheumatoid Arthritis Guidelines. Guidelines for the management of rheumatoid arthritis: 2002 Update.[see comment]. *Arthritis Rheum.* 2002;46(2):328–346.

4. Vliet Vlieland TP, Breedveld FC, Hazes JM. The 2-year follow-up of a randomized comparison of in-patient multidisciplinary team care and routine out-patient care for active rheumatoid arthritis. *Br J Rheum.* 1997;36(1):82–85.

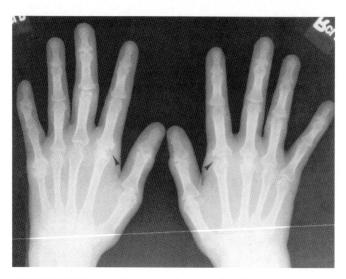

FIGURE 92-7 Hand radiographs in long-standing rheumatoid arthritis demonstrating carpal destruction, radiocarpal joint narrowing, bony erosion (arrowheads), and soft-tissue swelling. (*From Chen MYM, Pope TL, Jr., Ott DJ. Basic Radiology; Figure 7-42, p.194, Copyright 2004, McGraw-Hill.*)

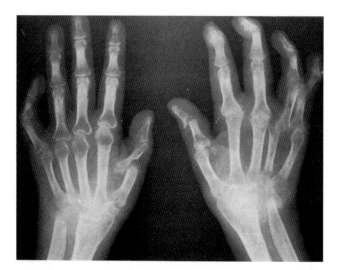

FIGURE 92-8 Severe changes of late rheumatoid arthritis including radiocarpal joint destruction, ulnar deviation, erosion of the ulnar styloid bilaterally, dislocation of the left thumb proximal interphalangeal joint, and dislocation of the right fourth and fifth metacarpophalangeal joints. (*From Brunicardi CF, Andersen, Billiar TR, et al. Schwartz's Principles of Surgery; Figure 42-40, p.1666, Copyright 2005, McGraw-Hill.*)

93 ANKYLOSING SPONDYLITIS

Heidi Chumley, MD

PATIENT STORY

A 25-year-old man has had thoracic and lumbar back pain for approximately 1 year. He feels stiff most mornings, and his pain decreases as he moves about. He gets good relief from ibuprofen. He feels he is too young to have chronic pain and wonders if something else is wrong. A work-up shows changes in his spine consistent with ankylosing spondylitis. A blood test reveals that he is HLA-B27 positive.

EPIDEMIOLOGY

- Prevalence in general population is approximately 0.25%.
- Five percent of patients in primary care with low back pain have a spondyloarthritis—a spectrum of diseases that includes ankylosing spondylitis.[1]
- More common in male versus females (~4:1).
- Ninety percent of patients are HLA-B27 positive.[2] However, many people with HLA-B27 do not develop the disease.

ETIOLOGY AND PATHOPHYSIOLOGY

- Inflammatory arthritis with a poorly understood pathology.
- Environment and genetic factors result in inflammation.
- Chronic inflammation causes in extensive new bone formation.

DIAGNOSIS

Mean delay of 7 to 8 years until diagnosis.

CLINICAL FEATURES

- Younger patient (less than 40 years of age).
- Pain in lower back and/or sacroiliac joints.
- Inflammatory (pain and stiffness worsen with immobility and improve with motion; symptoms are worse at night or early morning).
- Good response to NSAIDS: Sensitivity = 77%, specificity = 85%, LR+ 5.1.[1]

    Consider screening patients younger than 45 years of age with chronic low back pain for more than 3 months.[3]

- Symptoms of inflammatory back pain have fair sensitivity (75%) and specificity (75%). LR+ 3.1. Number needed to screen is 7.[1,3]

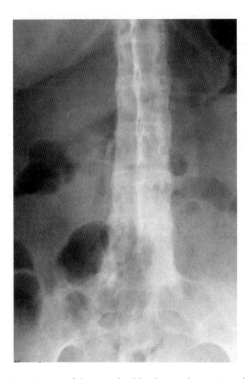

FIGURE 93-1 Fusion of the vertebral bodies and posterior elements gives the spine the classic "bamboo" appearance seen in ankylosing spondylitis. (*From Chen MYM, Pope TL, Jr., Ott DJ. Basic Radiology Copyright 2004, McGraw-Hill.*)

- HLA-B27 has good sensitivity (90%) and specificity (90%). LR +9.0. Number needed to screen is 3. Test is expensive.[1,3]

- May also consider HLA-B27 for patients with inflammatory back pain only.[1]

  Radiologic findings confirm the diagnosis; however, these may occur years after the onset of symptoms.

- Plain films: typical spinal features include erosions, squaring, sclerosis, syndesmophytes, and fractures (**Figures 93-1** and **93-2**); may also see sacroiliac joint fusion (**Figure 93-3**).

- MRI: detects inflammation, such as acute sacroiliitis, which occurs prior to bony change visible by radiographs.

DIFFERENTIAL DIAGNOSIS

Causes of back pain in patients younger than 45 years:

- Lumbar strain or muscle spasm—acute onset often with precipitating event.

- Herniated disc—acute onset with pain radiating below the knee into lower leg or foot with numbness, weakness and/or loss of ankle jerk reflex.

- Vertebral fractures—risk factors for osteoporosis or significant trauma.

- Abdominal pathology such as pancreatitis—associated with GI symptoms.

- Kidney diseases: Nephrolithiasis—pain radiating into groin; pyelonephritis—fever, nausea, and urinary symptoms.

- Osteoarthritis—worse after working; less commonly has inflammatory symptoms.

- Other spondyloarthritides (SpA) include psoriatic spondyloarthritis (**Figure 93-4**), SpA associated with inflammatory bowel disease, reactive SpA, and undifferentiated SpA.

MANAGEMENT

- NSAIDS and physical therapy reduce pain. Continuous NSAIDS reduce radiographic progression.[4]

- Disease modifying antirheumatic drugs (methotrexate, leflunomide) have not been demonstrated to have patient-oriented outcomes.[4]

- Tissue necrosis factor blockers are recommended for patients who fail NSAIDS and physical therapy. Consider treating or referring for treatment with shorter duration of symptoms, elevated acute phase reactants (i.e., c-reactive protein), or rapid radiographic progression. SOR **C**

  ○ Infliximab improves pain scores and quality of life within 2 weeks (61% vs. 19% placebo).[4] SOR **A** Many relapse; high cost, but economic analysis is favorable compared to estimated cost of loss of function.[4]

  ○ Etanercept improves pain scores (60% vs. 12%).[4] SOR **A** Relief within 2 weeks. Many relapse; reinitiation works.[4]

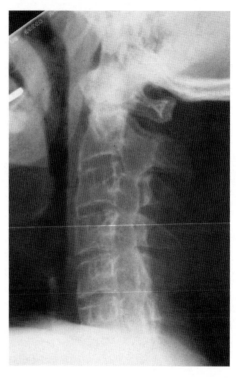

FIGURE 93-2 Syndesmophytes are the thin vertical connections between the anterior aspects of the vertebral bodies. They are located in the outer layers of the annulus fibrosis. (*From Chen MYM, Pope TL, Jr., Ott DJ. Basic Radiology; Copyright 2004, McGraw-Hill.*)

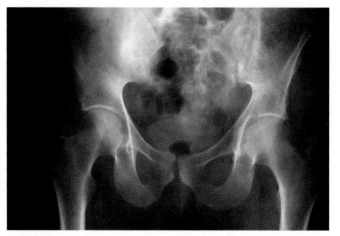

FIGURE 93-3 AS with near fusion of right SI joint, pseudowidening (from erosive changes) of the left SI joint. (*Courtesy of Everett Allen, MD.*)

PATIENT EDUCATION

Ankylosing spondylitis is a chronic disease. NSAIDS and physical therapy and exercise are important in controlling pain and slowing progression of disease. If these are ineffective, tissue necrosis factor blockers are effective; however, these are expensive and pain recurs when they are stopped.

FOLLOW-UP

Follow patients for progression of pain or decreased function using standard ankylosing spondylitis, such as the Bath Ankylosing Spondylitis Disease Activity Index or Functional Index.

PATIENT AND PROVIDER RESOURCES

The Spondylitis Association of America is found at **http://www.spondylitis.org/main.aspx** and contains downloadable brochures and the Bath Ankylosing Spondylitis Disease Activity Index and Bath Ankylosing Spondylitis Functional Index.

REFERENCES

1. Rudwaleit M, van der HD, Khan MA, Braun J, Sieper J. How to diagnose axial spondyloarthritis early. *Ann Rheum Dis*. 2004;63(5): 535–543.

2. Kim Th, Uhm WS, Inman RD. Pathogenesis of ankylosing spondylitis and reactive arthritis. [Review] [73 refs]. *Curr Opin Rheum*. 2005;17(4):400–405.

3. Sieper J, Rudwaleit M. Early referral recommendations for ankylosing spondylitis (including pre-radiographic and radiographic forms) in primary care. [Review] *Ann Rheum Dis*. 2005;64(5): 659–663.

4. Zochling J, Braun J. Management and treatment of ankylosing spondylitis. [Review]. *Curr Opin Rheum*. 2005;17(4):418–425.

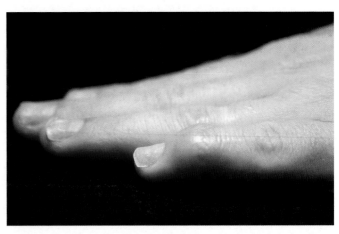

FIGURE 93-4 Psoriatic arthritis with DIP joint involvement and nail pitting. (*Courtesy of Everett Allen, MD.*)

94 GOUT

Mindy A. Smith, MD, MS
Heidi Chumley, MD

PATIENT STORY

A 91-year-old woman arrives by ambulance to the emergency department because she was experiencing severe pain in her right middle finger (**Figure 94-1**). History reveals that she has had swelling of her finger for approximately 1 year. Palpation of the distal interphalangeal joint demonstrated firmness rather than fluctuance. A radiograph of the finger was ordered and is shown in **Figure 94-2**. The radiograph and physical examination are consistent with acute gouty arthritis superimposed on tophaceous gout. The diagnosis was confirmed by an aspirate of the finger demonstrated negatively birefringent, needle-like crystals, both intracellularly and extracellularly. She was started on colchicine 0.6 mg every hour and her pain was markedly decreased in 4 hours. Her serum uric acid level was determined to be 10.7 mg/dL. The colchicine gave her diarrhea but was used in this case because the risk of using nonsteroidal anti-inflammatory drugs (NSAIDs) was considered to be high because of her previous history of gastric bleeding secondary to NSAIDs.

EPIDEMIOLOGY

- Gout affects 1% to 2% of the U.S. population and approximately 6% of men older than 80 years.[1]
- Gout is more prevalent in men than women.
- Gout usually begins after age 30 years in men and after menopause in women; it is familial in approximately 40% of patients.[1]

ETIOLOGY AND PATHOPHYSIOLOGY

Gout is characterized by an increased uric acid pool, hyperuricemia, episodic acute and chronic arthritis, and deposition of uric acid crystals in connective tissue and kidneys. Gout is caused by:

- Defective uric acid metabolism.
- Cancers (e.g., multiple myeloma, blood disorders).
- Chronic renal disease.
- Psoriasis.
- Alcoholism.
- Medications that reduce uric acid excretion including thiazide diuretics, loop diuretics, low-dose salicylates, cyclosporine, niacin, ethambutol, and pyrazinamide.

Gout is often associated with hyperuricemia from either overproduction or underexcretion. Eighty to ninety percent of gout patients with hyperuricemia are underexcreters.

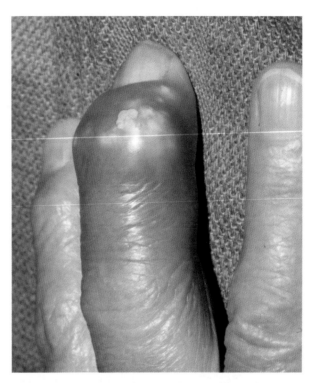

FIGURE 94-1 Acute gouty arthritis superimposed on tophaceous gout. (*Courtesy of West J Med and JM Geiderman, MD.*)

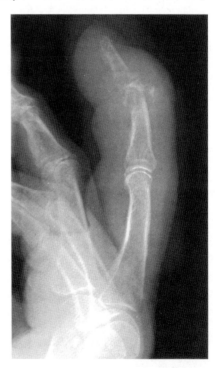

FIGURE 94-2 This x-ray of the finger in **Figure 94-1** shows several tophi [monosodium urate (MSU) deposits] in the soft tissue over the third distal interphalangeal joint. Note the typical punched out lesions under the tophi. This is subchondral bone destruction. (*Courtesy of West J Med and JM Geiderman, MD.*)

Gout's symptoms are caused by deposition of monosodium urate (MSU) crystals that cause local inflammation, tissue necrosis, fibrosis, and subchondral bone destruction.

DIAGNOSIS

CLINICAL FEATURES

- Gout usually begins at night as an acute attack over several hours.
- Fever, chills, and arthralgias sometimes precede gout. Initially only one joint may be affected but other joints commonly involved are fingers and toes (75%) and knees and ankles (50%).
- The most common site is the first MTP joint and the name for gout at this site is podagra (**Figure 94-3**).
- Joint involvement is often asymmetric.
- The affected joint is swollen, red, hot, and painful to touch and move (**Figures 94-1, 94-3,** and **94-4**). Symptoms subside in 3 to 10 days.
- Tophi may be seen at the metatarsophalangeal (MTP) joint, elbow, hands, and ears (**Figures 94-1** and **94-5**).
- Dietary or alcohol excess, trauma, surgery, and serious medical illness may precipitate gout attacks.

LABORATORY STUDIES

- Serum uric acid is often elevated, but is variable from week to week and normal in 25% of patients with gout.
- Measure 24-hour urine for excretion of uric acid.
- On microscopy, the presence of MSU crystals from synovial fluid or a tophus that are negatively birefringent in polarized light (yellow against a red background) helps to confirm the diagnosis, but there are limited data on the accuracy of crystal identification.
- Even with light microscopy refractile needle-shaped crystals of uric acid can be visualized in the joint fluid (**Figure 94-4**).
- Diagnostic characteristics useful in predicting gout, based on the 1977 criteria developed by the American College of Rheumatology, are:
  - Monoarthritis.
  - Redness over the joints.
  - First MTP joint involved (**Figure 94-3**).
  - Unilateral first MTP joint attack.
  - Unilateral tarsal joint attack.
  - Tophi identified (**Figures 94-1** and **94-5**).
  - Hyperuricemia.
  - Asymmetric swelling in joint on radiograph.
  - Subcortical cysts on radiograph.
  - MSU crystals in joint fluid (**Figure 94-5**).
  - Joint fluid culture negative.

The presence of 6 of these 11 criteria helps confirm gout (LR + 20, LR–0.02).[2]

IMAGING

Although radiographs are negative early in the disease, punched-out erosions ("rat bites") are seen later and can be diagnostic especially if seen adjacent to tophi (**Figure 94-2**).

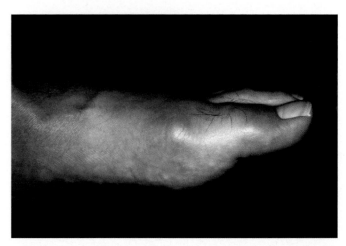

FIGURE 94-3 Podagra—typical inflammatory changes of gout at first metatarsal phalangeal joint. (*Courtesy of Richard P. Usatine, MD.*)

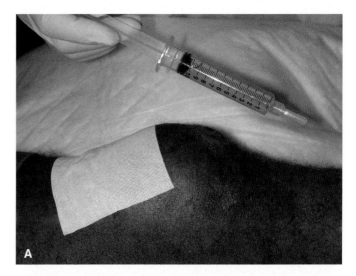

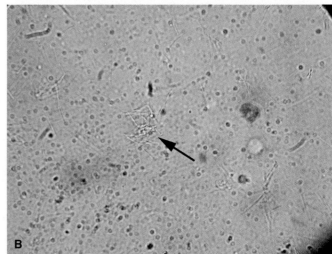

FIGURE 94-4 (A) A 52-year-old homeless man with acute monoarticular gouty arthritis presenting with knee pain and swelling. Knee aspiration revealed a straw-colored effusion. **(B)** With light microscopy numerous refractile needle-shaped crystals of uric acid were visualized in the joint fluid. The arrow points to a cluster of needle-shaped uric acid crystals. (*Reproduced with permission from A swollen knee. Journal of Family Practice, January 2003;52(1):53, Dowden Health Media.*)

DIFFERENTIAL DIAGNOSIS

In addition to gout, the differential diagnosis of inflammatory monoarthritis includes the following:

- Cellulitis—joint motion is not painful, synovial culture is negative (see Chapter 114, Cellulitis).
- Septic arthritis—fever, painful motion, synovial fluid has many white blood cells and a positive culture.
- Rheumatic arthritis—symmetric joint involvement (usually hands), slow onset, synovial culture is negative (see Chapter 92, Rheumatoid Arthritis).
- Pseudogout—findings like gout, synovial fluid with short rods, crystal refraction blue on red background (calcium pyrophosphate dihydrate).

MANAGEMENT

ACUTE GOUT

- NSAID, such as indomethacin 50 to 75 mg every 6 to 8 hours, in patients without renal impairment (serum creatinine should be less than 2.0) or peptic ulcer disease.[3] SOR **B**
- Colchicine 0.5 to 0.6 mg every hour up to 10 doses until symptoms decrease.[3] SOR **C** Most patients will have diarrhea before pain decreases.
- Intra-articular injection with long-acting steroid (e.g., triamcinolone acetonide, 10–40 mg, depending on the size of the joint).[3] SOR **C**
- Intramuscular or systemic corticosteroid for patients who cannot take oral medication.[3] SOR **C**

CHRONIC GOUT

The treatment of chronic gout includes modifications in diet and existing medications (if possible), medication to lower uric acid production, and/or medication to increase uric acid excretion (via blocking reabsorption).

The level of urinary uric acid helps to determine which medication should be used with levels ≥600 to 800 mg/24 hours indicating a need to halt production with allopurinol and levels <600 mg/24 hours indicating a need for uricosuric drugs. Treatment measures include:[1]

- Reducing the intake of certain purine-rich foods (e.g., organ meats, red meats and seafood).
- Increasing fluid intake to 2000 mL/d.
- Lowering alcohol intake.
- Changing medications: Discontinue aspirin (low dose up to 2 g/d causes uric acid retention) and consider stopping a thiazide diuretic.
- Giving allopurinol (100–300 mg/d for mild gout; for patients with moderate to severe tophaceous gout give 400–600 mg/d with a maximum daily dose of 800 mg/d).
  - Because this therapy may precipitate an acute gout attack, give colchicine (0.6 mg twice daily for the first 6 months of therapy) concomitantly during initiation of allopurinol to reduce the frequency and severity of acute flares.[4] SOR **B**

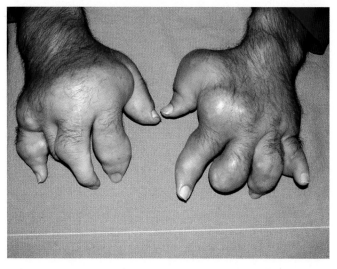

FIGURE 94-5 Severe tophaceous gout causing major deformities in the hands. (*Courtesy of Eric Kraus, MD.*)

- To optimize dosing, allopurinol may be titrated beginning with 100 mg/d to a serum uric acid less than 6.0.[5] SOR **B**
- Consider uricosuric agents (probenecid, 250 mg twice daily increasing to 2 to 3 g/d or sulfinpyrazone, 50 to100 mg twice daily increasing to 200 to 400 twice daily) in patients with uric acid excretion of less than 600 mg/24 hours, with normal renal function, younger than 60 years, and no history of renal calculi.[3] SOR **C** Consider giving the patient oral potassium citrate (10–20 m Eg three to 4 times a day) to prevent crystal precipitation in the urine since uricosuric agents increase urinary uric acid excretion.

PATIENT EDUCATION

Advise patients to lose weight, minimize alcohol use eat less meat and seafood and obtain more protein from dairy.[3]

FOLLOW-UP

- Untreated, recurrent, and more severe attacks are common with 60% of patients experiencing a recurrence in the first year and 25% in year two.
  - Colchicine 0.5 mg up to 3 times a day decreases attacks, but may not decrease joint destruction.[5] SOR **B**

ALTERNATIVE THERAPY

- Consuming diary products may be protective against gout.[1]
- A number of Chinese and Vietnamese medicinal plants and herbs have Xanthine oxidase inhibitory activity, but few have been tested for clinical effectiveness.

REFERENCES

1. Choi HK, Curhan G. Gout: Epidemiology and lifestyle choices. *Curr Opin Rheumatol.* 2005;17(3):341–345.

2. Silman AJ, Hochberg MC. *Epidemiology of the Rheumatic Diseases.* New York, NY: Oxford University Press, 1993.

3. Wortmann RL. Recent advances in the management of gout and hyperuricemia. *Curr Opin Rheumatol.* 2005;17(3):319–324.

4. Borstad GC, Bryant LR, Abel MP, et al. Colchicine for prophylaxis of acute flares when initiating allopurinol for chronic gouty arthritis. *J Rheumatol.* 2004;31(12):2429–2432.

5. Winklerprins VJ, Weismantel AM, Trinh TH. Clinical inquiries. How effective is prophylactic therapy for gout in people with prior attacks? *J Fam Pract.* 2004;53(10):837–838.

95 OLECRANON BURSITIS

Heidi Chumley, MD

PATIENT STORY

A 60-year-old man presents with swelling in his elbow for the last 2 months. He does not have pain unless he leans on his elbow. He denies any trauma. **Figure 95-1** demonstrates a "goose egg" swelling over the olecranon bursa that is not warm and tender only to palpation. He has full range of motion. His olecranon bursitis was treated with ice, rest, and NSAIDs and he was told to avoid leaning on his elbow.

EPIDEMIOLOGY

Prevalence of aseptic olecranon bursitis is unknown, but is estimated to be twice as common as septic olecranon bursitis.[1]

- Prevalence of septic olecranon bursitis is at least 10 per 100,000 in the general population.[2]
  - Peak age of onset is 40 to 50 years.
  - Eighty-one percent are male.
  - Fifty percent have antecedent trauma.

ETIOLOGY AND PATHOPHYSIOLOGY

Inflammation or degeneration of the sac overlying the olecranon bursa from:

- Repetitive motion or trauma, such as direct pressure on the elbow.
- Systemic diseases such as gout, pseudogout, or rheumatoid arthritis.
- Infection, typically by staphylococcus aureus or another gram-positive organism.

DIAGNOSIS

The diagnosis of olecranon bursitis is made clinically, by its typical appearance (**Figures 95-1** and **95-2**). When necessary, joint aspiration verifies the diagnosis and separates septic from aseptic bursitis.

CLINICAL FEATURES OF SEPTIC BURSITIS[2]

- Common symptoms: Pain (87%), redness (77%), and subjective fever or chills (45%).
- Common signs: Erythema (92%), swelling (85%), edema (75%), tenderness (59%), and fluctuance (50%).
- Less common signs: decreased range of motion (27%) and temperature $>$ or $=37.8°C$ (20%).

CLINICAL FEATURES OF ASEPTIC BURSITIS

- Swelling with minimal pain and tenderness.
- Erythema may be present (**Figure 95-2**).
- Fever is typically absent.

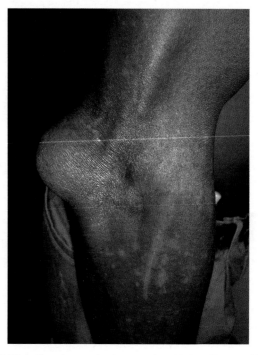

FIGURE 95-1 Chronic aseptic olecranon bursitis in a 60-year-old man showing typical swelling over the olecranon. There is no erythema or tenderness. (*Courtesy of Richard P. Usatine, MD.*)

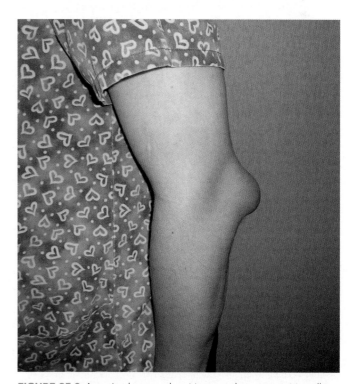

FIGURE 95-2 Aseptic olecranon bursitis secondary to repetitive elbow leaning in this computer programmer. There is some erythema and minimal tenderness. The aspirated fluid was clear. Most patients (70%) retain full extension in the elbow despite swelling over the olecranon. (*Courtesy of Richard P. Usatine, MD.*)

ASPIRATION

Aspirate when there is suspicion of infection or crystal disease (moderate pain, fever, warmth over the olecranon)[3] or for discomfort caused by extensive swelling.[4]

- Septic bursitis: Cloudy with increased neutrophils; more than 85% grow staphylococcus aureus; Gram stain positive approximately 65% of the time.
- Aseptic bursitis: typically clear; no bacterial growth.
- Elevated white blood cells: Infection, rheumatoid arthritis, or gout.
- Crystals: Gout or pseudogout.

IMAGING

- Usually not indicated.
- In traumatic bursitis, radiographs may identify a foreign body.
- In atypical cases, MRI may be needed to determine the extent of soft tissue involvement.

DIFFERENTIAL DIAGNOSIS

Pain and swelling around the elbow joint may be caused by:

- Gout or pseudogout (acute pain with signs of inflammation, prior history of gout (pseudogout).
- Rheumatoid arthritis (pain, inflammation, loss of range of motion, often involves other joints).
- Septic joint (acute pain, loss of range of motion, fever).
- Hemorrhage into the bursa (history of trauma, bruising).

Other causes of elbow pain typically without swelling include:

- Lateral or medial epicondylitis (pain lateral or medial, not over olecranon).
- Ulnar nerve entrapment (concurrent numbness in fingers).

MANAGEMENT

Aspirate fluid as follows:[4]

- Flex elbow to 45 degrees.
- Locate triangle formed by lateral olecranon, the head of the radius, and the lateral epicondyle.
- Using sterile technique, insert needle into the soft tissue in the middle of the triangle, pointing toward the medial epicondyle. (If there is a significant amount of fluid, it is hard to miss the fluid regardless of the direction of the needle as long as the needle gauge is sufficient for aspiration. Small gauge needles are wonderful for steroid injections and anesthesia but a larger gauge needle should be used for aspiration. Consider a 20- to 22-gauge needle and if an 18 gauge is to be used, give the patient some local anesthetic first.
- Aspirate fluid and send for CBC, Gram stain, culture, and evaluate for crystals if gout or pseudogout is expected.

- Consider injecting with steroid (see below) only if aspirate is clear and history does not suggest infection.

SEPTIC BURSITIS

- Identify organism using Gram stain and culture.
- If the WBC is slightly elevated and no organisms are seen on Gram stain, treat empirically with oral antibiotics active against gram positives until culture results are available (i.e., cephalexin 500 mg twice a day or levofloxacin 500 mg/d).[5] SOR **C**
- If WBCs are moderately elevated and organisms are seen on Gram stain, use intravenous medications such as oxacillin or nafcillin 2 g every 6 hours or cephazolin 1 to 2 g every 8 hours.[5] SOR **C**
- Vancomycin can be considered for penicillin or cephalosporin allergic patients or in communities with high rates of MRSA.[5] SOR **C**
- Home IV therapy is safe and effective for immunocompetent patients.[2] SOR **B**
- Hospitalize immunosuppressed patients or those who do not respond to therapy.[5] SOR **C**
- Aspirate after several days of treatment and continue antibiotics for 5 days after fluid is sterile.[5] SOR **C**
- Refer to an orthopedic specialist if incision and debridement of the bursa is needed. SOR **C**

ASEPTIC BURSITIS

- The first line of treatment should be wearing an elbow pad at all times in addition to modification of activities (no leaning on elbows) and NSAIDs as tolerated.
- Patient education about aggravating factors.
- Ice and rest.
- Consider corticosteroid injection for severe pain, persistent, or recurrent fluid accumulation.[5] SOR **C** There is a risk of converting an aseptic olecranon bursitis to a septic one with aspiration and steroid injection. Therefore, the treatment options noted above should be exhausted prior to consideration of steroid injection.
- Consider surgical referral for recalcitrant fluid accumulation.

PATIENT EDUCATION

Limit bursa aggravation by not leaning on elbows or pushing off on elbows when arising. Aseptic and septic bursitis may require multiple aspirations.

FOLLOW-UP

Follow septic bursitis until fluid is sterile. Reaspirate after 4 to 5 days of antibiotics and continue antibiotics for 5 days after fluid is sterile.

REFERENCES

1. Stell IM. Septic and non-septic olecranon bursitis in the accident and emergency department–an approach to management. *J Accid Emerg Med*. 1996;13(5):351–353.

2. Laupland KB, Davies HD. Calgary home parenteral therapy program study group. Olecranon septic bursitis managed in an ambulatory setting. The Calgary home parenteral therapy program study group. *Clin Invest Med.* 2001;24:171–178.

3. Work Loss Data Institute. Elbow (acute and chronic). National Guidelines Institute, http://www.guidelines.gov. Updated 2005. Accessed February 2, 2006.

4. Cardone DA, Tallia AF. Diagnostic and therapeutic injection of the elbow region. [review] [13 refs]. *Am Fam Physician.* 2002;66(11): 2097–2100.

5. Sheon RP. Kotton, CN. Septic Bursitis. UpToDate. http://www.utdol.com/utd/content/topic.do?topicKey=skin_inf/12648. Accessed February 24, 2008.

SECTION 2   FRACTURES

96 CLAVICLE FRACTURE

Heidi Chumley, MD

PATIENT STORY

A 17-year-old boy presents after falling off of his skateboard and landing directly on his lateral shoulder. He had immediate pain and swelling in the middle of his clavicle. His examination revealed a bump in the middle of his clavicle. A radiograph confirmed a midclavicular fracture (**Figure 96-1**). He was treated conservatively with a sling, which he wore for approximately 1 of the recommended 3 weeks. A follow-up radiograph demonstrated good healing. The bump on his clavicle is still palpable; however, this does not bother him.

EPIDEMIOLOGY

- 2.6% of all fractures in adults with an overall incidence of 64 per 100,000 per year; midshaft fractures account for approximately 69% to 81% of all clavicle fractures.[1]
- 10% to 15% of fractures in children; 90% are midshaft fractures.[2]

ETIOLOGY AND PATHOPHYSIOLOGY

- Most are caused by accidental trauma from fall against the lateral shoulder or an outstretched hand or direct blow to the clavicle; however stress fractures in gymnasts and divers have been reported.
- Pathologic fractures (uncommon) can result from lytic lesions, bony cancers or metastases, or radiation.
- Birth trauma (neonatal).
- Physical assaults, intimate partner violence and child abuse can cause clavicular fractures.

DIAGNOSIS

CLINICAL FEATURES

- History of trauma with a mechanism known to result in clavicle fractures (i.e., fall on an outstretched hand or lateral shoulder, or direct blow).
- Pain and swelling at the fracture site.
- Gross deformity at site of fracture.
- Radiographic evidence of fracture.
- For the typical distribution and classification of clavicular fractures, see **Table 96-1**.

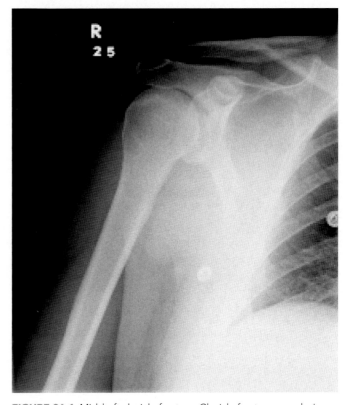

FIGURE 96-1 Midshaft clavicle fracture. Clavicle fractures are designated midshaft (in the middle third), distal (distal third), or medial (medial third). (*From Simon RR, Sherman SC, Koenigsknecht SJ. Emergency Orthopedics the Extremities, p. 286, Fig. 11-35, McGraw-Hill, Copyright 2007.*)

TABLE 96-1 Typical Distribution/Classification

Group (Approx. %)	Fracture Location	Radiographic Appearance
Group I (80%)	Middle third	Upward displacement (Figures 96-1 to 96-3)
Group II (15%)	Distal third	Medial side of fragment is displaced upward (Figure 96-4)
Type I		Minimal displacement
Type II		Fracture medial to coracoclavicular ligaments; some overlapping of fragments
Type III		Fracture at the articular surface of the acromioclavicular (AC) joint; can look like AC separation.
Group III (5%)	Medial third	Medial side of fragment up; distal side down

DIFFERENTIAL DIAGNOSIS

- Acromioclavicular (AC) separation: (**Figure 96-5**) fall directly on the "point" of the shoulder or a direct blow, pain with overhead movement, tenderness at the AC joint, and AC joint separation on radiographs.
- Sternoclavicular dislocation: fall on the shoulder, chest and shoulder pain exacerbated by arm movement or when lying down, and a prominence from the superomedial displacement of the clavicle (uncommon).
- Pseudoarthrosis of the clavicle: painless mass in the middle of the clavicle from failure of the central part of the clavicle to ossify (extremely rare).

MANAGEMENT

For all adults and children:

- Assess neurovascular status of injured extremity.
- Assess for damage to lungs (pneumothorax or hemothorax).
- Determine the classification and amount of displacement by radiograph (**Figure 96-1**). (See also **Table 96-1**).
- Treat pain as needed with acetaminophen or NSAIDs.

Most clavicular fractures can be treated nonoperatively, other options include fixation with plates or pins.

- Treat most children with any type of clavicle fracture conservatively, without immobilization.[2] SOR **C**
  - Treat children nonoperatively even with 90-degree displacement and several inches of overlap.[2] SOR **C**
  - Refer for surgical evaluation, children with impingement of soft tissue/muscle, instability of shoulder girdle, displacement with skin perforation/necrosis, or risk to mediastinal structures.[2] SOR **C**

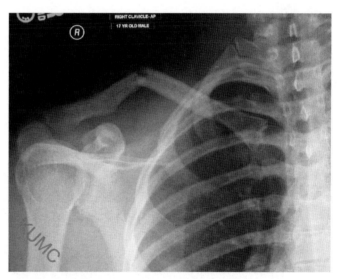

FIGURE 96-2 Mid-shaft clavicle fracture with angulation. (*From Simon RR, Sherman SC, Koenigsknecht SJ. Emergency Orthopedics the Extremities, p. 297, Fig. 11-54, McGraw-Hill, Copyright 2007.*)

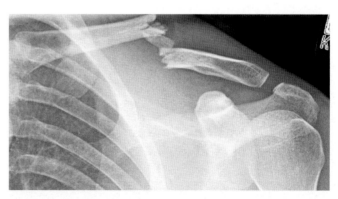

FIGURE 96-3 Mid-shaft clavicular fracture with proximal fragment displaced superiorly from the pull of the sternocleidomastoid muscle. (*From Simon RR, Sherman SC, Koenigsknecht SJ. Emergency Orthopedics the Extremities, p. 283, Fig. 11-32, McGraw-Hill, Copyright 2007.*)

- Treat most adults with midshaft clavicular fractures nonoperatively. SOR **B**
  - Place adults in a sling instead of a figure-of-eight. Patients treated with a sling had higher treatment satisfaction than those treated with a figure-of-eight bandage.[3] SOR **B**
  - Midclavicular fractures can be treated with a clavicle brace; treat until radiographic evidence of healing has occurred. SOR **C** Wearing the brace frees the upper extremities for activities of daily living. The clavicle brace may improve the alignment of the midclavicular fracture.
  - Discuss risk of nonunion with patients who have displaced fractures. Nonoperative treatment has a 5.9% nonunion rate, whereas operative rates are 0% to 2%.[1]
  - Consider referring patients with displaced fractures. Nonoperative treatment has a 15.1% nonunion rate, whereas operative rates are 0% to 2%.[1]

- Treat most middle age to elderly patients with distal (type II) clavicle fractures conservatively.

- Distal clavicle fractures are commonly treated by wearing a sling for 6 weeks to minimize the weight of the arm pulling on the distal clavicle fragment.
  - Discuss the risk of nonunion and the low rate of impaired function. Patients with distal clavicle fractures treated nonoperatively had nonunion rates of 21%; however, there was no difference in function between those who healed and those with a nonunion.[4] SOR **B**

- Consider consulting with a physician skilled in managing clavicular fractures in patients with a distal clavicle fracture. These fractures have a high rate of nonunion. They are commonly treated by having a patient wear a sling for 6 weeks. If the patient continues to have a symptomatic nonunion after many months, surgery may be considered.

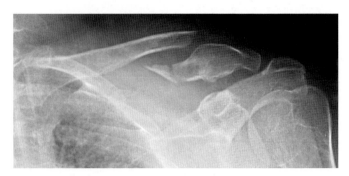

FIGURE 96-4 Distal clavicular fracture. (*From Simon RR, Sherman SC, Koenigsknecht SJ. Emergency Orthopedics the Extremities, p. 286, fig. 11-35, McGraw-Hill, Copyright 2007.*)

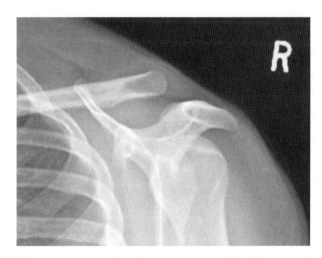

FIGURE 96-5 Acromioclavicular joint separation (third degree) with a wide AC joint and the clavicle displaced from the acromion. (*From Simon RR, Sherman SC, Koenigsknecht SJ. Emergency Orthopedics the Extremities, p. 297, fig. 11-54, McGraw-Hill, Copyright 2007.*)

PATIENT EDUCATION

Most clavicle fractures heal without surgery, especially if the fracture is not displaced. Fractures in adults take 6 to 8 weeks to heal and fractures in children take approximately 3 to 4 weeks to heal. Often, there will be a bump at the site of the healed fracture, which typically does not interfere with any activities.

FOLLOW-UP

Monitor with examination and radiographs until pain has resolved, any lost function has returned, and there is radiographic evidence of healing. Initially, repeat x-ray every 1 to 2 weeks to evaluate for any change in alignment. If the fracture is stable, repeat x-ray every 4 to 6 weeks until the clavicle has healed. If there is no evidence of healing after 2 to 3 months, referral should be considered.

PATIENT RESOURCES

The American Academy of Orthopedic Surgeons has a patient information handout under Broken Collarbone at **http://www. aaos.org.**

PROVIDER RESOURCES

Wheeless' Textbook of Orthopaedics from Duke University online: **http://www.wheelessonline.com/ortho/clavicle_fractures.**

REFERENCES

1. Zlowodzki M, Zelle BA, Cole PA, Jeray K, McKee MD. Evidence-Based Orthopaedic Trauma Working Group. Treatment of acute midshaft clavicle fractures: Systematic review of 2144 fractures: On behalf of the Evidence-Based Orthopaedic Trauma Working Group. *J Orthop Trauma.* 2005;19(7):504–507.

2. Kubiak R, Slongo T. Operative treatment of clavicle fractures in children: a review of 21 years. *J Pediatr Orthop.* 2002;22:736–739.

3. Andersen K, Jensen PO, Lauritzen J. Treatment of clavicular fractures. Figure-of-eight bandage versus a simple sling. *Acta Orthop Scand.* 1987;58(1):71–74.

4. Robinson CM, Cairns DA. Primary nonoperative treatment of displaced lateral fractures of the clavicle. *J Bone Joint Surg Am.* 2004; 86-A(4):778–782.

97 DISTAL RADIAL FRACTURE

Heidi Chumley, MD

PATIENT STORY

A 65-year-old woman tripped on a rug in her home and fell on her outstretched hand with her wrist dorsiflexed (extended). She felt immediate pain in her wrist and has difficulty in moving her wrist or hand. She has been postmenopausal for 15 years and has never taken hormone replacement therapy or bisphosphates. She presented with pain and swelling in her wrist. Her arm had a "dinner fork" deformity. Radiographs showed a distal radius fracture (Colles fracture) (**Figures 97-1** and **97-2**). There was dorsal angulation seen on the lateral view (**Figure 97-2**).

EPIDEMIOLOGY

- More common in older women: female-to-male ratio of 3.2:1.[1]

- Prevalence: 10.8% of women and 2.6% of men in a community study of 452 people older than 40 years in the United Kingdom had a prior distal radius fracture.[2]

- Incidence (Sweden): 115 per 100,000 women and 29 per 100,000 men.[1]

ETIOLOGY AND PATHOPHYSIOLOGY

- Classic history is a fall on an outstretched hand.

- In patients older than 40 years of age, there is a strong association with osteoporosis. Patients with low-impact distal radius fractures have higher rates of osteoporosis than age-matched controls without fractures by bone density measured at the wrist (60% vs. 35%, $p < 0.001$; OR 5.7, 95% CI 1.2–27.2) and lumbar spine (47% vs. 20%, $p < 0.005$, OR 3.9, 95% CI 1.1–14.3).[3]

- Postmenopausal women and older men with distal radius fractures have an increased risk for a future hip fracture (RR = 1.53; 95% CI, 1.34–1.74; $p < 0.001$; RR = 3.26; 95% CI, 2.08–5.11; $p < 0.001$, respectively).[4]

DIAGNOSIS

Diagnosis is suspected by a history of falling on a dorsiflexed wrist and confirmed with a plain radiograph showing the fracture of the distal radius (**Figures 97-1** and **97-2**).

CLINICAL FEATURES

Patients present with wrist pain and are not able to use the wrist or hand. The distal radius typically angles dorsally creating the "dinner fork" deformity (**Figure 97-2**). Swelling is usually present.

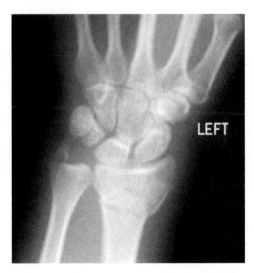

FIGURE 97-1 Anterior–posterior view demonstrating a transverse distal radius fracture (Colles fracture). (*From Simon RR, Sherman SC, Koenigsknecht SJ. Emergency Orthopedics, the Extremities, 5th ed, p. 204, Fig. 8-30 (left side), Copyright 2007, McGraw-Hill.*)

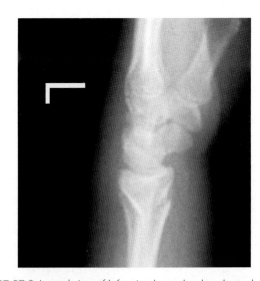

FIGURE 97-2 Lateral view of left wrist shows the dorsal angulation that gives the arm the "dinner fork" deformity. (*From Simon RR, Sherman SC, Koenigsknecht SJ. Emergency Orthopedics, the Extremities, 5th ed, p. 204, Fig. 8-30 (right side), Copyright 2007, McGraw-Hill.*)

DIFFERENTIAL DIAGNOSIS

Causes of pain at the wrist:

- Scaphoid fracture: forced hyperextension, tenderness in anatomic snuffbox, radiograph demonstrates scaphoid fracture (70%).
- Intra-articular dorsal or volar rim fractures (Barton's): forced wrist dorsiflexion with pronation, tenderness at distal radius, triangular fragment on radiograph (**Figure 97-3**).
- Radial styloid fracture (Hutchinson's): forced hyperextension, tenderness at the radial styloid, radiograph indicates styloid fracture (**Figure 97-4**).
- De Quervain's Tenosynovitis: no acute injury, pain on radial side of wrist from abductor pollicis longus and extensor pollicis brevis involvement, pain over the tendon when the thumb is placed into the patient's fist and the wrist is deviated to the ulnar side, radiographs (not usually done) are normal.

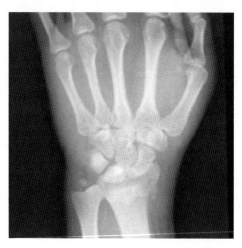

FIGURE 97-3 Barton's fracture: intra-articular radial rim fracture demonstrating a triangular fragment. (*From Simon RR, Sherman SC, Koenigsknecht SJ. Emergency Orthopedics, the Extremities, 5th ed, p. 207, Fig. 8-35 (left side), Copyright 2007, McGraw-Hill.*)

MANAGEMENT

Examine patients for the following associated complications:

- Flexor tendon injuries.
- Median and ulnar nerve injuries.

Examine radiographs for the following associated injuries:

- Ulnar styloid or neck fractures.
- Carpal fractures.
- Distal radioulnar subluxation.

Management is based on whether the fracture is non-articular or articular, displaced or nondisplaced, reducible or irreducible. There are multiple accepted classification schemes; however the Universal Classification of radial fractures, shown in **Table 97-1**, is the most straight-forward when determining management.[5]

- The patient's wrist in most cases is splinted for the first few days after injury to allow swelling to decrease prior to casting.
- On the basis of the type of fracture, the patient's wrist is typically cast from 4 to 6 weeks and followed with serial radiographs.
- The patient should be referred to a musculoskeletal or orthopedic specialist if a fracture requires reduction.
- All patients with a low-impact distal radius fracture are at a higher risk for osteoporosis and clinicians should consider screening for osteoporosis.

PATIENT EDUCATION

- Distal radial fractures may result in limitations of wrist function.
- Nontraumatic fractures, in patients older than 40 years of age, may indicate osteoporosis.

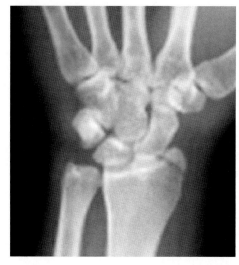

FIGURE 97-4 Hutchinson's fracture: radial styloid fracture. (*From Simon RR, Sherman SC, Koenigsknecht SJ. Emergency Orthopedics, the Extremities, 5th ed, p. 208, Fig. 8-36 (radiograph only), Copyright 2007, McGraw-Hill.*)

TABLE 97-1 Universal Classification of Radial Fractures

Fracture Classification	Management
I Nonarticular, nondisplaced	Immobilization with cast or splint[6] for 4–6 weeks
II Nonarticular, displaced	Reduction with cast or splint immobilization;[6] Surgical management if irreducible or unstable fracture
III Articular, nondisplaced	Immobilization; pinning if unstable
IV Articular, displaced	Surgical management

FOLLOW-UP

- Management and follow-up often involve a physician with expertise in managing distal radial fractures.
- Evaluate for osteoporosis.

REFERENCES

1. Masud T, Jordan D, Hosking DJ. Distal forearm fracture history in an older community-dwelling population: The Nottingham Community Osteoporosis (NOCOS) Study. *Age Ageing*. 2001;30: 255–258.

2. Mallmin H, Ljunghall S. Incidence of Colles' fracture in Uppsala. A prospective study of a quarter-million population. *Acta Orthop Scand*. 1992;63(2):213–215.

3. Kanterewicz E, Yanez A, Perez-Pons A, Codony I, Del RL, ez-Perez A. Association between Colles' fracture and low bone mass: Age-based differences in postmenopausal women. *Osteoporos Int*. 2002;13(10):824–828.

4. Haentjens P, Autier P, Collins J, Velkeniers B, Vanderschueren D, Boonen S. Colles fracture, spine fracture, and subsequent risk of hip fracture in men and women. A meta-analysis. *J Bone Joint Surg Am*. 2003;85-A(10):1936–1943.

5. Newport ML. Upper extremity disorders in women. *Clin Orthop*. 2000;(372):85–94.

6. Tumia N, Wardlaw D, Hallett J, Deutman R, Mattsson SA, Sanden B. Aberdeen Colles' fracture brace as a treatment for Colles' fracture. A multicentre, prospective, randomised, controlled trial. *J Bone Joint Surg Br*. 2003;85(1):78–82.

98 METATARSAL FRACTURE

Heidi Chumley, MD

PATIENT STORY

A 37-year-old man inverted his ankle while playing basketball with his teenagers in their driveway. He felt a pop and had immediate pain. He had tenderness over the base of his fifth metatarsal. Having met the Ottawa ankle rules for radiographs (see later), a radiograph was obtained, which revealed a nondisplaced fracture at the base of the fifth metatarsal (**Figure 98-1**).

EPIDEMIOLOGY

- Foot fractures are common injuries among recreational and serious athletes; however, incidence and prevalence in most populations is unknown.

- In women older than 70 years, the incidence of foot fractures is 3.1 per 1000 woman-years, and more than 50% of these are fifth metatarsal fractures.[1]

- Ninety percent of fifth metatarsal fractures are avulsion injuries (**Figure 98-1**). These are often called Dancer's fractures because this fracture is common in ballet dancers. It is also common in gymnasts and other athletes.

ETIOLOGY AND PATHOPHYSIOLOGY

- Avulsion fractures result when the peroneus brevis tendon and the lateral plantar fascia pull off the base of the fifth metatarsal, typically during an inversion injury.

- Jones fracture results from landing on the outside of the foot with the foot plantar flexed.

DIAGNOSIS

The diagnosis of avulsion or Jones fractures is made on plain radiographs in a patient with a history of injury and acute lateral foot pain. Diaphyseal stress fractures may require CT imaging.

CLINICAL FEATURES

- Avulsion injury—sudden onset of pain (and tenderness on examination) at the base of the fifth metatarsal after forced inversion with the foot and ankle in plantar flexion.

- Acute Jones fracture—sudden pain at the base of the fifth metatarsal, with difficulty bearing weight on the foot, after a laterally directed force on the forefoot during plantar flexion of the ankle.

- Stress fracture—history of chronic foot pain with repetitive motion.

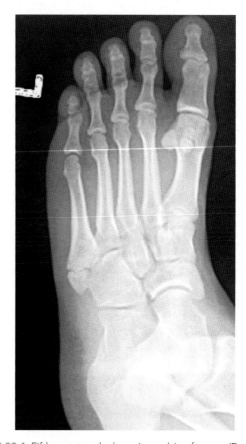

FIGURE 98-1 Fifth metatarsal tuberosity avulsion fracture (Dancer's fracture). (*From Simon RR, Sherman SC, Koenigsknecht SJ. Emergency Orthopedics, the Extremities, 5th ed, p. 488, Fig. 18-21B, McGraw-Hill, Copyright 2007.*)

RADIOGRAPHIC FINDINGS

- Avulsion fracture—fracture line at base of fifth metatarsal oriented perpendicularly to the metatarsal shaft (**Figure 98-1**).
- Acute Jones fractures (**Figure 98-2**) and stress fractures both have a fracture line through the proximal 1.5 cm of the fifth metatarsal shaft. These should be classified into type I, II, or III as below:[2]
  - Type I fractures have a sharp, narrow fracture line, no intramedullary sclerosis, and minimal cortical hypertrophy.
  - Type II fractures (delayed unions) have a widened fracture line with radiolucency, involve both cortices, and have intramedullary sclerosis.
  - Type III fractures (nonunions) have a wide fracture line, periosteal new bone and radiolucency, and obliteration of the medullary canal by sclerotic bone.

DIFFERENTIAL DIAGNOSIS

Pain at the fifth metatarsal can also be caused by:

- Diaphyseal stress fracture: may be radiographically similar to Jones fracture but are often seen more distally in the shaft; occur in patients with no injury and history of overuse (e.g., ballet dancing, marching, etc).
- Lisfranc injury: disruption of the tarsal metatarsal joints. This pain is typically in the midfoot and more commonly medial.

X-ray findings that can be confused with foot fractures include:

- Apophysis, a secondary center of ossification at the proximal end of the fifth metatarsal seen in girls, age 9 to 11, and boys, age 11 to 14. The apophysis is oblique to the metatarsal shaft, whereas avulsion fractures are perpendicular.
- Accessory Ossicles (i.e., os peroneum, located at the lateral border of the cuboid) have smooth edges, whereas avulsion fractures have rough edges.

MANAGEMENT

Apply the Ottawa ankle rules to determine which patients with an injury and ankle/foot pain should have an x-ray.[3] SOR **A** Ottawa rules: X-ray patients who cannot walk four steps immediately after the injury or have localized tenderness at the posterior edge or tip of either malleolus, the navicular, or the base of the fifth metatarsal.[3]

- Treat nondisplaced avulsion fractures with an ankle splint or walking boot with ambulation for 3 to 6 weeks.[4] SOR **B** Refer displaced avulsion fractures.
- Consider referring Jones fractures because of the high rate of nonunion caused by the poor blood supply. Type I or II may be treated with immobilization for at least 6 to 8 weeks. Type II can also be treated with surgery. Type III requires surgical repair. Elite athletes or patients needing a faster recovery are often surgically treated.[5] SOR **B**

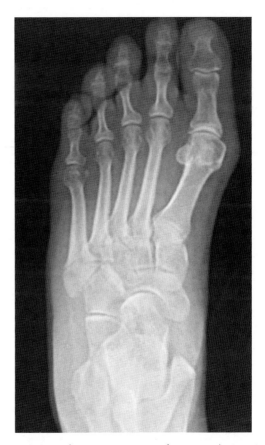

FIGURE 98-2 Jones fracture, a transverse fracture at the junction of the diaphysis and metaphysic. (*From Simon RR, Sherman SC, Koenigsknecht SJ. Emergency Orthopedics, the Extremities, 5th ed, p. 488, Fig. 18-21A, McGraw-Hill, Copyright 2007.*)

PATIENT EDUCATION

Patients with nondisplaced avulsion fractures require a splint or boot, but can remain ambulatory. Jones fractures have a poor blood supply and often do not reconnect, even with immobilization. Surgery may result in a faster return to activities in some cases.

PATIENT RESOURCES

Medline Plus has a section on all types of fractures: **http://www.nlm.nih.gov/medlineplus/fractures.html.**

PROVIDER RESOURCES

The Ottawa ankle and foot rules are part of MedRules© and can be downloaded (free) for use on a PDA from a number of web sites including **http://pbrain.hypermart.net** or **http://www.pdacortex.com.**

REFERENCES

1. Hasselman CT, Vogt MT, Stone KL, Cauley JA, Conti SF. Foot and ankle fractures in elderly white women. Incidence and risk factors. *J Bone Joint Surg Am.* 2003;85-A(5):820–824.

2. Lehman RC, Torg JS, Pavlov H, Delee JC. Fractures of the base of the fifth metatarsal distal to the tuberosity: A review. *Foot Ankle.* 1987;7:245–252.

3. Stiell IG, Greenberg GH, Mcknight RD, Nair RC, Mcdowell I, Reardon M. Decision rules for the use of radiography in acute ankle injuries. Refinement and prospective validation. *JAMA.* 1993; 269:1127–1132.

4. Konkel KF, Menger AG, Retzlaff SA. Nonoperative treatment of fifth metatarsal fractures in an orthopaedic suburban private multi-speciality practice. *Foot Ankle Int.* 2005;26:704–707.

5. Portland G, Kelikian A, Kodros S. Acute surgical management of jones' fractures. *Foot Ankle Int.* 2003;24:829–833.

99 HIP FRACTURE

Heidi Chumley, MD

PATIENT STORY

A 75-year-old woman with moderate dementia is brought to the office by her family because she is refusing to walk for the past 2 days. Her caretakers are not aware of a fall, but state she seemed unsteady since beginning a new depression medication 4 weeks ago. **Figure 99-1** shows that she has a nondisplaced, complete, femoral neck fracture. Undoubtedly she fell when unobserved approximately 3 days ago. She is referred to orthopedics for management of her hip fracture. Unfortunately, the dementia is a bad prognostic sign for recovery of ambulation.

EPIDEMIOLOGY

- Approximately 300,000 hip fractures per year in the United States of America.[1]

- 70% to 80% of hip fractures occur in women.[1]

- Average age is 70 to 80 years; risk increases with age.[1]

- Half of the patients with a hip fracture have osteoporosis.[2]

ETIOLOGY AND PATHOPHYSIOLOGY

- Approximately 95% of hip fractures are caused by a fall.

DIAGNOSIS

- In a population study, major risk factors for hip fracture include:
  - Low bone mineral density (3.6-fold [95% CI 2.6–4.5] in women and 3.4-fold [95% CI 2.5–4.6] in men for each SD [0.12 g/cm^2] reduction in bone mineral density).[3]
  - Postural instability and/or quadriceps weakness.
  - A history of falls.
  - Prior hip fracture.[3]

- Other factors associated with increased risk include: dementia, tobacco use, physical inactivity, impaired vision, and alcohol use.

- Physical examination: Abducted and externally rotated hip; limp or refusal to walk.

- Radiographs: Plain radiographs show most hip fractures. Consider MRI, bone scan, or CT for indeterminate radiographs.

- Types of fractures: Hip fractures are usually classified according to anatomic location as intracapsular (femoral neck fracture, **Figure 99-1**) or extracapsular (intertrochanteric or subtrochanteric fracture, **Figure 99-2**).[4]

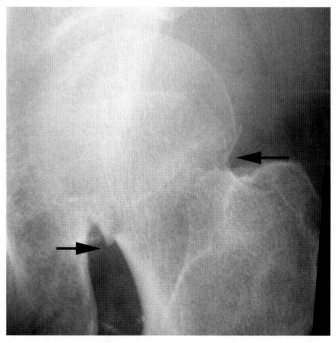

FIGURE 99-1 Nondisplaced, complete, femoral neck fracture (black arrows). Nondisplaced fractures can be incomplete (fracture through part of the femoral neck) or complete (fracture through the entire femoral neck). (*From Simon RR, Sherman SC, Koenigsknecht SJ. Emergency Orthopedics, the Extremities, 5th ed, p. 358, Fig. 13-8, Copyright 2007, McGraw-Hill.*)

DIFFERENTIAL DIAGNOSIS

Hip pain can be caused by bone or joint pathology, soft tissue injuries, spine pathology, or can be referred. Some causes include:[4]

- Pelvic fractures, bone cancers, or metastases; osteoarthritis, inflammatory, crystal, or septic arthritis.
- Iliotibial band syndrome, trochanteric bursitis, iliopsoas bursitis, pyriformis syndrome, muscle strain.
- Lumbar disc herniation, lumbar spinal stenosis, sciatica.
- Hernia, abdominal or pelvic pathology.

MANAGEMENT

Preventing hip fracture is important; 50% of patients with a hip fracture do not regain previous level of function; 20% die within a year.
   Lower risk of hip fracture by:

- Screening for osteoporosis.[5] SOR **B**
- Treating osteoporosis with bisphosphonates. SOR **A**
- Preventing falls by monitoring vision; assessing gait, strength, and balance, and minimizing the use of psychotropic medications in elderly. SOR **C**
- Encouraging exercise, such as Tai Chi for lower-body strengthening and balance.
- Calcium and vitamin D supplementation do not decrease risk of hip fracture, but should be part of an osteoporosis prevention and treatment strategy.[6] SOR **A**
- Hip pads have not decreased the risk of hip fracture in population studies, largely because of nonadherence, but are effective when worn.[7] SOR **A**

   Refer to an orthopedic surgeon unless the patient is not healthy enough to withstand surgery.

PATIENT EDUCATION

It is much easier to prevent hip fractures than to treat hip fractures. After a hip fracture, patients often need prolonged time (months) in a nursing care facility. Physical therapy is crucial in regaining as much function as possible.

FOLLOW-UP

Patients with hip fracture may benefit from multidisciplinary follow-up including monitoring for complications such as avascular necrosis, identifying and treating osteoporosis, modifying risk factors for further falls, and maximizing function through therapy.

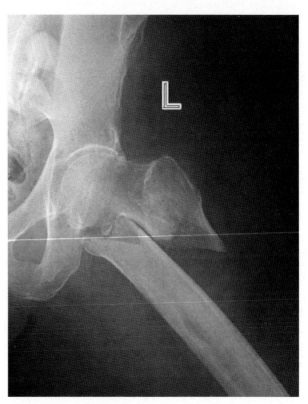

FIGURE 99-2 Unstable intertrochanteric fracture demonstrating displacement and a reverse oblique fracture line. Intertrochanteric fractures are unstable when there are multiple fracture lines, displacement between the femoral shaft and neck, or when the fracture line runs in an oblique reverse direction, with the most superior part of the fracture on the medial surface of the femur. The patient experience severe pain, hip swelling, and shortening of the involved leg. (*From Simon RR, Sherman SC, Koenigsknecht SJ. Emergency Orthopedics, the Extremities, 5th ed, p. 361, Fig. 13-12, Copyright 2007, McGraw-Hill.*)

REFERENCES

1. NHANES 2005–2006. National Center for Health Statistics. Center for Disease Control. Department of Health and Human Services. Available at: http://www.cdc.gov/nchs. Accessed June 2, 2008.

2. Robbins JA, Schott AM, Garnero P, Delmas PD, Hans D, Meunier PJ. Risk factors for hip fracture in women with high BMD: EPIDOS study. *Osteoporos Int.* 2005;16(2):149–154.

3. Nguyen ND, Pongchaiyakul C, Center JR, Eisman JA, Nguyen TV. Identification of high-risk individuals for hip fracture: A 14-year prospective study. *J Bone Miner Res.* 2005;20(11);1921–1928.

4. Brunner LC, Eshilian-Oates L, Kuo TY. Hip fractures in adults. *Am Fam Physician.* 2003;67(3):537–542.

5. Kern LM, Powe NR, Levine MA, et al. Association between screening for osteoporosis and the incidence of hip fracture. *Ann Intern Med.* 2005;142(3):173–181.

6. Porthouse J, Cockayne S, King C, et al. Randomised controlled trial of calcium and supplementation with cholecalciferol (vitamin D3) for prevention of fractures in primary care. *BMJ.* 2005; 330(7498):1003.

7. Parker MJ, Gillespie WJ, Gillespie LD. Hip protectors for preventing hip fractures in older people.[Update of *Cochrane Database Syst Rev.* 2004;(3):CD001255; PMID: 15266444]. *Cochrane Database of Syst Rev.* 2005;(3):CD001255.

SECTION 3 SOFT TISSUE

100 KNEE INJURIES

Heidi Chumley, MD

PATIENT STORY

A 33-year-old woman felt a pop in her knee while skiing around a tree. She felt immediate pain and had enough difficulty walking when paramedics removed her from the slopes. Within a couple of hours, her knee had a moderate effusion. On examination the next day, she was able to walk four steps with pain. She had a moderate effusion without gross deformity and full range of motion. She had no tenderness at the joint line, the head of the fibula, over the patella, or over the medial or lateral collateral ligaments. She had a positive Lachman's test, a negative McMurray's test, and no increased laxity with valgus or varus stress. The physician suspected an anterior cruciate ligament (ACL) tear and placed her in a long leg range of motion brace and advised to use crutches until an evaluation by her physician within the next several days. She was treated with acetaminophen for pain and advised to rest, apply ice, and keep her leg elevated. Later, an MRI confirmed an ACL tear (**Figure 100-1**).

EPIDEMIOLOGY

- Knee injuries are the second most common adolescent sporting injury (after ankle injuries)[1] and are seen typically in sports requiring pivoting such as basketball or football. See **Figure 100-2** for the normal anatomy of the knee.

- Most significant knee injuries are ligamentous and meniscal instead of fracture or dislocation.

- The risk of ACL injury was 3.79 times greater in girls in a prospective study of boy and girl high school basketball players in Texas.[1]

- Incidence of ACL injuries was approximately 3 per 1000 person-years in United States active military personnel with no difference in gender.[2]

- Meniscal injuries commonly occur with ACL tears (23%–65%).[3]

- Meniscal tears were seen on MRI in 91% of patients with symptomatic osteoarthritis, but also seen in 76% of age-matched controls without knee pain.[4]

- Collateral ligament injuries account for approximately 25% of acute knee injuries.

ETIOLOGY AND PATHOPHYSIOLOGY

- ACL injuries occur with sudden deceleration with a rotational maneuver, usually without contact.

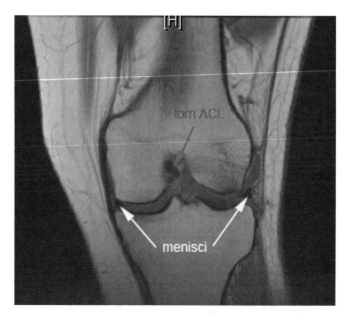

FIGURE 100-1 MRI of anterior cruciate ligament tear in the frontal view. Note the normal menisci, which are black throughout. (*Courtesy of Kansas University Medical Center, John E. Delzell, Jr., MD, MSPH.*)

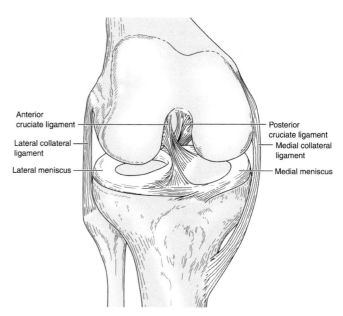

FIGURE 100-2 Anatomy of a normal knee. (*From Simon RR, Sherman SC, Koenigsknecht SJ. Emergency Orthopedics: The Extremities. Fig. 15-5 on p. 392. Copyright 2007. New York: McGraw-Hill.*)

- ACL injuries are thought to occur more commonly in women because of decreased leg strength and increased ligamentous laxity.

- Acute meniscal injuries occur with a twisting motion on the weight-bearing knee.

- Chronic meniscal tears occur from mechanical grinding of osteophytes on the meniscus in older patients with osteoarthritis.

- Medial collateral and lateral collateral injuries occur from valgus and varus stress, respectively.

DIAGNOSIS

CLINICAL FEATURES ON HISTORY

ACL:
- Rotational injury.
- "Pop" reported by patient.
- Unable to bear full weight.
- Effusion within the first few hours.

Meniscal injury:
- Foot planted with femur rotated internally with valgus stress (medial) or femur rotated externally with varus stress (lateral).
- Joint line pain.
- Effusion over the first several hours.
- Usually ambulatory with instability or locking (mechanical) symptoms.

Collateral injury:
- Valgus or varus stress injury.
- Usually ambulatory without instability or locking symptoms.

PHYSICAL EXAMINATION

- Inspect the knee for effusions—usually present for an ACL tear.

- Test range of motion—often normal; inability to extend fully can indicate either a medial meniscal tear or an ACL tear displaced posteriorly.

- Palpate for tenderness—joint line tenderness may indicate a meniscal tear (+LR=1.1; −LR=0.8).[5] Tenderness at the head of the fibula or at the patella are two of the five Ottawa rules for obtaining radiographs; tenderness along the medial or lateral collateral ligament may indicate damage to those ligaments.

- Perform tests for ACL tear—Lachmans' test (+LR=12.4; −LR=0.14),[5] anterior drawer test (+LR=3.7; −LR=0.6),[5] pivot shift test (+LR=20.3; −LR=0.4).[5]
  ○ Patients with ACL tears typically have a history of rotational injury; inability to bear weight; positive provocative tests; normal plain radiographs; and abnormal MRI.

- Perform tests for meniscal tears—McMurray test (+LR=17.3; −LR=0.5).[5]
  ○ Patients with meniscal tears typically have history of rotational injury with valgus/varus stress or history of osteoarthritis; able to bear weight, commonly with instability or locking; positive McMurray's test; normal plain radiographs; and abnormal MRI.

- Perform varus and valgus stress to test the lateral and medial collateral ligaments.
  ○ Patients with injuries to the collateral ligaments typically have a history of valgus/varus stress to extended knee; able to bear

weight without instability or locking; laxity with valgus or varus stress testing; normal plain radiographs and abnormal MRI.

RADIOGRAPHS

- Determine whether or not to obtain plain radiographs (anteroposterior, lateral, intercondylar notch, and sunrise views) to assess for a fracture based on either the Pittsburgh or Ottawa knee rules (the Ottawa rules may be less sensitive in children):
  - Pittsburg (99% sensitivity, 60% specificity; tested in population ages 6–96)[5]—obtain x-ray for:
    - Recent significant fall or blunt trauma.
    - Age less than 12 years or more than 50 years.
    - Unable to take 4 unaided steps.
  - Ottawa (98.5% sensitivity, 48.6% specificity; −LR=0.05; tested in 6 studies of 4249 adult patients),[6]—obtain x-ray for:
    - Age 55 years or older.
    - Tenderness at the head of the fibula.
    - Isolated tenderness of the patella.
    - Inability to flex knee to 90 degrees.
    - Inability to bear weight for four steps both immediately and in the examination room regardless of limping.
- MRI is 95% and 90% accurate in identifying ACL tears and meniscal injuries, respectively (**Figures 100-2** to **100-4**).[7]

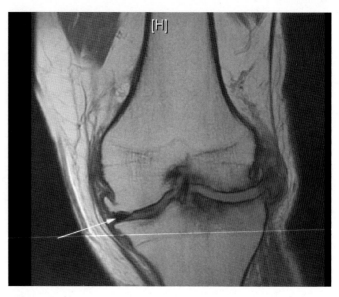

FIGURE 100-3 Medial meniscal tear on the frontal view, seen as a small white line through the black meniscus. (*Courtesy of Heidi Chumley, MD.*)

DIFFERENTIAL DIAGNOSIS

Acute knee pain can be caused by trauma affecting structures of the knee other than ligaments and menisci, arthritis, infection, or tumors including:

- Trauma.
  - Intra-articular fractures (patella, femoral condyles, tibial eminence, tibial tuberosity, and tibial plateau)—history of trauma or chronic overuse; edema, ecchymosis, point tenderness, or deformity may be present; visible on plain radiographs (**Figures 100-5** and **100-6**).
  - Patellar dislocation—severe hyperextension (anterior dislocation), fall on a bent knee or knee hitting the dashboard (posterior dislocation), valgus or varus stress (medial or lateral dislocation); visible deformity; effusion and immobility; neurovascular complications (peroneal nerve and popliteal artery); visible on plain radiographs.
- Arthritis: no history of trauma.
  - Reiter's syndrome—fever/malaise; oligoarthritis involving the knee, ankle, feet and/or wrist involvement, urethritis, conjunctivitis or iritis; elevated C-reactive protein or ESR; arthritic changes on radiographs.
  - Juvenile rheumatoid arthritis—children younger than 16 years; acute pain and swelling without trauma; fever or skin rashes (systemic JRA); knee is commonly involved; arthritic changes on plain radiographs.
  - Rheumatoid arthritis—adults aging 30 to 50 years, more commonly women; polyarthritis involving hands, wrists, feet, and knees; fever/malaise; positive rheumatoid factor; erosive

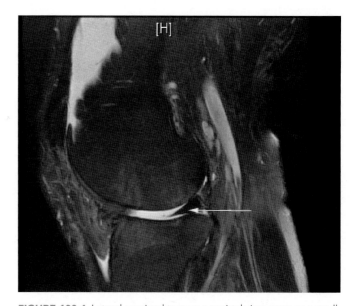

FIGURE 100-4 Lateral meniscal tear on a sagittal view, seen as a small white line in the black meniscus. (*Courtesy of Heidi Chumley, MD.*)

arthritis changes on radiographs (see Chapter 92, Rheumatoid Arthritis).

○ Gout or pseudogout—adults aging 30 to 60 years, more commonly men; single joint erythema, warmth and tenderness without trauma; abnormal joint fluid with elevated WBC; radiographs may be normal or abnormal (sclerotic regions, degenerative changes, or soft tissue calcifications) (see Chapter 94, Gout).

○ Osteoarthritis—older adults; gradual onset; symptoms worse after use; radiographic osteophytes (see Chapter 91, Osteoarthritis).

• Infections such as cellulitis, septic arthritis, osteomyelitis—May have history of skin break by bite or puncture wound; fever; erythema, warmth with cellulitis; decreased range of motion, inability to walk, abnormal fluid aspirate with septic arthritis; chronic symptoms and abnormal radiograph with osteomyelitis.

• Malignant tumors (e.g., osteosarcoma, chondroblastoma) or benign tumors (e.g., bone cysts, osteochondroma)—no (or insignificant) history of trauma; chronic symptoms or acute symptoms caused by pathologic fracture; abnormal radiographs and MRI.

MANAGEMENT

Initial management for traumatic knee pain includes rest, ice, compression, and elevation.

• Provide pain relief with acetaminophen. Add a nonsteroidal anti-inflammatory medication if needed.[8] SOR **C**

• Prevent further injury (e.g., limit activities to toe-touch weight bearing and place in a long leg range of motion brace)[7] until evaluation by a provider trained to manage acute knee injuries. SOR **C**

• Obtain plain radiographs if indicated by the Pittsburg or Ottawa rules.[6] SOR **A**

• Consider an MRI for suspected ACL, meniscal, or collateral ligament tear based on the mechanism of injury and physical examination findings.[7] SOR **C**

FOR ACL TEARS

• Refer to a physician trained in surgical repair as repair results in 80% to 95% return to normal activity in 4 to 6 months.[8] SOR **C**

• Surgical repair is typically done at least 3 weeks after the injury. Repair within the first 3 weeks results in a high incidence of arthrofibrosis.

• Refer to physical therapy if available to institute early knee range of motion (before surgery).[8] SOR **C**

FOR MENISCAL TEARS

• Refer to a physician for discussion of nonsurgical and surgical treatments as rates of healing vary by location of meniscal tear and associated injuries.[9] SOR **C**

For collateral tears, the treatment is based on the severity of the tear. SOR **C**

• For all grades, instruct in early range of motion exercises (or refer to physical therapy).

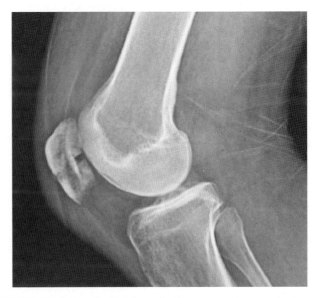

FIGURE 100-5 Nondisplaced patellar fracture seen best on the lateral view. (*From Simon RR, Sherman SC, Koenigsknecht SJ. Emergency Orthopedics: The Extremities. Fig. 15-26, bottom photo only, p. 405. Copyright 2007. New York: McGraw-Hill.*)

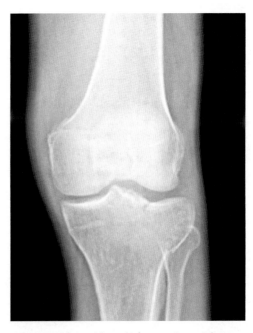

FIGURE 100-6 Lateral condylar split fracture (type 1) has no depression of the articular surface and is usually the result of low-impact trauma. More common in children. (*From Simon RR, Sherman SC, Koenigsknecht SJ. Emergency Orthopedics: The Extremities. Fig. 15-14, p. 398. Copyright 2007. New York: McGraw-Hill.*)

- Grade I MCL or LCL ($\leq$5 cm laxity on valgus or varus stress), weight-bearing as tolerated with early ambulation.
- Grade II MCL or LCL (5–10 cm laxity), place in a brace blocking the last 20 degrees of flexion, weight-bearing as tolerated.
- Grade III MCL (>10 cm laxity), place in a hinged brace, initially non-weight bearing, advancing to weight bearing over 4 weeks. Grade III LCL tears often require surgery.

PATIENT EDUCATION

- ACL tears often require surgery, take 4 to 6 months to heal, and require a commitment to rehabilitation for the best results.
- Meniscal tears may require surgery when mechanical symptoms are present. The location of the tear determines how likely surgical repair is to be effective because of the blood supply available for healing.
- Meniscal tears are commonly seen on MRI in patients with osteoarthritis who do not have pain and meniscal tears seen on MRI may not be contributing to arthritic pain.
- Collateral tears can often be treated conservatively, while protecting the knee in a brace and preserving range of motion. Complete tears to the lateral collateral ligament often require surgery.

FOLLOW-UP

Timing of follow-up is determined by the orthopedic surgeon or sports medicine specialist or other provider skilled in acute knee injury management.

PATIENT RESOURCES

The American Academy of Family Physicians has a patient algorithm for knee pain at **http://www.familydoctor.org.**

The National Institute of Health through the National Institute for Arthritis and Musculoskeletal and Skin Diseases has patient information on several types of knee problems at **http://www.niams.nih.gov.**

PROVIDER RESOURCES

MedRules has the Ottawa Knee Rules as part of their free package for PDAs at **http://pbrain.hypermart.net/medrules. html.**

Acute Knee Injuries: Use of Decision Rules for Selective Radiograph Ordering **http://www.aafp.org/afp/991201ap/ 2599.html.**

REFERENCES

1. Messina DF, Farney WC, DeLee JC. The incidence of injury in Texas high school basketball. A prospective study among male and female athletes. *Am J Sports Med.* 1999;27(3):294–299.

2. Owens BD, Mountcastle SB, Dunn WR, DeBerardino TM, Taylor DC. Incidence of anterior cruciate ligament injury among active duty U.S. military servicemen and servicewomen. *Mil Med.* 2007; 172(1):90–91.

3. Cimino PM. The incidence of meniscal tears associated with acute anterior cruciate ligament disruption secondary to snow skiing accidents. *Arthroscopy.* 1994;10(2):198–200.

4. Bhattacharya T, Gale D, Dewire P, et al. The clinical importance of meniscal tears demonstrated by magnetic resonance imaging in osteoarthritis of the knee. *J Bone Joint Surg Am* 2003;85-A:4–9.

5. Ebell MH. Evaluating the Patient with a Knee Injury. *Am Fam Physician.* 2005;71(6):1169–1172.

6. Bachmann KM, Haberzeth S, Steurer J, Ter Riet G. The accuracy of the Ottawa knee rule to rule out knee fractures: A systematic review. *Ann Intern Med.* 2004;140(2):121–124.

7. David K, Frank B. Anterior cruciate ligament rupture. *Br J Sports Med.* 2005;39:324–329.

8. New Zealand Guidelines Group (NZGG). *The Diagnosis and Management of Soft Tissue Knee Injuries: Internal Derangements.* Wellington (NZ): New Zealand Guidelines Group (NZGG), 2003:100.

9. Greis PE, Bardana DD, Holmstrom MC and Burks RT. Meniscal injury I: Basic science and evaluation. *J Am Acad Orthop Surg.* 2002; 10(2):168–176.

101 DUPUYTREN'S DISEASE

Heidi Chumley, MD

PATIENT STORY

A 53-year-old man presented with stiffness in his hands. He said his hand began to feel stiff several years ago, and now he finds that he cannot straighten many of his fingers (**Figure 101-1**). He delayed seeing a physician because he did not feel any pain in his hands. He recently began having difficulty holding his woodworking tools and wants to regain the function he has lost in his hands.

EPIDEMIOLOGY

- Dupuytren's disease is an autosomal dominant disease with incomplete penetrance.
- Higher prevalence among Caucasians with increasing incidence related to aging.
- More common in men than women.[1,2]
- Higher incidence in people who use tobacco and alcohol or have diabetes mellitus or epilepsy.[2]

ETIOLOGY AND PATHOPHYSIOLOGY

Dupuytren's contractures (**Figures 101-1** and **101-2**) form in three stages:

- Myofibroblasts in the palmar fascia proliferate to form nodules.
- Myofibroblasts then align along the lines of tension, forming cords.
- Tissue becomes acellular leaving thick cords of collagen that tighten resulting in flexion contractures at the metacarpal phalangeal joint, the proximal interphalangeal joint, and, occasionally, the distal interphalangeal joint.

DIAGNOSIS

- Clinical diagnosis based on the history and physical examination.
- Nodules with flexion contractures are considered diagnostic, particularly in older Caucasian males; however nodules may disappear late in the disease.[2]
- Early diagnosis or diagnosis in atypical populations such as children may require histological confirmation.

DIFFERENTIAL DIAGNOSIS

Consider the other causes of hand contractures and palmar nodules including:

- Hand contractures.

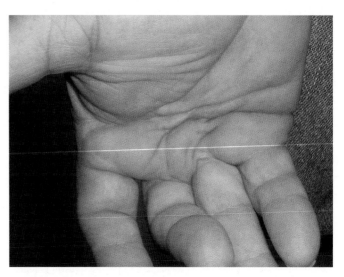

FIGURE 101-1 Dupuytren's contractures in a 53-year-old man showing flexion contractures at the proximal interphalangeal joints of the third digit and a palmar cord. (*Courtesy of Richard P. Usatine, MD.*)

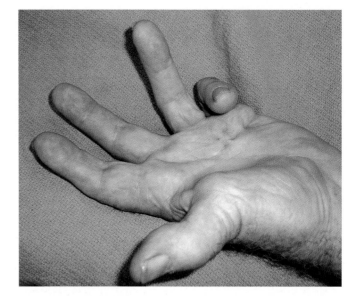

FIGURE 101-2 Dupuytren's contractures in a 58-year-old man showing flexion contractures of the fourth and fifth digits and a palmar cord. (*Courtesy of Richard P. Usatine, MD.*)

- ○ Intrinsic joint contractures—loss of range of motion from any primary joint disease.
- ○ Stenosing tenosynovitis—localized swelling of the hand limits tendon movement within the sheath with resulting "triggering"; digit catches, but can be straightened.
- ○ Rheumatoid arthritis—bony deformities resulting in ulnar deviation at the metacarpophalangeal joints and/or the wrist.
- Palmar nodules.
  - ○ Ganglionic cysts.
  - ○ Epidermal inclusion cysts.
  - ○ Occupational hyperkeratosis.
  - ○ Callous formation.
  - ○ Hand tumors including epitheloid sarcomas and soft-tissue giant cell tumors.

MANAGEMENT

The treatment goal of Dupuytren's contractures is to restore hand function by increasing range of motion at involved joints.

- Surgical fasciotomy decreases the degree of flexion deformity and results in modest improvements in hand function. Studies indicated that improvements in function are best correlated to changes at the proximal interphalangeal joint.[3]
- Collagenase injection, a nonsurgical treatment, showed promise in early trials.[4]

- Radiotherapy and hyperbaric oxygen are also being studied with mixed results.

PATIENT EDUCATION

- Initial decreases in joint deformity and improvements in hand function may be lost over time.
- Modifying risk factors (e.g., smoking, alcohol intake) known to contribute to the development of Dupuytren's Contractures are prudent, but are not shown to alter the course of the disease.

REFERENCES

1. Gudmundsson KG, Arngrimsson R, Sigfusson N, Bjornsson A, Jonsson T. Epidemiology of Dupuytren's disease: Clinical, serological, and social assessment. The Reykjavik study. *J Clin Epidemiol*. 2000;53(3):291–296.

2. Saar JD, Grothaus PC. Dupuytren's disease: An overview. *Plast Reconstr Surg*. 2000;106(1):125–134.

3. Draviaraj KP, Chakrabarti I. Functional outcome after surgery for Dupuytren's contracture: A prospective study. *J Hand Surg [Am]*. 2004;29(5):804–808.

4. Badalamente MA, Hurst LC, Hentz VR. Collagen as a clinical target: Nonoperative treatment of Dupuytren's disease. *J Hand Surg [Am]*. 2002;27(5):788–798.

PART 13

DERMATOLOGY

SECTION 1   CHILDHOOD DERMATOLOGY

102   NORMAL SKIN CHANGES

Cristina Fernandez, MD
Mindy A. Smith, MD, MS

PATIENT STORY

A 2-week-old infant is brought to the office for her first well-baby
check. The parents want to know about all the spots and bumps on
the baby's face. They are reassured to hear that the milia and neonatal
acne will go away without treatment (**Figures 102-1** and **102-2**).

EPIDEMIOLOGY

- Approximately 40% of newborn infants in the United States
  develop milia[1] (**Figure 102-1**). This condition is mainly associated
  with newborns carried to full term or near term.

- Acne neonatorum, seen in up to 20% of newborns, is an acne-like
  eruption of the cheeks, which occurs predominantly in baby boys in
  the first weeks of their life (**Figure 102-2**).

- The prevalence of mongolian spots varies among different ethnic
  groups. They have been reported in approximately 96% of black infants, 90% of Native American infants, 81% to 90% of Asian
  infants, 46% to 70% of Hispanic infants, and 1% to 10% of white
  infants[1,2] (**Figures 102-3** and **102-4**).

- Erythema toxicum neonatorum (ETN) occurs in 30% to 50% of
  full-term infants and in 5% of premature infants. The incidence
  rises with increasing gestational age and birth weight[3,4] (**Figures
  102-5** and **102-6**).

ETIOLOGY AND PATHOPHYSIOLOGY

- Milia are inclusion cysts that contain trapped keratinized stratum
  corneum. They may rarely be associated with other abnormalities in
  syndromes including epidermolysis bullosa and the oro-facial-digi-
  tal syndrome (type 1).[1,5]

- Maternal androgenic hormones that stimulate sebaceous glands
  cause neonatal acne.
  - Hyperactivity of sebaceous glands, stimulated by neonatal andro-
    gens, has been implicated as the underlying pathogenic
    mechanism.
  - Histologic examination shows hyperplastic sebaceous glands with
    keratin-plugged orifices.

- The mongolian spot is a hereditary, congenital, developmental condition exclusively involving the skin. It results from entrapment of

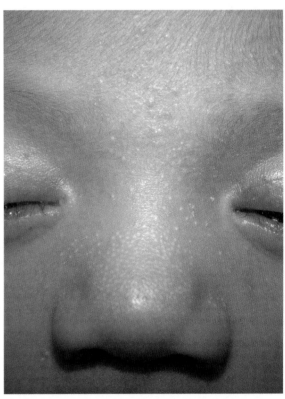

FIGURE 102-1 Milia on the face of a 2-week-old infant with greatest
number of milia on the nose. (*Courtesy of Richard P. Usatine, MD.*)

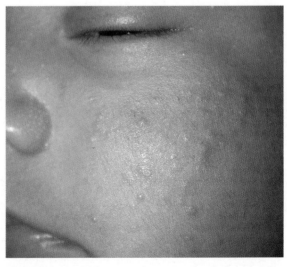

FIGURE 102-2 Neonatal acne on the same infant. (*Courtesy of
Richard P. Usatine, MD.*)

melanocytes in the dermis during their migration from the neural crest into the epidermis.

○ Mongolian spots have been associated with cleft lip, spinal meningeal tumor, melanoma, and phakomatosis pigmentovascularis types 2 and 5.[1,6]

○ A few cases of extensive mongolian spots have been reported with inborn errors of metabolism, the most common being Hurler syndrome, followed by gangliosidosis type 1, Niemann-Pick disease, Hunter syndrome, and mannosidosis. In such cases, they are likely to persist rather than resolve.[1,6]

• ETN is thought to be an immune system reaction; the condition is associated with increased levels of immunological and inflammatory mediators (e.g., interleukins 1 and 8, eotaxin).[7]

○ The eosinophilic infiltrate of ETN suggests an allergic-related or hypersensitivity-related etiology, but no allergens have been identified. Newborn skin appears to respond to any injury with an eosinophilic infiltrate.

○ Because ETN rarely is seen in premature infants, it is believed that mature newborn skin is required to produce this reaction pattern.

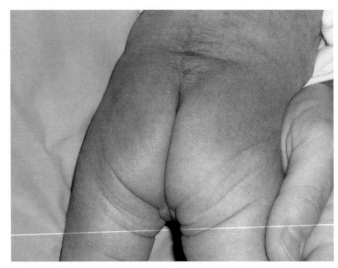

FIGURE 102-3 Large mongolian spots covering the buttocks and back of a Hispanic infant. (*Courtesy of Richard P. Usatine, MD.*)

DIAGNOSIS

CLINICAL FEATURES

• Milia are characterized as tiny, pearly white papules (**Figure 102-1**) that are actually small inclusion cysts ranging from 1–2 mm in diameter. No visible opening is present.[1]

○ Milia usually appear after 4 to 5 days of life in full-term newborns. Manifestations of milia may be delayed from days to weeks in infants born before term.[6,8]

• Neonatal acne (**Figure 102-2**) includes comedones (i.e., white heads), papules, and pustules.

○ Papules and pustules are the most frequent types of lesions (72.7%), followed by comedones only (22.7%).[1,5]

○ This condition may come and go until the baby is between 4 and 6 months old.

• A mongolian spot (**Figures 102-3** and **102-4**) is a bluish-black macule or patch typically a few centimeters in diameter, although much larger lesions can also occur. Lesions may be solitary or numerous.

○ Generalized mongolian spots involving large areas covering the entire posterior or anterior trunk and the extremities have been reported.

○ Several variants exist including:[1,2]

■ Persistent mongolian spots—these are larger, have sharper margins, and persist for many years (**Figure 102-4**).

■ Aberrant mongolian spots involve unusual sites such as the face or extremities.

■ Persistent aberrant mongolian spots also are referred to as macular-type blue nevi.

• ETN commonly presents with a blotchy, evanescent, macular erythema (**Figures 102-5** and **102-6**).

○ The macules are irregular, blanchable, and vary in size.

○ In more severe cases, pale yellow or white wheals or papules on an erythematous base may follow. In approximately 10% of patients, 2 to 4 mm pustules develop.[1,5]

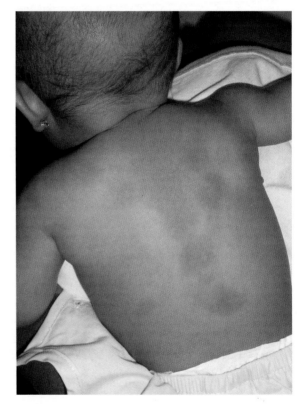

FIGURE 102-4 Prominent mongolian spots on the back of a 1-year-old black child. (*Courtesy of Richard P. Usatine, MD.*)

○ ETN occurs within the first 4 days of life in full-term infants, with the peak onset within the first 48 hours following birth. Rare cases have been reported at birth.

○ Delayed onset can rarely occur in full-term and preterm infants up to 14 days of age.

○ Infants with ETN otherwise are healthy and lack systemic symptoms.

TYPICAL DISTRIBUTION

• Milia are found on the forehead, nose, upper lip, cheeks, and scalp. They can, however, occur anywhere and may be present at birth or appear subsequently. The milia on the child in **Figure 102-1** were present at birth.

• Neonatal acne occurs on the face with the cheeks being the most common site (81.8%)[1] (**Figure 102-2**).

• Mongolian spots most commonly involve the lumbosacral area, but the buttocks, flanks, and shoulders may be affected with extensive lesions (**Figures 102-3** and **102-4**).

• ETN sites of predilection include the forehead, face, trunk, and proximal extremities, but lesions may occur anywhere, including the genitalia. Involvement of the mucous membranes and palms and soles rarely occurs (**Figures 102-5** and **102-6**).

LABORATORY STUDIES AND IMAGING

• No laboratory studies are required.

• In extensive mongolian spots involving the back, radiographic studies are needed to rule out a spinal meningeal tumor or anomaly.[9]

• ETN is often diagnosed clinically, based on history and physical examination, but a peripheral smear of intralesional contents can be done to confirm the diagnosis.[1,7]

○ A Tzanck smear or Gram stain shows inflammatory cells with greater than 90% eosinophils and variable numbers of neutrophils.

○ A complete blood count also shows eosinophilia (up to 18%) in approximately 15% of patients. Eosinophilia may be more pronounced when the eruption shows a marked pustular component.

DIFFERENTIAL DIAGNOSIS

Other diagnoses that may be confused with milia, neonatal acne, and ETN include:

• Miliaria—Heat rash (prickly heat) (**Figure 102-7**) with tiny papules that can be red (miliaria rubra) or clear (miliaria crystallina) or pustular (miliaria pustulosa). Warm and humid weather leads to a blockage of the eccrine sweat ducts and the papules are caused by leakage of sweat into the epidermis or dermis.

• Neonatal pustular melanosis—This eruption, present at birth, consists of 2- to 4-mm nonerythematous vesicles filled with a milky fluid. These vesicles rupture, leaving a collarette of white scales and a central pigmented macule typically lasting up to 3 months. The

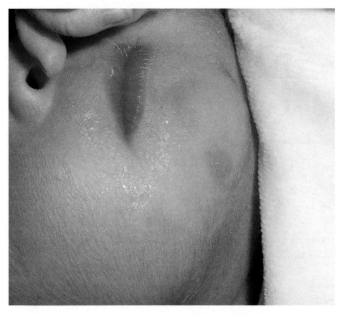

FIGURE 102-5 One small spot of erythema toxicum neonatorum (ETN) on a 2-day-old infant. (*Courtesy of Richard P. Usatine, MD.*)

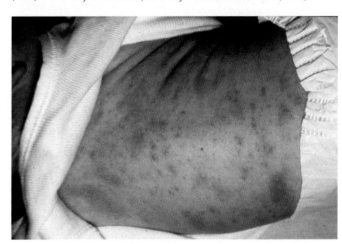

FIGURE 102-6 More widespread case of ETN covering the infant. ETN is completely benign and will resolve spontaneously. (*Courtesy of the University of Texas Health Sciences Center, Division of Dermatology.*)

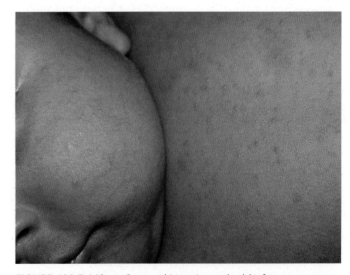

FIGURE 102-7 Miliaria (heat rash) in a 6-month-old infant on a warm summer day. (*Courtesy of Richard P. Usatine, MD.*)

lesions may be profuse or sparse and typically are found under the chin and on the neck, upper chest, lower back, and buttocks (see Chapter 104, Pustular Diseases of Childhood).

Mongolian spots may be confused with the following lesions also present at birth or shortly after:

- Congenital nevi—these lesions are much less common (1%–2% of newborns). They are of variable color from tan or brown to red or black, often within a single lesion and the pigment may fade off into surrounding skin. The borders are often irregular and the lesion can appear slightly raised over time (although a macular portion is usually found at the edges). There may be many lesions (more than 100) on a single person. A biopsy can confirm (see Chapter 156, Congenital Nevi).

- Melanocytic nevi – present in 1% of infants. Most moles are tan to brown, usually less than 6 mm with a round shape and sharp borders. In children, nevi are most often found on the outer forearms, followed by the outer upper arms, neck, and face. Biopsy is needed if a melanoma is suspected (see Chapter 155, Nevus, Melanocyfic).

- There are reports of mongolian spots being confused for the bruising that occurs in child abuse. A good history and a clear knowledge of the pattern of mongolian spots should help to differentiate between these two entities.

ETN can also be confused with the following:

- Miliaria—see information above.

- Folliculitis—primary lesion is a papule or pustule pierced by a central hair, although the hair may not always be visualized. Deeper lesions present as erythematous, often fluctuant, nodules. Folliculitis rarely occurs in the first few days of life when ETN is most commonly seen (see Chapter 111, Folliculitis).

- Chickenpox—the characteristic rash appears in crops of lesions beginning with red macules and passing through stages of papule, vesicle (on an erythematous base), pustule, and crust. Simultaneous presence of different stages of the rash is a hallmark. Infants are mostly born with adequate maternal antibodies to varicella, so that timing should differentiate between these two conditions (see Chapter 117, Chickenpox).

MANAGEMENT

- All these conditions are benign and self-limited. The most important treatment is to convince the parents to not be anxious because all of these conditions should resolve in time.

- No treatment is needed for milia, they usually resolve within a few months.

- No treatment is necessary for neonatal acne, it usually resolves in a few weeks.

- There is no treatment for mongolian spots, which often fade in the first year of life.

- ETN is a benign self-limited disorder requiring no treatment.

PARENT EDUCATION

Explain to the parents (or guardians) that:

- Milia is a benign self-limiting rash that disappears within a few months without leaving any scars. No drug therapy is required and use of any over-the-counter rash medications is not recommended.
- Neonatal acne resolves on its own in weeks. Oils and lotions do not help and may actually aggravate the acne.
- Mongolian spots are likely to fade over time and may disappear by age 7 to 13 years.
- ETN will usually disappear within 2 weeks.

PROVIDER RESOURCES

emedicine.com has helpful articles on these conditions.

Milia—**http://www.emedicine.com/ped/topic1457.htm.**

Mongolian spots—**http://www.emedicine.com/derm/topic271.htm.**

ETN—**http://www.emedicine.com/DERM/topic139.htm.**

Miliaria—**http://www.emedicine.com/derm/topic266.htm.**

Acne vulgaris—**http://www.emedicine.com/derm/topic2.htm.**

PATIENT RESOURCES

http://www.nlm.nih.gov/medlineplus/ency/article/003259.htm.

REFERENCES

1. Agrawal R. Milia. http://www.emedicine.com/ped/topic1457.htm. Accessed March 11, 2008.

2. Ashrafi MR, Shabanian R, Mohammadi M, Kavusi S. Extensive mongolian spots: A clinical sign merits special attention. *Pediatr Neurol.* 2006;34(2):143–145.

3. Cordova A. The mongolian spot: A study of ethnic differences and a literature review. *Clin Pediatr (Phila).* 1981;20(11):714–719.

4. Clemons RM. Issues in newborn care. *Prim Care.* 2000;27(1):251–267.

5. Liu C, Feng J, Qu R. Epidemiologic study of the predisposing factors in erythema toxicum neonatorum. *Dermatology.* 2005;210(4):269–272.

6. Johr RH, Schachner LA. Neonatal dermatologic challenges. *Pediatr Rev.* 1997;18(3):86–94.

7. Mallory SB. Neonatal skin disorders. *Pediatr Clin North Am.* 1991;38(4):745–761.

8. Keitel HG, Yadav V. Etiology of toxic erythema. Erythema toxicum neonatorum. *Am J Dis Child.* 1963;106:306–309.

9. Lorenz S, Maier C, Segerer H. Skin changes in newborn infants in the first 5 days of life. *Hautarzt.* 2000;51(6):396–400.

10. Ashrafi MR, Shabanian R, Mohammadi M, Kavusi S. Extensive mongolian spots: A clinical sign merits special attention. *Pediatr Neurol.* 2006;34(2):143–145.

103 CHILDHOOD HEMANGIOMAS

Megha Madhukar, BA
Richard P. Usatine, MD

PATIENT STORY

A baby girl is brought to the office because her mother is concerned over the growing strawberry hemangioma on her face. Her mother is reassured that most of these childhood hemangiomas regress over time and that there is no need for immediate treatment (**Figure 103-1**).

EPIDEMIOLOGY

- Hemangiomas are the most common benign tumors of infancy. Strawberry hemangiomas are also called superficial hemangiomas of infancy. Cavernous hemangiomas are also called deep hemangiomas of infancy.

- Hemangiomas consist of an abnormally dense group of dilated blood vessels.

- Hemangiomas are solitary and come in a wide range of sizes.

- Thirty percent are present at birth, while the other 70% appear within the first few weeks of life.[1]

- Occur more commonly in Caucasian infants (10%–12%), than African American (1.4%) and Asian American (0.8%) infants.[1]

- Females are affected more often than males (3:1).[1]

- Hemangiomas are much more common in premature infants.

ETIOLOGY AND PATHOPHYSIOLOGY

- Most childhood hemangiomas are thought to occur sporadically.

- Hemangiomas are characterized by an initial phase of rapid proliferation, followed by spontaneous and slow involution, often leading to complete regression. Most childhood hemangiomas are small and innocuous, but some grow to threaten a particular function (**Figure 103-2**) or even life.

- Rapid growth during the first month of life is the historical hallmark of hemangiomas, when rapidly dividing endothelial cells are responsible for the enlargement of these lesions. The hemangiomas become elevated and may take on numerous morphologies (dome-shaped, lobulated, plaquelike, and/or tumoral). The proliferation phase occurs during the first year, with most growth taking place during the first 6 months of life. Proliferation then slows and the hemangioma begins to involute.

- The involutional phase may be rapid or prolonged. No specific feature has been identified in explaining the rate or completeness of involution. However, in one type of hemangioma, the rapidly involuting congenital hemangioma, the proliferation phase occurs

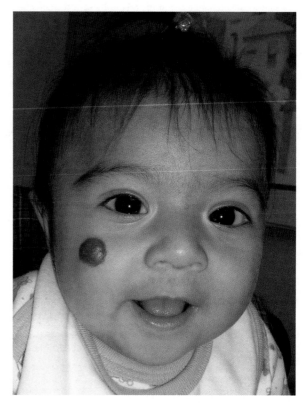

FIGURE 103-1 Strawberry hemangioma on the face causing no functional problems. Treatment is reassurance and watchful waiting. (*Courtesy of Richard P. Usatine, MD.*)

entirely in utero such that the lesion is fully developed at birth, followed by complete involution during the second year of life.[1]

- A good rule of thumb is: 50% of childhood hemangiomas will involute by age 5, 70% by age 7, and the remainder of childhood hemangiomas take an additional 3 to 5 years to complete the process of involution.[1]

- Of the lesions that have involuted by age 6, 38% will leave residual evidence of the hemangioma in the form of a scar, telangiectasia, or redundant, "bag-like" skin. The chance of a permanent scar increases the longer it takes to involute. For example, of the lesions that involute after age 6, 80% may exhibit a cosmetic deformity.[1]

- Infants born to mothers who have undergone chorionic villus sampling may be at an increased risk for developing hemangiomas.[1]

DIAGNOSIS

CLINICAL FEATURES

Early lesions may be subtle, resembling a scratch or bruise, or alternatively may look like a small patch of telangiectasias or an area of hypopigmentation. Hemangiomas can start off as a flat red mark, but as proliferation ensues, it grows to become a spongy mass protruding from the skin. The earliest sign of a hemangioma is blanching of the involved skin with a few fine telangiectasias followed by a red macule. Rarely, a shallow ulceration may be the first sign of an incipient hemangioma.[1] Hemangiomas are typically diagnosed based on appearance, rarely warranting further diagnostic tests.

Hemangiomas may be superficial, deep, or a combination of both. Superficial hemangiomas are well defined, bright red, appear as nodules or plaques located above clinically normal skin (**Figures 103-1** to **103-3**). Deep hemangiomas are raised flesh colored nodules, which often have a bluish hue and feel firm and rubbery (**Figure 103-4**).

Most are clinically insignificant unless they impinge on vital structures, ulcerate, bleed, incite a consumptive coagulopathy, or cause high output cardiac failure or structural abnormalities. Blocking vision is a common reason needed for treatment (**Figure 103-2**).

TYPICAL DISTRIBUTION

Anywhere on the body, most often on the face, scalp, back, or chest.

IMAGING

Most hemangiomas of infancy do not need imaging. If the hemangioma is very large, deep or undefined, MRI with and without IV gadolinium helps delineate the location and extent of the hemangioma while also differentiating them from high flow vascular lesions, like arteriovenous malformations.[1] Ultrasound is a useful tool to differentiate hemangiomas from other subcutaneous structures such as cysts and lymph nodes as well as from other soft tissue masses.[1]

Plain radiography may be useful for evaluating hemangiomas that impinge on an airway.[1]

BIOPSY

Biopsies are rarely needed and can be risky because vascular lesions may bleed profusely. If a biopsy is being considered, it might be best to refer to a specialist.

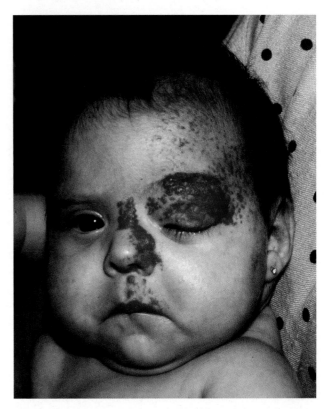

FIGURE 103-2 Large hemangioma on the face needing immediate treatment to prevent amblyopia in the right eye. While this hemangioma follows the V1 dermatome this is not a port wine stain and the patient does not have Sturge-Weber syndrome. (*Courtesy of Richard P. Usatine, MD.*)

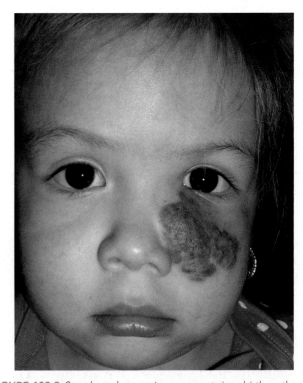

FIGURE 103-3 Strawberry hemangioma present since birth on the face of a 22-month-old girl. While it is close to her eye, her vision has never been occluded. She has been followed by ophthalmology and no active treatment was recommended. The hemangioma grew larger during the first year of life and is now beginning to involute without treatment. (*Courtesy of Richard P. Usatine, MD.*)

DIFFERENTIAL DIAGNOSIS

- Superficial capillary malformations that are frequently seen in infants include those above the eyelids and nape of the neck. These are called salmon patches and not dangerous. The "angel's kisses" on the eyelids usually disappear by age 2. The "stork bites" may last into adulthood but are rarely an issue because they often get covered by hair (**Figures 103-5** and **103-6**). These capillary malformations are a variant of nevus flammeus or port-wine stain. They are macular, sharply circumscribed, pink to purple, and varied in size (see Chapter 195, Hereditary and Congenital Vascular Skin Lesions).

- Blue rubber bleb nevus syndrome—Bluish cutaneous vascular malformations which empty with pressure, texture resembles rubbery nodules, similar to deep hemangiomas.[2]

- Maffucci syndrome—rare congenital non-hereditary mesodermal dysplasia characterized by multiple enchondromata, cutaneous hemangiomas, and more recently spindle cell hemangiomas.[3] It is important to identify Maffucci's early since it is associated with an increased risk of malignancy. May appear as multiple vascular malformations of the skin with a "grape-like" appearance (see Chapter 195, Hereditary and Congenital Vascular Skin Lesions).

- Angiosarcoma—rare, malignant endothelial tumor characterized as ill defined red patches, plaques, or nodules (see Chapter 194, Acquired Vascular Skin Lesions).[4]

- Arteriovenous malformation—benign, single red papules on head or neck, may be cutaneous or mucosal.[4]

- Infantile fibrosarcoma—a rare and highly malignant tumor of childhood that may take on the form of a highly vascularized mass, resembling a hemangioma, especially after a hemangioma has ulcerated as a result of rapid proliferation.[5]

MANAGEMENT

- The majority of hemangiomas will eventually involute without complications and require no treatment, but approximately 20% cause complications like ulcerations, irreversible cutaneous expansion or threaten vital structures such as the eyes, nose, or airways.[6]

- Systemic corticosteroids are the mainstay of therapy for function- and life-threatening hemangiomas while topical and intralesional administration remain first-line treatment for the more uncomplicated cases needing treatment.

- Prednisone 3–5 mg/kg per day has been shown to provide an effective and rapid way of treating hemangiomas.[7] SOR **B** In a study, 68% of patients receiving systemic corticosteroid treatment with oral prednisone experienced rapid and virtually complete involution of hemangiomas.[7] Another 25% experienced significant regression and treatment demonstrated no effect in 7% of patients. The authors recommended treating with oral prednisone for 6 to 8 weeks and in more severe cases for 12 weeks. Side effects include moon facies and irritability, which resolved once therapy was discontinued.[7] Growth may be retarded temporarily.

- Ultrapotent topical corticosteroids have been found especially helpful in the treatment of small hemangiomas, especially periocular

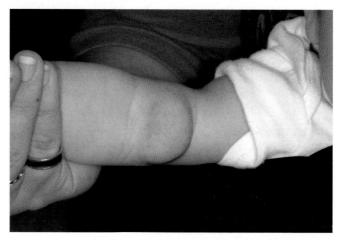

FIGURE 103-4 Deep (cavernous) hemangioma on the arm in a 9-month-old child. Treatment is watchful waiting. (*Courtesy of Richard P. Usatine, MD.*)

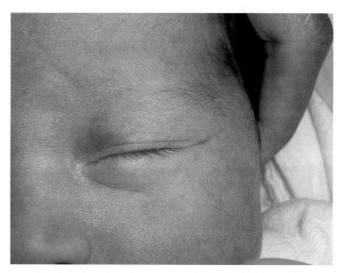

FIGURE 103-5 Salmon patch (a variant of nevus flammeus) on the upper eyelid called an angel's kiss. These resolve by age 2. (*Courtesy of Richard P. Usatine, MD.*)

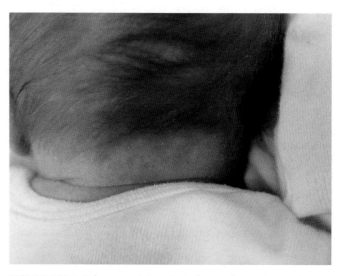

FIGURE 103-6 Salmon patch (a variant of nevus flammeus) on the neck of the new born called a stork bite. These vascular malformations persist into adulthood. (*Courtesy of Dan Stulberg, MD.*)

hemangiomas and those at sites prone to ulceration and disfigurement. Seventy-four percent of patients demonstrated good or at least partial response to treatment with the majority experiencing cessation of growth before what would have been expected for their age. Thinner, more superficial hemangiomas demonstrated better improvement than thicker, deeper lesions.[8] SOR **B**

- Intralesional corticosteroid injections, composed of a mixture containing triamcinolone acetonide (20 mg average dose) and betamethasone acetate (3 mg average dose) with varying number of injections, have been found to successfully treat head and neck childhood hemangiomas in properly selected infants. In a research study, 13% of the hemangiomas treated with intralesional injections almost completely involuted, 32% showed greater than 50% reduction in volume, 32% showed definite but less than 50% reduction in volume, and 23% showed little to no decrease in size.[9] SOR **B** Avoid intralesional steroids around eye.

- Second-line therapies include Interferon Alfa-2a or 2b, laser therapy, and surgery. SOR **C**

- If corticosteroid therapy fails to provide results, therapy with Interferon Alfa 2a may be considered. In one study, 90% of infants being treated with up to 3 mU/m^2/day of Interferon Alfa-2a experienced 50% or greater regression of their lesions by 8 months of treatment. Side effects were transient and included fever, neutropenia, and skin necrosis, with no long-term effects.[10] SOR **C** Interferon Alfa-2a appears to be well tolerated in pediatric patients, and effective in hastening involution of symptomatic hemangiomas. Daily use of 3 mU/m^2 of subcutaneous Interferon Alfa-2a for 3 or more months has been shown to demonstrate more than 50% reduction in size of lesions in some patients and 25% to 30% regression of lesion size in others.[11] SOR **C**

- Treatment with flashlamp-pumped pulsed dye laser has been found to be an effective treatment method for superficial cutaneous hemangiomas at sites of potential functional impairment and on the face. 76% of patients in a study were found to have excellent or good results with the flashlamp-pumped pulsed dye laser. Hemangiomas with a deep component do not seem to benefit from flashlamp-pumped pulsed dye laser therapy to the same degree as a truly superficial hemangioma, since the laser is limited by its depth of vascular injury.[12] SOR **B**

- Facial hemangiomas causing severe functional disturbance and serious psychological distress are strong reasons to consider surgical excision before the child reaches the expected age of spontaneous regression. SOR **C**

- Large periocular hemangiomas demand early surgery to prevent debilitating consequences such as amblyopia (**Figure 103-2**). Early surgical treatment is also recommended for proliferative labial tumors because not only do they have a tendency to bleed but also make eating difficult. Additionally, surgery is advised for hemangiomas located on the nasal tip since they regress slowly and may ultimately result in distortion of the nasal framework.[13]

- Laser surgery may be considered for selective ablation of vascular tissue, like ulcerated hemangiomas and thin superficial hemangiomas, especially when their locations may result in psychosocial distress for the patient, i.e., facial hemangiomas. The pulsed dye laser seems especially promising with its ability to selectively dam-

age blood vessels with minimal damage to surrounding tissues.[14] This procedure is also associated with decreased pain and increased healing. SOR **B**

- Surgical excision of proliferating hemangiomas is quite hazardous because of the risk of hemorrhage and damage to nearby vital structures. However, the benefits to early excision include saving vision, or life, when the hemangioma's growth and/or location is particularly threatening. Although risky, early excision will also decrease the negative psychosocial impact of having a disfiguring lesion during childhood.

- Surgical excision of involuted hemangiomas is not uncommon to remove the residual tissue that may be causing cosmetic or functional impairment. Excision is performed in late involution to reduce the risk of hemorrhage.

- Depending on the location and how complex the hemangioma is, consultations with ophthalmologists, otolaryngologists, plastic surgeons, and pediatric neurosurgeons may be necessary to ensure proper care.

PATIENT EDUCATION

- Parents must be educated about the variable natural history, prognosis, risks and benefits of different treatments, and possible complications related to childhood hemangiomas.

FOLLOW-UP

Watchful waiting and serial observations during well-child examinations is recommended for uncomplicated hemangiomas of infancy. Hemangiomas with complicating factors need close follow-up on an individual basis.

PATIENT AND PROVIDER RESOURCES

- Medline Plus article on Hemangiomas—**http://www.nlm. nih.gov/medlineplus/ency/article/001459.htm.**
- Hemangiomas and Vascular Anomalies—nonprofit educational Web site **http://www.birthmarks.us/.**

REFERENCES

1. Richard JA. Infantile Hemangiomas. http://www.emedicine. com/derm/topic201.htm. Accessed March 31, 2008.

2. Elewski BE, Hughey LC, Parsons ME. *Differential Diagnosis in Dermatology*. St. Louis: London, Elsevier 2005:545.

3. McDermott AL, Dutt SN, Shavda SV, DW Morgan. Maffucci's syndrome: Clinical and radiological features of a rare condition. *J Laryngol Otol*. 2001;115(10):845–847.

4. Barnhill RL. Vascular Tumors In: Hunt SJ, Santa Cruz DJ, Barnhill, RL eds. *Textbook of Dermatopathology*. New York: McGraw-Hill, 1998:821.

5. Yan AC, Chamlin SL, Liang MG, et al. Fibrosarcoma: A masquerader of ulcerated hemangioma. *Pediatr Dermatol.* 2006;23(4): 330–334.

6. Enjolras O, Wassef M, Mazoyer E, et al. Infants with kasabach-merrit syndrome do not have "true" hemangiomas. *J Pediatr.* 1997;130(4):631–640.

7. Sadan N, Wolach B. Treatment of hemangiomas of infants with high doses of prednisone. *J Pediatrics.* 1996;128 (1);141–146

8. Garzon MC, Lucky AW, Hawrot A, Frieden IJ. Ultrapotent topical corticosteroid treatment of hemangiomas of infancy. *J Am Acad Dermatol.* 2005;52:281–286.

9. Sloan G, Reinisch J, NIchter L, Saber W, Lew K, Morwood D. Intralesional corticosteroid therapy for infantile hemangiomas. *Plast Reconstr Surg.* 1989;83;459–466.

10. Ezekowitz RA, Mulliken JB, Follkman J. Interferon Alfa-2a therapy for life-threatening hemangiomas of infancy. *N Engl J Med.* 1992;326:1456–1463.

11. Bauman N, Burke D, Smith R. Treatment of massive or life-threatening hemangioms with recombinant alfa 2a interferon). *Otolaryngol Head Neck Surg.* 1997;117:99–110

12. Poetke M, Phillip C, Berlien HP. Flashlamp-pumped pulsed dye laser for hemangiomas in infancy: Treatment of superficial vs. mixed hemangiomas. *Arch Dermatol.* 2000;136(5):628–632.

13. Demiri EC, Pelissier P, Genin-Etcheberry T, Tsakoniatis N, Martin D, Baudet J. Treatment of facial haemangiomas: The present status of surgery. *Br J Plast Surg.* 2001;54(8):665–674.

14. Eedy DJ, Breathnach SM, Walker NPJ. *Surgical Dermatology.* Oxford: Blackwell Science. 1996:245.

104 PUSTULAR DISEASES OF CHILDHOOD

Andrew Shedd, MD
Richard P. Usatine, MD

PATIENT STORY

A 1-year-old boy is brought for a second opinion about the recurrent pruritic vesicles and pustules on his hands and feet. This is the third episode and in both previous episodes the physicians thought the child had scabies. The child was treated with permethrin both times and within 2 to 3 weeks the skin cleared. No other family members have had lesions or symptoms. **Figures 104-1** to **104-3** demonstrate a typical case of infantile acropustulosis that is often misdiagnosed as scabies. While the condition can be recurrent it is ultimately self-limited and will resolve.

EPIDEMIOLOGY

Acropustulosis:

- Rare, intensely pruritic, vesiculopustular disease of young children.[1]
- Typically begins in the second or third months[1] of life and as late as 10 months of age.[2]
- Occur slightly more often in darker skinned patients and males.[1]
- Typically spontaneously remits by 6 to 36 months of life.[2]

Transient neonatal pustular melanosis (TNPM):

- A disease of newborns.[3]
- Equal male-to-female ratio.[3]
- Seen in 4.4% of black infants and 0.6% of white infants.[4]
- Early, spontaneous remission.[3]

ETIOLOGY AND PATHOPHYSIOLOGY

Acropustulosis:

- The exact cause and mechanism have yet to be determined.[5]
- Some physicians speculate that it is a persistent reaction to scabies ("postscabies syndrome"). Suggestive of this infectious etiology, infantile acropustulosis will occasionally be concurrently present amongst siblings. Also, patients diagnosed with this disorder frequently have received prior treatment for scabies; which may either provide evidence of an infectious etiology or demonstrate the frequent misdiagnosis, as in the patient above. Odom et al. concludes that in some cases, this disease may represent a hypersensitivity reaction to *Sarcoptes scabiei*.[4]

TNPM:

- The etiology is uncertain[6]; however, it may result from an obstruction of the pilosebaceous orifice.[3]

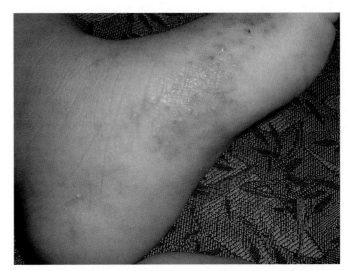

FIGURE 104-1 Infantile acropustulosis (acropustulosis of infancy) on the foot of a 1-year-old boy. (*Courtesy of Richard P. Usatine, MD.*)

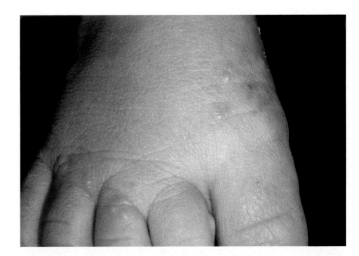

FIGURE 104-2 Acropustulosis with vesiculopustular eruption on the toes of the same boy (shown in Figure 104-1). (*Courtesy of Richard P. Usatine, MD.*)

DIAGNOSIS

Acropustulosis—A workup to rule out potentially serious infectious causes should be considered whenever confronted with a new pustular dermatosis early in a child's life. A workup might include a scraping for scabies, and KOH preparation as rapid diagnostic tests. If these studies are negative, the diagnosis may be made clinically as described below.

TNPM—This diagnosis can often be made clinically. However, if performed, a Wright stain of the exudate will reveal a predominance of neutrophils with an occasional eosinophil, and the Gram stain will be negative.[3]

CLINICAL FEATURES

Acropustulosis—These vesiculopustular lesions begin around the second or third months of life and are typically concentrated on the hands and feet[1] (**Figures 104-1 to 104-3**). They begin acutely as small pink papules and progress within 24 hours to pustules[1] of less than 5 mm in diameter.[2] Recurrent episodes of these intensely pruritic lesions typically last 10 days and may recur every 2–5 weeks,[1,2] decreasing in frequency and severity[2] until spontaneous remission around 3 years of age.[1] There may be a residual scale and post-inflammatory hyperpigmentation.[2]

TNPM—This condition is characterized by the presence at birth of 2 to 3 mm macules and pustules[4] on a nonerythematous base[7] (**Figures 104-4 and 104-5**). The lesions probably evolve prenatally[7] and subsequently rupture postnatally in 1 to 2 days. They heal with hyperpigmented macules that fade by 3 months of age,[3] with lighter-skinned patients experiencing less hyperpigmentation.[7] Sometimes, the only evidence of the disease is the presence of small, brown macules with a rim of scale at birth.[7]

TYPICAL DISTRIBUTION

Acropustulosis—Although most commonly found on the palms and soles, the pustules may also be found on the dorsal surfaces of the hands and feet and occasionally the face, scalp, and trunk.[5]

TNPM—They are most common on the face and chin; however, they may also be present on the neck, chest, sacrum, abdomen, and thighs.[7]

LABORATORY STUDIES

Acropustulosis—A blood count is not needed but might reveal a slight leukocytosis and frequently an eosinophilia. Stained smears of the lesions are also not needed but will demonstrate many neutrophils,[1] with some eosinophils possible early in the course.[2]

TNPM—A Wright stain will reveal numerous neutrophils and some eosinophils, with a negative Gram's stain.[3] Blood counts should be normal and no laboratory workup is generally indicated.

DIFFERENTIAL DIAGNOSIS

• Scabies infestation—Characterized by pruritic, intraepidermal burrows and vesicles with scale and crust, most commonly found in the web spaces of the digits, wrists, elbow, genitals, and lower extremities.

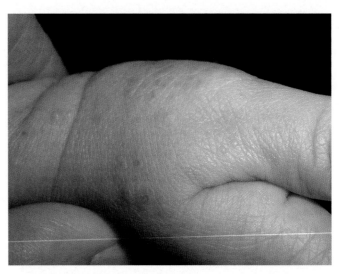

FIGURE 104-3 Acropustulosis with pruritic eruption on the hand and wrist of the same boy. (*Courtesy of Richard P. Usatine, MD.*)

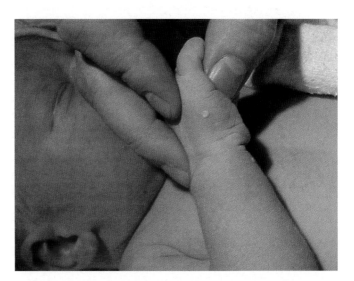

FIGURE 104-4 Neonatal pustular melanosis on the hand of a newborn. (*Courtesy of Dan Stulberg, MD.*)

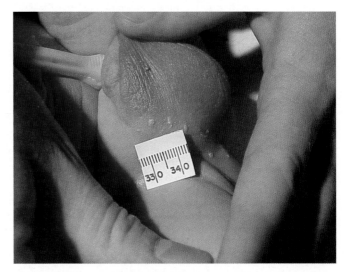

FIGURE 104-5 Neonatal pustular melanosis on scrotum of the same newborn. (*Courtesy of Dan Stulberg, MD.*)

May be present in other family members, and is not present at birth. Microscopic examination of the scrapings of the burrows may reveal mites, feces, eggs, or all of the above.[3] Acropustulosis will be refractory to all scabies therapies but scabies therapy may appear to work because each episode of acropuslulosis is self-limited (see Chapter 137, Scabies).

- Erythema toxicum neonatorum—Appearing on the neonate 1 to 2 days after birth, this disease of unknown etiology causes 2 to 3 cm diffuse blotchy macules with 1 to 4 mm central vesicles. The lesions, which spare the palms and soles, contain a predominance of eosinophils and resolve spontaneously by 2 weeks of age[3] (see Chapter 102, Normal Skin Changes of Infancy).

- Impetigo—A superficial infection of the skin with vesicles, bullae, and honey-colored crusts, caused by group A Streptococcus, or Staphylococcus aureus. Gram stain and culture should be positive[3] (see Chapter 110, Impetigo).

- Cutaneous candidiasis—Slightly pruritic areas of intensely erythematous papules, pustules, and plaques, possibly with white exudate, found around the genitals and folds of skin. *Candida* yeast forms present on KOH preparation or culture[3] (see Chapter 130, Mucocutaneous Candidiasis).

- Varicella—Characteristic "dew-drops on a rose-petal" that develop in childhood. Uniformly distributed, pruritic, with known contacts likely. Now less common because of immunization (see Chapter 117, Chickenpox).

- Herpes—Grouped, painful vesicles on an erythematous base. May occur as gingivostomatitis in young children but rarely seen in the distribution of the pustular diseases of childhood. More likely to be vesicular rather than pustular (see Chapter 123, Herpes Simplex).

- Hand-foot-and-mouth disease—This illness is caused by the Coxsackie virus and produces papules and macules of the hands and feet that progress to flat vesicles before ulceration and eventual resolution. They typically affect the dorsum of the hands and feet and are also accompanied by painful oral lesions[3] (see Chapter 122, Hand, Foot and Mouth Disease).

- Psoriasis, pustular—This severe form of psoriasis is rare in children and is characterized by the acute appearance of diffuse, painful, pinpoint pustules with high fever, fatigue, and anorexia[1] (see Chapter 145, Proriasis).

MANAGEMENT

Acropustulosis:

- Corticosteroids (topical and oral) generally are not effective,[1] and not necessary in management.[5] SOR **C**

- Oral antihistamines may be helpful in controlling pruritus.[1] SOR **C**

- Pramoxine, lotion or cream, may be used topically for control of itching as it works by a different mechanism than antihistamines.[5] SOR **C**

- Dapsone (1–2 mg/kg per day, maximum dose of 100 mg/day)[5] has been used with good results. However, the risks of complications

are generally considered to outweigh the benefits, unless the pruritus is debilitating.[1] SOR **C**

TNPM:

- No treatment is necessary. The parents should be reassured that the condition is benign and will resolve spontaneously with eventual normalization of any hyperpigmented macules.[6] SOR **B**

PATIENT EDUCATION

Once other conditions have been ruled out, reassurance that these diseases are self-limited is the most important piece of information to communicate to the family.

FOLLOW-UP

Regarding acropustulosis, initial follow-up may be appropriate for control of symptoms and assurance of a stable disease course. With symptoms controlled, follow-up may be unnecessary as the child ages and the disease decreases in severity and frequency. If dapsone is prescribed, proper monitoring is indicated.

TNPM will need no specific follow-up other than normal well-child care.

PATIENT AND PROVIDER RESOURCES

- **http://www.emedicine.com/derm/topic8.htm**
- **http://www.emedicine.com/ped/topic698.htm**

REFERENCES

1. Ruggero C, Gelmetti C. *Pediatric Dermatology and Dermatopathology: A Concise Atlas*. London, UK: Martin Dunitz, 2002.

2. Weinberg S, Prose NS, Leonard K. *Color Atlas of Pediatric Dermatology*. 3rd ed. New York, NY: McGraw-Hill, 1998.

3. Kay S. Kane, Jennifer Bissonette, Howard P. Baden, et al. *Color Atlas and Synopsis of Pediatric Dermatology*. New York, NY: McGraw-Hill, 2002.

4. Odom RB, James WD, Timothy GB. *Andrews' Diseases of the Skin, Clinical Dermatology*. 9th ed. Philadelphia, PA: WB Saunders Company, 2000.

5. Pride H. Acropustulosis of Infancy. eMedicine. http://www.emedicine.com/derm/topic8.htm. Accessed March 28, 2007.

6. St. John EB. Neonatal Pustular Melanosis. eMedicine. http://www.emedicine.com/ped/topic698.htm. Accessed March 28, 2006.

7. Cohen BA. *Pediatric Dermatology*. 3rd ed. Philadelphia, PA: Elsevier Mosby, 2005.

105 DIAPER RASH AND PERIANAL DERMATITIS

Julie Scott Taylor, MD, MSc

PATIENT STORY

A 2-month-old baby girl was brought to the office with a severe diaper rash that was not getting better with Desitin. Upon examination, the physician noted a white coating on the tongue and buccal mucosa. The diaper area was red with skin erosions and satellite lesions (**Figure 105-1**). The whole picture is consistent with candidiasis of the mouth (thrush) and the diaper region. The child was treated with oral nystatin suspension and topical clotrimazole cream in the diaper area with good results.

EPIDEMIOLOGY

- Diaper dermatitis is the most common dermatitis of infancy.
- Variability in prevalence of 7% to 35% among infants in different studies.[1]
- No differences in prevalence between genders or among races.
- One study showed an incidence of 19.4% in children ages 3 to 6 months.[1]
- Lower incidence among breast-fed infants.
- Typically begins around age 3 weeks, peaks at age 9 to 12 months, and then decreases with age until it resolves completely with toilet training.
- Individual episodes last from 1 day to 2 weeks.
- Aggravating factors include poor skin care, diarrhea, recent antibiotic use, and urinary tract abnormalities.
- Perianal streptococcal dermatitis occurs in children between 6 months and 10 years of age (**Figures 105-2** and **105-3**).
  ○ Incidence ranges from 1 in 218 to 1 in 2000 pediatric outpatient visits.[2]

ETIOLOGY AND PATHOPHYSIOLOGY

- Primary diaper dermatitis. An acute skin inflammation in the diaper area with an ill-defined and multifactorial etiology.
- Main cause is irritation of thin skin as a result of prolonged contact with moisture including feces and urine.[3]
  1. Occlusion/lack of exposure to air
  2. Friction and mechanical trauma
  3. Local irritants: fecal proteases and lipases
  4. Increased pH
  5. Maceration of the stratum corneum with loss of the protective barrier function of skin
  6. The ammonia in urine is NOT a direct cause

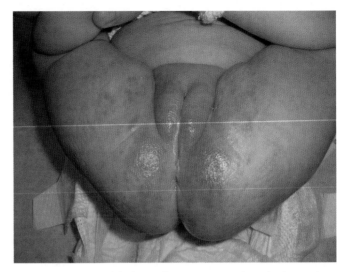

FIGURE 105-1 *Candida* diaper dermatitis in an infant who has oral thrush. (*Courtesy of Richard P. Usatine, MD.*)

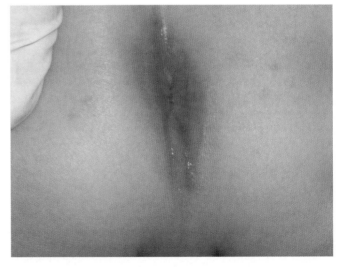

FIGURE 105-2 Perianal dermatitis caused by group A beta-hemolytic streptococci. (*Reproduced with permission from Photo Rounds: Itchy perianal erythema. The Journal of Family Practice, December 2007;56 (12):1025, Dowden Health Media.*)

- Irritant diaper dermatitis (IDD) or "napkin dermatitis." A combination of intertrigo (wet skin damaged from chafing) and miliaria (heat rash) when eccrine glands become obstructed from excessive hydration. It is a noninfectious, nonallergic, often asymptomatic contact dermatitis that typically lasts for less than 3 days after a change in diaper practices.

- Candidal diaper dermatitis. Within 3 days, 45% to 75% of diaper rashes are colonized with *Candida albicans* of fecal origin.

- Bacterial diaper dermatitis. Via secondary infections, usually *Staphylococcus* or *Streptococcus* species. Perianal streptococcal dermatitis is caused by group A beta-hemolytic *streptococci* (**Figures 105-2** and **105-3**). Other common bacterial isolates include *E. coli*, *Peptostreptococcus*, and *Bacteroides*. Usually occurs during the warm summer months.

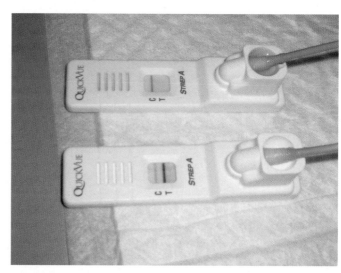

FIGURE 105-3 A positive rapid strep test taken from a swab of the perianal area of the infant in the previous photo. (*Reproduced with permission from Photo Rounds: Itchy perianal erythema. The Journal of Family Practice, December 2007;56(12):1027, Dowden Health Media.*)

DIAGNOSIS

CLINICAL FEATURES

IDD begins with shiny erythema with or without scale and poorly demarcated margins on the convex skin surfaces in areas covered by diapers. Moderate cases can have papules, plaques, vesicles, and small superficial erosions that can progress to well-demarcated ulcerated nodules typically with sparing of skin folds. Pustules or papules beyond the rash border (called "satellite lesions"), involvement of the skin folds, and white scaling all indicate a fungal infection with *Candida*. Secondary bacterial infections can have redness, honey-colored crusting, swelling, red streaking, and/or purulent discharge. With impetigo in the diaper area, bullae are not usually intact but instead present as superficial erosions. Perianal streptococcal dermatitis is a bright red, sharply demarcated rash sometimes associated with blood-streaked stools.

TYPICAL DISTRIBUTION

Diaper dermatitis is primarily found on the buttocks, the genitalia, the mons pubis and lower abdomen, and the medial thighs. Pay particular attention to the involvement or sparing of skin folds. Be sure to evaluate for rashes outside of the diaper area as well. If *Candida* is suspected, the oropharynx should be inspected for signs of thrush such as white plaques.

LABORATORY STUDIES

Clinical diagnosis is based primarily on the physical examination. Rarely indicated tests that are occasionally used in more complicated cases include a potassium hydroxide preparation for hyphae, a mineral oil preparation for scabies, a complete blood count with a differential, a gram stain of a bulla, a zinc level, or a skin biopsy. A rapid strep test can be used to diagnose perianal streptococcal dermatitis (**Figures 105-2** and **105-3**).

DIFFERENTIAL DIAGNOSIS

There are two distinctive severe variants of IDD.[4] Jacquet's diaper dermatitis (dermatitis syphiloides posterosiva or erosive variant) is a term used to describe severe noduloerosive lesions with heaped-up borders seen in children with persistent diarrhea. Granuloma gluteale infantum is a rare and poorly understood primary diaper dermatitis that presents with granulomatous nodules that can have large, raised, purple erosions with rolled margins. It resolves spontaneously over the course of a few months, often with residual scarring.

Perianal pseudoverrucous papules. Shiny, smooth, red, moist, flat-topped lesions commonly confused with genital warts that occur in the context of Hirschsprung's disease.

Secondary diaper dermatitis is an eruption in the diaper area with a defined etiology. Atopic dermatitis, seborrheic dermatitis, and psoriasis are examples of rashes that can appear anywhere on the body and can be exaggerated in the groin as a result of wearing diapers. Family history of atopy or psoriasis and rash in other locations besides the groin can be helpful. Congenital syphilis, scabies, HIV, Langerhans cell histiocytosis, and acrodermatitis enteropathica (caused by zinc deficiency) are examples of rashes in the diaper area regardless of diaper use. Allergic contact dermatitis as a result of an allergen in the diaper itself is possible but rare.

MANAGEMENT

TREATMENT

- Parental behavior change to keep the skin as exposed and dry as possible. SOR Ⓑ Frequent diaper changes (as soon as they are wet or soiled and at least every 3–4 hours); using super-absorbent disposable diapers. SOR Ⓑ Frequent gentle cleaning of the affected area with lukewarm tap water instead of commercial wipes containing alcohol. Pat dry.

- Barrier preparations including zinc oxide paste, petroleum jelly, or lanolin to affected area after each diaper change.[5] SOR Ⓑ Pastes are better than ointments which in turn are better than creams or lotions. Avoid products with fragrances or preservatives to minimize allergic potential. Apply thickly like "icing on a cake." These barrier preparations should be used *on top* of other indicated therapies.

- For moderate to severe inflammation, consider a non-fluorinated, low-potency topical steroid cream such as hydrocortisone 1% qid to the affected area until the rash is gone. To avoid skin erosions, atrophy, and striae, it is best to not go beyond 2 weeks of therapy with any topical steroid on a baby's bottom.

- For *Candida*, use topical OTC antifungal creams such as clotrimazole, miconazole after every diaper change until the rash resolves. SOR Ⓑ For concomitant oral thrush, treat with oral nystatin swish and swallow qid. There is little evidence to support the addition of oral antifungal therapy in patients without thrush.[6] SOR Ⓑ

- Avoid combination antifungal–steroid agents that contain steroids stronger than hydrocortisone. Potent topical steroids can cause striae and skin erosions, hypothalamus–pituitary–adrenal axis suppression, and Cushing's syndrome. Of note, in the National Ambulatory Medical Care Survey, these combined agents were prescribed inappropriately in 24.3% of visits for diaper dermatitis.[6]

- For mild bacterial infections, use topical antibiotic ointments such as bacitracin or mupirocin after every diaper change until the rash resolves. SOR Ⓑ

- For more severe bacterial infections, use oral antibiotics such as amoxicillin/clavulanate, cephalexin, or erythromycin.[1] Perianal streptococcal dermatitis can be treated with amoxicillin, penicillin VK or cephalexin.[2] SOR **B**

- Ciclopirox 0.77% topical suspension (Loprox), a broad-spectrum agent with antifungal, antibacterial, and anti-inflammatory properties was used safely and effectively in one trial of 44 children to treat diaper dermatitis caused by *Candida*.[6] SOR **B**

- Other therapies proven to work in small trials include a mixture of honey, olive, and beeswax (a pilot study with 12 subjects) and the orange-red dye eosin.[6] SOR **B**

- Dye-free diapers for allergic contact dermatitis. SOR **B**

PREVENTION AND ROUTINE SKIN CARE

- Keep skin as dry as possible.

- Promote the use of barrier preparations daily to maintain skin integrity.

- There is no evidence to suggest that topical vitamin A prevents diaper dermatitis.[7] SOR **B**

- Disposable diapers–Although many individual trials show benefits, a 2006 Cochrane Review found that there is not enough evidence from good quality randomized controlled trials to support or refute the use and type of disposable diapers for the prevention of diaper dermatitis in infants.[8] SOR **B**

PATIENT (PARENT) EDUCATION

Prevention and early treatment are the best strategies. Keep the child's diaper area as clean, cool, and dry as possible with frequent diaper changes. Do NOT use creams that contain boric acid, camphor, phenol, methyl salicylate, or compound of benzoin or talcum powder or cornstarch. Reassurance that while this common condition is sometimes distressing for parents and uncomfortable for children, it is rarely dangerous.

FOLLOW-UP

No follow-up needed unless the rash worsens or persists. The exception is perianal streptococcal dermatitis where follow-up is recommended because recurrences are common.

PATIENT RESOURCES

- Diaper Rash—Tips on Prevention and Treatment at **http://familydoctor.org/051.xml**
- Diaper Rash on eMedicine Health—**http://children. webmd.com/tc/Diaper-Rash-Topic-Overview**

PROVIDER RESOURCES

- Kazzi AA, Dib R. Pediatrics, Diaper Rash—**http://www. emedicine.com/emerg/topic374.htm**

REFERENCES

1. Kazzi AA, Dib R. Pediatrics, Diaper Rash. http://www. emedicine.com/emerg/topic374.htm. Accessed March 20, 2007.

2. Brilliant L. Perianal streptococcal dermatitis. *Am Fam Physician*. 2002;61(2):391–393.

3. Gupta AK, Skinner AR. Management of diaper dermatitis. *Int J Dermatol*. 2004;43(11):830–834.

4. Scheinfeld N. Diaper dermatitis: A review and brief survey of eruptions of the diaper area. *Am J Clin Dermatol*. 2005;6(5): 273–281.

5. Atherton DJ. A review of the pathophysiology, prevention, and treatment of irritant diaper dermatitis. *Curr Med Res Opin*. 2004; 20(5):645–649.

6. Humphrey S, Bergman JN. Practical management strategies for diaper dermatitis. *Skin Therapy Lett*. 2006;11(7):1–6.

7. Davies MW, Dore AJ, Perissinotto KL. Topical vitamin A, or its derivatives, for treating and preventing napkin dermatitis in infants. *Cochrane Database Syst Rev*. 2005;4:CD004300.

8. Baer EL, Davies MW, Easterbrook KJ. Disposable nappies for preventing napkin dermatitis in infants. *Cochrane Database Syst Rev*. 2006;3:CD004262.

SECTION 2 ACNEIFORM DISORDERS

106 ACNE VULGARIS

Richard P. Usatine, MD

PATIENT STORY

A 16-year-old boy (**Figure 106-1**) with severe nodulocystic acne and scarring presents for treatment. After trying oral antibiotics, topical retinoids, and topical benzyl peroxide with no significant benefit, the patient and his mother request isotretinoin (Accutane). After 4 months of isotretinoin, the nodules and cysts cleared and there remained only a few papules (**Figure 106-2**). He is much happier and more confident about his appearance. The skin cleared fully after the last month of isotretinoin.

EPIDEMIOLOGY

- Acne can occur from infancy to the end of life.
- Close to 100% of people have acne at some time in their life.

ETIOLOGY AND PATHOPHYSIOLOGY

The four most important steps in acne pathogenesis:

1. Sebum overproduction related to androgenic hormones and genetics.
2. Abnormal desquamation of the follicular epithelium (keratin plugging).
3. *Propionibacterium acnes* proliferation.
4. Follicular obstruction which can lead to inflammation and follicular disruption.

Neonatal acne is thought to be related to maternal hormones and is temporary (**Figure 106-3**).

Acne can be precipitated by mechanical pressure as with a helmet strap (**Figure 106-4**) and medications such as phenytoin and lithium (**Figure 106-5**).

DIAGNOSIS

CLINICAL FEATURES

Morphology of acne includes comedones, papules, pustules, nodules, and cysts.

- Obstructive acne = comedonal acne = noninflammatory acne and consists of only comedones (**Figure 106-6**).

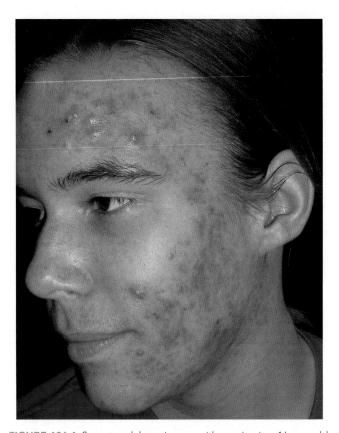

FIGURE 106-1 Severe nodulocystic acne with scarring in a 16-year-old boy. (*Courtesy of Richard P. Usatine, MD.*)

- Open comedones are blackheads and closed comedones are called whiteheads and look like small papules.

- Inflammatory acne has papules, pustules, nodules, and cysts in addition to comedones (**Figure 106-5**).

TYPICAL DISTRIBUTION

Face, back, chest, and neck.

LABORATORY STUDIES

None unless you suspect androgen excess and/or polycystic ovarian syndrome (PCOS).[1] SOR Ⓐ Obtain testosterone and DHEA-S levels if you suspect androgen excess and/or PCOS.

Consider FSH and LH levels if you suspect (PCOS).

DIFFERENTIAL DIAGNOSIS

- Acne conglobata is an uncommon and unusually severe form of acne characterized by burrowing and interconnecting abscesses and irregular scars, often producing pronounced disfigurement.[2] Sinus tracks can form with multiple openings that drain foul-smelling purulent material (**Figures 106-7** and **106-8**). The nodules are usually found on the chest, the shoulders, the back, the buttocks, the upper arms, the thighs, and the face.[2]

- Acne fulminans is characterized by sudden onset ulcerative crusting cystic acne, mostly on the chest and back[3] (**Figures 106-9** to **106-11**). Fever, malaise, nausea, arthralgia, myalgia, and weight loss are common. Leukocytosis and elevated erythrocyte sedimentation rate are usually found. There may also be focal osteolytic lesions. The term acne fulminans may also be used in cases of severe aggravation of acne without systemic features.[3]

- Rosacea can resemble acne by having papules and pustules on the face. It is usually seen in older adults with prominent erythema and telangiectasias. Rosacea does not include comedones and may have ocular or nasal manifestations (see Chapter 107, Rosacea). Rosacea fulminans or pyoderma faciale has features of severe acne and rosacea (**Figure 106-12**).

- Folliculitis on the back may be confused with acne. Look for hairs centrally located in the inflammatory papules of folliculitis to help distinguish it from acne. Acne on the back usually accompanies acne on the face as well (Chapter 111, Folliculitis).

- Acne keloidalis nuchae consists of papules, pustules, nodules, and keloidal tissue found at the posterior hairline. It is most often seen in men of color after shaving the hair at the nape of the neck (see Chapter 108, Pseudofolliculitis and Acne Keloidalis Nuchae).

- Actinic comedones (blackheads) are related to sun exposure and are seen later in life (**Figure 106-13**).

MANAGEMENT

Treatment is based on type of acne and severity. Categories to choose from are topical retinoids, topical antimicrobials, systemic antimicrobials, hormonal therapy, oral isotretinoin, and injection therapy.

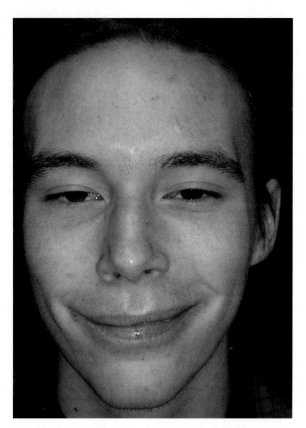

FIGURE 106-2 A happier boy now that his nodules and cysts have cleared at the start of the fifth month of isotretinoin treatment. (*Courtesy of Richard P. Usatine, MD.*)

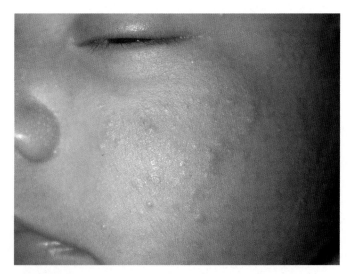

FIGURE 106-3 Neonatal acne in a healthy 2-week-old infant that resolved without treatment. (*Courtesy of Richard P. Usatine, MD.*)

MEDICATIONS FOR ACNE THERAPY

The Agency for Healthcare Research and Quality in a review of 250 comparisons found 14 had evidence of level A.[4] These comparisons demonstrated the efficacy over vehicle or placebo control of topical clindamycin, topical erythromycin, benzoyl peroxide, topical tretinoin, oral tetracycline, and norgestimate/ethinyl estradiol.[4] Level A conclusions demonstrating equivalence include: Benzoyl peroxide at various strengths was equally efficacious in mild/moderate acne; adapalene and tretinoin were equally efficacious.[4] SOR Ⓐ

Topical

- Benzoyl peroxide—antimicrobial effect (gel, cream, lotion) (2.5, 5, 10%) 10% causes more irritation and is not more effective.[4] SOR Ⓐ

- Topical antibiotics—clindamycin and erythromycin are the mainstays of treatment.
  - Erythromycin—solution, gel.[4] SOR Ⓐ
  - Clindamycin—solution, gel, lotion.[4] SOR Ⓐ
  - Benzamycin gel—erythromycin 3%, benzoyl peroxide 5%.[1] SOR Ⓐ
  - BenzaClin gel—clindamycin 1%, benzoyl peroxide 5%.[1] SOR Ⓐ
  - Dapsone 5% gel.[5] SOR Ⓑ

- Retinoids.
  - Tretinoin (Retin-A) gel, cream, liquid, micronized.[4] SOR Ⓐ
  - Adapalene gel—less irritating than tretinoin.[4] SOR Ⓐ
  - Tazarotene—strongest topical retinoid with greatest risk of irritation.[6] SOR Ⓐ

- Azelaic acid—useful to treat spotty hyperpigmentation and acne (**Figure 106-14**).[1] SOR Ⓑ

- Tea tree oil 5% gel.[7] SOR Ⓑ

Systemic

- Oral antibiotics.
  - Tetracycline 500 mg qd-bid—inexpensive, absorbed best on an empty stomach.[1,4] SOR Ⓐ
  - Doxycycline 40 to 100 mg qd bid—inexpensive, well tolerated, can take with food and increases sun sensitivity.[1] SOR Ⓐ
  - Minocycline 50 to 100 mg qd bid—expensive, not proven to be better than other systemic antibiotics including tetracycline.[1,8] SOR Ⓐ
  - Erythromycin 250 to 500 mg bid—inexpensive, frequent GI disturbance but can be used in pregnancy.[1] SOR Ⓐ
  - Trimethoprim/sulfamethoxazole DS bid—effective but risk of Stevens-Johnson syndrome is real. Reserve for short courses in particularly severe and resistant cases.[1] SOR Ⓐ

- Isotretinoin (Accutane) is the most powerful treatment for acne. It is especially useful for cystic and scarring acne that has not responded to other therapies. SOR Ⓐ Dosed at approximately 1 mg/kg/d for 5 months. Women of childbearing age must use two forms of contraception. Monitor for depression.

- The U.S. Food and Drug Administration requires that prescribers of isotretinoin, patients who take isotretinoin, and pharmacists who dispense isotretinoin all must register with the iPLEDGE system.[9] *www.ipledgeprogram.com*

- Hormonal treatments:
  - Oral contraceptives only for females—choose ones with low androgenic effect.[1,4] SOR Ⓐ FDA-approved oral contraceptives are

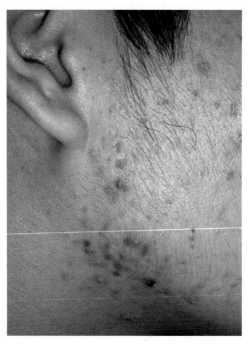

FIGURE 106-4 Inflammatory acne showing pustules and nodules in a 17-year-old boy that uses a helmet while playing football in high school. (*Courtesy of Richard P. Usatine, MD.*)

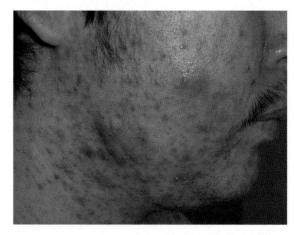

FIGURE 106-5 Severe inflammatory acne in a young adult. His acne worsened when this man was started on phenytoin for his seizure disorder. (*Courtesy of Richard P. Usatine, MD.*)

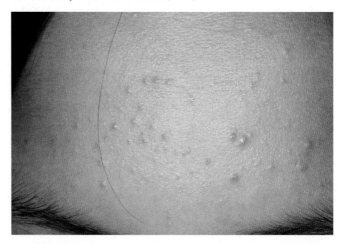

FIGURE 106-6 Comedonal acne in a 15-year-old girl. Open comedones (blackheads) and closed comedones (whiteheads) are visible on her forehead. (*Courtesy of Richard P. Usatine, MD.*)

Ortho Tri-cyclen, Yaz, and Estrostep. Other oral contraceptives with similar formulations also help acne in women even though these have not received FDA approval for this indication. Note Yaz and Yasmine have progestin drospirenone, which is derived from 17-alpha-spirolactone. It shares an antiandrogenic effect with spironolactone.

○ Spironolactone may be used for adult women when other therapies fail.[1,10,11] This may be especially useful if the patient has hirsutism. Standard dosing is 50 to 200 mg/d. May start with 25 mg bid and monitor for hyperkalemia. The risk of hyperkalemia increases with a higher dose. Titrate up as needed and tolerated.[1] SOR Ⓑ

○ One small prospective study of 27 women with severe papular and nodulocystic acne used a combination of EE/DRSP (Yasmin) and spironolactone 100 mg daily. Eighty-five percent of subjects were entirely clear of acne lesions or had excellent improvement and there was no significant elevation of serum potassium.[12]

Steroid injection therapy

For painful nodules and cysts:[1] SOR Ⓒ Be careful to avoid producing skin atrophy.

• Dilute 0.1 cc of 10 mg/cc triamcinolone acetonide (Kenalog) with 0.4 cc of sterile saline for a 2 mg/cc suspension.

• Inject 0.1 cc with a 1 cc tuberculin syringe into each nodule using a 30-gauge needle (**Figure 106-15**).

ACNE THERAPY BY SEVERITY

Comedonal acne (Figure 106-6).

• Topical retinoid or azelaic acid.

• No need for antibiotics or antimicrobials—do not need to kill *P. acnes.*

Mild papulopustular

• Topical antibiotics and benzoyl peroxide.

• Topical retinoid or azelaic acid.

• May add oral antibiotics if topical agents are not working.

Papulopustular or nodulocystic acne—moderate to severe—inflammatory

• Topical antibiotic, benzoyl peroxide, and oral antibiotic.

• Oral antibiotics are often essential at this stage.

• Topical retinoid or azelaic acid.

• Steroid injection therapy—for painful nodules and cysts.

Severe cystic or scarring acne

• Isotretinoin if there are no contraindications.

• Steroid injection therapy—for painful nodules and cysts.

Acne fulminans (Figures 106-9 to 106-11):

• Start with systemic steroids (prednisone 40 to 60 mg per day—approximately 1 mg/kg/day). SOR Ⓒ

• Systemic steroid treatment rapidly controls the skin lesions and systemic symptoms. The duration of steroid treatment in one Finnish series was 2 to 4 months to avoid relapses.[13] SOR Ⓒ

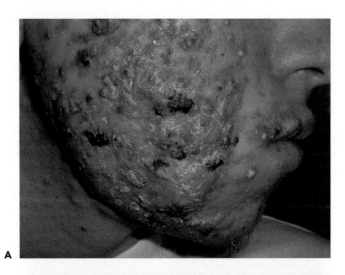

A

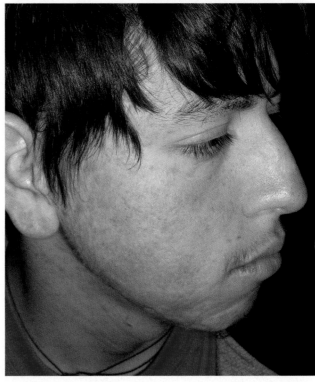

B

FIGURE 106-7 (A) Acne conglobata in a 16-year-old boy. He has severe cysts on his face with sinus tracks between them. He required many weeks of oral prednisone before isotretinoin was started. His acne cleared completely with his treatment. (B) Acne conglobata cleared with minimal scarring after oral prednisone and 5 months of isotretinoin therapy. (*Courtesy of Richard P. Usatine, MD.*)

- Therapy with isotretinoin, antibiotics, or both was often combined with steroids, but the role of these agents is still uncertain.[13] SOR **C**
- One British series used oral prednisolone 0.5 to 1 mg/kg daily for 4 to 6 weeks (thereafter slowly reduced to zero).[14] SOR **C**
- Oral isotretinoin was added to the regimen at the fourth week, initially at 0.5 mg/kg daily and gradually increased to achieve complete clearance.[14] SOR **C**
- Consider introducing isotretinoin at approximately 4 weeks into the oral prednisone if there are no contraindications. SOR **C**

Acne conglobata and pyoderma faciale may be treated like acne fulminans but the course of oral prednisone does not need to be as long. SOR **C**

COMBINATION THERAPIES

- Combination therapy with multiple topical agents can be more effective than single agents.[1] SOR **B**
- Topical retinoids and topical antibiotics are more effective when used in combination than either are used alone.[1] SOR **B**
- Benzoyl peroxide and topical antibiotics used in combination are effective treatment for acne by helping to minimize antibiotic resistance.[1] SOR **B**
- The adjunctive use of clindamycin/benzoyl peroxide gel with tazarotene cream promotes greater efficacy and may also enhance tolerability.[15]
- Combination therapy with topical retinoids and oral antibiotics can be helpful at the start of acne therapy. However, maintenance therapy with combination tazarotene and minocycline therapy showed a trend for greater efficacy but no statistical significance vs tazarotene alone.[16]

MOST AFFORDABLE MEDICATIONS

Topical benzoyl peroxide, erythromycin, clindamycin and oral tetracycline, and doxycycline.

NEWER EXPENSIVE MODES OF THERAPY

Intense pulsed light and photodynamic therapy use lasers, special lights, and topical chemicals to treat acne.[17–19] These therapies are very expensive and the data do not suggest that these should be first-line therapies at this time. Patients who have failed other therapies in whom isotretinoin is not an option may benefit from these options when they can afford these therapies. SOR **C** As more family doctors are now doing cosmetic dermatology, these options are available in their offices along with the offices of dermatologists.

PATIENT EDUCATION

Adequate face washing twice a day. Do not scrub the face with abrasive physical or chemical agents. There is no evidence that chocolate needs to be avoided or that other dietary changes need to be made.

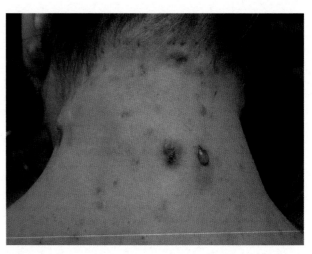

FIGURE 106-8 Acne conglobata in a 42-year-old woman showing communicating sinus tracks between cysts. There is pus draining from one of the sinus tracks on the right side of the neck. (*Courtesy of Richard P. Usatine, MD.*)

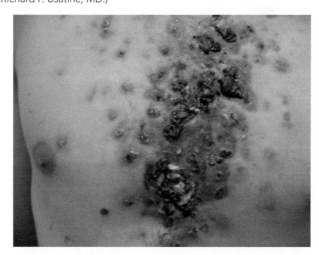

FIGURE 106-9 Acne fulminans in a 17-year-old boy. He was on isotretinoin when he developed worsening of his acne with polymyalgia and arthralgia. He presented with numerous nodules and cysts covered by hemorrhagic crusts on his chest and back. (*With permission from Grunwald MH, Amichai B. Nodulo-cystic eruption with musculoskeletal pain. J Fam Pract. 2007;56:205–206, Dowden Health Media.*)

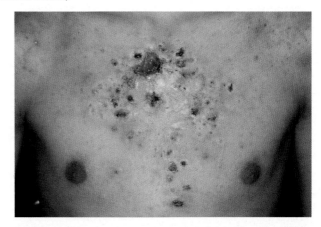

FIGURE 106-10 Acne fulminans with severe rapidly worsening truncal acne in a 15-year-old-boy. He did not have fever or bone pain but had a WBC of 17,000. He responded rapidly to prednisone and was started on isotretinoin. The ulcers and granulation tissue worsened initially on isotretinoin but prednisone helped to get this under control. (*Courtesy of Richard P. Usatine, MD.*)

FOLLOW-UP

Is completely dependent upon the acne severity and the treatments prescribed. Isotretinoin requires monthly follow-up visits but other therapies can be monitored every few months at first and then once to twice a year. Keep in mind that many treatments for acne take months to work, so quick follow-up visits may be disappointing to you and the patient.

PATIENT RESOURCES

• Medline Plus—**http://www.nlm.nih.gov/medlineplus/acne.html**

PROVIDER RESOURCES

• **http://www.emedicine.com/derm/topic2.htm**
• Management of Acne. Summary, Evidence Report(Technology Assessment: Number 17. AHRQ Publication No. 01-E018, March 2001. Agency for Healthcare Research and Quality, Rockville, MD—**http://www.ahrq.gov/clinic/epcsums/acnesum.htm**

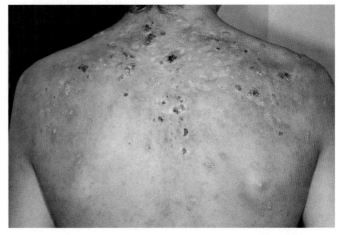

FIGURE 106-11 Acne fulminans on the back of the same boy. Ulcers and cysts are visible. (*Courtesy of Richard P. Usatine, MD.*)

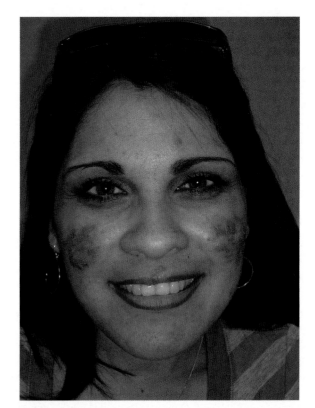

FIGURE 106-12 Pyoderma faciale is almost exclusively seen in adult women. It can present with severe cystic facial acne often in a malar distribution. It also is called rosacea fulminans. It started abruptly 6 months before and her ANA was normal. (*Courtesy of Richard P. Usatine, MD.*)

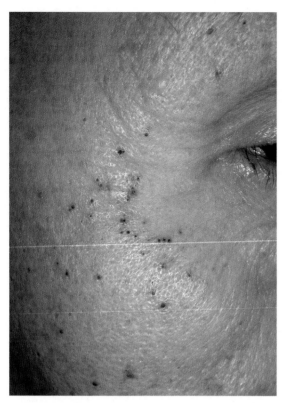

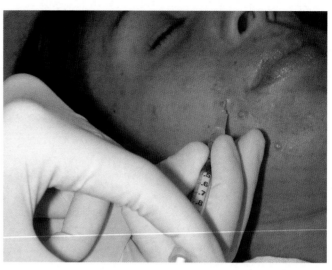

FIGURE 106-15 Injection of acne nodules with 2 mg per cc triamcinolone acetonide. (*Courtesy of Richard P. Usatine, MD.*)

FIGURE 106-13 Actinic comedones related to sun exposure in an older man. These are typically seen on the side of the face clustering around the eyes. (*Courtesy of Richard P. Usatine, MD.*)

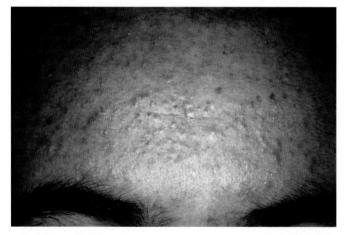

FIGURE 106-14 Obstructive or comedonal acne with spotty hyperpigmentation. Azelaic acid was helpful to treat the acne and the hyperpigmentation. (*Courtesy of Richard P. Usatine, MD.*)

REFERENCES

1. Strauss JS, Krowchuk DP, Leyden JJ, et al. Guidelines of care for acne vulgaris management. *J Am Acad Dermatol.* 2007;56:651–663.

2. Schwartz, R. A. and Zaba, R. Acne Conglobata. http://www.emedicine.com/derm/topic756.htm. Accessed May 15, 2007.

3. Grunwald MH, Amichai B. Nodulo-cystic eruption with musculoskeletal pain. *J Fam Pract.* 2007;56:205–206.

4. Agency for Healthcare Research and Quality (AHRQ). *Management of Acne.* http://www.ahrq.gov/clinic/epcsums/acnesum.htm. 2001. Accessed May 15, 2007.

5. Draelos ZD, Carter E, Maloney JM, et al. Two randomized studies demonstrate the efficacy and safety of dapsone gel, 5% for the treatment of acne vulgaris. *J Am Acad Dermatol.* 2007;56:439–410.

6. Webster GF, Guenther L, Poulin YP, Solomon BA, Loven K, Lee J. A multicenter, double-blind, randomized comparison study of the efficacy and tolerability of once-daily tazarotene 0.1% gel and adapalene 0.1% gel for the treatment of facial acne vulgaris. *Cutis.* 2002;69(2 Suppl):4–11.

7. Enshaieh S, Jooya A, Siadat AH, Iraji F. The efficacy of 5% topical tea tree oil gel in mild to moderate acne vulgaris: A randomized, double-blind placebo-controlled study. *Indian J Dermatol Venereol Leprol.* 2007;73:22–25.

8. Garner SE, Eady EA, Popescu C, Newton J, Li WA. Minocycline for acne vulgaris: Efficacy and safety. *Cochrane Database Syst Rev.* 2003;CD002086.

9. Harper JC, Fulton J. Acne Vulgaris. http://www.emedicine.com/derm/topic2.htm. Accessed January 23, 2007.

10. Sato K, Matsumoto D, Iizuka F, et al. Anti-androgenic therapy using oral spironolactone for acne vulgaris in Asians. *Aesthetic Plast Surg.* 2006;30:689–694.

11. Shaw JC. Low-dose adjunctive spironolactone in the treatment of acne in women: a retrospective analysis of 85 consecutively treated patients. *J Am Acad Dermatol.* 2000;43:498–502.

12. Krunic A, Ciurea A, Scheman A. Efficacy and tolerance of acne treatment using both spironolactone and a combined contraceptive containing drospirenone. *J Am Acad Dermatol.* 2008;58:60–62.

13. Karvonen SL. Acne fulminans: Report of clinical findings and treatment of twenty-four patients. *J Am Acad Dermatol.* 1993;28:572–579.

14. Seukeran DC, Cunliffe WJ. The treatment of acne fulminans: A review of 25 cases. *Br J Dermatol.* 1999;141:307–309.

15. Tanghetti E, Abramovits W, Solomon B, Loven K, Shalita A. Tazarotene versus tazarotene plus clindamycin(benzoyl peroxide in the treatment of acne vulgaris: A multicenter, double-blind, randomized parallel-group trial. *J Drugs Dermatol.* 2006;5:256–261.

16. Leyden J, Thiboutot DM, Shalita AR, et al. Comparison of tazarotene and minocycline maintenance therapies in acne vulgaris: A multicenter, double-blind, randomized, parallel-group study. *Arch Dermatol.* 2006;142:605–612.

17. Yeung CK, Shek SY, Bjerring P, Yu CS, Kono T, Chan HH. A comparative study of intense pulsed light alone and its combination with photodynamic therapy for the treatment of facial acne in Asian skin. *Lasers Surg Med.* 2007;39:1–6.

18. Horfelt C, Funk J, Frohm-Nilsson M, Wiegleb ED, Wennberg AM. Topical methyl aminolaevulinate photodynamic therapy for treatment of facial acne vulgaris: Results of a randomized, controlled study. *Br J Dermatol.* 2006;155:608–613.

19. Wiegell SR, Wulf HC. Photodynamic therapy of acne vulgaris using 5-aminolevulinic acid versus methyl aminolevulinate. *J Am Acad Dermatol.* 2006;54:647–651.

107 ROSACEA

Richard P. Usatine, MD

PATIENT STORY

A 34-year-old woman with extensive papulopustular rosacea (**Figures 107-1** to **107-3**) has a history of easy facial flushing since her teen years. Her face has been persistently redder in the past 5 years and she is bothered by this. She acknowledges that her mom has similar redness in her face and that she is from northern European heritage. In the last 6 months, since her daughter was born, she has developed many "pimples." Physical examination reveals papules, pustules and telangiectasias. No comedones are seen. She knows that the sun makes it worse but finds that many sunscreens are irritating to her skin. The patient is started on oral tetracycline daily and 1% metronidazole cream to use once daily. She agrees to wear a hat and stay out of the sun during the middle of the day. She will continue to look for a sunscreen she can tolerate. She knows that precipitating factors for her include hot and humid weather, alcohol, hot beverages and spicy foods. She will do her best to avoid those factors but knows she cannot control the weather.

EPIDEMIOLOGY

- Presents in the second or third decade of life.

- Common in fair-skinned people of Celtic and northern European heritage.

- Women are more often affected than men.

- Men are more prone to the extreme forms of hyperplasia, which causes rhinophymatous rosacea (**Figures 107-4** and **107-5**).

ETIOLOGY AND PATHOPHYSIOLOGY

- While the exact etiology is unknown, the pathophysiology involves nonspecific inflammation followed by dilation around follicles and hyperreactive capillaries. These dilated capillaries become telangiectasias (**Figures 107-6** and **107-7**).

- As rosacea progresses, diffuse hypertrophy of the connective tissue and sebaceous glands ensues (**Figures 107-4** and **107-5**).

- Alcohol may accentuate erythema, but does not cause the disease. Rosacea runs in families.

- Sun exposure may precipitate an acute rosacea flare, but flare-ups can happen without sun exposure.

- A significant increase in the hair follicle mite *Demadex folliculorum* is sometimes found in rosacea. It is theorized that these mites play a role because they incite an inflammatory or allergic reaction by mechanical blockage of follicles.

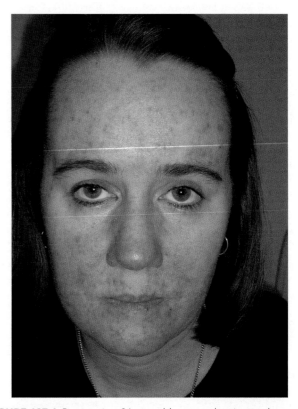

FIGURE 107-1 Rosacea in a 34-year-old woman showing erythema, papules and pustules covering much of the face. Note her fair skin and blue eyes from her Northern European heritage. (*Courtesy of Richard P. Usatine, MD.*)

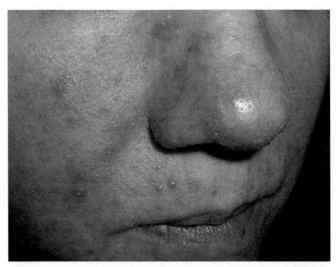

FIGURE 107-2 Close-up of papules and pustules in the same woman. Note the absence of comedones. This is not acne. This is predominantly papulopustular rosacea. (*Courtesy of Richard P. Usatine, MD.*)

DIAGNOSIS

CLINICAL FEATURES

Rosacea has 4 stages or subtypes:

1. Erythematotelangiectatic rosacea (**Figures 107-6** and **107-7**). This stage is characterized by frequent mild to severe blushing with persistent central facial erythema.

2. Papulopustular rosacea (**Figures 107-1** to **107-3, 107-8** and **107-9**). This is a highly vascular stage that involves longer periods of flushing than the first stage—often lasting from days to weeks. Minute telangiectasias and papules start to form by this stage, and some patients begin having very mild ocular complaints such as ocular grittiness or conjunctivitis. These patients may have many unsightly pustules with severe facial erythema. They are more prone to develop a hordeolum (stye) (see Chapter 12, Hordeolum and Chalazion).

3. Phymatous or Rhinophymatous rosacea (**Figures 107-4** and **107-5**). Characterized by hyperplasia of the sebaceous glands which form thickened confluent plaques on the nose known as rhinophyma. This hyperplasia can cause significant disfigurement to the forehead, eyelids, chin, and nose. The nasal disfiguration is seen more commonly in men than women. W. C. Fields is famous for his rhinophyma and intake of alcohol. Rhinophyma can occur without any alcohol use as seen in the patient in **Figure 107-5.**

4. Ocular rosacea (**Figures 107-10** to **107-12**). An advanced subtype of rosacea that is characterized by impressive, severe flushing with persistent telangiectasias, papules, and pustules. The patient may complain of watery eyes, a foreign body sensation, burning, dryness, vision changes, and lid or periocular erythema. The eyelids are most commonly involved with telangiectasias, blepharitis, and recurrent hordeola and chalazia (**Figures 107-10** and **107-11**). Conjunctivitis may be chronic. While corneal involvement is least common, it can have the most devastating consequences. Corneal findings may include punctate erosions, corneal infiltrates, and corneal neovascularization. In the most severe cases, blood vessels may grow over the cornea and lead to blindness (**Figure 107-12**).

TYPICAL DISTRIBUTION

Rosacea occurs on the face especially on the cheeks and nose. However, the forehead, eyelids, and chin can also be involved (**Figure 107-13**).

LABORATORY STUDIES

Not needed when the clinical picture is clear. If you are considering lupus or sarcoid, an ANA, CXR or punch biopsy may be needed.

DIFFERENTIAL DIAGNOSIS

- Acne—the age of onset for rosacea tends to be 30 to 50 years, much later than the onset for acne vulgaris. Comedones are prominent in most cases of acne and generally absent in rosacea (see Chapter 106, Acne).

- Sarcoidosis on the face is much less common than rosacea but the inflamed plaques can be red and resemble the inflammation of rosacea (see Chapter 168, Sarcoidosis).

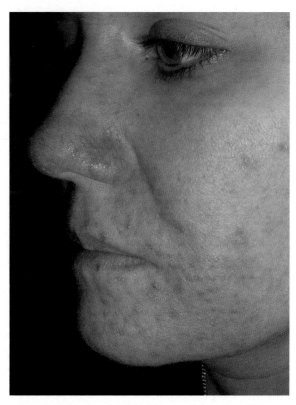

FIGURE 107-3 Close-up showing telangiectasias on the nose and papules around the mouth and chin. (*Courtesy of Richard P. Usatine, MD.*)

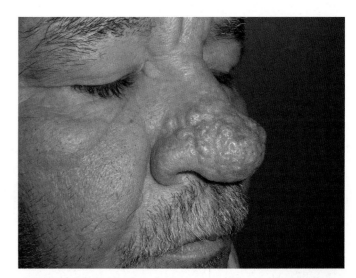

FIGURE 107-4 Rhinophymatous rosacea with hypertrophy of the skin of the nose of a 51-year-old Hispanic man. The patient acknowledges previous heavy alcohol intake. (*Courtesy of Richard P. Usatine, MD.*)

- Seborrheic dermatitis tends to produce scale while rosacea does not. While both cause central facial erythema, papules and telangiectasias are present in rosacea and are not part of seborrheic dermatitis (see Chapter 144, Seborrheic Dermatitis).

- SLE can be scarring, does not usually produce papules or pustules, and it spares the nasolabial folds and nose (see Chapter 173, Lupus–Systemic and Cutaneous). The patient in **Figure 107-13** has a butterfly distribution of her rosacea but her right nasolabial fold is involved along with her chin.

MANAGEMENT

- A systematic review by Van Zuuren et al. examined the efficacy of metronidazole, tetracycline, and azelaic acid in treating rosacea. The best evidence supports the topical use of metronidazole (0.75% or 1%) and azelaic acid (15 or 20%).[1] SOR Ⓐ

- When there are a limited number of papules and pustules, start with metronidazole (0.75% or 1%) and azelaic acid (15 or 20%).[1]

- If the skin lesions are more extensive, oral antibiotics, such as tetracycline and metronidazole are recommended.[1] SOR Ⓒ

- Oral tetracycline may be prescribed in doses ranging from 250–500 mg daily to twice daily.

- Both 0.75% metronidazole cream and 1.0% metronidazole cream are equally effective when used once daily for moderate to severe rosacea.[2] However, the prescribing information still suggests twice daily for the 0.75% cream. One percent gel and cream preparations are suggested to be applied once daily.

- Patient that are started on oral antibiotics alone and improve may be switched to topical agents such as metronidazole or azelaic acid for maintenance.

- Azelaic acid in a 15% gel appeared to offer some modest benefits over 0.75% metronidazole gel in a manufacturer sponsored study.[3] Azelaic acid was not as well tolerated, so both medications are reasonable options with the choice depending on patient preference and tolerance.[3] SOR Ⓑ

- The *Demadex* mite may be one causative agent in rosacea. One study found Permethrin 5% cream to be as effective as metronidazole 0.75% gel and superior to placebo in the treatment of rosacea.[4] SOR Ⓑ

- Severe papulopustular disease refractory to antibiotics and topical treatments can be treated with oral isotretinoin at a low dose of 0.1 to 0.5 mg/kg. SOR Ⓒ

- Simple electrosurgery or laser without anesthesia can be used to treat the telangiectasias associated with rosacea.[1] SOR Ⓒ

- Rhinophyma can be excised with radiofrequency electrosurgery or laser. Isotretinoin is also used to treat rhinophyma.[1] SOR Ⓒ

- Traditional therapies for mild ocular rosacea include oral tetracyclines, lid hygiene, and warm compresses.[1] SOR Ⓒ Ocular rosacea that involves the cornea should be immediately referred to an ophthalmologist to prevent blindness (**Figure 107-12**).

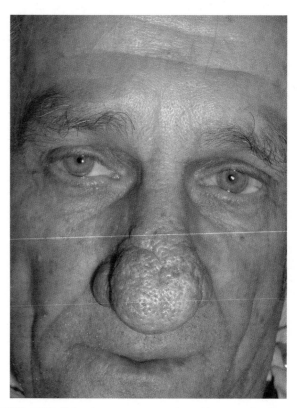

FIGURE 107-5 Rhinophymatous rosacea in a older man who does not drink alcohol. While this is often called a WC Field's nose, it is not necessarily related to heavy alcohol use. (*Courtesy of Richard P. Usatine, MD.*)

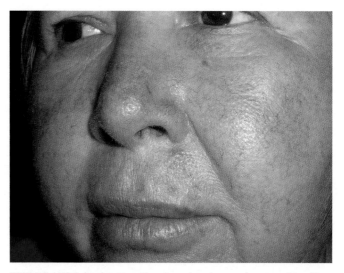

FIGURE 107-6 Erythematotelangiectatic subtype of rosacea in a middle-aged Hispanic woman. (*Courtesy of Richard P. Usatine, MD.*)

PATIENT EDUCATION

Sun protection including use of a hat and daily application of sunscreen should be emphasized. Choose a sunscreen that is nonirritating and protects against UVA and UVB rays. Advise patients to keep a diary to identify and avoid precipitating factors such as hot and humid weather, alcohol, hot beverages, spicy foods, and large hot meals.

FOLLOW-UP

Follow-up can be in 1 to 3 months as needed.

PATIENT RESOURCES

National Rosacea Society **(www.rosacea.org)**.

PROVIDER RESOURCES

http://www.emedicine.com/derm/topic377.htm

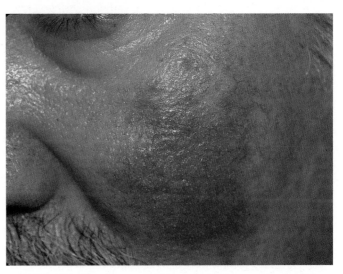

FIGURE 107-7 Rosacea in a middle-aged man showing deep erythema and many telangiectasias. (*Courtesy of Richard P. Usatine, MD.*)

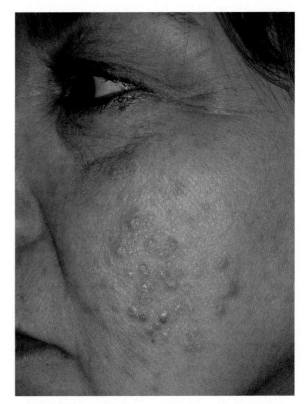

FIGURE 107-8 Papulopustular rosacea in a middle-aged woman. (*Courtesy of Richard P. Usatine, MD.*)

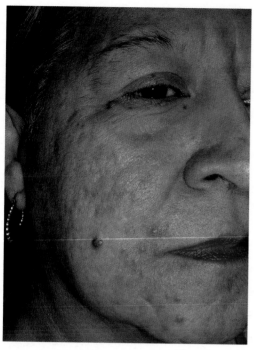

FIGURE 107-9 Papulopustular rosacea in a woman who has a history of recurrent hordeola. (*Courtesy of Richard P. Usatine, MD.*)

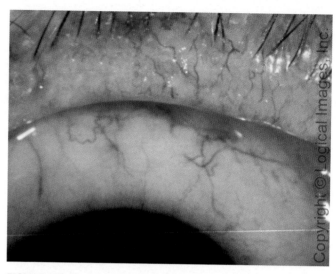

FIGURE 107-11 Ocular rosacea with Meibomian gland dysfunction leading to thick viscous discharge and plugging of meibomian gland orifices. Conjunctivitis and blepharitis are both present. (*Copyright © and Courtesy of Logical Images, Inc.*)

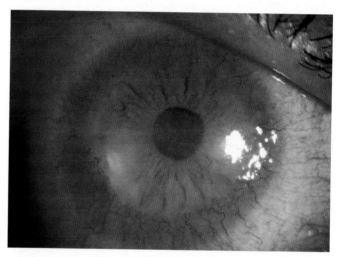

FIGURE 107-12 Neovascularization involving the cornea in a patient with severe ocular rosacea. This type of corneal involvement can lead to blindness. (*Courtesy of Paul Comeau.*)

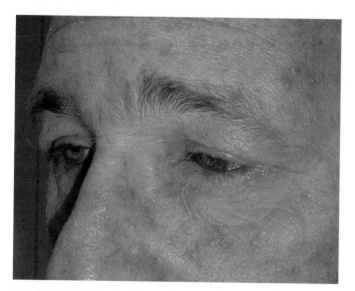

FIGURE 107-10 Ocular rosacea showing blepharitis, and conjunctival hyperemia, telangiectasias of the lid. (*Courtesy of Richard P. Usatine, MD.*)

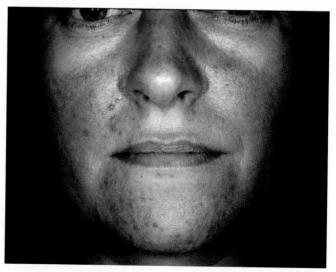

FIGURE 107-13 Rosacea in a young woman with a butterfly pattern along with chin involvement. This is not lupus. (*Courtesy of Richard P. Usatine, MD.*)

REFERENCES

1. van Zuuren EJ, Graber MA, Hollis S, Chaudhry M, Gupta AK, Gover M. Interventions for rosacea. *Cochrane Database of Syst Rev*. 2005;(3):):CD003262.

2. Dahl MV, Jarratt M, Kaplan D, Tuley MR, Baker MD. Once-daily topical metronidazole cream formulations in the treatment of the papules and pustules of rosacea. *J Am Acad Dermatol*. 2001;45(5):723–730.

3. Elewski BE, Fleischer AB, Pariser DM. A comparison of 15% azelaic acid gel and 0.75% metronidazole gel in the topical treatment of papulopustular rosacea. *Arch Dermatol*. 2003;139:1444–1450.

4. Kocak M, Yagli S, Vahapoglu G, Eksioglu M. Permethrin 5% cream versus metronidazole 0.75% gel for the treatment of papulopustular rosacea: A randomized double-blind placebo-controlled study. *Dermatology*. 2002;205:265–270.

108 PSEUDOFOLLICULITIS AND ACNE KELOIDALIS NUCHAE

E.J. Mayeaux, Jr., MD

PATIENT STORY

This 17-year-old young African-American man comes to the office because he is bothered by the uncomfortable bumps on the back of his neck for the last 2 years (**Figure 108-1**). He is an athletic young man more than 6 feet tall and likes to keep his hair short for his sports. He notices the bumps get irritated and larger when he shaves his hair. He also has bumps on his face that get worse when he shaves his face (**Figure 108-2**). He is diagnosed with pseudofolliculitis barbae and acne keloidalis nuchae. His treatment consisted of patient education and twice-daily tretinoin cream and 0.1% triamcinolone cream to neck area and nightly tretinoin cream to the beard area. He was told he could use 1% hydrocortisone cream to the face as needed. It was suggested that he minimize shaving if possible.

EPIDEMIOLOGY

- Pseudofolliculitis (razor bumps or shave bumps) is a common skin condition affecting the hair-bearing areas of the body that are shaved (**Figures 108-2 to 108-4**). It is most common in black men, with at least 50% of black men who shave being prone to the condition.[1] In the beard area it is called pseudofolliculitis barbae, and when it occurs after pubic hair is shaved it is referred to as pseudofolliculitis pubis.

- Acne keloidalis nuchae occurs most often in black men but can be seen in all ethnicities (**Figures 108-1 and 108-5**). The lesions are often painful and cosmetically disfiguring.

- Both conditions can be seen in women but far less often than men.

ETIOLOGY AND PATHOPHYSIOLOGY

- Pseudofolliculitis develops when, after shaving, the free end of tightly coiled hair reenters the skin, causing a foreign-body-like inflammatory reaction. Shaving produces a sharp free end below the skin surface. Tightly curled hair has a greater tendency for the tip to pierce the the surface of the skin and form ingrown hairs. This explains, the relative predominance of this condition in patients of African descent. The hair eventually forms a loop and if the embedded tip is pulled out there may be spontaneous resolution of symptoms.

- The exact cause of acne keloidalis is uncertain. It often develops in areas of pseudofolliculitis or folliculitis. It may be associated with haircuts where the posterior hairline is shaved with a razor and with tightly curved hair shafts. Other possible etiologies include irritation from shirt collars, chronic bacterial infections, and an autoimmune process. Based on histologic changes, it may be a form of primary scarring alopecia.[2]

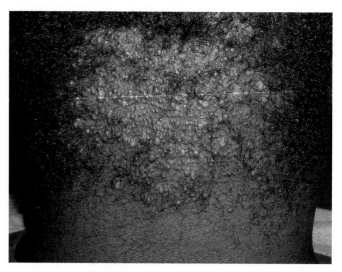

FIGURE 108-1 Acne keloidalis nuchae in a 17-year-old African American man. (*Courtesy of Richard P. Usatine, MD.*)

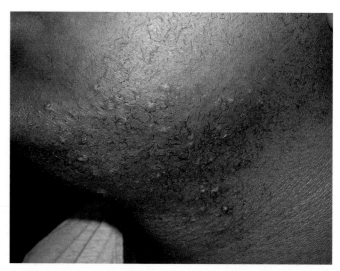

FIGURE 108-2 Pseudofolliculitis barbae along the jaw-line and neck in the patient in **Figure 108-1**. (*Courtesy of Richard P. Usatine, MD.*)

DIAGNOSIS

CLINICAL FEATURES

- The diagnosis of pseudofolliculitis is based upon clinical appearance. A piece of hair often may be identified protruding from a lesion. Inflammation results in the formation of firm, skin-colored, erythematous or hyperpigmented papules that occur after shaving (**Figures 108-2** to **108-4**). Pustules may develop secondarily. The severity varies from a few papules or pustules to hundreds of lesions.

- Patients with acne keloidalis initially develop a folliculitis or pseudofolliculitis, which heal with keloid-like lesions, sometimes with discharging sinuses. It starts after puberty as 2 to 4 mm firm, follicular papules (**Figure 108-1**). More papules appear and enlarge over time. Papules may coalesce to form keloid-like plaques, which are usually arranged in a band-like distribution along the posterior part of the hairline (**Figures 108-5** and **108-6**).

TYPICAL DISTRIBUTION

- Pseudofolliculitis affects the hair bearing area of the body that are shaved, especially the face, neck, and pubic area (**Figures 108-2** to **108-4**).

- Acne keloidalis occurs on the occipital scalp and the posterior part of the neck (**Figures 108-1, 108-5,** and **108-6**).

LABORATORY STUDIES

Histologic evaluation of a biopsy may confirm the clinical diagnosis but is usually not necessary.

DIFFERENTIAL DIAGNOSIS

- True folliculitis which is an acute pustular infection of a hair follicle with more localized inflammation (see Chapter 111, Folliculitis).

- Impetigo which presents with yellowish pustules or bullae that rupture and develop honey crusts, sometimes with adenopathy (see Chapter 110, Impetigo).

- Acne Vulgaris which presents with comedones and pustules usually including the forehead (see Chapter 106, Acne).

MANAGEMENT

- Avoiding close shaving, avoiding all shaving, or permanently removing hair may cure pseudofolliculitis and prevents worsening of acne keloidalis nuchae.[3] However, some occupations such as the military and law enforcement require facial shaving. Occasionally, a doctor's note will allow these men to go without shaving. In mild cases, shaving should be discontinued for a month. The beard can be coarsely trimmed with scissors or electric clippers during this time. Shaving should not resume until all inflammatory lesions have resolved. Warm Burow's solution compresses may be applied to the lesions for ten minutes, three times per day. Instruct the patient to search for ingrown hairs each day using a magnifying mirror and release them gently using a sterilized needle or tweezers. The hairs

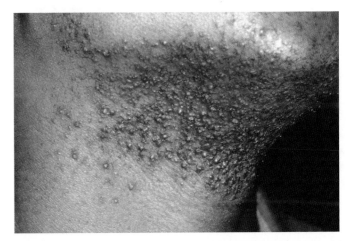

FIGURE 108-3 Longstanding pseudofolliculitis barbae in a 47-year-old African-American man. (*Courtesy of Jeffrey Meffert, MD.*)

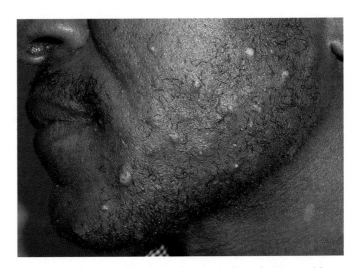

FIGURE 108-4 Pseudofolliculitis barbae on the face of a 28-year-old African man who works providing aid to Darfur refugees. The painful nodules become worse every time he shaves. (*Courtesy of Richard P. Usatine, MD.*)

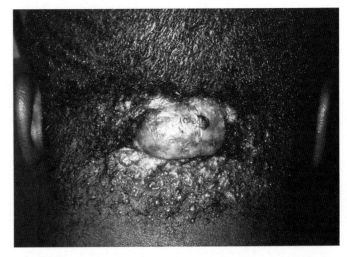

FIGURE 108-5 Severe acne keloidalis with large keloidal mass. (*Courtesy of Jeffrey Meffert, MD.*)

should not be plucked since this may cause recurrence of symptoms with hair regrowth. SOR Ⓒ

○ Hydrocortisone 1% cream can be applied as necessary to reduce inflammation. SOR Ⓒ

○ Topical erythromycin, clindamycin, and combination clindamycin/benzoyl peroxide (BenzaClin, Duac) and erythromycin/benzoyl peroxide (Benzamycin) may be used once or twice daily.[4] SOR Ⓑ

○ Oral erythromycin or tetracycline 500 mg twice daily may be used for patients with more severe secondary inflammation. SOR Ⓒ

○ Tretinoin cream, 0.025%, may be a useful in patients with mild disease, but is rarely helpful in moderate to severe cases.[5] It is applied nightly for a week then reduced to every second or third night. Tretinoin may be used in conjunction with a midpotency topical corticosteroid applied each morning. The mechanism of action is thought to be by relieving hyperkeratosis and "toughening" the skin. Topical combination cream (tretinoin 0.05%, fluocinolone acetonide 0.01%, and hydroquinone 4%) (Tri-Luma) adds an additional postinflammatory hyperpigmentation treatment. SOR Ⓒ

○ Chemical depilatories (Ali, Royal Crown, Magic Shave, and others) cause less symptoms than shaving.[6] SOR Ⓑ However, these creams can cause severe irritation, so testing a small amount on the forearm is important. They work by breaking the disulfide bonds in hair, which results in the hair being bluntly broken at the follicular opening instead of sharply cut below the surface. They should be used every second or third day to avoid skin irritation, although this can be controlled with hydrocortisone cream. Barium sulfide 2% powder depilatories can be made into a paste with water, applied to the beard, and removed after 3 to 5 minutes. Calcium thioglycolate preparations are left on 10 to 15 minutes, but the fragrances can cause an allergic reaction and chemical burns can result if it is left for too long.

○ Topical eflornithine HCL 13.9% cream (Vaniqa) may be used to inhibit hair growth. It decreases the rate of hair growth and may make the hair finer and lighter. Unfortunately, this treatment requires daily application for continued efficacy.

○ The only definitive cure is permanent hair removal. Electrolysis is expensive, painful, and sometimes unsuccessful. Laser hair removal is fairly successful for treating pseudofolliculitis.[7] SOR Ⓑ

• People who have acne keloidalis nuchae should avoid anything that causes folliculitis or pseudofolliculitis such as getting their neck or hairline shaved with a razor.

○ Twice-daily treatment with tretinoin (Retin-A) and a class 2 or 3 corticosteroid may be sufficient to shrink lesions and relieve all symptoms (see Use of Topical Corticosteroids in appendix).

○ When pustules, crust formation, or drainage is present, use topical clindamycin or erythromycin. Unresponsive patients may be changed to a systemic antibiotic. SOR Ⓒ

○ Intralesional steroid injections (10–20 mg/mL) may be used to soften and shrink keloids. Warn patients that this therapy may cause hypopigmentation. SOR Ⓒ

○ Other therapies that may be considered are laser therapy (carbon dioxide or ND:YAG) followed by intralesional triamcinolone injections or cryotherapy for two 20 seconds bursts, allowed to thaw and is then frozen again a minute later. These methods may produce more pain and hypopigmentation. SOR Ⓒ

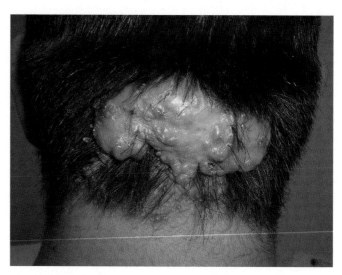

FIGURE 108-6 Severe acne keloidalis in a Hispanic man. Surgery is the only treatment that can remove this keloidal mass. (*Courtesy of Aaron Moon, MD.*)

○ Recalcitrant keloidal lesions may be treated with removing individual papules with a small punch, or large keloids (**Figure 108-5**) with an elliptical excision closed with sutures. After removal, the wound edges should be injected with a mixture of equal amount of triamcinolone acetonide 40 mg/mL and sterile saline. Remove the sutures in 1 to 2 weeks and inject the edges every month with the above mixture for 3 to 4 times. SOR ⓒ

○ In severe cases (**Figure 108-6**), some trained physicians will excise the large keloids after using tissue expanders to stretch the scalp, and steroid injections after removal. SOR ⓒ

PATIENT EDUCATION

• For those who must shave, have the patient clip hairs no shorter than needed for maintenance. Use fine scissors or facial hair clippers if possible. When shaving, have the patient rinse with warm tap water for several minutes, use generous amounts of a highly lubricating shaving gel, and allow it to soften the skin for five to ten minutes before shaving. The patient should always use sharp razors and shave in the direction of hair growth. Specialized guarded razors (e.g., "PFB Bump Fighter") are available in pharmacies and by mail order. After shaving rinse the face with tap water, and then apply cold water compresses.

• With acne keloidalis, instruct males who play football to make sure their helmets fit properly and do not cause irritation on the posterior part of the scalp. They should avoid having the posterior part of the hairline shaved with a razor as part of a haircut, and discontinue wearing garments that rub or irritate the posterior parts of the scalp and the neck.

REFERENCES

1. Coquilla BH, Lewis CW. Management of pseudofolliculitis barbae. *Mil Med.* 1995;160:263.

2. Sperling LC, Homoky C, Pratt L, Sau P. Acne keloidalis is a form of primary scarring alopecia. *Arch Dermatol.* 2000;136(4):479–484.

3. Chui CT, Berger TG, Price VH, Zachary CB. Recalcitrant scarring follicular disorders treated by laser-assisted hair removal: A preliminary report. *Dermatol Surg.* 1999;25:34.

4. Cook-Bolden FE, Barba A, Halder R, Taylor S. Twice-daily applications of benzoyl peroxide 5% clindamycin 1% gel versus vehicle in the treatment of pseudofolliculitis barbae. *Cutis.* 2004;73:18.

5. Brown LA, Jr., Pathogenesis and treatment of pseudofolliculitis barbae. *Cutis.* 1983;32:373.

6. Hage JJ, Bowman FG. Surgical depilation for the treatment of pseudofolliculitis or local hirsutism of the face: experience in the first 40 patients. *Plast Reconstr Surg.* 1991;88:446–451.

7. Ross EV, Cooke LM, Timko AL, et al. Treatment of pseudofolliculitis barbae in skin types IV, V, and VI with a long-pulsed neodymium: yttrium aluminum garnet laser. *J Am Acad Dermatol.* 2002;47:263.

109 HIDRADENITIS SUPPURATIVA (ACNE INVERSA)

Richard P. Usatine, MD

PATIENT STORY

A 25-year-old woman presents with new tender lesions in her axilla (**Figure 109-1**). She admits to years of similar outbreaks in both axilla and occasional painful bumps in the groin. She states that it is painful to have them opened and just wants to get some relief without surgery. We elected to inject the nodules with triamcinolone and start the patient on doxycycline 100 mg twice daily. Smoking cessation was emphasized and the patient agreed to start on a nicotine patch that evening. She had relief within 24 hours and no recurrences reported in the time since she was seen.

EPIDEMIOLOGY

- Occurs after puberty in about 1% of population.[1]
- Incidence is higher in females in the range of 4:1 to 5:1. Flare-ups may be associated with menses.[1]

ETIOLOGY AND PATHOPHYSIOLOGY

- Disorder of the terminal follicular epithelium in the apocrine gland-bearing skin.[1]
- Starts with occlusion of hair follicles that lead to occlusion of surrounding apocrine glands.
- Chronic relapsing inflammation with mucopurulent discharge (**Figures 109-2 to 109-7**).
- Can lead to sinus tracts, draining fistulas and progressive scarring (**Figures 109-2 to 109-7**).
- It is called acne inversa because it involves intertriginous areas and not the regions affected by acne (similar to inverse psoriasis).

DIAGNOSIS

CLINICAL FEATURES

- Most common presentation is painful, tender, firm, nodular lesions in axillae (**Figures 109-1 to 109-3**).
- Nodules may open and drain pus spontaneously and heal slowly, with or without drainage, over 10 to 30 days.[1]
- Nodules may recur several times yearly or in severe cases new lesions form as old ones heal.

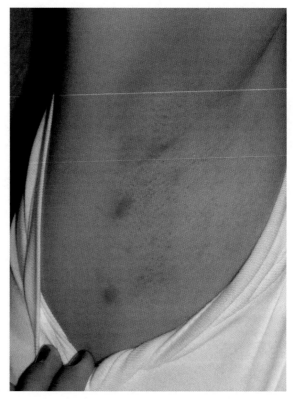

FIGURE 109-1 Mild HS in the axilla of a young woman. She has a history of recurrent lesions in her axilla. (*Courtesy of Richard P. Usatine, MD.*)

- Surrounding cellulitis may be present and require systemic antibiotic treatment.

- Chronic recurrences result in thickened sinus tracts, which may become draining fistulas (**Figures 109-3** to **109-7**).

- Hidradenitis suppurativa (HS) can cause disabling pain, diminished range of motion, and social isolation (**Figure 109-5**).

TYPICAL DISTRIBUTION

- Axillary, inguinal, periareolar, intermammary zones, pubic area, infraumbilical midline, gluteal folds, top of the anterior thighs, and the perianal region.[1]

LABORATORY STUDIES

Culture of purulence is likely to yield staphylococci and streptococci and is usually unnecessary to determine treatment. Culture may be useful if you suspect methicillin-resistant *Staphylococcus aureus.*

DIFFERENTIAL DIAGNOSIS

- Bacterial infections including folliculitis, carbuncles, furuncles, abscess, and cellulitis may resemble HS but are less likely to be recurrent in the intertriginous areas.

- Epidermal cysts in the intertriginous regions may resemble HS. Theses cysts contain a typical malodorous keratin core.

- Granuloma inguinale and lymphogranuloma venereum are sexually transmitted infections that can produce inguinal adenopathy that could be mistaken for HS.

MANAGEMENT

- Lifestyle changes are recommended including weight loss if obesity is present. SOR **C**

- Smoking is a risk factor for HS and cessation is highly recommended for many reasons.[1] SOR **B** for HS and SOR **A** for other health reasons.

- Frequent bathing and wearing loose-fitting clothing may help.

Medical treatment is similar to acne treatment:

- Oral antibiotics are used in acute and chronic treatment. Oral tetracyclines are standardly used but cephalexin may be best if there is evidence of cellulitis. If there is methicillin-resistant *Staphylococcus aureus* present, trimethoprim/sulfamethoxazole or clindamycin are alternatives.

- Tetracycline 500 mg bid and Doxycycline 100 mg bid can be used acutely and to prevent new lesions. SOR **B**

- Topical clindamycin bid may be used. In one RCT, systemic therapy with tetracyclines did not show better results than topical therapy with clindamycin.[2] SOR **B**

- Isotretinoin can reduce the severity of attacks in some patients but is not a reliable cure for HS.[1] SOR **C**

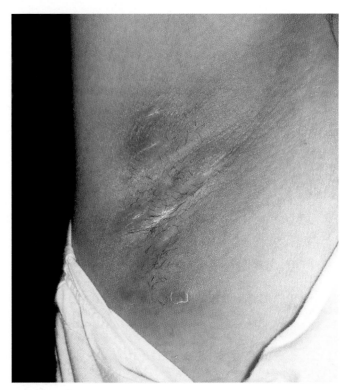

FIGURE 109-2 Moderate HS in a young woman. The lesions are deeper and there have been some chronic changes with scarring and fibrosis from previous lesions. (*Courtesy of Richard P. Usatine, MD.*)

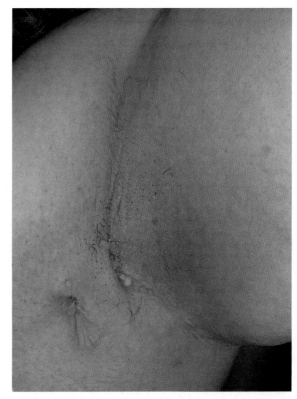

FIGURE 109-3 33-year-old Hispanic woman with sinus tracts, draining fistulas, and scarring secondary to her chronic HS. Note the mucopurulent discharge. (*Courtesy of Richard P. Usatine, MD.*)

- Anti-TNF agents are being studied for severe, recalcitrant HS. Etanercept (25 mg subcutaneously twice weekly) has shown efficacy in a small study of 6 patients.[3] SOR **C**

Surgical treatments include the following:

- Intralesional steroids with 5 to 10 mg/cc of triamcinolone may help to decrease inflammation and pain within 24 to 48 hours. SOR **C**

- Incision and drainage of acute lesions is suggested for large fluctuant abscesses that can occur in HS. While this may give some relief of the pressure, the surgical treatment and repacking of the wound is painful, and there is no evidence that it speeds healing. SOR **C**

- Lancing small nodules is more painful than helpful and is not recommended.

- Surgical excision of affected area with or without skin grafting is used for recalcitrant disabling disease and should be individualized based on the stage and location of the disease.[4] SOR **B**

PATIENT EDUCATION

Smoking cessation, weight loss if overweight, and avoid tight-fitting clothes.

FOLLOW-UP

If there is cellulitis or a large abscess that was drained, follow-up should be within days. Chronic relapsing disease can ultimately be managed with appointments every 3 to 6 months depending upon the treatment and its success.

PATIENT RESOURCES

Hidradenitis Suppurativa Foundation—
http://www.hs-foundation.org/.

PROVIDER RESOURCES

http://www.emedicine.com/med/topic2717.htm.

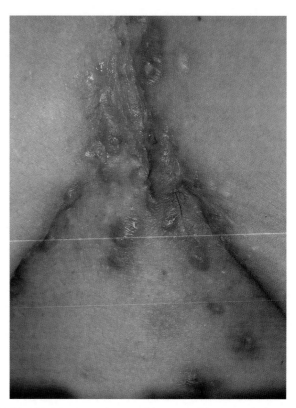

FIGURE 109-4 Longstanding painful severe HS between the breasts of a 45-year-old woman. (*Courtesy of Richard P. Usatine, MD.*)

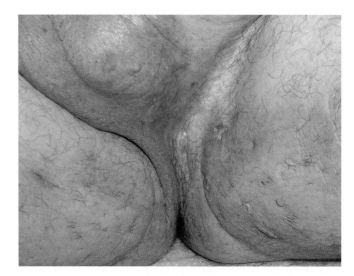

FIGURE 109-5 Severe disabling HS in a 34-year-old white man who is morbidly obese. He finds it painful to walk. (*Courtesy of Richard P. Usatine, MD.*)

REFERENCES

1. Fite D. Hidradenitis Suppurativa. http://www.emedicine.com/emerg/topic259.htm. Accessed 5, 2006.

2. Jemec GB, Wendelboe P. Topical clindamycin versus systemic tetracycline in the treatment of hidradenitis suppurativa. *J Am Acad Dermatol.* 1998;39:971–974.

3. Cusack C, Buckley C. Etanercept: Effective in the management of hidradenitis suppurativa. *Br J Dermatol.* 2006;154:726–729.

4. Kagan RJ, Yakuboff KP, Warner P, Warden GD. Surgical treatment of hidradenitis suppurativa: A 10-year experience. *Surgery.* 2005; 138:734–740.

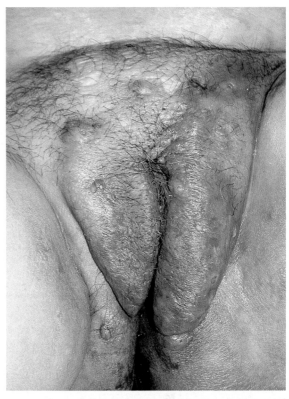

FIGURE 109-6 Severe HS in the vulva and on the Mons pubis. The skin is thickened and hyperpigmented from the ongoing inflammatory lesions present in the area. (*Courtesy of Suraj Reddy, MD.*)

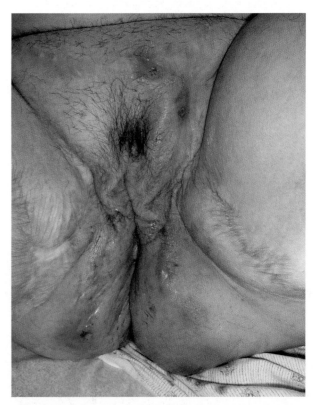

FIGURE 109-7 Thirty-year history of severe hidradenitis in a 54-year-old woman. Note the scars from previous plastic surgeries. Note the draining cysts, fistulas, and the acute abscess on her left buttocks. (*Courtesy of Richard P. Usatine, MD.*)

110 IMPETIGO

Richard P. Usatine, MD

PATIENT STORIES

A young woman presented to the office with a 3-day history of an uncomfortable rash on her lip and chin (**Figure 110-1**). She denied any trauma or previous history of oral herpes. This case of impetigo resolved quickly with oral cephalexin.

An 11-year-old-child presented with a 5-day history of a skin lesion that started after a hiking trip (**Figure 110-2**). This episode of bullous impetigo was found to be secondary to methicillin-resistant *Staphylococcus aureus* (MRSA). The lesion was rapidly progressive and was developing a surrounding cellulitis. She was admitted to a hospital and treated with intravenous clindamycin with good results.[1]

EPIDEMIOLOGY

- Most frequent in children aged 2 to 6 years, but it can be seen in patients of any age.
- Common among homeless people living on the streets.
- Contagious and can be spread within a household.

ETIOLOGY AND PATHOPHYSIOLOGY

- Impetigo is caused by *Staphlococcus aureus* and/or group A beta-hemolytic *Streptococcus* (GABHS).
- Bullous impetigo is almost always caused by *S. aureus* and is less common that the typical crusted impetigo.
- Impetigo may occur after minor skin injury, such as an insect bite, abrasion, or dermatitis.

DIAGNOSIS

CLINICAL FEATURES

- Vesicles, pustules, honey-colored (**Figure 110-1**), brown or dark crusts, erythematous erosions (**Figure 110-3**), ulcers in ecthyma (**Figure 110-4**), bullae in bullous impetigo (**Figures 110-5** to **110-7**).

TYPICAL DISTRIBUTION

- Face (**Figures 110-1, 110-4** to **110-6** and **110-8**) is most common, followed by hands, legs (**Figures 110-2** and **110-9**), trunk, and buttocks.

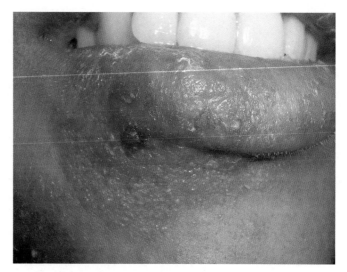

FIGURE 110-1 Typical honey crusted plaque on the lip of an adult with impetigo. (*Courtesy of Richard P. Usatine, MD.*)

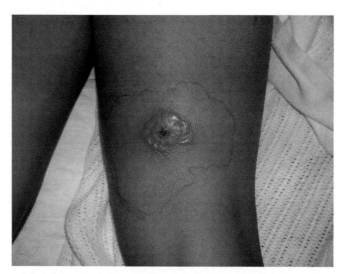

FIGURE 110-2 Bullous impetigo secondary to MRSA on the leg of an 11-year-old child. Note the surrounding cellulitis. (*With permission from Studdiford J, Stonehouse A. Bullous eruption on the posterior thigh 1. J Fam Pract. 2005;54:1041–1044.*)

CULTURE

• Culture is important because of the rising incidence of MRSA-causing impetigo.

DIFFERENTIAL DIAGNOSIS

Many of the conditions below can become impetigo after being secondarily infected (**Figures 110-10** and **110-11**) with bacteria. This process is called impetiginization.

• Atopic dermatitis—a common inflammatory skin disorder characterized by itching and inflamed skin. It can become secondarily infected with bacteria (see Chapter 139, Atopic Dermatitis).

• Herpes simplex virus infection anywhere on the skin or mucus membranes can become secondarily infected (see Chapter 123, Herpes Simplex).

• Eczema herpeticum is eczema superinfected with herpes rather than bacteria (see **Figure 139-4**).

• Scabies—pruritic contagious disease caused by a mite that burrows in skin (see Chapter 137, Scabies).

• Folliculitis—inflammation and/or infection of hair follicles that may be bacterial (see Chapter 111, Folliculitis).

• Tinea corporis—a cutaneous fungal infection caused by dermatophytes, frequently with ring-like scale (see Chapter 132, Tinea Corporis).

• Pemphigus vulgaris—somewhat rare bullous autoimmune condition with flaccid vesicles and bullae that rupture easily affecting people between 40 and 60 years of age (see Chapter 178, Pemphigus).

• Bullous pemphigoid—an autoimmune condition with multiple tense bullae that primarily affects people more than 60 years of age (see Chapter 177, Bullous Pemphigoid).

• Acute allergic contact dermatitis—dermatitis from direct cutaneous exposure to allergens such as poison ivy. Acute lesions are erythematous papules and vesicles in a linear pattern (see Chapter 140, Contact Dermatitis).

• Insect bites—scratched, open lesions can become secondarily infected with bacteria (impetiginized) (**Figure 110-9**).

• Second-degree burn or sunburn—the blisters when opened leave the skin susceptible to secondary infection (**Figure 110-10**).

• Seborrheic dermatitis—on the face or scalp can become secondarily infected (**Figure 110-11**).

• Staphylococcal scalded skin syndrome—life-threatening syndrome of acute exfoliation of the skin caused by an exotoxin from a staphylococcal infection. This condition is seen almost entirely in infants and young children (**Figure 110-12**).

MANAGEMENT

• There is good evidence that topical mupirocin is equally or more effective than oral treatment for people with limited impetigo SOR Ⓐ Mupirocin also covers MRSA.[2]

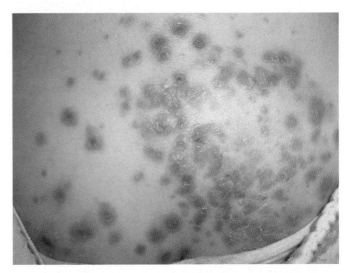

FIGURE 110-3 Widespread impetigo with honey crusted erythematous lesions on the back of a 7-year-old child. (*Courtesy of Richard P. Usatine, MD.*)

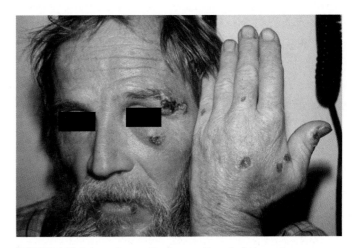

FIGURE 110-4 Impetigo on the face and hand of a homeless man. Note the ecthyma (ulcerated impetigo) on the dorsum of the hand. (*Courtesy of Richard P. Usatine, MD.*)

- In this day of increasing community-acquired MRSA, it is probably best to culture all but the most limited cases of impetigo. SOR **C**

- Extensive impetigo could be treated for 7 days with antibiotics that cover group A beta-hemolytic *Streptococcus* and *S. aureus* such as cephalexin or dicloxacillin.[3] SOR **A**

- Community-acquired MRSA can present as bullous impetigo in children (**Figure 110-2**) or adults.

- If you suspect MRSA, culture the lesions and start one of the following oral antibiotics: trimethoprim/sulfamethoxazole, clindamycin, tetracycline, or doxycycline.[4] SOR **A** Clindamycin has the advantage of covering GABHS and most MRSA. Trimethoprim/sulfamethoxazole has good MRSA coverage but is not recommended for GABHS.

- If there are recurrent MRSA infections, one might choose to prescribe intranasal mupirocin ointment and chlorhexidine bathing to decrease MRSA colonization.[5] SOR **B**

PATIENT EDUCATION

Discuss hygiene issues and how to avoid spread within the household or other living situations such as homeless shelters.

FOLLOW-UP

Arrange follow-up based on severity of case and the age and immune status of the patient. Follow-up on culture results and make sure that the patient is on an antibiotic that covers the cultured organism. This is especially important for MRSA. Be aware of inducible MRSA resistance to clindamycin. If the MRSA susceptibility studies show erythromycin resistance and no resistance to clindamycin, make sure your lab does a disk diffusion induction test (D-test) for clindamycin (if that is the antibiotic you have chosen to use). This will determine a more accurate susceptibility for the clindamycin and can avoid the development of clindamycin resistance during treatment.[6]

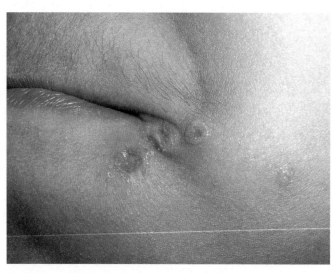

FIGURE 110-5 Bullous impetigo around the mouth of a young boy that progressed to desquamation of the skin on his hands and feet. (*Courtesy of Richard P. Usatine, MD.*)

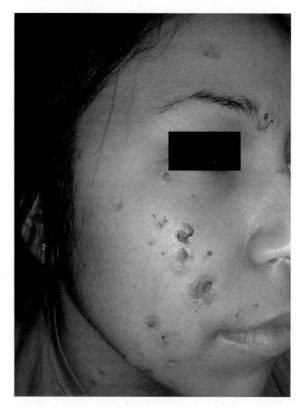

FIGURE 110-6 Bullous impetigo on the face of a 14-year-old girl. MSSA was cultured from the impetigo. (*Courtesy of Richard P. Usatine, MD.*)

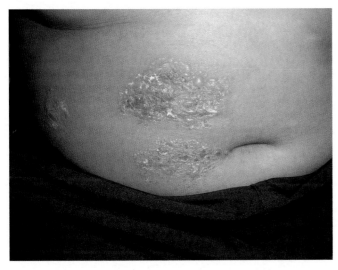

FIGURE 110-7 Bullous impetigo on the abdomen of an 8-year-old boy. (*Courtesy of Richard P. Usatine, MD.*)

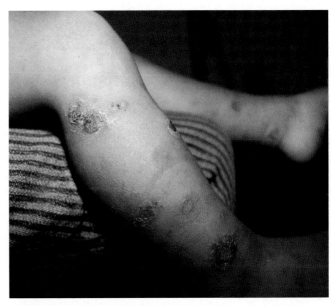

FIGURE 110-9 Impetigo secondary to flea bites on the legs of a young girl. (*Courtesy of Richard P. Usatine, MD, Previously published in the Western Journal of Medicine.*)

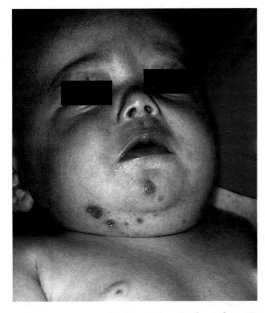

FIGURE 110-8 Impetigo on the face and neck of an infant. (*Courtesy of Richard P. Usatine, MD.*)

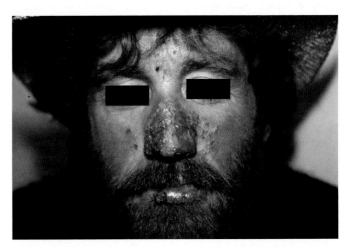

FIGURE 110-10 Secondary impetiginization of a second-degree sunburn in a homeless man. (*Courtesy of Richard P. Usatine, MD.*)

REFERENCES

1. Studdiford J, Stonehouse A. Bullous eruption on the posterior thigh 1. *J Fam Pract.* 2005;54:1041–1044.

2. Koning S, Verhagen AP, van-Suijlekom-Smit LWA, Morris A, Butler CC, van-der-Wouden JC. Interventions for impetigo. The Cochrane Database of Systematic Reviews, 2003, Issue 2. Chichester, UK: John Wiley & Sons. DOI: 10 1002/14651858 CD00326

3. Stevens DL, Bisno AL, Chambers HF, et al. Practice guidelines for the diagnosis and management of skin and soft-tissue infections. *Clin Infect Dis.* 2005;41:1373–1406.

4. Naimi TS, LeDell KH, Como-Sabetti K, et al. Comparison of community- and health care-associated methicillin-resistant *Staphylococcus aureus* infection. *JAMA.* 2003;290:2976–2984.

5. Wendt C, Schinke S, Württemberger M, Oberdorfer K, Bock-Hensley O, von Baum H. Value of whole-body washing with chlorhexidine for the eradication of methicillin-resistant *Staphylococcus aureus:* A randomized, placebo-controlled, double-blind clinical trial. *Infect Control Hosp Epidemiol.* 2007;28(9):1036–1043.

6. Schreckenberger PC, Ilendo E, Ristow KL. Incidence of constitutive and inducible clindamycin resistance in *Staphylococcus aureus* and coagulase-negative *staphylococci* in a community and a tertiary care hospital. *J Clin Microbiol.* 2004;42(6):2777–2779.

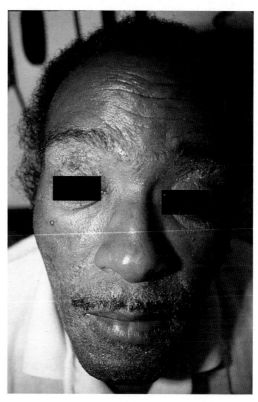

FIGURE 110-11 Seborrheic dermatitis complicated by secondary impetiginization on the eyelids. (*Courtesy of Richard P. Usatine, MD.*)

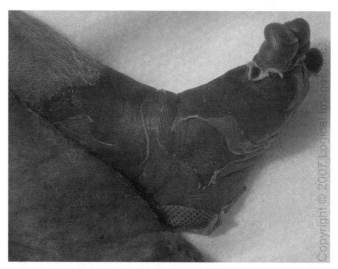

FIGURE 110-12 Staphylococcal scalded skin syndrome in an infant. A severe form of bullous impetigo with large areas of skin exfoliation. (*Courtesy of Logical Images.*)

111 FOLLICULITIS

Khalilah Hunter-Anderson, MD
Richard P. Usatine, MD

PATIENT STORY

A 42-year-old woman is seen for multiple papules and pustules on her back (**Figure 111-1**). Further questioning demonstrates that she was in a friend's hot tub twice over the previous weekend. The outbreak on her back started after she went into the hot tub the second time. This is a case of pseudomonas folliculitis or "hot-tub" folliculitis. The patient avoided this hot tub and the folliculitis disappeared spontaneously. Another option is to treat with an oral fluoroquinolone that covers pseudomonas.

EPIDEMIOLOGY

- Folliculitis is a cutaneous disorder that affects all age groups, race, and gender.

- It can be infectious or noninfectious. It is most commonly of bacterial origin (**Figures 111-2** and **111-3**).

- Pseudofolliculitis or sycosis barbae is most frequently seen in males as a result of shaving (**Figure 111-4**).[1]

- Acne keloidalis nuchae or keloidal folliculitis is commonly seen in black patients but can be seen in patients of any ethnic background (**Figures 111-5** and **111-6**).[2]

- Eosinophilic folliculitis is described in patients with HIV infection (**Figure 111-7**).

- Methicillin-resistant staphylococcus or MRSA can pose a significant challenge to the treatment of folliculitis (**Figure 111-8**).

ETIOLOGY AND PATHOPHYSIOLOGY

- Folliculitis is an infection of the hair follicle and can be superficial in which it is confined to the upper hair follicle; or deep in which inflammation spans the entire depth of the follicle.

- Infection can be of bacterial, viral, or fungal origin. *Staphylococcus aureus* is by far the most common bacterial causative agent.

- The noninfectious form of folliculitis is often seen in adolescents and young adults who wear tight fitting clothes. Folliculitis can also be caused by chemical irritants or physical injury.

- Topical steroid use, ointments, lotions, or makeup can swell the opening to the pilosebaceous unit and cause folliculitis.

- Bacterial folliculitis or staphylococcus folliculitis typically presents as infected pustules most prominent on the face, buttocks, trunk, or extremities. It can progress to a deeper infection with the development of furuncles or boils (**Figure 111-9**). Infection can occur as a result of mechanical injury or via local spread from nearby infected wounds. An area of desquamation is frequently seen surrounding infected pustules in *S. aureus* folliculitis.[1-3]

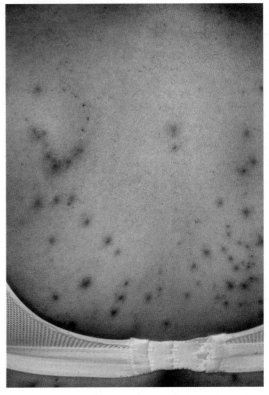

FIGURE 111-1 Pseudofolliculitis from *pseudomonas aeruginosa* in a hot tub. (*Courtesy of Richard P. Usatine, MD.*)

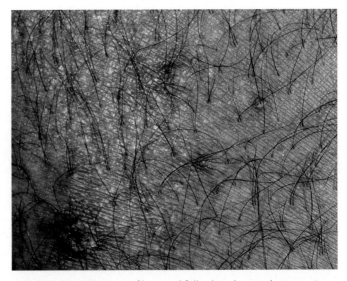

FIGURE 111-2 Close-up of bacterial folliculitis showing hairs coming through pustules. (*Courtesy of Richard P. Usatine, MD.*)

- Parasitic folliculitis usually occurs as a result of mite infestation (Demodex). These are usually seen on the face, nose, and back and typically cause an eosinophilic pustular-like folliculitis.[1]

- Folliculitis decalvans is a chronic form of folliculitis involving the scalp, leading to hair loss or alopecia (**Figure 111-10**). Staphylococci infection is the usual causative agent, but there has also been a suggested genetic component to this condition.[1] It is also called tufted folliculitis because some of the hair follicles will have many hairs growing from them simultaneously (**Figure 111-11**) (see Chapter 182, Scarring Alopecia).

- Acne keloidalis nuchae is a chronic form of folliculitis found on the posterior neck that can be extensive and lead to keloidal tissue and alopecia.[1-3] While it is often thought to occur almost exclusively in black men, it can be seen in men of all ethnic backgrounds and occasionally in women (**Figures 111-5** and **111-6**) (see Chapter 108, Pseudofolliculitis and Acne Keloidalis Nuchae).

- Fungal folliculitis is epidermal fungal infections that are seen frequently. Tinea capitis infections are a form of dermatophytic folliculitis (see Chapter 131, Tinea Capitis). Pityrosporum folliculitis is caused by yeast infection, seen in a similar distribution as bacterial folliculitis on the back, chest, and shoulders (**Figure 111-12**) (see Chapter 135, Tinea Versicolor). Candidal infection is less common and is usually seen in individuals who are immunosuppressed, present in hairy areas that are moist, and unlike most cases of folliculitis, may present with systemic signs and symptoms.[1-4]

- Pseudomonas folliculitis or "hot tub" folliculitis is usually a self-limited infection that follows exposure to water or objects that are contaminated with *pseudomonas aeruginosa* (**Figure 111-1**). This occurs when hot tubs are not adequately chlorinated or brominated. This also occurs when loofah sponges or other items used for bathing become a host for pseudomonal growth. Onset of symptoms is usually within 6 to 72 hours after exposure with the complete resolution of symptoms in a couple of days provided that the individual avoids further exposure.[4]

- Gram-negative folliculitis is an infection with gram-negative bacteria that most typically occurs in individuals who have been on long-term antibiotic therapy usually those taking oral antibiotics for acne. The most frequently encountered infective agents include *Klebsiella*, *Escherichia coli*, *Enterobacter*, and *Proteus*.[5]

- Pseudofolliculitis barbae (razor bumps) is most commonly seen in black males who shave. Papules develop when the sharp edge of the hair shaft reenters the skin (ingrown hairs); seen on the cheeks and neck as a result of curled ingrown hair.[2] It can also occur in women with hirsutism who shave or pluck their hairs (**Figure 111-4**) (see Chapter 108, Pseudofolliculitis and Acne Keloidalis Nuchae).[6]

- Viral folliculitis seen is primarily caused by herpes simplex virus and molluscum contagiosum.[4] Herpetic folliculitis is seen primarily in individuals with a history of herpes simplex infections type I or II. But most notably may be a sign of immunosuppression as is the case with HIV infection.[7] The expression of herpes folliculitis in HIV infection ranges from simple to necrotizing folliculitis and ulcerative lesions. Molluscum is a pox virus and molluscum contagiosum has been well documented in similar patient populations (HIV and AIDS) and also in children (see Chapters 123, Herpes Simplex and 124, Molluscum Contagiosum).[7-9]

FIGURE 111-3 Chronic bacterial folliculitis on the back with scarring and hyperpigmentation. (*Courtesy of E.J. Mayeaux, Jr., MD.*)

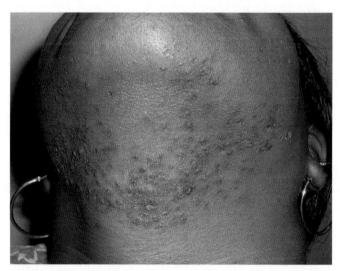

FIGURE 111-4 Pseudofolliculitis and hyperpigmented scars on the neck of a black woman who shaves and plucks out her facial hair. (*Courtesy of Richard P. Usatine, MD.*)

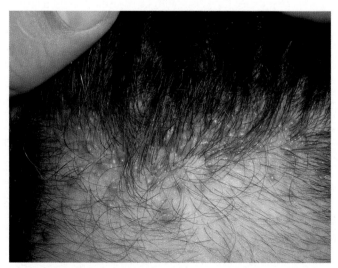

FIGURE 111-5 Acne Keloidalis Nuchae with inflamed papules and pustules on the neck of a young Hispanic man. (*Courtesy of Richard P. Usatine, MD.*)

- Actinic superficial folliculitis is a sterile form of folliculitis seen predominantly in warm climates or during hot or summer months. Pustules occur primarily on the neck, over the shoulders, upper trunk, and upper arms usually within 6 to 36 hours after sun exposure.[10]

- Eosinophilic folliculitis is associated with HIV infection and can occur as a result of the viral infection itself in which case the exact mechanism by which this occurs is uncertain (though felt to be autoimmune) (**Figure 111-7**).[9,11–12,14] It is associated with diminished CD4 cell counts. Eosinophilic folliculitis, generally improves with the initiation of highly active antiretroviral therapy (HAART), but can occur during the restoration of immune function with HAART.[12]

DIAGNOSIS

Often the diagnosis of folliculitis is based on a good history and physical.

CLINICAL FEATURES

Folliculitis has its characteristic presentation as the development of papules or pustules that are thin-walled surrounded by margin of erythema or inflammation. Look for a hair at the center of the lesions (**Figure 111-2**). There is usually an absence of systemic signs and patients symptoms range from mild discomfort and pruritus to severe pain with extensive involvement.

TYPICAL DISTRIBUTION

Any area of the skin may be affected and often location may be related to the pathogen or cause of folliculitis. The face, scalp, neck trunk, axillae, extremities, and groin are some of the more common areas affected.

LABORATORY TESTS

Laboratory testing may be unnecessary in simple superficial folliculitis and where the history is clear and quick resolution occurs. Clinical diagnosis of herpes and fungal folliculitis may be difficult and diagnosis may be made based on strong clinical suspicion or as a result of failed antimicrobial therapy. KOH preps can be used to look for tinea versicolor or other fungal organisms. Herpes culture or a quick test for herpes can be used when herpes is suspected.[1] SOR **A**

DIFFERENTIAL DIAGNOSIS

- *Grover's disease* is very pruritic condition of unknown cause that produces reddish papules and slight scale on the back of middle-aged men. It is also called "transient acantholytic dermatosis" and may resolve spontaneously in a period of years. It resembles folliculitis but the papules are not centered on hair follicles (**Figure 111-13**).

- *Miliaria* is blockage of the sweat glands that can resemble the small papules of folliculitis. The eccrine sweat glands become blocked so that sweat leaks into the dermis and epidermis. Clinically, skin

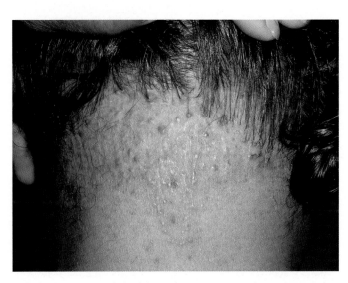

FIGURE 111-6 Acne keloidalis nuchae in a woman demonstrating the folliculitis around the hair follicles and the scarring alopecia that has occurred. (*Courtesy of Richard P. Usatine, MD.*)

FIGURE 111-7 Eosinophilic folliculitis on the chest of an HIV positive woman. (*Courtesy of Richard P. Usatine, MD.*)

lesions may range from clear vesicles to pustules. These skin lesions primarily occur in times of increased heat and humidity, and are self-limited (see Chapter 102, Normal Skin Changes of Infancy).[1]

- *Impetigo* is a bacterial infection of the skin that affects the superficial layers of the epidermis as opposed to hair follicles. It is contagious unlike folliculitis. It has a bullous and nonbullous form, and honey-crusted lesions frequently predominate as opposed to the usual pustules seen in folliculitis (see Chapter 110, Impetigo).[4,6]

- *Keratosis pilaris* consists of papules that occur as a result of a build-up of keratin in the openings of hair follicles especially on the lateral upper arms and thighs. It is not an infection but can develop into folliculitis if lesions become infected (see Chapter 139, Atopic Dermatitis).[1,6]

- *Acne vulgaris* is characterized by the presence of comedones, papules, pustules, and nodules that are as a result of follicular hyperproliferation and plugging with excessive sebum. Inflammation occurs when *Propionibacterium acnes* and other inflammatory substances get extruded from the blocked pilosebaceous unit.[15] While acne on the face is rarely confused with folliculitis, acne on the trunk can resemble folliculitis. To distinguish between them look for facial involvement and comedones seen in acne (see Chapter 106, Acne Vulgaris).

MANAGEMENT

- Management of folliculitis varies by causative agent and underlying pathophysiology.

- Antiviral, antibiotic, and antifungal are used as topical and/or systemic agents. Approaches to nonpharmacologic therapy include patient education on the prevention of chemical and mechanical skin irritation. Glycemic control in diabetic patients may help treat folliculitis.[1–3] Good hygiene helps to control symptoms and prevent recurrence.

- With superficial bacterial folliculitis, treatment with topical preparations such as mupirocin (Bactroban) or fusidic acid may be sufficient.[1] SOR Ⓐ Additionally, topical clindamycin may be considered in the mildest cases in which MRSA is involved.[1] SOR Ⓐ

- Deep or extensive bacterial folliculitis warrants oral therapy with first-generation cephalosporins (cephalexin), penicillins (amoxicillin-clavulanate and dicloxacillin), macrolides, or fluoroquinolones.[1,4,6] SOR Ⓐ

- Pseudomonas or "hot tub" folliculitis will usually resolve untreated within a week of onset (**Figure 111-1**). For severe cases treatment with ciprofloxacin provides adequate antipseudomonal coverage.[1,4] SOR Ⓑ Application of warm compress to affected areas also provides symptomatic relief.

- Pityrosporum folliculitis and/or tinea versicolor can be treated with systemic antifungals, topical azoles, and/or with shampoos containing azoles, selenium, or zinc (**Figure 111-12**) (see Chapter 135, Tinea Versicolor).

- Candidal folliculitis in immunosuppressed persons may be treated with oral itraconazole (see Chapter 130, Mucocutaneous Candidiasis).[1] SOR Ⓐ

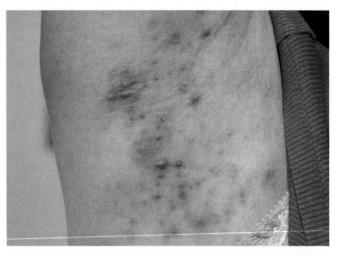

FIGURE 111-8 MRSA folliculitis in the axilla of a 29-year-old woman. The lesions were present for 4 weeks in the axilla, left forearm, and right thigh. The MRSA was sensitive to tetracyclines and resolved with oral doxycycline. (*Courtesy of Alisha N. Plotner, MD and Robert T. Brodell, MD and with permission from J Fam Pract. 2008;57(4):253–255, Dowden Health Media.*)

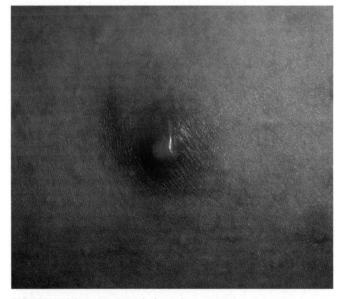

FIGURE 111-9 Isolated single furuncle in an adult woman. (*Courtesy of Richard P. Usatine, MD.*)

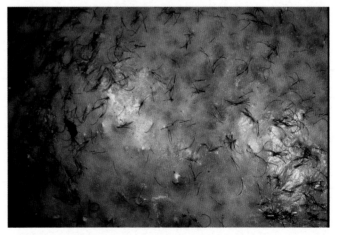

FIGURE 111-10 Close-up of folliculitis decalvans showing inflammation of hair follicles with visible pustules and atrophic scarred areas of the scalp. (*Courtesy of Jeffrey Meffert, MD.*)

- Demodex folliculitis can be treated with Ivermectin or topically with 5% permethrin cream.[4] SOR Ⓐ

- Herpes folliculitis can be treated with acyclovir, valacyclovir, and famciclovir. Regimen may frequently include acyclovir 200 mg 5 times a day for 5 days (see Chapter 123, Herpes Simplex).[1] SOR Ⓐ

- Eosinophilic folliculitis associated with HIV is treated with HAART, topical steroids, antihistamines, itraconazole, metronidazole, oral retinoids, and UV light therapy.[11] Topical steroids and nonsteroidal anti-inflammatory agents (NSAIDs) and isotretinoin are treatments of choice for HIV associated eosinophilic folliculitis.[9–13] SOR Ⓑ Relief with systemic antihistamines are variable and UV therapy is time consuming and expensive.[11,12] SOR Ⓒ

PATIENT EDUCATION

Prevention is most important, and centers on good personal hygiene and proper laundering of clothing. Patients should be encouraged to avoid tight fitting clothing. Hot tubs should be properly cleaned and the chemicals should be maintained appropriately. Electric razors for shaving can help prevent pseudofolliculitis barbae and should be cleaned regularly with alcohol. Patients with acne keloidalis nuchae should avoid shaving the hair in the involved area.

FOLLOW-UP

Most cases of folliculitis are superficial and resolve easily with treatment. Dermatologic and surgical consultation may be required in cases of chronic folliculitis with scarring.

PATIENT RESOURCES

- http://www.mayoclinic.com/health/folliculitis/DS00512.

PROVIDER RESOURCES

- http://www.emedicine.com/derm/topic159.htm.

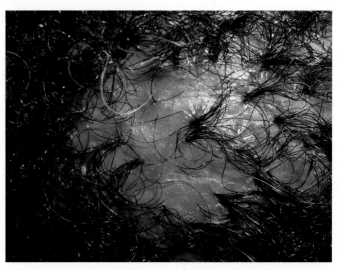

FIGURE 111-11 Tufted folliculitis in a 34-year-old black man with visible tufts of hair (multiple hairs from one follicle) growing from a number of abnormal follicles. There are crusts and hair loss. (*Courtesy of Richard P. Usatine, MD.*)

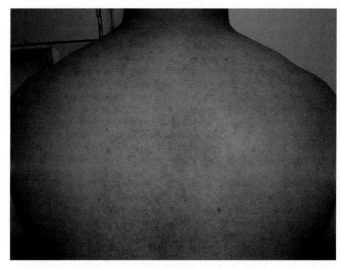

FIGURE 111-12 Pityrosporum folliculitis on the back of a young black man. KOH preparation showed Pityrosporum looking like ziti and meatballs. (*Courtesy of Richard P. Usatine, MD.*)

REFERENCES

1. Luelmo-Aguilar J, Santandreu MS. Folliculitis recognition and management. *Am J Clin Dermatol.* 2004;5(5):301–310.

2. Habif T. *Clinical Dermatology*, 4th ed St Louis: Mosby, 2004.

3. Levy AL, Simpson G, Skinner RB Jr., Medical pearl: Circle of desquamation, a clue to the diagnosis of folliculitis and furunculosis caused by Staphylococcus aureus. *J Am Acad Dermatol.* 2006; 55(6):1079–1080.

4. Stulberg DL, Penrod MA, Blatny RA. Common bacterial skin infections. *Am Fam Physician.* 2002;66(1):119–124.

5. Neubert U, Jansen T, Plewig G. Bacteriologic and immunologic aspects of gram-negative folliculitis: A study of 46 patients. *Int J Dermatol.* 1999;38(4):270–274.

6. *Ferri's Clinical Advisor 2007: Instant Diagnosis and Treatment*. 9th ed. www.clinderm.com.

7. Boer A, Herder N, Winter K, Falk T. Herpes folliculitis: Clinical histopathological, and molecular pathologic observations. *Br J Dermatol.* 2006;154(4):743–746.

8. Weinberg JM. Mysliwiec A, Turiansky GW, Redfield R, James WD. Viral folliculitis. Atypical presentations of herpes simplex, herpes zoster, and molluscum contagiosum. *Arch Dermatol.* 1997;133(8):983–986.

9. Fearfield LA, Rowe A, Francis N, et al. Itchy folliculitis and human immunodeficiency virus infection: Clinicopathological and immunological features, pathogenesis and treatment. *Br J Dermatol.* 1999;141(1):3–11.

10. Labandeira J, Suarez-Campos A, Toribio J. Actinic superficial folliculitis. *Br J Dermatol.* 1998;138(6):1070–1074.

11. Nervi SJ, Schwartz RA, Dmochowski M. Eosinophilic pustular folliculitis: A 40 years retrospect. *J Am Acad Dermatol.* 2006;55(2): 285–289.

12. Rajendran PM, Dolev JC, et al. Eosinophilic folliculits: Before and after the introduction of antiretroviral therapy. *Arch Dermatol.* 2005;141(10):1227–1231.

13. Jang KA, Kim SH, Choi JH, Sung KJ, Moon KC, Koh JK. Viral folliculitis on the face. *Br J Dermatol.* 2000;142(3):555–559.

14. Toutous-Trellu L, Abraham S, Pechère M, et al. Topical tacrolimus for effective treatment of eosinophilic folliculitis associated with human immunodeficiency virus infection. *Arch Dermatol.* 2005; 141(10):1203–1208.

15. Strauss JS, Krowchuk DP, Leyden JJ, et al. Guidelines of care for acne vulgaris management. *J Am Acad Dermatol.* 2007;56(4): 651–663.

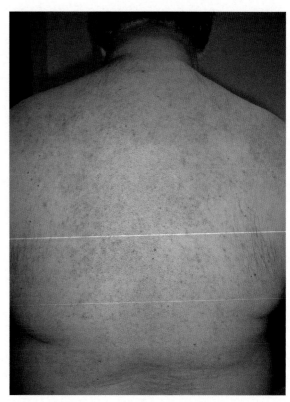

FIGURE 111-13 Grover's disease on the back of a middle-age man. This is also called "transient acantholytic dermatosis." It is very pruritic with reddish papules and slight scale. (*Courtesy of Richard P. Usatine, MD.*)

112 PITTED KERATOLYSIS

Michael Babcock, MD
Richard P. Usatine, MD

PATIENT STORY

A 34-year-old man comes to the office with a terrible foot odor problem. He is wearing cowboy boots and he says that his feet are always sweaty. He is embarrassed to remove his boots, but when the physician convinces him to do so the odor is overwhelming. While breathing through the mouth, the physician sees the typical pits of pitted keratolysis. His socks are moist and the skin is somewhat macerated from the hyperhidrosis. His foot has many crateriform pits on the heel (**Figure 112-1**). He is prescribed topical erythromycin solution for the pitted keratolysis and topical aluminum chloride for the hyperhidrosis. It is suggested that he wear a lighter and more breathable shoe until this problem improves.

EPIDEMIOLOGY

- Seen more commonly in men.
- Often a complication of hyperhidrosis.
- Seen more often in hot and humid climates.

ETIOLOGY AND PATHOPHYSIOLOGY

- Pitted keratolysis is the result of a gram-positive bacterial infection of the stratum corneum.
- *Kytococcus sedentarius* (formerly *Micrococcus* spp.), *Corynebacterium* species, and *Dermatophilus congolensis* have all been shown to cause pitted keratolysis.[1]
- Proteases produced by the bacteria degrade keratins to give the clinical appearance.[2]
- The associated malodor is likely secondary to the production of sulfur by-products.[1]

DIAGNOSIS

CLINICAL FEATURES

Pitted keratolysis usually presents as painless, malodorous, slimy crateriform pits coalescing into larger superficial erosions of the stratum corneum (**Figures 112-1 to 112-4**). It may be associated with itching and a burning sensation in some patients (**Figure 112-2**).

TYPICAL DISTRIBUTION

Pitted keratolysis usually involves the callused pressure-bearing areas of the foot, such as heel, ball of the foot, and plantar great toe. It can also be found in friction areas between the toes.[3]

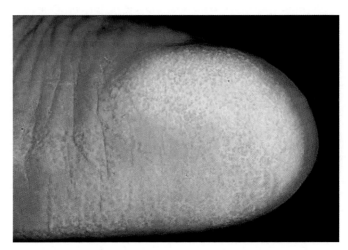

FIGURE 112-1 Many crateriform pits on the heel of a foot in a man with pitted keratolysis and hyperhidrosis. (*Courtesy of Richard P. Usatine, MD.*)

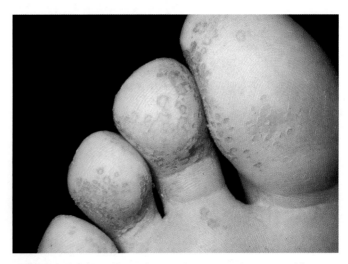

FIGURE 112-2 Pitted keratolysis on the pressure-bearing and friction areas of the toes. This 17-year-old male athlete noticed that his feet had an itchy, burning sensation at the heels and toes. His foot odor had become so malodorous (somewhat akin to rotting fish) that he would not remove his shoes except immediately before washing his feet. (*Reprinted with permission from Meffert JJ. "Toxic Sock" Syndrome. May 1, 1998, American Family Physician 1998;57(9): 2215–2216. Copyright © 1998 American Academy of Family Physicians. All Rights Reserved.*)

LABORATORY STUDIES

Typically a clinical diagnosis but biopsy will reveal keratin pits lined by bacteria.

DIFFERENTIAL DIAGNOSIS

• Characteristic clinical features make the diagnosis easy, but it is possible to have other diseases causing plantar pits, which can be included in the differential. These include plantar warts, basal cell nevus syndrome, and arsenic toxicity.

• Plantar warts are typically not as numerous. They have a firm callus ring around a soft core with small black dots from thrombosed capillaries (see Chapter 128, Plantar Warts).

• Basal cell nevus syndrome will typically have pits involving the palms and soles, bone abnormalities, a history of many basal cell carcinomas, and a characteristic facies with frontal bossing, hypoplastic maxilla, and hypertelorism (wide set eyes) (see Chapter 163, Basal Cell Carcinoma).

• Arsenic toxicity can result in pits on the palms and soles, but it can also have hyperpigmentation, many skin cancers, Mee's lines (white lines on the fingernails), or other nail disorders.

MANAGEMENT

• Treatment is based on bacterial elimination and reducing the moist environment in which the bacteria thrive. Various topical antibiotics are effective for pitted keratolysis.

• Topical erythromycin or clindamycin solution or gel can be applied twice daily until the condition resolves. SOR Ⓒ Generic 2% erythromycin solution with and applicator top is a very inexpensive and effective preparation. It may take 3 to 4 weeks to clear the odor and skin lesions.

• Topical mupirocin is more expensive but also effective. SOR Ⓒ

• Oral erythromycin is effective and may be considered if topical therapy fails. SOR Ⓒ

• Treating underlying hyperhidrosis is also important to prevent recurrence. This can be done with topical aluminum chloride of varying concentrations. SOR Ⓒ Drysol is 20% aluminum chloride solution and can be prescribed with an applicator top.

• Botulinum toxin injections is an expensive and effective treatment for hyperhidrosis.[4] SOR Ⓒ It should be reserved for treatment failures because of the cost, the discomfort of the multiple injections, and the need to repeat the treatment every 3 to 4 months.

PATIENT EDUCATION

Patients should be taught about the etiology of this disorder to help avoid recurrence. Helpful preventative strategies include avoiding occlusive footwear and use moisture-wicking socks or changing sweaty socks frequently.

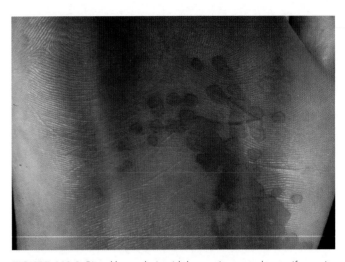

FIGURE 112-3 Pitted keratolysis with hyperpigmented crateriform pits coalescing into superficial erosions on the pressure-bearing areas of the foot. (*Courtesy of Jeffrey Meffert, MD.*)

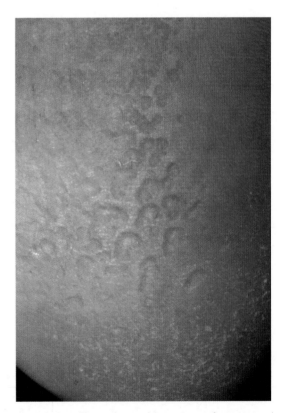

FIGURE 112-4 Pitted keratolysis with many crateriform pits coalescing into superficial erosions on the heel. (*Courtesy of Jeffrey Meffert, MD.*)

FOLLOW-UP

Follow-up is needed for treatment failures, recurrences, and the treatment of underlying hyperhidrosis if present. This can be annually for prescription aluminum chloride or approximately every 3 to 4 months for botulinum toxin injections.

PATIENT RESOURCES

http://www.sweathelp.org

http://www.aad.org/public/publications/pamphlets/
common_hyperhidrosis.html

PROVIDER RESOURCES

http://www.emedicine.com/derm/topic332.htm

REFERENCES

1. Bolognia J, Jorizzo J, Rapini R. *Dermatology*. 2nd ed. Mosby, Philadelphia, 2008;1088–1089.

2. Takama H, Tamada Y, Yano K, et al. Pitted Keratolysis: Clinical manifestations in 53 cases. *Br J Dermatol*. 1997;137(2):282–285.

3. Longshaw C, Wright J, Farrell A, et al. *Kytococcus sedentarius*, the organism associated with pitted keratolysis, produces two keratin-degrading enzymes. *J Appl Microbiol*. 2002;93(5):810–816.

4. Vadoud-Seyedi J. Treatment of plantar hyperhidrosis with botulinum toxin type A. *Int J Dermatol*. 2004;43(12):969–971.

113 ERYTHRASMA

Anna Allred, MD
Richard P. Usatine, MD

PATIENT STORY

A 12-year-old Hispanic girl, accompanied by her mother, presents with a 1-year history of a red irritated rash in both axilla (**Figure 113-1**). She has been seen by multiple physicians and many antifungal creams had been tried with no results. Even hydrocortisone did not help. She had stopped wearing deodorant for fear that she was allergic to all deodorants. While the rash barely fluoresced at all, the physical examination and history were most consistent with erythrasma. The patient was given a prescription for oral erythromycin and the erythrasma cleared to the great delight of the patient and her mother.

EPIDEMIOLOGY

- Erythrasma is caused by the diphtheroid *Corynebacterium minutissimum* organism, which is present in the normal skin flora and favors heat and humidity.
- As a result, erythrasma is also more commonly found in warmer climate regions.
- Erythrasma is more commonly found in those with diabetes, immunocompromised states, obesity, hyperhidrosis, poor hygiene, and advanced age.
- Both sexes are equally affected.
- The inguinal location is more common in men.

ETIOLOGY AND PATHOPHYSIOLOGY

- *Corynebacterium minutissimum*, a lipophilic gram-positive nonspore forming rod-shaped organism, is the causative agent.
- Under favorable conditions, such as heat and humidity, this organism invades and proliferates the upper one-third of the stratum corneum.
- The organism produces porphyrins which result in the coral red fluorescence seen under a Wood's lamp (**Figure 113-2**).

DIAGNOSIS

CLINICAL FEATURES

- Erythrasma is a sharply delineated, dry, red-brown patch with slightly scaling patches. Some lesions appear redder while others have a browner color (**Figures 113-3** and **113-4**).
- The lesions may appear with central clearing and be slightly raised from the surrounding skin (**Figure 113-5**).
- The lesions are typically asymptomatic; however, patients complain of itching and burning when lesions occur in the groin (**Figure 113-6**).

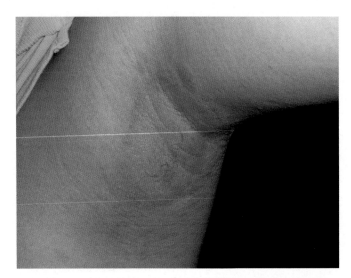

FIGURE 113-1 Erythrasma in the axilla of a 12-year-old Hispanic girl. (*Courtesy of Richard P. Usatine, MD.*)

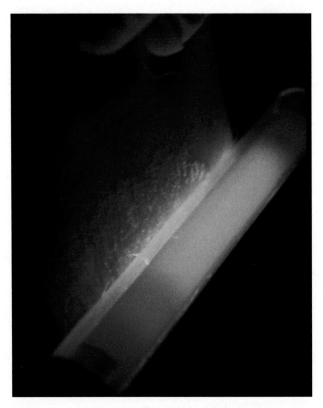

FIGURE 113-2 Coral red fluorescence seen with a Wood's lamp held in the axilla of a patient with erythrasma. (*Courtesy of the University of Texas Health Sciences Center, Division of Dermatology.*)

TYPICAL DISTRIBUTION

Erythrasma is characteristically found in the intertriginous areas especially the axilla and the groin. Patches of erythrasma may also be found in the interspaces of the toes, intergluteal cleft, perianal skin, and inframammary area.

LABORATORY STUDIES

Illumination of the plaque with a Wood's lamp reveals coral-red fluorescence. It should be noted, that washing the area before examination may eliminate the fluorescence. The diagnosis may be confirmed by applying Gram stain or methylene blue stain to scrapings from the skin to reveal gram-positive rods and dark blue granules, respectively. However, if the presentation is typical and the plaque reveals fluorescence then microscopic examination and cultures are not needed. Microscopic examination is useful if erythrasma is suspected but the plaque does not fluoresce.

DIFFERENTIAL DIAGNOSIS

- Psoriasis—inverse psoriasis occurs in the same areas as erythrasma and also causes pink to red plaques with well-demarcated borders. The best way to distinguish psoriasis from erythrasma is to look for other clues of psoriasis in the patient, including nail pitting or onycholysis and hyperkeratotic plaques on the elbows, knees, or scalp. Also, inverse psoriasis may be seen in the intergluteal cleft as well as below the breasts or pannus in overweight individuals (see Chapter 145, Psoriasis). The Wood's lamp may help differentiate between these diagnoses.

- Dermatophytosis—cutaneous fungal infections also closely resemble erythrasma when they occur in the axillary and inguinal areas. Tinea infections also have well-demarcated borders that can be raised with central clearing. This distinctive ringworm look is more obvious with tinea than erythrasma but a scraping for microscopic examination should be able to distinguish between the two conditions. Examination of the feet will frequently show tinea pedis and onychomycosis when there are tinea infections elsewhere on the body (see Chapter 132, Tinea Corposis and Chapter 133, Tinea Crusis).

- Candidiasis—look for satellite lesions to help distinguish candidiasis from erythrasma. Candidiasis will not fluoresce and a microscopic examination with *Candida* infections should show branching pseudohyphae (see Chapter 130, Mucocutaneous Candidiasis).

- Intertrigo—is a term for inflammation in intertriginous areas (skin folds). It is caused or exacerbated by heat, moisture, maceration, friction, and lack of air circulation. It is frequently made worse by infection with *Candida*, bacteria, or dermatophytes and therefore overlaps with the erythrasma, candida, and dermatophytosis. Obesity and diabetes especially predispose to this condition. All efforts should be made to find coexisting infections and treat them.

- Contact dermatitis to deodorants can mimic erythrasma. The history and Wood's lamp should help to differentiate the two conditions (see Chapter 140, Contact Dermatitis).

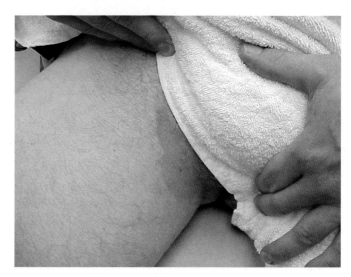

FIGURE 113-3 Light brown erythrasma in the groin of a young man. It does not have the degree of scaling usually seen with tinea cruris. (*Courtesy of Dan Stulberg, MD.*)

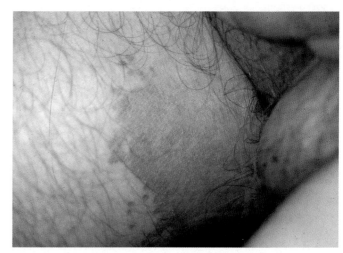

FIGURE 113-4 Brown erythrasma in the groin of a man with diabetes. (*Courtesy of the University of Texas Health Sciences Center, Division of Dermatology.*)

MANAGEMENT

- The treatment of choice is oral erythromycin 250 mg 4 times a day for 14 days, showing cure rates as high as 100%.[1,2,3] SOR **B**
  - However, some advocate that oral erythromycin is only required for the treatment of extensive or resistant cases.[4] SOR **C**
  - Topical therapy has been recommended in addition to oral therapy in patients with hidden reservoirs of infection (i.e., interdigital involvement.) SOR **C**
    - Topical clindamycin may be applied once daily during the course of oral erythromycin therapy and for 2 weeks after physical clearance of the lesions for treatment and prophylaxis.[3,5] SOR **C**
- Topical erythromycin 2% solution applied twice daily.[2,4,6] SOR **C**
  - It has been advocated that the areas should be vigorously washed with soap and water prior to application of topical antibiotics.[4] SOR **C**
  - The patient may also wear loose-fitting cotton undergarments during treatment and to help prevent recurrence.[4] SOR **C**
- Tight blood glucose control is recommended in the management of a diabetic patient with erythrasma.[1] SOR **C**

PATIENT EDUCATION

Reassure that erythrasma is curable with antibiotic treatment.

FOLLOW-UP

Have the patient follow up in 2 to 4 weeks as needed to determine if erythrasma resolved.

PATIENT RESOURCES

http://www.dermnetnz.org/bacterial/erythrasma.html.

PROVIDER RESOURCES

http://www.emedicine.com/derm/topic140.htm.

REFERENCES

1. Ahmed I, Goldstein B. Diabetes mellitus. *Clin Dermatol.* 2006; 24(4):237–246.

2. James WD, Berger TG, Elston DM. *Andrew's Diseases of the Skin Clinical Dermatology.* 10th ed. London: Saunders/Elsevier, 2006.

3. Holdiness MR. Management of cutaneous erythrasma. *Drugs.* 2002;62(8):1131–1141.

4. Karakatsanis G, Vakirlis E, Kastoridou C, Devliotou-Panagiotidou D. Coexistence of pityriasis versicolor and erythrasma. *Mycoses.* 2004;47(7):343–345.

5. Holdiness MR. Erythrasma and common bacterial skin infections. *Am Fam Physician.* 2003;15;67(2):254.

6. Miller SD, David-Bajar K. Images in clinical medicine. A brilliant case of erythrasma. *N Engl J Med.* 2004;14;351(16):1666.

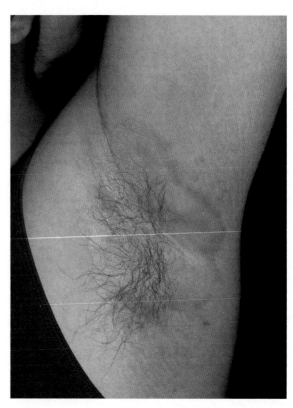

FIGURE 113-5 Pinkish erythrasma in the axilla of a 32-year-old man with some central clearing and elevated borders. (*Courtesy of Richard P. Usatine, MD.*)

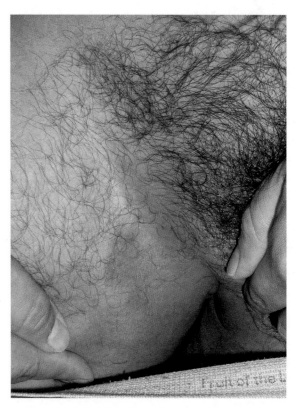

FIGURE 113-6 Pinkish erythrasma in the groin of the man in **Figure 113-5**. Men are more likely to have erythrasma in the crural region. (*Courtesy of Richard P. Usatine, MD.*)

114 CELLULITIS

Richard P. Usatine, MD

PATIENT STORY

A 4-year-old child presents with a fever and a red and swollen foot (**Figure 114-1**). The patient injured her foot 3 days before with a door. On physical examination, the foot was warm, tender, red, and swollen, and the child's temperature was 103°F. This is classic cellulitis and the child was admitted for IV antibiotics.

EPIDEMIOLOGY

- Facial cellulitis occurs more often in adults aged 50 years or older, or children aged 6 months to 3 years.
- Perianal cellulitis occurs more commonly in young children but can be seen in adults as well (see Chapter 105, Diaper and Perianal Dermatitis).

ETIOLOGY AND PATHOPHYSIOLOGY

- An acute infection of the skin that involves the dermis and subcutaneous tissues.
- Often begins with a break in the skin caused by trauma, a bite, or an underlying dermatosis (e.g., tinea pedis, stasis dermatitis) (**Figures 114-2 to 114-4**).
- Is most often caused by group A beta-hemolytic *Streptococcus* (GABHS) or *Staphylococcus aureus.* May also be caused by beta-hemolytic *Streptococcus* from groups B, C, or G.
- After a cat or dog bite, is often caused by *Pasteurella multocida.*
- After saltwater exposure, cellulitis can be secondary to *Vibrio vulnificus* in warm climates.

Erysipelas is a specific type of superficial cellulitis with prominent lymphatic involvement and leading to a sharply defined and elevated border (**Figure 144-5**).

DIAGNOSIS

CLINICAL FEATURES

Rubor (red), calor (warm), tumor (swollen), and dolor (painful).

TYPICAL DISTRIBUTION

Can occur on any part of the body, but is most often seen on the extremities and face (**Figures 114-1 to 114-7**). Periorbital cellulitis can be life-threatening (**Figure 114-8**). Cellulitis can also occur around the anus. This is called perianal cellulitis (**Figure 114-9**).

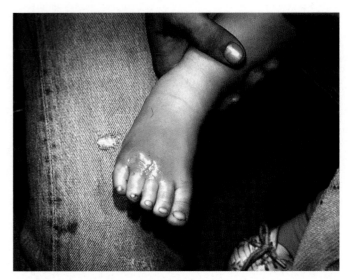

FIGURE 114-1 Cellulitis of the foot after an injury with a door in a 4-year-old girl. (*Courtesy of Richard P. Usatine, MD.*)

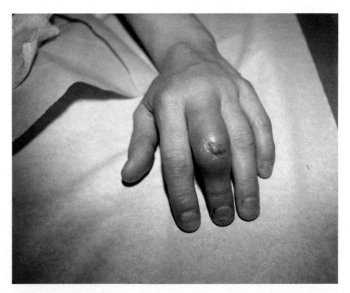

FIGURE 114-2 Cellulitis of the finger after a clenched fist injury in which the patient cut his finger on the tooth of the man he assaulted. (*Courtesy of Richard P. Usatine, MD.*)

BLOOD CULTURE

Results are positive in only 5% of cases and the results of culture of needle aspirations of the inflamed skin are variable and not recommended.[1]

DIFFERENTIAL DIAGNOSIS

- Thrombophlebitis—inflammation of a vein caused by a blood clot. The pain and tenderness are over the involved vein.

- Venous stasis—swelling, discoloration, and pain of the lower extremities that can lead to cellulitis. Venous stasis dermatitis can add erythema and scaling to the picture and resemble cellulitis (**Figure 114-4**) (see Chapter 50, Venous Stasis).

- Allergic reactions—allergic reactions to vaccines or bug bites may resemble cellulitis because of the erythema and swelling. (**Figure 114-10**).

- Acute gout—may resemble cellulitis if there is significant cutaneous inflammation beyond the involved joint (see Chapter 94, Gout).

- Necrotizing fasciitis—deep infection of the subcutaneous tissues and fascia with diffuse swelling, severe pain, and bullae in a toxic-appearing patient. It is important to recognize the difference between standard cellulitis and necrotizing fasciitis. Imaging procedures can detect gas in the soft tissues. Rapid progression from mild erythema to violaceous or necrotic lesions and/or bullae in a number of hours is a red flag for necrotizing fasciitis. The toxicity of the patient and the other physical findings should encourage rapid surgical consultation (see Chapter 116, Necrotizing Fasciitis).

MANAGEMENT

- The first decision is whether or not the patient needs hospitalization and IV antibiotics. It is often best to hospitalize any immunocompromised patients (HIV, transplant, chronic renal or liver disease, on prednisone, diabetes out of control) with cellulitis because they may decompensate quickly.

- Evidence comparing different durations of treatment, oral versus intravenous antibiotics is lacking.[2] RCTs comparing different antibiotic regimens found clinical cure in 50% to 100% of people, but provided insufficient information on differences between regimens.[2] SOR **A**

- One quasirandomized trial in 73 hospitalized people with erysipelas, but excluding patients with clinical signs of septicemia comparing oral versus intravenous penicillin, found no significant difference in clinical efficacy.[2] SOR **B**

- Standard oral therapy for cellulitis not requiring hospitalization involves covering GABHS and *S. aureus* with cephalexin or dicloxacillin.[1] SOR **A** The standard dose is 500 mg orally every 6 hours for each antibiotic and the typical duration is 7 to 10 days. SOR **C**

- Penicillin allergic patients may be treated with clindamycin rather than erythromycin because of the growing macrolide resistance in the United States.[1] SOR **A**

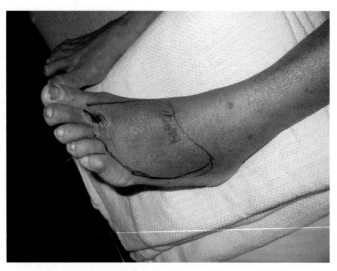

FIGURE 114-3 Cellulitis of the foot of a diabetic person in which there is possible necrosis and gangrene of the second toe, requiring hospitalization and a podiatry consult. (*Courtesy of Richard P. Usatine, MD.*)

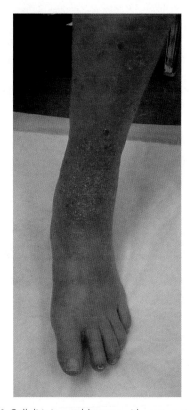

FIGURE 114-4 Cellulitis in an older man with venous stasis dermatitis. (*Courtesy of Richard P. Usatine, MD.*)

- Parenteral treatment is usually done with penicillinase-resistant penicillins or first-generation cephalosporins such as cefazolin, or, for patients with life-threatening penicillin allergies, clindamycin, or vancomycin.[1] SOR **A**

- In cases of uncomplicated cellulitis, 5 days of antibiotic treatment with levofloxacin is as effective as a 10-day course.[3] SOR **B** This is not a good choice if MRSA is suspected.

- Treat underlying conditions (e.g., tinea pedis, lymphedema) that predispose the patient to the infection.

- While MRSA is increasing in its prevalence in skin and soft tissue infections,[4] the difficulty in obtaining microbiological cultures for cellulitis makes it difficult to know how much MRSA is a problem in cellulitis. If there is a coexisting abscess or crusting lesion, it is best to obtain a culture to guide therapy. Consider treating empirically for MRSA based on your local community data and lack of response to initial treatment with antibiotics known not to cover MRSA. SOR **C**

- When MRSA is suspected, clindamycin may be a good empirical choice because it covers GABHS and most MRSA. Trimethoprim/ sulfamethoxazole has good MRSA coverage but is not recommended for GABHS which is a common organism in cellulitis. If clindamycin is chosen, be aware of inducible MRSA resistance to clindamycin. If the MRSA susceptibility studies show erythromycin resistance and no resistance to clindamycin, make sure your lab does a disk diffusion induction test (D-test) for clindamycin. This will determine a more accurate susceptibility for the clindamycin and can avoid the development of clindamycin resistance during treatment.[5]

- Do not miss necrotizing fasciitis. Patients with severe pain, bullae, crepitus, skin necrosis, or significant toxicity merit imaging and immediate surgical consultation (see Chapter 116, Necrotizing Fasciitis).

PATIENT EDUCATION

Recommend that the patient rest and elevate the involved extremity. If outpatient therapy is followed, then provide precautions (e.g., vomiting and unable to hold medicine down) for which the patient should seek more immediate follow-up.

FOLLOW-UP

If prescribing oral outpatient therapy, consider follow-up in 1 to 2 days to assess response to the antibiotic and to determine the adequacy of outpatient therapy.

PATIENT RESOURCES

Medline Plus for patients—**http://www.nlm.nih.gov/ medlineplus/cellulitis.html.**

http://en.wikipedia.org/wiki/Cellulitis.

PROVIDER RESOURCES

http://www.emedicine.com/derm/topic464.htm.

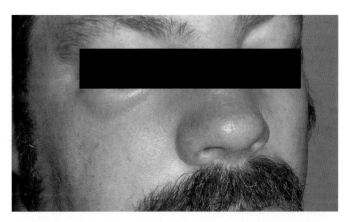

FIGURE 114-5 Erysipelas of the central face that responded well to oral antibiotic therapy. (*Courtesy of Ernesto Samano Ayon, MD.*)

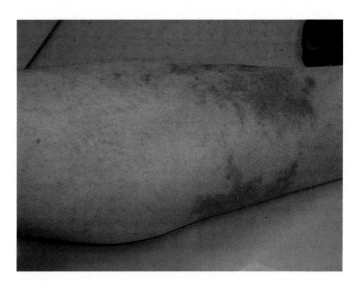

FIGURE 114-6 Cellulitis of the leg in a 55-year-old man that developed after a minor abrasion and a long plane flight. Petechiae and ecchymoses are visible and not infrequently seen in cellulitis. (*Courtesy of Richard P. Usatine, MD.*)

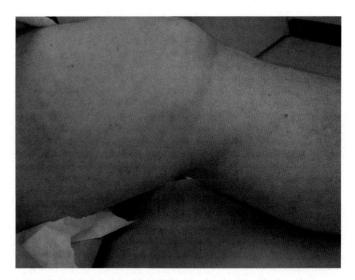

FIGURE 114-7 Ascending lymphangitis characterized by lymphatic streaking up the leg in the same patient. (*Courtesy of Richard P. Usatine, MD.*)

REFERENCES

1. Stevens DL, Bisno AL, Chambers HF, et al. Practice guidelines for the diagnosis and management of skin and soft-tissue infections. *Clin Infect Dis.* 2005;41:1373–1406.

2. Morris A. Cellulitis and erysipelas. *Clin Evid.* 2004;2271–2277.

3. Hepburn MJ, Dooley DP, Skidmore PJ, Ellis MW, Starnes WF, Hasewinkle WC. Comparison of short-course (5 days) and standard (10 days) treatment for uncomplicated cellulitis. *Arch Intern Med.* 2004;164:1669–1674.

4. Moran GJ, Krishnadasan A, Gorwitz RJ, et al. For the Emergency ID Net Study Group. Methicillin-resistant S. aureus infections among patients in the emergency department. *N Engl J Med.* 2006;355:666–674.

5. Schreckenberger PC, Ilendo E, Ristow KL. Incidence of constitutive and inducible clindamycin resistance in Staphylococcus aureus and coagulase-negative staphylococci in a community and a tertiary care hospital. *J Clin Microbiol.* 2004;42(6):2777–2779.

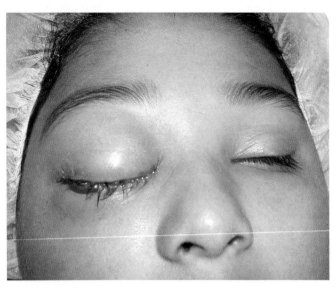

FIGURE 114-8 Life-threatening staphylococcal periorbital cellulitis requiring operative intervention. (*Courtesy of Frank Miller, MD.*)

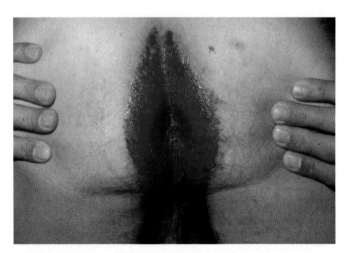

FIGURE 114-9 Severe perianal cellulitis in an adult man. (*Courtesy of Jack Resneck Sr., MD.*)

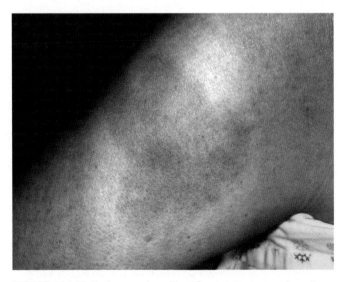

FIGURE 114-10 Redness and swelling after a pneumococcal vaccine the day before in a 66-year-old woman. This allergic reaction looks like bacterial cellulitis. It resolved with oral diphenhydramine. (*Courtesy of Richard P. Usatine, MD.*)

115 ABSCESS

Richard P. Usatine, MD

PATIENT STORY

A young man is seen in a shelter in San Antonio after being evacuated from New Orleans after the devastating floods of Hurricane Katrina (**Figure 115-1**). He has facial pain and swelling and noticeable pus near the eye. His vision is normal. The area is anesthetized with lidocaine and epinephrine. The abscess is drained with a #11 blade. The patient is started on an oral antibiotic because of the proximity to the eye and the local swelling that could represent early cellulitis. A culture to look for methicillin-resistant *Staphylococcus aureus* (MRSA) was not available in the shelter, but close follow-up was set for the next day and patient was doing much better.

EPIDEMIOLOGY

- Changing resistance patterns of *S. aureus* requires consideration that the abscess is caused by MRSA.
- Risk factors for MRSA infection and other abscesses—IVDA, homelessness, dental disease, contact sports, incarceration, and high prevalence in the community.

ETIOLOGY AND PATHOPHYSIOLOGY

- Most cutaneous abscesses are caused by *S. aureus*.
- Community acquired MRSA can cause single or multiple abscesses, especially in persons using IV drugs, living on the streets, or in prisons.
- A dental abscess can spread into tissue outside the mouth as in the homeless person in **Figure 115-2**.
- Community acquired MRSA has become so prevalent in our community that both the patients shown in **Figures 115-3** and **115-4** had no special risk factors and both had abscesses that grew out MRSA.

DIAGNOSIS

CLINICAL FEATURES

Collection of pus in or below the skin. Patients often feel pain and have tenderness at the involved site. There is swelling, erythema, warmth, and fluctuance in most cases (**Figures 115-1** to **115-4**).

TYPICAL DISTRIBUTION

Skin abscesses can be found anywhere from head to feet. Frequent sites include the hands, feet, extremities, head, neck, buttocks, and breast.

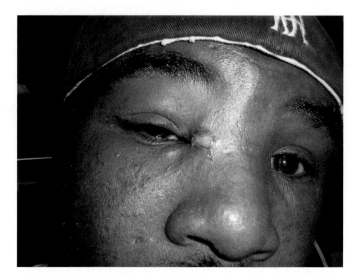

FIGURE 115-1 Abscess seen on the face of a man after evacuation from the flood waters of New Orleans following Hurricane Katrina. (*Courtesy of Richard P. Usatine, MD.*)

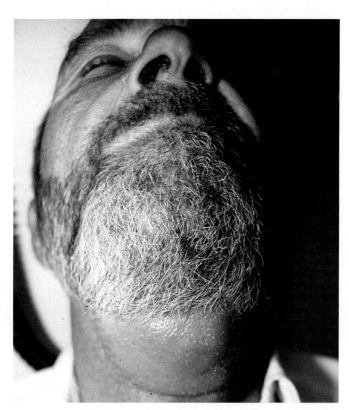

FIGURE 115-2 Neck abscess secondary to dental abscess in a homeless man. This was drained in the OR by ENT. (*Courtesy of Richard P. Usatine, MD.*)

LABORATORY STUDIES

Culture to determine if the organism is MRSA to guide antibiotic treatment when needed.

DIFFERENTIAL DIAGNOSIS

- Epidermal inclusion cyst with inflammation/infection—these cysts (AKA sebaceous cysts) can become inflamed, swollen, and superinfected. While the initial erythema may be sterile inflammation, these cysts can become infected with *S. aureus*. The treatment consists of incision and drainage and antibiotics if cellulitis is also present. If these are removed before they become inflamed, the cyst may come out intact (**Figure 115-5**).

- Cellulitis with swelling and no pocket of pus—when it is unclear if an area of infected skin has an abscess, needle aspiration with a large gauge needle may be helpful to determine whether to incise the skin. Cellulitis alone should have no area of fluctuance (see Chapter 114, Cellulitis).

- Hidradenitis suppurativa—recurrent inflammation surrounding the apocrine glands of the axilla and inguinal areas (see Chapter 109, Hidradenitis Suppurativa [Acne Inversa]).

- Furuncles and carbuncles—A furuncle or boil is an abscess that starts in hair follicle or sweat gland. A carbuncle occurs when the furuncle extends into the subcutaneous tissue.

- Acne cysts—more sterile inflammation than true abscess, often better to inject with steroid rather than incise and drain (see Chapter 106, Acne Vulgaris).

MANAGEMENT

- The time-honored and best treatment for an abscess is incision and drainage.[1-4] SOR **A** Inject 1% lidocaine with epinephrine into the skin at the site you plan to open using a 27- or 30-gauge needle. Open the abscess with a linear incision using a #11 blade scalpel following skin lines if possible. Drain the pus and pack with gauze.

- With the current epidemic of MRSA, it may be judicious to culture all abscesses and infected epidermal cysts. While antibiotics may not be necessary at first, if they come back worse, the culture can then guide your choice of antibiotic. SOR **C**

- If there is no surrounding cellulitis, an antibiotic should not be needed.[2] SOR **A**

- If you suspect MRSA and there are signs of cellulitis as well, culture the purulent discharge and start one of the following oral antibiotics: Trimethoprim-sulfamethoxazole, clindamycin, tetracycline, or doxycycline.[5] SOR **A** Note that there is inducible MRSA resistance to clindamycin. If the MRSA susceptibility studies show erythromycin resistance and no resistance to clindamycin, make sure your lab does a disk diffusion induction test (D-test) for clindamycin (if that is the antibiotic you have chosen to use). This will determine a more accurate susceptibility for the clindamycin and can avoid the development of clindamycin resistance during treatment.[6]

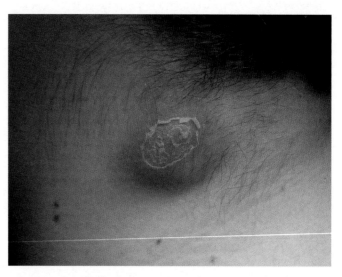

FIGURE 115-3 MRSA abscess on the neck that patient thought was a spider bite. (*Courtesy of Edward Wright, MD.*)

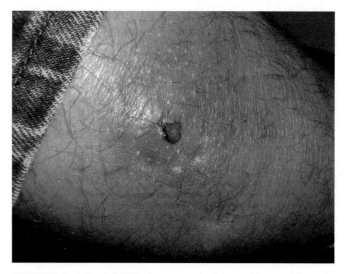

FIGURE 115-4 Large MRSA abscess on the leg in a 62-year-old man beginning to drain spontaneously. The abscess cavity was large and patient was placed on TMP/SX to cover any surrounding cellulitis. (*Courtesy of Richard P. Usatine, MD.*)

- Incision and drainage without adjunctive antibiotic therapy was found to be effective management of community-acquired MRSA skin and soft tissue abscesses with a diameter of less than 5 cm in immunocompetent children.[7] SOR **B**

PATIENT EDUCATION

Patients may shower daily and reapply outer gauze. They should not take a bath or swim and immerse the wound in water until the incision is closed.

FOLLOW-UP

Follow-up visits and removal of packing can be handled in many different ways. There is no evidence to support one practice over another. Patients or family members can be taught to change the packing at home.

PATIENT RESOURCES

VisualDxHealth article on abscess—**http://www.visualdxhealth.com/adult/abscess.htm.**

PROVIDER RESOURCES

Practice guidelines for the diagnosis and management of skin and soft-tissue infections. *Clin Infect Dis.* 2005;41:1373–1406.[8]

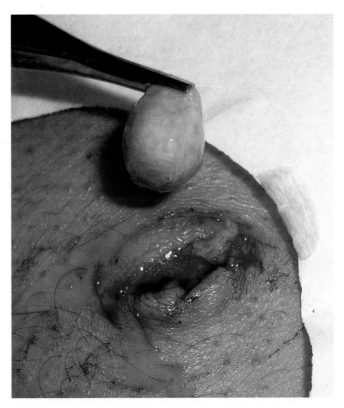

FIGURE 115-5 Epidermal inclusion cyst removed intact. There is no need for antibiotics in this case. (*Courtesy of Richard P. Usatine, MD.*)

REFERENCES

1. Usatine R, Moy R, Tobinick E, Siegel D. *Skin Surgery: A Practical Guide*. St. Louis: Mosby, 1998.

2. Llera JL, Levy RC. Treatment of cutaneous abscess: A double-blind clinical study. *Ann Emerg Med.* 1985;14:15–19.

3. Simms MH, Curran F, Johnson RA, et al. Treatment of acute abscesses in the casualty department. *Br Med J (Clin Res Ed).* 1982; 284:1827–1829.

4. Sorensen C, Hjortrup A, Moesgaard F, Lykkegaard-Nielsen M. Linear incision and curettage vs. deroofing and drainage in subcutaneous abscess. A randomized clinical trial. *Acta Chir Scand.* 1987; 153:659–660.

5. Naimi TS, LeDell KH, Como-Sabetti K, et al. Comparison of community- and health care-associated methicillin-resistant Staphylococcus aureus infection. *JAMA.* 2003;290:2976–2984.

6. Schreckenberger PC, Ilendo E, Ristow KL. Incidence of constitutive and inducible clindamycin resistance in Staphylococcus aureus and coagulase-negative staphylococci in a community and a tertiary care hospital. *J Clin Microbiol.* 2004;42(6):2777–2779.

7. Lee MC, Rios AM, Aten MF, et al. Management and outcome of children with skin and soft tissue abscesses caused by community-acquired methicillin-resistant Staphylococcus aureus 2. *Pediatr Infect Dis J.* 2004;23:123–127.

8. Stevens DL, Bisno AL, Chambers HF, et al. Practice guidelines for the diagnosis and management of skin and soft-tissue infections. *Clin Infect Dis.* 2005;41:1373–1406.

116 NECROTIZING FASCIITIS

Jeremy A. Franklin, MD

PATIENT STORY

A 54-year-old woman with diabetes was brought to the emergency department with right leg swelling, fever, and altered mental status.[1] The patient noted a pimple in her groin 5 days earlier and over the past few days had increasing leg pain. Her right leg was tender, red, hot, and swollen (**Figure 116-1**). Large bullae were present. Her temperature was 102°F and her blood sugar was 573. The skin had a "woody" feel and a radiograph of her leg showed gas in the muscles and soft tissues (**Figure 116-2**). She was taken to the operating room for debridement of her necrotizing fasciitis. Broad-spectrum antibiotics were also started but the infection continued to advance quickly. The patient died the following day; her wound culture later grew *Escherichia coli*, *Proteus vulgaris*, *Corynebacterium*, *Enterococcus*, *Staphylococcus sp.*, and *Peptostreptococcus.*[1]

EPIDEMIOLOGY

- Historical background:
  - First described by Hippocrates in fifth century BC, the first case described in the United States occurred in 1871.[2]
  - Term "necrotizing fasciitis" was first used in 1952.[2]
- Incidence in adults is 0.40 cases per 100,000 population.[3]
- Incidence in children is 0.08 cases per 100,000 population.[3]
- Overall incidence has increased fivefold over the last decade.[3]
- Type I necrotizing fasciitis is the most common form of necrotizing fasciitis.[4]
- Risk factors for type I necrotizing fasciitis:
  - Diabetes mellitus.
  - Severe peripheral vascular disease.
  - Obesity.
  - Alcoholism and cirrhosis.
  - Intravenous drug use.
  - Decubitus ulcers.
  - Poor nutritional status.
  - Postoperative patients or those with penetrating trauma.
  - Abscess of the female genital tract.
- Risk factors of type II necrotizing fasciitis:
  - Diabetes mellitus.
  - Severe peripheral vascular disease.
  - Recent parturition.
  - Trauma.
  - Muscle strain.
  - Varicella.
  - Use of nonsteroidal anti-inflammatory drugs is controversial.[4,5]

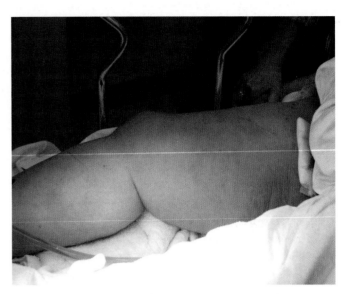

FIGURE 116-1 Necrotizing fasciitis on the leg and groin showing erythema, swelling, and bullae. (*With permission from Dufel S, Martino M. Simple cellulitis or a more serious infection? J Fam Pract. 2006; 55(5):396–400.*)

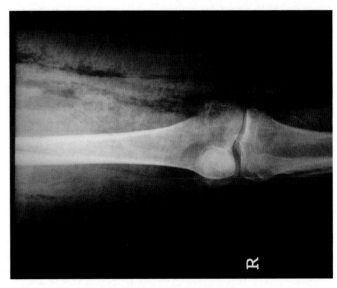

FIGURE 116-2 Radiograph of the patient's leg showing gas in the soft tissues and muscles. (*Courtesy of Susan Dufel, MD.*)[1]

ETIOLOGY AND PATHOPHYSIOLOGY

- Type I necrotizing fasciitis:
  - Polymicrobial infection with aerobic and anaerobic bacteria.
    - Up to 15 pathogens have been isolated in a single wound.[6]
    - Average of five different isolates per wound.[5]
  - Most common organisms:
    - Non-group A streptococci.[2,6]
    - *Enterobacteriaceae* organisms.[2]
    - *Bacteroides.*[5]
    - *Peptostreptococcus.*[5]
  - Saltwater variant:
    - Penetrating trauma or open wound contaminated with saltwater.
    - Caused by marine vibrios with *Vibrio vulnificus* being most virulent.[2,5]
- Type II necrotizing fasciitis:
  - Generally a monomicrobial infection caused by *Streptococcus pyogenes:*
    - May occur in combination with *Staphylococcus aureus.*[5]
    - Methicillin-resistant *Staphylococcus aureus* very rarely implicated.[6,7]
  - *S. pyogenes* strains may produce pyrogenic exotoxins, which act as superantigens to stimulate production of TNF-α, TNF-β, IL-1, IL-6, and IL-2.[4]

DIAGNOSIS

Examination by an experienced surgeon is critical for early diagnosis and treatment.

CLINICAL FEATURES

- Rapid progression of erythema (**Figure 116-3**) to bullae (**Figure 116-4**), ecchymosis, and necrosis or gangrene (**Figure 116-5**).
- Edematous, wooden feel of subcutaneous tissues extending beyond the margin of erythema.
- Unresponsive to empiric antimicrobial therapy.
- High fevers and severe systemic toxicity.
- Unrelenting intense pain out of proportion to cutaneous findings.
  - Pain progresses to cutaneous anesthesia as disease evolves.
- Crepitus in type I necrotizing fasciitis.[4,6]

TYPICAL DISTRIBUTION

- May occur at any anatomic location.
- Majority of cases occur on lower extremities (**Figures 116-1** to **116-5**).
- Also common on abdominal wall and in perineum.

LABORATORY AND IMAGING

- Routine laboratory tests are nonspecific.
- Cultures are best obtained from deep tissue biopsies.[6]

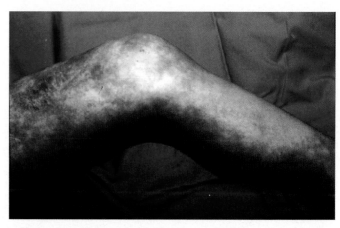

FIGURE 116-3 Necrotizing fasciitis with violaceous color of the skin on the affected leg. (*Courtesy of Fred Bongard, MD.*)

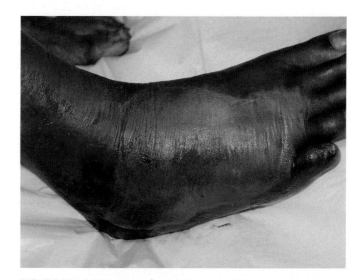

FIGURE 116-4 Necrotizing fasciitis that started when patient stepped on a nail. A large flaccid bulla is visible along with swelling and erythema. A rapid below the knee amputation allowed this patient to survive. (*Courtesy of Ramesh Subramaniam, MD.*)

- Standard radiographs are of little value unless air is demonstrated in the tissues.
- MRI may help delineate the extent of disease but should not delay surgical consultation.

BIOPSY

- Gross examination reveals swollen, dull, gray fascia with stringy areas of necrosis.[6]
- Necrosis of superficial fascia and fat produces watery, foul-smelling "dishwater pus."[2]
- Histology demonstrates subcutaneous fat necrosis, vasculitis, and local hemorrhage.[2]

DIFFERENTIAL DIAGNOSIS

- Cellulitis—Acute spreading infection of skin and soft tissues characterized by erythema, edema, pain, and calor. Rapid progression of disease despite antibiotics, systemic toxicity, intense pain, and skin necrosis suggest necrotizing fasciitis rather than cellulitis (see Chapter 114, Cellulitis).
- Pyomyositis—Suppuration within individual skeletal muscle groups. Pain localized to a specific muscle group and lack of systemic toxicity suggests pyomyositis rather than necrotizing fasciitis. Imaging of the muscle will confirm the diagnosis.
- Erythema induratum—Tender, erythematous subcutaneous nodules occurring on the lower legs (especially the calves). Lack of fever, systemic toxicity, and skin necrosis suggest erythema induratum rather than necrotizing fasciitis. Lesions of erythema induratum may have a chronic, recurrent course and the patient frequently has a history of tuberculosis or a positive PPD test.
- Clostridial myonecrosis—Acute necrotizing infection of muscle tissue caused by clostridial organisms. Surgical exploration and cultures are required to differentiate from necrotizing fasciitis.
- Streptococcal or staphylococcal toxic shock syndrome—Systemic inflammatory response to a toxin-producing bacteria characterized by fever, hypotension, generalized erythroderma, myalgia, and multisystem organ involvement. Necrotizing fasciitis may occur as part of the toxic shock syndrome. Consultation with infectious disease and surgery is essential.

MANAGEMENT

- Surgical debridement is the primary therapeutic modality.[2–7] SOR **A**
  - Extensive, definitive debridement should be the goal with the first surgery.
  - May require amputation of extremity to control disease.
  - Daily surgical debridement until no further need identified.
  - All other treatment modalities should be considered adjunctive.
- Antibiotics
  - Type I necrotizing fasciitis:
    - Initial antibiotic regimen must include coverage of gram-positive, gram-negative, and anaerobic organisms.[6] SOR **B**

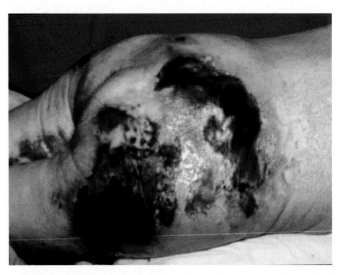

FIGURE 116-5 Necrotizing fasciitis with gangrene. Even with a radical hemipelvectomy this patient did not survive. (*Courtesy of Fred Bongard, MD.*)

- First-line antimicrobial regimens:
  - Ampicillin-sulbactam *plus* clindamycin *plus* ciprofloxacin.[6]
  - Piperacillin-tazobactam *plus* clindamycin *plus* ciprofloxacin.[6]
  - Carbapenem monotherapy (imipenem/cilastin *or* meropenem *or* ertapenem).[6]
  - Cefotaxime *plus* metronidazole.[6]
  - Cefotaxime *plus* clindamycin.[6]
- Type II necrotizing fasciitis:
  - Antibiotic regimen of choice is penicillin *plus* clindamycin.[6] SOR **A**
  - Presence of *S. aureus* necessitates use of penicillinase-resistant penicillin (i.e., nafcillin or oxacillin) or first-generation intravenous cephalosporin (e.g., cefazolin).
  - Presence of methicillin-resistant *Staphylococcus aureus* necessitates use of vancomycin.
  - Alternative agents for patients with severe penicillin hypersensitivity include vancomycin, linezolid, daptomycin, and quinupristin/dalfopristin.
- Hyperbaric oxygen.
  - Controversial adjunctive therapy.
  - Recent study demonstrated decreased morbidity (50% vs. 0%) and mortality (34% vs. 11.9%).[8] SOR **B**
  - Enhances the bactericidal activity of neutrophils, is lethal to certain anaerobes, and reduces tissue edema.[2]
- Immune globulin intravenous.
  - Controversial adjunctive therapy.[4,6] SOR **B**
- Aggressive fluid resuscitation.
  - Often necessary because of massive capillary leak syndrome.[2,4]

PROGNOSIS AND FOLLOW-UP

- Overall case fatality rate remains 20% to 47% despite aggressive, modern therapy.[5,6]
- Early diagnosis and treatment can reduce case fatality rate to 12%.[5]
- Risk of a secondary case of necrotizing fasciitis is 50-fold higher than in the general population.[4]

REFERENCES

1. Dufel S, Martino M. Simple cellulitis or a more serious infection? *J Fam Pract*. 2006;55(5):396–400.

2. Green RJ, Dafoe DC, Raffin TA. Necrotizing fasciitis. *Chest*. 1996;110:219–229.

3. Trent JT, Kirsner RS. Necrotizing fasciitis. Wounds compendium. *Clin Res Pract*. 2002;14:284–292.

4. Stevens DL, Bisno AL, Chambers HF, et al. Practice guidelines for the diagnosis and management of skin and soft-tissue infections. *Clin Infect Dis*. 2005;41:1373–1406.

5. Cheng N, Chang S, Kuo Y, Wang J, Tang Y. Necrotizing fasciitis caused by methicillin-resistant Staphylococcus aureus resulting in death. A report of three cases. *J Bone Joint Surg Am*. 2006;88:1107–1110.

6. Swartz MN, Pasternack MS. Cellulitis and subcutaneous tissue infections. In: Mandell GL, Bennett JE, Dolin R eds. *Principles and Practice of Infectious Diseases*. Philadelphia, PA: Churchill Livingstone, 2005:1189–1191.

7. Stevens DL. Necrotizing fasciitis, gas gangrene, myositis, and myonecrosis. In: Cohen J, Powderly WG, Berkeley SF, Calandra T, et al. eds. *Infectious Diseases*. New York, NY: Mosby, 2004:145–155.

8. Escobar SJ, Slade JB Jr., Hunt TK, Cianci P. Adjunctive hyperbaric oxygen therapy (HBO₂) for treatment of necrotizing fasciitis reduces mortality and amputation rate. *Undersea Hyperb Med*. 2005;32:437–443.

SECTION 4 VIRAL INFECTION

117 CHICKENPOX

E.J. Mayeaux, Jr., MD

PATIENT STORY

A 12-year-old girl presents with a 3-day history of a body-wide pruritic vesicular rash (**Figure 117-1**). The episode started 24 hours before the rash with fever and malaise. The patient is diagnosed with varicella and no antiviral medications are given.

EPIDEMIOLOGY

- Chickenpox is a highly contagious viral infection.

- The rate of secondary household attack is more than 90% in susceptible individuals (**Figure 117-2**).[1]

- Adults and immunocompromised patients generally develop more severe disease than normal children.

- Traditionally, primary infection with varicella-zoster virus (VZV) occurred during childhood (**Figure 117-3**). In childhood, it is usually a benign self-limited illness in immunocompetent hosts. It occurs throughout the year in temperate regions, but the incidence peaks in the late spring and summer months.

- Prior to the introduction of the varicella vaccine in 1995, the yearly incidence of chickenpox in the United States was approximately four million cases with around 11,000 hospital admissions and 100 deaths.[2]

- As the vaccination rates steadily increased in the United States, there has been a corresponding fourfold decrease in the number of cases of chickenpox cases down to disease rates of from 0.3 to 1.0 per 1000 population in 2001.[2]

ETIOLOGY AND PATHOPHYSIOLOGY

- Chickenpox is caused by a primary infection with the VZV, which is a double-stranded, linear DNA herpesvirus.

- Transmission occurs via contact with aerosolized droplets from nasopharyngeal secretions or by direct cutaneous contact with vesicle fluid from skin lesions.

- The incubation period for VZV is approximately 15 days where the virus undergoes replication in regional lymph nodes, followed by two viremic phases, the second of which persists through the development of skin lesions generally by day 14.[3]

- The vesicular rash appears in crops for several days. The lesions start as vesicle on a red base, which is classically described as a

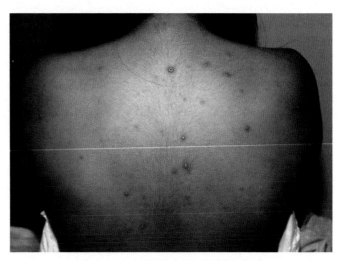

FIGURE 117-1 Chickenpox in a child. Note lesions in various stages (papules, intact vesicles, pustules, and crusted papules) caused by multiple crops of lesions. The vesicles are on a red base. (*Courtesy of Richard P. Usatine, MD.*)

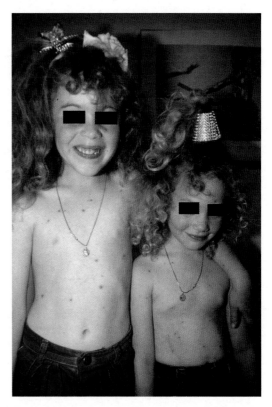

FIGURE 117-2 Chickenpox in sisters seen before the varicella vaccine was available. The girls are feeling better now that the disease is resolving. (*Courtesy of Richard P. Usatine, MD.*)

dew-drop on a rose petal (**Figure 117-4**). The lesions gradually develop a pustular component (**Figure 117-5**) followed by the evolution of crusted papules (**Figure 117-6**). The period of infectivity is generally considered to last from 48 hours prior to the onset of rash until skin lesions have fully crusted.

- The most frequent complication in healthy children is bacterial skin superinfection (**Figure 117-3**). Less common skin complications (seen more frequently in immunosuppressed hosts) include bullous varicella, purpura fulminans, or necrotizing fasciitis.

- Encephalitis is a serious potential complication of chickenpox that develops toward the end of the first week of the exanthema. One form, acute cerebellar ataxia, occurs mostly in children and is generally followed by complete recovery. A more diffuse encephalitis most often occurs in adults and may produce delirium, seizures, and focal neurologic signs. It has significant rates of long-term neurologic sequelae and death.

- Pneumonia is rare in healthy children but accounts for the majority of hospitalizations in adults, where it has up to a 30% mortality rate.[4] It usually develops insidiously within a few days after the rash has appeared with progressive tachypnea, dyspnea, and dry cough. Chest x-rays reveal diffuse bilateral infiltrates. Treat with prompt administration of intravenous acyclovir. The use of adjunctive steroids therapy is controversial.

- Varicella hepatitis is rare, and typically only occurs in immunosuppressed individuals. It is frequently fatal.

- Reactivation of latent VZV results in herpes zoster or shingles.

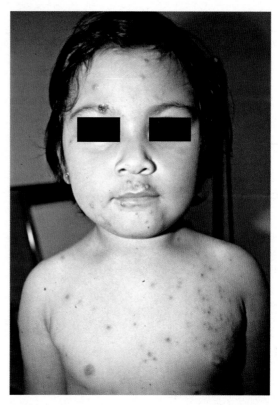

FIGURE 117-3 Chickenpox in a child. Note the widespread distribution of the lesions. The honey-crusted lesion on the eyebrow suggests a secondary bacterial infection (impetigo). (*Courtesy of Richard P. Usatine, MD.*)

DIAGNOSIS

CLINICAL FEATURES

- The typical clinical manifestations of chickenpox include a prodrome of fever, malaise, or pharyngitis, followed in 24 hours by the development of a generalized vesicular rash.

- The lesions are pruritic and appear as successive crops of vesicles more than 3 to 4 days.

- Coexisting lesions in different stages of development on the face, trunk, and extremities are common.

- New lesion stop forming in approximately 4 days, and most lesions have fully crusted by 7 days.

TYPICAL DISTRIBUTION

Body-wide—No laboratory tests are needed unless the diagnosis is uncertain. For children or adults in which there is uncertainty about previous disease and it is important to establish a quick diagnosis, a direct fluorescent antibody test can be done on a scraping of a lesion. In many laboratories a result can be obtained within 24 hours (**Figure 117-7**).

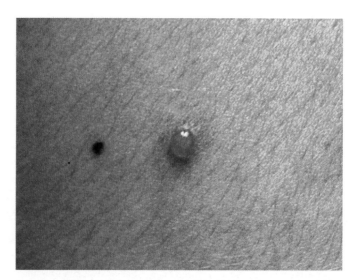

FIGURE 117-4 Dew-drop on a rose petal—the classic description of a varicella vesicle on a red base. (*Courtesy of Richard P. Usatine, MD.*)

DIFFERENTIAL DIAGNOSIS

- Pemphigus and bullous pemphigoid are usually seen in adults while varicella is a disease of children.

- Dermatitis herpetiformis is characterized by pruritic papulovesicles over the extremities and on the trunk, and granular IgA deposits on the basement membrane (see Chapter 179, Other Bullous Disease).

- Herpes Simplex infection presents with similar lesions but is generally restricted to the genital and oral areas. The vesicles of herpes simplex tend to be more clustered in a group rather than the wide distribution of varicella (see Chapter 123, Herpes Simplex).

- Impetigo can have bullous or crusted lesions anywhere on the body. The lesions often have mild erythema and a yellowish color to the crusts (see Chapter 110, Impetigo).

- Insect bites are often suspected by history and can occur on the entire body.

MANAGEMENT

- Superinfection may be treated with topical or oral antibiotics.

- Prophylactic use of varicella zoster immune globulin (125 U/10 kg, up to 625 U intramuscularly) in recently exposed susceptible individuals can prevent or attenuate the disease. However, the immune globulin is extremely hard to obtain at times.[5]

- Acyclovir is U.S. Food and Drug Administration approved for treatment of varicella in healthy children. It should be given during the first 24 hours of rash.[1] However, the Committee on Infectious Disease of the American Academy of Pediatrics issued a statement saying they did not consider the routine administration of acyclovir to all healthy children with varicella to be justified.[6] SOR **C**

- For adults, acyclovir 20 mg/kg po four times daily (800 mg maximum) for 5 days may be used for treatment if started in the first 24 hours of the rash.[5] SOR **A**

- Early treatment with intravenous acyclovir may be effective for treatment of varicella hepatitis and pneumonia, and may also be useful in the treatment of immunosuppressed patients. SOR **B**

- Adults who get varicella should be assessed for neurologic and pulmonary disease.

- Varicella immunization (Varivax) can be used to prevent chickenpox. SOR **A** For children age 12 months to 12 years, inject 0.5 mL SQ. For children older than 12 years of age and adults inject two doses SQ of 0.5 mL separated by 4 to 8 weeks. It is contraindication in individuals allergic to gelatin or neomycin, and in immunosuppressed individuals (it is a live vaccine). In 2006, the Advisory Committee on Immunization Practices recommended that all children younger than 13 years of age should be administered routinely two doses of varicella-containing vaccine, with the first dose administered at 12 to 15 months of age and the second dose at 4 to 6 years of age (i.e., before first grade). The second dose can be administered at an earlier age provided the interval between the first and second dose is at least 3 months.[7]

PATIENT EDUCATION

- Avoid scratching the blisters and keep fingernails short. Scratching may lead to superinfection.

- Calamine lotion and oatmeal (Aveeno) baths may help relieve itching.

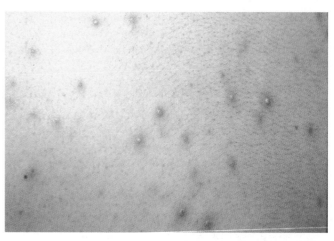

FIGURE 117-5 Varicella with pustular lesions. (*Courtesy of the University of Texas Health Sciences Center, Division of Dermatology.*)

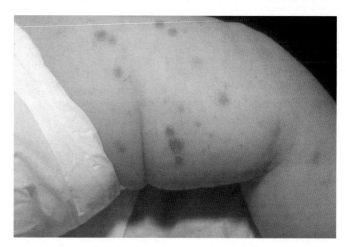

FIGURE 117-6 Rash after all of the lesions have crusted over. The patient is usually considered not contagious at this time. (*Courtesy of the University of Texas Health Sciences Center, Division of Dermatology.*)

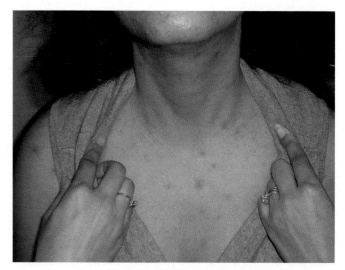

FIGURE 117-7 A 29-year-old woman with mild case of varicella in 2007. Her previous history of varicella in childhood was uncertain so a direct scraping of a lesion was performed and the varicella virus was identified quickly with a direct fluorescent antibody test. (*Courtesy of Richard P. Usatine, MD.*)

- Do not use aspirin or aspirin-containing products to relieve fever. The use of aspirin has been associated with development of Reye syndrome that may cause death.

FOLLOW-UP

- Follow-up is unnecessary for immunocompetent children and adults who are having no complications. All patients or parents should report any respiratory or neurologic problems immediately.

PATIENT RESOURCES

- KidsHealth: Chickenpox—**http://www.kidshealth.org/ parent/infections/skin/chicken_pox.html.**
- Wikipedia—**http://en.wikipedia.org/wiki/ Chickenpox.**

PROVIDER RESOURCES

- Centers for Disease Control and Prevention National Immunization Program—**http://www.cdc.gov/nip/diseases/ varicella/.**
- MedlinePlus Medical Encyclopedia—**http://www.nlm.nih. gov/medlineplus/chickenpox.html.**
- Advisory Committee on Immunization Practices Provisional Recommendations for Prevention of Varicella—**http://www. cdc.gov/nip/vaccine/varicella/ varicella_acip_recs_prov_june_2006.pdf.**

REFERENCES

1. Wharton M. The epidemiology of varicella-zoster infections. *Infect Dis Clin North Am*. 1996;10:571.
2. Decline in annual incidence of varicella—Selected states, 1990–2001. *MMWR Morb Mortal Wkly Rep*. 2003;52:884.
3. Grose C. Variation on a theme by Fenner: The pathogenesis of chickenpox. *Pediatrics*. 1981;68:735.
4. Schlossberg D, Littman M. Varicella pneumonia. *Arch Intern Med*. 1988;148:1613.
5. Ogilvie MM. Antiviral prophylaxis and treatment in chickenpox. A review prepared for the uk advisory group on chickenpox on behalf of the british society for the study of infection. *J Infect*. 1998;36(Suppl 1):31.
6. Centers for Disease Control: Prevention of varicella: Recommendations of the advisory committee on immunization practices. *MMWR Morb Mortal Wkly Rep*. 1996;45(RR-11):1.
7. Advisory Committee on Immunization Practices Provisional Recommendations for Prevention of Varicella. http://www.cdc.gov/ nip/vaccine/varicella/varicella_acip_recs_prov_june_2006.pdf. Accessed October 6, 2006.

118 HERPES ZOSTER—SKIN

E.J. Mayeaux, Jr., MD
Richard P. Usatine, MD

PATIENT STORY

A 14-year-old boy presents with deep burning pain and a vesicular eruption in a band starting at the left chest and ending just across the midline of the back (**Figure 118-1**). The varicella-zoster virus (VZV) leaves the dorsal root ganglion to travel down the spinal nerves to the cutaneous nerves of the skin. The vesicles do cross the midline by a few centimeters because the posterior primary ramus of the spinal nerve includes a small cutaneous medial branch that reaches across the midline.[1] The boy was treated with analgesics and an antiviral medication. The zoster healed with scarring.

EPIDEMIOLOGY

- Herpes zoster (shingles) is a syndrome characterized by a painful, usually unilateral vesicular eruption that develops in a restricted dermatomal distribution (**Figures 118-1** and **118-2**).[2,3] The lifetime incidence is 10% to 20% of the population. Older age groups account for the highest incidence of zoster. Approximately 4% of patients will experience a second episode of herpes zoster.[4]

- Both genders are affected equally.

- Herpes zoster occurs more frequently and more severely in immunosuppressed patients, including transplant patients.

ETIOLOGY AND PATHOPHYSIOLOGY

- After primary infection with either chickenpox or vaccine-type VZV a latent infection is established in the sensory dorsal root ganglia. Reactivation of this latent VZV infection results in herpes zoster (shingles).

- Both sensory ganglia neurons and satellite cells surrounding the neurons serve as sites of VZV latent infection. During latency, the virus only expresses a small number of viral proteins.

- How the virus emerges from latency is not clearly understood. Once reactivated, virus spreads to other cells within the ganglion. The dermatomal distribution of the rash corresponds to the sensory fields of the infected neurons within the specific ganglion.[3]

- Loss of VZV-specific cell mediated immune response is responsible for reactivation.[3]

- The pain associated with zoster infections and postherpetic neuralgia (PHN) is thought to result from injury to the peripheral nerves and altered central nervous system processing.

- The most common complications are PHN and bacterial superinfection that can delay healing and cause scarring of the zoster lesions.

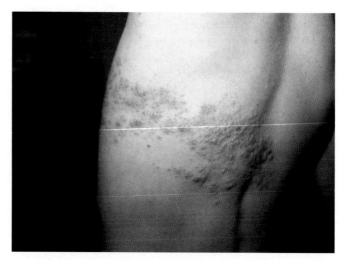

FIGURE 118-1 A 14-year-old boy with severe case of herpes zoster in a thoracic distribution. (*Courtesy of Richard P. Usatine, MD.*)

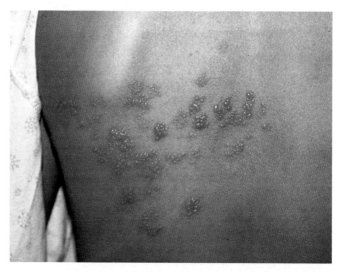

FIGURE 118-2 Close-up of Herpes zoster lesions. Note grouped vesicles on a red base. (*Courtesy of Richard P. Usatine, MD.*)

Approximately 19% of patients develop complications that may include:[5]

- ○ Postherpetic neuralgia (PHN)-the most common complication seen in 10% at 90 days[5] (see below).
- ○ Ocular complications including uveitis and keratitis 4%[5] (See Chapter 119, Zoster Ophthalmicus).
- ○ Bell's palsy and other motor nerve plastic, 3%.[5]
- ○ Bacterial skin infection 2%.[5]
- ○ Meningitis caused by central extension of the infection.
- ○ Herpes zoster oticus (Ramsay Hunt syndrome) (**Figure 118-3**) includes the triad of ipsilateral facial paralysis, ear pain, and vesicles in the auditory canal and auricle.[6] Disturbances in taste perception, hearing (tinnitus, hyperacusis), lacrimation, and vestibular function (vertigo) may occur.
- ○ Other rare complications may include acute retinal necrosis, transverse myelitis, encephalitis, leukoencephalitis, contralateral thrombotic stroke syndrome, and granulomatous vasculitis.[7]

- Immunosuppressed patients are at increased risk for complications, including severe complications such as disseminated infection, visceral involvement, pneumonitis, and/or meningoencephalitis.

- PHN is the persistence of pain, numbness, and/or dysesthesias precipitated by movement or in response to non-noxious stimuli in the affected dermatome for more than 1 month after the onset of zoster. The incidence of PHN in the general population is 1.38 per 1000 person years, and it occurs more commonly in individuals older than 60 years and immunosuppressed individuals.[3]

- In a large study, rates of zoster-association pain (PHN) persisting at least 90 days were:
  - ○ 10% overall, 12% in women and 7% in men.
  - ○ ages 22–59 years - 5% overall, 6% in women and 5% in men.
  - ○ ages 60–69 years - 10% overall, 14% in women and 5% in men.
  - ○ ages 70–79 years - 17% overall, 18% in women and 15% in men.
  - ○ age ≥80 years - 20% overall, 23% in women and 13% in men.[5]

DIAGNOSIS

- Clinical features: A deep burning pain is the most common first symptom and can precede the rash by days to weeks. A prodrome of fever, dysesthesias, malaise, and headache leads in several days to a dermatomal vesicular eruption. The rash starts as grouped vesicles or bullae which evolve into pustular or hemorrhagic lesions within three to four days (**Figures 118-1** to **118-4**). The lesions typically crust in approximately a week, with complete resolution within 3 to 4 weeks.[4]

- Typical distribution: Generally limited to one dermatome in immunocompetent patients, but sometimes affects neighboring dermatomes. Rarely, a few scattered vesicles located away from the involved dermatome as a result of release of VZV from the infected ganglion into the bloodstream.[3] If there are more than 20 lesions distributed outside the dermatome affected, the patient has disseminated zoster. The thoracic and lumbar dermatomes are the most commonly involved. Occasionally zoster will be seen on the extremities (**Figure 118-4**).

- Meningitis associated with VZV infection can be diagnosed by cerebrospinal fluid showing pleocytosis.

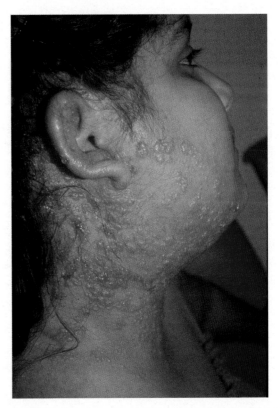

FIGURE 118-3 Herpes zoster oticus (Ramsay Hunt syndrome) with the classic presentation of vesicles on the auricle. (*Courtesy of the University of Texas Health Sciences Center, Division of Dermatology.*)

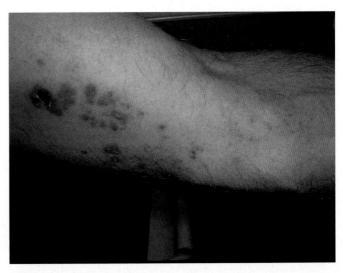

FIGURE 118-4 Herpes zoster on the arm that follows a dermatomal pattern. (*Courtesy of E.J. Mayeaux, Jr., MD.*)

DIFFERENTIAL DIAGNOSIS

- Pemphigus and other bullous diseases present with blisters but not the classic dermatomal distribution (see Chapter 176, Overview of Bullous Disease and Chapter 178, Pemphigus).
- Molluscum contagiosum presents with white or yellow flat toped papules with central umbilication caused by a pox virus. The lesions are more firm and unless irritated do not have a red base as seen with zoster (see Chapter 124, Molluscum Contagiosum).
- Scabies may present as a pustular rash that is not confined to dermatomes and usually has characteristic lesions in the webs of the fingers (see Chapter 137, Scabies).
- Insect bites are often suspected by history and can occur over the entire body.
- Folliculitis presents with characteristic pustules arising from hair shafts (see Chapter 111, Folliculitis).
- Zoster mimics coronary artery disease when it presents with chest pain before the vesicles are visible.
- Herpes Simplex infection presents with similar lesions but is usually restricted to the perioral region, genital area, buttocks, and fingers (see Chapter 122, Herpes Simplex).

MANAGEMENT

- The objectives of treatment of herpes zoster include (1) hastening the resolution of the acute viral infection, (2) treatment of the associated pain, and (3) prevention of PHN.
- Antiviral agents used in the treatment of herpes zoster include Acyclovir (Zovirax), Famciclovir (Famvir), and Valacyclovir (Valtrex) all started within 72 hours of the onset of the rash (**Table 118-1**).[8] SOR Ⓐ
- Adding corticosteroids to acyclovir therapy may accelerate times to crusting and healing, return to uninterrupted sleep, resuming full activity, and to discontinue analgesic. Data is lacking for combining corticosteroids with other antivirals.
- Pain can be managed with over-the-counter analgesics or narcotics. Pain should be treated aggressively. This may actually prevent or lessen the severity of post-herpetic neuralgia. Narcotic analgesics with hydrocodone are appropriate when needed. SOR Ⓒ
- Calamine lotion and topically administered lidocaine may be used to reduce pain and itching. SOR Ⓒ
- Treatment of herpes zoster with steroids does not reduce the prevalence of PHN.
- Treatment of herpes zoster early with valacyclovir, famciclovir or amitriptyline does reduce pain of PHN at 6 months.
- Treatment of PHN includes tricyclic antidepressants, gabapentin (Neurontin), pregabalin (Lyrica) and/or opioid analgesics. (**Table 118-2**).
- Use of varicella (chickenpox) vaccine has not led to an increase in vaccine-associated herpes zoster in immunized patients or in the general population, and has led to an overall decrease in herpes zoster.[6]

TABLE 118-1 Treatments for Herpes Zoster

Medication	Dosage
Acyclovir (Zovirax)	800 mg orally five times daily for 7–10 d or 10 mg/kg intravenously every 8 hours for 7–10 d
Famciclovir (Famvir)	500 mg orally three times daily for 7 d
Valacyclovir (Valtrex)	1000 mg orally three times daily for 7 d
Prednisone (Deltasone)	30 mg orally twice daily for 1 week followed by a tapering dose for approximately 2 wk

TABLE 118-2 Effective Treatments for Postherpetic Neuralgia

Treatment	Benefit/risk	Risks	NNT for >=50% pain reduction	Dose/Duration
Lidocaine patch 5%	Reduces pain and acts as mechanical barrier	Application site sensitivity	4.4	Apply up to 3 patches for up to 12 hours
Tricyclic antidepressants (including amitriptyline) (strongest evidence)	Reduces pain, better sleep, decreases anxiety and depression	Multiple side effects including sedation and dry mouth	2.7	25–150 mg qhs
Gabapentin (Neurontin) (strongest evidence)	Reduces pain, improves sleep, mood and quality of life	Somnolence, dizziness, decreased memory	3.2 to 4.3	300–600 mg tid (can go as high as 1200 mg tid)
Pregabalin (Lyrica)	May reduce pain	Peripheral edema and weight gain	Not known	75 mg bid
Opioids (Morphine, Oxycodone, methadone)	Reduces pain	Somnolence, constipation, tolerance	Variable	Start low and titrate to effective dose
Tramadol	Reduces pain and is not a true narcotic	Dizziness, nausea, somnolence, constipation,	3.8	50–100 mg qid

*NNT (numbers needed to treat)
Information from DynaMed Editorial Team. Postherpetic Neuralgia. Last updated 2008 March 17. Available from DynaMed: http://www.ebscohost.com/dynamed. Accessed March 22, 2008

- The herpes zoster vaccine contains a much higher dose of the live attenuated virus than the varicella vaccine. In adults 60 years of age or older, immunization reduces the incidence of herpes zoster by 51% compared with placebo.[3] In those who do develop zoster, the duration of pain and discomfort is shorter and the incidence of PHN is greatly reduced. It reduces the incidence of PHN from 1.38 to 0.46 per 1000 person years.[3]

PATIENT EDUCATION

- Herpes zoster in an immunocompetent host is only contagious from contact with open lesions.
- Patients with disseminated zoster or with zoster and are immunocompromised should be isolated from nonimmune individuals like with primary varicella infection (in which airborne spread is possible).
- Individuals who have not had varicella and are exposed to a patient with herpes zoster are only at risk of developing primary varicella and not herpes zoster.

FOLLOW-UP

- Follow-up is based on the severity of the case and the immune status of the patient.

PATIENT RESOURCES

- Centers for Disease Control and Prevention National Immunization Program—**http://www.cdc.gov/nip/diseases/varicella/faqs-gen-shingles.htm**
- Medinfo UK—**http://www.medinfo.co.uk/conditions/shingles.html**
- The Skin Site—**http://www.skinsite.com/info_herpes_zoster.htm**

PROVIDER RESOURCES

- MedlinePlus Medical Encyclopedia: Herpes zoster—**http://www.nlm.nih.gov/medlineplus/ency/article/000858.htm**
- eMedicine-Herpes Zoster: **http://www.emedicine.com/EMERG/topic823.htm**
- DynaMed Editorial Team. Postherpetic Neuralgia. Last updated 2008 March 17. Available from DynaMed: **http://www.ebscohost.com/dynamed.** Accessed March 22, 2008.
- Management of Herpes Zoster (Shingles) and Postherpetic Neuralgia. *Am Fam Physician.* 2000;61:2437–2444,2447–2448. Available online—**http://www.aafp.org/afp/20000415/2437.html**

REFERENCES

1. Usatine RP, Clemente C. Is Herpes Zoster Unilateral? *West J Med* 1999;170:263.

2. Gnann JW, Jr., Whitley RJ. Herpes zoster. *N Engl J Med*. 2002;347: 340.

3. Oxman MN. Immunization to reduce the frequency and severity of herpes zoster and its complications. *Neurology*. 1995;45:S41.

4. Stankus SJ, Dlugopolski M, Packer D. Management of herpes zoster (shingles) and postherpetic neuralgia. *Am Fam Physician*. 2000;61:2437–2444,2447–2448.

5. Yawn BP, Saddier P, Wollan PC, St Sauver JL, Kurland MJ, Sy LS. A population-based study of the incidence and complication rates of herpes zoster before zoster vaccine introduction. *Mayo Clin Proc*. 2007;82(11):1341–1349.

6. Adour KK. Otological complications of herpes zoster. *Ann Neurol*. 1994;35(Suppl):S62.

7. Arvin AM, Pollard RB, Rasmussen LE, Merigan TC. Cellular and humoral immunity in the pathogenesis of recurrent herpes viral infections in patients with lymphoma. *J Clin Invest*. 1980;65:869.

8. Tyring SK, Beutner KR, Tucker BA, Anderson WC, Crooks RJ. Antiviral therapy for herpes zoster: randomized, controlled clinical trial of valacyclovir and famciclovir therapy in immunocompetent patients 50 years and older. *Arch Fam Med*. 2000;9:863–869.

119 ZOSTER OPHTHALMICUS

E.J. Mayeaux, Jr., MD
Richard P. Usatine, MD

PATIENT STORY

A 44-year-old HIV-positive Hispanic man presented with painful herpes zoster of his right forehead (**Figure 119-1**). He was particularly worried because his right eye was red, painful, and very sensitive to light (**Figure 119-2**). On physical examination there was significant conjunctival injection, corneal punctation and clouding, and a small layer of blood in the anterior chamber (hyphema). The pupil was somewhat irregular, and along with the hyphema and ciliary flushing, this indicated an anterior uveitis. The patient had a unilateral ptosis on the right side with limitations in elevation, depression, and adduction of the eye secondary to cranial nerve III palsy from the zoster. The patient was immediately referred to ophthalmology and the anterior uveitis, corneal involvement, and cranial nerve III palsy were confirmed. The ophthalmologist started the patient on topical ophthalmic preparations of erythromycin, moxifloxacin, prednisolone, and atropine. Oral acyclovir was also prescribed. Unfortunately, the patient did not return for follow-up until 6 months later when he returned to the ophthalmologist with significant corneal scarring (**Figure 119-3**). The patient is currently on a waiting list for a corneal transplant.

EPIDEMIOLOGY

- Incidence rates of herpes zoster ophthalmicus complicating herpes zoster range from 8% to 56%.[1]

- Ocular involvement is not correlated with age, gender, or severity of disease.

- Immunocompromised persons, especially when caused by human immunodeficiency virus infection, have a much higher risk of developing zoster complications, including herpes zoster ophthalmicus.

ETIOLOGY AND PATHOPHYSIOLOGY

- Herpes zoster is a common infection caused by varicella-zoster virus, the same virus that causes chickenpox. Reactivation of the latent virus in neurosensory ganglia produces the characteristic manifestations of herpes zoster (shingles).

- Herpes zoster outbreaks may be precipitated by aging, poor nutrition, immunocompromised status, physical or emotional stress, and excessive fatigue.

- Although zoster most commonly involves the thoracic and lumbar dermatomes, reactivation of the latent virus in the trigeminal ganglia may results in herpes zoster ophthalmicus (**Figures 119-1** to **119-6**).

- Serious sequelae may occur including chronic ocular inflammation, vision loss, and disabling pain. Early diagnosis is important to prevent progressive corneal involvement and potential loss of vision.[2]

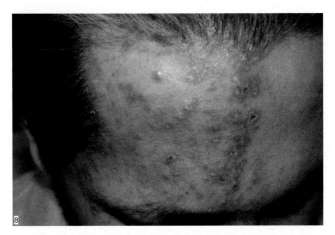

FIGURE 119-1 A 44-year-old HIV-positive Hispanic man with painful herpes zoster of his right forehead.

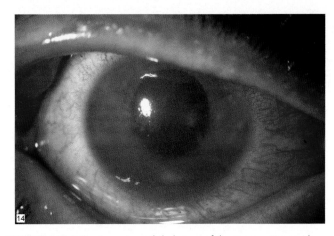

FIGURE 119-2 Acute zoster ophthalmicus of the same patient with conjunctival injection, corneal punctation (keratitis), and a small layer of blood in the anterior chamber (hyphema). A diagnosis of anterior uveitis was suspected based on the irregularly shaped pupil, the hyphema, and ciliary flush. A slit-lamp exam confirmed the anterior uveitis (iritis).

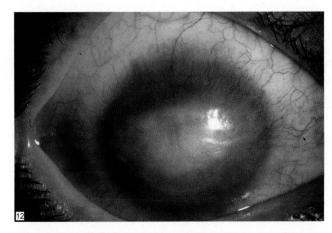

FIGURE 119-3 Corneal scarring and conjunctival injection of the same patient 6 months later after being lost to follow-up.

- Since the nasociliary branch of the first (ophthalmic) division of the trigeminal (fifth cranial) nerve innervates the globe (**Figure 119-7**), the most serious ocular involvement develops if this branch is involved.

- Classically, involvement of the tip of the nose (Hutchinson's sign) has been thought to be a clinical predictor of ocular involvement via the external nasal nerve (**Figures 119-4** and **119-5**). Hutchinson's sign is a powerful predictor of ocular inflammation and corneal denervation with relative risks of 3.35 and 4.02, respectively. The manifestation of herpes zoster skin lesions at the dermatomes of both nasociliary branches (at the tip, the side, and the root of the nose) was invariably associated with the development of ocular inflammation in one study.[3]

- Epithelial keratitis is the earliest potential corneal finding (**Figure 119-2**). On slit lamp examination, it appears as multiple, focal, swollen spots on the cornea that stain with fluorescein dye. They may either resolve or progress to dendrite formation. Herpes zoster virus dendrites form branching or frond-like patterns that have tapered ends and stain with fluorescein dye. These lesions can lead to anterior stromal corneal infiltrates.

- Stromal keratitis occurs in 25% to 30% of patients with herpes zoster ophthalmicus, and is characterized by multiple fine granular infiltrates in the anterior corneal stroma. The infiltrates probably arise from antigen–antibody reaction and may be prolonged and recurrent.[4]

- Anterior uveitis evolves to inflammation of the iris and ciliary body and occurs frequently with herpes zoster ophthalmicus (**Figure 119-2**). The inflammation is usually mild, but may cause a mild intraocular pressure elevation. The course of disease may be prolonged, especially without timely treatment, and may lead to glaucoma and cataract formation.

- Herpes zoster virus is the most common cause of acute retinal necrosis. Symptoms include blurred vision and/or pain in one or both eyes and signs include peripheral patches of retinal necrosis that rapidly coalesce, occlusive vasculitis, and vitreous inflammation. It commonly causes retinal detachment. Bilateral involvement is observed in one-third of patients but may be as high as 70% in patients with untreated disease. Treatment includes long courses of oral and intravenous acyclovir (Zovirax), and corticosteroids.[5]

- Varicella-zoster virus is a member of the same family (Herpesviridae) as herpes simplex virus, Epstein-Barr virus, and cytomegalovirus.

- The virus damages the eye and surrounding structures by neural and secondary perineural inflammation of the sensory nerves.

- Conjunctivitis, usually with *Staphylococcus aureus*, is a common complication of herpes zoster ophthalmicus.

DIAGNOSIS

CLINICAL FEATURES

- The syndrome usually begins with a prodrome of low-grade fever, headache, and malaise that may start up to 1 week before the rash appears.

- Unilateral pain or hypesthesia in the affected eye, forehead, top of the head, and or nose may precede or follow the prodrome. The

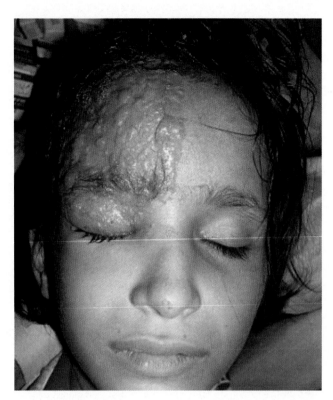

FIGURE 119-4 This 5-year-old girl had herpes zoster involving the ophthalmic branch of the trigeminal nerve. Note the vesicles and bullae on the forehead and eyelid and the crust on the nasal tip (Hutchinson's sign). Fortunately she did not have ocular complications and her case of zoster fully healed with oral acyclovir and acyclovir eye ointment. (*Courtesy of Amor Khachemoune, MD.*)

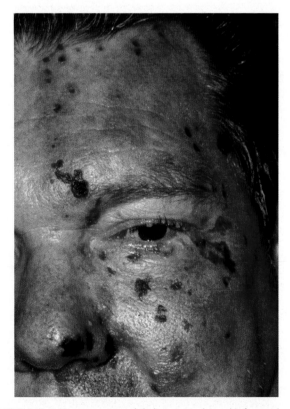

FIGURE 119-5 Herpes zoster ophthalmicus involving the first and second branch of the trigeminal nerve and the eyelids There is conjunctival hyperemia and purulent left eye discharge. The nasociliary branch of the ophthalmic branch of the trigeminal nerve is involved, producing the black crusting on the tip of the nose. (*Courtesy of Richard P. Usatine, MD.*)

rash starts with erythematous macules along the involved dermatome, then rapidly progresses over several days to papules, vesicles and pustules (**Figures 119-4** to **119-6**). The lesions rupture and typically crust over, requiring several weeks to heal completely.

- With the onset of a vesicular rash along the trigeminal dermatome, hyperemic conjunctivitis, episcleritis, and lid droop (ptosis) can occur (**Figure 119-6**).

- Approximately two-thirds of patients with herpes zoster ophthalmicus develop corneal involvement (keratitis).[1] The epithelial keratitis may feature punctate or dendriform lesions (**Figure 119-2**). Complications of corneal involvement can lead to corneal scarring (**Figure 119-3**).[6]

- Iritis (uveitis) occurs in approximately 40% of patients and can be associated with hyphema and an irregular pupil (**Figure 119-2**).[1]

TYPICAL DISTRIBUTION

- The frontal branch of the first division of the trigeminal nerve (which include the Supraorbital, Supratrochlear and External Nasal Peripheral nerves) is most frequently involved, and 50% to 72% of patients experience direct eye involvement (**Figure 119-7**).[1]

- Although herpes zoster ophthalmicus most often produces a classic dermatomal rash in the trigeminal distribution, a minority of patients may have only cornea findings.

DIFFERENTIAL DIAGNOSIS

- Bacterial or viral conjunctivitis presents as eye pain and foreign body sensation associated with discharge but no rash (see Chapter 15, Conjunctivitis).

- Trigeminal neuralgia presents with facial pain but without the rash or conjunctiva findings.

- Glaucoma which presents as inflammation, pain, and injection, but without the rash or conjunctiva findings (see Chapter 18, Glaucoma).

- Traumatic abrasions usually present with a history of trauma and corneal findings but no other zoster findings (see Chapter 14, Corneal Foreign Body/Abrasion).

- Pemphigus and other bullous diseases present with blisters but not in a dermatomal distribution (see Chapter 176, Overview of Bullous Disease).

MANAGEMENT

- Referral to an ophthalmologist urgently should be initiated when eye involvement is seen or suspected.SOR **C**

- The standard treatment for Herpes zoster ophthalmicus is to initiate antiviral therapy with acyclovir (800 mg, five times daily for 7–10 days), valacyclovir (1000 mg three times daily for 7 or 14 days), or famciclovir (500 mg orally three times a day for 7 days), as soon as possible in order to decrease the incidence of dendritic and stromal keratitis as well as anterior uveitis.[7] SOR **A**

- Oral acyclovir, valacyclovir, and famciclovir in patients with ophthalmic involvement have comparable outcomes. Treatment is

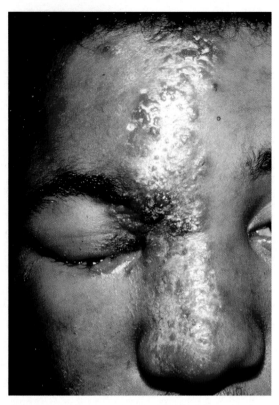

FIGURE 119-6 Herpes zoster ophthalmicus causing eyelid swelling and ptosis. Note the positive Hutchinson's sign. (*Courtesy of Richard P. Usatine, MD.*)

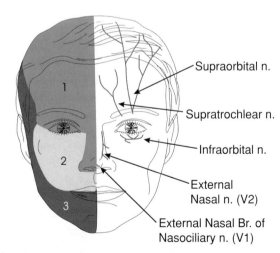

FIGURE 119-7 Diagram demonstrating the sensory distribution of the trigeminal (fifth cranial) nerve, and major peripheral nerves of the first (ophthalmic) division that may be involved with Herpes zoster ophthalmicus. The infraorbital nerve from the second division is also shown. (*Courtesy of. E.J. Mayeaux, Jr., MD.*)

most commonly oral acyclovir but intravenous acyclovir (10 mg/kg three times daily for 7 days) may be considered in immunocompromised patients or the rare patient who is extremely ill.[8] SOR Ⓐ

- Topical steroid ophthalmic drops are applied to the involved eye to reduce the inflammatory response and control immune keratitis and iritis.[1,2] SOR Ⓑ

- The ophthalmologist may prescribe a topical cycloplegic (such as atropine) to treat the ciliary muscle spasm that is painful in iritis. SOR Ⓒ

- Topical ophthalmic antibiotics may also be prescribed to prevent secondary infection of the eye. SOR Ⓒ

- As in all cases of zoster, pain should be treated effectively with oral analgesics and other appropriate medications. Early and effective treatment of pain may help to prevent postherpetic neuralgia (see Chapter 118, Herpes Zoster—Skin).

- Topical anesthetics should never be used with ocular involvement because of their corneal toxicity. SOR Ⓑ

- Secondary infection, usually *S. aureus*, may develop and should be treated with broad-spectrum topical and/or systemic antibiotics.

PATIENT EDUCATION

- Zoster of the eye is a very serious vision threatening illness that requires strict adherence to medical therapy and close follow-up.

- Viral transmission to nonimmune individuals from patients with herpes zoster can occur, but it is less frequent than with chickenpox. Virus can be transmitted through contact with secretions.

- Zoster vaccine decreases the incidence of zoster in the ophthalmic division of the trigeminal nerve but it is not indicated for persons that have already had a recent case of zoster.[9]

FOLLOW-UP

- Early diagnosis is critical to prevent progressive corneal involvement and potential loss of vision. Patients with herpes zoster should be informed that they should present for medical care with any zoster involving the first (ophthalmic) division of the trigeminal nerve or the eye itself.

PATIENT RESOURCES

- Steen-Hall Eye Institute—**http://www.steen-hall.com/zoster.html**
- EyeMDLink.com—**http://www.eyemdlink.com/Condition.asp?ConditionID=223**

PROVIDER RESOURCES

- Shaikh S, Christopher N. Evaluation and Management of Herpes Zoster Ophthalmicus. *Am Fam Physician* 2002;66:1723–1730, 1732. Available online at—**http://www.aafp.org/afp/20021101/1723.html**

- eMedicine: Herpes Zoster—**http://www.emedicine.com/OPH/topic257.htm**

REFERENCES

1. Pavan-Langston D. Herpes zoster ophthalmicus. *Neurology*. 1995; 45:S50.

2. Severson EA, Baratz KH, Hodge DO, Burke JP. Herpes zoster ophthalmicus in olmsted county, minnesota: Have systemic antivirals made a difference?. *Arch Ophthalmol*. 2003;121:386.

3. Zaal MJ, Völker-Dieben HJ, D'Amaro J. Prognostic value of Hutchinson's sign in acute herpes zoster ophthalmicus. *Graefes Arch Clin Exp Ophthalmol*. 2003;241(3):187–191.

4. Liesegang TJ. Corneal complications from herpes zoster ophthalmicus. *Ophthalmology*. 1985;92:316–324.

5. Liesegang TJ. Herpes zoster ophthalmicus natural history, risk factors, clinical presentation, and morbidity. *Ophthalmology*. 2008; 115(2 Suppl):S3-12.

6. Albrecht Ma. Clinical features of varicella-zoster virus infection: Herpes zoster. http://www.uptodate.com. Accessed March 27, 2008.

7. McGill J, Chapman C, Mahakasingam M. Acyclovir therapy in herpes zoster infection. A practical guide. *Trans Ophthalmol Soc U K*. 1983;103(pt 1):111–114.

8. Gnann JW, Jr., Whitley RJ. Herpes zoster. *N Engl J Med*. 2002;347: 340.

9. Gelb LD. Preventing herpes zoster through vaccination. *Ophthalmology*. 2008;115(2 Suppl):S35-8.

120 MEASLES

E.J. Mayeaux, Jr., MD

PATIENT STORY

An 18-month-old boy, who is visiting family in San Antonio with his parents from Central America, presents with a 3-day history of fever, malaise, conjunctivitis, coryza, and cough. He had been exposed to a child with similar symptoms approximately 2 weeks prior. A day before, he developed a maculopapular rash that blanches under pressure (**Figures 120-1** and **120-2**). His shot records are unavailable but his mother states that his last vaccine was before age 1. He is diagnosed with measles and supportive care is provided.

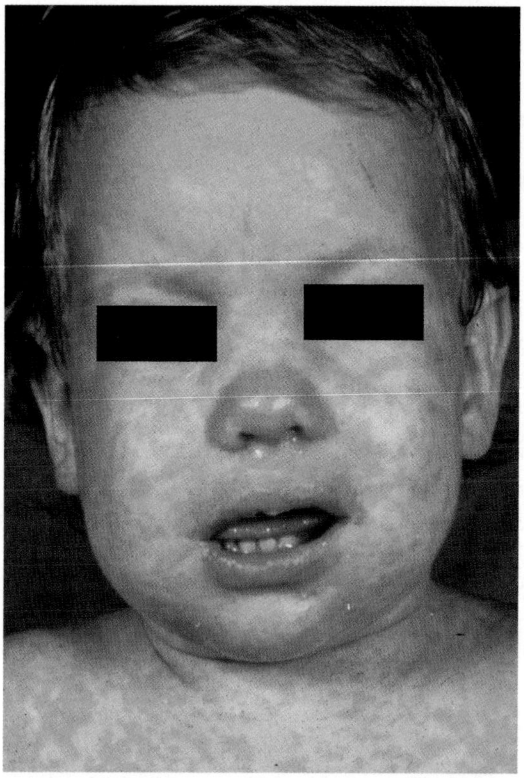

EPIDEMIOLOGY

- Last major outbreak in the United States was during 1989 to 1990 and prompted a change in immunization policy in 1991, so that all children are to have 2 MMR vaccines before starting kindergarten.

- This practice interrupted the transmission of indigenous measles in the United States by 1993 and reduced incidence of measles to an historic low (<0.5 cases per million persons) by 1997 to 1999.[1]

- Approximately 30 million measles cases are reported annually worldwide. Most reported cases are from Africa. In 1998, the reported cases of measles per 100,000 total population reported to the World Health Organization was 1.6 in the Americas, 8.2 in Europe, 11.1 in the Eastern Mediterranean region, 4.2 in South East Asia, 5.0 in the Western Pacific region, and 61.7 in Africa.[1]

ETIOLOGY AND PATHOPHYSIOLOGY

- Measles is caused by the measles virus, a member of the family paramyxoviridae, genus *Morbillivirus* (hence the name, morbilliform rash).

- It is highly contagious, transmitted by airborne droplets, and commonly causes outbreaks.

- Classic measles infection starts with the incubation phase that is usually asymptomatic and lasts for 10 to 14 days. It starts after entry of the virus into the respiratory mucosa with local viral replication. The infection then spreads to regional lymphatic tissues, and then throughout the body through the bloodstream.

- The prodrome phase starts with the appearance of systemic symptoms including fever, malaise, anorexia, conjunctivitis, coryza, and cough. The respiratory symptoms are caused by mucosal inflammation from viral infection of epithelial cells. Patients may develop Koplik's spots, which are small whitish, grayish, or bluish papules with erythematous bases that develop on the buccal mucosa usually near the molar teeth (**Figure 120-3**). The prodrome usually lasts for 2 to 3 days.

- The classic measles rash (**Figures 120-1** and **120-2**) is maculopapular and blanches under pressure. Clinical improvement in

FIGURE 120-1 Typical measles rash that began on the face and became confluent. (*Courtesy of the University of Texas Health Sciences Center, Division of Dermatology.*)

symptoms typically ensues within 2 days. Three to four days after the rash first appears, it begins to fade to a brownish color which is followed by fine flaking. The cough may persist for up to 2 weeks.

- Fever persisting beyond the third day of rash suggests a measles-associated complication.

- Immunity after measles infection is thought to be life-long in most cases. Measles reinfection occasionally occurs, but it is extremely rare.

- Atypical measles is a measles variant that occurs in previously-vaccinated persons. Patients develop high fever and headache 7 to 14 days after exposure, and often present with a dry cough and pleuritic chest pain. Two to three days later, a rash develops that spreads from the extremities to the trunk. The rash may be vesicular, petechial, purpuric, or urticarial. Patients may develop respiratory distress, peripheral edema, hepatosplenomegaly, paresthesias, or hyperesthesia.

- The measles virus can cause a variety of clinical syndromes including the classic childhood illness and a less intense form in persons with suboptimal levels of anti-measles antibodies.

- Measles virus infection can also result in more severe illness, including lymphadenopathy, splenomegaly, laryngotracheobronchitis (croup), giant cell pneumonia, and measles inclusion body encephalitis in immunocompromised patients.[2] This form occurs in the very old and young, those with vitamin A deficiency, and in pregnant women.

- Postinfection neurologic syndromes can occur. Postinfectious encephalomyelitis is a demyelinating disease that presents during the recovery phase, and is thought to be caused by a postinfectious autoimmune response.[3] The major manifestations include fever, headache, neck stiffness, ataxia, mental status changes, and seizures. CSF analysis demonstrates lymphocytosis and elevated proteins. Postinfectious encephalomyelitis has a 10% to 20% mortality rate, and residual neurologic abnormalities are common.[3]

- Subacute sclerosing panencephalitis (SSPE) is a progressive, fatal, neurological degenerative disease that may represent a persistent infection of the central nervous system with a variant of the virus. It usually occurs in patients younger than 20 years of age and 7 to 10 years after natural measles.[4] Patients develop neurologic symptoms, myoclonus, dementia, and eventually flaccidity or decorticate rigidity.

- Measles in pregnancy is a rare entity in areas that practice vaccination. Premature births may be more common in gravid women with measles, but there is no clear evidence of teratogenicity.[5]

DIAGNOSIS

Measles is a distinct disease characterized by fever, malaise, conjunctivitis, coryza, cough, rash, and Koplik's spots.

CLINICAL FEATURES

Koplik's spots appear during the prodrome phase and are pathognomonic for measles infection and occur approximately 48 hours before the characteristic measles exanthem. The classic blanching rash is

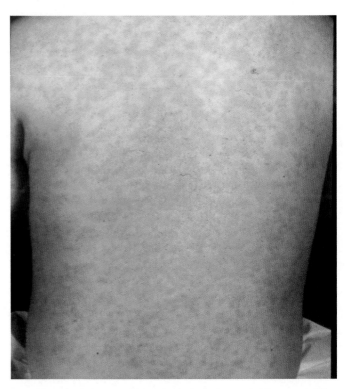

FIGURE 120-2 The typical measles rash on the trunk. (*Courtesy of the University of Texas Health Sciences Center, Division of Dermatology.*)

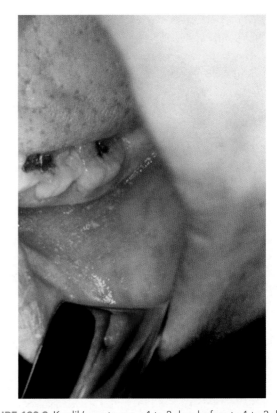

FIGURE 120-3 Koplik's spots occur 1 to 2 days before to 1 to 2 days after the cutaneous rash. Their presence is considered to be pathognomonic for measles, and appear as punctate blue-white spots on the bright red background of the oral buccal (cheek) mucosa. (*Courtesy of the Centers for Disease Control and Prevention.*)

usually adequate to make a tentative diagnosis. The most rapid and accurate test to confirm acute measles is a blood test for measles specific IgM antibodies. By waiting until the third day of the rash, a false-negative IgM result can be avoided.[1]

TYPICAL DISTRIBUTION

The rash begins on the face and spreads centrifugally to involve the neck, trunk, and finally the extremities. The lesions may become confluent, especially on the face. This cranial-to-caudal rash progression is characteristic of measles.

DIFFERENTIAL DIAGNOSIS

• Upper respiratory tract infections—The prodrome stage of measles can be confused with a URI except that significant fever is typically present with measles infection.

• Fordyce spots—Tiny yellow-white granules on the buccal or lip mucosa caused by benign ectopic sebaceous glands, may be mistaken for Koplik's spots. Fordyce spots do not have an erythematous base.

• Alternative diagnoses that may be confused with the measles rash include Rocky Mountain spotted fever, infectious mononucleosis, scarlet fever, Kawasaki disease, toxic shock syndrome, dengue fever, and simple drug eruption (see Chapter 196, Cutaneous Drug Reactions).

• Measles can usually be distinguished clinically from rubella, erythema infectiosum (parvovirus B19 infection), roseola, and enteroviral infection by the intensity of the measles rash, its subsequent brownish coloration, and the disease course.

MANAGEMENT

• The treatment of measles is mostly supportive and includes antipyretics, fluids, and treatment of superinfections such as bacterial pneumonia and otitis.

• When outbreaks of measles occur, it is important to prevent spread of the disease. Suspected cases of measles should be immediately reported to the local or state department of health.

• Measures to control spread of infection should not be delayed for laboratory confirmation. Vaccine should be promptly administered to all susceptible persons, or they should be removed from the outbreak setting for a minimum of 3 weeks.

• Giving serum immune globulin 0.25 mL/kg of body weight to a maximum dose of 15 mL to a susceptible person within 6 days of exposure to measles, can prevent or modify disease. This is especially important in patients in whom the risk of complications of measles is higher such as pregnant women, children younger than 1 year of age, and immunocompromised patients.

PATIENT RESOURCES

• KidsHealth—**http://www.kidshealth.org/parent/ infections/bacterial_viral/measles.html.**
• Wikipedia—**http://en.wikipedia.org/wiki/Measles.**

PROVIDER RESOURCES

- MedlinePlus-Measles—**http://www.nlm.nih.gov/ medlineplus/measles.html.**
- CDC Measles—**http://www.cdc.gov/nip/publications/ ink/meas.pdf.**

REFERENCES

1. Chen S, Fennelly G. Measles. http://www.emedicine.com/PED/ topic1388.htm. Accessed March 22, 2008.

2. Kaplan LJ, Daum RS, Smaron M, McCarthy CA. Severe measles in immunocompromised patients. *JAMA.* 1992;267:1237.

3. Johnson RT, Griffin DE, Hirsch RL, et al. Measles encephalomyelitis—clinical and immunologic studies. *N Engl J Med.* 1984;310:137.

4. Bellini WJ, Rota JS, Lowe LE, et al. Subacute sclerosing panencephalitis: More cases of this fatal disease are prevented by measles immunization than was previously recognized. *J Infect Dis.* 2005; 192:1686.

5. Siegel M, Fuerst HT. Low birth weight and maternal virus diseases. A prospective study of rubella, measles, mumps, chickenpox, and hepatitis. *JAMA.* 1966;197:680.

121 FIFTH DISEASE (ERYTHEMA INFECTIOSUM)

E.J. Mayeaux, Jr., MD

PATIENT STORY

A 2-year-old boy presents with mild flu-like symptoms and a rash. He had erythematous malar rash and a "lace-like" erythematous rash on the trunk and extremities (**Figures 121-1** and **121-2**). The "slapped cheek" appearance made the diagnosis easy for fifth disease. The parents were reassured that this would go away on its own. The child returned to day care the next day.

Erythema infectiosum (EI) is also commonly referred to as "fifth disease" since it represents the fifth of the six common childhood viral exanthems described.

EPIDEMIOLOGY

- EI is common throughout the world. Most individuals become infected during their school years.

- EI is very contagious via the respiratory route and occurs more frequently between late winter and early summer. In some communities, there are cycles of local epidemics every 4 to 10 years.[1]

- 30% to 40% of pregnant women lack measurable IgG to the infecting agent and are, therefore, presumed to be susceptible to infection. Infection during pregnancy can in some cases lead to fetal death.

ETIOLOGY AND PATHOPHYSIOLOGY

- EI is a mild viral febrile illness with an associated rash caused by parvovirus B19 (**Figure 121-3**).

- Most persons with parvovirus B19 infection never develop the clinical picture of EI.

- Parvovirus B19 infects rapidly dividing cells and is cytotoxic for erythroid progenitor cells.

- After initial infection, a viremia occurs with an associated precipitous drop in the reticulocyte count and anemia. The anemia is rarely clinically apparent in healthy patients but can cause serious anemia if the red blood cell count is already low. Patients with a chronic anemia such as sickle cell or thalassemia may experience a transient aplastic crisis.[2]

- Vertical transmission can result in congenital infection if a woman becomes infected during her pregnancy.[3] The risk of a fetal loss or hydrops fetalis is greatest (loss rate of 11%) when the infection occurs within the first 20 weeks of gestation.[4]

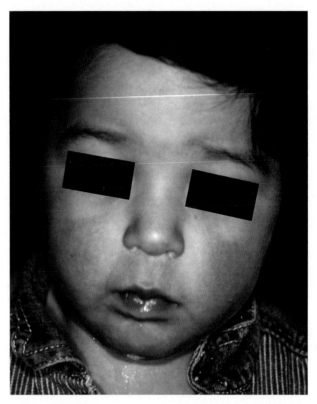

FIGURE 121-1 Classic erythematous malar rash with "slapped cheek" appearance of fifth disease (Erythema infectiosum). (*Courtesy of Richard P. Usatine, MD.*)

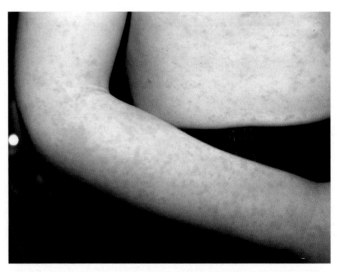

FIGURE 121-2 Classic fifth disease "lace-like" erythematous rash on the trunk and extremities. (*Courtesy of Richard P. Usatine, MD.*)

DIAGNOSIS

CLINICAL FEATURES

Fifth disease is characterized by a classic erythematous malar rash with relative circumoral pallor or "slapped cheek" appearance in children (**Figure 121-1**) and a "lace-like" erythematous rash on the trunk and extremities (**Figures 121-2** and **121-4**). Children and adults may experience up to 4 or more days of specific flu-like symptoms prior to the appearance of the rash. Arthropathy affecting the hands, wrists, knees, and ankles may precede the development of a rash in adults. The course is usually self-limited.

TYPICAL DISTRIBUTION

The rash starts with the classic slapped-cheek appearance (**Figure 121-1**). Then an erythematous macular rash occurs on the extremities. After several days, the extremities rash fades into a lacy pattern (**Figures 121-2** and **121-4**). The exanthem may recur over several weeks in association with exercise, sun exposure, bathing in hot water, or stress.

LABORATORY STUDIES

Laboratory studies are not usually needed since the diagnosis can be made by history and PE. Serum B19-specific IgM may be ordered in pregnant women exposed to fifth disease. After 3 weeks, infection is also indicated by a fourfold or greater rise in serum B19-specific IgG antibody titers.

Patients with symptoms of anemia, a history of increased RBC destruction (e.g., sickle cell disease, hereditary spherocytosis), or with decreased RBC production (e.g., iron deficiency anemia) should be tested for anemia.

DIFFERENTIAL DIAGNOSIS

- Acute rheumatic fever presents as a fine papular (sandpaper) rash in association with a streptococcus infection (see Chapter 33, Strawberry Tongue and Scarlet Fever).

- Allergic-hypersensitivity reaction presents with a body-wide vasculitic rash (see Section 14, Hypersensitivity Syndromes).

- Lyme disease presents with an expanding rash with central clearing (see Chapter 211, Lyme Disease).

MANAGEMENT

- EI (fifth disease) is usually self-limited and requires no specific therapy.

- NSAID or acetaminophen therapy may alleviate fevers and arthralgias. SOR **C**

- Transient aplastic anemia may be severe enough to require transfusion until the patient's red cell production recovers. SOR **C**

- Pregnant women who are exposed to or have symptoms of parvovirus infection should have serologic testing. SOR **C** Prior to 20 weeks gestation, women testing positive for acute infection

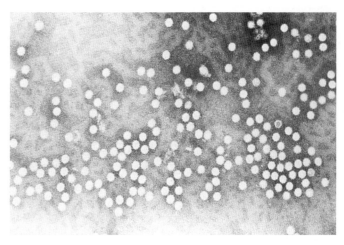

FIGURE 121-3 Transmission electron microscopy of parvovirus B19. (*Courtesy of the Centers for Disease Control and Prevention.*)

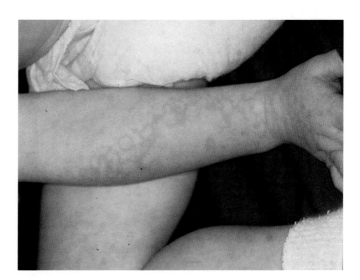

FIGURE 121-4 Classic reticular eruption on the extremities. (*Courtesy of Jeffrey Meffert, MD.*)

(i.e., positive IgM and negative IgG) should be counseled concerning the low risk of fetal loss and congenital anomalies. If positive, some experts recommend that the patient should receive ultrasounds to look for signs of fetal hydrops. SOR **C** Intrauterine transfusion is currently the only effective treatment to alleviate fetal anemia.[5]

PATIENT EDUCATION

- Explain to parents that the disease is usually self-limited. Normal activities may be pursued as tolerated with sun protection or avoidance.

- Children who present with the classic findings of EI are past the infectious state and can attend school and day care.

- During pregnancy, a woman who has an acute infection prior to 20 weeks gestation should be counseled concerning the low risks of fetal loss and congenital anomalies. Beyond 20 weeks gestation, some physicians my recommend repeated ultrasounds to look for signs of fetal hydrops.

PATIENT RESOURCES

- KidsHealth: Fifth Disease—**http://www.kidshealth.org/ parent/infections/bacterial_viral/fifth.html**

- Centers for Disease Control and Prevention, National Center for Infectious Diseases—**http://www.cdc.gov/ncidod/ dvrd/revb/respiratory/parvo_b19.htm**

- Parvovirus and pregnancy—**http://www.cdc.gov/ncidod/ dvrd/revb/respiratory/B19&preg.htm**

PROVIDER RESOURCES

- eMedicine—**http://www.emedicine.com/derm/ topic136.htm**

- AFP Parvovirus B19 Infections. 1999;60:1455–60— **http://www.aafp.org/afp/991001ap/1455.html**

REFERENCES

1. Naides SJ. Erythema infectiosum (fifth disease) occurrence in Iowa. *Am J Public Health*. 1988;78:1230.

2. Serjeant GR, Serjeant GE, Thomas PW, et al. Human parvovirus infection in homozygous sickle cell disease. *Lancet*. 1993;341:1237.

3. Jordan JA. Identification of human parvovirus B19 infection in idiopathic nonimmune hydrops fetalis. *Am J Obstet Gynecol*. 1996; 174:37.

4. Enders M, Weidner A, Zoellner I, et al. Fetal morbidity and mortality after acute human parvovirus B19 infection in pregnancy: Prospective evaluation of 1018 cases. *Prenat Diagn*. 2004;24:513.

5. de Jong EP, de Haan TR, Kroes ACM, Beersma MFC, Oepkes D, Walther FJ. Parvovirus B19 infection in pregnancy. *J Clin Virol*. 2006;36(1):1–7.

122 HAND, FOOT, AND MOUTH DISEASE

E.J. Mayeaux, Jr., MD

PATIENT STORY

A 4-year-old boy presents to a free clinic for homeless families with a low-grade fever and lesions on his hands and feet (**Figures 122-1** and **122-2**). The mother notes that two other kids in the transitional living center also have a similar rash. Upon further investigation, the mouth lesions are noted (**Figure 122-3**). The mother is reassured that this is nothing more than hand, foot, and mouth disease and will go away on its own. Treatment includes fluids and antipyretics as needed.

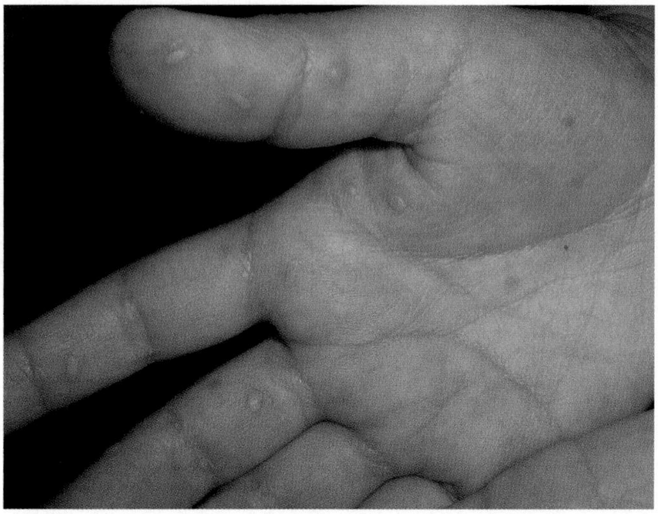

EPIDEMIOLOGY

- Hand, foot, and mouth disease (HFMD) is a viral illness that may affect humans and some animals, and presents with a distinct clinical presentation. The disease occurs worldwide.

- Epidemics tend to occur every 3 years in the United States. In temperate climates, the peak incidence is in late summer and early fall.

- HFMD generally has a mild course, but it may be more severe in infants and young children.[1,2]

- There is no racial or gender predilection. Most cases affect children younger than 10-year-old.

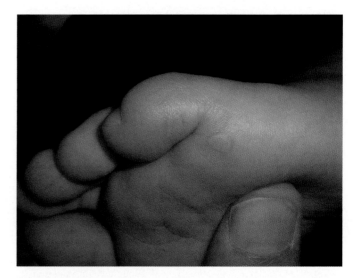

FIGURE 122-1 Typical flat vesicular lesions on the hand of a 4-year-old boy with hand, foot, and mouth disease. (*Courtesy of Richard P. Usatine, MD.*)

ETIOLOGY AND PATHOPHYSIOLOGY

- HFMD is most commonly caused by members of the Enterovirus genus, especially coxsackie viruses. Epidemic infections are usually caused by coxsackievirus A16 or enterovirus 71.[2] Sporadic cases occur caused by other coxsackie viruses.

- Coxsackievirus infections are highly contagious. Transmission occurs via aerosolized droplets of nasal and/or oral secretions or direct contact with fecal material. During epidemics, the virus is spread from child to child and from mother to fetus.

- The incubation period averages 3 to 6 days. Initial viral implantation is in the GI tract mucosa, and it then spreads to lymph nodes within 24 hours. Viremia rapidly ensues, with spread to the oral mucosa and skin. Usually by day 7, a neutralizing antibody response develops, and the virus is cleared from the body.

- When HFMD is caused by Enteroviruses, it may also result in myocarditis, pneumonia, meningoencephalitis, and death.

- Infection in the first trimester of pregnancy may lead to spontaneous abortion or intrauterine growth retardation.

FIGURE 122-2 Foot of the boy in **Figure 122-1**. Lesions tend to be on palms and soles, fingers, and toes. (*Courtesy of Richard P. Usatine, MD.*)

DIAGNOSIS

CLINICAL FEATURES

A prodrome lasting 12 to 36 hours is usually the first sign of HFMD, and it usually consists of typical general viral infection symptoms with anorexia, abdominal pain, and sore mouth. Lesions are present for 5 to 10 days, and heal spontaneously in 5 to 7 days. Each lesion begins as a 2 to 10 mm erythematous macule, which develops a gray, oval vesicle that parallels the skin tension lines in its long axis (**Figures 122-1** and **122-2**). The oral lesions (**Figure 122-3**) begin as erythematous macules, evolve into 2 to 3 mm vesicles on an erythematous base, and then rapidly become ulcerated. The vesicles are painful and may interfere with eating. Cervical or submandibular lymphadenopathy may be present.

TYPICAL DISTRIBUTION

Skin lesions develop on the hands, feet, and/or buttocks and oral lesions may involve the palate, buccal mucosa, gingiva, and/or tongue.

LABORATORY STUDIES

Laboratory tests are not needed.

DIFFERENTIAL DIAGNOSIS

- Aphthous stomatitis presents as single or multiple painful ulcers in the mouth without skin eruptions (see Chapter 40, Aphthous Ulcer).

- Chickenpox present with body-wide vesicular lesions in multiple crops (see Chapter 117, Chickenpox).

- Erythema multiforme demonstrates body-wide target lesions that also involve the skin of the palms and soles (see Chapter 170, Erythema Multiforme).

- Herpes simplex presents with painful recurrent ulcerations of the lips or genitals without simultaneous hand or foot lesions unless there is herpetic whitlow on the hand (see Chapter 123, Herpes Simplex).

MANAGEMENT

- Usually the mouth lesions are not as painful as in herpes gingivostomatitis. If there is a lot of mouth pain leading to poor oral intake, the following medications may be considered. Topical oral anesthetics such as 2% viscous lidocaine by prescription or 20% topical benzocaine (Orabase) OTC may be used to treat painful oral ulcers. SOR Ⓒ A solution combining aluminum and magnesium hydroxide (liquid antacid) and 2% viscous lidocaine has been reported as helpful when swished and spit out several times a day as needed for pain. SOR Ⓒ

- Acetaminophen or NSAIDs/COX-2 s may be used to manage fever, and analgesics may be used to treat arthralgias. SOR Ⓒ Aspirin should not be used in viral illnesses in children younger than 12 years of age to prevent Reyes syndrome. SOR Ⓒ

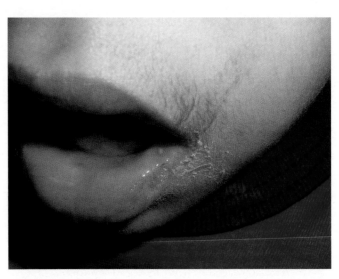

FIGURE 122-3 Mouth lesions in same boy appear as small ulcers on the lips and oral mucosa. (*Courtesy of Richard P. Usatine, MD.*)

• A case report of enterovirus HFMD in an immunocompromised patient reported a faster resolution of symptoms and lesions with oral acyclovir.[3] SOR Ⓒ

PATIENT EDUCATION

Educate parents of young children to watch for signs of dehydration owing to decreased oral intake secondary to mouth pain. The patient may attend school once symptoms subside, but good hand-washing should be encouraged to reduce the spread of disease. Report any neurological symptoms to healthcare providers immediately.

PATIENT RESOURCES

Mayo Clinic: Hand, foot, and mouth disease—**http://www.mayoclinic.com/health/hand-foot-and-mouth-disease/DS00599.**

Centers for Disease Control and Prevention: Hand, foot, and mouth disease—**http://www.cdc.gov/ncidod/dvrd/revb/enterovirus/hfhf.htm.**

PROVIDER RESOURCES

eMedicine: Hand, foot, and mouth disease—**http://www.emedicine.com/derm/topic175.htm.**

Medline Plus: Hand, foot, and mouth disease—**http://www.nlm.nih.gov/medlineplus/ency/article/000965.htm.**

REFERENCES

1. Chang LY, King CC, Hsu KH, et al. Risk factors of enterovirus 71 infection and associated hand, foot, and mouth disease/herpangina in children during an epidemic in Taiwan. *Pediatrics.* 2002;109(6): e88

2. Chong CY, Chan KP, Shah VA, et al. Hand, foot and mouth disease in Singapore: A comparison of fatal and non-fatal cases. *Acta Paediatr.* 2003;92(10):1163–1169.

3. Faulkner CF, Godbolt AM, DeAmbrosis B, Triscott J. Hand, foot and mouth disease in an immunocompromised adult treated with aciclovir. *Australas J Dermatol.* 2003;44(3):203–206.

123 HERPES SIMPLEX

E.J. Mayeaux, Jr., MD

PATIENT STORY

A 32-year-old man presents with complains of a 1-week history of multiple painful vesicles on the shaft of his penis associated with tender groin adenopathy (**Figure 123-1**). The vesicles broke 2 days ago and the pain has increased. He had similar lesions 1 year ago but never went for health care at that time. He has had three different female sexual partners in the last 2 years but has no knowledge of them having any sores or diseases. He was given the presumptive diagnosis of genital herpes and a course of acyclovir. His herpes culture came back positive and his RPR and HIV tests were negative.

EPIDEMIOLOGY

- Herpes simplex virus (HSV) affects more than one-third of the world's population, with the two most common cutaneous manifestations being genital (**Figures 123-1 to 123-4**) and orolabial herpes (**Figures 123-5 to 123-7**).[1]

- Orolabial herpes is the most prevalent form of herpes infection and often affects children younger than 5 years of age (**Figure 121-7**). The duration of the illness is 2 to 3 weeks, and oral shedding of virus may continue for as long as 23 days.[1]

- Herpetic whitlow is an intense painful infection of the hand involving the terminal phalanx of one or more digits. In the United States, the estimated annual incidence is 2.4 cases per 100 000 persons.[2]

ETIOLOGY AND PATHOPHYSIOLOGY

- HSV belongs to the family Herpesviridae and is a double-stranded DNA virus.

- HSV exists as two separate types (types 1 and 2), which have affinities for different epithelia.[2] 90% of HSV-2 infections are genital, whereas 90% of those caused by HSV-1 are oral–labial.

- HSV enters through abraded skin or intact mucous membranes. Once infected, the epithelial cells die forming vesicles and creating multinucleated giant cells.

- Retrograde transport into sensory ganglia leads to lifelong latent infection.[1] Reactivation of the virus may be triggered by immunodeficiency, trauma, fever, and ultraviolet light.

- Genital HSV infection is usually transmitted through sexual contact. When it occurs in a preadolescent, the possibility of abuse must be considered.

- Evidence indicates that 21.9% of all persons in the United States, 12 years or older, have serologic evidence of HSV-2 infection, which is more commonly associated with genital infections.[3]

- As many as 90% of those infected are unaware that they have herpes infection and may unknowingly shed virus and transmit infection.[4]

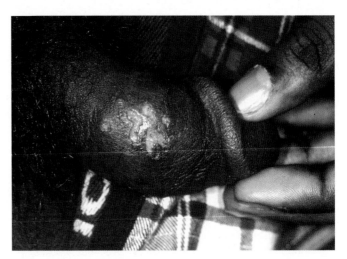

FIGURE 123-1 Recurrent Genital HSV on the penis showing grouped ulcers (deroofed vesicles). (*Courtesy of Richard P. Usatine, MD.*)

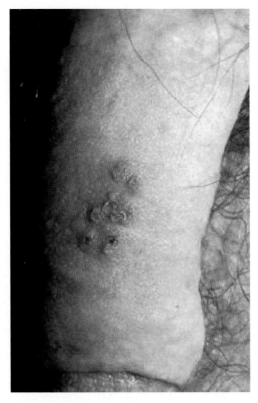

FIGURE 123-2 Herpes simplex on the penis with intact vesicles and visible crusts. (*Courtesy of Jack Rezneck, Sr., MD.*)

- Primary genital herpes has an average incubation period of 4 days, followed by a prodrome of itching, burning or erythema.

- With both types, systemic symptoms are common in primary disease and include fever, headache, malaise, abdominal pain, and myalgia.[5] Recurrences are usually less severe and shorter in duration than the initial outbreak.[1,5]

- Maternal–fetal transmission of HSV is associated with significant morbidity and mortality. Manifestations of neonatal HSV include localized infection of the skin, eyes, and mouth, CNS disease, or disseminated multiple organ disease (**Figure 123-8**). The CDC and the American College of Obstetricians and Gynecologists recommend that cesarean delivery should be offered as soon as possible to women who have active HSV lesions or, in those with a history of genital herpes, symptoms of vulvar pain or burning at the time of delivery.

- Herpetic whitlow occurs as a complication of oral or genital HSV infection and in medical personnel who have contact with oral secretions (**Figures 123-9** and **123-10**).

- Toddlers and preschool children are susceptible to herpetic whitlow if they have herpes labialis and engage in thumb-sucking or finger-sucking behavior.

- Like all HSV infections, herpetic whitlow usually has a primary infection, which may be followed by subsequent recurrences. The virus migrates to the peripheral ganglia and Schwann cells where it lies dormant. Recurrences observed in 20% to 50% of cases are usually milder and shorter in duration.

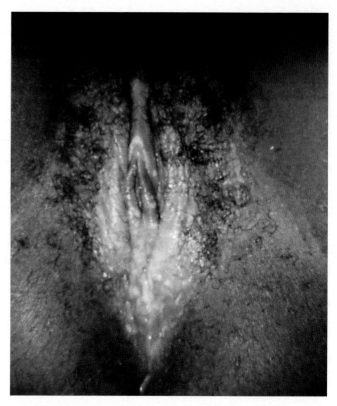

FIGURE 123-3 Vulvar HSV at the introitus showing small punched out ulcers. (*Courtesy of the CDC and Susan Lindsley.*)

DIAGNOSIS

CLINICAL FEATURES

- The diagnosis of HSV infection may be made by clinical appearance. Many patients have systemic symptoms, including fever, headache, malaise, and myalgias.

- Orolabial herpes typically takes the form of painful vesicles and ulcerative erosions on the tongue, palate, gingiva, buccal mucosa, and lips (**Figures 123-5** to **123-7**).

- Genital herpes presents with multiple transient, painful vesicles that appear on the penis (**Figures 123-1** and **123-2**), vulva (**Figure 123-3**) buttocks (**Figure 123-4**), perineum, vagina or cervix, and tender inguinal lymphadenopathy.[5] The vesicles break down and become ulcers which develop crusts while these are healing.

- Recurrences typically occur two to three times a year. The duration is shorter and less painful than in primary infections. The lesions are often single and the vesicles heal completely by 8 to 10 days.

- UV radiation in the form of sunlight. Another reason to use sun protection when outdoors triggers recurrence of orolabial HSV-1, an effect which is not fully suppressed by acyclovir.

LABORATORY STUDIES

- The gold standard of diagnosis is viral isolation by tissue culture.[1] The sensitivity rate is only 70% to 80% and depends upon the stage at which the specimen is collected. The sensitivity is highest at first in the vesicular stage and declines with ulceration and crusting. The tissue culture assay can be positive within 48 hours but may take

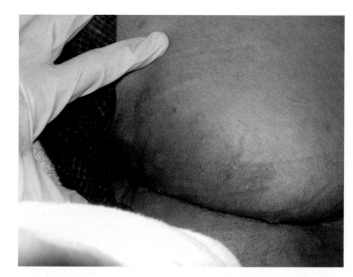

FIGURE 123-4 Recurrent HSV on the buttocks of a woman. Women are prone to getting buttocks involvement owing to sleeping with partners that have genital involvement. (*Courtesy of Richard P. Usatine, MD.*)

longer. The Tzanck test and antigen detection tests have lower sensitivity rates (50%–70%) than viral culture.[5] Serologic testing is extremely sensitive but is only helpful in diagnosing recurrent infections. The direct fluorescent-antibody (DFA) assay can simultaneously detect herpes simplex virus types 1 and 2 faster than the culture but is less sensitive.

- Polymerase chain reaction enzyme-linked immunosorbent assay (PCR-ELISA) is extremely sensitive (96%) and specific (99%).[1] This test is generally reserved for CSF testing in suspected HSV encephalitis or meningitis.

- If the herpes was acquired by sexual contact, screening should be performed for other STDs such as syphilis and HIV.

- Biopsy is usually unnecessary unless no infectious etiology is found for a genital lesion and a malignancy is suspected.

DIFFERENTIAL DIAGNOSIS

- Syphilis produces a painless or mildly painful, indurated, clean-based ulcer (chancre) at the site of exposure. It is best to investigate for syphilis or co-existing syphilis in any patient presenting for the first time with a genital ulcer of unproven etiology (see Chapter 209, Syphilis).

- Chancroid produces a painful deep, undermined, purulent ulcer that may be associated with painful inguinal lymphadenitis (see Chapter 209, Syphilis).

- Drug eruptions produce pruritic papules or blisters without associated viral symptoms (see Chapter 196, Cutaneous Drug Reactions).

- Behcet's disease produces ulcerative disease around the mouth and genitals, possibly before onset of sexual activity.

- Acute paronychia which presents as a localized abscess in a nail fold and is the main differential diagnosis in the consideration of herpetic whitlow (see Chapter 187, Paronychia).

- Felon—a red, painful infection, usually bacterial, of the fingertip pulp. It is important to distinguish whitlow from a felon (where the pulp space usually is tensely swollen) since incision and drainage of a felon is needed, but should be avoided in herpetic whitlow because it may lead to an unnecessary secondary bacterial infections.

MANAGEMENT

- Acyclovir is a guanosine analog that acts as a DNA chain terminator which, when incorporated, ends viral DNA replication. Valacyclovir is the l-valine ester prodrug of acyclovir. Famciclovir is the oral form of penciclovir, a purine analog similar to acyclovir. They must be administered early in the outbreak to be effective, but are safe and extremely well-tolerated.[5] SOR Ⓐ

- HSV strains resistent to acyclovir have been detected in immuncompromised patients so that other antivirals (e.g. famciclovir) need to be considered in these patients. SOR Ⓒ

- Topical medication for HSV infection is generally not very effective. Topical penciclovir applied every 2 hours for 4 days, reduces clinical healing time by approximately 1 day.[1]

- In the treatment of primary orolabial herpes, oral acyclovir (200 mg 5 times daily for 5 days) accelerates healing by 1 day and can

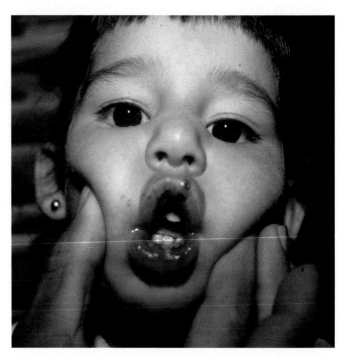

FIGURE 123-5 Primary herpes gingivostomatitis in a young girl. Her mom has painted gentian violet on her lips and gums. (*Courtesy of Richard P. Usatine, MD.*)

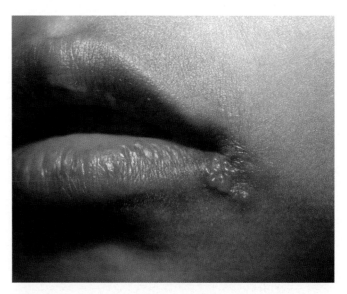

FIGURE 123-6 Close-up of recurrent HSV-1 showing vesicles on a red base at the vermillion border in a young girl. (*Courtesy of Richard P. Usatine, MD.*)

reduce the mean duration of pain by 36%.[6] SOR Ⓐ The clinical importance of these effects is questionable.

- The oral lesions in primary herpes gingivostomatitis can lead to poor oral intake especially in children (**Figure 123-5**). To prevent dehydration, the following medications may be considered. Topical oral anesthetics such as 2% viscous lidocaine by prescription or 20% topical benzocaine (Orabase) OTC may be used to treat painful oral ulcers. SOR Ⓒ A solution combining aluminum and magnesium hydroxide (liquid antacid) and 2% viscous lidocaine has been reported as helpful when swished and spit out several times a day as needed for pain. SOR Ⓒ

- Short-term prophylactic therapy with acyclovir for orolabial HSV may be used in patients who anticipate intense exposure to UV light. Early treatment of recurrent orolabial HSV infection with Famciclovir 250 mg 3 times daily for 5 days can markedly decrease the size and duration of lesions.[7] SOR Ⓐ

- Antiviral therapy is recommended for an initial genital herpes outbreak. Dosing for anti-herpes drugs are shown in **Table 123-1**.

- The same 3 antiviral medications can be used to prevent recurrences. Traditionally this is reserved for use in patients who have more than 4–6 outbreaks per year (see **Table 123-1**).

PATIENT EDUCATION

- Measures to prevent genital HSV infection:
  - Abstain from sexual activity or limit number of sexual partners to prevent exposure to the disease.
  - Use condoms to protect against transmission, but this is not foolproof since ulcers can occur on areas not covered by condoms.
  - Prevent autoinoculation by patting dry affected areas, not rubbing with towel.

- Studies have shown that patients may shed virus when they are otherwise asymptomatic. A link between HSV genital ulcer disease and sexual transmission of human immunodeficiency virus (HIV) has been established. Safer sex practices should be strongly encouraged to prevent transmission of HSV to others and acquiring HIV by the patient.

FOLLOW-UP

- The patient should return for follow-up if pain is uncontrolled or superinfection is suspected. The patient should be periodically evaluated for the need for suppressive therapy based on the number of recurrences per year.

PATIENT RESOURCES

National Institute of Allergy and Infectious Diseases—
http://www.niaid.nih.gov/factsheets/stdherp.htm

Centers for Disease Control and Prevention—**http://www.cdc.gov/std/Herpes/STDFact-Herpes.htm**

American Academy of Family Physicians—
http://familydoctor.org/891.xml

University of Michigan Pediatric Advisor: Herpetic Whitlow—
http://www.med.umich.edu/1libr/pa/pa_herpwhit_hhg.htm

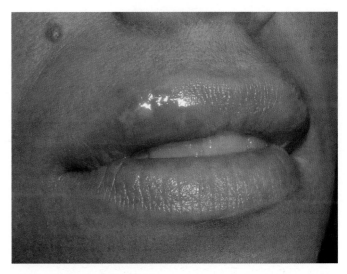

FIGURE 123-7 Orolabial HSV in an adult woman showing deroofed blisters (ulcer). (*Courtesy of Richard P. Usatine, MD.*)

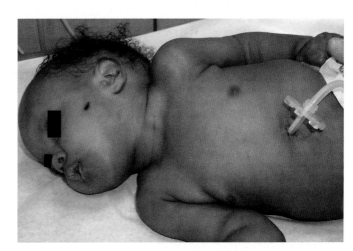

FIGURE 123-8 Hospitalized baby with a recurrence of skin lesions after neonatal HSV-2 infection and CNS involvement. (*Courtesy of Jack Resneck, Sr., MD.*)

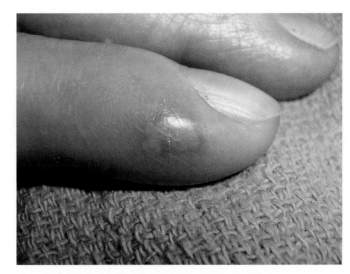

FIGURE 123-9 Herpetic whitlow lesion on distal index finger. (*Courtesy of Richard P. Usatine, MD.*)

TABLE 123-1 Dosage of Treatments for Genital Herpes Infection

Drug	Primary Infection Dosage	Recurrent Infection Dosage	Chronic Suppressive Therapy
Acyclovir (Zovirax)	200 mg 5 times daily or 400 mg three times daily for 7–10 d	200 mg 5 times daily for 5 d or 800 mg twice daily for 5 d	400 mg twice daily or 200 mg 3–5 times daily
Famciclovir (Famvir)*	250 mg 3 times daily for 10 d	125 mg twice daily for 5 d	250 mg po twice daily
Valacyclovir (Valtrex)	1 g twice daily for 10 d	500 mg twice daily for 5 d	500 mg to 1 g once daily

*Famciclovir is not FDA-labeled for this indication.

PROVIDER RESOURCES

MedlinePlus Medical Encyclopedia: Herpes simplex— **http://www. nlm.nih.gov/medlineplus/ency/ article/001324.htm**

eMedicine: Herpes Simplex—**http://www.emedicine.com/ MED/topic1006.htm**

Treatment of Common Cutaneous Herpes Simplex Virus Infections. *Am Fam Physician.* 2000;61:1697–7041705–61708. Also available at—**http://www.aafp.org/afp/20000315/ 1697.html**

REFERENCES

1. Whitley RJ, Kimberlin DW, Roizman B. Herpes simplex viruses. *Clin Infect Dis.* 1998;26:541–555.

2. Gill MJ, Arlette J, Buchan K. Herpes simplex virus infection of the hand. A profile of 79 cases. *Am J Med.* 1988;84:89–93.

3. Fleming DT, McQuillan GM, Johnson RE, et al. Herpes simplex virus type 2 in the United States, 1976 to 1994. *N Engl J Med.* 1997;337:1105–1111.

4. Mertz GJ. Epidemiology of genital herpes infections. *Infect Dis Clin North Am.* 1993;7:825–839.

5. Clark JL, Tatum NO, Noble SL. Management of genital herpes. *Am Fam Physician.* 1995;51:175–182,187–188.

6. Spruance SL, Stewart JC, Rowe NH, McKeough MB, Wenerstrom G, Freeman DJ. Treatment of recurrent herpes simplex labialis with oral acyclovir. *J Infect Dis.* 1990;161:185–190.

7. Spruance SL, Rowe NH, Raborn GW, Thibodeau EA, D'Ambrosio JA, Bernstein DI. Perioral famciclovir in the treatment of experimental ultraviolet radiation-induced herpes simplex labialis: A double-blind, dose-ranging, placebo-controlled, multicenter trial. *J Infect Dis.* 1999;179:303–310.

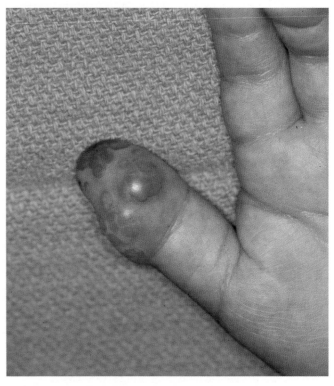

FIGURE 123-10 Severely painful herpetic whitlow on the thumb. (*Courtesy of Eric Kraus, MD.*)

124 MOLLUSCUM CONTAGIOSUM

E.J. Mayeaux, Jr., MD

PATIENT STORIES

An 8-year-old girl is brought to the office because of an outbreak of bumps on her face for the past 3 months (**Figure 124-1**). Occasionally she scratches them but she is otherwise asymptomatic. The mother and child are unhappy with the appearance of the molluscum contagiosum and chose to try topical imiquimod 5% cream. Fortunately her health insurance covered this expensive treatment. A topical treatment was chosen to avoid the risk of hypopigmentation that can occur in dark skinned individuals with cryotherapy.

An 11-year-old girl was also seen with molluscum on her face. The child and her parent decided to try cryotherapy as her treatment. She very bravely tolerated the treatment with liquid nitrogen in a Cryo-Gun (**Figure 124-2**). The molluscum disappeared without scarring or hypopigmentation after two treatments.

EPIDEMIOLOGY

- Up to 5% of children in the United States have clinical evidence of molluscum contagiosum infection.[1] It is a common non-sexually transmitted condition in children (**Figures 124-1 to 124-6**).

- In adults, molluscum occurs most commonly in the genital region (**Figure 124-7**). In this case, it is considered a sexually transmitted disease. Prevalence of molluscum contagiosum in patients who are HIV positive may be as high as 5% to 18% (**Figure 124-6**).[2]

- Subclinical cases may occur and may be more common in the general community than is generally recognized.

ETIOLOGY AND PATHOPHYSIOLOGY

- Molluscum contagiosum is a benign condition that is often transmitted through close contact in children and through sexual contact in adults.

- Molluscum contagiosum is a large DNA virus of the Poxviridae family of poxvirus. It is related to the orthopoxviruses (variola, vaccinia, smallpox, and monkeypox viruses).

- Molluscum replicates in the cytoplasm of epithelial cells.

- It causes a chronic localized skin infection consisting of dome shaped papules on the skin (**Figure 124-3**).

- Like most of the viruses in the poxvirus family, molluscum is spread by direct skin-to-skin contact. It can also spread by autoinoculation when scratching, touching, or treating lesions.

- Any one single lesion is usually present for approximately 2 months, but autoinoculation often causes continuous crops of lesions.

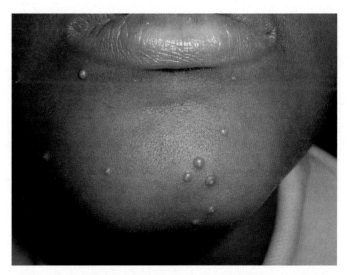

FIGURE 124-1 Molluscum contagiosum on the face of an 8-year-old girl. (*Courtesy of Richard P. Usatine, MD.*)

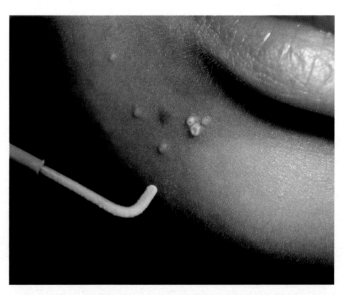

FIGURE 124-2 Cryotherapy of molluscum on the face of an 11-year-old girl. The central umbilication is easily seen in the two papules that were just frozen. (*Courtesy of Richard P. Usatine, MD.*)

DIAGNOSIS

CLINICAL FEATURES

- Firm, multiple, 2 to 5 mm pearly dome shaped papules with a characteristic umbilicated center (**Figure 124-3**). Not all the papules have a central umbilication, so it helps to take a moment and look for a papule that has this characteristic morphology. If all features point to molluscum and no single lesion has central umbilication, do not rule out molluscum as the diagnosis.

- The lesions range in color from pearly white, to flesh-colored, to pink or yellow.

TYPICAL DISTRIBUTION

The lesions may appear anywhere on the body except the palms and soles. The number of lesions may be greater in an HIV-infected individual (**Figure 124-6**). In adults, they are often found around the genitalia, inguinal area, buttocks, or inner thighs (**Figure 124-7**). In children, the lesions are often on the trunk or face (**Figures 124-1** to **124-6**). If a child is found to have molluscum contagiosum in the genital area, a history and physical exam should be directed at looking for other clues of sexual abuse (see Chapter 8, Child Sexual Abuse). Not all cases of molluscum in this area will be secondary to sexual abuse (**Figure 124-8**).

BIOPSY

If confirmation is needed, smears of the caseous material expressed from the lesions can be examined. Hematoxylin and eosin staining from a shave biopsy usually reveals keratinocytes that contain eosinophilic cytoplasmic inclusion bodies.[3] If a single lesion is suspicious for BCC, perform a shave biopsy.

DIFFERENTIAL DIAGNOSIS

- Scabies is caused by Sarcoptes scabiei mite and can be transmitted through close or sexual contact. Early lesions are flesh colored to red papules that produce significant itching. The itching and excoriations are greater than seen with molluscum. Scabies lesions also usually appear in the finger webs, ventral wrist fold, and underneath the breasts in women (see Chapter 137, Scabies).

- Dermatofibromas—firm to hard nodules ranging in color from flesh to black that typically dimples downward when compressed laterally. Usually not seen in crops as in molluscum. These nodules are deeper in the dermis and don't appear stuck on like molluscum (see Chapter 153, Dermatofibroma).

- Basal cell carcinomas are also pearly and raised. Usually not seen in crops as in molluscum. If a single lesion could be a BCC or molluscum, a biopsy is warranted (see Chapter 163, Basal Cell Carcinoma).

MANAGEMENT

- Treatment of nongenital lesions is usually not medically necessary since the infection is usually self-limited and spontaneously resolves

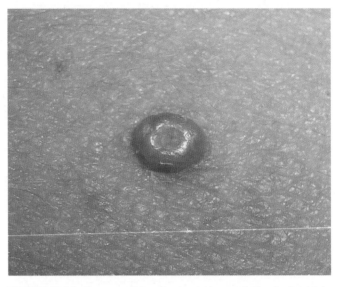

FIGURE 124-3 Close-up of a molluscum lesion on the back of a child showing a dome shaped pearly papule with a characteristic umbilicated center. (*Courtesy of Richard P. Usatine, MD.*)

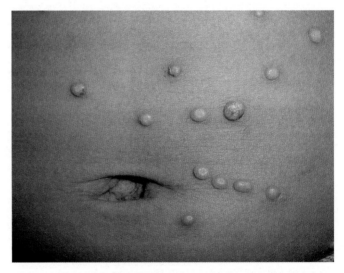

FIGURE 124-4 A group of molluscum contagiosum lesions on the abdomen of a 4-year-old boy. (*Courtesy of Richard P. Usatine, MD.*)

after a few months. Treatment may be performed in an attempt to decrease autoinoculation. Patients and parents of children often want treatment for cosmetic reasons and when watchful waiting fails.

- Excisional curettage or cryotherapy can effectively remove molluscum if the patient will allow treatment. SOR **B** Many children will fear treatment with a curette or with any form of cryotherapy.

- Genital lesions should be treated to prevent spread by sexual contact.

- Curettage and cryotherapy[5] are physical methods used to eradicate molluscum.[4] SOR ? Cantharidin[6] and trichloroacetic acid[7] are topical chemicals that can be applied by the physician in the office. SOR ?

- Tretinoin cream[8] 0.1% or gel 0.025% applied daily are commonly used but not FDA-approved for this indication. SOR **B**

- Topical imiquimod 5% (Aldara) cream has been shown (not FDA approved) to be better than vehicle alone to treat molluscum.[9] SOR **B** It can be well tolerated, although application site irritation can be uncomfortable and lead to discontinuation of therapy. It has been shown not to have systemic or toxic effects in children.[10] In one study, 23 children ranging in age from 1 to 9 years with MC infection were randomized to either imiquimod cream 5% (12 patients) or vehicle (11 patients). Parents applied study drug to patient's lesions 3 times a week for 12 weeks. Complete clearance at week 12 was noted in 33.3% (4/12) of imiquimod patients and in 9.1% (1/11) of vehicle patients.[11]

- In the HIV-infected patient, molluscum may resolve after control of HIV disease with highly active antiretroviral therapy. SOR **B**

PATIENT EDUCATION

- Instruct patients to avoid scratching to prevent autoinoculation.

FOLLOW-UP

- Have patients watch for complications that may include irritation, inflammation, and secondary infections. Lesions on eyelids may be associated with follicular or papillary conjunctivitis, so eye irritation should prompt a visit to an eye care specialist.

PATIENT RESOURCES

American Academy of Dermatology—**http://www.aad.org/ public/Publications/pamphlets/ MolluscumContagiosum.htm.**

Medline plus—**http://www.nlm.nih.gov/medlineplus/ ency/article/000826.htm.**

PROVIDER RESOURCES

EMedicine by WebMD—**http://www.emedicine. com/derm/topic270.htm.**

Dermatology Online Journal—**http://dermatology.cdlib. org/92/reviews/molluscum/diven.html.**

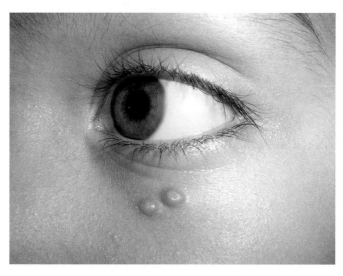

FIGURE 124-5 Molluscum contagiosum under the eye of a young girl with central umbilication. (*Courtesy of Richard P. Usatine, MD.*)

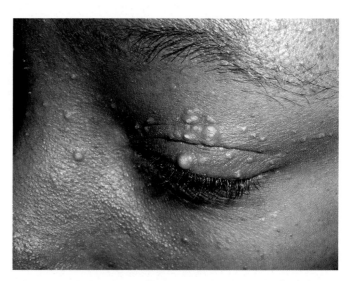

FIGURE 124-6 Extensive molluscum contagiosum on the face of a young girl HIV-positive from birth. (*Courtesy of Richard P. Usatine, MD.*)

REFERENCES

1. Dohil MA, Lin P, Lee J, et al. The epidemiology of molluscum contagiosum in children. *J Am Acad Dermatol*. 2006;54:47.

2. Schwartz JJ, Myskowski PL. Molluscum contagiosum in patients with human immunodeficiency virus infection. *J Am Acad Dermatol*. 1992;27:583.

3. Cotell SL, Roholt NS. Images in clinical medicine. Molluscum contagiosum in a patient with the acquired immunodeficiency syndrome. *N Engl J Med*. 1998;338:888.

4. Hanna D, Hatami A, Powell J, et al. A prospective randomized trial comparing the efficacy and adverse effects of four recognized treatments of molluscum contagiosum in children. *Pediatr Dermatol*. 2006;23(6):574–579.

5. Silverberg NB, Sidbury R, Mancini AJ. Childhood molluscum contagiosum: Experience with cantharidin therapy in 300 patients. *J Am Acad Dermatol*. 2000;43(3):503–507.

6. Yoshinaga IG, Conrado LA, Schainberg SC, Grinblat M. Recalcitrant molluscum contagiosum in a patient with AIDS: Combined treatment with CO(2) laser, trichloroacetic acid, and pulsed dye laser. *Lasers Surg Med*. 2000;27(4):291–294.

7. Wetmore SJ. Cryosurgery for common skin lesions. Treatment in family physicians' offices. *Can Fam Physician*. 1999;45:964–974.

8. Papa CM, Berger RS. Venereal herpes-like molluscum contagiosum: Treatment with tretinoin. *Cutis*. 1976;18(4):537–540.

9. Hengge UR, Esser S, Schultewolter T, et al. Self administered topical 5% imiquimod for the treatment of common warts and molluscum contagiosum. *Br J Dermatol*. 2000;143:1026–1031.

10. Barba Ar, Kapoor S, Berman B. An open label safety study of topical imiquimod 5% cream in the treatment of Molluscum contagiosum in children. *Dermatol Online J*. 2001;7(1):20.

11. Theos AU, Cummins R, Silverberg NB, Paller AS. Effectiveness of imiquimod cream 5% for treating childhood molluscum contagiosum in a double-blind, randomized pilot trial. *Cutis*. 2004;74(2): 134–138, 141–142.

12. Calista D, Boschini A, Landi G. Resolution of disseminated molluscum contagiosum with Highly Active Anti-Retroviral Therapy (HAART) in patients with AIDS. *Eur J Dermatol*. 1999;9:211.

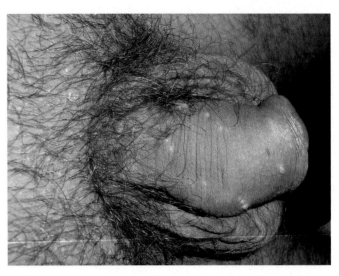

FIGURE 124-7 Molluscum contagiosum on and around the penis. His girlfriend has them on the buttocks. (*Courtesy of Richard P. Usatine, MD.*)

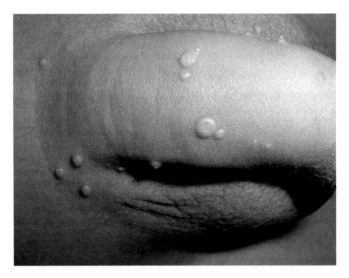

FIGURE 124-8 Molluscum contagiosum on the penis of a young boy. There was no history of sexual abuse. (*Courtesy of Richard P. Usatine, MD.*)

125 COMMON WART

E.J. Mayeaux, Jr., MD

PATIENT STORY

An 11-year-old girl presents with warts on her fingers that have not responded to OTC wart medications (**Figure 125-1**). It causes her and her mother some social embarrassment and they would like to be rid of them. Her mother is also worried that it is affecting her daughter's nails. The girl was able to tolerate the discomfort of liquid nitrogen treatment and wanted all her warts treated. The mother was instructed to purchase 40% salicylic acid to continue treatment of any residual warts at home.

INTRODUCTION

Human papillomaviruses (HPV) are DNA viruses that infect skin and mucous membranes. The most common clinical manifestation of these viruses is warts (verrucae). There are more than 150 distinct HPV subtypes based on DNA testing. Some tend to infect specific body sites or types of epithelium. Some HPV types have a potential to cause malignant change but transformation is rare on keratinized skin.

EPIDEMIOLOGY

- Warts are estimated to occur in up to 10% of children, adolescents, and young adults. They are most common between 12 to 16 years of age.

ETIOLOGY AND PATHOPHYSIOLOGY

- Cutaneous verrucae (warts) occur most commonly in children and young adults (**Figures 125-1** and **125-2**).[1] They are also more common among meat handlers. Other possible predisposing conditions include atopic dermatitis and conditions that decrease cell-mediated immunity such as AIDS and immunosuppressant drugs.

- Infection with HPV occurs by skin-to-skin contact. It starts with a break in the integrity of the epithelium caused by maceration or trauma that allows the virus to infect the basal layers.

- Warts may infect the skin on opposing digits causing "kissing warts" (**Figure 125-3**).

- Individuals with subclinical infection may serve as a reservoir for HPV.

- An incubation period following inoculation lasts for approximately 2 to 6 months.

- Sixty to seventy percent of cutaneous warts resolve in 3 to 24 months without treatment.[2,3]

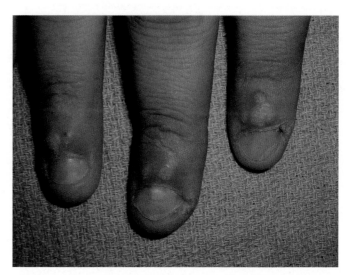

FIGURE 125-1 Common warts on the hands of an 11-year-old girl. These periungual warts are particularly difficult to eradicate. (*Courtesy of Richard P. Usatine, MD.*)

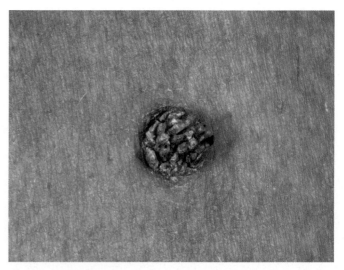

FIGURE 125-2 Close-up of common wart on the thigh of a young adult. Note the cylindrical projections on the wart surface. (*Courtesy of Richard P. Usatine, MD.*)

DIAGNOSIS

CLINICAL FEATURES

- The diagnosis of warts is based upon clinical appearance. The wart will obscure normal skin markings.
- Common warts (verruca vulgaris) are well-demarcated, rough, hard papules with irregular papillary surface. They are usually asymptomatic unless located on a pressure point.
- Warts may form cylindrical projections (**Figure 125-2**). These projections may be seen clearly in digitate warts. The projections often become fused together and form a highly organized mosaic pattern on the surface of common warts.

TYPICAL DISTRIBUTION

- Common anatomic locations include the dorsum of the hand, between the fingers, flexor surfaces, and adjacent to the nails (peri-ungual) (**Figures 125-1** and **125-3**).

BIOPSY

- Paring the surface with a surgical blade may expose punctate hemorrhagic capillaries, or black dots which are thrombosed capillaries. If the diagnosis is doubt, a shave biopsy is indicated to confirm the diagnosis.

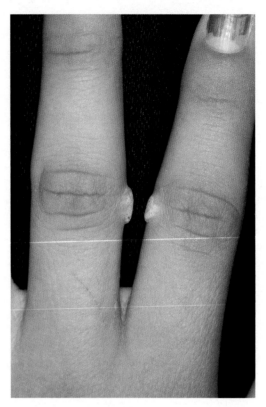

FIGURE 125-3 Warts may infect the skin on opposing digits causing "kissing warts." (*Courtesy of Richard P. Usatine, MD.*)

DIFFERENTIAL DIAGNOSIS

- Seborrheic keratosis are usually more darkly pigmented, have a stuck-on appearance, and "horn cysts" may be visible on close examination. They also have a wide distribution on the body (see Chapter 151, Seborrheic Keratosis).
- Acrochordon (skin tags) are pedunculated flesh-colored papules that are ore common in diabetics. They lack the surface roughness of common warts. Filiform warts also may be pedunculated but typically have a characteristic filiform appearance (see Chapter 150, Skin Tag).
- Squamous cell carcinoma should be considered when lesions have irregular growth, pigmentation, ulceration, or resist therapy, particularly in sun-exposed areas and in immunosuppressed patients (see Chapter 164, Squamous Cell Carcinoma).
- Amelanotic melanoma—Although extremely rare, lesions that are treatment resistant or atypical should be monitored closely or biopsied to establish the diagnosis (see Chapter 165, Melanoma).

MANAGEMENT

- Therapies for common warts do not specifically treat the HPV virus. They work by destruction of virus-containing skin while preserving uninvolved tissue. This usually exposes the blood and its immune cells to the virus, which may promote an immune response against the virus.
- The least painful methods should be used first, especially in children. SOR **C**

- A Cochrane review found that there is a considerable lack of evidence on which to base the rational use of the local treatments for common warts.[4] The trials are highly variable in method and quality. There is evidence that simple topical treatments containing salicylic acid have a therapeutic effect.[4] SOR **A** There is less evidence for the efficacy of cryotherapy and no convincing evidence that it is any more effective than simple topical treatments.

- *Cryotherapy* using liquid nitrogen is useful but is painful for younger children.[4] SOR **B** It must be used cautiously where nerves are located superficially (such as on the fingers) to prevent pain and neuropathy. Overfreezing in the periungual region can result in permanent nail dystrophy. Anesthesia is usually unnecessary but may be achieved with 1% lidocaine or EMLA cream. Liquid nitrogen is applied for 10–20 seconds so that the freeze ball extends 2 mm beyond the lesion (**Figure 125-4**). Two freeze cycles may improve resolution, but it is better to under-freeze than over-freeze since over-freezing may lead to permanent scarring or hypopigmentation. After cryotherapy, the skin shows erythema and may progress to hemorrhagic blistering. Healing occurs in approximately a week and hypopigmentation may occur. Ring warts may result from an inadequate margin of treatment of a common wart (**Figure 125-5**).

- *Salicylic acid* is a useful agent, especially for thick or multiple warts.[4] SOR **A** It is safe in children. The cure rate associated with this therapy is in the range of 60% to 80%.[5] A number of preparations are available without a prescription. Forty percent salicylic acid plasters (Mediplast®) are available over the counter. The 40% salicylic acid plasters are cut to fit and then applied a few millimeters beyond the wart for 48 hours. Then the patch is removed, the wart pared down with a nail file, pumice stone or scalpel, and the process repeated as needed. DuoFilm is 17% salicyclic acid and lactic acid in a flexible collodion with an applicator brush for easy application to multiple warts. This over the counter solution is applied overnight.

- Treating warts with *duct tape* appear to be at least as effective as cryotherapy in one study.[6] The wart is covered with duct tape for 6 days, then the tape is removed, the wart is debrided with an emery board or pumice stone, and the duct tape was reapplied the next morning. Treatment is repeated up to 8 weeks or until the wart resolves. Treatment with duct tape is safe in children, cheap, and essentially pain free. However, a randomized controlled trial in adults showed it to be no better than moleskin and both groups only had a 21% to 22% success rate.[7] SOR **B**

- *Simple excision* is used for small or filiform warts. The area is injected with lidocaine and the wart is excised with sharp scissors or a scalpel blade. SOR **C**

- *Imiquimod* is a topical immunomodulator that is indicated for treatment of anogenital warts but is also used on nongenital warts. SOR **B** It is nonscarring and painless, although local irritation is common. Debriding heavily keratinized warts may enhance penetration of the medication. The cream is applied in a thin layer to the lesions three times a week (every other night) and covered with a adhesive bandage or tape. The medication is removed with soap and water in the morning.

- Treatments for resistant lesions are often carried out in referral practices that have a high enough volume to use more expensive or

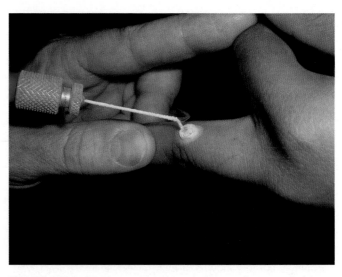

FIGURE 125-4 Cryotherapy showing an adequate free zone (halo) around the wart. (*Courtesy of Richard P. Usatine, MD.*)

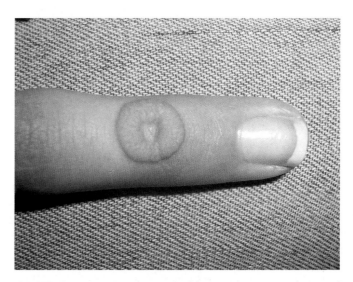

FIGURE 125-5 Ring wart that resulted from inadequate cryotherapy of a common wart. (*Courtesy of Richard P. Usatine, MD.*)

specialized therapy. Cantharidin is an extract of the blister beetle that is applied to the wart after which blistering occurs. Intralesional bleomycin or laser therapy are also useful for recalcitrant warts. Intralesional immunotherapy with skin test antigens (i.e., mumps, *Candida*, or *Trichophyton* antigens) may lead to the resolution both of the injected wart and other warts that were not injected. Contact immunotherapy using dinitrochlorobenzene, squaric acid dibutylester, and diphenylcyclopropenone may be applied to the skin to sensitize the patient and then to the lesion to induce an immune response. SOR **C**

- Early open-label, uncontrolled studies indicate cimetidine might be useful in treating warts. However, three placebo-controlled, double-blind studies and two open-label comparative trials demonstrate that its efficacy is equal to placebo.

PATIENT EDUCATION

- Since spontaneous regression occurs in two-thirds of warts within 2 years, observation without treatment is always an option.

- New warts may appear while others are regressing. This is not a treatment failure but part of the natural disease process with HPV.

- Therapy often takes weeks to months, so patience and perseverance are essential for successful therapy.

- Tools used for paring down warts, such as nail files and pumice stones, should not be used on normal skin or by other people. Similarly, hair-bearing areas with warts should be shaved with depilatories, electric razors, or not at all to help limit spread of warts.

FOLLOW-UP

- Schedule patients for return visits after treatment to limit loss of follow-up and to assess therapy.

- Follow-up visits can be left to the patient's discretion when self-applied therapy is being used.

PATIENT RESOURCES

American Academy of Family Physicians—
http://familydoctor.org/209.xml

MayoClinic.com—**http://www.mayoclinic.com/health/common-warts/DS00370**

PROVIDER RESOURCES

Cutaneous warts: An evidence-based approach to therapy. *Am Fam Physician*. 2005;72:647–652. Available online at **http://www.aafp.org/afp/20050815/647.html**

Medline Plus—**http://www.nlm.nih.gov/medlineplus/ency/article/000885.htm**

Cochrane review: Topical treatments for cutaneous warts—
http://www.cochrane.org/reviews/en/ab001781.html

REFERENCES

1. Kilkenny M, Marks R. The descriptive epidemiology of warts in the community. *Australas J Dermatol.* 1996;37:80–86.

2. Allen AL, Siegfried EC. What's new in human papillomavirus infection. *Curr Opin Pediatr.* 2000; 12:365–369.

3. Sterling JC, Handfield-Jones S, Hudson PM. Guidelines for the management of cutaneous warts. *Br J Dermatol.* 2001;144:4–11.

4. Gibbs S, Harvey I, Sterling JC, Stark R. Local treatments for cutaneous warts. *Cochrane Database Syst Rev.* 2001; 2:CD001781.

5. Parish LC, Monroe E, Rex IH, Jr. Treatment of common warts with high-potency (26%) salicylic acid. *Clin Ther.* 1988;10:462–466.

6. Focht DR, III, Spicer C, Fairchok MP. The efficacy of duct tape vs cryotherapy in the treatment of verruca vulgaris (the common wart). *Arch Pediatr Adolesc Med.* 2002;156:971–974.

7. Wenner R, Askari SK, Cham PM, Kedrowski DA, Liu A, Warshaw EM. Duct tape for the treatment of common warts in adults: A double-blind randomized controlled trial. *Arch Dermatol.* 2007;143(3):309–313.

126 FLAT WARTS

E.J. Mayeaux, Jr., MD

PATIENT STORY

A 16-year-old girl presents with multiple flat lesions on her forehead (**Figure 126-1**). It started with just a few lesions but has spread over the past 3 months. She is diagnosed with flat warts and topical imiquimod is prescribed as the initial treatment.

EPIDEMIOLOGY

- Flat (or juvenile) warts (verruca plana) are most commonly found in children and young adults (**Figures 126-1** to **126-4**).

- Flat warts are the least common variety of wart, but are generally numerous on an individual.[1]

ETIOLOGY AND PATHOPHYSIOLOGY

- Like all warts, flat warts are caused by HPV.

- Flat warts may spread in a linear pattern secondary to spread by scratching or trauma, such as shaving.

- Flat warts present a special treatment problem because they persist for a long time, they are generally located in cosmetically important areas, and they are resistant to therapy.

DIAGNOSIS

CLINICAL FEATURES

Multiple small, flat-topped papules that may be pink, light brown, or light yellow colored (**Figures 126-1** to **126-4**).

TYPICAL DISTRIBUTION

Flat warts typical involve the forehead, around the mouth, the backs of the hands (**Figures 126-1** and **126-2**), and shaved areas, such as the lower face in men and the lower legs in women (**Figure 126-4**).

BIOPSY

Although usually not necessary, a shave biopsy can confirm the diagnosis.

DIFFERENTIAL DIAGNOSIS

- Lichen planus produces flat-topped papules that may be confused with flat warts. Look for characteristic signs of lichen planus such as the symmetric distribution, purplish coloration, and oral lacy lesions. (Wickham's striae are white fine reticular scale seen on the lesions.) The distribution of lichen planus is different with most

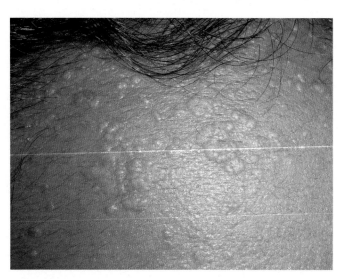

FIGURE 126-1 Flat warts on a patient's forehead. (*Courtesy of Richard P. Usatine, MD.*)

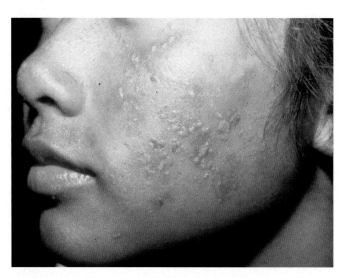

FIGURE 126-2 Flat warts on the cheek. (*With permission from Usatine RP, Moy RL, Tobinick EL, Siegel DM. Skin Surgery: A Practical Guide. 1998, Mosby-Year Book Inc. St. Louis.*)

common sites being the ankles, wrists and back (see Chapter 147, Lichen Planus).

- Seborrheic keratosis are often more darkly pigmented, have a stuck-on appearance, and 'horn cysts' may be visible on close examination (see Chapter 151, Seborrheic Keratosis).

- Squamous cell carcinoma should be considered when lesions have irregular growth or pigmentation, ulceration, or resist therapy, particularly in sun-exposed areas and in immunosuppressed patients (see Chapter 164, Squamous Cell Carcinoma).

MANAGEMENT

- There are no current therapies for HPV that are virus specific.

- Flat warts may be treated with salicylates, 5-fluorouracil, or cryotherapy or tretinoin.

- Topical salicylic acid treatments by topical liquid or patch are the most effective treatment for all types of warts with a success rate average of 73% from 5 pooled placebo controlled trials.[2] NNT = 4 SOR Ⓐ Salicylic acid may be more acceptable on the legs than the face.

- 5-Fluorouracil (Efudex 5% cream, Fluoroplex 1%) may be used to treat flat warts. Apply the cream to affected areas twice daily for 3 to 5 weeks. Sun protection is essential because the drug is photosensitizing. Persistent hypo- or hyperpigmentation may occur following use, but applying it with a cotton-tipped applicator to individual lesions instead of to the area may minimize this adverse reaction.[3,4] SOR Ⓑ

- Cryosurgery may be applied to flat warts. Areas treated with cryotherapy usually heal well, and no additional anesthesia is required which is important when flat warts cover large areas. Liquid nitrogen is applied until the freeze ball extends 1-2 mm into normal tissue, usually approximately 5 to 10 seconds for flat warts. Hypopigmentation, hair loss, and sweat gland destruction may occur in the freeze area. The technique and response are similar to that described in the chapter on common warts. SOR Ⓒ

- Imiquimod (Aldara) cream is an immune modifier that has shown some efficacy in treating flat warts.[5,6] It is nonscarring and painless to apply. There are rare reports of systemic side effects. The cream is applied to the lesions three times a week (every other day). The cream may be applied to the affected area, not strictly to the lesion itself.[7] It can be used on all external HPV infected sites, but not on occluded mucous membranes. The drug causes minimal pain when used correctly, and has almost no systemic side effects. Therapy can be temporarily halted if symptoms become problematic. Imiquimod has the advantage of having almost no risk of scarring.[5,6] SOR Ⓑ

- Tretinoin cream, 0.025%, 0.05%, or 0.1%, applied at bedtime over the entire involved area is one accepted treatment. The frequency of application is then adjusted in order to produce a mild fine scaling and erythema. Sun protection is important. Treatment may be required for weeks or months and may not be effective. No published studies were found to support this treatment. SOR Ⓒ

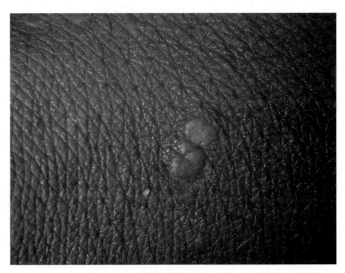

FIGURE 126-3 Closeup of a flat wart. Note typical small, flat-topped papule. (*Courtesy of Richard P. Usatine, MD.*)

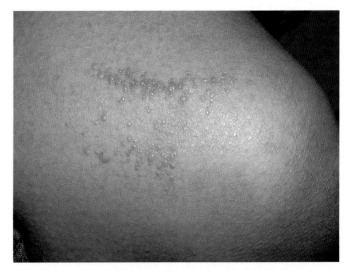

FIGURE 126-4 Flat warts just above the knee of a young woman. Probably spread by shaving. (*Courtesy of Richard P. Usatine, MD.*)

PATIENT EDUCATION

• To help avoid spreading warts, patients should avoid touching or scratching the lesions.

• Razors that are used in areas where warts are located should not be used on normal skin or by other people to prevent spread.

FOLLOW-UP

• Schedule patients for a return visit in 2 to 3 weeks after therapy to assess efficacy.

PATIENT RESOURCES

KidsHealth—**http://www.kidshealth.org/parent/ infections/skin/wart.html.**

American Academy of Dermatology—**http://www.aad.org/ public/Publications/pamphlets/Warts.htm.**

PROVIDER RESOURCES

Cutaneous warts. An evidence-based approach to therapy. *Am Fam Physician.* 2005;72:647–52. **http://www.aafp.org/afp/ 20050815/647.html.**

Medline Plus—**http://www.nlm.nih.gov/medlineplus/ ency/article/000885.htm.**

Cochrane review: Topical treatments for cutaneous warts— **http://www.cochrane.org/reviews/en/ab001781.html.**

REFERENCES

1. Williams H, Pottier A, Strachan D. Are viral warts seen more commonly in children with eczema? *Arch Dermatol.* 1993;129:717–720.

2. Gibbs S, Harvey I. Topical treatments for cutaneous warts. Cochrane Database of Systematic Reviews 2006, Issue 3. Art. No.: CD001781. DOI: 10.1002/14651858.CD001781.pub2.

3. Lockshin NA. Flat facial warts treated with fluorouracil. *Arch Dermatol.* 1979;115:929–1030.

4. Lee S, Kim J-G, Chun SI. Treatment of verruca plana with 5% 5-fluorouracil ointment. *Dermatologica.* 1980;160:383–389.

5. Cutler K, Kagen MH, Don PC, McAeer P, Weinberg JM. Treatment of facial verrucae with topical imiquimod cream in a patient with human immunodeficiency virus. *Acta Derm Venereol.* 2000;80: 134–135.

6. Kim MB. Treatment of flat warts with 5% imiquimod cream. *J Eur Acad Dermatol Venereol* 2006;20(10):1349–1350.

7. Schwab RA, Elston DM. Topical imiquimod for recalcitrant facial flat warts. *Cutis.* 2000;65:160–162.

127 GENITAL WARTS

E.J. Mayeaux, Jr., MD
Richard P. Usatine, MD

PATIENT STORY

An 18-year old woman presents with a concern that she might have genital warts (**Figure 127-1**). She has never had a sexually transmitted disease (STD) but admits to two new sexual partners in the last 6 months. The patient is told that her concern is accurate and she has condyloma caused by HPV (an STD). The treatment options are discussed and she chooses to have cryotherapy with liquid nitrogen followed by imiquimod self-applied beginning 2 weeks afterwards. A Pap smear is performed with testing for gonorrhea and chlamydia before doing the cryotherapy and the patient is sent to the lab to have blood tests for syphilis and HIV. Fortunately all the additional tests are negative and her Pap smear is normal. Further patient education is performed and follow-up is arranged.

EPIDEMIOLOGY

- Anogenital warts (condylomata acuminata) are the most common viral sexually transmitted disease in the United States. There are approximately 1 million new cases of genital warts per year in the United States.[1]
- Most infections are transient and cleared within 2 years.[1]
- Many infections persist and recur and cause much distress for the patients.

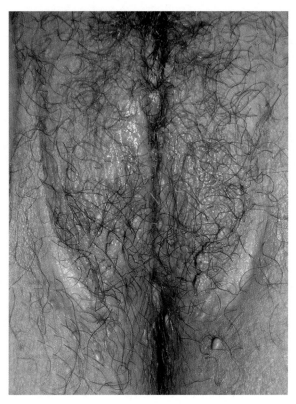

FIGURE 127-1 Multiple vulvar exophytic condyloma in an 18-year-old woman. (*Courtesy of Richard P. Usatine, MD.*)

ETIOLOGY AND PATHOPHYSIOLOGY

- Condyloma acuminatum is caused by human papilloma virus (HPV) infection. HPV encompasses a family of primarily sexually transmitted double-stranded DNA viruses. The incubation period after exposure ranges from three weeks to 8 months.
- There are over 70 distinct HPV subtypes, approximately 35 types are specific for the anogenital epithelium. Most lesions are caused by HPV types 6 and 11, which rarely are associated with invasive carcinoma of the external genitalia.[2] Coinfection with HPV types associated with squamous intraepithelial neoplasia can occur.
- Acquisition of condylomata is related to sexual intercourse and other types of sexual activity. Digital/anal, oral/anal, and digital/vaginal contact probably can also spread the virus, as may fomites.[3]
- The disease is also more common in immunosuppressed individuals.

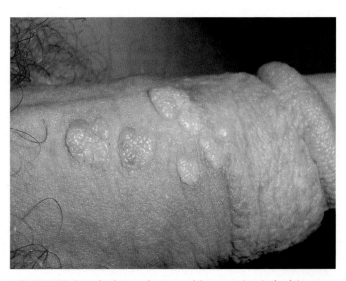

FIGURE 127-2 Multiple exophytic condyloma on the shaft of the penis. (*Courtesy of Richard P. Usatine, MD.*)

DIAGNOSIS

CLINICAL FEATURES

- Genital warts typically present as flesh-colored, exophytic lesions on the genitalia, including the penis, vulva, vagina, scrotum, perineum, and perianal skin.

- External warts can appear as small bumps, or they may be flat, verrucous, or pedunculated.

- Less commonly, warts can appear as reddish or brown smooth, raised papules, or as dome-shaped lesions on keratinized skin.

LABORATORY STUDIES

- HPV viral typing is not recommended.[2]

TYPICAL DISTRIBUTION

- In women, the most common sites of infection are the vulva (85%) (**Figure 127-1**), perianal area (58%), and the vagina (42%).

- In men, the most common sites of infection are the penis (**Figures 127-2** to **127-4**) and scrotum.

- Perianal warts (**Figure 127-5**) can occur in men or women who have a history of anal intercourse and those who do not have any such history (**Figure 127-6**).

BIOPSY

Diagnosis may be confirmed by shave biopsy if necessary. Biopsy is indicated if:

- The diagnosis is uncertain.

- The patient has a poor response to appropriate therapy.

- Warts are atypical in appearance (pigmented, indurated, fixed, or ulcerated).

- Patient is at high risk for HPV-related malignancy.

DIFFERENTIAL DIAGNOSIS

- Pearly penile papules which are small papules around the edge of the glans penis (**Figure 127-7**).

- Common skin lesions such as seborrheic keratoses and nevi—these are rare in the genital area (**Figure 127-8**) (see Chapters 151, Seborrheic Keratosis and 155, Nevus).

- Giant condyloma or Buschke-Lowenstein tumor is a low grade, locally invasive malignancy that can appear as a fungating condyloma (**Figure 127-9**). Persons with HIV/AIDS have a higher risk of giant condyloma and malignant transformation (**Figure 127-10**).

- Molluscum contagiosum—waxy umbilicated papules around the genitals and lower abdomen (see Chapter 124, Molluscum Contagiosum).

- Malignant neoplasms such as basal cell carcinoma and squamous cell carcinomas (see Chapters 163, Basal Cell Carcinoma and 164, Squamous Cell Carcinoma).

- Condyloma lata is caused by secondary syphilis infection, lesions appear flat and velvety (see Chapter 209, Syphilis).

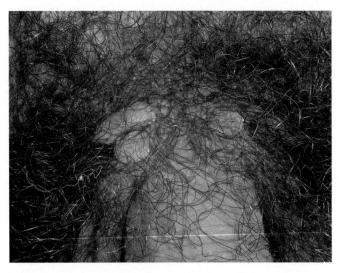

FIGURE 127-3 Multiple exophytic condyloma at the base of the penis. (*Courtesy of Richard P. Usatine, MD.*)

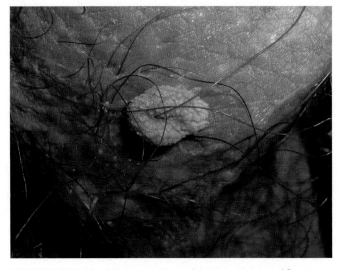

FIGURE 127-4 Condyloma acuminata demonstrating a cauliflower appearance with typical papillary surface. (*Courtesy of Richard P. Usatine, MD.*)

- Micropapillomatosis of the vulva is a normal variant and appear as distinct individual papillary projections from the labia.

MANAGEMENT (TABLE 127-1)

- The primary treatment goal is removal of symptomatic warts.
- The choice of therapy is based on the number, size, site, and morphology of lesions, as well as patient preference, treatment cost, convenience, adverse effects, and physician experience.
- Treatment with 5% fluorouracil cream (Efudex) is no longer recommended because of severe local side effects and teratogenicity.[2]

PATIENT EDUCATION

HPV is transmitted mainly by skin to skin contact. Although condoms may decrease the levels of transmission, they are imperfect barriers at best since they can fail, and they do not cover the scrotum or vulva, where infection may reside.

FOLLOW-UP

- Patients should be offered a follow-up evaluation 2 to 3 months after treatment to check for new lesions.[2] SOR Ⓒ

PATIENT RESOURCES

HPV and genital warts: Patient information—**http://lib-sh.lsuhsc.edu/fammed/pted/hpv.html.**

HPV.com—**http://hpv.com/genital-warts.html.**

PROVIDER RESOURCES

Zuber T, Mayeaux EJ, Jr. *Atlas of Primary Care Procedures*. Philadelphia, PA: Lippincott, Williams, & Wilkins, 2003.

Mayeaux EJ, Jr., Harper MB, Barksdale W, Pope JB. External HPV infections. *Am Fam Physician*. 1995;53:1137–1150.

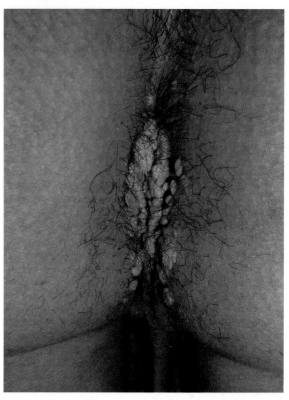

FIGURE 127-5 Perianal warts in a gay man with history of anal receptive intercourse. These lesion responded to cryotherapy. (*Courtesy of Richard P. Usatine, MD.*)

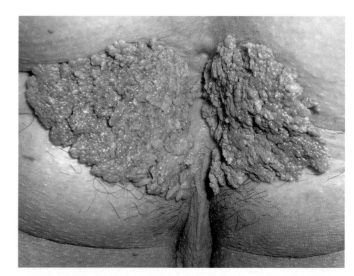

FIGURE 127-6 Extensive perianal warts in a 17-year-old boy who denies sexual abuse and anal intercourse. Patient failed imiquimod therapy and was referred to surgery. (*Courtesy of Richard P. Usatine, MD.*)

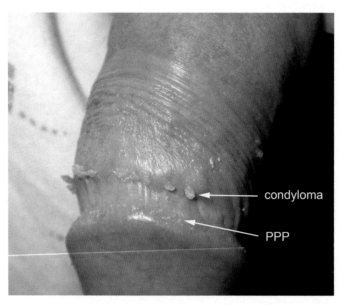

FIGURE 127-7 Condyloma coexisting with pearly penile papules (PPP), which are a normal variant. (*Courtesy of Richard P. Usatine, MD.*)

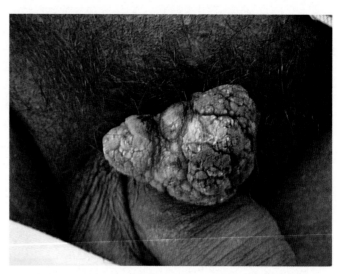

FIGURE 127-9 Buschke-Lowenstein tumor (giant condylomata acuminata) at the base of the penis. This was treated with surgical resection. The margins were clear and there was no squamous cell carcinoma found. (*Courtesy of Suraj Reddy, MD.*)

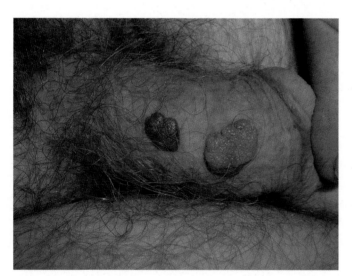

FIGURE 127-8 Two large Condyloma that resemble seborrheic keratoses. Shave biopsy was positive for HPV. (*Courtesy of Richard P. Usatine, MD.*)

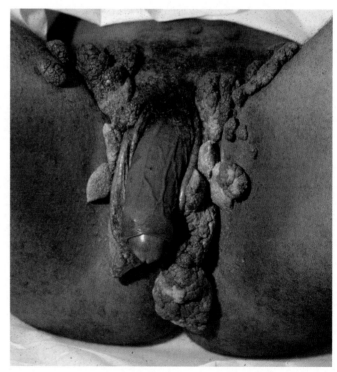

FIGURE 127-10 Giant condylomata acuminata in a man with AIDS. (*Courtesy of Jack Resneck, Sr., MD.*)

TABLE 127-1 Treatments for External Genital Warts

Treatment	Possible Adverse Effects	Clearance (%)	Recurrence (%)
Patient Applied Therapy			
Imiquimod (Aldara®) is applied at bedtime for 3 days, then[4] rest 4 days; alternatively, apply every other day for 3 applications; may repeat weekly cycles up to 16 weeks. SOR Ⓐ	Erythema, irritation, ulceration, pain and pigmentary changes; minimal systemic absorption.	30–50	15
Podofilox (Condylox®) is applied twice daily for 3 days, then rest[5] 4 days; may repeat for 4 cycles. SOR Ⓐ	Burning, pain, inflammation; low risk for systemic toxicity unless applied to occluded membranes.	45–80	5–30
Physician Applied Therapy			
Cryotherapy performed with liquid nitrogen or a cryoprobe. SOR Ⓑ	Pain or blisters at application site, scaring	60–90	20–40
Interferon (intralesional) is rarely used for recalcitrant lesions.[6] SOR Ⓐ	Local burning, itching, and irritation at injection site. Flu-like symptoms, elevated transaminase levels, thrombocytopenia	20–60	50–62
Podophyllin resin is applied to each wart and allow to[7] dry, and is repeated weekly as needed. SOR Ⓐ	Local irritation, erythema, burning, and soreness at application site; neurotoxic and oncogenic if absorbed.	30–80	20–65
Surgical treatment for warts involves removal to the dermal-epidermal junction. Options include scissor excision, shave excision, laser vaporization, and loop electrosurgical excision procedure excision. SOR Ⓑ	Pain, bleeding, scarring; risk for burning and allergic reaction from local anesthetic. Laser and LEEP have risk for spreading HPV in plume.	35–70	5–50
Trichloroacetic acid (TCA) and bichloracetic acid (BCA) are applied to each wart and allow to dry, and is repeated weekly. SOR Ⓑ	Local pain and irritation. No systemic side effects.	50–80	35

REFERENCES

1. Burk RD, Kelly P, Feldman J, et al. Declining prevalence of cervicovaginal human papillomavirus infection with age is independent of other risk factors. *Sex Transm Dis.* 1996;23:333–341.

2. Sexually transmitted diseases treatment guidelines 2002. Centers for Disease Control and Prevention. *MMWR Recomm Rep.* 2002;51: 1–78.

3. Palefsky JM. Cutaneous and genital HPV-associated lesions in HIV-infected patients. *Clin Dermatol.* 1997;15:439–447.

4. Gotovtseva EP, Kapadia AS, Smolensky MH, Lairson DR. Optimal frequency of imiquimod (Aldara) 5% cream for the treatment of external genital warts in immunocompetent adults: a meta-analysis. *Sex Transm Dis.* 2008;35(4):346–351.

5. Langley PC, Tyring SK, Smith MH. The cost effectiveness of patient-applied versus provider-administered intervention strategies for the treatment of external genital warts. *Am J Manag Care.* 1999;5(1):69–77.

6. Welander CE, Homesley HD, Smiles KA, Peets EA. Intralesional interferon alfa-2b for the treatment of genital warts. *Am J Obstet Gynecol.* 1990;162(2):348–354.

7. Hellberg D, Svarrer T, Nilsson S, Valentin J. Self-treatment of female external genital warts with 0.5% podophyllotoxin cream (Condyline) vs weekly applications of 20% podophyllin solution. *Int J STD AIDS.* 1995;6(4):257–261.

128 PLANTAR WART

E.J. Mayeaux, Jr., MD

PATIENT STORY

A 15-year-old boy presents with painful growths on his right heel for about 6 months (**Figure 128-1**). It is painful to walk on and he would like it treated. He was diagnosed with multiple large plantar warts called mosaic warts. The lesions were treated with gentle paring with a No. 15 blade scalpel and liquid nitrogen therapy over a number of sessions. He and his mom were instructed on how to use salicylic acid plasters on the remaining warts.

EPIDEMIOLOGY

- Plantar warts (verruca plantaris) are human papilloma virus (HPV) lesions that occur on the soles of the feet (**Figures 128-1** to **128-5**) and palms of the hands (**Figure 128-6**).
- Plantar warts affect mostly adolescents and young adults, affecting up to 10% of people in this age group.[1]

ETIOLOGY AND PATHOPHYSIOLOGY

- Plantar warts are caused by human papillomavirus.
- They usually occur at points of maximum pressure, such as on the heels (**Figures 128-1** to **128-4**) or over the heads of the metatarsal bones (**Figure 128-5**), but may appear anywhere on the plantar surface.
- A thick, painful callus forms in response to pressure induced as the size of the lesion increases. Even a minor wart can cause a lot of pain.
- A cluster of many warts that appear to fuse is referred to as a mosaic wart (**Figures 128-1** and **128-4**).

DIAGNOSIS

CLINICAL FEATURES

Plantar warts present as thick painful endophytic plaques located on the soles and/or palms. Warts have the following features:

- They lack skin lines crossing their surface (**Figure 128-3**).
- Have a highly organized mosaic pattern on the surface when examined with a hand lens.
- Painful when compressed laterally.
- Have centrally located black dots (thrombosed vessels) that may bleed with paring (**Figures 128-1** to **128-6**).

TYPICAL DISTRIBUTION

They occur on the palms of the hands and soles of the feet.

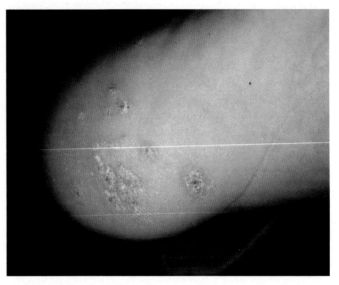

FIGURE 128-1 Plantar warts: Note small black dots in wart that represent thrombosed vessels. Large plantar warts such as this one are called mosaic warts. (*Courtesy of Richard P. Usatine, MD.*)

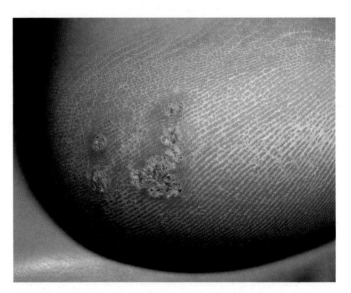

FIGURE 128-2 Close-up of plantar wart on the side of the heel. Note the disruption of skin lines and black dots. (*Courtesy of Richard P. Usatine, MD.*)

BIOPSY

If the diagnosis is doubtful, a shave biopsy is indicated to confirm the diagnosis.[2]

DIFFERENTIAL DIAGNOSIS

- Corns and callus are pressure induced skin thickenings that occur on the feet and can be mistaken for plantar warts. Callus are generally found on the sole and corns are usually on the toes. Callus and corns have skin lines crossing the surface, and are painless with lateral pressure (see Chapter 200, Corn and Callus).

- Black heel presents as a cluster of blue-black dots that result from ruptured capillaries. They appear on the plantar surface of the heel following the shearing trauma of sports that involve sudden stops or position changes. Examination reveals normal skin lines, and paring does not cause additional bleeding. The condition resolves spontaneously in a few weeks.

- Black warts are plantar warts undergoing spontaneous resolution, which may turn black and feel soft when pared with a blade.[3]

- Squamous cell carcinoma should be considered when lesions have irregular growth or pigmentation, ulceration, or resist therapy, particularly in immunosuppressed patients (see Chapter 164, Squamous Cell Carcinoma).

- Amelanotic melanoma, although extremely rare, can look similar to HPV lesions. Lesions that are treatment resistant or atypical, particularly on the palms or soles, should be monitored closely. A biopsy is required to establish the diagnosis (see Chapter 165, Melanoma).

MANAGEMENT

- Painless plantar warts do not require therapy. Minimal discomfort can be relieved by periodically removing the hyperkeratosis with a blade or pumice stone.

- Painful warts should be treated using a technique that causes minimal scarring since scars on the soles of the feet are usually permanent and painful.

- Patients with diabetes must be treated with the utmost care to minimize complications.

- *Topical Salicylic acid* solutions are available over-the-counter and provide conservative keratolytic therapy. These preparations are nonscarring, minimally painful, and relatively effective, but require persistent application of medication once each day for weeks to months. The wart is first pared with a blade, pumice stone, or emery board, and the area soaked in warm water. The solution is then applied, allowed to dry, reapplied, and occluded with adhesive tape.[4] White pliable keratin forms and should be pared away carefully until pink skin is exposed.[5] SOR **B**

- *40% salicylic acid plasters* are available OTC and by prescription. The treatment is similar to the previous process, except that the salicylic acid has been incorporated into a pad. They are particularly useful in treating mosaic warts covering a large area. Pain is quickly

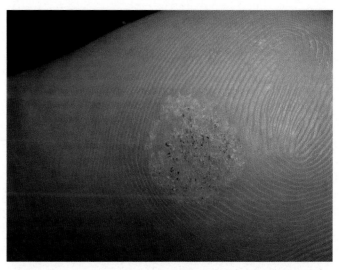

FIGURE 128-3 Close up of a different plantar wart demonstrating disruption of normal skin lines. Corns and callus do not tend to disrupt normal skin lines. The black dots are thrombosed vessels frequently seen in plantar warts. (*Courtesy of Richard P. Usatine, MD.*)

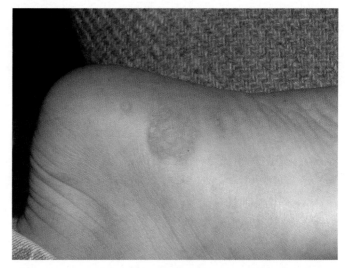

FIGURE 128-4 Demonstrates a mosaic wart that is formed when several plantar warts become confluent. (*Courtesy of Richard P. Usatine, MD.*)

relieved in plantar warts, because a large amount of keratin is removed during the first few days of treatment.[5] SOR **B**

- *Acid chemotherapy* with Trichloroacetic Acid (TCA) or Bichloracetic Acid (BCA) is commonly employed to treat plantar warts in the office. They are considered safe during pregnancy for external lesions. The excess keratin is first pared with a scalpel, then the entire lesion is coated with acid, and the acid is worked into the wart with a sharp toothpick. The process is repeated every 7 to 10 days. SOR **C**

- *Cryotherapy* with liquid nitrogen therapy is commonly used, but plantar warts are more resistant than other HPV lesions. The liquid nitrogen is applied to form a freeze ball that covers the lesion and 2 mm of surrounding normal tissue, usually 10 to 20 seconds per freeze. SOR **C** There is no evidence that two freezing episodes are better than one other than it allows for more freeze time in a way that is more acceptable to the patient. It is always better to under-freeze than over-freeze in areas where scarring can produce permanent disability.

- Treatments for resistant lesions are often carried out in referral practices that have a high enough volume to use more expensive or specialized therapy. Cantharidin is an extract of the blister beetle that is applied to the wart after which blistering occurs. Intralesional immunotherapy with skin test antigens (i.e., mumps, *Candida*, or *Trichophyton* antigens) may lead to the resolution both of the injected wart and other warts that were not injected. Contact immunotherapy using dinitrochlorobenzene, squaric acid dibutylester, and diphenylcyclopropenone may be applied to the skin to sensitize the patient and then to the lesion to induce an immune response. Intralesional bleomycin or laser therapy are also useful for recalcitrant warts. SOR **C**

PATIENT EDUCATION

- Because spontaneous regression occurs, observation of painless lesions without treatment is preferable.

- Therapy often takes weeks to months, so patience and perseverance are essential for successful therapy.

- Tools used for paring down warts, such as nail files and pumice stones, should not be used on normal skin or by other people.

FOLLOW-UP

- Regular follow-up to assess treatment efficacy, adverse reactions, and patient tolerance are recommended to minimize treatment drop-outs.

PATIENT RESOURCES

MayoClinic.com—**http://www.mayoclinic.com/health/plantar-warts/DS00509**

American Academy of Orthopaedic Surgeons—**http://www.orthoinfo.aaos.org/fact/thr_report.cfm?Thread_ID/225**

Healthcommunities.com—**http://www.podiatrychannel.com/plantarwarts/**

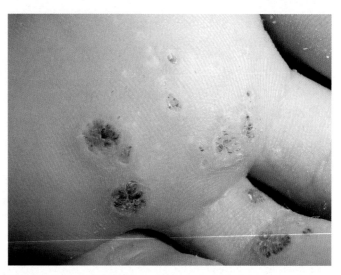

FIGURE 128-5 Multiple plantar warts on the ball of the foot and toes. The thrombosed vessels within the warts appear as black dots. (*Courtesy of Richard P. Usatine, MD.*)

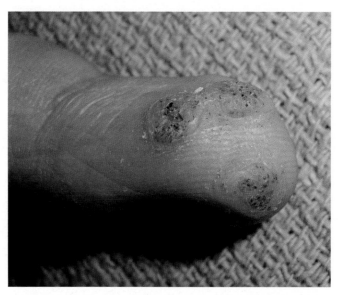

FIGURE 128-6 Close up of plantar wart on a finger also showing disruption of skin lines and black dots. (*Courtesy of Richard P. Usatine, MD.*)

PROVIDER RESOURCES

Cutaneous warts: An evidence-based approach to therapy. *Am Fam Physician*. 2005;72:647–652. **http://www.aafp.org/afp/20050815/647.html**

Medline Plus—**http://www.nlm.nih.gov/medlineplus/ency/article/000885.htm**

REFERENCES

1. Laurent R, Kienzler JL. Epidemiology of HPV infections. *Clin Dermatol*. 1985;3(4):64–70.

2. Beutner, KR. Nongenital human papillomavirus infections. *Clin Lab Med*. 2000;20:423–430.

3. Berman A, Domnitz JM, Winkelmann RK. Plantar warts recently turned black. *Arch Dermatol*. 1982;118:47–51.

4. Landsman MJ, Mancuso JE, Abramow SP. Diagnosis, pathophysiology, and treatment of plantar verruca. *Clin Podiatr Med Surg*. 1996; 13(1):55–71.

5. Cochrane review: Topical treatments for cutaneous warts— http://www.cochrane.org/reviews/en/ab001781.html. Accessed April 1, 2008.

129 CUTANEOUS FUNGAL INFECTIONS—OVERVIEW

Richard P. Usatine, MD

PATIENT STORY

A 55-year-old woman presents with a red pruritic area on her face for 3 months (**Figure 129-1**). The annular distribution immediately is suspicious for a dermatophyte infection. Further investigation demonstrates that the patient has severe tinea pedis in a moccasin distribution. The patient is treated with an oral antifungal agent and her fungal infection clears over the coming month.

EPIDEMIOLOGY

- Fungal infections of the human body are ubiquitous and common.
- More detailed epidemiology is found in the sections on the specific infections.

PATHOPHYSIOLOGY

Mucocutaneous fungal infections are caused by:

- Dermatophytes in three genera: *Microsporum*, *Epidermophyton,* and *Trichophyton*. There are approximately 40 species in the three genera and these fungi cause: tinea pedis and manus, tinea capitis, tinea corporis, tinea cruris, tinea faciei and onychomycosis (**Figures 129-1** to **129-6**).
- Yeasts in the genera of *Candida* and *Pityrosporum (Malassezia)*—There are also multiple types of species and the *Pityrosporum* cause seborrhea and tinea versicolor (**Figures 129-7** and **129-8**). While tinea versicolor has the name tinea in it, it is not a true dermatophyte.

DIAGNOSIS

CLINICAL FEATURES OF TINEA INFECTIONS

Scaling, erythema, pruritus, central clearing, concentric rings, and maceration (see **Table 129-1**). Changes in pigmentation are not uncommon in various types of tinea especially tinea versicolor.

- **Figure 129-1** shows tinea faciei on the face with typical scaling and ringlike pattern, hence, the name ringworm. There is also erythema and central clearing. The patient was experiencing pruritus.
- **Figure 129-2** shows annular pruritic lesion with concentric rings in the axilla of a young woman caused by tinea corporis. The concentric rings have a high specificity (80%) for tinea infections.

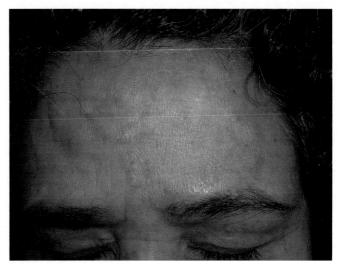

FIGURE 129-1 Tinea faciei on the face of a 55-year-old woman with typical scaling and ringlike pattern (ringworm). Note the well-demarcated raised border and central clearing. (*Courtesy of Richard P. Usatine, MD.*)

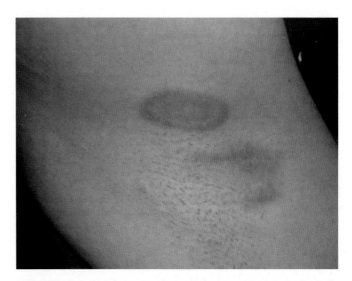

FIGURE 129-2 Annular pruritic lesion with concentric rings in the axilla of a young woman caused by tinea corporis. The concentric rings have a high specificity for tinea infections. (*Courtesy of Richard P. Usatine, MD.*)

- Note that tinea infections will not show central clearing in 58% of cases as in **Figure 129-3** in which tinea cruris has no central clearing.

- Hyperpigmentation is common in dark-skinned individuals as seen in **Figure 129-4** on the abdomen of an aboriginal female. Note the hyperpigmentation is seen in the tinea corporis as well as in the tribal scarification lines.

- Hypopigmentation is frequently seen in tinea versicolor (**Figure 129-8**).

TYPICAL DISTRIBUTION

Literally found from head to toes:

- **Figure 129-5** shows tinea capitis in a 5-year-old black girl with hair loss and an inflammatory response. Her kerion is healing after initiating oral griseofulvin.

- The two-foot one-hand syndrome is a curious phenomenon with tinea manus of one hand and tinea pedis of both feet (**Figure 129-6**). It is not clear why only one hand is involved in these cases. In this case it was the nondominant hand.

LABORATORY STUDIES

Creating a KOH Prep:

- Scrape the leading edge of the lesion on to a slide using the side of a No. 15 scalpel or another microscope slide (**Figure 129-9**).

- Use your coverslip to push the scale into the center of the slide.

- Add two drops of KOH (or fungal stain) to the slide and place coverslip on top.

- Gently heat with flame from an alcohol lamp or lighter if you are using KOH without stain or dimethyl sulfoxide (DMSO). Avoid boiling.

- If you use KOH with DMSO or a fungal stain you may not need to heat the slide. You can purchase fungal stains that come with KOH and DMSO in the solution. These inexpensive stains come conveniently in small plastic squeeze bottles that have a shelf life from 1 to 3 years. Two useful stains that can help increase your ability to identify fungus are Chlorazol and Swartz Lamkins stains. These are available at http://www.delasco.com/pcat/1/Chemicals/

- Examine with microscope starting with 10 power to look for the cells and hyphae and then switch to 40 power to confirm your findings (**Figures 129-10** to **129-13**). The fungal stain helps the hyphae to stand out among the epithelial cells.

- It helps to start with 10 power to find the clumps of cells and look for groups of cells that appear to have fungal elements within them (**Figure 129-10**).

- Do not be fooled by cell borders which look linear and branching. You should see true fungal morphology at 40 power that should confirm that you are looking at real fungus and not artifact. The fungal stains bring out these characteristics including cell walls, nuclei and Arthroconidia (**Figures 129-11** to **129-13**).

- KOH test characteristics[1] (without fungal stains): sensitivity 77% to 88%, specificity 62% to 95% (**Table 129-2**). The sensitivity and specificity should be higher with fungal stains and the experience of the person performing the test.

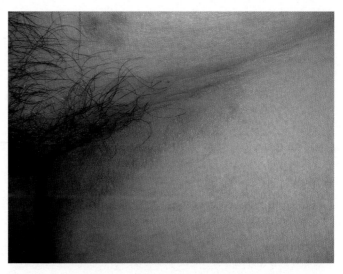

FIGURE 129-3 Tinea cruris with well-demarcated raised border and no central clearing. (*Courtesy of Richard P. Usatine, MD.*)

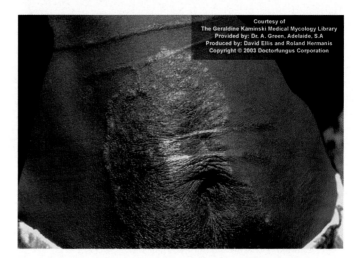

FIGURE 129-4 Tinea corporis on the abdomen of an aboriginal female. Note that hyperpigmentation is seen in the tinea corporis as well as in the tribal scarification lines. (*Courtesy of www.doctorfungus. org © 2006.*)

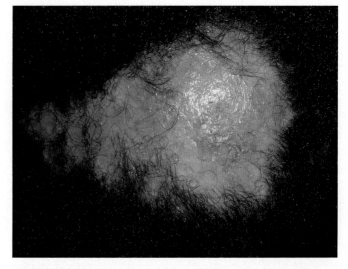

FIGURE 129-5 Tinea capitis in a 5-year-old black girl with hair loss and an inflammatory response. Her kerion is healing after initiating oral griseofulvin. (*Courtesy of Richard P. Usatine, MD.*)

OTHER LABORATORY STUDIES

- Fungal culture—send skin scrapings, hair, or nail clippings to your laboratory in a sterile container such as a urine cup. These will be plated out on fungal agar and the laboratory can report the species to you if positive.

- Biopsy specimens can be sent in formalin for periodic acid Schiff (PAS) staining when KOH and fungal cultures seem to be falsely negative.

- UV light (Woods lamp), looking for fluorescence. The microsporum species are most likely to fluoresce. However, the majority of tinea infections are caused by trichophyton species that do not fluoresce.

MANAGEMENT

There is a wide variety of topical antifungal medications (**Table 129-3**). A Cochrane systematic review of 70 trials of topical antifungals for tinea pedis showed good evidence for efficacy compared to placebo[2] for:

- Allylamines (naftifine, terbinafine, butenafine).

- Azoles (clotrimazole, miconazole, econazole).

- Allylamines cure slightly more infections than azoles but are more expensive.[2]

- No differences in efficacy found between individual allylamines or individual azoles.[2] SOR **A**

Oral antifungals are needed for all tinea capitis infections and more severe infections of the rest of the body. True dermatophyte infections that do not respond to topical antifungals may need an oral agent.

- A Cochrane systematic review of 12 trials of oral antifungals for tinea pedis showed oral terbinafine for 2 weeks cures 52% more patients than oral griseofulvin.[3] SOR **A**

- Terbinafine is equal to itraconazole in patient outcomes.[3]

- No significant differences in comparisons between a number of other oral agents.[3]

Oral antifungals used for fungal infections of the skin, nails or mucus membranes:

- Itraconazole (Sporanox).

- Fluconazole (Diflucan).

- Griseofulvin.

- Ketoconazole (Nizoral).

- Terbinafine (Lamisil).

PROVIDER RESOURCES

Fungal skin from New Zealand—**http://www.dermnetnz.org/fungal/**.

Doctor fungus from the USA—**http://www.doctorfungus.org/**.

World of dermatophytes from Canada—**http://www.provlab.ab.ca/mycol/tutorials/derm/dermhome.htm**.

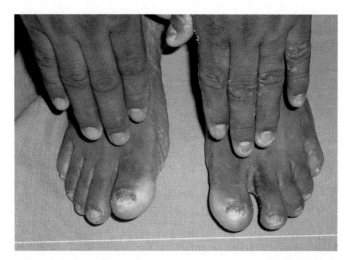

FIGURE 129-6 Two foot, one hand syndrome with tinea manus of one hand and tinea pedis of both feet. (*Courtesy of Richard P. Usatine, MD.*)

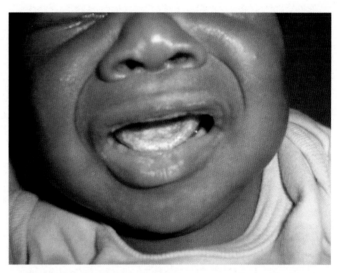

FIGURE 129-7 Thrush in the mouth of an infant caused by *Candida*. (*Courtesy of Richard P. Usatine, MD.*)

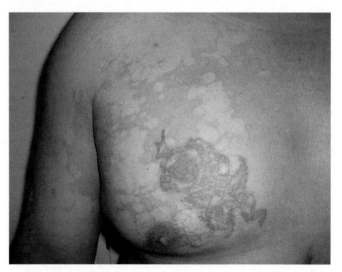

FIGURE 129-8 Tinea versicolor showing hypopigmentation on the chest. (*Courtesy of Richard P. Usatine, MD.*)

TABLE 129-1 Diagnostic Value of Selected Signs and Symptoms in Tinea Infection*

Sign/Symptom	Sensitivity (%)	Specificity (%)	PV+ (%)	PV− (%)	LR+	LR−
Scaling	77	20	17	80	0.96	1.15
Erythema	69	31	18	83	1.00	1.00
Pruritus	54	40	16	80	0.90	1.15
Central clearing	42	65	20	84	1.20	0.89
Concentric rings	27	80	23	84	1.35	0.91
Maceration	27	84	26	84	1.69	0.87

*Signs and symptoms were compiled by 27 general practitioners prior to submission of skin for fungal culture. Specimens were taken from 148 consecutive patients with erythematosquamous lesions of glabrous skin. Culture results were considered the gold standard; level of evidence = 2b.

PV+, positive predictive value; PV−, negative predictive value; LR+, positive likelihood ratio; LR−, negative likelihood ratio. From Thomas B. Clear choices in managing epidermal tinea infectios. *J Fam Pract.* 2003;52:850–862. Adapted from Lousbergh et al. *J Fam Pract* 1999;16:611–615, Dowden Health Media.

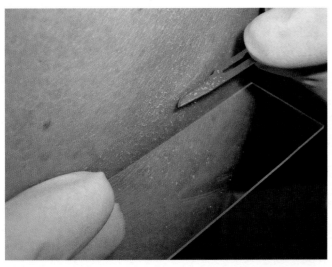

FIGURE 129-9 Making a KOH preparation by scraping in area of scale with a No. 15 blade. This was a case of tinea versicolor. (*Courtesy of Richard P. Usatine, MD.*)

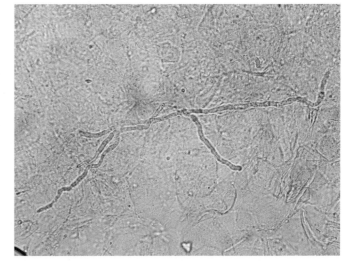

FIGURE 129-11 Trichophyton rubrum from tinea cruris using Swartz Lamkins fungal stain at 40 power. Straight hyphae with visible septae. (*Courtesy of Richard P. Usatine, MD.*)

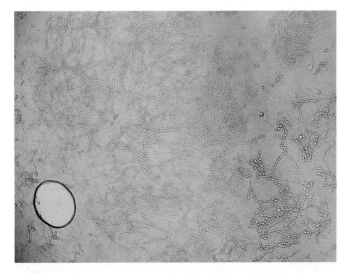

FIGURE 129-10 Trichophyton rubrum from tinea cruris visible among skin cells using light microscopy at 10 power and Swartz Lamkins fungal stain. Start your search on 10 power and move to 40 power to confirm your findings. (*Courtesy of Richard P. Usatine, MD.*)

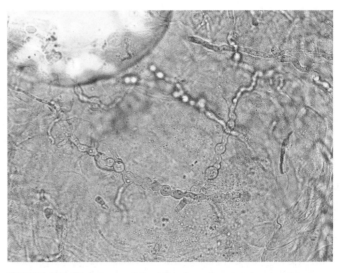

FIGURE 129-12 Arthroconidia visible from tinea cruris using Swartz Lamkins fungal stain at 40 power. (*Courtesy of Richard P. Usatine, MD.*)

TABLE 129-2 Diagnostic Value of Clinical Diagnosis and KOH Prep in Tinea Infection

Test	Sensitivity (%)	Specificity (%)	PV+ (%)	PV− (%)	LR+	LR−
Clinical diagnosis*	81	45	24	92	1.47	0.42
KOH prep (study one)[†]	88	95	73	98	17.6	0.13
KOH prep (study two)[†]	77	62	59	79	2.02	0.37

*The clinical diagnosis set was compiled by 27 general practitioners prior to submission of skin for fungal culture. Specimens were taken from consecutive patients with erythrosquamous lesions. Culture results were considered the gold standard; study quality = 2b.
[†]Both studies of KOH preps were open analyses of patients with suspicious lesions. Paired fungal culture was initiated simultaneously with KOH prep and was considered the gold standard; study quality = 2b.
From Thomas B. Clear choices in managing epidermal tinea infectios. *J Fam Pract*, Dowden Health Media.

TABLE 129-3 Topical Antifungal Preparations

Generic Name	Brand Name	OTC or R_x	Class	Price ($)/30 g or mL, Unless Specified*
Butenafine	Mentax Lotrimin Ultra	R_x OTC	Allylamine	55 per 15 g 15 per 25.5 g
Ciclopirox	Loprox Generic	R_x	Pyridone	95 45
Clotrimazole	Lotrimin AF Cream Lotrimin AF Spray Generic	OTC	Azole	15 7 for 4.6 oz spray 8
Econazole	Spectazole Generic	R_x	Azole	40 20
Ketoconazole	Nizoral	2% R_x	Azole	28
Miconazole	Micatin Generic	OTC	Azole	15 4
Naftifine	Naftin	R_x	Allylamine	47
Oxiconazole	Oxistat	R_x	Azole	51
Sertaconazole	Ertaczo	R_x	Azole	57
Terbinafine	Lamisil AT	OTC	Allylamine	17
Tolnaftate[†]	Tinactin cream Lamisil AF defense and Tinactin powder spray Generic cream	OTC	Miscellaneous	12 7 for 4.6 oz spray 8

*Prices from: www.drugstore.com. Accessed September 3, 2006.
[†]All the above antifungals will treat dermatophytes and Candida. Tolnaftate is effective only for dermatophytes and not Candida. Nystatin is effective only for Candida and not the dermatophytes.

REFERENCES

1. Thomas B. Clear choices in managing epidermal tinea infections. *J Fam Pract.* 2003;52:850–862.

2. Crawford F, Hart R, Bell-Syer S, Torgerson D, Young P, Russell I. Topical treatments for fungal infections of the skin and nails of the foot. *Cochrane Database Syst Rev.* 2000;CD001434.

3. Bell-Syer SE, Hart R, Crawford F, Torgerson DJ, Tyrrell W, Russell I. Oral treatments for fungal infections of the skin of the foot. *Cochrane Database Syst Rev.* 2002;CD003584.

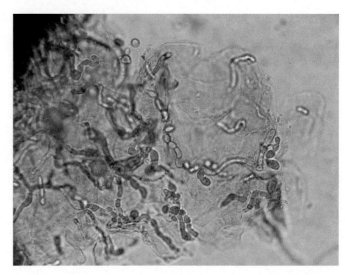

FIGURE 129-13 Trichophyton rubrum from tinea cruris using Chlorazol black fungal stain at 40 power. (*Courtesy of Richard P. Usatine, MD.*)

130 MUCOCUTANEOUS CANDIDIASIS

Richard P. Usatine, MD

PATIENT STORY

The 42-year-old man (**Figure 130-1**) was admitted to the hospital for community-acquired pneumonia and type 2 diabetes out of control. On the second day of admission, when he was feeling a bit better, he asked about the itching he was having on his penis. Physical examination revealed an uncircumcised penis with white discharge on the glans and the inside the foreskin consistent with candida balanitis. KOH prep was positive for the pseudohyphae of candida. The patient was treated with a topical azole and the balanitis resolved.

EPIDEMIOLOGY

Cutaneous and mucosal candida infections are seen commonly in persons with obesity, diabetes, hyperhidrosis, and/or immunodeficiency.

ETIOLOGY AND PATHOPHYSIOLOGY

- Infections caused by *Candida* species are primarily *Candida albicans*.[1]
- *C. albicans* has the ability to exist in both hyphal and yeast forms (termed dimorphism). If pinched cells do not separate, a chain of cells is produced and is termed pseudohyphae.[1]
- Risk factors include obesity, diabetes, hyperhidrosis, immunodeficiency, HIV, heat, use of oral antibiotics, and use of inhaled or systemic steroids.[1]

DIAGNOSIS

CLINICAL FEATURES

- Typical distribution: groin, glans penis, vulva, inframammary, under abdominal pannus, between fingers, in creases of neck, corners of mouth, nail folds in chronic paronychia.
- Morphology: macules, patches, plaques that are pink to bright red with small peripheral satellite lesions.
- Candidiasis of the nipple in the nursing mother is associated with infantile thrush (**Figures 130-2** and **130-3**). Nipple candidiasis is almost always bilateral, with the nipples appearing bright red and inflamed. In this case, the inflammation was made worse by the application of a topical antibiotic that caused a secondary contact dermatitis.
- The candida infection in the corners of the mouth are called perlèche or angular cheilitis (**Figure 130-4**).

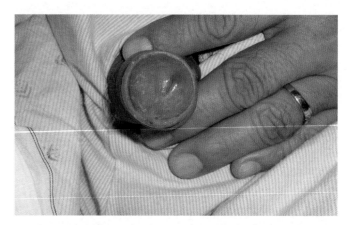

FIGURE 130-1 Candida balanitis in a man with uncontrolled diabetes. (*Courtesy of Richard P. Usatine, MD.*)

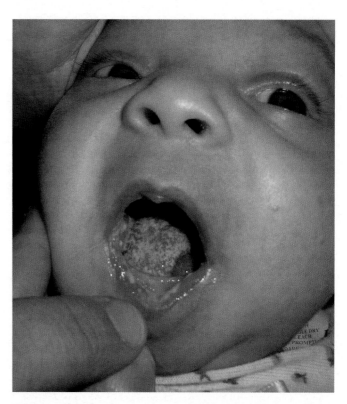

FIGURE 130-2 Thrush in an otherwise healthy infant. (*Courtesy of Richard P. Usatine, MD.*)

LABORATORY STUDIES

Scrape involved area and add to a slide with KOH (DMSO optional). *C. albicans* exist in both hyphal and yeast forms (dimorphism). Look for pseudohyphae and/or budding yeast (**Figure 130-5**).

DIFFERENTIAL DIAGNOSIS

- Intertrigo is a nonspecific inflammatory condition of the skin folds. It is induced or aggravated by heat, moisture, maceration, and friction. The condition frequently is worsened by infection with candida or dermatophytes (**Figures 130-6** and **130-7**). In **Figure 130-6** there is significant hyperpigmentation secondary to the inflammation.

- Tinea corporis or cruris—can be distinguished from Candida when you see an annular pattern or concentric circles in the tinea (**Figure 130-7**). There is no scrotal involvement in tinea cruris. Candida intertrigo may have scrotal involvement (see Chapters 132, Tinea Corporis and 133, Tinea Cruris).

- Erythrasma—may be brown and glows a coral red with UV light (see Chapter 113, Erythrasma).

- Inverse psoriasis—psoriasis in the intertriginous areas as seen in **Figure 130-8** (see Chapter 145, Psoriasis).

- Seborrhea—inflammation related to overgrowth of Pityrosporum, yeast like organism (see Chapter 144, Seborrheic Dermatitis).

MANAGEMENT

PRIMARY CANDIDAL SKIN INFECTIONS

- Topical azoles including clotrimazole, miconazole, and nystatin (polyenes), are effective.[3] SOR **B**

- Keeping the infected area dry is important.[2] SOR **C**

- For more details of the topical antifungals (see Table 129-3 in Chapter 129, Cutaneous Fungal Infections—Overview).

- In one study, miconazole ointment was well tolerated and significantly more effective than the zinc oxide/petrolatum vehicle control for treatment of diaper dermatitis complicated by candidiasis.[3]

- Do not use tolnaftate which is active against dermatophytes but not candida.

- If recurrent or recalcitrant, consider fluconazole 150 mg qwk × 2 or ketoconazole 200 mg qd for 1 to 2 weeks.

OROPHARYNGEAL CANDIDIASIS

- Treat initial episodes with clotrimazole troches (one 10-mg troche 5 times per day for adults) or nystatin (available as a suspension of 100,000 U/mL [dosage, 4–6 mL qid] or as flavored 200,000 U pastilles [dosage, 1 or 2 pastilles 4–5 times per day for 7–14 days]).[2] SOR **B**

- Oral fluconazole (100 mg/d for 7–14 days) is as effective as—and, in some studies, superior to—topical therapy.[2] SOR **A**

- Itraconazole solution (200 mg/d for 7–14 days) is as effective as fluconazole.[2] SOR **A**

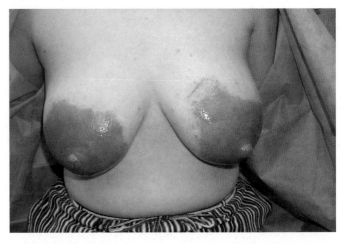

FIGURE 130-3 Candida rash with superimposed contact dermatitis in a breast-feeding woman. Her baby has thrush and both need treatment to eradicate the infection. The contact dermatitis was to the neomycin containing topical antibiotic she applied to her sore breasts. (*Courtesy of Jack Resneck, Sr., MD.*)

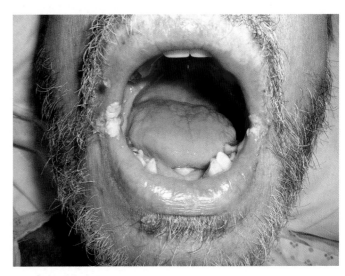

FIGURE 130-4 Thrush and perlèche in a man with AIDS. The candida infection in the corners of the mouth are called perlèche or angular cheilitis. (*Courtesy of Richard P. Usatine, MD.*)

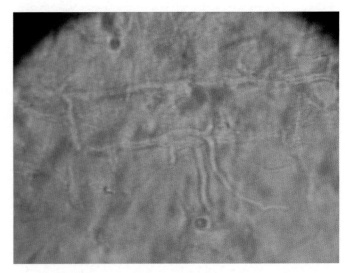

FIGURE 130-5 The branching pseudohyphae of Candida under the microscope. (*Courtesy of Richard P. Usatine, MD.*)

- Ketoconazole and itraconazole capsules are less effective than fluconazole, because of variable absorption.[2] SOR **A**

- Fluconazole-refractory oropharyngeal candidiasis will respond to oral itraconazole therapy (>200 mg/day, preferably in solution form) approximately two-thirds of the time.[2] SOR **A**

- Children with thrush are usually treated with oral nystatin suspension.[2] SOR **B**

- HIV/AIDS patients with oral candidiasis may be treated with clotrimazole troches. If unresponsive to topical therapy, fluconazole may be needed.[2] SOR **A**

- Denture-related disease may require extensive and aggressive disinfection of the denture for definitive cure.[2] SOR **C**

MAMMARY CANDIDIASIS IN BREAST-FEEDING

- Most mammary candidiasis does not present with red breasts as seen in **Figure 130-3**.

- Nipple pain and discomfort along with thrush is adequate data to treat the mother and child.

- Topical nystatin and oral fluconazole are safe for infants and the mother.[2]

CHRONIC MUCOCUTANEOUS CANDIDIASIS

- Chronic mucocutaneous candidiasis (**Figure 130-9**) requires a long-term approach that is analogous to that used in patients with AIDS.[2]

- Systemic therapy is needed, and azole antifungal agents (ketoconazole, fluconazole, and itraconazole) have been used successfully.[2]

- As with HIV-infected patients, development of resistance to these agents has been described.[2]

PATIENT EDUCATION

Keep the infected area clean and dry. For thrush in a baby, treat sources of infection such as the mother's breasts and bottle nipples. If the baby is bottle fed, boil the nipples between uses.

PATIENT AND PROVIDER RESOURCES

Cutaneous Candidiasis—**http://www.emedicine.com/DERM/topic67.htm** (Accessed June 24, 2007).

Intertrigo—**http://www.emedicine.com/DERM/topic198.htm** (Accessed September 2, 2006).

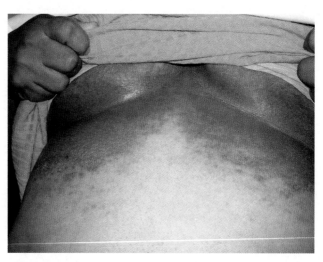

FIGURE 130-6 Candida under the breasts of an overweight Hispanic woman showing hyperpigmentation. The border is not well-demarcated and there are satellite lesions. (*Courtesy of Richard P. Usatine, MD.*)

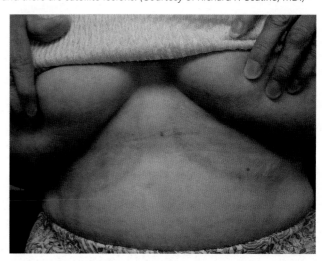

FIGURE 130-7 Tinea corporis under the breasts of a 55-year-old woman. Note the annular pattern with well-demarcated borders. KOH was positive for dermatophytes and not Candida. (*Courtesy of Richard P. Usatine, MD.*)

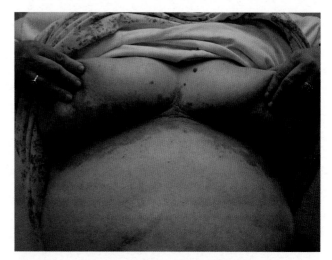

FIGURE 130-8 Inverse psoriasis that closely resembles Candida intertrigo in the submammary folds. This patient did not improve with topical antifungals and finally a biopsy showed that this was inverse psoriasis. Inverse psoriasis is often mistaken for a fungal infection unless the physician is aware of this condition. Frequently there are other clues to the diagnosis of psoriasis in the skin and nails so that a biopsy is not needed. (*Courtesy of Richard P. Usatine, MD.*)

REFERENCES

1. Scheinfeld, N. Cutaneous. Candidiasis. Updated June 18, 2007. http://www.emedicine.com/DERM/topic67.htm. Accessed June 24, 2007.

2. Pappas PG, Rex JH, Sobel JD et al. Guidelines for treatment of candidiasis. *Clin Infect Dis.* 2004;38:161–189.

3. Spraker MK, Gisoldi EM, Siegfried EC et al. Topical miconazole nitrate ointment in the treatment of diaper dermatitis complicated by candidiasis. *Cutis.* 2006;77(2):113–120.

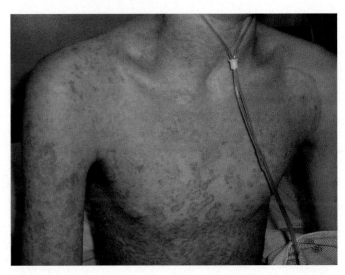

FIGURE 130-9 Severe chronic cutaneous candidiasis in a 22-year-old man with immunosuppression. (*Courtesy of Richard P. Usatine, MD.*)

131 TINEA CAPITIS

Richard P. Usatine, MD

An 11-year-old boy has a history of 2 months of progressive patchy hair loss (**Figure 131-1**). He has some itching of the scalp but his mother is worried about his hair loss. Physical examination reveals alopecia with scaling of the scalp and broken hairs looking like black dots in the areas of hair loss. A KOH preparation is created by scraping an area of alopecia on to a slide. A few loose hairs are added to the slide before the KOH and cover slip are placed. Fungal elements are seen under the microscope. After 6 weeks of griseofulvin, the tinea capitis is fully resolved.

EPIDEMIOLOGY

• Tinea capitis is more common in young, black boys.

• Tinea capitis is the most common type of dermatophytoses in children younger than 10 years (**Figures 131-1 to 131-5**). It rarely occurs after puberty or in adults.[1]

• Combs, brushes, couches, and sheets may harbor the live dermatophyte for a long period of time.

• Spread from person to person with direct contact or through fomites.

• Occasionally spread from cats and dogs to humans.

ETIOLOGY AND PATHOPHYSIOLOGY

• Tinea capitis is a superficial fungal infection affecting hair shafts and follicles on the scalp but could involve the eyebrows and eyelashes.

• Caused by *Trichophyton* and *Microsporum* dermatophytes. The most common organism in the United States is *Trichophyton tonsurans* which is associated with black dot alopecia. *Microsporum canis* is less common now than decades ago. The natural reservoir of *Microsporum canis* is dogs and cats.

DIAGNOSIS

• The clinical appearance is often adequate to make the diagnosis.

• Confirm the diagnosis by scraping the scaling areas on the scalp and placing a few loose hairs on a microscope slide with KOH. (DMSO and a fungal stain will help). Look for Hyphae and spores (**Figure 131-6**). Look for endoectothrix invasion of the hair shaft with fungus.

CLINICAL FEATURES

• Alopecia and scaling of the scalp (**Figures 131-1** and **131-2**).

• A kerion occurs when there is an inflammatory response to the tinea. The scalp gets red, swollen, and boggy. There may be serosanguineous discharge and some crusting as this dries (**Figure 131-3**).

• There may be broken hairs that look like black dots in the areas of hair loss (**Figure 131-4**).

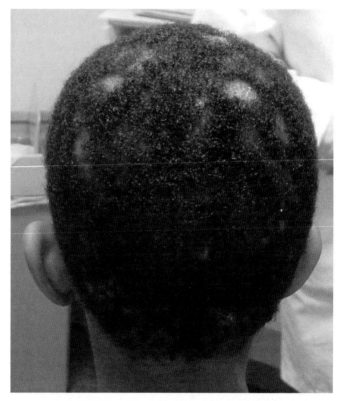

FIGURE 131-1 Tinea capitis in a young black boy. The most likely organism is *Trichophyton tonsurans*. (*Courtesy of Richard P. Usatine, MD.*)

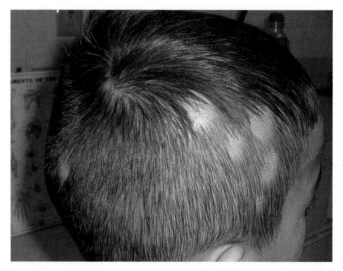

FIGURE 131-2 Tinea capitis with patchy hair loss and scaling of the scalp in a young boy. (*Courtesy of Richard P. Usatine, MD.*)

- Cervical lymphadenopathy is common from the tinea capitis (**Figure 131-5**).
- Tinea capitis in an infant can even have the rings of ringworm.

TYPICAL DISTRIBUTION

By definition it occurs on the head but usually is found on the scalp. Rarely involves the eyebrows and eyelashes.

LABORATORY STUDIES

- Scrape the scale and treat with KOH/DMSO to dissolve the keratin to look for septate, branching hyphae (**Figure 131-6**).
- If the diagnosis is uncertain, send a few loose hairs and a scraping of the scalp scale for a fungal culture.
- You may look at the scalp with an UV light (Woods lamp), looking for fluorescence, but the yield is low. Only the microsporum species will fluoresce (**Figures 131-7** and **131-8**) and this organism is the involved dermatophyte less than 30% of the time.

DIFFERENTIAL DIAGNOSIS

- Alopecia areata—produces areas of hair loss with no scaling, inflammation, or scarring in the underlying scalp. It is an autoimmune process in which the immune system attacks the person's own hair follicles (see Chapter 180, Alopecia Areata).
- Seborrhea of the scalp (dandruff)—is caused by the Pityrosporum yeast resulting in scaling and inflammation but rarely causes hair loss. The scalp involvement tends to be more widespread than patchy and localized as seen in tinea capitis (see Chapter 144, Seborrheic Dermatitis).
- Trichotillomania—self-inflicted alopecia caused when the patient pulls and twists her/his own hair (see Chapter 181, Traction Alopecia and a Trichotillomania).
- Traction alopecia—alopecia that occurs when the patient or parent pulls the hair to style it into braids and pony-tails. There should be no scaling of the scalp and the pattern of hair loss should match the hair style (**Figure 130-9**) (see Chapter 181, Traction Alopecia and a Trichotillomania).
- Scarring alopecia—seen with SLE and discoid lupus. Scarring and hypopigmentation should differentiate this from tinea capitis (see Chapter 182, Scarring Alopecia).
- Tinea barbae (**Figure 131-10**) is a type of tinea infection of the hair follicles of the beard.

MANAGEMENT

- Topical antifungal therapy is not adequate and oral treatment is needed.
- Griseofulvin remains the treatment of choice for tinea capitis even if it requires a somewhat longer course than the newer antifungal agents.[2–5] SOR **B** Most importantly, it is less expensive and available in a liquid form for children. Prescribe a 6- to 8-week course of griseofulvin for tinea capitis.

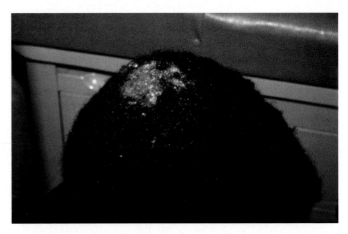

FIGURE 131-3 A kerion resulting from inflammation of the tinea capitis on this young boy. The kerion looks superinfected but it is nothing more than an exuberant inflammatory response to the dermatophyte. (*Courtesy of Richard P. Usatine, MD.*)

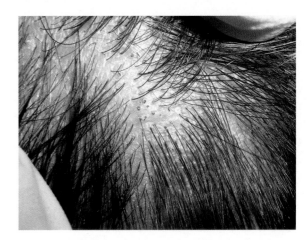

FIGURE 131-4 Close-up of black dot alopecia in a 7 year-old girl showing the black dots where infected hairs have broken off. (*Courtesy of www.doctorfungus.org © 2006.*)

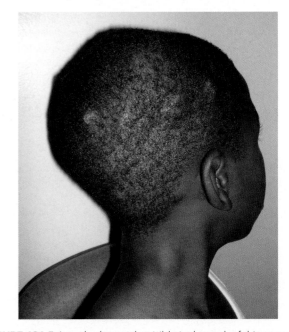

FIGURE 131-5 Lymphadenopathy visible in the neck of this young boy with tinea capitis. The fungal infection shows more scaling and crusting than actual hair loss. The lymphadenopathy is a reaction to the tinea and not a bacterial superinfection. (*Courtesy of Heather Goff, MD.*)

- A 2- to 4-week course of terbinafine is at least as effective as a 6- to 8-week course of griseofulvin for the treatment of Trichophyton infections of the scalp. Griseofulvin is likely to be superior to terbinafine for the rare cases caused by Microsporum species. SOR Ⓑ

- For the treatment of tinea capitis caused by the Trichophyton species griseofulvin given for 6 weeks is similar in efficacy to terbinafine, itraconazole, and fluconazole given for 2 to 3 weeks. SOR Ⓑ

- In a single study in Peru, 4 weeks of terbinafine was as effective as 8 weeks of griseofulvin at the end of the 8 weeks but at week 12, the efficacy of griseofulvin decreased to 44%, whereas the efficacy of terbinafine was 76%. SOR Ⓑ

- Terbinafine is effective and offers a shorter course of therapy than griseofulvin. It is not available in liquid form.

- Fluconazole is available in liquid form and appears to be effective and safe to treat cutaneous fungal infections, but fewer clinical trials have been published about it for tinea capitis.[1]

- Griseofulvin is available in many forms including liquid (125 mg microsize/5cc) for children. The dose for microsize griseofulvin is 20 mg/kg per day and ultramicrosize griseofulvin is 10 mg/kg per day. Ultramicrosize preparations are stronger per mg than the microsize, but do not come in liquid form. The tablets are less expensive than the liquids and can be used for children that can swallow a pill. The standard course should be 6 to 8 weeks for tinea capitis to deal with increasing resistance patterns.

- None of these agents require laboratory monitoring at the recommended lengths of treatment for tinea capitis.[1]

- A kerion may resolve with oral antifungal treatment alone. If it is severe and painful, consider a short pulse of oral steroids to speed up resolution. SOR Ⓒ

- While oral therapy is still the recommended treatment for tinea capitis, there is one study using 2% ketoconazole shampoo in which 33% of the young black children were cured clinically and mycologically with follow-up for one year.[6] SOR Ⓑ It also may be used as an adjunct for oral therapy to reduce fungal load. Another use for this antifungal shampoo is empirical treatment while waiting for a culture to come back in an equivocal case. SOR Ⓒ

PATIENT EDUCATION

Patients and parents need to exercise care to avoid spreading the infection to others. Explain the importance of not sharing combs, brushes, and towels.

FOLLOW-UP

Follow-up may be scheduled to check for full resolution of the infection.

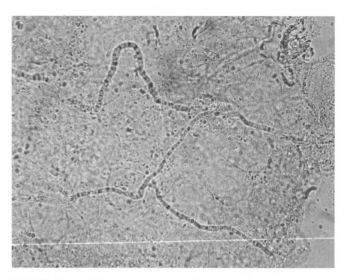

FIGURE 131-6 Trichophyton tonsurans from tinea capitis visible among skin cells at 40 power after adding Swartz Lamkins fungal stain. (*Courtesy of Richard P. Usatine, MD.*)

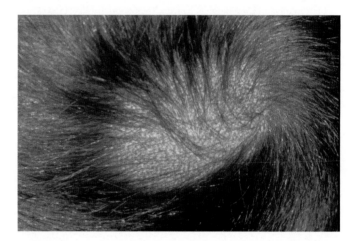

FIGURE 131-7 Tinea capitis in a young boy. (*Courtesy of Jeff Meffert, MD.*)

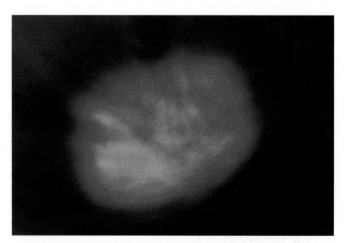

FIGURE 131-8 Fluorescence in the boy in **Figure 131-7** indicating that this is a microsporum species causing the tinea capitis. (*Courtesy of Jeff Meffert, MD.*)

REFERENCES

1. Johnston KL, Chambliss ML, DeSpain J. Clinical inquiries. What is the best oral antifungal medication for tinea capitis? *J Fam Pract.* 2001;50:206–207.

2. Caceres-Rios H, Rueda M, Ballona R, Bustamante B. Comparison of terbinafine and griseofulvin in the treatment of tinea capitis. *J Am Acad Dermatol.* 2000;42:80–84.

3. Fleece D, Gaughan JP, Aronoff SC. Griseofulvin versus terbinafine in the treatment of tinea capitis: A meta-analysis of randomized, clinical trials. *Pediatrics.* 2004;114:1312–1315.

4. Foster KW, Friedlander SF, Panzer H, Ghannoum MA, Elewski BE. A randomized controlled trial assessing the efficacy of fluconazole in the treatment of pediatric tinea capitis. *J Am Acad Dermatol.* 2005;53:798–809.

5. Gupta AK, Adam P, Dlova N et al. Therapeutic options for the treatment of tinea capitis caused by Trichophyton species: griseofulvin versus the new oral antifungal agents, terbinafine, itraconazole, and fluconazole. *Pediatr Dermatol.* 2001;18:433–438.

6. Greer DL. Successful treatment of tinea capitis with 2% ketoconazole shampoo. *Int J Dermatol.* 2000;39(4):302–304.

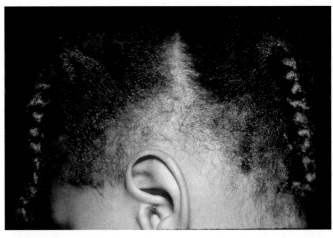

FIGURE 131-9 Traction alopecia that is related to the tight braids that put pressure on the hair follicle. The slight scaling was caused by seborrhea but tinea capitis must be in the differential diagnosis. (*Courtesy of Richard P. Usatine, MD.*)

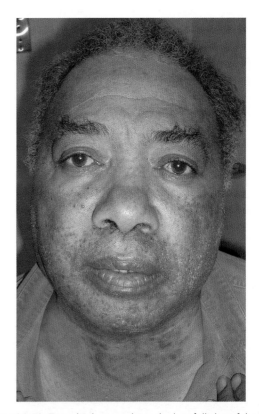

FIGURE 131-10 Tinea barbae involving the hair follicles of the beard in a 63-year-old man with cutaneous lupus. The annular eruption on the neck was initially confused for his lupus until a KOH scraping confirmed a fungal infection. The tinea barbae became inflammatory like a kerion with swelling of the upper lip before it was cured with oral terbinafine. (*Courtesy of Richard P. Usatine, MD.*)

132 TINEA CORPORIS

Richard P. Usatine, MD

PATIENT STORY

A 6-year-old girl is brought to the office for a round, itchy rash on her body (**Figure 132-1**). It was first noted 2 weeks ago. The family cat does have some patches of hair loss. Note the concentric rings with scaling, erythema, and central sparing. Ultraviolet (UV) light showed green fluorescence and the KOH is positive for branching and septate hyphae. The child is treated with a topical antifungal cream bid and the tinea resolved in 3–4 weeks.

EPIDEMIOLOGY

- Excessive heat and humidity make a good environment for fungal growth.
- Dermatophytes are spread by exposure to infected animals or persons and contact with contaminated items.

ETIOLOGY AND PATHOPHYSIOLOGY

- Tinea corporis is a common superficial fungal infection of the body characterized by well-demarcated, annular lesions with central clearing, erythema, and scaling of the periphery.
- Dermatophytes: *Trichophyton*, *Microsporum*, and *Epidermophyton* species.

DIAGNOSIS

Diagnosis is made based on clinical history, physical examination, and microscopy.

CLINICAL FEATURES

- Morphology: Well-demarcated, annular lesion with central clearing, erythema, and scaling of the periphery. Concentric rings are highly specific (80%) for tinea infections (**Figure 132-1**).
- Other characteristics: Pruritus of affected area.

TYPICAL DISTRIBUTION

Any part of the body including the face and axilla (**Figures 132-1** to **132-3**).

Tinea incognito is a type of tinea infection that was previously not recognized by the physician/patient and topical steroids were used on the site. While applying the steroid the dermatophyte continues to grow and can be cosmetically problematic (**Figure 132-4**). In some cases the infection may cause hyperpigmentation as in **Figures 132-4** to **132-6**. Note the concentric rings in (**Figures 132-5** and **132-6**).

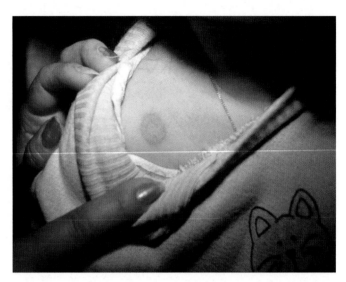

FIGURE 132-1 Tinea corporis on the shoulder of this young girl. This is a very typical annular pattern and the cat on a sweat shirt may be a clue to an infected pet at home spreading a *Microsporum* dermatophyte to its owner. Note the concentric rings with scaling, erythema, and central sparing. (*Courtesy of Richard P. Usatine, MD.*)

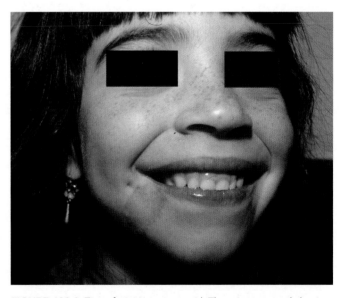

FIGURE 132-2 Tinea faciei in a young girl. There is no central clearing or annular pattern here but this was a cutaneous dermatophyte infection that resolved with a topical antifungal medicine. (*Courtesy of Richard P. Usatine, MD.*)

Tinea corporis can cover large parts of the body as in **Figure 132-7**.

LABORATORY STUDIES

- KOH prep of skin scraping can be very useful to confirm a clinical impression or when the diagnosis is not certain. Scrape the skin with the side of a slide or scalpel making sure to scrape the periphery and the erythematous part. Scrape hard enough to get some stratum corneum without causing bleeding. False negatives can occur secondary to inadequate scraping, patient using topical antifungals or inexperienced viewer.

- Use KOH with dimethyl sulfoxide (DMSO) to dissolve the epithelial cells more rapidly without heating. Use fungal stain when available (Chapter 129, Cutaneous Fungal Infections—Overview).

- Skin scraping and culture: gold standard, but more costly and may take up to two weeks for the culture to grow.

- Skin biopsy sent in formalin for periodic acid Schiff (PAS) staining when the KOH and culture remain negative but the clinical picture is consistent with a fungal infection.

DIFFERENTIAL DIAGNOSIS

- Granuloma Annulare: Inflammatory, benign dermatosis of unknown cause, characterized by both dermal and annular papules (**Figure 132-8**) (see Chapter 166, Granuloma Annulare).

- Psoriasis: Plaque with scale on extensor surfaces and trunk. Occasionally the plaques can have an annular appearance (**Figure 132-9**). Inverse psoriasis in intertriginous areas can also mimic tinea corporis (see Chapter 145, Psoriasis).

- Erythema annulare centrifugum (EAC): scaly red rings with normal skin in the center of the rings. The scale is trailing the erythema as the ring expands while the scale is leading in tinea corporis (**Figure 132-10**) (see Chapter 199, Erythema Annulare Centrifugum).

- Cutaneous larva migrans has serpiginous burrows made by the hookworm larvae and these burrows can look annular and be confused with tinea corporis (see Chapter 138, Cutaneous Larva Migrans).

- Nummular eczema: round coin-like red scaly plaques without central clearing (see Chapter 139, Atopic Dermatitis).

- Erythrasma: found in the axilla and groin without an annular configuration and central clearing. Fluoresces coral red under UV lamp (see Chapter 113, Erythrasma).

MANAGEMENT

- Use topical antifungal medications for tinea corporis that involves small areas of the body such as seen in **Figures 132-1** and **132-2**.

- While all the topical antifungal agents may be effective, the evidence supports the greater effectiveness of the allylamines (terbinafine) over the less expensive azoles for tinea pedis and corporis.[1,2] SOR **A**

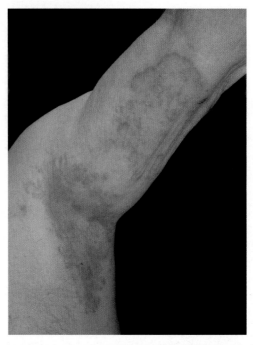

FIGURE 132-3 Extensive tinea corporis in the axilla and arm of this older adult. (*Courtesy of Richard P. Usatine, MD.*)

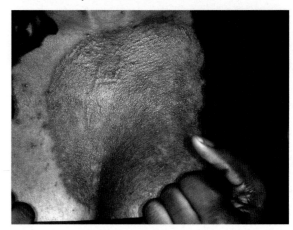

FIGURE 132-4 Tinea incognito on the chest of this black woman. This tinea infection continued to grow as the patient applied the topical steroids given to her by her physician. There is an extensive amount of postinflammatory hyperpigmentation. (*Courtesy of Richard P. Usatine, MD.*)

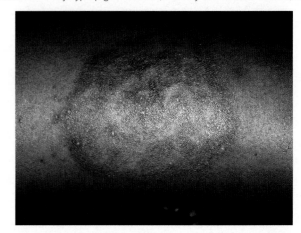

FIGURE 132-5 Tinea incognito on the arm of the same patient in the previous figure. Concentric rings are seen as this dermatophyte infection continued to grow under the influence of the topical steroids. (*Courtesy of Richard P. Usatine, MD.*)

- Studies show that terbinafine 1% cream or solution applied once daily for 7 days is highly effective for tinea corporis/cruris.[3,4] The 1% cream (which is available OTC as Lamisil AF) produced a mycological cure of 84.2% vs 23.3% with placebo. Number needed to treat (NNT) = 1.6.[3] SOR Ⓐ

- Oral antifungal agents should be considered for first line therapy for tinea corporis covering large areas of the body as seen in **Figures 132-6** and **132-7**. However, it is not wrong to attempt topical treatment if the size of the area infected is on the borderline. The patient with tinea incognito in **Figures 132-4** and **132-5** did need oral therapy to resolve her infection. Unfortunately, the postinflammatory hyperpigmentation did not resolve well.

- One randomized controlled trial (RCT) showed that oral itraconazole 200 mg daily for 1 week is similarly effective, equally well tolerated and at least as safe as itraconazole 100 mg for 2 weeks in the treatment of tinea corporis or cruris.[5] SOR Ⓑ

- In one study, patients with mycologically-diagnosed tinea corporis and tinea cruris were randomly allocated to receive either 250 mg of oral terbinafine once daily or 500 mg of griseofulvin once daily for 2 weeks. The cure rates were higher for terbinafine at 6 weeks.[6] SOR Ⓑ

- In summary, if an oral agent is needed, the evidence is greatest for the use of:
  ○ Terbinafine 250 mg daily for 2 weeks.[6] SOR Ⓑ
  ○ Itraconazole 200 mg daily for 1 week.[5] SOR Ⓑ
  ○ Itraconazole 100 mg daily for 2 weeks.[5] SOR Ⓑ

PATIENT EDUCATION

Keep the skin clean and dry. Infected pets should be treated.

FOLLOW-UP

Consider follow-up appointments in 4 to 6 weeks for difficult and more widespread cases. If there are concerns about bacterial superinfection, follow-up should be sooner.

PATIENT RESOURCES

VisualDxHealth article on Ringworm—**http://www.visualdxhealth.com/adult/tineaCorporis.htm**

Medline Plus Medical Encyclopedia—**http://www.nlm.nih.gov/medlineplus/ency/article/000877.htm**

http://www.nlm.nih.gov/medlineplus/ency/article/000877.htm

http://www.emedicine.com/DERM/topic421.htm

http://www.doctorfungus.org/

PROVIDER RESOURCES

eMedicine topic—**http://www.emedicine.com/DERM/topic421.htm**

Doctor Fungus Web site—**http://www.doctorfungus.org/**

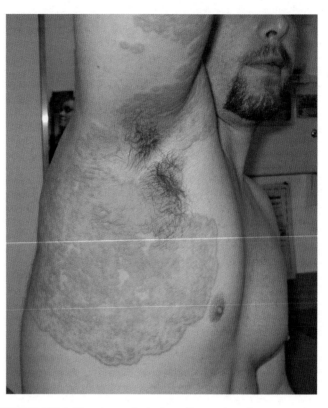

FIGURE 132-6 Tinea incognito in the axillary region of a young man who was prescribed topical steroids. While there is some hyperpigmentation, erythema is most prominent. (*Courtesy of Chris Wenner, MD.*)

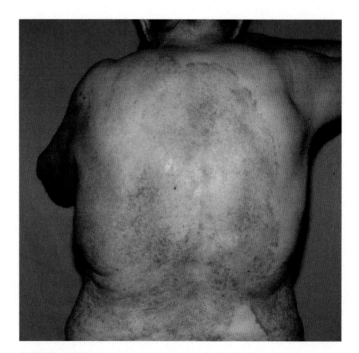

FIGURE 132-7 Tinea corporis covering the back of an elderly woman. (*Courtesy of Jack Resneck, Sr., MD.*)

REFERENCES

1. Thomas B. Clear choices in managing epidermal tinea infections. *J Fam Pract*. 2003;52:850–862.

2. Crawford F, Hart R, Bell-Syer S, Torgerson D, Young P, Russell I. Topical treatments for fungal infections of the skin and nails of the foot. *Cochrane Database Syst Rev*. 2000;CD001434.

3. Budimulja U, Bramono K, Urip KS et al. Once daily treatment with terbinafine 1% cream (Lamisil) for one week is effective in the treatment of tinea corporis and cruris. A placebo-controlled study. *Mycoses*. 2001;44:300–306.

4. Lebwohl M, Elewski B, Eisen D, Savin RC. Efficacy and safety of terbinafine 1% solution in the treatment of interdigital tinea pedis and tinea corporis or tinea cruris. *Cutis*. 2001;67:261–266.

5. Boonk W, de GD, de KE, Remme J, van HB. Itraconazole in the treatment of tinea corporis and tinea cruris: Comparison of two treatment schedules. *Mycoses*. 1998;41:509–514.

6. Voravutinon V. Oral treatment of tinea corporis and tinea cruris with terbinafine and griseofulvin: A randomized double blind comparative study. *J Med Assoc Thai*. 1993;76:388–393.

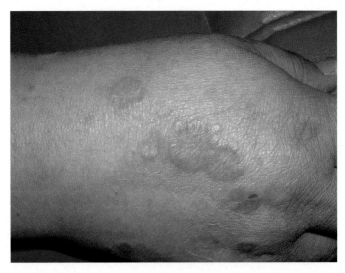

FIGURE 132-8 Multiple annular lesions caused by granuloma annulare. No scale is visible. (*Courtesy of Richard P. Usatine, MD.*)

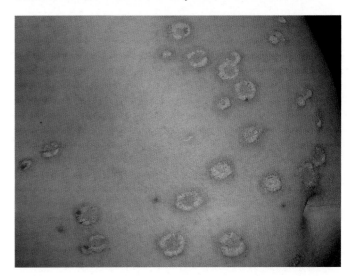

FIGURE 132-9 Widespread annular lesions caused by psoriasis. Not all lesions that are annular with scale are tinea corporis. (*Courtesy of Richard P. Usatine, MD.*)

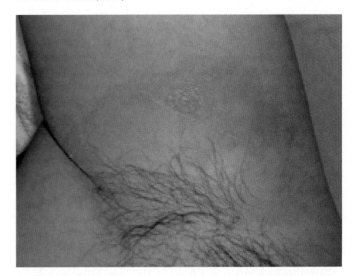

FIGURE 132-10 Erythema annulare centrifugum (EAC) in the axilla of a 28-year-old man. After multiple failed trials of antifungal medicines, a punch biopsy showed this to be EAC. Note the trailing scale rather than leading scale seen in tinea corporis. (*Courtesy of Richard P. Usatine, MD.*)

133 TINEA CRURIS

Richard P. Usatine, MD

PATIENT STORY

A 59-year-old man presents with itching in the groin **Figure 133-1**. On examination, he was found to have scaly erythematous plaques in the inguinal area. A skin scraping was treated with Swartz–Lamkins stain and the dermatophyte was highly visible under the microscope (**Figure 133-2**). He was treated with a topical antifungal medicine until his tinea cruris resolved.

EPIDEMIOLOGY

More common in men than women and rare in children.

ETIOLOGY AND PATHOPHYSIOLOGY

- Most commonly caused by the dermatophytes: *Trichophyton rubrum, Epidermophyton floccosum,* and *Trichophyton mentagrophytes. T. rubrum* is the most likely organism.[1]
- Can be spread by fomites, such as contaminated towels.
- Autoinoculation can occur from fungus on the feet or hands.

DIAGNOSIS

CLINICAL FEATURES

The cardinal features are scale and signs of inflammation. In light-skinned persons inflammation often appears red and in dark-skinned persons the inflammation often leads to hyperpigmentation as seen in **Figures 133-3** and **133-4**.

TYPICAL DISTRIBUTION

By definition it is in the inguinal area. However, the fungus can grow outside of this area to involve the abdomen as seen in **Figure 133-4**. Tinea can be present in multiple locations as in the patient in **Figure 133-5** that had tinea in the groin, on her feet, face and under her breasts.

LABORATORY STUDIES

Diagnosis is often made based on clinical presentation but a skin scraping treated with KOH and a fungal stain analyzed under the microscope can be helpful (**Figure 133-2**). False negatives may occur if scraping is inadequate, patient is using topical antifungals, or the viewer is inexperienced.

Skin scraping and culture: Definitive, but expensive and may take up to 2 weeks for the culture to grow.

UV lamp can be used to look for the coral red fluorescence of erythrasma. Most tinea cruris is caused by trichophyton rubrum so will not fluoresce.

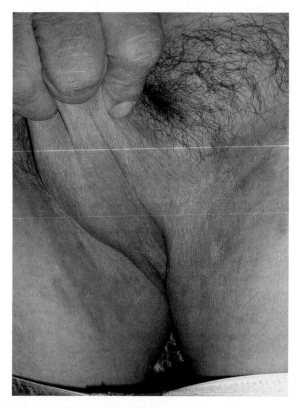

FIGURE 133-1 Tinea cruris in a 59-year-old Hispanic man present for 1 year. (*Courtesy of Richard P. Usatine, MD.*)

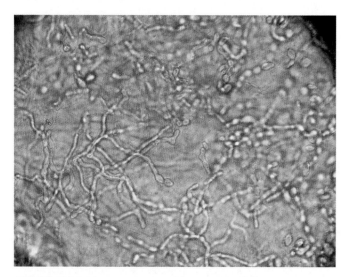

FIGURE 133-2 Microscopic view of the scraping of the groin in a man with tinea cruris. The hyphae are easy to see under 40 power with Swartz–Lamkin stain. (*Courtesy of Richard P. Usatine, MD.*)

DIFFERENTIAL DIAGNOSIS

- Cutaneous candida in the groin can become red and have scaling that extends to the thigh and scrotum. Tinea cruris does not involve the scrotum. Candida often has satellite lesions. However, tinea cruris can have a few satellite lesions too (see Chapter 130, Mucocutaneous Candidiasis).

- Erythrasma in the groin appears similar to tinea cruris. It is not uncommon and may show coral red fluorescence with an ultraviolet light (**Figure 133-6**) (see Chapter 113, Erythrasma).

- Contact dermatitis can occur anywhere on the body. If the contact is near the groin this can be mistaken for tinea cruris (see Chapter 140, Contact Dermatitis).

- Inverse psoriasis causes inflammation in the intertriginous areas of the body. It does not have the thick plaques of plaque psoriasis. Inverse psoriasis is frequently misdiagnosed as a fungal infection until an astute clinician recognizes the pattern or does a biopsy (**Figure 133-7**) (see Chapter 145, Psoriasis).

- Intertrigo is an inflammatory condition of the skin folds. It induced or aggravated by heat, moisture, maceration, and friction.[2] The condition frequently is worsened by infection with candida or dermatophytes so there is some overlap with tinea cruris.

MANAGEMENT

- Tinea cruris is best treated with a topical allylamine or an azole antifungal (SOR **A**, based on multiple RCTs). Differences in current comparison data are insufficient to stratify the two groups of topical antifungals.[3]

- The fungicidal allylamines (naftifine and terbinafine) and butenafine (allylamine derivative) are a more costly group of topical tinea treatments, yet they are more convenient as they allow for a shorter duration of treatment compared with fungistatic azoles (clotrimazole, econazole, ketoconazole, oxiconazole, miconazole, and sulconazole).[3]

- Fluconazole 150 mg once weekly for 2 to 4 weeks appears to be effective in the treatment of tinea cruris.[4] SOR **B**

- One randomized controlled trial (RCT) showed that itraconazole 200 mg for 1 week is similarly effective, equally well tolerated and at least as safe as itraconazole 100 mg for 2 weeks in the treatment of tinea corporis or cruris.[5] SOR **B**

- Patients with mycologically-diagnosed tinea corporis and tinea cruris were randomly allocated to receive either 250 mg of oral terbinafine once daily or 500 mg of griseofulvin once daily for 2 weeks. The cure rates were higher for terbinafine at 6 weeks.[6] SOR **B**

- If there are multiple sites infected with fungus, treat all active areas of infection simultaneously to prevent reinfection of the groin from other body sites. If the tinea is widespread as in the patient in **Figure 133-5**, an oral agent is warranted.

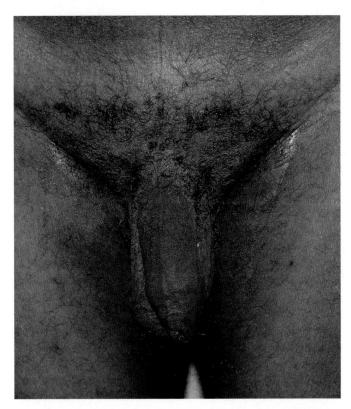

FIGURE 133-3 Tinea cruris in an older black man with hyperpigmentation secondary to the inflammatory response. A silvery scale is also seen but this is not psoriasis. (*Courtesy of Richard P. Usatine, MD.*)

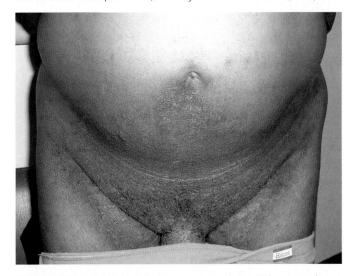

FIGURE 133-4 Tinea cruris that has expanded beyond the inguinal area in this 35-year-old black man. Postinflammatory hyperpigmentation is visible throughout the infected area. (*Courtesy of Richard P. Usatine, MD.*)

PATIENT EDUCATION

- Advise patients with tinea pedis to put on their socks before their undershorts to reduce the possibility of direct contamination. SOR **C**
- Dry the groin completely after bathing. SOR **C**

FOLLOW-UP

As needed.

PATIENT RESOURCES

VisualDxHealth—**http://www.visualdxhealth.com/adult/tineaCruris.htm.**

eMedicineHealth—**http://www.emedicinehealth.com/jock_itch/article_em.htm.**

PROVIDER RESOURCES

Fungal Skin from New Zealand—**http://www.dermnetnz.org/fungal/.**

Doctor Fungus from the USA—**http://www.doctorfungus.org/.**

World of Dermatophytes from Canada—**http://www.provlab.ab.ca/mycol/tutorials/derm/dermhome.htm.**

REFERENCES

1. http://www.emedicine.com/DERM/topic471.htm. Accessed September 2, 2006.

2. http://www.emedicine.com/DERM/topic198.htm. Accessed September 2, 2006.

3. Nadalo D, Montoya C, Hunter-Smith D. What is the best way to treat tinea cruris? *J Fam Pract.* 2006;55:256–258.

4. Nozickova M, Koudelkova V, Kulikova Z, Malina L, Urbanowski S, Silny W. A comparison of the efficacy of oral fluconazole, 150 mg/week versus 50 mg/day, in the treatment of tinea corporis, tinea cruris, tinea pedis, and cutaneous candidosis. *Int J Dermatol.* 1998;37:703–705.

5. Boonk W, de GD, de KE, Remme J, van HB. Itraconazole in the treatment of tinea corporis and tinea cruris: Comparison of two treatment schedules. *Mycoses.* 1998;41:509–514.

6. Voravutinon V. Oral treatment of tinea corporis and tinea cruris with terbinafine and griseofulvin: A randomized double blind comparative study. *J Med Assoc Thai.* 1993;76:388–393.

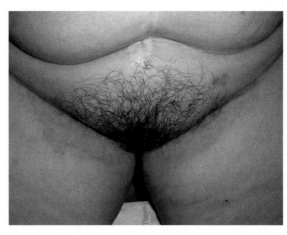

FIGURE 133-5 A 55-year-old woman with tinea cruris showing erythema and scale. Although less common in women, women do get tinea cruris. This patient had tinea on her feet, face and under her breasts. She was treated with oral terbinafine for 3 weeks. (*Courtesy of Richard P. Usatine, MD.*)

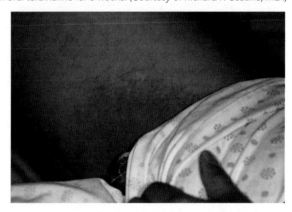

FIGURE 133-6 Erythrasma in the groin can be mistaken for tinea cruris. This erythrasma fluoresced coral red with an ultraviolet light. (*Courtesy of Richard P. Usatine, MD.*)

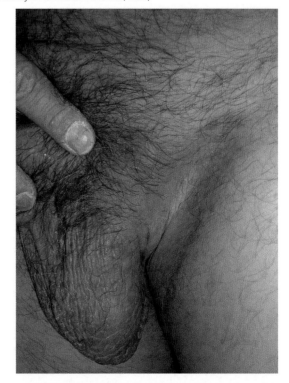

FIGURE 133-7 Inverse psoriasis in a man who also has the nail changes of psoriasis. (*Courtesy of Richard P. Usatine, MD.*)

134 TINEA PEDIS

Richard P. Usatine, MD

A 38-year-old man presents with an itchy rash on his hands and blisters on his feet for 1 week duration (**Figure 134-1**). Vesicular tinea pedis with bullae were present. The papules and vesicles between the fingers were typical of an autosensitization reaction (ID reaction) (**Figure 134-2**). The patient was treated with an oral antifungal medication and a short burst of oral prednisone for the autosensitization reaction.

EPIDEMIOLOGY

- Tinea pedis is thought to be the world's most common dermatophytosis.[1]
- 70% of the population will be infected with tinea pedis at some time.[1]
- More commonly affects males than females.[1]
- Prevalence increases with age and it is rare before adolescence.[1]

ETIOLOGY AND PATHOPHYSIOLOGY

- A cutaneous fungal infection most commonly caused by *Trichophyton rubrum*.[1]
- *Trichophyton mentagrophytes* and *Epidermophyton floccosum* follow in that order.
- *T. rubrum* causes most tinea pedis and onychomycosis.

DIAGNOSIS

TYPICAL DISTRIBUTION/MORPHOLOGY

Three types of tinea pedis

- Interdigital type—most common (**Figure 134-3**).
- Moccasin type (**Figures 134-4** and **134-5**).
- Inflammatory/vesicular type—least common (**Figure 134-1**).

Some authors describe an ulcerative type (**Figure 134-6**).

CLINICAL FEATURES

- Interdigital—white or green fungal growth between toes with erythema, maceration, cracks, and fissures—especially between 4th and 5th digits (**Figure 134-3**). The dry type has more scale and the moist type becomes macerated.
- Moccasin—scale on sides and soles of feet (**Figures 134-4** and **134-5**).
- Vesicular—vesicles and bullae on feet (**Figure 134-1**).

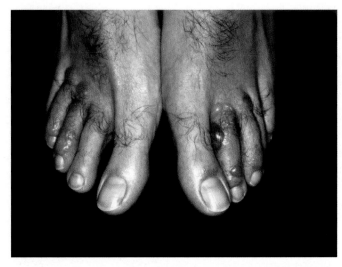

FIGURE 134-1 Vesicular tinea pedis with bullae present. This is an inflammatory reaction to the tinea pedis. (*Courtesy of Richard P. Usatine, MD.*)

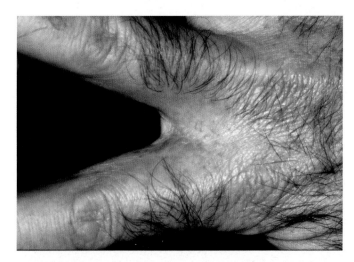

FIGURE 134-2 The hand shows an autosensitization reaction to the inflammatory tinea pedis in the previous figure. The vesicles between the fingers are typical of an autosensitization reaction, also known as an ID reaction. (*Courtesy of Richard P. Usatine, MD.*)

- Ulcerative tinea pedis is characterized by rapidly spreading vesiculopustular lesions, ulcers, and erosions, typically in the web spaces (**Figure 134-6**). It is accompanied by a secondary bacterial infection. This can lead to cellulitis or lymphangitis.

- Autosensitization (dermatophytid reaction) (ID reaction) is a hypersensitivity response to the fungal infection causing papules on the hands (**Figure 134-2**).

- Examine nails for evidence of onychomycosis—fungal infections of nails may include subungual keratosis, yellow or white discolorations, dysmorphic nails (see Chapter 186, Onychomycosis).

- Examine to exclude cellulitis that may show erythema, swelling, tenderness with red streaks tracking up the foot and lower leg (see Chapter 114, Cellulitis).

TYPICAL DISTRIBUTION

Between the toes, on the soles, and lateral aspects of the feet

LABORATORY STUDIES

Diagnosis is often made based on clinical presentation but a skin scraping treated with KOH and a fungal stain analyzed under the microscope can be helpful (**Figure 134-7**).

In the patient with tinea incognito on his foot and lower leg, the physicians were set astray by his diagnosis of systemic lupus erthematosus (SLE) (**Figure 134-8**). It took a skin scraping to demonstrate that this was tinea and not lupus to get the patient the treatment he needed (**Figure 134-7**).

Skin scraping and culture: definitive, but expensive and may take up to 2 weeks for the culture to grow.

DIFFERENTIAL DIAGNOSIS

- Pitted keratolysis: well-demarcated pits or erosions in the sole of the foot caused by bacteria (**Figure 134-9**) (see Chapter 112, Pitted Keratolysis).

- Contact dermatitis: tends to be seen on the dorsum and sides of the foot (**Figure 134-10**) (see Chapter 140, Contact Dermatitis).

- Keratodermas: thickening of the soles of the feet that can be caused by a number of etiologies including menopause (**Figure 134-11**). This condition looks a lot like tinea pedis in the moccasin distribution.

- Dyshidrotic eczema is characterized by scale and tapioca-like vesicles on the hands and feet (**Figure 134-12**) (see Chapter 141, Hand Eczema).

- Friction blisters: blisters on the feet of persons leading an active athletic lifestyle.

- Psoriasis: can mimic tinea pedis but will usually be present in other areas as well (**Figure 134-13**) (see Chapter 145, Psoriasis).

MANAGEMENT (TABLE 134-1)

TOPICAL ANTIFUNGALS

- Systematic review of 70 trials of topical antifungals showed good evidence for efficacy compared to placebo for the following:

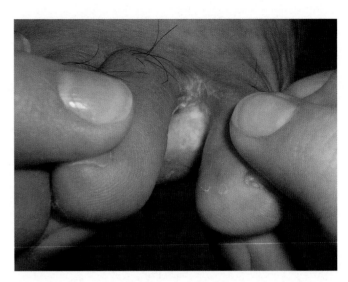

FIGURE 134-3 Tinea pedis seen in the interdigital space between the 4th and 5th digits. This is the most common area to see tinea pedis. (*Courtesy of Richard P. Usatine, MD.*)

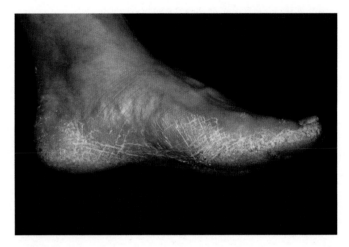

FIGURE 134-4 Tinea pedis in the moccasin distribution. (*Courtesy of Richard P. Usatine, MD.*)

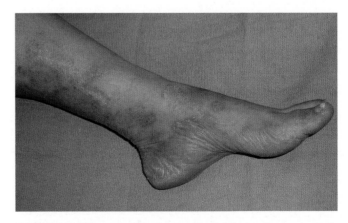

FIGURE 134-5 Tinea pedis in a moccasin distribution that has spread up the leg. (*Courtesy of Richard P. Usatine, MD.*)

- ○ Allylamines (naftifine, terbinafine, butenafine)[2] SOR **A**
- ○ Azoles (clotrimazole, miconazole, econazole)[2] SOR **A**
- ○ Allylamines cure slightly more infections than azoles but are more expensive[2] SOR **A**
- ○ No differences in efficacy found between individual allylamines or individual azoles (**Table 134-2**) SOR **A**

ORAL ANTIFUNGALS

- Systematic review of 12 trials, involving 700 participants: oral terbinafine for 2 weeks cures 52% more patients than oral griseofulvin.[3] SOR **A**
- Terbinafine is equal to itraconazole in patient outcomes.[3] SOR **A**
- No significant differences in comparisons between a number of oral agents.[3] SOR **A**

Dosing for tinea pedis needing oral therapy:

- Itraconazole two 100 mg tablets daily for 1 week.[4]
- Terbinafine 250 mg po daily for 1 to 2 weeks.[4]

   Patients with onychomycosis may have recurrences of the skin infection related to the fungus that remains in the nails and, therefore, may need oral treatment for 3 months to achieve better results.

   Topical urea (Carmol, Keralac) may be useful to decrease scaling in patients with hyperkeratotic soles.[3] Available in 10% to 40% concentrations.

PATIENT EDUCATION

- Do not go barefoot in public showers and locker rooms. SOR **C**
- Keep feet dry and clean, use clean socks and shoes that allow the feet to get fresh air. SOR **C**
- Use the topical medication beyond the time in which the feet look clear to prevent relapse.

PATIENT RESOURCES

eMedicineHealth—**http://www.emedicinehealth.com/athletes_foot/article_em.htm**

PROVIDER RESOURCES

http://www.emedicine.com/DERM/topic470.htm

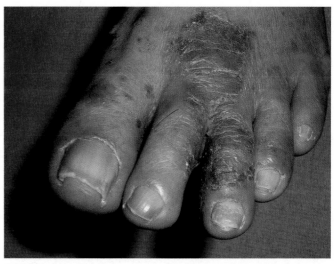

FIGURE 134-6 Ulcerative tinea pedis with spreading vesicles related to a bacterial superinfection. The patient was treated with antifungals and antibiotics. (*Courtesy of Richard P. Usatine, MD.*)

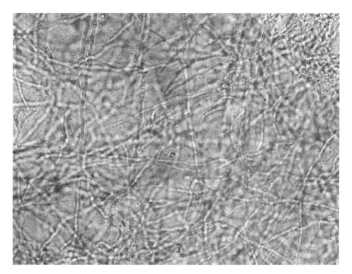

FIGURE 134-7 Microscopic view of the scraping of the foot in the man with tinea incognito in the next figure. The hyphae have proliferated and are easy to see under 40 power with Swartz–Lamkins stain. (*Courtesy of Richard P. Usatine, MD.*)

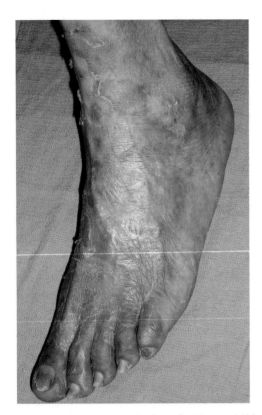

FIGURE 134-8 Tinea incognito on the foot of a 63-year-old black man with lupus. He was given topical steroids that allowed this fungus to spread and thrive. (*Courtesy of Richard P. Usatine, MD.*)

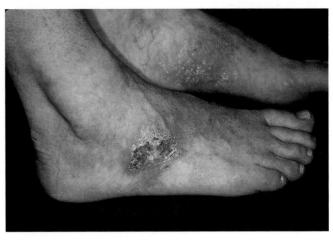

FIGURE 134-10 Contact dermatitis to tennis shoes with typical distribution that crosses the dorsum of the foot. (*Courtesy of Richard P. Usatine, MD.*)

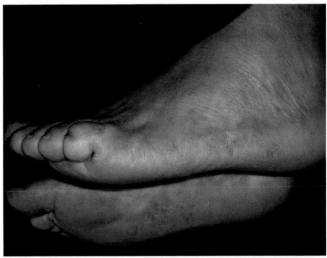

FIGURE 134-11 Keratoderma climactericum, which started when this woman entered menopause. (*Courtesy of Richard P. Usatine, MD.*)

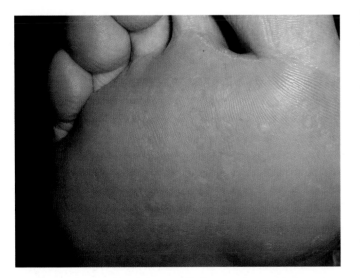

FIGURE 134-9 Pitted keratolysis on the foot causing a malodorous foot that is sometimes mistaken for tinea pedis. Look closely to see the subtle pits on the ball of the foot. (*Courtesy of Richard P. Usatine, MD.*)

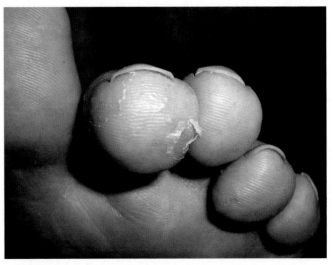

FIGURE 134-12 Dyshidrotic eczema on the foot showing tapioca vesicles with peeling of skin on the tip of the second toe. The patient also has typical tapioca vesicles between the fingers. (*Courtesy of Richard P. Usatine, MD.*)

TABLE 134-1 Management

Tinea Pedis Type	Treatment for Mild Cases	Treatment for Recalcitrant Cases	SOR
Interdigital type	Topical antifungal	Another topical antifungal or an oral antifungal	A
Moccasin type	Topical antifungal	Oral antifungal	A
Inflammatory/vesicular type	Oral antifungal	Oral antifungal	A

Reprinted with permission from Clear choices in managing epidermal tinea infections. *The Journal of Family Practice, November 2003;52(11):857, Dowden Health Media.*

TABLE 134-2 Topical Antifungal Medications

Agent	Formulation	Frequency*	Duration*	NNT[†]
IMIDAZOLES				
Clotrimazole	1% cream	Twice daily	2–4 (wk)	2.9
	1% solution			
	1% swabs			
Econazole	1% cream	Twice daily	2–4 (wk)	2.6
Ketoconazole	2% cream	Once daily	2–4 (wk)	No data available
Miconazole	2% cream	Twice daily	2–4 (wk)	2.8 (at 8 wk)
	2% spray			
	2% powder			
Oxiconazole	1% cream	Once to twice daily	2–4 (wk)	2.9
	1% lotion			
Sulconazole	1% cream	Once to twice daily	2–4 (wk)	2.5
	1% solution			
ALLYLAMINES				
Naftifine	1% cream	Once to twice daily	1–4 (wk)	1.9
	1% gel			
Terbinafine	1% cream	Once to twice daily	1–4 (wk)	1.6 (1.7 for tinea cruris/tinea corporis at 8 wk)
	1% solution			
BENZYLAMINE				
Butenafine	1% cream	Once to twice daily	1–4 (wk)	1.9 (1.4 for tinea corporis and 1.5 for tinea cruris)
OTHER				
Ciclopirox	0.77% cream	Twice daily	2–4 (wk)	2.1
	0.77% lotion			
Tolnaftate	1% powder	Twice daily	4 (wk)	3.6 (at 8 wk)
	1% spray			
	1% swabs			

*Manufacturer guidelines.

[†]NNT, number needed to treat. NNT is calculated from systematic review of all randomized controlled trials for tinea pedis at 6 weeks after the initiation of treatment except where otherwise noted. (*With permission from Clear choices in managing epidermal tinea infections. J Fam Pract. 2003;52(11):857, Dowden Health Media.*)

REFERENCES

1. Robbins C. Tinea Pedis. http://www.emedicine.com/DERM/topic470.htm. Accessed June 24, 2007.

2. Crawford F, Hart R, Bell-Syer S, Torgerson D, Young P, Russell I. Topical treatments for fungal infections of the skin and nails of the foot. *Cochrane Database Syst Rev.* 2000;CD001434.

3. Bell-Syer SE, Hart R, Crawford F, Torgerson DJ, Tyrrell W, Russell I. Oral treatments for fungal infections of the skin of the foot. *Cochrane Database Syst Rev.* 2002;CD003584.

4. Thomas B. Clear choices in managing epidermal tinea infections. *J Fam Pract.* 2003;52:850–862.

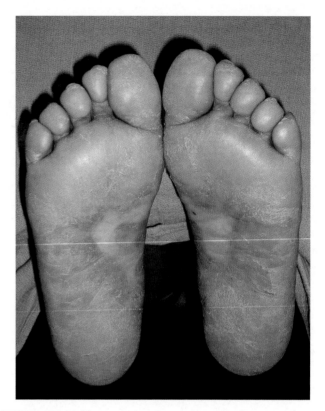

FIGURE 134-13 Plantar psoriasis in a patient with other areas of psoriasis also present. (*Courtesy of Richard P. Usatine, MD.*)

135 TINEA VERSICOLOR

Richard P. Usatine, MD

PATIENT STORY

A young black man presents to the office with a 5-year history of white spots on his trunk (**Figure 135-1**). He has no symptoms with this but is worried that this could be a disease that he could spread to his girlfriend. These spots get worse during the summer months but never go away completely. He was relieved to receive a treatment for his tinea versicolor and to find out that it is rarely spread to others through contact.

EPIDEMIOLOGY

- Common superficial skin infection caused by the dimorphic lipophilic yeast *Pityrosporum* (Malassezia furfur).

- Seen more commonly in men than women as is true for other tinea infections.

- Seen more often during the summer.

ETIOLOGY AND PATHOPHYSIOLOGY

- Tinea versicolor is caused by *Pityrosporum* (Malassezia furfur), which is a lipophilic yeast that can be normal human cutaneous flora.

- *Pityrosporum* exists in two shapes—*Pityrosporum ovale* (oval) and *Pityrosporum orbiculare* (round). Tinea versicolor is also called pityriasis versicolor after the organism that causes it.

- Tinea versicolor starts when the yeast that normally colonizes the skin changes from the round form to the pathologic mycelial form and then invade the stratum corneum.[1]

- *Pityrosporum* is also associated with seborrhea and Pityrosporum folliculitis.

- The white and brown colors are secondary to damage caused by the Pityrosporum to the melanocytes, while the pink is an inflammatory reaction to the organism.

- *Pityrosporum* thrive on sebum and moisture and tend to grow on the skin in areas where there are sebaceous follicles secreting sebum.

DIAGNOSIS

CLINICAL FEATURES

The pattern of hypopigmented and brown macules on the trunk with a fine scale points to tinea versicolor. Versicolor means a variety of or variation in colors and tinea versicolor tends to come in white, pink, and brown colors (**Figures 135-1 to 135-5**).

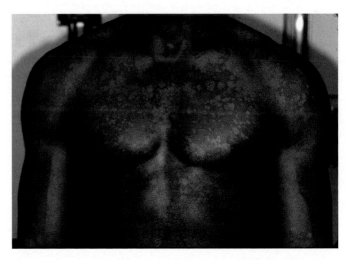

FIGURE 135-1 Tinea versicolor showing areas of hypopigmentation. (*From the Western Journal of Medicine and Richard P. Usatine, MD.*)

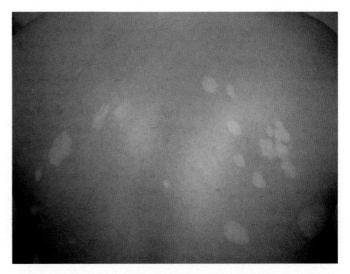

FIGURE 135-2 Patches of hypopigmentation across the back caused by tinea versicolor in a young Latino man. Vitiligo is on the differential diagnosis in this case. A KOH preparation confirmed tinea versicolor. (*Courtesy of Richard P. Usatine, MD.*)

TYPICAL DISTRIBUTION

Tinea versicolor is found on the chest, abdomen, upper arms, and back while seborrhea tends to be seen on the scalp, face, and anterior chest.

LABORATORY STUDIES

A scraping of the scaling portions of the skin can be performed onto a slide using the side of another slide or a scalpel. KOH with DMSO (DMSO helps the KOH dissolve the keratinocytes faster and reduces the need for heating the slide) is placed on the slide and covered with a coverslip. Microscopic examination reveals the typical "spaghetti and meatballs" pattern of tinea versicolor. The spaghetti or more accurately "ziti" is the short mycelial form and the meatballs are the round yeast form (**Figures 135-6** and **135-7**). Fungal stains such as the Swartz Lamkins stain help make the identification of the fungal elements easier.

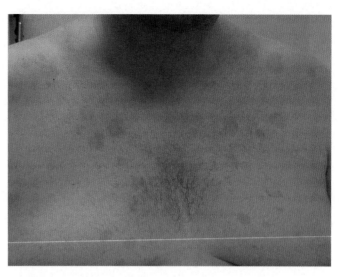

FIGURE 135-3 Pink scaly patches caused by tinea versicolor. Seborrhea may be seen in this location but tends to be worse in the presternal region. (*Courtesy of Richard P. Usatine, MD.*)

DIFFERENTIAL DIAGNOSIS

- Pityriasis rosea has a fine collarette scale around the border of the lesions and is frequently seen with a herald patch. Negative KOH (see Chapter 146, Pityriasis Rosea).

- Secondary syphilis is usually not scaling and tends to have macules on the palms and soles. Negative KOH (see Chapter 209, Syphilis).

- Tinea corporis is rarely as widespread as tinea versicolor and each individual lesion usually has central clearing and a well-defined raised scaling border. The KOH preparation in tinea corporis shows hyphae with multiple branch points and not the "ziti and meatballs" pattern of tinea versicolor (see Chapter 132, Tinea Corporis).

- Vitiligo—the degree of hypopigmentation is greater and the distribution is frequently different with vitiligo involving the hands and face (see Chapter 191, Vitiligo).

- Pityriasis alba—lightly hypopigmented areas with slight scale that tend to be found on the face and trunk of children with atopy. These patches are frequently smaller and rounder than tinea versicolor (see Chapter 139, Atopic Dermatitis).

- Pityrosporum folliculitis is caused by the same organism but presents with pink or brown papules on the back. The patient complains of itchy rough skin and the KOH is positive (**Figure 135-8**).

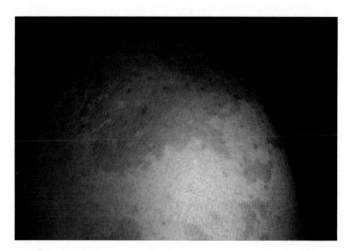

FIGURE 135-4 Large areas of pink tinea versicolor on the shoulder in a cape like distribution. (*Courtesy of Richard P. Usatine, MD.*)

MANAGEMENT

Topical

- Because tinea versicolor is usually asymptomatic the treatment is mostly for cosmetic reasons.

- The mainstay of treatment has been topical therapy using antidandruff shampoos, because the same Pityrosporum species that cause seborrhea and dandruff also cause tinea versicolor.[1]

- Patients may apply selenium sulfide 2½% lotion or shampoo, or zinc pyrithione shampoo to the involved areas daily from 1 to 2 weeks. Various amounts of time are suggested to allow the preparations to work, but there are no studies that show a minimum exposure time needed. A typical regimen involves applying the lotion or shampoo to the involved areas for 10 minutes and then washing it off in the shower. SOR **C**

- One study used ketoconazole 2% shampoo (Nizoral) as a single application or daily for 3 days and found it safe and highly effective in treating tinea versicolor.[2] SOR **B**

- Topical antifungal creams for smaller areas of involvement can include ketoconazole and clotrimazole. SOR **C**

ORAL TREATMENT AND PREVENTION

- A single dose 400 mg oral fluconazole provided the best clinical as well as mycological cure rate with no relapse during 12 months of follow-up.[3] SOR **B**

- A single dose of 300 mg of oral fluconazole repeated weekly for 2 weeks was equal to 400 mg of ketoconazole in a single dose repeated weekly for 2 weeks. No significant differences in efficacy, safety, and tolerability between the two treatment regimens were found.[4] SOR **B**

- A single dose 400 mg oral ketoconazole to treat tinea versicolor is safe and cost-effective compared to using the newer more expensive oral antifungal agents such as itraconazole.[5] SOR **B**

- Oral itraconazole 200 mg given twice a day for 1 day a month has been shown to be safe and effective as a prophylactic treatment for tinea versicolor.[6] SOR **B**

- There is no evidence that establishes the need to sweat after taking oral antifungals to treat tinea versicolor.

PATIENT EDUCATION

Patients should be told that the change in skin color will not reverse immediately. The first sign of successful treatment is the lack of scale. The yeast acts like a sunscreen in the hypopigmented macules. Sun exposure will hasten the normalization of the skin color in the patients with hypopigmentation.

FOLLOW-UP

None needed unless it is a stubborn or recurrent case. Recurrent cases can be treated with monthly topical or oral therapy.

PATIENT AND PROVIDER RESOURCES

VisualDxHealth—**http://www.visualdxhealth.com/adult/tineaVersicolor.htm.**

http://www.emedicine.com/DERM/topic423.htm.

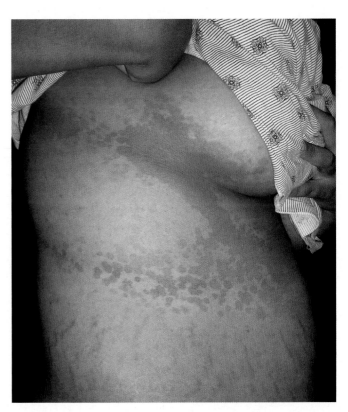

FIGURE 135-5 Hyperpigmented variant of tinea versicolor in a Hispanic woman. (*Courtesy of Richard P. Usatine, MD.*)

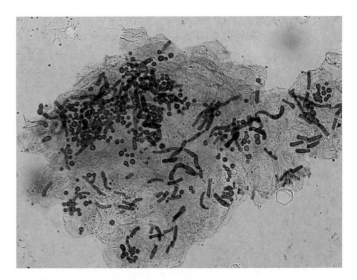

FIGURE 135-6 Microscopic examination of scrapings done from previous patient showing short mycelial forms and round yeast forms suggestive of spaghetti and meatballs. Swartz–Lamkins stain was used. (*Courtesy of Richard P. Usatine, MD.*)

REFERENCES

1. Bolognia J, Jorizzo J, Rapini R. *Dermatology*. St. Louis: Mosby, 2003.

2. Lange DS, Richards HM, Guarnieri J, et al. Ketoconazole 2% shampoo in the treatment of tinea versicolor: A multicenter, randomized, double-blind, placebo-controlled trial. *J Am Acad Dermatol*. 1998;39(6):944–950.

3. Bhogal CS, Singal A, Baruah MC. Comparative efficacy of ketoconazole and fluconazole in the treatment of pityriasis versicolor: A one year follow-up study. *J Dermatol*. 2001;28(10):535–539.

4. Farschian M, Yaghoobi R, Samadi K. Fluconazole versus ketoconazole in the treatment of tinea versicolor. *J Dermatolog Treat*. 2002;13(2):73–76.

5. Gupta, Aditya K, Del Rosso, James Q. An evaluation of intermittent therapies used to treat onychomycosis and other dermatomycoses with the oral antifungal agents. *Int J Dermatol*. 2000;39(6):401–411

6. Faergemann J, Gupta AK, Mofadi AA, et al. Efficacy of itraconazole in the prophylactic treatment of pityriasis (tinea) versicolor. *Arch Dermatol*. 2002;138:69–73.

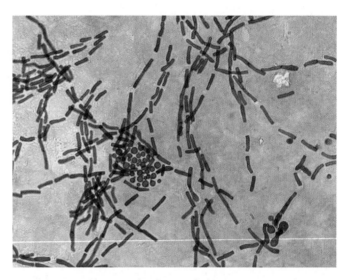

FIGURE 135-7 Close-up of Malassezia furfur (Pityrosporum) showing the ziti and meatball appearance after Swartz–Lamkins stain was applied to the scraping of tinea versicolor in a young woman. (*Courtesy of Richard P. Usatine, MD.*)

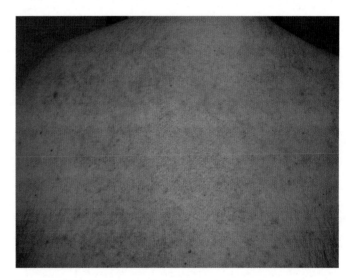

FIGURE 135-8 Pityrosporum folliculitis on the back of man with pruritus. (*Courtesy of Richard P. Usatine, MD.*)

136 LICE

Lesa Brookes, MD
Richard P. Usatine, MD

PATIENT STORY

A 64-year-old schizophrenic homeless woman presented to a homeless clinic for itching all over her body. She stated that she could see creatures feed on her and move in and out of her skin. The physical examination revealed that she was unwashed and had multiple excoriations over her body (**Figure 136-1**). Body lice and their progeny were visible along the seams of her pants (**Figure 136-2**). Treatment of this lousy infestation required giving her new clothes and a shower.[1]

EPIDEMIOLOGY

- Head lice are most common among school-aged children. Each year, approximately 6 to 12 million children of ages 3 to 12 years have infestations.[2]

- Head lice infestation is seen across all socioeconomic groups and is not a sign of poor hygiene.[3]

- In the United States, black children are affected less often as a result of their oval-shaped hair shafts that are difficult for lice to grasp.[2]

- Body lice infest the seams of clothing (**Figure 136-2**) and bed linen. Infestations are associated with poor hygiene and conditions of crowding.

- Pubic lice are most common in sexually active adolescents and adults. Young children with pubic lice typically have infestations of the eyelashes. Although infestations in this age group may be an indication of sexual abuse, children generally acquire the crab lice from their parents.[4]

ETIOLOGY AND PATHOPHYSIOLOGY

- Lice are parasites that have six legs with terminal claws that enable them to attach to hair and clothing. There are three types of lice responsible for human infestation. All three kinds of lice must feed daily on human blood and can only survive a day or two away from the host. The three types of lice are as follows:
  - Head lice (*Pediculus humanus capitis*)—Measure 2 to 4 mm in length (**Figure 136-3**).
  - Body lice (*Pediculus humanus corporis*)—Body lice similarly measure 2 to 4 mm in length (**Figure 136-4**).
  - Pubic or crab lice (*Phthirus pubis*)—Pubic lice are shorter, with a broader body and have an average length of 1 to 2 mm (**Figure 136-5**).

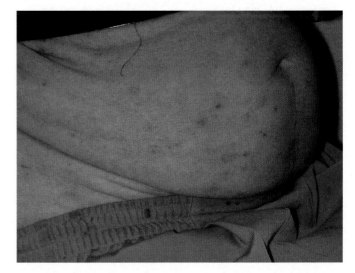

FIGURE 136-1 A 64-year-old schizophrenic homeless woman with body lice and visible excoriations. (*Courtesy of Richard P. Usatine, MD and Usatine RP, Halem L. A terrible itch. J Fam Pract. 2003;52(5): 377–379, Dowden Health Media.*)

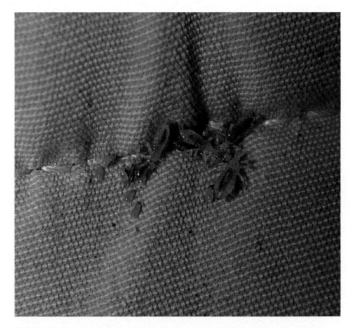

FIGURE 136-2 Adult body lice and nymphs visible along the pant seams of the woman in **Figure 136-1** (*Courtesy of Richard P. Usatine, MD.*)

- Female lice have a lifespan of aproximately 30 days and can lay approximately 10 eggs (nits) a day.[2]
- Nits are firmly attached to the hair shaft or clothing seams by a glue-like substance produced by the louse (**Figures 136-6 to 136-8**).
  - Nits are incubated by body heat.
  - The incubation period from laying eggs to hatching of the first nymph is 7 to 14 days.
  - Mature adult lice capable of reproducing appear 2 to 3 weeks later.[3]
- Transmission of head lice occurs through direct contact with the hair of infested individuals. The role of fomites (e.g., hats, combs, brushes) in transmission is negligible.[4] Head lice do not serve as vectors for transmission of disease among humans.
- Transmission of body lice occurs through direct human contact or contact with infested material. Unlike head lice, body lice are well-recognized vectors for transmission of the pathogens responsible for epidemic typhus, trench fever, and relapsing fever.[3]
- Pubic or crab lice are transmitted primarily through sexual contact. In addition to pubic hair (**Figure 136-9**), infestations of eyelashes, eyebrows, beard, upper thighs, abdominal, and axillary hairs may also occur.

DIAGNOSIS

CLINICAL FEATURES

- Head lice: Look for nits and lice in the hair especially above the ears, behind the ears and at the nape of the neck. There are many more nits present than live adults. Finding nits without an adult louse does not mean that the infestation has resolved (**Figures 136-6 and 136-7**).
- Body lice: Looks for the lice and larvae in the seams of the clothing (**Figure 136-2**).
- Pubic lice: Look for nits and lice on the pubic hairs (**Figure 136-9**). These lice and their nits may also be seen on the hairs of the upper thighs, abdomen, axilla, beard, eyebrows, and eyelashes. Little specks of dried blood may be seen in the underwear as a clue to the infestation.
- Nits can be seen in active disease or treated disease. Nits closer to the base of the hairs are generally newer and more likely to be live and unhatched. Unfortunately, nits that were not killed by pediculicides can hatch and start the infestation cycle over again. Note that nits are glued to the hairs and flakes of dandruff can be easily brushed off.

  Pruritus is the hallmark of lice infestation. It is the result of an allergic response to louse saliva.[5]

- Therefore, head lice are associated with excoriated lesions that appear on the scalp, ears, neck, and back.
- Occipital and cervical adenopathy may develop, especially when lesions become super-infected.
- Body lice result in small maculopapular eruptions that are predominantly found on the trunk (**Figure 136-1**).

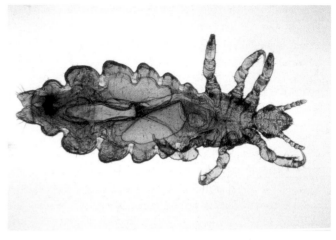

FIGURE 136-3 Adult head louse with elongated body. (*Courtesy of CDC/Dennis D. Juranek.*)

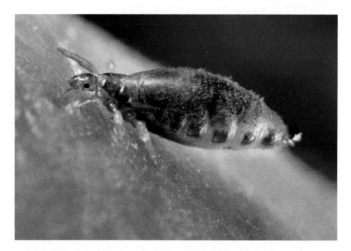

FIGURE 136-4 A body louse feeding on the blood of the photographer. The dark mass inside the abdomen is a previously ingested blood meal. (*Courtesy of CDC/Frank Collins, PhD.*)

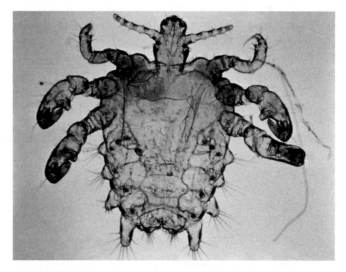

FIGURE 136-5 The crab louse has a short body and its large claws are responsible for the "crab" in its name. (*Courtesy of CDC/WHO.*)

- Chronic infestations often result in hyperpigmented, lichenified plaques known as "vagabond's skin."[6]
- Pubic lice produce bluish-gray spots (macula cerulea) that can be found on the chest, abdomen, and thighs.[6]

LABORATORY AND IMAGING

Direct visualization and identification of live lice or nits are sufficient to make a diagnosis (**Figures 136-2** to **136-7** and **136-9**).

- The use of a magnification lens, Wood's lamp, or louse comb may also aid in the detection or confirmation of lice infestation.
- If you find an adult louse put it on a slide with a cover slip loosely above it. Look at it under the microscope on the lowest power (**Figures 136-4** and **136-5**). You will be amazed to see the internal workings of the live organs. If the louse was not found in a typical location, you can use the morphology of the body and legs to determine the type of louse causing the infestation. Show it to others in your office to see their amazement.
- In cases of pubic lice infestations, individuals should be screened for other sexually transmitted diseases.[3]

DIFFERENTIAL DIAGNOSIS

- Dandruff, hair casts, and debris should be ruled out in cases of suspected lice infestations. Unlike nits, these particles are easily removed from the hair shaft. In addition, adult lice are absent.
- Scabies is also characterized by intense pruritus and papular eruptions. Unlike lice infestations, scabies may be associated with vesicles, and the presence of burrows is pathognomonic. Diagnosis is confirmed by microscopic examination of the scrapings from lesions for the presence of mites or eggs (see Chapter 137, Scabies).

MANAGEMENT

- *Pediculus humanus capitis* (head lice):
  - Routinely treated using a nonprescription 1% permethrin cream rinse (Nix) or pyrethrins with piperonyl butoxide (RID) shampoo that is applied to the hair and left on for 10 minutes. A Cochrane review found no evidence that any one pediculicide was better than another; permethrin, synergised pyrethrin, and malathion were all effective in the treatment of head lice.[7] SOR Ⓐ Pyrethrins are only pediculicidal, while permethrin is both pediculicidal and ovicidal. It is important to note that treatment failure is common with these agents owing to the emergence of resistant strains of lice. Overall treatment efficacy also depends on the removal of nits from the hair shafts.[8]
  - After 7 to 10 days repeat application is an option when permethrin is used, however, it is a necessity for pyrethrin.
  - Nits are removed with a fine-toothed comb following the application of all treatments. This step is critical in achieving resolution.
    - A 1:1 vinegar:water rinse (left under a conditioning cap or towel for 15–20 min) or 8% formic acid crème rinse may enhance removal of tenacious nits.[6]

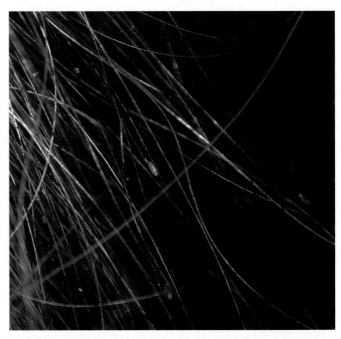

FIGURE 136-6 Pearly nits on the hair of a schoolgirl. (*Courtesy of Richard P. Usatine, MD.*)

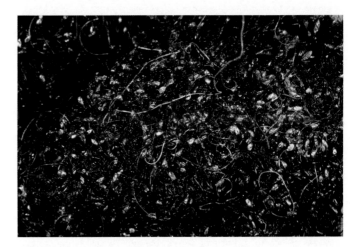

FIGURE 136-7 Massive infestation of head lice on a mentally ill homeless person. (*Courtesy of Richard P. Usatine, MD.*)

- Combs and hairbrushes should be discarded, soaked in hot water (temperature >55°C) for 5 minutes, or treated with pediculicides.[9]
  - Lice persisting after treatment with a pyrethroid may be an indication of resistance.
    - Malathion 0.5% (Ovide) is available by prescription only, and is a highly effective therapeutic agent for resistant lice. Malathion may have greater efficacy than pyrethrins.[8] It is approved for use in children age 6 years and older. The lotion is applied to dry hair for 8 to 12 hours and then washed. Repeat application is recommended after 7 to 10 days if live lice are still present. When used appropriately, malathion is 78% to 95% effective.[8]
    - Other therapeutic options include permethrin 5% cream and lindane 1% shampoo.
      - Permethrin 5% is conventionally used to treat scabies, however it is anecdotally recommended for treatment of recalcitrant head lice.[3] SOR Ⓒ
      - Lindane is considered a second-line treatment option owing to the possibility of central nervous system toxicity, which is most severe in children.
    - Oral therapy options include a 10-days course of trimethoprim-sulfamethoxazole or two doses of Ivermectin (200 μg/kg) 7 to 10 days apart. SOR Ⓒ Trimethoprim-sulfamethoxazole is postulated to kill the symbiotic bacteria in the gut of the louse.[2] Combination therapy with 1% permethrin and trimethoprim-sulfamethoxazole is recommended in cases of multiple treatment failure or suspected cases of resistance to therapy.[3,10] SOR Ⓒ

- *Pediculus humanus corporis* (body lice):
  - Improving hygiene, and laundering clothing and bed linen at temperatures of 65°C for 15 to 30 minutes will eliminate body lice.[6]
  - In settings where individuals cannot change clothing (e.g., indigent population), a monthly application of 10% lindane powder can be used to dust the lining of all clothing.[6]
  - Additionally, lindane lotion or permethrin cream may be applied to the body for 8 to 12 hours to eradicate body lice.

- *Phthirus pubis* (pubic lice):
  - Pubic lice infestations are treated with a 10-minute application of the same topical pediculicides used to treat head lice.
  - Retreatment is recommended 7 to 10 days later.
  - Petroleum ointment applied two to four times a day for 8 to 10 days will eradicate eyelash infestations.
  - Clothing, towels, and bed linen should also be laundered to eliminate nit-bearing hairs.[6]

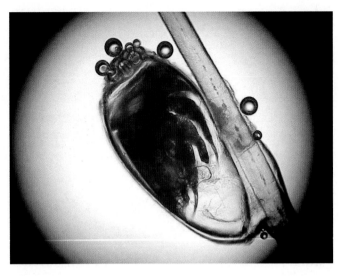

FIGURE 136-8 Microscopic view of a nit cemented to the hair and about to hatch. (*Courtesy of Dan Stulberg, MD.*)

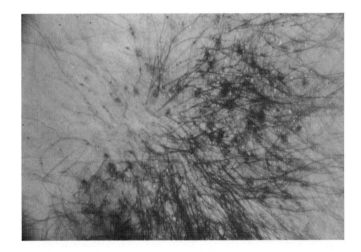

FIGURE 136-9 Crab lice infesting pubic hair. (*Courtesy of the University of Texas Health Sciences Center, Division of Dermatology.*)

PATIENT EDUCATION

- Patients should be instructed to wash potentially contaminated articles of clothing, bed linen, combs, brushes, and hats. Any item that cannot be washed or drycleaned may be vacuumed.

- Nit removal is important in preventing continued infestation as a result of new progeny. Careful examination of close contacts, with appropriate treatment for infested individuals is important in avoiding recurrence.

- In cases of pubic lice, all sexual contacts should be treated.

FOLLOW-UP

- Patients should be re-examined upon completion of therapy to confirm eradication of lice.

PATIENT RESOURCES

http://www.emedicinehealth.com/lice/article_em.htm.

http://www.cdc.gov/ncidod/dpd/parasites/lice/default.htm.

PROVIDER RESOURCES

http://www.cdc.gov/ncidod/dpd/parasites/lice/default.htm.

http://www.emedicine.com/med/topic1769.htm.

http://home.mdconsult.com/das/search/openres/68927844-2?searchId=573657804.

REFERENCES

1. Usatine RP, Halem L. A terrible itch. *J Fam Pract*. 2003;52(5):377–379.

2. Frankowski BL, Weiner LB. Head Lice. *Pediatrics*. 2002;110(3):638–643.

3. Pickering LK, Baker CJ, Long SS, McMillan JA. Red Book: 2006 Report of the Committee on Infectious Diseases. 27th ed. Elk Grove Village, American Academy of Pediatrics, 2006:488–493.

4. Maguire JH, Pollack RJ, Spielman A. Ectoparasite infestations and arthropod bites and stings. In: Kasper DL, Fauci AS, Longo DL, Braunwald EB, Hauser SL, Jameson JL, eds. *Harrison's Principles of Internal Medicine* 16th ed. New York, NY: McGraw-Hill, 2005:2601–2602.

5. Flinders DC, De Schweinitz P. Pediculosis and scabies. *Am Fam Physician*. 2004;69(2):341–348.

6. Darmstadt GL. Arthropod Bites and Infestations. In: Behrman RE, Kliegman RM, Jenson HB eds. *Nelson Textbook of Pediatrics*. 16th ed. Philadelphia, PA: WB Saunders, 2000:2046–2047.

7. Dodd CS. Interventions for treating headlice (Cochrane Review). In Cochrane Library Issue 2. Chichester, UK: John Wiley and Sons, LTD, 2006.

8. Baustian GH, Jones RC, Opal SM, et al. Pediculosis. Updated June 8, 2005. http://www.mdconsult.com/das/pdxmd/body/90172329-2/0?type=med&eid=9-u1.0-1_mt_1014574. Accessed April 4, 2007.

9. Rubeiz N, Kibbi AG. Pediculosis. Updated May 10, 2006. http//www.emedicine.com/emerg/TOPIC409.HTM. Accessed April 4, 2007.

10. Hipolito RB, Mallorca FG, Zuniga-Macaraig ZO, Apolinario PC, Wheeler-Sherman J. Head lice infestation: single drug versus combination therapy with one percent permethrin and trimethoprim/sulfamethoxazole. *Pediatrics*. 2001 Mar;107(3):E30.

137 SCABIES

Pierre Chanoine, MD
Richard P. Usatine, MD

PATIENT STORY

A 2-year-old boy is seen with severe itching and crusting of his hands (**Figures 137-1** and **137-2**). He also has a pruritic rash over the rest of his body. The child has had this problem since 2 months of age and has had a number of treatments for scabies. Other adults and children in the house have itching and rash. Various attempts at treatment have only included topical preparations. A scraping was done and scabies mites and scybala (feces) were seen (**Figures 137-3** and **137-4**). The child and all the family members were put on ivermectin simultaneously and the Norwegian scabies cleared from the child. The family cleared as well and the child was given a repeat dose of ivermectin to avoid relapse.

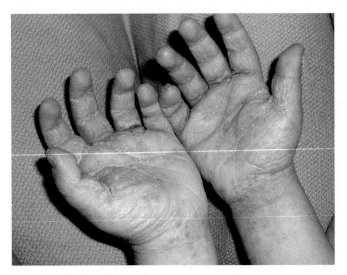

FIGURE 137-1 Crusted scabies (Norwegian scabies) in a 2-year-old boy. (*Courtesy of Richard P. Usatine, MD.*)

EPIDEMIOLOGY

- Three hundred million cases per year are estimated worldwide.[1] In some tropical countries, scabies is endemic.

- Scabies is more common in children, homeless persons, and individuals who are immunocompromised.

- Institutionalized individuals also have a higher incidence of the infestation.

ETIOLOGY AND PATHOPHYSIOLOGY

- Human scabies is caused by the mite *Sarcoptes scabei*, an obligate human parasite (**Figure 137-3**).[1,2]
  - Adult mites spend their entire life cycle, around 30 days, within the epidermis. After copulation the male mite dies and the female mite burrows through the superficial layers of the skin excreting feces (**Figure 137-4**) and laying eggs (**Figure 137-5**).
  - Mites move through the superficial layers of skin by secreting proteases that degrade the stratum corneum.
  - Infected individuals usually have less than 100 mites. In contrast, immunocompromised hosts can have up to 1 million mites, and are susceptible to crusted scabies also called Norwegian Scabies (**Figures 137-1, 137-2, 137-6** to **137-8**).[1]

- Transmission usually occurs via direct skin contact.

- Mites can also survive for 3 days outside of the human epidermis allowing for infrequent transmission through bedding and clothing.

- The incubation period is on average 3 to 4 weeks for an initial infestation. Sensitized individuals can have symptoms within hours of re-exposure.

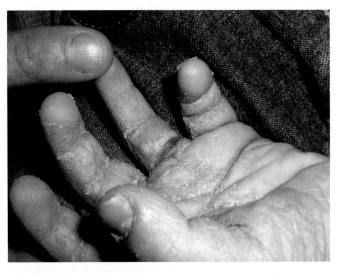

FIGURE 137-2 The boy in **Figure 137-1** with a close-up of his hand showing crusting and a fissure. (*Courtesy of Richard P. Usatine, MD.*)

DIAGNOSIS

CLINICAL FEATURES

- Pruritus is a hallmark of the disease.[1]
- Skin findings include papules (**Figures 137-9** to **137-14**), nodules (**Figures 137-10** and **137-11**), burrows (**Figure 137-9**), and rarely vesiculopustules (**Figure 137-14**).
- Infants and young children can also exhibit irritability and poor feeding.
- Pruritic papules/nodules around the axillae (**Figure 137-11**), umbilicus, or on the penis and scrotum (**Figure 137-12**) are highly suggestive of scabies.

TYPICAL DISTRIBUTION

- Classic distribution in scabies includes the interdigital spaces (**Figures 137-9** and **137-15**), wrists (**Figure 137-1**), ankles, waist (**Figure 137-10**), groin, axillae (**Figure 137-11**), palms, and soles (**Figures 137-1, 137-2, 137-6,** and **137-8**).
  - Genital involvement can also occur (**Figure 137-12**).
  - In children, the head can also be involved (**Figure 137-16**).

LABORATORY STUDIES AND IMAGING

- Mineral oil examination using light microscopy provides a definitive diagnosis with identification of mites, eggs, or feces (**Figures 137-3** to **137-5**). This can be challenging to do and may be time consuming to find mites, eggs, or feces even when these items are there. The inability to find these items should not be used to rule out scabies in a clinically suspicious case. In what is believed to be a recurrent case, it is helpful to find definitive evidence that your diagnosis is correct.
- Dermatoscopy can be used to look for the arrowhead sign. A small arrowhead looking mite at the end of a burrow.[3]
- Videodermatoscopy can also be used to diagnose scabies.[4] Videodermatoscopy allows for skin magnification with incidental lighting at magnifications of 100 to 600 times affording better visualization of mites and eggs. The technique is noninvasive and does not cause pain.

BIOPSY

Rarely necessary unless you have reasons to suspect another diagnosis.

DIFFERENTIAL DIAGNOSIS

- Atopic dermatitis—Itching is a prominent symptom in AD and scabies. The distribution of involved skin can help to differentiate the two diagnoses. Look for burrows in scabies and a history of involved family members. In children, atopic dermatitis is often confined to the flexural and extensor surfaces of the body. In adults, the hands are a primary site of involvement (see Chapter 139, Atopic Dermatitis).
- Contact dermatitis—Characterized by vesicles and papules on bright red skin, which are rare in scabies. Chronic contact dermatitis often leads to scaling and lichenification and may not be as pruritic as scabies (see Chapter 140, Contact Dermatitis).

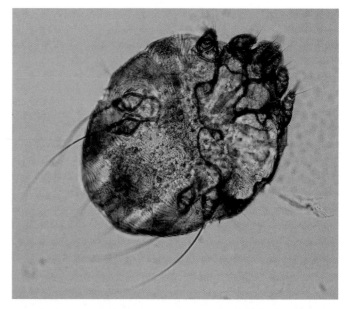

FIGURE 137-3 Microscopic view of the scabies mite from a patient with crusted scabies. (*Courtesy of Richard P. Usatine, MD.*)

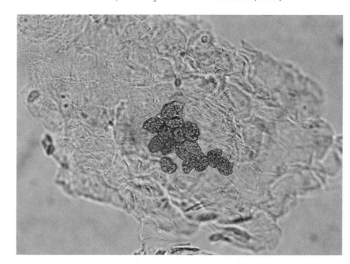

FIGURE 137-4 Scraping of the patient's hand produced a good view of the scybala (the mites' feces). (*Courtesy of Richard P. Usatine, MD.*)

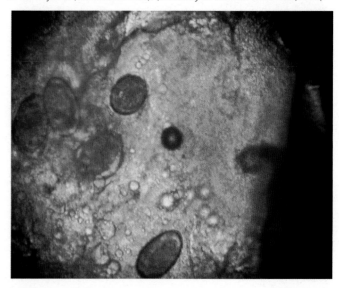

FIGURE 137-5 Scabies eggs from a scraping. (*Courtesy of Eric Kraus, MD.*)

- Seborrheic dermatitis—A papulosquamous eruption with scales and crusts which is limited to the sebum rich areas of the body; namely, the scalp, the face the postauricular areas, and the intertriginous areas. Pruritus is usually mild or absent (see Chapter 144, Seborrheic Dermatitis).

- Non-bullous impetigo—Honey-crusted plaques are a hallmark of non-bullous impetigo. Scabies can become secondarily infected so consider that both diagnoses can occur concomitantly (see Chapter 110, Impetigo).

- Arthropod bites—Bites may exhibit puncta that allow for differentiation from scabies.

- Acropustulosis of infancy (**Figure 137-17**)—A vesico-pustular recurrent eruption limited to the hands, wrists, feet, and ankles. It is rare after 2 years of age (see Chapter 104, Pustular Diseases of Childhood).

MANAGEMENT

Treatment includes administration of an antiscabicide and an antipruritic.[1,5]

- Permethrin 5% cream (Elimite, Acticin) is the most effective treatment based upon a systematic review in the Cochrane Database.[5] SOR Ⓐ The cream is applied from the neck down (include the head when it is involved) and rinsed off 8 to 14 hours later. Usually, this is done overnight. Repeating the treatment in 1 to 2 weeks may be more effective. SOR Ⓒ Unfortunately, scabies resistance to permethrin is increasing.

- Ivermectin is an oral treatment for resistant or crusted scabies. Studies have demonstrated its safety and efficacy. Most studies used a single dose of ivermectin at 200 mcg/kg.[5] SOR Ⓐ Some experts advocate repeating a dose 1 week later. It is worth noting that the FDA has not labeled this drug for use in children weighing <15 kg.

- Diphenhydramine, hydroxyzine, and mid-potency steroid creams can be used for symptomatic relief of itching. SOR Ⓒ. It is important to note that pruritus may persist for 1 to 2 weeks after successful treatment because the dead scabies mites and eggs still have antigenic qualities that may cause persistent inflammation.

- Environmental decontamination is a standard component of all therapies. SOR Ⓒ
  - Clothing, bed linens, and towels should be machine washed in hot water.
  - Clothing or other items (e.g., stuffed animals) that cannot be washed may be dry cleaned or stored in bags for 1 week.

- All household or family members living in the infested home should be treated. SOR Ⓒ Failure to treat all involved individuals often results in recurrences within the family.

- Other less effective medications include topical benzyl benzoate, crotamiton, lindane, and synergized natural pyrethrins.[5] SOR Ⓐ

- Antibiotics are needed if there is evidence of a bacterial superinfection. SOR Ⓒ

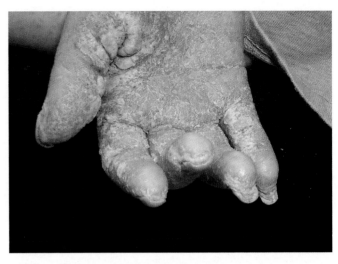

FIGURE 137-6 Norwegian scabies with crusting on the hand. (*Courtesy of Jack Resneck, Sr., MD.*)

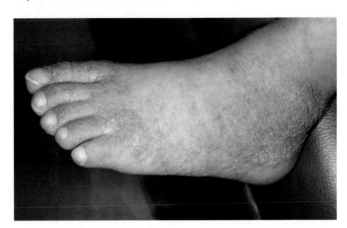

FIGURE 137-7 Crusted scabies on the foot of a 5-year-old boy with Down's syndrome. (*Courtesy of Richard P. Usatine, MD.*)

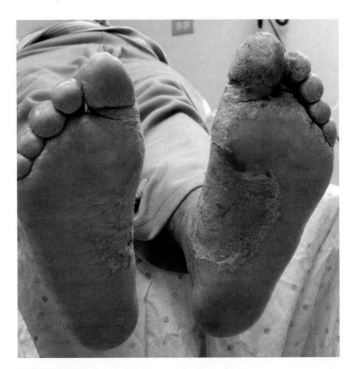

FIGURE 137-8 Crusted scabies on the feet of an immunosuppressed transplant patient in the hospital. (*Courtesy of Deborah Henderson, MD.*)

PATIENT EDUCATION

- Patients should avoid direct contact including sleeping with others until they have completed the first application of the medicine.
- Patients may return to school and work 24 hours after first treatment.
- Patients should be warned that itching may persist for 1 to 2 weeks after successful treatment but that if symptoms are still present by the third week, the patient should return for further evaluation.

FOLLOW-UP

- Routine follow-up is indicated when symptoms do not resolve.
- Consider an immunologic work-up for individuals with crusted scabies.

PATIENT RESOURCES

http://www.cdc.gov/ncidod/dpd/parasites/scabies/factsht_scabies.htm.

PROVIDER RESOURCES

http://www.emedicine.com/ped/topic2047.htm.

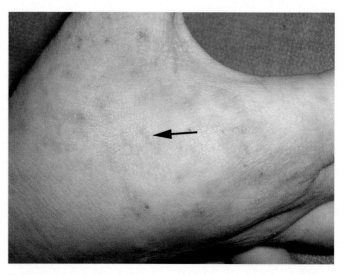

FIGURE 137-9 Scabies infestation on the hand of an incarcerated woman. Arrow points to one burrow. (*Courtesy of Richard P. Usatine, MD.*)

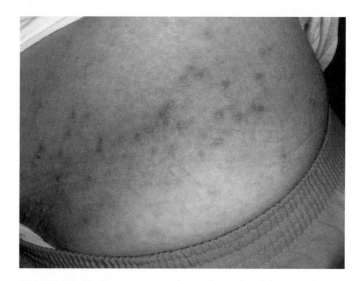

FIGURE 137-10 Same women with papules and nodules around waist. (*Courtesy of Richard P. Usatine, MD.*)

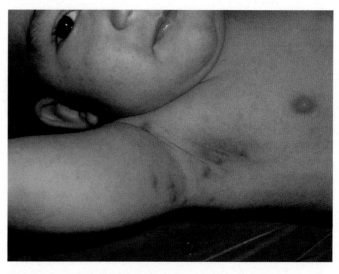

FIGURE 137-11 Scabetic nodules in the axilla of a toddler with scabies. (*Courtesy of Richard P. Usatine, MD.*)

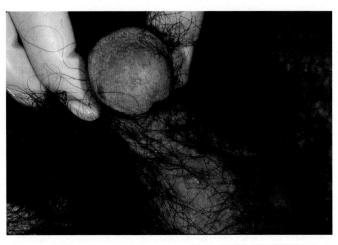

FIGURE 137-12 Pruritic papules on the glans of the penis and scrotum secondary to sexually transmitted scabies in a gay man. (*Courtesy of Richard P. Usatine, MD.*)

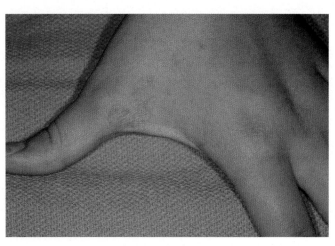

FIGURE 137-15 Mother of the child in the previous figure with scabies. Note that she has small papules in the first interdigital space. (*Courtesy of Richard P. Usatine, MD.*)

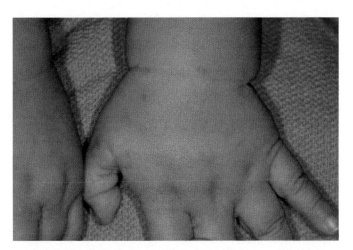

FIGURE 137-13 Scabies on the hand and wrist of a 9-month-old child. (*Courtesy of Richard P. Usatine, MD.*)

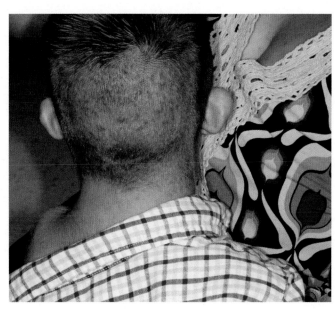

FIGURE 137-16 Scabies on the head of a 5-year-old boy with Down's syndrome. The papules of scabies can be seen on the chest of his mother. (*Courtesy of Richard P. Usatine, MD.*)

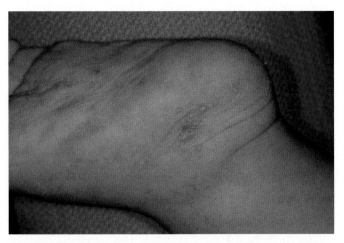

FIGURE 137-14 Scabies on the foot of the same child (**Figure** 137-13) showing pustules. While this also looks like acropustulosis, the mother also had scabies. (*Courtesy of Richard P. Usatine, MD.*)

REFERENCES

1. Hengge UR, Currie B, Jäger G, et al. Scabies: A ubiquitous neglected skin disease. *Lancet Infect Dis*. 2006;6(12):769–779.

2. Paller AS, Mancini AJ. Scabies. In: Paller AS, Mancini AJ eds. *Hurwitz Clinical Pediatric Dermatology: A Textbook of Skin Disorders of Childhood and Adolescence*. Philadelphia, PA: WB Saunders, 2006: 479–488.

3. Fox GN, Usatine RP. Itching and rash in a boy and his grandmother. *J Fam Pract*. 2006;55(8):679–684.

4. Lacarruba F, Letizia M, Caltabiano R, et al. High-Magnification Videodermatoscopy: A new noninvasive diagnostic tool for scabies in children. *Pediatr Dermatol*. 2001;18(5):439–441.

5. Strong M, Johnstone PW. Interventions for treating scabies. *Cochrane Database of Syst Rev*. 2007;3:CD000320.

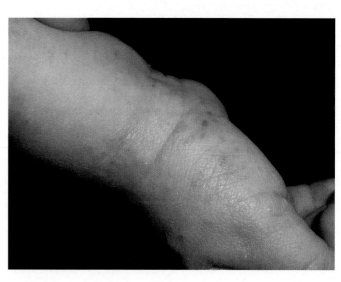

FIGURE 137-17 Infantile acropustulosis in a 9-month-old child that was mistakenly treated for scabies. No one else in the household had lesions and the scabies treatment did not lead to resolution of the pustules and vesicles. (*Courtesy of Richard P. Usatine, MD.*)

138 CUTANEOUS LARVA MIGRANS

Jennifer A. Keehbauch, MD

PATIENT STORY

A mother brought her 18-month-old son to the physician's office for an itchy rash on his feet and buttocks (**Figures 138-1** and **138-2**).[1] The first physician examined the child and made the incorrect diagnosis of tinea corporis. The topical clotrimazole cream failed. The child was unable to sleep because of the intense itching and was losing weight secondary to his poor appetite. He was taken to an urgent care clinic where the physician learned that the family had returned from a trip to the Caribbean prior to the visit to the first physician. The child had played on beaches that were frequented by local dogs. The physician recognized the serpiginous pattern of cutaneous larva migrans (CLM) and successfully treated the child with topical thiabendazole.

EPIDEMIOLOGY

- Most common skin disease of travelers from tropical countries.[2]

- The exact incidence is unknown in the United States because it is not a reportable condition. A survey by the CDC found that 35% to 52% of dogs in shelters harbor helminths capable of producing disease in humans. CLM is the second most common helminthic infection.[3]

- In the United States, it is found predominantly in Florida and the Gulf Coast.[4]

- Children are more frequently affected than adults.

ETIOLOGY AND PATHOPHYSIOLOGY

- Caused most commonly by dog and cat hookworms (i.e., ancylostoma braziliense, ancylostoma caninum).[5]

- Eggs are passed in cat or dog feces.

- Larvae are hatched in moist, warm, sand/soil.

- Infective stage larvae penetrate the skin.

DIAGNOSIS

The diagnosis is based on history and clinical findings.

CLINICAL FEATURES

- Elevated, serpiginous, or linear reddish brown tracks 1 to 5 cm long (**Figures 138-1** to **138-3**).[2,5]

- Intense pruritus.

- Symptoms last for weeks to months.

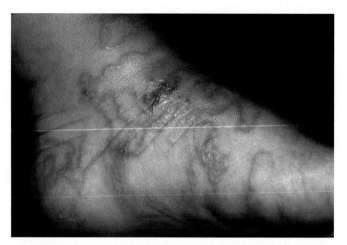

FIGURE 138-1 The serpiginous rash of cutaneous larva migrans on the foot of an 18-month-old boy after a family trip to the beaches of the Caribbean. (*Courtesy of Richard P. Usatine, MD. Usatine RP. A rash on the feet and buttocks. West J Med. 1999;170(6):344–335.*)

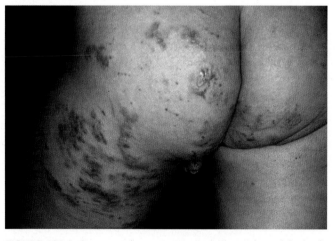

FIGURE 138-2 Cutaneous larva migrans on the buttocks and thigh of the same boy showing significant excoriations. (*Courtesy of Richard P. Usatine, MD. Usatine RP. A rash on the feet and buttocks. West J Med. 1999;170(6):344–335.*)

TYPICAL DISTRIBUTION

- Feet and lower extremities (73%), buttocks (13% to 18%), and abdomen (16%).[4,6]

LABORATORY AND IMAGING

- Not indicated, but rarely blood tests shows—eosinophilia or elevated immunoglobulin E levels.[5]

DIFFERENTIAL DIAGNOSIS

May be confused with the following conditions:

- Cutaneous fungal infections—lesions are typically scaling plaques and annular macules with central clearing. If the serpiginous track of CLM is circular, this can lead to the incorrect diagnosis of "ringworm." The irony is that ringworm is a dermatophyte fungus while CLM really is a worm (see Chapter 132, Tinea Corporis).

- Contact dermatitis—differentiate by distribution of lesions, presence of vesicles, and absence of classical serpiginous tracks (see Chapter 140, Contact Dermatitis).

- Erythema migrans of Lyme disease—lesions are usually annular macules or patches and are not raised and serpiginous (see Chapter 211, Lyme Disease).

- Phytophotodermatitis—the acute phase of phytophotodermatitis is erythematous with vesicles; this later develops into postinflammatory hyperpigmented lesions. This may be acquired while preparing drinks with lime on the beach and not from the sandy beach infested with larvae (see Chapter 192, Photosensitivity).

MANAGEMENT

- Oral thiabendazole is the only FDA approved medication for CLM. It can also be compounded to form a topical cream (15%) from 500 mg tablets in a water-soluble base. The original trials that proved effectiveness for the oral and topical forms were small and performed in the 1960s.[2] The cream is a good choice for children who cannot swallow the tablets.
  - The recommended dose for the oral form is 25 mg/kg every 12 hours for 2 to 5 days (not to exceed 3g/d). SOR B The cream is applied topically bid to tid for 5 days to the larval track and 2 to 3 cm above the lesions.[2] SOR B
  - Cure rates of 75% to 89% with the oral form and 96% to 98% with topical treatment.[2]
  - Less well tolerated as an oral treatment; adverse reactions include nausea (49%), vomiting (16%), and headache (7%). There are no reported side effects for the topical preparation.[2]
- Ivermectin (Stromectol) lacks FDA indication, but has been well studied.
  - A single dose of 0.2 mg/kg (12–24 mg) is recommended.[7] SOR B
  - Cure rates of 100% with a single dose.[2]
  - No adverse events were reported in a series of 6 studies.[2]
  - Considered the drug of choice by many.
- Albendazole has been successfully prescribed for more than 25 years, but also lacks FDA indication.[2]
  - The recommended dose is 400 to 800 mg/d for 3 to 5 days.[2] SOR B

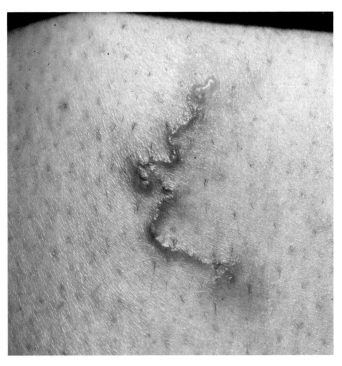

FIGURE 138-3 Close-up of a serpiginous burrow from cutaneous larva migrans on the leg. The actual larva is 2–3 cm beyond the visible tracks. (*Courtesy of John Gonzalez, MD.*)

○ Cure rates exceed 92%.[2]

○ Up to 27% will experience gastrointestinal side effects when the 800 mg dose is used for more than 3 days.[2]

• Cryotherapy is ineffective and harmful and should be avoided.[2] SOR Ⓑ

• Antihistamines may relieve itching.

• Antibiotics may be used if secondary infection occurs.

PATIENT EDUCATION

• Wear shoes on beaches where animals are allowed.

• Keep covers on sand boxes.

• For pet owners: Keep pets off the beaches, deworm pets, and dispose of feces properly.

FOLLOW-UP

• Follow-up if lesions persist.

PATIENT AND PROVIDER RESOURCES

eMedicine article on CLM—**http://www.emedicine.com/ derm/topic91.htm**

REFERENCES

1. Usatine RP. A rash on the feet and buttocks. *West J Med*. 1999;170 (6):334–335.

2. Caumes E. Treatment of cutaneous larva migrans. *Clin Infect Dis*. 2000;30:811–814.

3. Center for Disease Control. http://www.cdc.gov/ncidod/dpd/ parasites/ascaris/prevention.pdf. Accessed June 5, 2007.

4. Hotez P, Brooker S, Bethony J, et al. Hookworm Infection. *N Engl J Med*. 2004;351(8):799–807.

5. Le E, Hsu S. A serpiginous eruption on the buttocks. *Am Fam Physician*. 2000;62(11):2493–2494.

6. Jelinek T, Maiwald H, Nothdurft H, Loscher T. Cutaneous larva migrans in travelers: Synopsis of histories, symptoms and treating 98 patients. *Clin Infect Dis*. 1994;19:1062–1066.

7. Caumes E, Carriere J, Datry A, et al. A randomized trial of ivermectin versus albendazole for the treatment of cutaneous larva migrans. *J Trop Med Hyg*. 1993;49(5):641–644.

139 ATOPIC DERMATITIS

Richard P. Usatine, MD

PATIENT STORY

A 1-year-old Asian American girl is brought to her family physician for a new rash on her face and legs (**Figures 139-1** and **139-2**). The child is scratching both areas but is otherwise healthy. There is a family history of asthma, allergic rhinitis, and atopic dermatitis (AD) on the father's side. The child responded well to low-dose topical corticosteroids and emollients.

EPIDEMIOLOGY

- AD is the most frequent inflammatory skin disorder in the United States and the most common skin condition in children.[1]
- Prevalence is 7% to 15% in the United States and Europe.[1]
- 60% of cases begin during the first year of life and 90% by 5 years of age.[1]
- 60% of adults with AD have children with AD (**Figure 139-3**).[1]

ETIOLOGY AND PATHOPHYSIOLOGY

- Common inflammatory skin disorder that is characterized by itching and inflamed skin that is be triggered by the interplay of genetic, immunologic, and environmental factors.
- Vicious cycle of dermatitis associated with elevated T-lymphocyte activation, hyperstimulatory Langerhans' cells, defective cell mediated immunity, and B-cell IgE overproduction.
- Exotoxins of Staphylococcal aureus act as superantigens and stimulate activation of T-cells and macrophages.
- Patients may have a primary T-cell defect. This may be why they can get more severe skin infections caused by herpes simplex virus (eczema herpeticum as seen in **Figure 139-4**) or bacteria (widespread impetigo). They are also at risk of a bad reaction to the smallpox vaccine with dissemination of the attenuated virus beyond the vaccination site. Eczema vaccinatum is a potentially deadly complication of smallpox vaccination (**Figure 139-5**).

DIAGNOSIS

- History: If it does not itch it is not AD. It is the itch that rashes. Persons with AD often have other allergic conditions such as asthma and allergic rhinitis. These allergic conditions often run in their families.

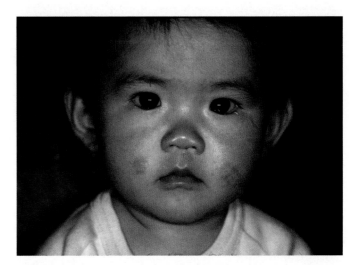

FIGURE 139-1 AD on the cheeks of an infant. (*With permission from Milgrom EC, Usatine RP, Tan RA, Spector SL. Practical Allergy. 2004, Elsevier, Inc. Philadelphia.*)

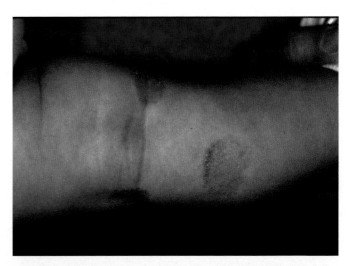

FIGURE 139-2 AD on the leg of the infant in **Figure 139-1**. The coinlike pattern is that of nummular eczema. (*With permission from Milgrom EC, Usatine RP, Tan RA, Spector SL. Practical Allergy. 2004, Elsevier, Inc. Philadelphia.*)

- The atopic triad is AD, allergic rhinitis, and asthma. Atopic persons have an exaggerated inflammatory response to factors that irritate the skin.

- Physical examination: Primary lesions include: vesicles, scale, papules and plaques.

- Secondary (or sequential) lesions include: lichenification that is thickened skin with accentuation of skin lines, crusts when a secondary infection has occurred, nodules in prurigo nodularis, excoriations from scratching, follicular hyperaccentuation (more prominent hyperkeratotic follicles) (**Figure 139-6**), fissures, and postinflammatory hyperpigmentation.

TYPICAL DISTRIBUTION

- AD often starts on the face in infancy and childhood (**Figures 139-1** and **139-7**).

- Flexural folds—especially the antecubital and popliteal fossa (**Figures 139-8** to **139-10**).

- Children will often have AD in the antecubital and popliteal fossa. Involvement of the neck, wrists, and ankles also may occur (**Figures 139-11** and **139-12**).

- AD in adults can occur on the hands, around the mouth, or eyelids as well as all the other areas (**Figures 139-13** and **139-14**).

- In one series, the prevalence of hand involvement in patients with active AD was 58.9%. There was a significant trend toward an increasing prevalence of hand involvement with increasing age.[2]

OTHER FEATURES OR CONDITIONS ASSOCIATED WITH AD ARE

- Keratosis pilaris (**Figure 139-15**).

- Ichthyosis (**Figure 139-16**).

- Pityriasis alba (**Figures 139-17** and **139-18**).

- Palmar or plantar hyperlinearity.

- Dennie-Morgan lines (infraorbital fold) (**Figure 139-14**).

- Hand or foot dermatitis (see Chapter 141, Hand Eczema).

- Cheilitis (see Chapter 31, Angular Cheilitis).

- Susceptibility to cutaneous infections (**Figures 139-4** and **139-5**).

- Xerosis (dry skin) (**Figure 139-19**).

LABORATORY STUDIES

Labs are rarely needed if the history and physical examination support the diagnosis. Occasionally a KOH preparation may be needed to rule out tinea or a skin scraping to rule out scabies. Of course, both of these conditions can occur on top of AD.

DIFFERENTIAL DIAGNOSIS

- Dyshidrotic eczema—Dry inflamed scaling skin on the hands and feet with tapioca like vesicles especially seen between the fingers (see Chapter 141, Hand Eczema).

- Seborrheic dermatitis—Greasy, scaly lesions on scalp, face, and chest (see Chapter 144, Seborrheic Dermatitis).

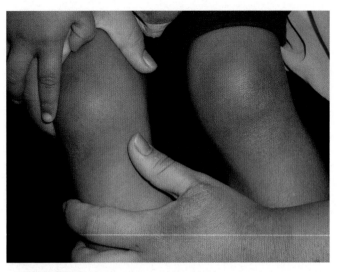

FIGURE 139-3 The child and his mother both have AD but not in the most typical distribution. (*Courtesy of Richard P. Usatine, MD.*)

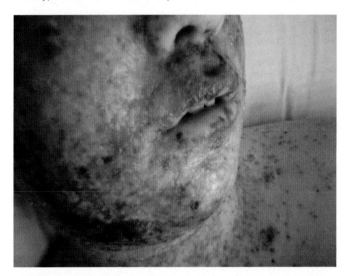

FIGURE 139-4 An 18-year-old woman with AD superinfected by herpes (eczema herpeticum). (*Reproduced with permission from Photo Rounds: Severe rash after dermatitis. The Journal of Family Practice, August 2004;53(8):613, Dowden Health Media.*)

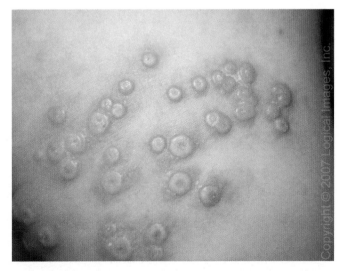

FIGURE 139-5 Eczema vaccinatum in a person with AD that was given the smallpox vaccine. (*With permission from Logical Images, Inc.*)

- Psoriasis—thickened plaques on extensor surfaces, scalp, and buttocks; pitted nails (see Chapter 145, Psoriasis).

- Lichen simplex chronicus (sometimes called neurodermatitis)—Usually, a single patch in an area accessible to scratching such as the ankle, wrist, and neck (see Chapter 142, Self-Inflicted Dermatoses).

- Contact dermatitis—Positive exposure history, rash in area of exposure; absence of family history (see Chapter 140, Contact Dermatitis).

- Scabies—Papules, burrows, finger web involvement, positive skin scraping (see Chapter 137, Scabies).

- Dermatophyte infection—on the hands or feet can look just like hand or foot dermatitis, a positive KOH preparation for hyphae can help make the diagnosis (see Chapter 134, Tinea Pedis).

MANAGEMENT

- Topical steroids and emollients are beneficial.[1] SOR **A**

- There is some evidence suggesting that controlling house dust mites reduces severity of symptoms in patients with the atopic triad. Bedding covers were found to be the most effective method to control dust mites and AD symptoms in this subgroup of AD patients. Unfortunately, dust mite interventions are not proven to be effective for patients with AD that do not have the full atopic triad.[1] SOR **B**

- Dietary restriction is useful only for infants with proven egg allergies. SOR **B** Egg-free diet was associated with an improvement in severity of AD in infants with a positive radioallergosorbent (RAST) test to eggs.[1]

- There is insufficient evidence that dietary manipulation in adults or children reduces symptom severity.

- Topical steroids have been proven to work for AD and are the mainstay of treatment.[1] SOR **A**
  - The ointments are best for dry and cracked skin.
  - Creams are easier to apply and are better tolerated by some patients.
  - Use weaker steroids for the face and the groin.
  - Use weaker steroids for babies and small children to avoid systemic absorption.
  - Use stronger steroids for thicker skin such as on the hands and feet.
  - Use stronger steroids for more severe outbreaks or lesions that have not responded to weaker steroids.
  - To avoid adverse effects, the highest potency steroids (clobetasol) should not be used for longer than 2 weeks continuously. However, they can be used intermittently for recurring AD in a pulse-therapy mode (e.g., apply every weekend, with no application on weekdays).

- For extensive flares consider oral prednisone or an intramuscular (IM) shot of triamcinolone (40 mg in 1 cc).[1] SOR **C**

- Topical and systemic antibiotics are used for AD that has become secondarily infected with bacteria. The most common infecting organism is *staphylococcus aureus*. Weeping fluid and crusting during an exacerbation should prompt consideration of antibiotic use[1] (**Figures 139-7** and **139-8**). SOR **A**

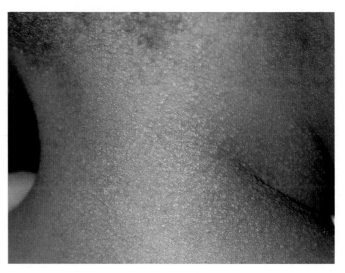

FIGURE 139-6 A young black girl with AD showing follicular hyper-accentuation on the neck. (*With permission from Milgrom EC, Usatine RP, Tan RA, Spector SL. Practical Allergy. 2004, Elsevier, Inc. Philadelphia.*)

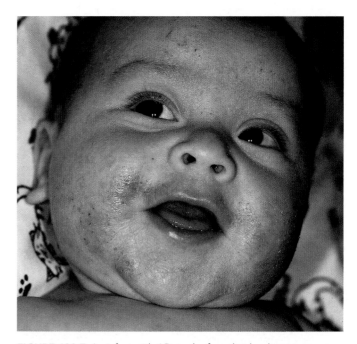

FIGURE 139-7 An infant with AD on the face that has become super-infected. (*With permission from Milgrom EC, Usatine RP, Tan RA, Spector SL. Practical Allergy. 2004, Elsevier, Inc. Philadelphia.*)

- The value of antihistamines in AD is controversial. If antihistamines are to be used, the sedating agents are most effective and can be given at night.[1] SOR **B**

- Short-term adjunctive use of topical doxepin may aid in the reduction of pruritus.[1] SOR **A**

- Topical calcineurin inhibitors (immunomodulators, such as pimecrolimus and tacrolimus) reduce the rash severity and symptoms in children and adults.[1] SOR **A** These work by suppressing antigen-specific T-cell activation and inhibiting inflammatory cytokine release. These are steroid-sparing medications that are helpful for eyelid eczema and in other areas when steroids may thin the skin (**Figure 139-20**). These agents are now only approved for persons more than 2 years of age and the FDA states that they should not be as first-line agents because of a possible risk of causing cancer. The American Academy of Dermatology (AAD) has released a statement that the "data does not prove that the proper topical use of pimecrolimus and tacrolimus is dangerous."

- Cyclosporine for severe refractory AD can be used in long-term maintenance therapy to treat and avoid remissions.[1] SOR **A**

- UV phototherapy may also be used in severe refractory AD with some success.[1] SOR **A**

PATIENT EDUCATION

Patients need to know that scratching their AD makes is worse and they should apply emollients or steroids when their skin is dry and/or pruritic. Regular use of the appropriate medications can control AD but can not cure it.

FOLLOW-UP

Regular follow-up should be given to patients with chronic and difficult to control AD. Establishing a good regimen is crucial to good control and then visits may be adjusted to longer intervals between visits.

PATIENT RESOURCES

American Academy of Family Physicians—**www.familydoctor. org/handouts/176.html.**

American Academy of Dermatology—**www.skincarephysicians. com/eczemanet/.**

The National Eczema Association—**www.nationaleczema.org/.**

PROVIDER RESOURCES

Hanifin JM, Cooper KD, Ho VC, et al. Guidelines of care for atopic dermatitis. *J Am Acad Dermatol.* 2004;50:391–404.

Disease management of atopic dermatitis: an updated practice parameter. Joint Task Force on Practice Parameters. *Ann Allergy Asthma Immunol.* 2004 Sep;93(3 Suppl 2):S1–21.

http://www.guidelines.gov/summary/summary. aspx?doc_id=6872.

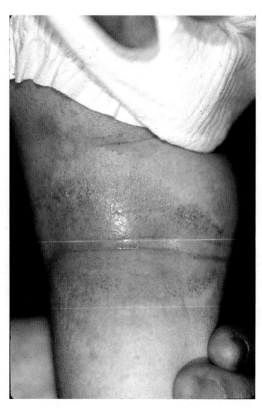

FIGURE 139-8 The same infant with superinfected AD of the popliteal fossa. (*With permission from Milgrom EC, Usatine RP, Tan RA, Spector SL. Practical Allergy. 2004, Elsevier, Inc. Philadelphia.*)

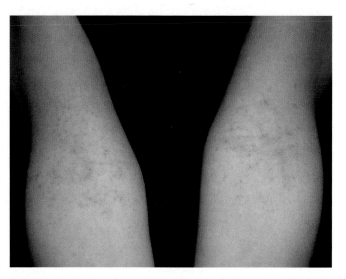

FIGURE 139-9 AD in the antecubital fossae of a 7-year-old girl. Note the prominent red papules with some excoriations. (*Courtesy of Richard P. Usatine, MD.*)

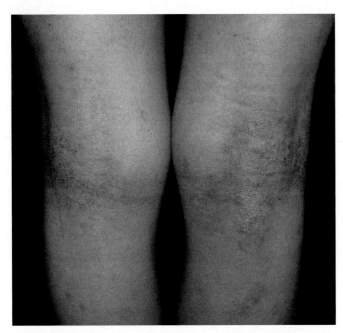

FIGURE 139-10 A 20-year-old young woman with severe chronic AD showing lichenification and hyperpigmentation in the popliteal fossa. (*Courtesy of Richard P. Usatine, MD.*)

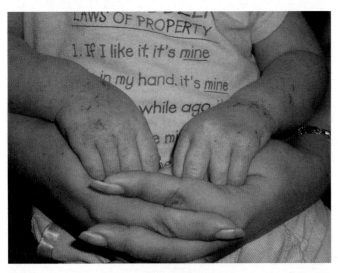

FIGURE 139-11 A 2-year-old girl with AD visible on her hands, wrists, and arms. (*Courtesy of Richard P. Usatine, MD.*)

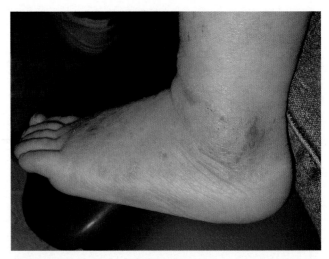

FIGURE 139-12 The girl in **Figure 139-11** with an exacerbation of her AD on the ankle showing many excoriations. (*Courtesy of Richard P. Usatine, MD.*)

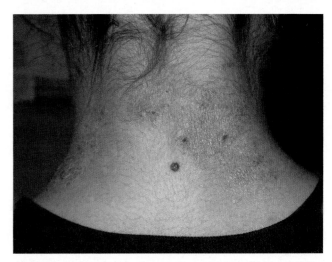

FIGURE 139-13 A young nurse with AD made worse by wearing the stethoscope around her neck. (*With permission from Milgrom EC, Usatine RP, Tan RA, Spector SL. Practical Allergy. 2004, Elsevier, Inc. Philadelphia.*)

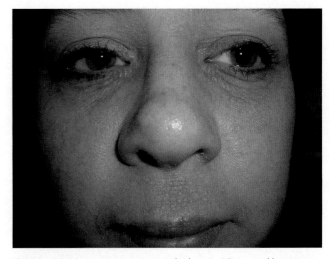

FIGURE 139-14 A young woman with chronic AD around her eyes and mouth. In addition to the eyelid involvement the patient has Denny Morgan lines visible on the lower eyelids. (*Courtesy of Richard P. Usatine, MD.*)

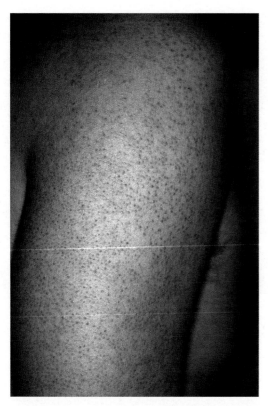

FIGURE 139-15 Keratosis pilaris on the lateral upper arm. (*With permission from Milgrom EC, Usatine RP, Tan RA, Spector SL. Practical Allergy. 2004, Elsevier, Inc. Philadelphia.*)

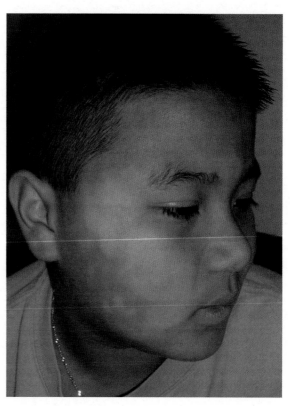

FIGURE 139-17 Pityriasis alba on the face of a young boy. (*Courtesy of Richard P. Usatine, MD.*)

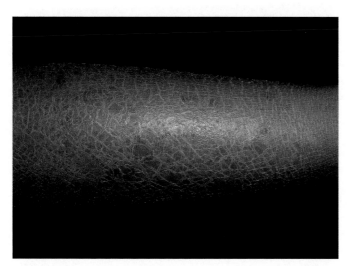

FIGURE 139-16 Acquired ichthyosis on the leg of a 9-year-old boy with AD. Note the fishscale appearance along with the dry skin. (*Courtesy of Richard P. Usatine, MD.*)

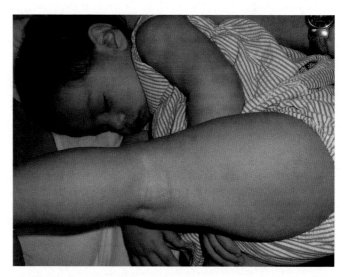

FIGURE 139-18 An 18-month-old girl with AD visible in her popliteal fossa and pityriasis alba on her arm. (*Courtesy of Richard P. Usatine, MD.*)

REFERENCES

1. Hanifin JM, Cooper KD, Ho VC, et al. Guidelines of care for atopic dermatitis. *J Am Acad Dermatol.* 2004;50:391–404.

2. Simpson EL. Prevalence and morphology of hand eczema in patients with atopic dermatitis. *Dermatitis.* 2006;17:123–127.

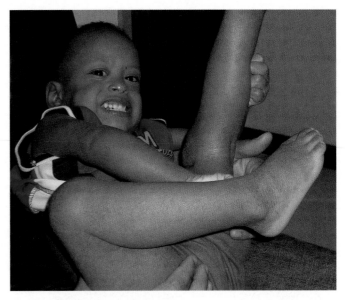

FIGURE 139-19 Severe AD in a 2-year-old black boy with very dry (xerotic) skin. He is spontaneously scratching and crying out in discomfort. (*Courtesy of Richard P. Usatine, MD.*)

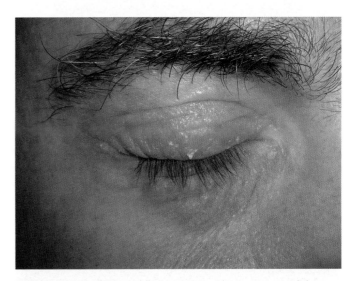

FIGURE 139-20 AD in middle-aged man with prominent eyelid involvement. The patient responded well to topical pimecrolimus and a low-potency topical steroid ointment. (*Courtesy of Richard P. Usatine, MD.*)

140 CONTACT DERMATITIS

Richard P. Usatine, MD

PATIENT STORY

A 38-year-old woman twisted her right ankle and applied a Chinese medicine patch to relieve the pain. The following day the patient developed a severe contact dermatitis (CD) with many small vesicles (<5 mm) and bullae (>5 mm) (**Figure 140-1**). The erythema was well-demarcated border and has been traced by the doctor's pen. Cold compresses and a highly potency topical steroid were prescribed. When the patient showed little improvement a 2-week course of oral prednisone was given starting with 60 mg daily and tapering down to 5 mg daily. The patient responded rapidly and the CD fully resolved.[1,2]

EPIDEMIOLOGY

- Some of the most common types of CD are secondary to exposures to poison ivy, nickel, and fragrances.[3]

- Patch testing data, indicate that the five most prevalent contact allergens out of more than 3700 known contact allergens are nickel (14.3% of patients' tested), fragrance mix (14%), neomycin (11.6%), balsam of Peru (10.4%), and thimerosal (10.4%).[4]

- Occupational skin diseases (chiefly CD) rank second only to traumatic injuries as the most common type of occupational disease. Chemical irritants such as solvents and cutting fluids account for most irritant contact dermatitis (ICD) cases. Sixty percent were allergic contact dermatitis (ACD) and 32% were ICD. Hands were primarily affected in 64% of ACD and 80% of ICD[3] (**Figure 140-2**).

ETIOLOGY AND PATHOPHYSIOLOGY

- CD is a common inflammatory skin condition characterized by erythematous and pruritic skin lesions resulting from the contact of skin with a foreign substance.

- ICD is caused by the nonimmune modulated irritation of the skin by a substance, resulting in a skin rash.

- ACD is a delayed-type hypersensitivity reaction in which a foreign substance comes into contact with the skin, and is linked to skin protein forming an antigen complex that leads to sensitization. Upon reexposure of the epidermis to the antigen, the sensitized T-cells initiate an inflammatory cascade, leading to the skin changes seen in ACD.

DIAGNOSIS

HISTORY

Ask about contact with known allergens (i.e., nickel, fragrances, neomycin, and poison ivy/oak).

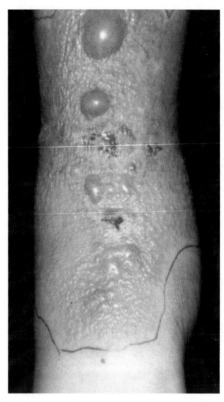

FIGURE 140-1 Severe acute ACD on the ankle of a woman after application of a Chinese topical medicine for a sprained ankle. (*With permission from Milgrom EC, Usatine RP, Tan RA, Spector SL. Practical Allergy. 2004, Elsevier, Inc. Philadelphia.*)

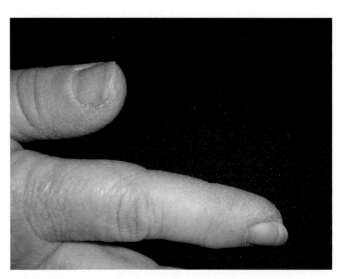

FIGURE 140-2 Occupational ICD in a woman whose hands are exposed to chemicals while making cowboy hats in Texas. (*With permission from Milgrom EC, Usatine RP, Tan RA, Spector SL. Practical Allergy. 2004, Elsevier, Inc. Philadelphia.*)

- Nickel exposure is often related to the wearing of rings, jewelry, and metal belt buckles (**Figures 140-3** to **140-6**).
- Fragrances in the forms of deodorants and perfumes (**Figure 140-7**).
- Neomycin applied as a triple antibiotic ointment by patients (**Figures 140-8** and **140-9**).
- Poison ivy/oak in outdoor settings. Especially ask when the distribution of the reaction is linear (**Figures 140-10** and **140-11**).
- Ask about occupational exposures especially solvents. For example, chemicals used in hat making can cause ICD on the hands (**Figure 140-2**).
- Tapes applied to skin after cuts or surgery are frequent causes of CD (**Figure 140-12**).
- If the CD is on the feet, ask about new shoes (**Figures 140-13** and **140-14**).

CLINICAL FEATURES

All types of CD have erythema. While it is not always possible to distinguish between ICD and ACD, here are some features that might help:

A. ICD:
- Location—usually the hands.
- Symptoms—burning, pruritus, pain.
- Dry and fissured skin (**Figure 140-2**).
- Indistinct borders.

B. ACD:
- Location—usually exposed area of skin, often the hands.
- Pruritus is the dominant symptom.
- Vesicles and bulla (**Figures 140-1** and **140-8**).
- Distinct angles, lines, and borders (**Figures 140-8** to **140-12**).

Both ICD and ACD may be complicated by bacterial superinfection showing signs of exudate, weeping, and crusts.

Toxicodendron (Rhus) dermatitis (poison ivy, poison oak, and poison sumac) is caused by urushiol, which is found in the saps of this plant family. Clinically, a line of vesicles can occur from brushing against one of the plants. Also, the linear pattern occurs from scratching oneself and dragging the oleoresin across the skin with the fingernails (**Figures 140-10** and **140-11**).

LABORATORY STUDIES

The diagnosis is most often made by history and physical examination. Consider culture if there are signs of superinfection and there is a concern for methicillin-resistant *Staphylococcus aureus* (MRSA). The following tests may be considered when the diagnosis is not clear.

- KOH preparation and/or fungal culture if tinea is suspected.
- Microscopy for scabies mites and eggs.
- Latex allergy testing—This type of reaction is neither ICD (nonimmunologic) nor ACD. The latex allergy type of reaction is a type I, or IgE-mediated response to the latex allergen.
- Patch testing—common antigens are placed on the skin of a patient. There are prefabricated kits for this testing that make this test an option for the family physician. The recent meta-analysis of

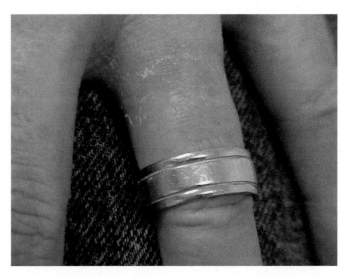

FIGURE 140-3 Patient moved up his ring to show the ACD secondary to a nickel allergy to the ring. (*With permission from Milgrom EC, Usatine RP, Tan RA, Spector SL. Practical Allergy. 2004, Elsevier, Inc. Philadelphia.*)

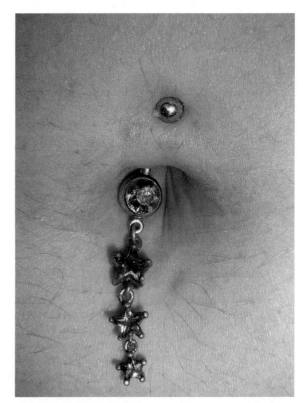

FIGURE 140-4 ACD to the metal in the belly-button ring of a young woman. (*Courtesy of Richard P. Usatine, MD.*)

the T.R.U.E. Test shows that nickel (14.7% of tested patients), thimerosal (5.0%), cobalt (4.8%), fragrance mix (3.4%), and balsam of Peru (3.0%) are the most prevalent allergens detected using this system.[4]

- Punch biopsy—when another underlying disorder is suspected that is best diagnosed with histology (e.g., psoriasis).

DIFFERENTIAL DIAGNOSIS

- Atopic dermatitis is usually more widespread than a CD. There is often a history of other atopic conditions such as allergic rhinitis and asthma. There may be family history of allergies. However, persons with atopic dermatitis are more prone to CD (**Figure 140-6**) (Chapter 139, Atopic Dermatitis).

- Dyshidrotic eczema: Seen on the hands and feet with tapioca vesicles, erythema, and scale. While this is not primarily caused by contact to allergens, various irritating substances can make it worse (Chapter 141, Hand Eczema).

- Immediate IgE contact reaction (e.g., latex glove allergy): Immediate erythema, itching, and possibly systemic reaction after contact with a known (or suspected) allergen.

- Fungal infections: A dermatophyte infection that can closely resemble CD when it occurs on the hands and feet. Tinea pedis is usually seen between the toes, on the soles or on the sides of the feet. CD of the feet is often on the dorsum of the foot and related to rubber or other chemicals in the shoes (**Figures 140-13** and **140-14**) (Chapter 134, Tinea Pedis).

- Scabies on the hands can be mistaken for CD. Look for burrows and for the typical distribution of the scabies infestation to distinguish this from CD (Chapter 137, Scabies).

- Allergies to the dyes used in tatoos can occur. While this is not strictly a contact dermatitis because the dye is injected below the skin, the allergic process is similar (**Figure 140-15**).

MANAGEMENT

- Identify and avoid the offending agent(s).[3] SOR **A**

- Cool compresses can soothe the symptoms of acute cases of CD.[3] SOR **C**

- Calamine and colloidal oatmeal baths may help to dry and soothe acute, oozing lesions.[3] SOR **C**

- Localized acute ACD lesions respond best with midpotency to high-potency topical steroids such as 0.1% triamcinolone to 0.05% clobetasol, respectively.[3] SOR **A**

- On areas of thinner skin (e.g., flexural surfaces, eyelids, face, anogenital region) lower-potency steroids can avoid skin atrophy.[3]

- There is insufficient data to support the use of topical steroids for ICD, but since it is difficult to distinguish clinically between ACD and ICD, these agents are frequently tried.

- If ACD involves extensive skin areas (>20%), systemic steroid therapy is often required and offers relief within 12 to 24 hours. The recommended dose is 0.5 to 1 mg/kg daily for 5 to 7 days, and

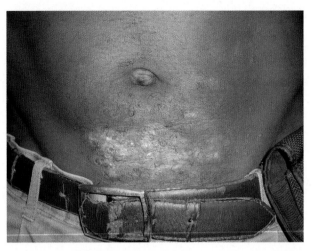

FIGURE 140-5 ACD to the metal in the belt buckle causing erythema, scaling, and hyperpigmentation. (*Courtesy of Richard P. Usatine, MD.*)

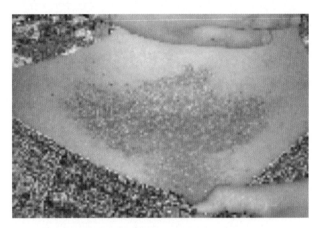

FIGURE 140-6 A 14-year-old girl with atopic dermatitis and allergy to the metal in her pants buckle. (*Courtesy of Richard P. Usatine, MD.*)

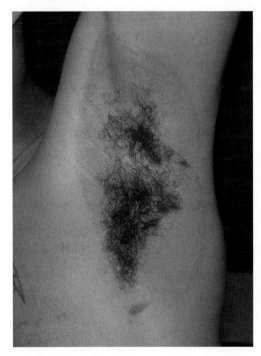

FIGURE 140-7 ACD to the fragrance in a new deodorant. (*With permission from Milgrom EC, Usatine RP, Tan RA, Spector SL. Practical Allergy. 2004, Elsevier, Inc. Philadelphia.*)

if the patient is comfortable at that time the dose may be reduced by 50% for the next 5 to 7 days. The rate of reduction of steroid dosage depends on factors such as severity, duration of ACD, and how effectively the allergen can be avoided.[3] SOR Ⓐ

- Oral steroids should be tapered over 2 weeks because rapid discontinuance of steroids can result in rebound dermatitis. Severe poison ivy/oak is often treated with oral prednisone for 2 to 3 weeks. Avoid using a Medrol dose-pack which has insufficient dosing and duration.

- The efficacy of topical immunomodulators (tacrolimus and pimecrolimus) in ACD or ICD has not been established.[3] SOR Ⓐ

- Although antihistamines are generally not effective for pruritus associated with ACD, they are commonly used. Sedation from more soporific antihistamines may offer some degree of palliation (diphenhydramine, hydroxyzine).[3] SOR Ⓒ

- Bacterial superinfection should be treated with an appropriate antibiotic that will cover *Streptococcus pyogenes* and *Staphylococcus aureus*. Treat for MRSA if suspected.

- Once the diagnosis of any CD is established, emollients, moisturizers, and/or barrier creams may be instituted as secondary prevention strategies for continued exposure.[3] SOR Ⓒ

For ICD and occupational CD of the hands:

- Wear gloves when working with potentially irritating substances such as solvents, soaps, and detergents.

- Use cotton liners under the gloves for both comfort and the absorption of sweat.

- Keep hands clean, dry, and well moisturized whenever possible.

- Petrolatum applied twice a day is a great way to moisturize dry and cracked skin without exposing the patient to new irritants.

PATIENT EDUCATION

Avoid the offending agent and take the medications as prescribed to relieve symptoms.

FOLLOW-UP

Depends upon severity of the CD and the duration.

PATIENT RESOURCES

Good online information for patients can be accessed at Medline-Plus and **www.emedicinehealth.com.**

PROVIDER RESOURCES

Beltrani VS, Bernstein IL, Cohen DE, Fonacier L. Contact dermatitis: A practice parameter. *Ann Allergy Asthma Immunol.* 2006;97:S1–38.

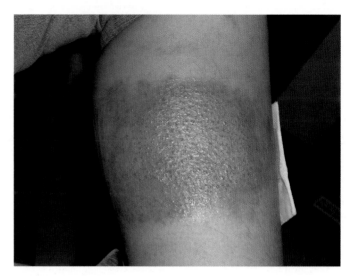

FIGURE 140-8 ACD to neomycin applied to the leg of a young woman. Her mom gave her triple antibiotic ointment to place over a bug bite with a large nonstick pad. The contact allergy follows the exact size of the pad and only occurs where the antibiotic was applied. (*Courtesy of Richard P. Usatine, MD.*)

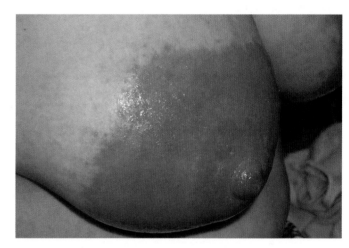

FIGURE 140-9 ACD to a neomycin containing topical antibiotic on the breasts. This woman applied this medicine to treat her breast discomfort that began when her breast-feeding baby developed thrush. (*Courtesy of Jack Resneck, Sr., MD.*)

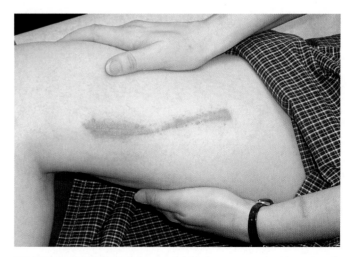

FIGURE 140-10 A linear pattern of ACD from poison ivy. (*Courtesy of Jack Resneck, Sr., MD.*)

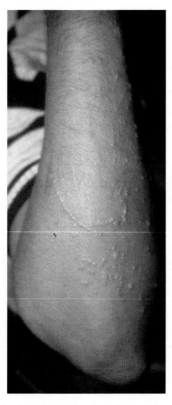

FIGURE 140-11 Multiple lines of vesicles from poison oak on the arm. (*With permission from Milgrom EC, Usatine RP, Tan RA, Spector SL. Practical Allergy. 2004, Elsevier, Philadelphia.*)

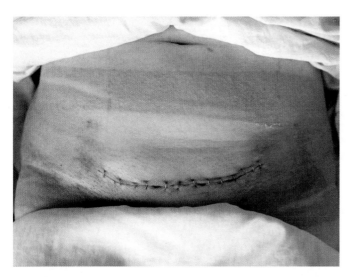

FIGURE 140-12 ACD to the tape used after an abdominal hysterectomy. (*With permission from Milgrom EC, Usatine RP, Tan RA, Spector SL. Practical Allergy. 2004, Elsevier, Inc. Philadelphia.*)

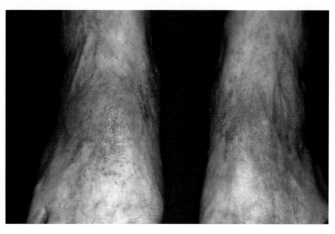

FIGURE 140-13 ACD from new shoes. This is the typical distribution found on the dorsum of the feet. (*With permission from Milgrom EC, Usatine RP, Tan RA, Spector SL. Practical Allergy. 2004, Elsevier, Inc. Philadelphia.*)

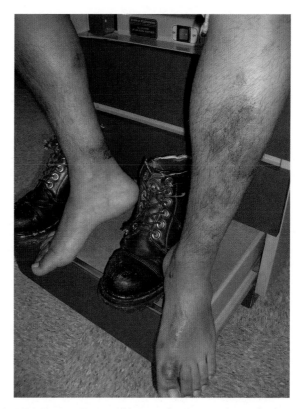

FIGURE 140-14 A 25-year-old man with ACD to a chemical in his boots. His boots were higher but he cut them down to try to alleviate the discomfort coming from the boots higher on his leg. (*With permission from Milgrom EC, Usatine RP, Tan RA, Spector SL. Practical Allergy. 2004, Elsevier, Inc. Philadelphia.*)

REFERENCES

1. Halstater B, Usatine RP. Contact Dermatitis. In: Milgrom E, Usatine RP, Tan R, Spector S, eds. *Practical Allergy*. Philadelphia, PA: Elsevier, 2003.

2. Usatine RP. A red twisted ankle. *West J Med.* 1999;171:361–362.

3. Beltrani VS, Bernstein IL, Cohen DE, Fonacier L. Contact dermatitis: A practice parameter. *Ann Allergy Asthma Immunol.* 2006;97: S1–S38.

4. Krob HA, Fleischer AB, Jr., D'Agostino R, Jr., Haverstock CL, Feldman S. Prevalence and relevance of contact dermatitis allergens: A meta-analysis of 15 years of published T.R.U.E. test data. *J Am Acad Dermatol.* 2004;51:349–353.

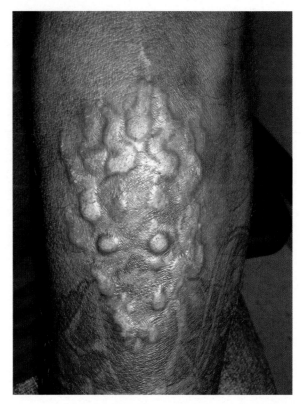

FIGURE 140-15 Man with allergy to red dye in tattoo. Everywhere that the red dye was used, the patient developed pain and swelling. (*Courtesy of Richard P. Usatine, MD.*)

141 HAND ECZEMA

Richard P. Usatine, MD

PATIENT STORY

An Asian American physician presents with dry scaling on her hands. Frequent hand washing makes it worse and it sometimes cracks. She has allergic rhinitis and she had more widespread atopic dermatitis in her youth. This is a case of chronic atopic hand dermatitis (**Figure 141-1**). The treatment suggested was use of Cetaphil (or equivalent nonsoap cleanser) instead of soap and water. She was directed to soak her hands 3 to 5 minutes in warm water every night, apply triamcinolone 0.1% ointment, and cover with cotton gloves overnight. Her hands cleared 90% with this treatment and she was pleased with the results.

EPIDEMIOLOGY

- The prevalence of hand dermatitis is estimated at approximately 2 to 8.9% in the general population.[1]

ETIOLOGY AND PATHOPHYSIOLOGY

- There are many clinical variants of hand dermatitis and a number of different classification schemas. Here is one accepted classification scheme:
    1. Contact (i.e., allergic and irritant) **Figure 141-2**.
    2. Hyperkeratotic (i.e., psoriasiform) **Figure 141-3**.
    3. Frictional (**Figure 141-4**).
    4. Nummular (**Figure 141-5**).
    5. Atopic (**Figure 141-6**).
    6. Pompholyx (i.e., dyshidrosis) (**Figure 141-7**).
    7. Chronic vesicular hand dermatitis[1] (**Figure 141-8**).
- Another way of looking at hand dermatitis is to break it down into three categories[2]:
    1. Endogenous—atopic, psoriasis, dyshidrotic.
    2. Exogenous—allergic and irritant contact dermatitis
    3. Infectious—tinea, candida, and/or superimposed *Staphylococcus aureus* (**Figure 141-9**)
- Most contact dermatitis of the hands is secondary to irritants such as soap, water, and chemicals.
- Allergic contact dermatitis is a type IV, delayed-type, cell-mediated, hypersensitivity reaction.
- Nine most frequent allergens related to hand contact dermatitis were identified by patch testing from 1994 to 2004.[3] These are quaternium-15 (16.5%), formaldehyde (13.0%), nickel sulfate (12.2%), fragrance mix (11.3%), thiuram mix (10.2%), balsam of

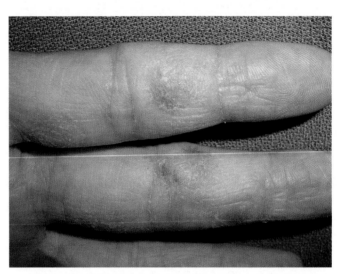

FIGURE 141-1 An Asian American physician with chronic atopic hand dermatitis. She has allergic rhinitis and she had more widespread atopic dermatitis in her youth. (*Courtesy of Richard P. Usatine, MD.*)

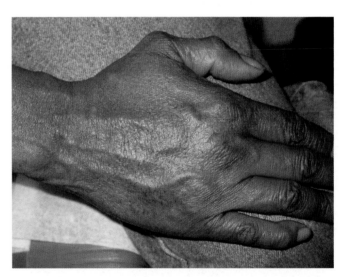

FIGURE 141-2 Contact dermatitis on the dorsum of the hand secondary to using the back of the hand to apply perfume to neck. (*With permission from the J Fam Pract. 2003;52(11):863, Dowden Health Media.*)

Peru (9.6%), carba mix (7.8%), neomycin sulfate (7.7%), and bacitracin (7.4%).[3]

- Rubber allergens were commonly associated with occupation. One-third of patients with allergic contact dermatitis had identifiable relevant irritants.[3]
- Most common allergens are preservatives, metals, fragrances, topical antibiotics, or rubber additives.[3]

DIAGNOSIS

CLINICAL FEATURES[1]

- Contact (i.e., allergic and irritant) (**Figure 141-2**).
  - Symptoms include burning, stinging, itching, and tenderness at the site of exposure to the irritant or allergen.[1]
  - Acute signs include papules, vesicles, bullae, and edema.
  - Weeping and crusting can occur with or without superinfection.
  - Chronic signs include plaques with fissuring, hyperpigmentation, and/or lichenification.
  - Irritant contact dermatitis may predispose to allergic contact dermatitis.

- Hyperkeratotic (i.e., psoriasiform) (**Figure 141-3**).
  - Symmetric hyperkeratotic plaques.
  - May be localized to the proximal or middle part of the palms.
  - Painful fissures are common.

- Frictional (**Figure 141-4**).
  - Mechanical factors often from work such as trauma, friction, pressure, and vibration induce skin changes with erythema and scale.
  - "Wear-and-tear dermatitis."[1]
  - Can be caused by contact with paper and fabrics.

- Nummular (**Figure 141-5**).
  - Nummular hand dermatitis (also called discoid hand dermatitis).
  - Tiny papules, papulovesicles, or "coin-shaped" eczematous plaques.
  - Dorsal hands and distal fingers are often involved.

- Atopic.
  - Patients with childhood atopic dermatitis are predisposed to develop hand dermatitis as adults (**Figure 141-6**).
  - There is no characteristic pattern and it can occur on any part of the hand.
  - Extension to or involvement of the wrist is common (**Figure 141-10**).

- Pompholyx (i.e., dyshidrosis, dyshidrotic eczema).
  - Has recurrent crops of papules, vesicles, and bullae on the lateral aspects of the fingers, as well as the palms and soles on a background of nonerythematous skin (**Figure 141-7**).
  - These are described as tapioca vesicles as they look like the small spheres in tapioca (**Figure 141-7**).
  - The vesicles open and the skin then peels (mild desquamation).
  - There may be pruritus or pain.
  - While some use the names pompholyx and dyshidrotic eczema interchangeably, others only use the name pompholyx to describe an explosive onset of large bullae, usually on the palms and dyshidrotic eczema to mainly describe chronic small tapioca vesicles on the sides of the fingers.

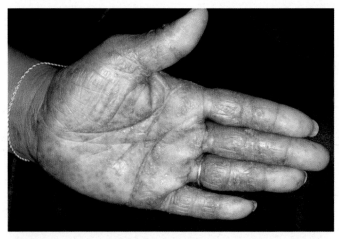

FIGURE 141-3 Hyperkeratotic hand dermatitis in a black woman. (*Courtesy of Richard P. Usatine, MD.*)

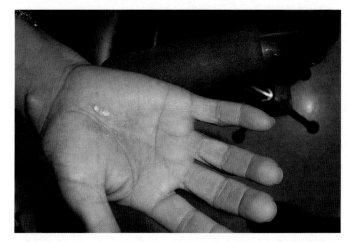

FIGURE 141-4 Frictional hand eczema that is worse on the hand that is used for the cane. The other side was affected by a stroke so only one hand is usable for ambulating with a cane. (*Courtesy of Richard P. Usatine, MD.*)

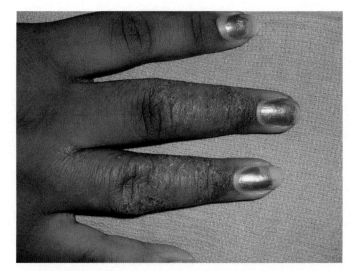

FIGURE 141-5 Nummular hand dermatitis with tiny papules, papulovesicles, and "coin-shaped" eczematous plaques on the distal fingers of a 14-year-old girl. (*Courtesy of Richard P. Usatine, MD.*)

○ Both conditions last 2 to 3 weeks and resolve, leaving normal skin, only to recur again at varying intervals.

○ Both conditions are idiopathic and closely related, if not identical

○ Symptoms may be associated with exogenous factors (e.g., nickel or hot weather) or endogenous factors (e.g., atopy or stress).

- Chronic vesicular hand dermatitis (**Figure 141-8**).

○ Chronic vesicles that are mostly palmar and pruritic.

○ Differentiated from pompholyx by a more chronic course and the presence of vesicles with an erythematous base.

○ The soles of the feet may also be involved.

○ Poorly responsive to treatments.

○ In one series, 55% of patients with this type of hand dermatitis were found to have positive patch test results.[4]

TYPICAL DISTRIBUTION

Of course, hand dermatitis is on the hands but both hands and feet can be involved in pompholyx and chronic vesicular hand dermatitis.

LABORATORY STUDIES

Scraping and using microscopy with KOH (with or without a fungal stain) to look for dermatophytes is helpful (see Chapter 129, Cutaneous Fungal Infections).

DIFFERENTIAL DIAGNOSIS

- Tinea manus is often found as part of the two-foot-one-hand syndrome in which both feet have scaling tinea pedis and one hand has scale as well (**Figure 141-11**) (see Chapter 129, Cutaneous Fungal Infections, and Chapter 134, Tinea Pedis).

- Candida can be seen in between the fingers with erythema and scale over the fingers and hand (**Figure 141-9**) (see Chapter 130, Mucocutaneous Candidiasis).

- Psoriasis often involves the hand. It can present with plaques on the dorsum of hand and over the knuckles of the fingers or on the palm of the hand. Palmoplantar psoriasis will involve the hands and feet (see Chapter 145, Psoriasis).

- Knuckle pads are thickening of the skin over the knuckles. These can be accompanied by hyperpigmentation.

MANAGEMENT

- Life-style modifying factors, as listed in **Table 141-1**, are essential.

- Avoid irritants and "wet work" at home and at work as much as possible. SOR **C**

- Avoid exposure to irritants by eliminating their use, substituting products, creating a physical barrier with cotton gloves under vinyl or nitrile gloves, or by changing jobs. SOR **C**

- Avoid latex gloves because of a high risk of latex allergy among patients with hand dermatitis. SOR **C**

- Frequent and liberal use of emollients can help restore normal skin-barrier function. Simple, inexpensive, petrolatum-based emollients were found to be equally as effective as an emollient containing skin-related lipids in a 2-month study of 30 patients with mild to moderate hand dermatitis.[5] SOR **B**

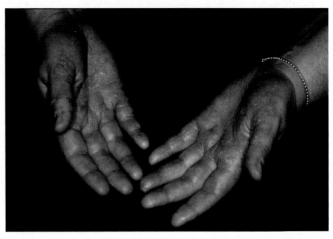

FIGURE 141-6 Atopic hand dermatitis on palms in Asian American woman with long history of atopic dermatitis. (*Courtesy of Richard P. Usatine, MD. Previously published in Practical Allergy.*)

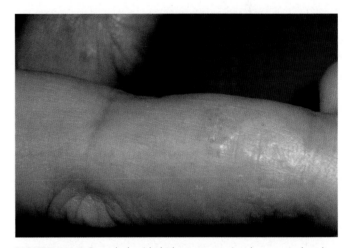

FIGURE 141-7 Pompholyx (dyshidrotic eczema) with acute outbreak of tapioca vesicles on the sides of the fingers. (*Courtesy of Richard P. Usatine, MD.*)

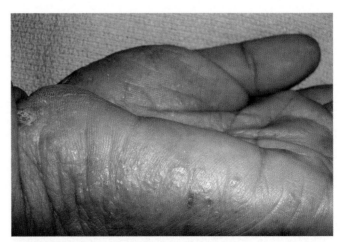

FIGURE 141-8 Chronic vesicular hand dermatitis going on for decades in this 51-year-old Hispanic woman. It is particularly bad in the hypothenar area. (*Courtesy of Richard P. Usatine, MD.*)

- Soak hands 3 to 5 minutes in warm water every night, apply triamcinolone 0.1% ointment and cover with cotton gloves overnight. The cotton gloves may be used repeatedly even though they will soak up some of the ointment. SOR Ⓒ

- Wear nitrile gloves over cotton gloves while washing dishes or cleaning with fluids. SOR Ⓒ

- Do not wash hands with soap or use only the mildest of soaps (e.g. Dove). Use Cetaphil, a nonsoap cleanser. SOR Ⓒ

See **Table 141-2** for a summary of the recommended therapeutic agents for different types of hand dermatitis.

TOPICAL AGENTS

- Topical steroids are first-line agents for inflammatory hand dermatitis. Ointments are considered more effective and contain fewer preservatives and additives than creams. Some patients will prefer a cream vehicle so that patient preference should be considered in prescribing topical steroids. It is better to have a patient use a cream than not use an ointment.

- Start with 0.1% triamcinolone ointment bid as it is inexpensive and effective. SOR Ⓒ Cut back on use when possible to avoid skin atrophy, striae, and telangiectasias.

- Topical calcineurin inhibitors, tacrolimus and pimecrolimus, are effective in the treatment of atopic and other allergic types of hand dermatitis.[6] SOR Ⓑ Skin burning or an unpleasant sensation of warmth is reported by approximately 50% of patients using topical tacrolimus and 10% with pimecrolimus.[6]

PHOTOTHERAPY AND IONIZING RADIATION

- Psoralen and UVA irradiation (PUVA) has been used to treat patients with all forms of hand dermatitis.[6] SOR Ⓒ

- Grenz rays (ionizing radiation with ultrasoft X-rays or Bucky rays) usually requires 200 to 400 rad (2–4 Gy) can be used every 1 to 3 weeks for up to a total of six treatments, followed by a 6-month hiatus.[6] SOR Ⓒ

SYSTEMIC STEROIDS AND IMMUNOMODULATORS

- Oral prednisone may be used to treat the most severe and recalcitrant case of hand dermatitis. Pulse dosing of 40 to 60 mg daily for 3 to 4 days may be valuable.[6] SOR Ⓒ

- Cyclosporine is a potent immunomodulating agent used to treat the severe and recalcitrant case of atopic and hand dermatitis. Unfortunately, relapse rates are high after discontinuation of the cyclosporine.[6] SOR Ⓑ

- Mycophenolate mofetil and methotrexate have been reported to be beneficial in case reports.[6] SOR Ⓒ

PATIENT EDUCATION

See **Table 141-1**.

FOLLOW-UP

Patients with chronic hand dermatitis are often desperately looking for help and often appreciate frequent follow-up until the dermatitis is controlled.

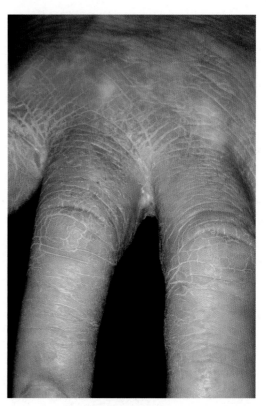

FIGURE 141-9 Contact hand dermatitis in a Chinese cook superinfected with Candida. See white scale between the fingers. The Candida in the interdigital space is also called erosio interdigitalis blastomycetica and is seen in patients with diabetes. (*Courtesy of Richard P. Usatine, MD.*)

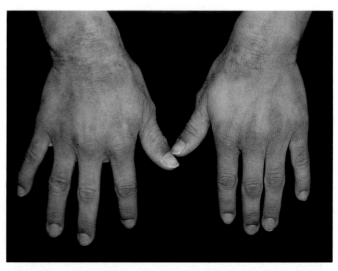

FIGURE 141-10 Hand dermatitis with prominent wrist involvement in a 20-year-old Hispanic woman with moderately severe widespread atopic dermatitis. (*Courtesy of Richard P. Usatine, MD.*)

TABLE 141-1 Sample Patient Handout on Lifestyle Management of Hand Dermatitis

Hand washing and moisturizing:

- Use lukewarm or cool water, and mild cleansers without perfume, coloring, or antibacterial agents, and with minimal preservatives. In general, bar soaps tend to have fewer preservatives than liquid soaps (Cetaphil or Aquanil liquid cleansers or generic equivalents are exceptions to this statement).

- Pat hands dry, especially between fingers.

- Immediately following partial drying of hands (e.g., within 3 minutes), apply a generous amount of a heavy cream or ointment (not lotion); petroleum jelly, a one-ingredient lubricant, works well.

- It is helpful to have containers of creams or ointments next to every sink in your home (next to the bed, next to the TV, in the car, and at multiple places at work).

- Moisturizing should be repeated as often as possible throughout the day, ideally 15 times per day.

- Avoid using washcloths, rubbing, scrubbing, or overuse of soap or water.

Occlusive therapy at night for intensive therapy:

- Apply a generous amount of your doctor's recommended emollient or prescribed medicine on your hands.

- Then put on cotton gloves and wear overnight.

When performing "wet work":

- Wear cotton gloves under vinyl or other nonlatex gloves.

- Try not to use hot water and decrease exposure to water to less than 15 minutes at a time, if possible.

- Use running water rather than immersing hands, if possible.

- Remove rings before wet or dry work.

- Wear protective gloves in cold weather and for dusty work. For frictional exposures, wear tight-fitting leather gloves (e.g., riding, or golfing gloves).

Avoid direct contact with the following, if possible:

- Shampoo

- Peeling fruits and vegetables, especially citrus fruits

- Polishes of all kinds

- Solvents (e.g., white spirit, thinners, and turpentine)

- Hair lotions, creams, and dyes

- Detergents and strong cleansing agents

- Fragranced chemicals

- "Unknown" chemicals

Heavy-duty vinyl gloves are better than rubber, nitrile, or other synthetic gloves because vinyl is less likely to cause allergic reactions.
Reprinted with permission from Fig. 9 in: Decker BC, Warshaw E, Lee G, Storrs FJ. Hand dermatitis: A review of clinical features, therapeutic options, and long-term outcomes. *Am J Contact Dermat.* 2003;14:126.

TABLE 141-2 Recommended Therapies for Hand Dermatitis Variants

Therapeutic Agent	Hand Dermatitis Variant						
	Irritant Contact	Allergic Contact	Hyperkeratotic	Nummular	Pompholyx (Dyshidrosis)	Frictional	Chronic Vesicular
Corticosteroids:							
Topicala	✓	✓		✓	✓	✓	✓
Oral		✓			✓*		✓
Cyclosporine		✓			✓		✓
Methotrexate		✓	✓		✓		✓
Mycophenolate		✓		✓	✓		✓
Tacrolimus pimecrolimus (topical)	✓	✓		✓	✓		✓
Phototherapy (UVB, PUVA and Grenz)	✓	✓	✓	✓	✓	✓	✓
Retinoids (topical and/or oral)			✓			✓	✓
Calcipotriene (topical)			✓			✓	✓

*Acute flares.
Reprinted with permission from Decker BC, Warshaw E, Lee G, Storrs FJ. Hand dermatitis: A review of clinical features, therapeutic options, and long-term outcomes. *Am J Contact Dermat*. 2003;14:128.

REFERENCE

1. Warshaw E, Lee G, Storrs FJ. Hand dermatitis: A review of clinical features, therapeutic options, and long-term outcomes. *Am J Contact Dermat*. 2003;14:119–137.

2. Bolognia J. *Dermatology*. Mosby, London, 2003.

3. Warshaw EM, Ahmed RL, Belsito DV, et al. Contact dermatitis of the hands: Cross-sectional analyses of North American Contact Dermatitis Group Data, 1994–2004. *J Am Acad Dermatol*. 2007; 57(2):301–314.

4. Li LF, Wang J. Contact hypersensitivity in hand dermatitis. *Contact Dermatitis*. 2002;47:206–209.

5. Kucharekova M, Van De Kerkhof PC, Van Der Valk PG. A randomized comparison of an emollient containing skin-related lipids with a petrolatum-based emollient as adjunct in the treatment of chronic hand dermatitis. *Contact Dermatitis*. 2003;48:293–299.

6. Warshaw EM. Therapeutic options for chronic hand dermatitis. *Dermatol Ther*. 2004;17:240–250.

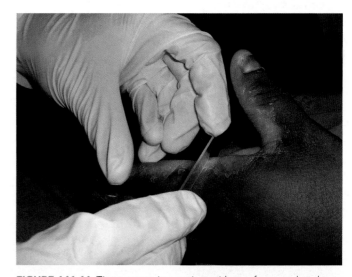

FIGURE 141-11 Tinea manus in a patient with two-foot one-hand syndrome. The scraping showed hyphae under the microscope with a KOH preparation. (*Courtesy of Richard P. Usatine, MD.*)

142 SELF-INFLICTED DERMATOSES

Richard P. Usatine, MD

PATIENT STORY

A 55-year-old woman presents with severe itching on her arms and legs. The itching disrupts her sleep and she sometimes scratches her arms and legs until exhaustion (**Figures 142-1** and **142-2**). She had used moisturizers, emollients, and topical corticosteroids, but they only alleviated the itching temporarily. The itching began 10 months earlier after finalizing the divorce from her husband of 20 years. The patient's right leg had been amputated above the knee after a car accident, and she now wore a prosthetic leg. The patient readily admitted to a great deal of psychological distress. She described feeling depressed since her divorce, and the loss of her leg further aggravated her situation. She has had difficulty securing a job and had high anxiety about being able to pay for rent and bills. The diagnosis made was neurotic excoriations (neurodermatitis) and the patient understood that she was doing this to her own skin. The patient improved with nail cutting, acknowledging the self-inflicted nature of her excoriations and topical clobetasol. One year later, the patient was working in the hospital laboratory with a tremendous improvement in her skin condition (**Figure 142-3**).

SYNONYMS

- Neurotic excoriations—neurodermatitis.

- Lichen simplex chronicus—neurodermatitis circumscripta.

- Prurigo nodularis—picker's nodules; lichen simplex chronicus, prurigo nodularis type; atypical nodular form of neurodermatitis circumscripta.

EPIDEMIOLOGY

- Studies show that neurotic excoriations primarily affects females with a mean onset between the ages of 30 to 45 years[1] (**Figures 142-1** to **142-5**).

- Lichen simplex chronicus (LSC) is observed more commonly in females than in males (**Figures 142-6** to **142-9**). Lichen nuchae is a form of lichen simplex that occurs on the midposterior neck and is observed almost exclusively in women (**Figures 142-8** and **142-9**).

- LSC occurs mostly in mid-to-late adulthood, with highest prevalence in persons aged 30 to 50 years.[2]

- For prurigo nodularis (PN) there is no documented difference in frequency between males and females. PN most often occurs in middle-aged and older persons[3] (**Figures 142-10** to **142-15**).

ETIOLOGY AND PATHOPHYSIOLOGY

- All three conditions are found on the skin in regions accessible to scratching.

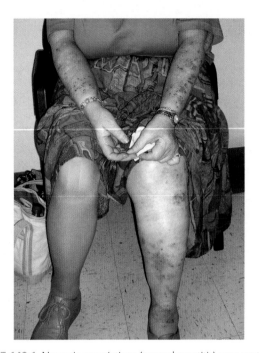

FIGURE 142-1 Neurotic excoriations (neurodermatitis) seen on three of four extremities. The fourth extremity is a prosthetic leg. (*With permission from Usatine RP, Saldana-Arregui MA. Photo Rounds: Ecoriations and ulcers and legs. The J Fam Pract 2004;53(9):713–716, Dowden Health Media.*)[1]

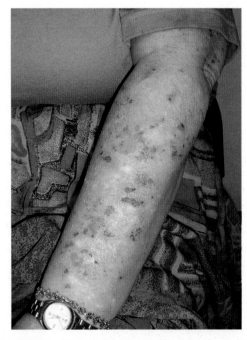

FIGURE 142-2 Neurotic excoriations with close-up of arm. (*With permission from Usatine RP, Saldana-Arregui MA. Photo Rounds: Ecoriations and ulcers and legs. The J Fam Pract 2004;53(9):713–716, Dowden Health Media.*)

- Pruritus provokes scratching that produces clinical lesions.

- The underlying pathophysiology is unknown for all three conditions.

- Some skin types are more prone to lichenification, such as skin that tends toward eczematous conditions (i.e., atopic dermatitis).[2]

- Neurotic excoriations (neurodermatitis) is a result of a psychodermatologic disorder in which patients inflict excoriations and ulcers on their skin and admit to their involvement.

- The pathogenesis of PN is still unknown. PN shares some histologic features (epidermal proliferation) with psoriasis and ichthyosis but is largely self-inflicted.[3]

DIAGNOSIS

CLINICAL FEATURES

Itching is the common historical theme for all three self-inflicted dermatoses.

Common psychiatric problems associated with all self-inflicted dermatoses include significant social stress, depression, anxiety, and obsessive–compulsive disorder.

Patients are often observed scratching and rubbing their skin. This results in:

- Lichenification of the skin (skin thickening with exaggerated skin lines) (**Figures 142-6** and **142-9**).

- Pigmentary changes (especially hyperpigmentation) (**Figures 142-4, 142-5, 142-9, 142-11,** and **142-15**).

- Excoriations, erosions, and ulcerations.

Common physical examination findings for all three disorders include:

- Neurotic excoriations—may vary from dug-out erosions, to ulcers covered with crusts and surrounded by erythema to areas receding into hypopigmented depressed scars (**Figure 142-5**).
- LSC—One or more slightly erythematous, scaly, well-demarcated, lichenified, firm, rough plaques[2] (**Figures 142-6 to 142-9**).
- Prurigo nodularis—raised nodules from 2 to 20 mm, colors vary from shades of red to brown (**Figures 142-10 to 142-15**).

Excoriations are almost always present on initial presentation. With treatment the excoriations may subside and the nodules may remain.

TYPICAL DISTRIBUTION

- Neurotic excoriations occur on areas easily reached by the patient, such as the arms, legs, and upper back (**Figures 142-1 to 142-5**).

- LSC occurs on:

  ○ Hands, wrists, extensor forearms, and elbows (**Figure 142-6**).

  ○ Knees, lower legs, and ankles (**Figure 142-7**).

  ○ Nape of neck (**Figures 142-8** and **142-9**).

  ○ Vulva and scrotum.

- In PN, nodules occur on the extensor surfaces of the arms, the legs, and sometimes the trunk (**Figures 142-10 to 142-15**).

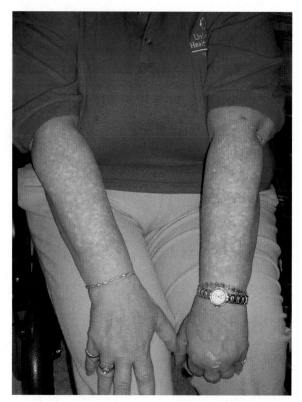

FIGURE 142-3 Same patient 1 year later after successful therapy. Hypopigmented scarring remains. (*Courtesy of Richard P. Usatine, MD.*)

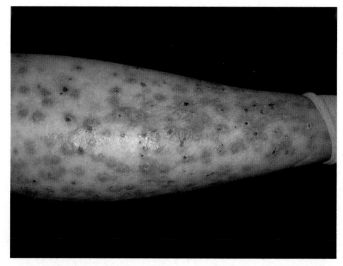

FIGURE 142-4 Neurotic excoriations on the leg with significant postinflammatory hyperpigmentation. (*Courtesy of Richard P. Usatine, MD.*)

LABORATORY STUDIES

Punch biopsy may be helpful when the diagnosis is uncertain.

DIFFERENTIAL DIAGNOSIS

- Acne keloidalis nuchae—acneiform eruption at the hairline from ingrown hairs, worse with shaving and short haircuts (see Chapter 108, Pseudofolliculitis and Acne Keloidalis Nuchae).

- Atopic dermatitis—an allergic skin disorder in patients with a personal or family history of atopic conditions. Patients with atopic dermatitis are more likely to get lichen simplex chronicus (see Chapter 139, Atopic Dermatitis).

- Contact dermatitis—a common inflammatory skin condition characterized by erythematous and pruritic skin lesions resulting from the contact of skin with a foreign substance (see Chapter 140, Contact Dermatitis).

- Delusions of parasitosis—delusions that tiny bugs or parasites are living on or below the patient's skin leading them to try to dig them out with their nails and fingers. This condition looks just like neurotic excoriations; however, the patient believes there are parasites causing the pruritus and it is very difficult to convince them otherwise.

- Nummular eczema—eczematous lesions in the shape of coins seen most often on the legs.

- Scabies—look for burrows between the fingers and the typical distribution of scabies on the hands, feet, wrists, waist, and axillae to differentiate scabies from a self-inflicted dermatosis. If you do a scraping and find evidence of the scabies mite that is the best way to confirm a true scabies infestation. Often family members have itching and lesions as well when the real diagnosis is scabies (see Chapter 137, Scabies).

MANAGEMENT

For all three self-inflicted dermatoses there is little evidence to guide therapy. The following three treatments can be used in all three conditions and are based on expert opinion and a few small studies: SOR ⓒ

- Topical corticosteroids—use mid-to-high potency steroids except in areas of thin skin.

- Oral antihistamines—sedating H1 blockers and consider doxepin (start with 10–25 mg PO qhs and titrate to response) for refractory cases.

- Oral antibiotics, if secondary infection is present.

- One small study of three patients with inflammatory skin diseases and severe nocturnal pruritus who underwent treatment with mirtazapine (Remeron) suggests that this may be an effective alternative for the treatment of nocturnal pruritus.[4] SOR ⓒ

Get a good psychosocial history and offer the patient treatment for any problems uncovered. It may help for patients to understand the connection between their self-inflicted lesions and their stressors. Some patients will have anxiety disorders or depression while others will be suffering with great psychosocial stressors like loss of work,

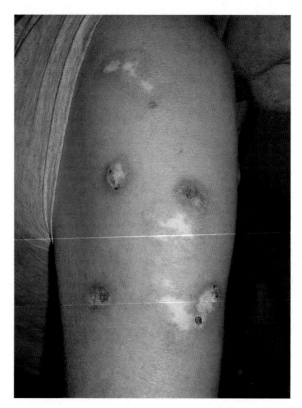

FIGURE 142-5 Neurotic excoriations on the upper arm with hypopigmented scarring. (*Courtesy of Richard P. Usatine, MD.*)

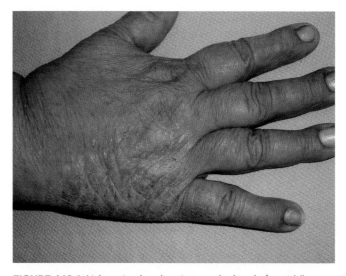

FIGURE 142-6 Lichen simplex chronicus on the hand of a middleaged woman with thick lichenification, erythema, and hyperpigmentation. She was continually scratching at her hand. (*Courtesy of Richard P. Usatine, MD.*)

homelessness or grief. Offer pharmacotherapy (including SSRIs) and counseling if indicated. Refer as needed for these therapies.

Other specific treatments to consider are as follows:

LSC—5% doxepin cream has been studied in patients with LSC, nummular eczema, and contact dermatitis. Applied four times per day for a period of 7 days led to an 84% response rate in reduction of pruritus (not lesions).[5] SOR **B**

Prurigo nodularis—a difficult condition to treat with mild-to-moderate success at best. Here are some treatments to consider:

- Intralesional steroids—triamcinolone 5 to 10 mg/cc. SOR **C**

- Cryotherapy—applied to each nodule to flatten the nodules and decrease pruritus. SOR **C**

- Calcipotriol—after 8 weeks of calcipotriol treatment, the reduction in the number and size of nodules was 49% and 56%, respectively, compared with 18% and 25% for the betamethasone valerate.[6] SOR **B**

- Ultraviolet light (narrow-band UVB) is sometimes useful when the condition is widespread. SOR **C**

- Dapsone has been tried with some reported success in this difficult condition. SOR **C**

PATIENT EDUCATION

Help patients to understand that they are unintentionally hurting their own skin. Patients need to minimize touching, scratching, and rubbing affected areas. Suggest that patients gently apply their medication or a moisturizer instead of scratching the pruritic areas. Give patients hope and show them **Figures 142-1 to 142-3** to demonstrate that even the most severe cases can heal if they stop manipulating their skin.

FOLLOW-UP

Follow-up is essential because these problems are chronic and difficult to treat. Patients need to know that you will not abandon them and continue to work with them to get relief. This is especially important when the patient is suffering from anxiety, depression, or other psychological problems.

PATIENT RESOURCES

http://www.aafp.org/afp/20011215/neurph.html.

PROVIDER RESOURCES

LSC—http://www.emedicine.com/DERM/topic236.htm.

PN—http://www.emedicine.com/derm/topic350.htm.

NE—http://www.emedicine.com/derm/topic941.htm.

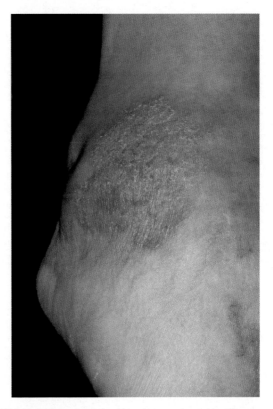

FIGURE 142-7 Lichen simplex chronicus on the ankle. (*Courtesy of Richard P. Usatine, MD.*)

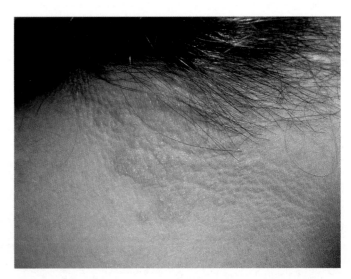

FIGURE 142-8 Lichen simplex chronicus on the neck of a Hispanic woman who also has acanthosis nigricans. (*Courtesy of Richard P. Usatine, MD.*)

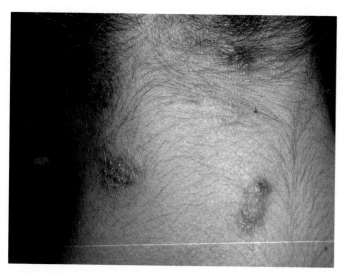

FIGURE 142-9 Lichen simplex chronicus on the neck of a Hispanic woman with thick plaque formation that resembles prurigo nodularis. (*Courtesy of Richard P. Usatine, MD.*)

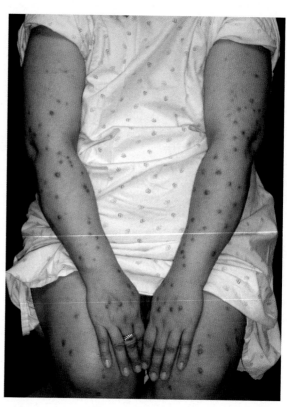

FIGURE 142-11 Prurigo nodularis on the arms and legs after 9 months of unsuccessful treatment in the patient in **Figure 142-10**. (*Courtesy of Richard P. Usatine, MD.*)

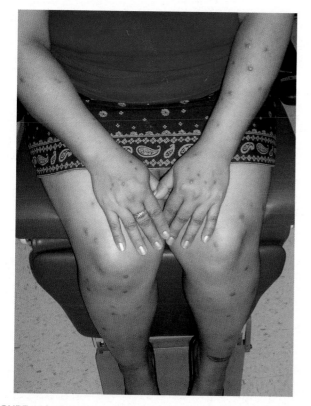

FIGURE 142-10 Prurigo nodularis on the arms and legs of a 42-year-old Hispanic woman. (*Courtesy of Richard P. Usatine, MD.*)

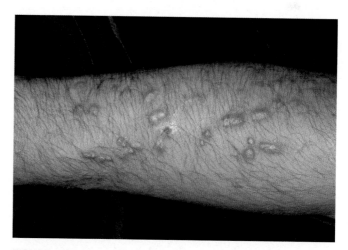

FIGURE 142-12 Severe prurigo nodularis on the arm. The nodules are somewhat linear from years of scratching. (*Courtesy of Richard P. Usatine, MD.*)

REFERENCES

1. Usatine RP, Saldana-Arregui MA. Excoriations and ulcers on the arms and legs. *J Fam Pract.* 2004;53:713–716.

2. Hogan, D. Lichen simplex chronicus. http://www.emedicine.com/DERM/topic236.htm. Updated June 12, 2006. Accessed December 26, 2006.

3. Hogan, D. Prurigo Nodularis. http://www.emedicine.com/derm/topic350.htm. Updated May 17, 2006. Accessed December 26, 2006.

4. Hundley JL, Yosipovitch G. Mirtazapine for reducing nocturnal itch in patients with chronic pruritus: A pilot study. *J Am Acad Dermatol.* 2004;50:889–891.

5. Drake LA, Millikan LE. The antipruritic effect of 5% doxepin cream in patients with eczematous dermatitis. Doxepin Study Group. *Arch Dermatol.* 1995;131:1403–1408.

6. Wong SS, Goh CL. Double-blind, right/left comparison of calcipotriol ointment and betamethasone ointment in the treatment of prurigo nodularis. *Arch Dermatol.* 2000;136:807–808.

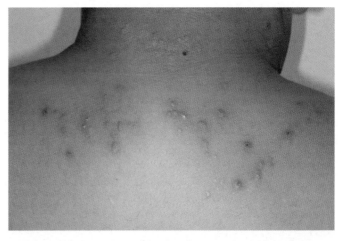

FIGURE 142-13 Prurigo nodularis on the upper back of a man. (*Courtesy of Richard P. Usatine, MD.*)

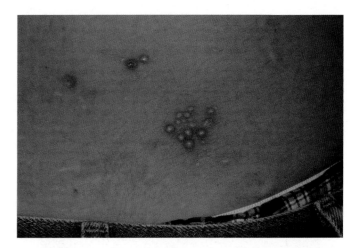

FIGURE 142-14 A cluster of nodules on the back of the same patient with prurigo nodularis. (*Courtesy of Richard P. Usatine, MD.*)

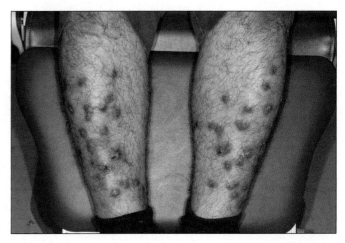

FIGURE 142-15 Severe prurigo nodularis on the legs with prominent hyperpigmentation of the nodules and some secondary infection. (*Courtesy of Richard P. Usatine, MD.*)

143 URTICARIA AND ANGIOEDEMA

Richard P. Usatine, MD

PATIENT STORY

A 26-year-old man was given trimethoprim/sulfamethoxazole for sinusitis and broke out in hives 1 week later. The hives were all over his trunk and arms (**Figures 143-1** and **143-2**). He had no airway compromise and had only urticaria without angioedema. His sinus symptoms were mostly resolved so he was told to stop the antibiotic and take an oral antihistamine. The H1 blocker gave him relief of symptoms and the wheals disappeared over the next 2 days.

EPIDEMIOLOGY

- It is estimated that 15% to 25% of the population may have urticaria sometime during their lifetime.[1]

- Urticaria affects 6% to 7% of preschool children and 17% of children with atopic dermatitis.[1]

- Among all age groups, approximately 50% have both urticaria and angioedema, 40% have isolated urticaria, and 10% have angioedema alone.[1]

- Acute urticaria is defined as less than 6 weeks' duration. A specific cause is more likely to be identified in acute urticaria.[1]

- The cause of chronic urticaria is determined in less than 20% of cases.[1]

- Chronic urticaria is twice as common in women as in men.[2]

- Chronic urticaria predominantly affects adults.[2]

- Up to 40% of patients with chronic urticaria for more than 6 months duration still have urticaria 10 years later.[2]

ETIOLOGY AND PATHOPHYSIOLOGY

- The pathophysiology of angioedema and urticaria can be IGE mediated, complement mediated, related to physical stimuli, autoantibody mediated, or idiopathic.

- These mechanisms lead to mast cell degranulation resulting in the release of histamine. The histamine and other inflammatory mediators produce the wheals, edema, and pruritus.

- Urticaria is a dynamic process in which wheals evolve as old ones resolve. These wheals result from localized capillary vasodilation, followed by transudation of protein-rich fluid into the surrounding skin. The wheals resolve when the fluid is slowly reabsorbed.

- Angioedema is an edematous area that involves transudation of fluid into the dermis and subcutaneous tissue (**Figures 143-3** and **143-4**).

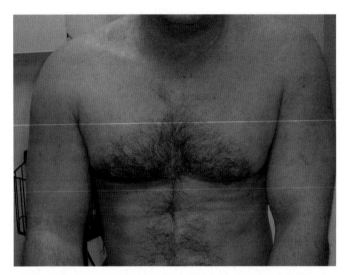

FIGURE 143-1 A 26-year-old man with acute urticaria to trimethoprim/sulfamethoxazole. (*Courtesy of Richard P. Usatine, MD.*)

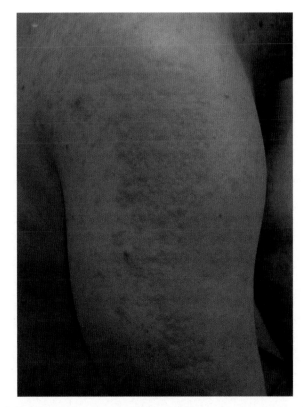

FIGURE 143-2 The patient in **Figure 143-2** showing a confluence of wheals with a well-demarcated border on his arm. (*Courtesy of Richard P. Usatine, MD.*)

The following etiologic types exist:

- Immunologic—IGE mediated, complement mediated. Occurs more often in patients with an atopic background. Antigens are most commonly foods or medications. The most common foods are milk, nuts, wheat, and shellfish.

- Physical urticaria—dermatographism, cold, cholinergic, solar, pressure, vibratory urticaria (**Figures 143-5** and **143-6**).

- Urticaria caused by mast cell releasing agents—mastocytosis, urticaria pigmentosa (**Figures 143-7** and **143-8**).

- Urticaria associated with vascular/connective tissue autoimmune disease.

- Hereditary angioedema is a potentially life-threatening disorder that is inherited in an autosomal dominant manner. In this disease, angioedema occurs without urticaria (**Figure 143-9**).

DIAGNOSIS

CLINICAL FEATURES

- Symptoms include itching, burning, or stinging.

- Wheals vary in size from small 2 mm papules of cholinergic urticaria (**Figure 143-8**) to giant hives where a single wheal may cover a large portion of the trunk.

- The wheal may be all red or white, or the border may be red with the remainder of the surface white.

- Wheals may be annular (**Figures 143-9** and **143-12**).

- If dermatographism is present, one can write on the skin and be able to see the resulting words or shapes (**Figure 143-10**).

- If you suspect urticaria pigmentosa, stroke a lesion with the wooden end of a cotton-tipped applicator. This induces erythema of the plaque and the wheal is confined to the stroke site. This is called Darier's sign.

TYPICAL DISTRIBUTION

- Angioedema is seen more often on the face and is especially found around the mouth and eyes (**Figures 143-3** and **143-4**). Sometimes angioedema can occur on the genitals or the trunk (**Figure 143-11**).

- Urticaria can be found anywhere on the body and is often on the trunk and extremities (**Figures 143-1** and **143-2**).

LABORATORY STUDIES

Consider tests that might help reveal the cause of the urticaria and/or angioedema.

- Order complement studies to investigate for hereditary or acquired C1 esterase inhibitor deficiency when angioedema occurs repeatedly without urticaria (**Figure 143-9**).

- Consider allergen skin testing and/or in vitro tests for when the history reveals that urticaria/angioedema occurs after direct contact with a suspected allergen.

- Punch biopsy of the involved area may be used to diagnose urticarial vasculitis or mastocytosis.

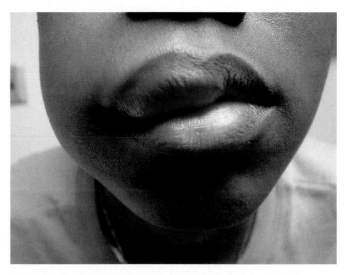

FIGURE 143-3 Young black woman with angioedema after being started on an ACE inhibitor for essential hypertension. (*Courtesy of Adrian Casillas, MD.*)

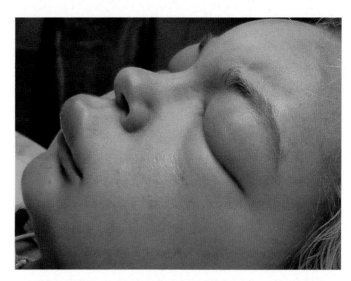

FIGURE 143-4 Severe angioedema around the eyes and mouth in a high school girl. (*Courtesy of Dan Stulberg, MD.*)

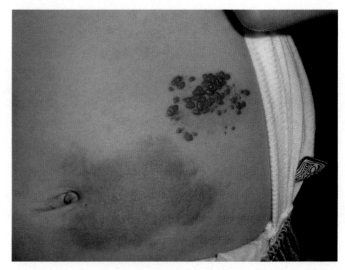

FIGURE 143-5 Urticaria pigmentosa on the abdomen of a 9-month-old child who also has a congenital hemangioma. (*Courtesy of Richard P. Usatine, MD.*)

DIFFERENTIAL DIAGNOSIS

- Insect bites—A good history and physical examination should help to distinguish between insect bites and urticaria.

- Erythema multiforme like urticaria can occur in response to an allergic/immunologic reaction to medications, infections, and neoplasms. The classic lesion of erythema multiforme is the target lesion in which there is disruption of the epithelium in the center. This disruption may be a vesicle, bulla, or erosion. Do not confuse annular lesions or concentric rings with erythema multiforme if the epidermis is intact, (**Figure 143-12** is not EM) (see Chapter 170, Erythema Multiforme).

- Urticarial vasculitis typically has lesions that last longer than 24 hours. The lesions are found more commonly on the lower extremities and when they heal they often leave a hyperpigmented areas. Causes range from a hypersensitivity vasculitis, such as Henoch–Schönlein purpura, to underlying connective tissue disease (**Figure 143-13**).[1]

- Mast cell releasability syndromes are syndromes in which there are too many mast cells in the skin or other organs of the body. These include cutaneous mastocytosis and urticaria pigmentosa (**Figures 143-5** and **143-6**).

- Pruritic urticarial papules and plaques of pregnancy can be differentiated from urticaria in pregnancy because the eruption remains fixed and increases in intensity until delivery (**Figure 143-14**) (see Chapter 71, Pruritic Urticarial Papules and Plaques of Pregnancy).

- Pemphigoid gestationis can have lesions that are urticarial. However it also has bullae that distinguish it from urticaria and of course the patient is pregnant or postpartum (see Chapter 72, Pemphigoid Gestationis).

MANAGEMENT

- Nonpharmacologic therapy
  - Avoid any causative agent, medication, stimulus, or antigen if found. SOR **B**
  - This may include an elimination diet or stopping a suspicious medication. ACE inhibitors are especially prone to causing angioedema (**Figure 143-3**).
  - In chronic urticaria, patients may benefit from avoidance of potential urticarial precipitants such as aspirin, NSAIDS, opiates, and alcohol.
  - Look for sources of chronic infections such as dental infections and tinea pedis. Treat these as it is possible, but unproven, that these could contribute to the chronic urticaria. SOR **C**
  - Stop all unnecessary OTC medications, supplements, and vitamins in chronic urticaria.
  - Stress reduction techniques may help in chronic urticaria but this is unproven. SOR **C**

- Antihistamines
  - There are a number of studies that show that nonsedating H1 antagonists do help control chronic idiopathic urticaria.[3,4] SOR **A**

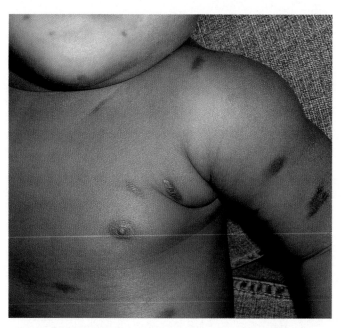

FIGURE 143-6 Urticaria pigmentosa in a 4-month-old black boy. His lesions started on day two of life and have proliferated. He has a positive Darier's sign in which stroking a lesion results in edema. (*Courtesy of Richard P. Usatine, MD.*)

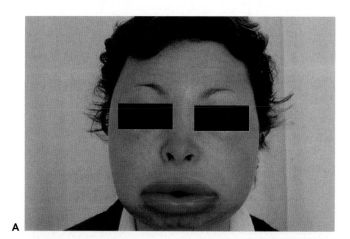

A

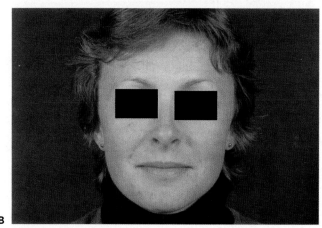

B

FIGURE 143-7 Hereditary angioedema: (A) Severe edema of the face during an episode, leading to grotesque disfigurement. (B) Angioedema will subside within hours. The patient had a positive family history and had multiple similar episodes including colicky abdominal pain. (*With permission from Fitzpatrick's Color Atlas and Synopsis of Clinical Dermatology, 5th ed, 2005. New York: McGraw-Hill.*)

- All patients should be offered the choice of at least two nonsedating H1 antagonists because responses and tolerance vary between individuals.[5] SOR Ⓐ
- A sedating antihistamine at night may help patients sleep better, although they probably add little to existing H1 receptor blockade.[5]
- The addition of an H2 antagonist may give better control of urticaria than H1 antagonists alone, although a benefit is not always seen.[5] SOR Ⓑ In one study, adding H2 blockers to H1 antagonists resulted in improvement of certain cutaneous outcomes for patients presenting with acute allergic syndromes to an emergency department.[6] SOR Ⓑ
- When initial antihistamines are not working, consider doxepin, an antidepressant and potent H1 antagonist.[7] SOR Ⓑ Its use is limited by the side effects of sedation and dry mouth. Start with 10 mg of doxepin in the evening and titrate up as needed and tolerated.

- Corticosteroids
  - Oral corticosteroids should be restricted to short courses for severe acute urticaria or angioedema affecting the mouth (e.g., prednisone 60 mg/d for 3–4 days in adults).[5,8] SOR Ⓑ
  - Short tapering courses of oral steroids over 3 to 4 weeks may be necessary for urticarial vasculitis and severe delayed pressure urticaria.
  - Long-term oral corticosteroids should not be used in chronic urticaria except in very selected cases under specialist supervision.[5]
  - A randomized controlled trial showed that clobetasol 0.05% in a foam formulation was safe and effective in the short-term treatment of patients with delayed pressure urticaria.[9] SOR Ⓑ

- Others
  - Epinephrine is valuable in severe acute urticaria or angioedema especially if there is a suspicion of airway compromise or anaphylaxis.
  - Immunosuppressive therapies for autoimmune urticaria should be restricted to patients with disabling disease who have not responded to optimal conventional treatments.[5]
  - The evidence for leukotriene modifiers in the treatment of urticaria is poor. SOR Ⓒ

PATIENT EDUCATION

In most cases we are not able to find the cause of urticaria. This is especially true for chronic urticaria. Fortunately, most chronic urticaria will subside over time and there are medicines to treat the condition until it runs its course. If one medication does not work, keep your follow-up visits to try other medications. Carefully observe for causative agents.

FIGURE 143-8 Cholinergic urticaria showing small wheals. (*Courtesy of Philip C. Anderson, MD.*)

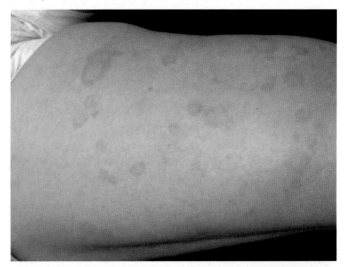

FIGURE 143-9 Chronic urticaria with annular urticarial plaques. (*Courtesy of Richard P. Usatine, MD.*)

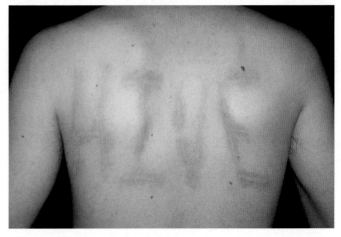

FIGURE 143-10 Dermatographism in a 21-year-old man with chronic urticaria. Note the exaggerated triple reaction. (*Courtesy of Richard P. Usatine, MD.*)

FOLLOW-UP

Follow-up is especially needed when the urticaria/angioedema persists or recurs.

PATIENT RESOURCES

eMedicineHealth.com is a consumer health information site with this information—**http://www.emedicinehealth.com/hives_and_angioedema/article_em.htm.**

PROVIDER RESOURCES

Allergy Resource Center by emedicine—**http://www.emedicine.com/rc/rc/pfeatured/i25/allergy.htm.**

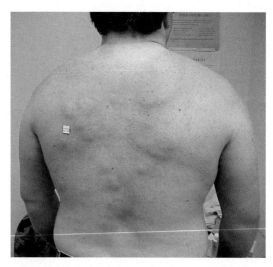

FIGURE 143-11 Angioedema and urticaria of the back. The thicker deeper wheals are angioedema. (*With permission from Milgrom EC, Usatine RP, Tan RA, Spector SL. Practical Allergy 2003, Philadelphia: Elsevier Dan Stulberg, MD.*)

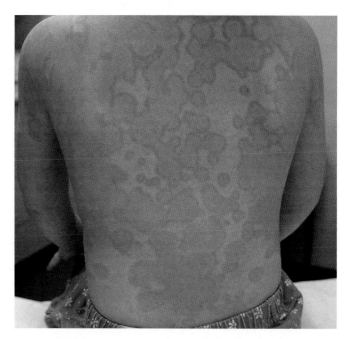

FIGURE 143-12 Giant urticaria. While this appears to have targets the real target lesions of erythema multiforme have a central lesion and have a scaling or bullous component affecting the epidermis. The history suggests that this may have been a serum sickness type reaction. (*With permission from Milgrom EC, Usatine RP, Tan RA, Spector SL. Practical Allergy, Elsevier, Inc. Philadelphia and Dan Stulberg, MD.*)

REFERENCES

1. Baxi S, Dinakar C. Urticaria and angioedema. *Immunol Allergy Clin North Am.* 2005;25:353–367, vii.

2. Usatine RP. Urticaria and Angioedema. In: Milgrom E, Usatine RP, Tan R, Spector S, eds. *Practical Allergy*. Philadelphia, PA: Elsevier, 2003.

3. Finn AF, Jr., Kaplan AP, Fretwell R, Qu R, Long J. A double-blind, placebo-controlled trial of fexofenadine HCl in the treatment of chronic idiopathic urticaria. *J Allergy Clin Immunol.* 1999;104: 1071–1078.

4. Ortonne JP, Grob JJ, Auquier P, Dreyfus I. Efficacy and safety of desloratadine in adults with chronic idiopathic urticaria: A randomized, double-blind, placebo-controlled, multicenter trial. *Am J Clin Dermatol.* 2007;8:37–42.

5. Grattan C, Powell S, Humphreys F. Management and diagnostic guidelines for urticaria and angio-oedema. *Br J Dermatol.* 2001; 144:708–714.

6. Lin RY, Curry A, Pesola GR, et al. Improved outcomes in patients with acute allergic syndromes who are treated with combined H1 and H2 antagonists. *Ann Emerg Med.* 2000;36:462–468.

7. Goldsobel AB, Rohr AS, Siegel SC, et al. Efficacy of doxepin in the treatment of chronic idiopathic urticaria. *J Allergy Clin Immunol.* 1986;78:867–873.

8. Pollack CV, Jr., Romano TJ. Outpatient management of acute urticaria: The role of prednisone. *Ann Emerg Med.* 1995;26:547–551.

9. Vena GA, Cassano N, D'Argento V, Milani M. Clobetasol propionate 0.05% in a novel foam formulation is safe and effective in the short-term treatment of patients with delayed pressure urticaria: A randomized, double-blind, placebo-controlled trial. *Br J Dermatol.* 2006;154:353–356.

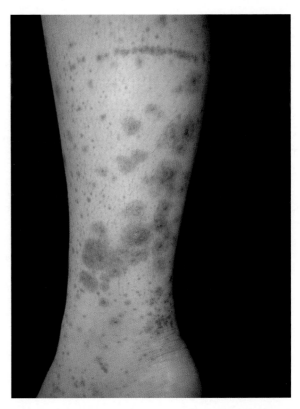

FIGURE 143-13 Henoch Schönlein purpura on the leg of a 20-year-old woman. This is a type of urticarial vasculitis. (*With permission from Milgrom EC, Usatine RP, Tan RA, Spector SL. Practical Allergy. 2003, Philadelphia: Elsevier.*)

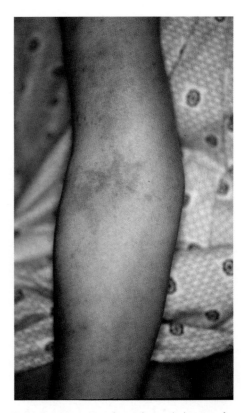

FIGURE 143-14 Pruritic urticarial papules and plaques of pregnancy on the arm of a pregnant woman. The wheals are indistinguishable from other types of urticaria. (*With permission from Milgrom EC, Usatine RP, Tan RA, Spector SL. Practical Allergy. 2003, Philadelphia: Elsevier.*)

144 SEBORRHEIC DERMATITIS

Richard P. Usatine, MD

PATIENT STORY

A 59-year-old man presents with a 3-month history of an itchy rash on his face (**Figures 144-1** and **144-2**). He states that he has had this rash on and off for many years but this is his worst case. He denies any major risk factors for HIV and does not have Parkinson's disease. He has been under more stress lately and has noticed that this rash has flared up in the past when under increased stress. Note the scale visible on the forehead and under the eyebrows and beard. There is also some mild erythema on the cheeks and around the nasolabial folds. The diagnosis of seborrheic dermatitis is made and treatment is begun with appropriate topical agents to treat the inflammation and the malassezia. On the following visit the patient has complete clearance of his seborrheic dermatitis.

EPIDEMIOLOGY

- Seborrhea is most commonly seen in patients aged 20 to 50 years, and mostly in males. The prevalence of seborrhea is approximately 3% to 5% in young adults who are HIV-negative.[1] The prevalence of seborrhea is higher in HIV-positive persons, although the vast majority of persons with seborrhea have a normal immune system.
- Seborrhea is more common in persons with Parkinson's disease.
- Babies can have seborrhea of the scalp (cradle cap).

ETIOLOGY AND PATHOPHYSIOLOGY

Seborrhea (seborrheic dermatitis) is a superficial inflammatory dermatitis that is found in regions with a greater number of pilosebaceous units, which produce sebum. Seborrhea is thought to be caused by an inflammatory hypersensitivity to epidermal, bacterial, or yeast antigens. Persons with seborrhea have a profusion of *Pityrosporum* yeast on the skin. *Pityrosporum* is also called *Malassezia* (e.g., *Malassezia furfur*, *Malassezia ovalis*). This yeast can be a normal part of skin flora; seborrhea is an inflammatory reaction to its presence. Seborrhea is characterized by remissions and exacerbations. The most common precipitating factors are stress, immunosuppression, and cold weather. The treatment of seborrhea should be directed at the inflammation and the *Pityrosporum*.

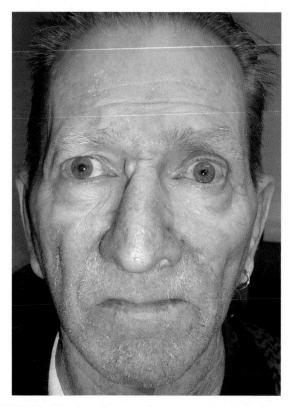

FIGURE 144-1 Seborrheic dermatitis following the typical distribution on the face of a 59-year-old man. Note the prominent scale and erythema on his forehead, glabella, and beard region. (*Courtesy of Richard P. Usatine, MD.*)

DIAGNOSIS

The diagnosis is made on history and physical examination. **Figures 144-1** and **144-2** reveal erythema and scale across the eyebrows, cheeks, and under beard.

CLINICAL FEATURES

* Seborrhea on the face and scalp can be very pruritic.
* Plaques of greasy scale are visible in the seborrheic distribution.
* In dark-skinned individuals, the involved skin and scale may become hyperpigmented (**Figure 144-3**).
* The more severe the seborrhea, the thicker and greasier the scale (**Figure 144-4**).
* Infants may develop seborrhea on the scalp, known as cradle cap (**Figure 144-5**). They may also have seborrhea on the face around the eyebrows (**Figure 144-6**). Some infants have a wider distribution involving the neck creases, armpits, or groin.

TYPICAL DISTRIBUTION

Scalp (i.e., dandruff), eyebrows (**Figures 144-6** and **144-7**), nasolabial creases, forehead, cheeks, around the nose, behind the ears (**Figure 144-8**), and under facial hair (**Figure 144-9**). Seborrhea can also occur over the sternum and in the axillae, submammary folds, umbilicus, groin, and gluteal creases.

LABORATORY STUDIES

HIV test if history is suspicious.

DIFFERENTIAL DIAGNOSIS

* SLE with butterfly rash—rash across bridge of nose in patient with other systemic abnormalities and abnormal blood tests (Chapter 173, Lupus Erythematosus - Systemic and Cutaneous).
* Rosacea—the erythema on the face is often associated with papules, pustules and possibly chalazia or hordeola (Chapter 107, Rosacea).
* Psoriasis —the scale of psoriasis tends to be thicker and distributed over extensor surfaces along with the scalp. Look for signs of nail involvement that support the diagnosis of psoriasis. (Chapter 145, Psoriasis).
* Tinea capitis—usually has hair loss with the scale and erythema. KOH and/or culture can help make the distinction (Chapter 131, Tinea Capitis).

MANAGEMENT

* Treat the *Malassezia* with antifungals:
  ○ Shampoos containing ketoconazole, selenium sulfide or zinc pyrithione (ZPT) are active against the *Malassezia* and are effective in the treatment of moderate to severe dandruff.[2,3] SOR Ⓐ
  ○ Ketoconazole 2% shampoo was found to be superior to zinc pyrithione 1% shampoo when used twice weekly. Ketoconazole

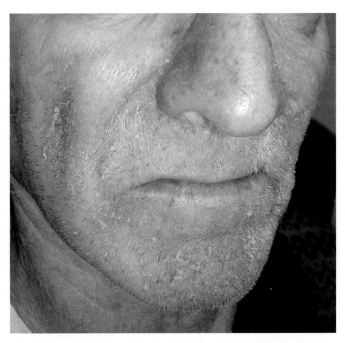

FIGURE 144-2 Close-up of seborrheic dermatitis showing the flaking scale and erythema around the beard region. (*Courtesy of Richard P. Usatine, MD.*)

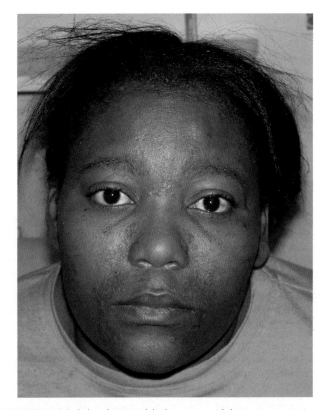

FIGURE 144-3 Seborrhea in a black woman with hyperpigmentation related to the inflammation. Note the prominent involvement in the nasolabial folds. (*Courtesy of Richard P. Usatine, MD.*)

led to a 73% improvement in the total dandruff severity score compared with 67% for ZPT 1% at 4 weeks.[3] SOR **B**

○ Ciclopirox shampoo 1% is effective and safe in the treatment of seborrheic dermatitis of the scalp.[4,5] SOR **A** It is by prescription only and is very expensive.

○ 2% ketoconazole cream, gel, or emulsion is safe and effective for facial seborrheic dermatitis.[6–8] SOR **B**

○ 1% ciclopirox cream is also safe and effective for facial seborrheic dermatitis and is equivalent to 2% ketoconazole cream.[6,9] SOR **B**

○ Oral terbinafine 250 mg daily for 4 weeks is effective for moderate to severe seborrhea.[10,11] SOR **A**

• Treat the inflammation using topical steroids

○ Lotion or solution is preferable on hair-covered area for patient comfort and usability.

○ 1% Hydrocortisone cream or lotion can be used bid to face, scalp, or other affected areas.[8,12] SOR **B**

○ Desonide 0.05% lotion is safe and effective for short-term treatment of seborrheic dermatitis of the face.[13] SOR **B** It is a nonfluorinated low to mid-potency steroid that is higher in potency than 1% hydrocortisone.

○ For moderate to severe seborrhea on the scalp.

■ 0.05% Fluocinonide solution once daily is affordable and beneficial. SOR **C**

■ 0.05% Clobetasol shampoo, solution, spray, or foam work well but are more costly. SOR **C**

OTHER TREATMENTS

• Pimecrolimus cream 1% is an effective and well-tolerated treatment for facial seborrheic dermatitis.[12,14,15] SOR **B** In one study, there was more burning noted with the pimecrolimus than the betamethasone 17-valerate 0.1% cream.[14]

• Metronidazole Gel—two small studies have found different results in the treatment of seborrheic dermatitis on the face. One suggests it works better than the vehicle alone and the other found no statistically significant difference from the placebo.[16,17] SOR **B**

• Tea tree oil 5% shampoo showed a 41% improvement in the quadrant-area-severity score compared with 11% in the placebo. Statistically significant improvements were also observed in the total area of involvement score, the total severity score, and the itchiness and greasiness components of the patients' self-assessments.[18] SOR **B**

• One small RCT (with high drop-out rate) using homeopathic medication consisting of potassium bromide, sodium bromide, nickel sulfate, and sodium chloride for 10 weeks showed significant improvement over placebo.[19] SOR **C**

PATIENT EDUCATION

For improved treatment results, encourage patients to wash the hair and scalp daily with an antifungal shampoo. Some patients fear that washing their hair too often will cause a "dry" scalp and need to understand that the scaling and flaking will improve rather than worsen with more frequent hair washing.

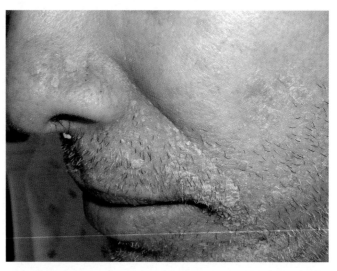

FIGURE 144-4 Severe seborrheic dermatitis on the face of a hospitalized man. The stress of his illness has worsened his otherwise mild seborrhea. (*Courtesy of Richard P. Usatine, MD.*)

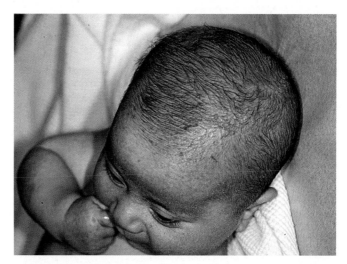

FIGURE 144-5 Cradle cap in an infant that also has atopic dermatitis. (*Courtesy of Richard P. Usatine, MD.*)

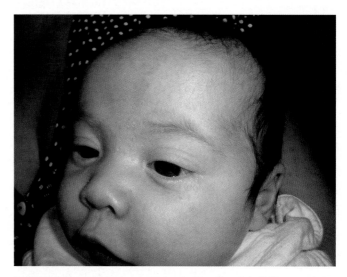

FIGURE 144-6 Mild seborrheic dermatitis with subtle flaking around the eyebrows of a 2-month-old girl who also has cradle cap. (*Courtesy of Richard P. Usatine, MD.*)

FOLLOW-UP

Patients with long-standing and severe seborrhea will appreciate a follow-up visit in most cases. Milder cases can be followed as needed.

PATIENT RESOURCES

VisualDxHealth - good information and photographs:
http://www.visualdxhealth.com/adult/seborrheicDermatitis.htm.
http://www.visualdxhealth.com/adult/dandruff.htm.

PROVIDER RESOURCES

eMedicine
http://www.emedicine.com/derm/topic396.htm.
DermNet NZ
http://dermnetnz.org/dermatitis/seborrhoeic-dermatitis.htm.

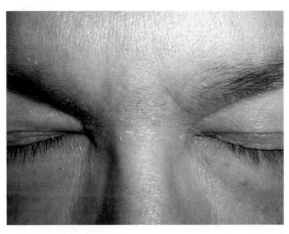

FIGURE 144-7 Seborrheic dermatitis with erythema and scale under the eyebrows and in the glabella region on a young man. (*Courtesy of Richard P. Usatine, MD.*)

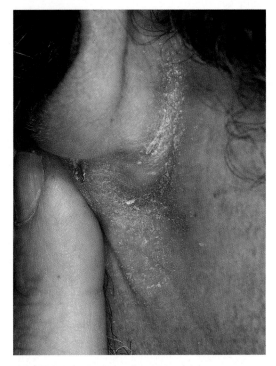

FIGURE 144-8 Seborrheic dermatitis behind the ear in a young woman. This is a good place to look for evidence of seborrhea. (*Courtesy of Richard P. Usatine, MD.*)

REFERENCE

1. Usatine RP. A red rash on the face. *J Fam Pract.* 2003;52:697–699.

2. Danby FW, Maddin WS, Margesson LJ, Rosenthal D. A randomized, double-blind, placebo-controlled trial of ketoconazole 2% shampoo versus selenium sulfide 2.5% shampoo in the treatment of moderate to severe dandruff. *J Am Acad Dermatol.* 1993;29:1008–1012.

3. Pierard-Franchimont C. A multicenter randomized trial of ketoconazole 2% and zinc pyrithione 1% shampoos in severe dandruff and seborrheic dermatitis. *Skin Pharmacol Appl Skin Physiol.* 2002;15(6):434–441.

4. Aly R. Ciclopirox gel for seborrheic dermatitis of the scalp. *Int J Dermatol.* 2003;42(Suppl 1):19–22.

5. Lebwohl M, Plott T. Safety and efficacy of ciclopirox 1% shampoo for the treatment of seborrheic dermatitis of the scalp in the US population: Results of a double-blind, vehicle-controlled trial. *Int J Dermatol.* 2004;43(Suppl 1):17–20.

6. Chosidow O, Maurette C, Dupuy P. Randomized, open-labeled, non-inferiority study between ciclopiroxolamine 1% cream and ketoconazole 2% foaming gel in mild to moderate facial seborrheic dermatitis. *Dermatology.* 2003;206:233–240.

7. Pierard GE, Pierard-Franchimont C, Van CJ, Rurangirwa A, Hoppenbrouwers ML, Schrooten P. Ketoconazole 2% emulsion in the treatment of seborrheic dermatitis. *Int J Dermatol.* 1991;30:806–809.

8. Katsambas A, Antoniou C, Frangouli E, Avgerinou G, Michailidis D, Stratigos J. A double-blind trial of treatment of seborrhoeic dermatitis with 2% ketoconazole cream compared with 1% hydrocortisone cream. *Br J Dermatol.* 1989;121:353–357.

9. Dupuy P, Maurette C, Amoric JC, Chosidow O. Randomized, placebo-controlled, double-blind study on clinical efficacy of ciclopiroxolamine 1% cream in facial seborrhoeic dermatitis. *Br J Dermatol.* 2001;144:1033–1037.

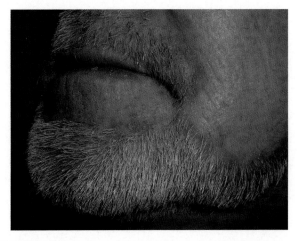

FIGURE 144-9 Seborrhea of the beard and mustache distribution with prominent erythema. (*Courtesy of Richard P. Usatine, MD.*)

10. Vena GA, Micali G, Santoianni P, Cassano N, Peruzzi E. Oral terbinafine in the treatment of multi-site seborrhoic dermatitis: A multicenter, double-blind placebo-controlled study. *Int J Immunopathol Pharmacol.* 2005;18:745–753.

11. Scaparro E, Quadri G, Virno G, Orifici C, Milani M. Evaluation of the efficacy and tolerability of oral terbinafine (Daskil) in patients with seborrhoeic dermatitis. A multicentre, randomized, investigator-blinded, placebo-controlled trial. *Br J Dermatol.* 2001; 144(4):854–857.

12. Firooz A, Solhpour A, Gorouhi F, et al. Pimecrolimus cream, 1%, vs hydrocortisone acetate cream, 1%, in the treatment of facial seborrheic dermatitis: A randomized, investigator-blind, clinical trial. *Arch Dermatol.* 2006;142:1066–1067.

13. Freeman SH. Efficacy, cutaneous tolerance and cosmetic acceptability of desonide 0.05% lotion (Desowen) versus vehicle in the short-term treatment of facial atopic or seborrhoeic dermatitis. *Australas J Dermatol.* 2002;43(3):186–189.

14. Rigopoulos D, Ioannides D, Kalogeromitros D, Gregoriou S, Katsambas A. Pimecrolimus cream 1% vs. betamethasone 17-valerate 0.1% cream in the treatment of seborrhoeic dermatitis. A randomized open-label clinical trial. *Br J Dermatol.* 2004;151: 1071–1075.

15. Warshaw EM, Wohlhuter RJ, Liu A, et al. Results of a randomized, double-blind, vehicle-controlled efficacy trial of pimecrolimus cream 1% for the treatment of moderate to severe facial seborrheic dermatitis. *J Am Acad Dermatol.* 2007;57(2): 257–264.

16. Parsad D, Pandhi R, Negi KS, Kumar B. Topical metronidazole in seborrheic dermatitis—a double-blind study. *Dermatology.* 2001; 202:35–37.

17. Koca R. Is topical metronidazole effective in seborrheic dermatitis? A double-blind study. *Int J Dermatol.* 2003;42(8):632–635.

18. Satchell AC, Saurajen A, Bell C, Barnetson RS. Treatment of dandruff with 5% tea tree oil shampoo. *J Am Acad Dermatol.* 2002; 47(6):852–855.

19. Smith SA BAW J. Effective treatment of seborrheic dermatitis using a low dose, oral homeopathic medication consisting of potassium bromide, sodium bromide, nickel sulfate, and sodium chloride in a double-blind, placebo-controlled study. *Altern Med Rev.* 2002;7(1):59–67.

145 PSORIASIS

Richard P. Usatine, MD

PATIENT STORY

A 33-year-old woman presents with uncontrolled psoriasis for 20 years. In addition to the plaque psoriasis (**Figure 145-1**), she has inverse psoriasis (**Figure 145-2**). Topical ultrahigh-potency steroids and topical calcipotriol have not controlled her psoriasis. The patient was referred for narrowband UVB treatment.

EPIDEMIOLOGY

- 1% to 2% of the American population has plaque psoriasis. Family history has been shown to predict disease occurrence. When both parents are affected by psoriasis, the rate of psoriasis is as high as 50%. When one parent is affected, the rate is 16.4%. Other studies have shown that 36% to 71% of patients with psoriasis have one relative who is also affected by psoriasis.[1]

- Race: higher prevalence in western European and Scandinavian populations.[1]

- Sex: no gender preference.[1]

- Age: Plaque psoriasis first appears during 2 peak age ranges. The first peak occurs in persons aged 16 to 22 years, and the second occurs in persons aged 57 to 60 years.[1]

- Risk factors: family history, smoking, and alcohol.[1]

ETIOLOGY AND PATHOPHYSIOLOGY

- Immune-mediated skin disease, where the T cell plays a pivotal role in the pathogenesis of the disease.

- Langerhans cell (antigen-presenting cells in the skin) migrate from the skin to regional lymph nodes, where they activate T cells that migrate to the skin and release cytokines.

- Cytokines are responsible for epidermal and vascular hyperproliferation and proinflammatory effects.[2]

DIAGNOSIS

Psoriasis has many forms and locations. These nine categories were used to describe psoriasis in a consensus statement of the American Academy of Dermatology (AAD).[3]

- Plaque (80–90% of patients with psoriasis) (**Figures 145-1** and **145-3** to **145-8**).

- Scalp psoriasis (**Figure 145-9**).

- Guttate psoriasis (**Figures 145-10** to **145-12**).

- Inverse psoriasis (**Figures 145-2, 145-13,** and **145-14**).

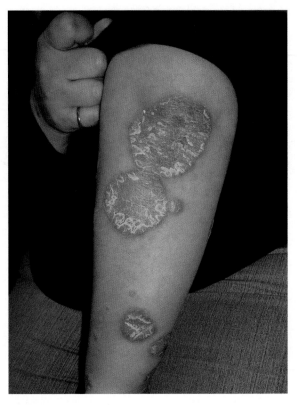

FIGURE 145-1 Typical plaque psoriasis on the elbow and arm. (*Courtesy of Richard P. Usatine, MD.*)

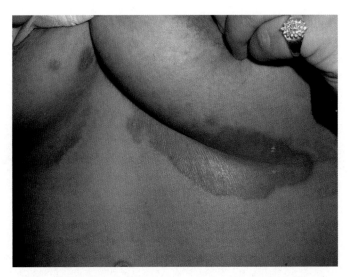

FIGURE 145-2 Inverse psoriasis in the inframammary folds of the patient in **Figure 145-1**. This is not a candida infection. (*Courtesy of Richard P. Usatine, MD.*)

- Palmar-plantar psoriasis (**Figures 145-15** and **145-16**). Also known as palmoplantar psoriasis.
- Erythrodermic psoriasis (**Figure 145-17**).
- Pustular psoriasis—localized and generalized (**Figures 145-18** to **145-20**).
- Nail psoriasis (**Figure 145-21**) (see Chapter 188, Psoriatic Nails).
- Psoriatic arthritis (see Chapter 93, Ankylosing Spondylitis).

Typical distribution in general: elbows, knees, extremities, trunk, scalp, face, ears, hands, feet, genitalia and intertriginous areas, and nails.

Plaque psoriasis:

- White scale on an erythematous raised base with well demarcated borders (**Figure 145-1**). The thickness and extent of the scale is variable.
- Silvery scale with a hyperpigmented base is seen in patients with darker skin (**Figure 145-5**).
- Positive Auspitz sign in which the peeling of the scale produces pinpoint bleeding on the plaque below
- Typical distribution includes the elbows and knees and other extensor surfaces. The plaques can be found from head to toe including the trunk.
- Plaques tend to be symmetrically distributed.
- Plaques can be annular with central clearing (**Figure 145-3**).
- When plaques occur at a site of injury it is known as the Koebner phenomenon (**Figure 145-22**).

Scalp psoriasis:

- Plaque on the scalp that may be seen at the hairline and around the ears (**Figure 145-9**).
- The thickness and extent of the plaques are variable as seen in plaque psoriasis.

Guttate psoriasis:

- Small round plaques that resemble water drops (guttate means like a water drop) (**Figures 145-10** and **145-12**).
- Typical distribution: the trunk and extremities but may include the face and neck.
- Classically described as occurring after strep pharyngitis or another bacterial infection. This is one type of psoriasis that occurs in childhood.

Inverse psoriasis:

- Found in the intertriginous areas of the axilla, groin, inframammary folds, and intergluteal fold. It can also be seen below the pannus or within adipose folds in obese individuals (**Figures 145-2, 145-3, and 145-14**).
- The name inverse refers to the fact that the distribution is not on extensor surfaces but in areas of body folds.
- Morphologically the lesions have little to no visible scale (**Figures 145-2, 145-13,** and **14**).
- Color is generally pink to red but can be hyperpigmented in dark-skinned individuals.

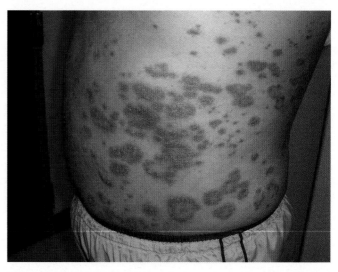

FIGURE 145-3 Plaque psoriasis with an annular configuration. (*Courtesy of Richard P. Usatine, MD.*)

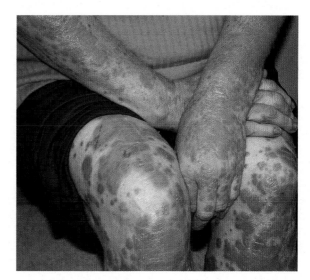

FIGURE 145-4 Inflamed plaque psoriasis with striking erythema. (*Courtesy of Suraj Reddy, MD.*)

Palmar-plantar (palmoplantar) psoriasis:

- Psoriasis that occurs on the plantar aspects of the hands and feet (palms and soles). The psoriasis can also be seen on other parts of the hands and feet.

- Morphologically this can be plaque-like, vesicular, or pustular (**Figures 145-15** and **145-16**). Exfoliation of the skin can occur on the palms and soles.

Erythrodermic psoriasis:

- Erythrodermic psoriasis is generally widespread and erythematosus (**Figure 145-17**).

- Morphologically it can have plaques and erythema or the erythroderma can appears with the desquamation of pustular psoriasis.

- Widespread distribution can impair the important functions of the skin and this can be a dermatologic urgency requiring hospitalization and IV fluids.

Pustular psoriasis:

- Pustular psoriasis comes in localized and generalized types.

- In the generalized type, the skin initially becomes fiery red and tender and the patient experiences constitutional signs and symptoms such as headache, fever, chills, arthralgia, malaise, anorexia, and nausea[1] (**Figure 145-20**). The desquamation that occurs in the generalized form can impair the important functions of the skin predisposing to dehydration and sepsis. This is a dermatologic emergency requiring hospitalization and IV fluids, preferably in a monitored bed with good nursing care.

- Typical distribution: flexural and anogenital (**Figure 145-19**). Less often, facial lesions occur. Pustules may occur on the tongue and subungually, resulting in dysphagia and nail shedding, respectively.

- Time course: within hours, clusters of nonfollicular, superficial 2- to 3-mm pustules may appear in a generalized pattern (**Figure 145-18**). These pustules coalesce within 1 day to form lakes of pus that dry and desquamate in sheets, leaving behind a smooth erythematous surface on which new crops of pustules may appear (**Figure 145-19**). These episodes of pustulation may occur for days to weeks causing the patient severe discomfort and exhaustion. Upon remission of the pustular component, most systemic symptoms disappear; however, the patient may be in an erythrodermic state or may have residual lesions.[1]

Nail psoriasis:

- Nail involvement in psoriasis can lead to pitting, onycholysis, subungual keratosis, splinter hemorrhages, oil spots, and nail loss (**Figure 145-22**) (see Chapter 188, Psoriatic Nails).

Psoriatic arthritis:

- Asymmetric oligoarthritis typically involving the hands, feet, and knees. The arthritis can also be symmetric resembling rheumatoid arthritis. Distal interphalangeal joint involvement may occur but is present only in the minority of cases. There may be inflammation at the insertion of tendons on to bone (enthesopathy).

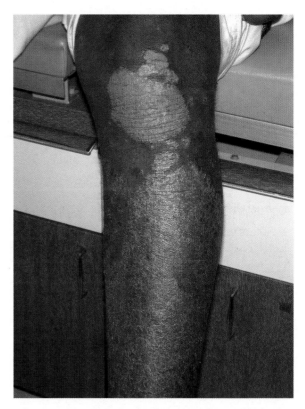

FIGURE 145-5 Plaque psoriasis with silvery scale on a black man. (*Courtesy of Richard P. Usatine, MD.*)

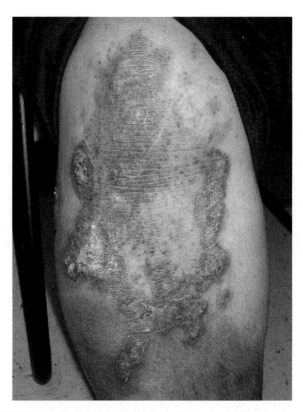

FIGURE 145-6 Psoriasis on the knee of a Hispanic man showing postinflammatory hyperpigmentation. (*Courtesy of Richard P. Usatine, MD.*)

DISEASE SEVERITY

- Moderate-to-severe disease is defined by psoriasis of the palms, soles, head, and neck, or genitalia, and in patients with more than 5% body surface area (BSA) involvement. A person's palm is approximately 1% body surface area and can be used to estimate BSA.

- Patients with psoriatic arthritis may have limited skin disease but require more aggressive systemic therapies.

LABORATORY STUDIES

Laboratory studies are rarely needed. Punch biopsy is used for evaluating atypical cases. Shave biopsy is not adequate for histology. For pustular psoriasis, a 4 mm punch around an intact pustule is preferred.

DIFFERENTIAL DIAGNOSIS

- Cutaneous T-Cell lymphoma can have plaques that resemble psoriasis. In most cases of psoriasis the distribution and nail changes will help to differentiate between these diseases. If needed, a punch biopsy can differentiate between these two conditions (see Chapter 169, Mycosis Fungoides).

- Lichen planus is another papulosquamous disease. Its distribution is more on flexor surfaces and around the wrists and ankles than the elbows and knees (see Chapter 147, Lichen Planus).

- Lichen simplex chronicus is a hyperkeratotic plaque with lichenification. It usually presents with less plaques than psoriasis and is typically found on the posterior neck, ankle, wrist, or lower leg. There is usually more lichenification than thick scale and it is always pruritic (see Chapter 142, Self-Inflicted Dermatoses).

- Nummular eczema presents with coin-like plaques. These are most commonly found on the legs and are usually not as thick as the plaques of psoriasis. Nummular eczema may also have vesicles and bullae. Psoriasis has a different distribution and often includes nail changes (see Chapter 139, Atopic Dermatitis).

- Pityriasis rosea is a self-limited process that has papulosquamous plaques. These plaques are less keratotic and have a collarette scale. Pityriasis rosea frequently has a herald patch (see Chapter 146, Pityriasis Rosea).

- Seborrheic dermatitis of the scalp can closely resemble psoriasis of the scalp especially when it is severe. Psoriasis generally has thicker plaques on the scalp and the plaques often cross the hairline. Seborrhea and psoriasis can both involve the ear. Both conditions respond to topical steroids (see Chapter 144, Seborrhea).

- Syphilis is the great imitator and secondary syphilis can be a papulosquamous eruption that has features similar to psoriasis. Secondary syphilis often involves the palms and soles and the RPR will be positive (see Chapter 209, Syphilis).

- Tinea corporis typically presents with annular plaques with central clearing. Psoriasis can do this as seen in **Figure 145-3**. Tinea corporis usually does not have as many plaques as psoriasis but a KOH preparation can be used to look for fungal elements to distinguish between these two conditions. Tinea corporis or cruris can

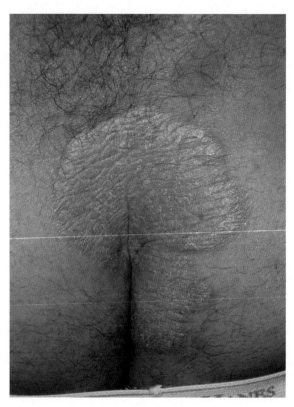

FIGURE 145-7 Plaque psoriasis in the sacral region and intergluteal fold. (*Courtesy of Richard P. Usatine, MD.*)

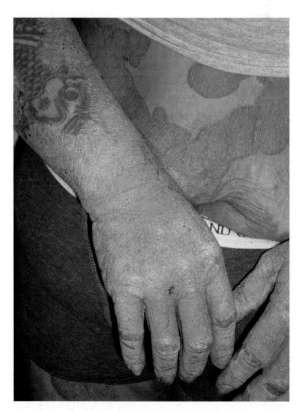

FIGURE 145-8 Thick plaques of psoriasis on the hands and abdomen. (*Courtesy of Richard P. Usatine, MD.*)

resemble inverse psoriasis in the intertriginous areas (see Chapter 132, Tinea corporis).

• Cutaneous candidiasis appears similar to inverse psoriasis when found in intertriginous areas (see Chapter 130, Mucocutaneous Candidiasis).

MANAGEMENT

Treat precipitating and underlying factors when these are known. Treat bacterial superinfection when present, with antibiotics. Encourage smoking cessation to all who smoke. Avoid or minimize alcohol use. Stress management techniques can be suggested in patients whom admit that stress is an important factor in worsening their condition. Use preventive techniques as much as possible by avoiding known precipitants.

Patient perception of their disease and expectations for therapy are as important as the evidence and recommendations that follow. Some patients are willing to live with some skin changes rather than go on systemic treatment while others want everything done with a goal of 100% clearance. Therefore, therapeutic choices are made in conjunction with patient's values and their life situation (economics and time issues surrounding treatment options).

Choice of topical vehicles:

• An ointment has a petrolatum base and will penetrate thick scale best.

• An emollient cream has some of the advantages of an ointment but is cosmetically more appealing to patients who find a basic ointment to be too greasy.

• Some patients prefer cream to avoid the oily feel of ointment even though it is less effective in general than an ointment.

• Lotions and foams are good for hair-bearing areas but where some moisturizing is desired.

• Steroid solutions work well for psoriasis of the scalp.

• New foam preparations have rapid absorption and are cosmetically appealing. These tend to be more expensive at this time.

Topical treatments:

• Research supports potent topical steroids as first-line therapy. [4] SOR Ⓐ Clobetasol is an ultra high potency steroid that is generic and comes in many vehicles for use on the body and scalp. A meta-analysis of the studies with clobetasol demonstrated 68% to 89% of patients had clear improvement or complete healing. [5] SOR Ⓐ

• Comparable efficacy has been shown for topical calcipotriene (vitamin D analogue) and tazarotene (retinoid) with a slight increase in adverse effects for tazarotene. [4] SOR Ⓐ

• Combination of topical steroids and calcipotriene or tazarotene is the most promising current topical treatment. It seems to have increased efficacy and fewer side effects. [4,5] SOR Ⓐ

  ○ One new expensive topical preparation combines betamethasone and calcipotriene to be applied once daily.

  ○ Another option is to prescribe clobetasol in the morning and calcipotriene in the evening for 2 to 4 weeks and then switch to clobetasol qd to bid on the weekends and calcipotriene qd to bid on the weekdays.

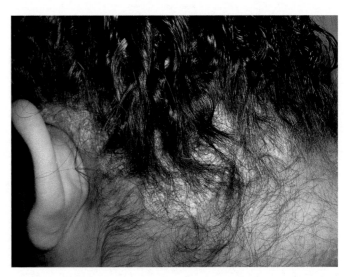

FIGURE 145-9 Scalp psoriasis. (*Courtesy of Richard P. Usatine, MD.*)

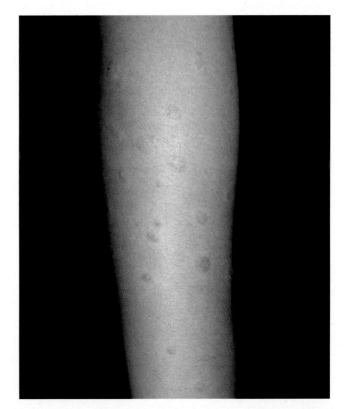

FIGURE 145-10 Guttate psoriasis in a 11-year-old girl that started 2 weeks after a strep pharyngitis. Note the typical drop-like (guttate) lesions on the arm. (*Courtesy of Richard P. Usatine, MD.*)

- The same pattern of clobetasol qd to bid on the weekends can be prescribed with tazarotene qd to bid on the weekdays.
- Clobetasol in the morning and tazarotene in the evening is a good combination to reduce irritation and increased efficacy.[5] SOR **A**

- Two trials randomized potent steroid treatment responders to either an intermittent maintenance regime (three applications each weekend) or to no maintenance. The results of more than 6 months indicate that patients receiving maintenance therapy were more than three times as likely to stay in remission.[6] SOR **B**

- Older treatments still in use include topical coal tar and topical anthralin.[1,5] Evidence does not support the use of coal tar alone or in combination at this time.[5] SOR **A** Topical anthralin is messy and not practical for long-term use.[5]

- Topical calcineurin inhibitors previously approved for eczema are being studied for use in psoriasis. Tacrolimus ointment seems most effective in treating psoriasis of the face and intertriginous areas where the skin is thin. Clinical trials suggest that tacrolimus (0.1 %) ointment twice a day produces a good response in a majority of patients with facial and intertriginous (inverse) psoriasis.[7–9] SOR **B**

- Emollients and keratolytics are safe and probably beneficial as adjunctive treatment. SOR **C**

- Intralesional steroids may help small plaques resolve. Use triamcinolone acetonide 5 to 10 mg/cc injected with a 27-gauge needle into the plaque. SOR **C**

Phototherapy:

- Is indicated in the presence of extensive and widespread disease (practically defined as more lesions than can be easily counted) and psoriasis not responding to topical therapy.[1]

- Narrowband UVB is more effective than broadband UVB and approaches psoralen and UVA (PUVA) in efficacy for the treatment of psoriasis in patients with skin types I–III.[10] SOR **A**

- At present, there are no predictors of the type(s) of psoriasis most responsive to narrowband UVB.[10]

- 63% to 80% of patients with psoriasis will clear with a course of narrowband UVB with equivalent relapse rates compared with PUVA.[10]

- Lack of requirement for psoralen and convenience suggests that narrowband UVB could be considered as the first-line phototherapy option with PUVA reserved for treatment failures.[10]

- Methotrexate pretreatment (15 mg per week × 3) allowed physicians to clear psoriasis in fewer phototherapy sessions than when phototherapy was administered alone in one study.[11]

Systemic:

- When topical agents and phototherapy fail, systemic agents or biologic agents are the next step.

- These agents are especially valuable in patients with psoriatic arthritis and cutaneous findings and may be started early in the course of treatment.

- Do not use systemic corticosteroid therapy for psoriasis. Pustular flares of disease may be provoked and these flares can be fatal[1] (**Figure 145-18**).

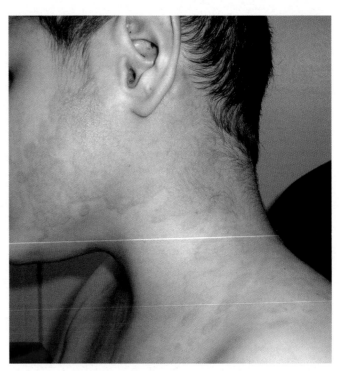

FIGURE 145-11 The salmon patches of guttate psoriasis in a 7-year-old boy with prominent neck, ear, and scalp involvement. This started 2 weeks after a strep pharyngitis. (*Courtesy of Richard P. Usatine, MD.*)

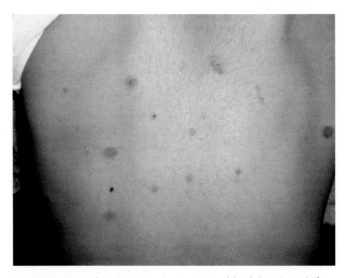

FIGURE 145-12 Guttate psoriasis in a 6-year-old girl that started after she recovered from a strep pharyngitis. Note the drop-like plaques on the back. (*Courtesy of Richard P. Usatine, MD.*)

- Methotrexate, cyclosporine and oral retinoids can cause birth defects so appropriate counseling, contraception, and testing should accompany therapy with these agents.

- Methotrexate (oral): Given as a weekly dose of 5 to 15 mg per week depending upon response and side effects.[12] SOR **A** Pretreatment laboratories should include Hepatitis B and C serologies. Need to follow CBC, differential, LFT's, chemistry profile, UA regularly. Patients should take folic acid 1 mg/day to prevent some of the possible adverse effects of methotrexate. May switch patient to another agent as the cumulative dose of methotrexate approaches 1.5 g to avoid performing a liver biopsy.[12] In one study, no significant differences in efficacy were found between methotrexate and cyclosporine for the treatment of moderate-to-severe psoriasis.[13] For methotrexate, reliable contraceptive methods should be used during and for at least 3 months after therapy in both men and women.[5]

- Cyclosporine (oral): For severe psoriasis, 1.25 mg/kg per day proved to be significantly more effective than placebo. An increase in serum creatinine level that required intervention occurred in 3.4% of cyclosporine treatment cycles; 2.5 and 5 mg/kg per day was significantly superior to etretinate.[14] SOR **A** Cyclosporine can be used for long-term therapy in patients with severe psoriasis for up to 2 years maximum.[5]

- Oral retinoids: Acitretin (Soriatane) is a potent systemic retinoid used for psoriasis.[15] SOR **A** Low-dose acitretin therapy (25 mg/d) seems to be better tolerated and associated with fewer abnormalities found after laboratory testing and fewer adverse effects than the 50 mg/d dosage.[15] Best to avoid use in women capable of pregnancy.

Biologic agents

- Before starting therapy, obtain a PPD. These agents can reactivate dormant TB.

- Etanercept (subcutaneous): For adults the dose is 50 mg twice weekly for 3 months then 50 mg weekly thereafter.[5] SOR **A** This agent is especially valuable in patients with psoriatic arthritis as well as psoriasis vulgaris.[5] SOR **A**.

- Other biologic agents to consider include alefacept (intramuscular or intravenous push), efalizumab (subcutaneous), infliximab (intravenous 2- to 3-hour infusion). All these agents can be beneficial but carry risks of severe infections.[5] SOR **A**

- Recommendations for the use of etanercept in psoriasis have been made by a European dermatology expert group consensus. They recommend patients are initiated on the 50 mg twice-weekly dose until remission is achieved (maximum 24 weeks). Before commencing treatment, contraindications, such as infection or previous malignancy (within 5 years), should be ruled out.[16]

- While the biologic agents are all very expensive, insurance often pays and there are patient assistance programs for uninsured patients with limited resources.

Methotrexate versus biologic agents:[12]

- Methotrexate is a very inexpensive medication with more than 40-year track record, but with known potential for hepatotoxicity requiring liver biopsy after 2 to 3 years of continued use (1.5 g) to assess liver damage.

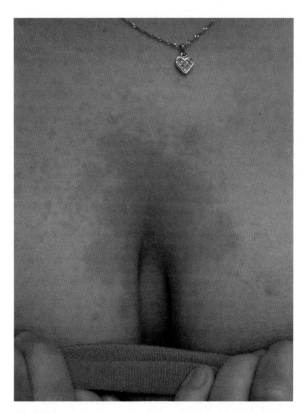

FIGURE 145-13 Inverse psoriasis between the breasts. (*Courtesy of Richard P. Usatine, MD.*)

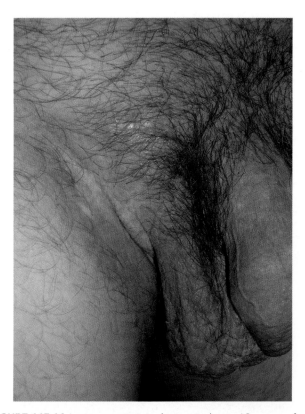

FIGURE 145-14 Inverse psoriasis in the inguinal area. (*Courtesy of Richard P. Usatine, MD.*)

- New biologic agents are engineered proteins with a safer profile than methotrexate; however, they are much more expensive and require parenteral administration. Biologics have the added advantage of longer remissions. The biologic agents are not side effect free and some of the potential side effects, while rare, are quite dangerous.

THERAPY BY TYPE OF PSORIASIS

PLAQUE TYPE

Mild-to-moderate plaque psoriasis: Clobetasol twice daily for 2 weeks. Then clobetasol twice daily on weekends only and calcipotriene twice daily during the weekdays.

Severe plaque form psoriasis: One systematic review found 665 studies dealing with the treatment of severe plaque psoriasis.[17] Photochemotherapy showed the highest average proportion of patients with clearance (70% [6947/9925]) and good response (83% [8238/9925]), followed by UV-B (67.9% [620/913]) and cyclosporine (64% [1030/1609]) therapy.[17] SOR Ⓐ Expert consensus in a meeting following data analysis supported the following sequence for the treatments: UV-B, photochemotherapy, methotrexate, acitretin, and cyclosporine.[17] SOR Ⓒ

SCALP

One head-to-head trial (no pun intended) in scalp psoriasis demonstrated no therapeutic difference between a topical vitamin D derivative and topical potent steroid.[6] Generic fluocinonide solution daily to the scalp is effective and affordable. Calcipotriene daily to scalp also helps but is more expensive. Mineral oil may be used to moisturize and remove scale. Shampoos with tar and/or salicylic acid can help to dissolve and wash away some of the scale.

GUTTATE PSORIASIS

Phototherapy (with or without tar) or photochemotherapy; topical therapies; systemic therapies as needed.[3] SOR Ⓒ Although both antibiotics and tonsillectomy have frequently been advocated for patients with guttate psoriasis, there is no good evidence that either intervention is beneficial.[18]

INVERSE PSORIASIS

High potency topical steroids can be used for inverse psoriasis even though the disease occurs in skinfolds. Topical tacrolimus before bedtime is an alternative alone or with a high potency topical steroid in the morning.

PALMAR-PLANTAR PSORIASIS

For mild disease you may start with topical treatments as in plaque psoriasis. See Chapter 141 for treatment suggestions used for hand dermatitis. For moderate to severe cases, systemic therapy such as oral acitretin or efalizumab (Raptiva) SQ may be needed.

ERYTHRODERMIC/GENERALIZED PSORIASIS

Treatment considerations include hospitalization for dehydration and close monitoring, cyclosporine, methotrexate, oral retinoids, phototherapy, or photochemotherapy.[3] SOR Ⓒ

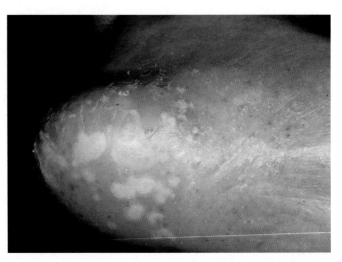

FIGURE 145-15 Palmoplantar psoriasis in a 31-year-old man with erythema, pustules and lakes of pus. Note the brown macules and papules, peeling skin and pustules that are typical of this condition. High-potency topical steroids did not help at all. It is painful for him to walk and systemic therapy has just been started. This is a localized form of pustular psoriasis. (*Courtesy of Jeff Meffert, MD.*)

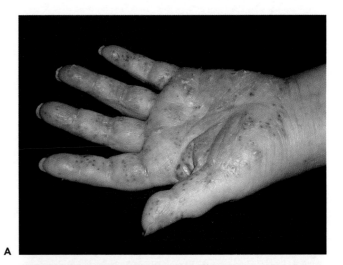

A

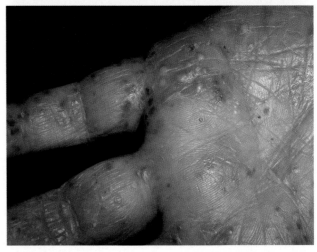

B

FIGURE 145-16 (A) Palmoplantar psoriasis with pustulosis that started 3 months ago on the hands of a 62-year-old woman. (B) Note the erythema, desquamation, brown papules and pustules that are typical of this condition. This is considered to be a localized form of pustular psoriasis. (*Courtesy of Richard P. Usatine, MD.*)

PUSTULAR PSORIASIS

Options include oral retinoids such as isotretinoin or acitretin (depends on sex and age of the patient), methotrexate, cyclosporine, phototherapy, and hospitalization as needed.[3] SOR ⓒ

PATIENT EDUCATION

This is a chronic disease that cannot be cured. There are many methods to control psoriasis. Patients need to develop a relationship with a family physician or dermatologist to control the psoriasis for maximum quality of life.

FOLLOW-UP

Follow-up may need to be frequent for various therapies including cytotoxic drugs, the biologics and light therapy. Well-controlled psoriasis on topical agents does not require frequent follow-up.

PATIENT RESOURCES

The National Psoriasis Foundation—**www.psoriasis.org/**.

PROVIDER RESOURCES

German evidence-based guidelines for the treatment of Psoriasis vulgaris (short version), published in 2007 and free on PubMed Central in English—**http://www.pubmedcentral.nih.gov/articlerender.fcgi?tool=pubmed&pubmedid=17497162.**

Finnish Medical Society Duodecim. Psoriasis. In: EBM Guidelines. Evidence-Based Medicine [Internet]. Helsinki, Finland: Wiley Interscience. John Wiley & Sons; 2005. Available on **http://www.guidelines.gov.**

REFERENCES

1. Lui, H and Mamelak, A. Plaque Psoriasis. http://www.emedicine.com/derm/topic365.htm. Accessed February 1, 2007.

2. Lee MR, Cooper AJ. Immunopathogenesis of psoriasis. *Australas J Dermatol.* 2006;47:151–159.

3. Callen JP, Krueger GG, Lebwohl M, et al. AAD consensus statement on psoriasis therapies. *J Am Acad Dermatol.* 2003;49:897–899.

4. Afifi T, de GG, Huang C, Zhou Y. Topical therapies for psoriasis: Evidence-based review. *Can Fam Physician.* 2005;51:519–525.

5. Nast A, Kopp I, Augustin M, et al. German evidence-based guidelines for the treatment of Psoriasis vulgaris (short version). *Arch Dermatol Res.* 2007;299:111–138.

6. Mason J, Mason AR, Cork MJ. Topical preparations for the treatment of psoriasis: A systematic review. *Br J Dermatol.* 2002;146:351–364.

7. Brune A, Miller DW, Lin P, Cotrim-Russi D, Paller AS. Tacrolimus ointment is effective for psoriasis on the face and intertriginous areas in pediatric patients. *Pediatr Dermatol.* 2007;24:76–80.

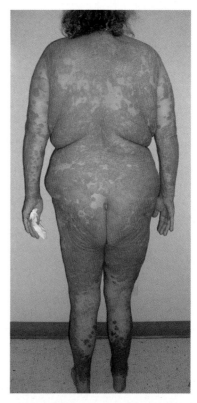

FIGURE 145-17 Erythrodermic psoriasis covering most of the body surface. (*Courtesy of Richard P. Usatine, MD.*)

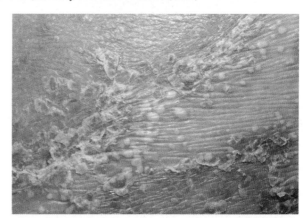

FIGURE 145-18 Pustular psoriasis on the back that occurred when oral prednisone was stopped. (*Courtesy of Jack Resneck, Sr., MD.*)

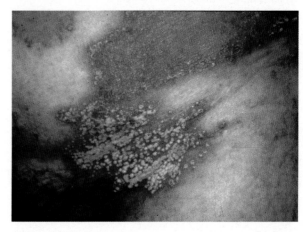

FIGURE 145-19 Localized pustular psoriasis in the groin. (*Courtesy of Jeffrey Meffert, MD.*)

8. Martin EG, Sanchez RM, Herrera AE, Umbert MP. Topical tacrolimus for the treatment of psoriasis on the face, genitalia, intertriginous areas and corporal plaques. *J Drugs Dermatol.* 2006;5: 334–336.

9. Lebwohl M, Freeman AK, Chapman MS, Feldman SR, Hartle JE, Henning A. Tacrolimus ointment is effective for facial and intertriginous psoriasis. *J Am Acad Dermatol.* 2004;51:723–730.

10. Ibbotson SH, Bilsland D, Cox NH, et al. An update and guidance on narrowband ultraviolet B phototherapy: A British Photodermatology Group Workshop Report. *Br J Dermatol.* 2004;151: 283–297.

11. Asawanonda P, Nateetongrungsak Y. Methotrexate plus narrowband UVB phototherapy versus narrowband UVB phototherapy alone in the treatment of plaque-type psoriasis: A randomized, placebo-controlled study. *J Am Acad Dermatol.* 2006;54: 1013–1018.

12. Saporito FC, Menter MA. Methotrexate and psoriasis in the era of new biologic agents. *J Am Acad Dermatol.* 2004;50:301–309.

13. Heydendael VM, Spuls PI, Opmeer BC, et al. Methotrexate versus cyclosporine in moderate-to-severe chronic plaque psoriasis. *N Engl J Med.* 2003;349:658–665.

14. Faerber L, Braeutigam M, Weidinger G, et al. Cyclosporine in severe psoriasis. Results of a meta-analysis in 579 patients. *Am J Clin Dermatol.* 2001;2:41–47.

15. Pearce DJ, Klinger S, Ziel KK, Murad EJ, Rowell R, Feldman SR. Low-dose acitretin is associated with fewer adverse events than high-dose acitretin in the treatment of psoriasis. *Arch Dermatol.* 2006;142:1000–1004.

16. Boehncke WH, Brasie RA, Barker J, et al. Recommendations for the use of etanercept in psoriasis: A European dermatology expert group consensus. *J Eur Acad Dermatol Venereol.* 2006;20: 988–998.

17. Spuls PI, Bossuyt PM, van Everdingen JJ, Witkamp L, Bos JD. The development of practice guidelines for the treatment of severe plaque form psoriasis. *Arch Dermatol.* 1998;134:1591–1596.

18. Owen CM, Chalmers RJ, O'Sullivan T, Griffiths CE. A systematic review of antistreptococcal interventions for guttate and chronic plaque psoriasis. *Br J Dermatol.* 2001;145:886–890.

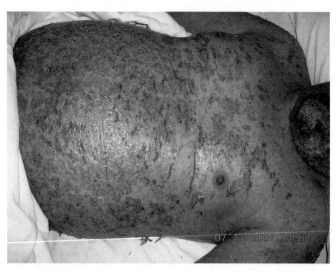

FIGURE 145-20 Generalized pustular psoriasis in a 47-year-old man with fever, exfoliation, and dehydration. This is the 20th time for this patient in his life. His siblings also get severe generalized pustular psoriasis. (*Courtesy of Meng Lu, MD.*)

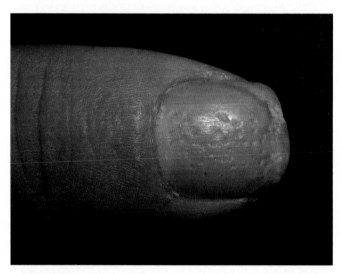

FIGURE 145-21 Nail pitting from psoriasis. (*Courtesy of Richard P. Usatine, MD.*)

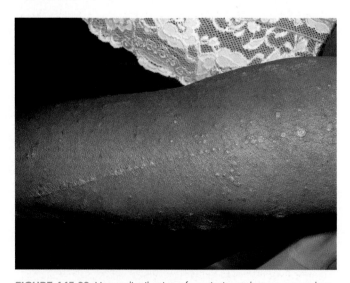

FIGURE 145-22 Linear distribution of psoriasis on the arm secondary to the Koebner phenomenon. (*Courtesy of Richard P. Usatine, MD.*)

146 PITYRIASIS ROSEA

David Henderson, MD
Richard P. Usatine, MD

PATIENT STORY

A 17-year-old young woman is brought to the office by her mom because of a rash that appeared 3 weeks ago for no apparent reason (**Figures 146-1** to **146-3**). She was feeling well and the rash is only occasionally pruritic. With and without mom in the room, the young woman denied sexual activity. The diagnosis of pityriasis rosea was made by the clinical appearance even though there was no obvious herald patch. The collarette scale was visible and the distribution was consistent with pityriasis rosea. The young woman and her mom were reassured that this would resolve spontaneously. At a subsequent visit for a college physical the skin was found to be completely clear with no scarring.

EPIDEMIOLOGY

- Pityriasis rosea is a papulosquamous eruption of unknown etiology.[1]

- It occurs throughout the life cycle. It is most commonly seen between the ages of 10 and 35 years.[2]

- The peak incidence is between 20 and 29 years of age.[1]

- The gender distribution is essentially equal.[1]

- The rash is most prevalent in winter months.[3]

ETIOLOGY AND PATHOPHYSIOLOGY

- The cause of pityriasis rosea is unknown, although numerous causes have been proposed.

- It has long been suspected that it may have a viral etiology because a viral-like prodrome often occurs prior to the onset of the rash. Human herpesvirus 7 has been proposed as a cause, but numerous studies have failed to demonstrate conclusive supportive evidence.[1]

- *Chlamydia pneumoniae, mycoplasma pneumoniae,* and *Legionella pneumophila* have been proposed as potential etiologic agents, but studies have not demonstrated any significant rise in antibody levels against any of these pathogens in patients with pityriasis rosea.[1]

- Pityriasis rosea may rarely occur as the result of a drug reaction. Documented drug reactions that have produced a pityriasis rosea-like eruption include barbiturates, captopril, clonidine, interferon, and the Hepatitis B vaccine.[1]

DIAGNOSIS

CLINICAL FEATURES

- In approximately 20% to 50% of cases, the rash of pityriasis rosea is preceded by a viral-like illness consisting of upper respiratory or gastrointestinal symptoms.

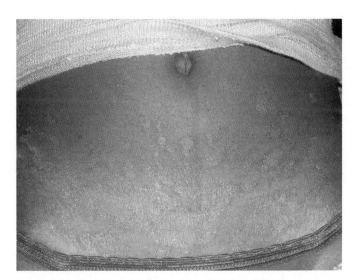

FIGURE 146-1 Pityriasis rosea in a 17-year-old young woman. Lesions are often concentrated in the lower abdominal area. (*Courtesy of Richard P. Usatine, MD.*)

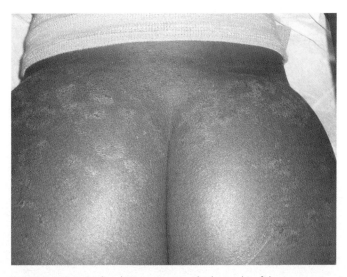

FIGURE 146-2 Scaling lesions seen on the buttocks of the same young woman. Note how some of the lesions are annular. (*Courtesy of Richard P. Usatine, MD.*)

- This is followed by the appearance of a *herald patch* in 17% of cases[3] (**Figure 146-4**).

- The herald patch is a solitary, oval, flesh-colored to salmon-colored lesion with scaling at the border. It often occurs on the trunk, and is generally 2 to 10 cm in diameter (**Figure 146-4**).

- One to two weeks after the appearance of the herald patch, other lesions appear on the trunk (**Figures 146-5 to 146-7**) and upper extremities (**Figure 146-8**).

- These lesions vary from oval macules to slightly raised plaques, 0.5 to 2 cm in size. They are salmon colored (or hyperpigmented in individuals with dark skin), and typically have a collarette of scaling at the border (**Figure 146-3**). It is common for some of the lesions to appear annular with central clearing.

- In many cases, the herald patch has resolved by the time the rest of the exanthem erupts which can make the diagnosis more difficult.

- There are no systemic symptoms.

- Itching occurs in approximately 25% of patients.

- The exanthem resolves in 8 weeks in 80% of patients.[1] However, it can last up to 3 to 5 months.[2]

TYPICAL DISTRIBUTION

- The rash is bilaterally symmetrical, generally most dense on the trunk, but also involves the upper and lower extremities.

- The lesions follow the cleavage, or Langer's lines, and may create the typical *fir* or *Christmas tree* pattern over the back (**Figure 146-5**). Do not expect to always see a Christmas tree pattern.

- Over the chest, the lesions create a V-shaped pattern, and run transversely over the abdomen (**Figure 146-6**).

- An inverse form has been described, characterized by more intense involvement of the extremities and relative sparing of the trunk (**Figure 146-8**).

LABORATORY STUDIES

Pityriasis rosea is a clinical diagnosis. There are no lab tests that aid in the diagnosis. Biopsy of lesions typically reveals only nonspecific inflammatory changes. It should be noted that secondary syphilis is also a papulosquamous eruption and can be difficult to distinguish from pityriasis rosea on clinical grounds. Therefore, taking a sexual history is important when a diagnosis of pityriasis rosea is being considered. In patients with a history of sexually transmitted diseases, or sexual practices that place them at risk, a blood test for syphilis should be considered (**Figure 146-7**) (see Chapter 209, Syphilis).

DIFFERENTIAL DIAGNOSIS

- Tinea corporis is usually more localized than pityriasis rosea. However, the annular patterns, scale and central clearing of some lesions in pityriasis rosea can mislead the clinician to misdiagnose tinea corporis. Tinea corporis tends to have fewer annular lesions and may have concentric circles rather than a single ring. Microscopy with KOH usually demonstrates branching hyphae (see Chapter 132, Tinea Corporis).

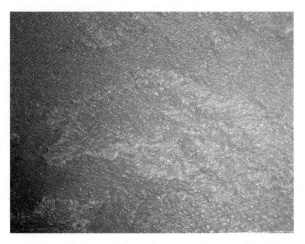

FIGURE 146-3 Close-up of lesion showing collarette scale. Note how the lesions can be annular with some central clearing. (*Courtesy of Richard P. Usatine, MD.*)

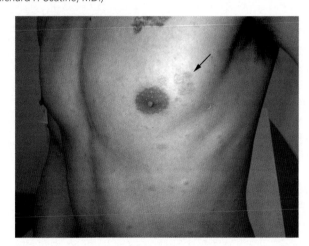

FIGURE 146-4 Pityriasis rosea in a 25-year-old Hispanic man. Arrow points to herald patch. (*Courtesy of Scott Youngquist, MD., Previously published in the Western Journal of Medicine, Reference 2.*)

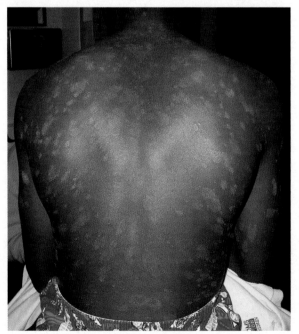

FIGURE 146-5 Pityriasis rosea in a 16-year-old boy. The scaling lesions follow skin lines and resemble a Christmas tree. (*Courtesy of E.J. Mayeaux, Jr., MD.*)

- Tinea versicolor has a distribution similar to pityriasis rosea, but is not associated with a herald patch. The pattern of scaling noted is generally more diffuse and not annular. Microscopy with KOH demonstrates the *spaghetti and meatball* pattern typical of Pityrosporum (see Chapter 135, Tinea Versicolor).

- Secondary syphilis is also a papulosquamous eruption. Lesions are often found on the palms and soles which is not the case in pityriasis rosea; however, the two conditions cannot always be accurately distinguished on clinical grounds and so a blood test for syphilis is indicated if there is a significant doubt in the diagnosis (**Figure 146-7**) (see Chapter 209, Syphilis).

- Nummular eczema has coin-like areas of scale that can resemble pityriasis rosea. The scale is not collarette and nummular eczema has a predilection for the legs, an area that is less often involved with pityriasis rosea (see Chapter 139, Atopic Dermatitis).

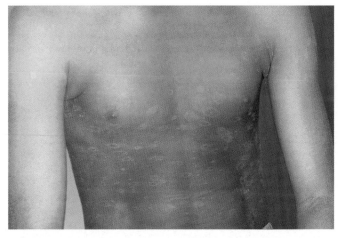

FIGURE 146-6 Pityriasis rosea in a 12-year-old boy showing classic scaling lesions across the chest and abdomen. Small annular lesions are visible. (*Courtesy of Jeffrey Meffert, MD.*)

MANAGEMENT

- Pityriasis rosea often requires no treatment at all other than reassurance.

- Topical steroids and oral diphenhydramine may be used to relieve itching when there is pruritus involved. SOR **C**

- One study found oral erythromycin to be effective in treating patients with pityriasis rosea,[4] while another study did not find erythromycin to be better than placebo.[5] SOR **B**

- Azithromycin did not cure pityriasis rosea in a study of children with this condition.[6]

- A Cochrane systematic review found inadequate evidence for efficacy for most treatments for pityriasis rosea.[7] Based on one small RCT, they noted that oral erythromycin may be effective in treating the rash and decreasing the itch.[4,7] The authors stated that this result should be treated with caution since it comes from only one small RCT.[4,7] SOR **B**

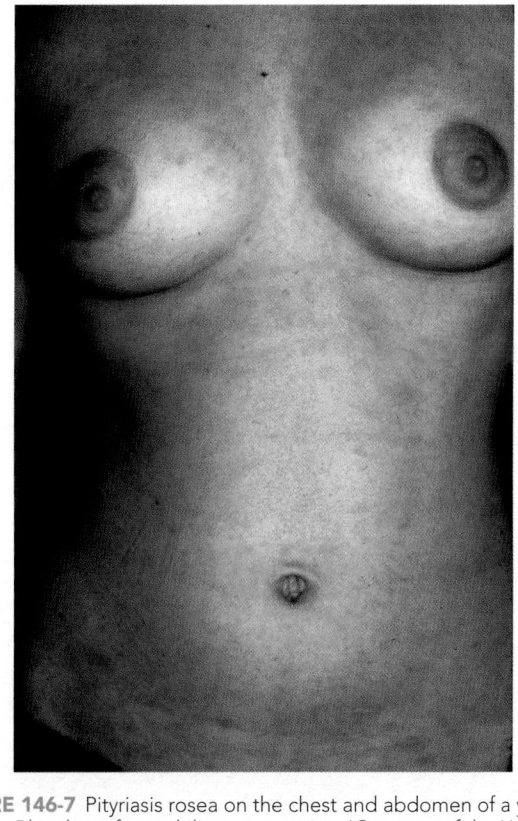

PATIENT EDUCATION

- Patients are often concerned about the duration of the rash and whether they are contagious. They should be reassured that pityriasis rosea is self-limited and not truly contagious. Although there have been reported clusters of pityriasis rosea in settings where people are living in close quarters (e.g., dormitories), it is not considered to be contagious. It has a reported recurrence rate of only 2%.[4]

FIGURE 146-7 Pityriasis rosea on the chest and abdomen of a young woman. Blood test for syphilis was negative. (*Courtesy of the University of Texas Health Sciences Center, Division of Dermatology.*)

FOLLOW-UP

- Patients should be instructed to follow up if the rash persists for longer than 3 months as reevaluation and consideration of an alternate diagnosis may be prudent.

REFERENCES

1. Stulberg DH, Wolfrey J, Pityriasis rosea. *Am Fam Physician*. 2004;69:87–92,94.

2. Youngquist S, Usatine R. It's beginning to look a lot like Christmas. *West J Med*. 2001;175(4):227–228.

3. Habif TP, Clinical Dermatology, 4th ed. St Louis, MO: Mosby; 2004:246–248.

4. Sharma PK, Yadav TP, Gautam RK, Taneja N, Satyanarayana L. Erythromycin in pityriasis rosea: A double-blind, placebo-controlled clinical trial. *J Am Acad Dermatol*. 2000;42(2 Pt 1):241–244.

5. Rasi A, Tajziehchi L, Savabi-Nasab S. Oral erythromycin is ineffective in the treatment of pityriasis rosea. *J Drugs Dermatol*. 2008;7(1):35–38.

6. Amer H, Fischer H. Azithromycin does not cure pityriasis rosea. *Pediatrics*. 2006;117(4):1702–1705.

7. Chuh AA, Dofitas BL, Comisel GG, Reveiz L, Sharma V, Garner SE, et al. Interventions for pityriasis rosea. *Cochrane Database Syst Rev*. 2007;(2):CD005068.

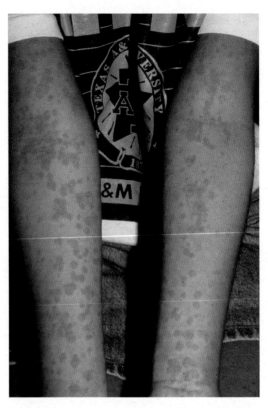

FIGURE 146-8 Pityriasis rosea on the arms with prominent erythematous lesions. (*Courtesy of the University of Texas Health Sciences Center, Division of Dermatology.*)

147 LICHEN PLANUS

Robert Kraft, MD
Richard P. Usatine, MD

PATIENT STORY

A 38-year-old Hispanic woman presents with a rash on her forearms, wrists, ankle, and back (**Figures 147-1 to 147-4**). She states the rash is mildly itchy and she does not like the way it looks. She would like some medication to make this better. Lichen planus (LP) was diagnosed and clobetasol was prescribed to keep the LP under better control.

EPIDEMIOLOGY

- LP is an inflammatory dermatosis of skin or mucous membranes that occurs in approximately 1% of all new patients seen at health care clinics.[1]
- Most cases occur between ages 30 and 60; LP can occur at any age.[1,2]
- There may be a slight female predominance.[2–4]

ETIOLOGY AND PATHOPHYSIOLOGY

- Usually idiopathic, thought to be a cell-mediated immune response to an unknown antigen.[2,3,5]
- Possible HLA-associated genetic predisposition.[2]
- Lichenoid-type reaction may be associated with medications (e.g., ACE inhibitors, thiazide-type diuretics, tetracycline, chloroquine), metals (e.g., gold, mercury), or infections (e.g., secondary syphilis).[2,5]
- Associated with liver disease, especially related to hepatitis C virus.[2,5]
- LP may be found with other diseases of altered immunity (e.g., ulcerative colitis, alopecia areata, myasthenia gravis).[1]
- Malignant transformation has been reported in ulcerative oral lesions in men.[1]

DIAGNOSIS

CLINICAL FEATURES[2,5]

- Classically, the five Ps of LP are planar, purple, polygonal, pruritic, and papular (**Figures 147-1 to 147-5**).
- These well-demarcated flat-topped violaceous lesions are often covered by lacy, reticular white lines (called Wickham's striae or Wickham's lines) (**Figure 147-4B**).
- An initial lesion is usually located on the flexor surface of the limbs, such as the wrists, followed by a generalized eruption with maximal spreading within 2 to 16 weeks.[1]
- Lesions are more often hyperpigmented rather than purple or pink in dark-skinned persons (**Figures 147-6** and **147-7**).
- Skin variants
  - Hypertrophic—typical papules develop into thicker reddish-brown to purple plaques (**Figures 147-5** and **147-7 to 147-10**)

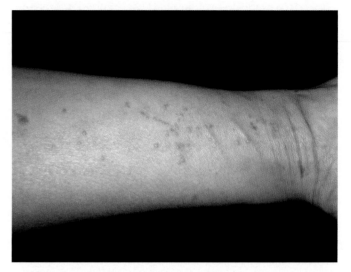

FIGURE 147-1 A 38-year-old Hispanic woman with lichen planus on her wrist. (*Courtesy of Richard P. Usatine, MD.*)

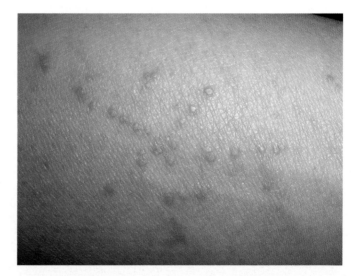

FIGURE 147-2 Close-up of wrist showing linearity of the lesions on the flexor surface. Lesions may be pink rather than purple. (*Courtesy of Richard P. Usatine, MD.*)

most commonly on the foot and shins. Seen more often in black men with hyperpigmented and hypertrophic lesions (**Figure 147-7**).

○ Follicular—pinpoint hyperkeratotic projections often on scalp, may lead to cicatricial alopecia.

○ Vesicular—vesicles or bullae occur alongside the more typical lichen planus lesions.

○ Actinic—typical lesions in sun-exposed areas, such as back of hands and arms.

○ Ulcerative—ulcers develop within typical lesions or start as waxy semitranslucent plaques on palms and soles; may require skin grafting.

• Mucous membrane variants

○ May be reticular (netlike; **Figure 147-11**), atrophic, erosive (**Figures 147-12** and **147-13**), or bullous. It is almost always bilateral.

○ Oral lesions may be asymptomatic or have a burning sensation; pain occurs with ulceration.[1,4,6]

• Genitalia variants

○ Reticular, annular (**Figure 147-14**), papular (**Figure 147-15**), or erosive lesions on penis, scrotum, labia, or vagina.

○ Vulvar/vaginal lesions may be associated with dyspareunia, a burning sensation, and/or pruritus.[1]

○ Vulvar and urethral stenosis can also be present.[1]

• Hair and nail variants; the latter present in 10% of patients.[1]

○ Violaceous, scaly, pruritic papules on the scalp can progress to scarring alopecia. Lichen planopilaris (lichen planus of the scalp) can cause widespread hair loss. (see Chapter 182, Scarring Alopecia).

○ Nail plate thinning results in longitudinal grooving and ridging; rarely destruction of nail fold and nail bed with splintering (**Figure 147-8**).

○ Hyperpigmentation, subungual hyperkeratosis, onycholysis, and longitudinal melanonychia can result from LP.[1]

TYPICAL DISTRIBUTION

Wrists, ankles, lower back, eyelids, shins, scalp, penis, mouth (i.e., buccal mucosa, lateral tongue, and gingival).[2,5]

LABORATORY STUDIES

• Wickham's striae can be accentuated by a drop of oil on the skin plaque and magnification.[5] Not all LP has visible Wickham's striae. This study is rarely needed. If the diagnosis is uncertain, a punch biopsy should be performed.

PUNCH BIOPSY

• Is a valuable method to make as initial diagnosis if the clinical picture is not certain. A biopsy is rarely needed to evaluate for malignant transformation.[5,7]

• Mainly lymphocytic immunoinflammatory infiltrate with hyperkeratosis, increased granular layer and liquefaction of basal cell layer.[2,5]

• Linear fibrin and fibrinogen deposits along basement membrane.[2,5]

• Direct immunofluorescence on biopsy specimen reveals globular deposits of IgM and complement at dermal–epidermal junction.[5]

DIFFERENTIAL DIAGNOSIS

Skin lesions that may be confused with LP:

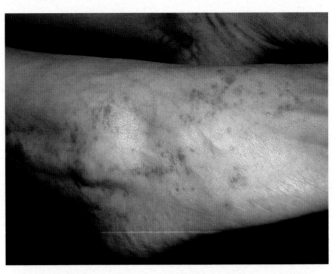

FIGURE 147-3 Ankle of the woman in **Figure 147-1** with typical lichen planus eruption. (*Courtesy of Richard P. Usatine, MD.*)

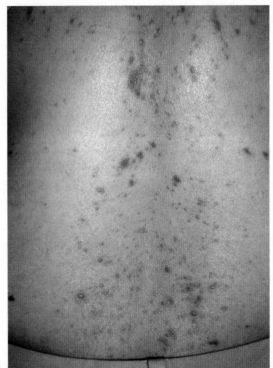

A

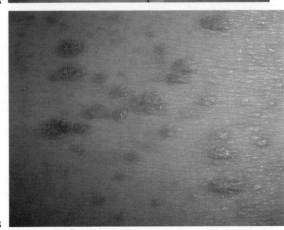

B

FIGURE 147-4 (A) Lichen planus on the back of the woman in **Figure 147-1**. (B) Close up of lesions on the back showing Wickham's striae crossing the flat papules of lichen planus. These lines are white and reticular like a net. (*Courtesy of Richard P. Usatine, MD.*)

- Eczematous dermatitis—"The itch that rashes"; dry skin, itching, often excoriations and lichenification of skin with predilection for flexor surfaces (see Chapter 139, Atopic Dermatitis).

- Psoriasis has more prominent silvery scale and generally located on extensor surfaces.[5] A punch biopsy can be used to distinguish between these two when the clinical picture is not clear (see Chapter 145, Psoriasis).

- Stasis dermatitis—Lower extremity eczematous dermatitis with inflammatory papules and often ulceration, in the setting of chronic venous insufficiency with dependent edema (see Chapter 50, Venous Insufficiency).

- Pityriasis rosea—Herald patch and subsequent pink papules and plaques with long axes along skin lines (Christmas tree pattern) (see Chapter 146, Pityriasis Rosea).

- Chronic cutaneous lupus erythematosus—Bright red sharply demarcated papules with adherent scale. Tend to regress centrally and can be light induced. Generally located on face, scalp, or forearms and hands. Biopsy may be necessary to differentiate (see Chapter 173, Lupus).[5]

- Bowen's disease—Sharply demarcated pink, red, brown, or black scaling or hyperkeratotic macule, papule, or plaque, usually mistaken for eczema or psoriasis, associated with ultraviolet radiation, human papilloma virus (HPV), chemicals, and chronic heat exposure. Biopsy is needed to make the diagnosis (see Chapter 159, Actinic Keratosis and Bowen's Disease).

- Lichen simplex chronicus—Localized confluence of lichenification from excoriation, patients have a strong urge to scratch their skin (see Chapter 142, Self-Inflicted Dermatoses).

- Prurigo nodularis—nodular form of lichen simplex chronicus, brown to red hard, domed nodules from scratching and picking of intense pruritus. Lichen planus is not usually so pruritic (see Chapter 142, Self-Inflicted Dermatoses).

Other mucous membrane lesions that may appear similar:[5]

- Leukoplakia—white adherent patch or plaque to oral mucosa. Less net-like pattern. Biopsy warranted because of the risk of malignancy (see Chapter 41, Leukoplakia).

- Thrush—Removable whitish plaques over an erythematous mucosal surface caused by candida infection, confirmed by potassium hydroxide (KOH) preparation (see Chapter 130, Mucocutaneous Candidiasis).

- Bite trauma in the mouth—May result in white areas of the lip or buccal mucosa; Persons may have a white bite line where the upper and lower molars occlude and this can be confused with oral lichen planus. If in doubt, a biopsy may be needed.

Genital lesions that may be differentiated from LP:[5]

- Psoriasis on the penis can look like LP on the penis. A shave biopsy can be used to differentiate between these two diagnoses (see Chapter 145, Psoriasis).

- Syphilis—Primary infection manifests as painless shallow ulcer (chancre) at site of inoculation, if untreated secondary syphilis presents with macular and then papular, pustular, or acneiform eruption on trunk, neck, palms, and soles, condyloma lata (soft, moist, flat-topped pink to tan papules) in the anogenital region (see Chapter 209, Syphilis).

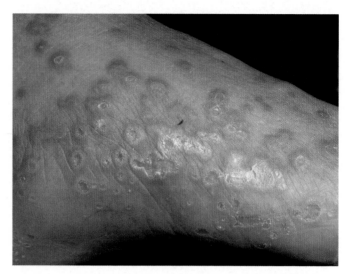

FIGURE 147-5 Hypertrophic lichen planus on the foot of a man. Purple polygonal lesions are seen. All five Ps are present—planar, purple, polygonal, pruritic and papular. (*Courtesy of M. Craven, MD.*)

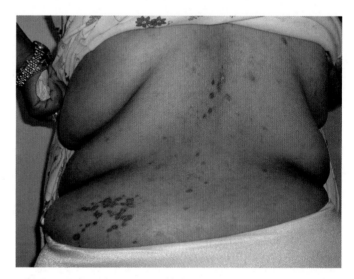

FIGURE 147-6 Hyperpigmented lichen planus on the back proven by punch biopsy. (*Courtesy of Richard P. Usatine, MD.*)

MANAGEMENT

LP may persist for months to years. Hypertrophic LP and oral LP can last for decades.[2] Any type of LP can recur. Antihistamines can be used for symptomatic pruritus.[5] SOR Ⓒ Symptomatic and severe cases can be treated as follows:

- Localized/topical treatment
  - Topical corticosteroids twice a day.[2,5] SOR Ⓑ Mid to high-potency steroids are usually needed.
  - Intralesional triamcinolone (3 mg/mL) for hypertrophic or mucous membrane lesions, may repeat every 3 to 4 weeks.[2,5,7] SOR Ⓑ
  - Steroids, cyclosporine, retinoids, tacrolimus, or pimecrolimus in mouthwash or adhesive base for oral disease.[2–9] SOR Ⓑ
- Systemic treatment can be considered for resistant or severe cases.
  - Oral steroids may be used starting with a three-week tapered course of oral prednisone (60 mg/d starting dose).[2,7] SOR Ⓑ
  - Systemic retinoids, e.g., acitretin 25 mg/d. Monitor Cr, LFTs, fasting lipids.[3,7] SOR Ⓑ Contraindicated in women of childbearing potential.
  - Cyclosporine (5 mg/kg/d). Monitor complete blood count, serum creatinine, liver function tests (LFTs), and blood pressure.[2] SOR Ⓑ
  - Azathioprine may be used as a steroid-sparing agent (50 mg po daily to start and titrate to 100 to 250 mg po daily). Monitor complete blood count and LFTs.[5,7] SOR Ⓒ
  - PUVA phototherapy may be effective but can cause phototoxic reactions and has long term risks including the development of squamous cell carcinoma. SOR Ⓒ

PATIENT EDUCATION

- Patients should understand that LP is often self-limiting and may resolve in 12 to 18 months.
- There is a significant chance of recurrence.
- Generally, LP is not dangerous and malignant transformation is so rare it is best not to scare them with this issue unless the patient has a severe case that is non-responsive to treatment.

FOLLOW-UP

- Follow-up depends on severity and treatment course.
- Oral and vaginal disease may be most challenging to treat.
  - Follow oral or vaginal lesions for possible malignant transformation. Because of low risk of transformation even with oral LP (best estimate 0.2% per year), routine screening and biopsy is not recommended.[7] Biopsy if suspecting malignancy; lesion becomes larger, ulcerated, nodular, or lose reticular pattern.

PATIENT RESOURCES

http://www.familydoctor.org/600.xml.

PROVIDER RESOURCES

http://www.emedicine.com/derm/topic233.htm.

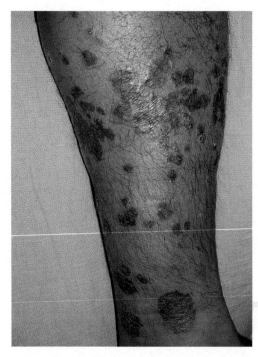

FIGURE 147-7 Close-up of hypertrophic lichen planus on the leg of a black man. Note the hyperpigmentation that is common when lichen planus occurs in a person with dark skin. (*Courtesy of Richard P. Usatine, MD.*)

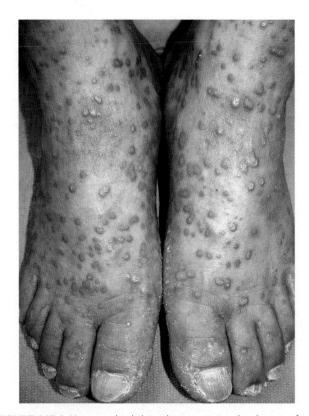

FIGURE 147-8 Hypertrophic lichen planus covering the dorsum of both feet with nail splintering. Note the purple color and Wickham's lines. (*Courtesy of Eric Kraus, MD.*)

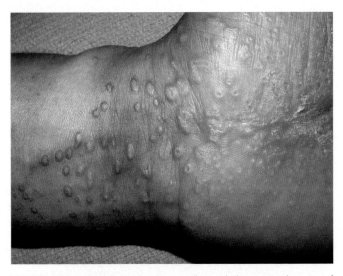

FIGURE 147-9 Thick hypertrophic papules and plaques on the wrist of the man in **Figure 147-8**. (*Courtesy of Eric Kraus, MD.*)

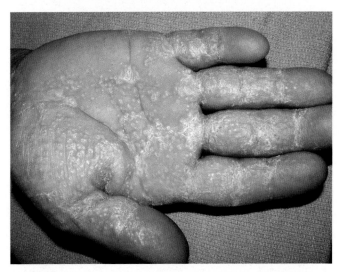

FIGURE 147-10 Palmar hypertrophic lichen planus in the man in **Figure 147-8**. (*Courtesy of Eric Kraus, MD.*)

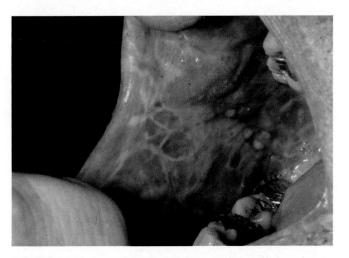

FIGURE 147-11 Asymptomatic white keratotic striae of lichen planus on right buccal mucosa of a 57-year-old man. The patient had similar involvement of the left buccal mucosa and gingivae. Lichen planus in the mouth is bilateral. (*Courtesy of Ellen Eisenberg, DMD.*)

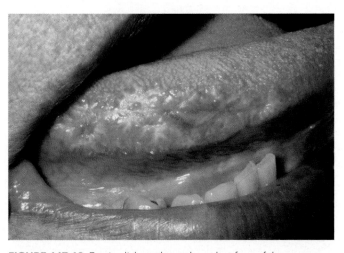

FIGURE 147-12 Erosive lichen planus, lateral surface of the tongue. This 62-year-old woman experiences tongue discomfort while eating acidic or spicy foods. She had been diagnosed with lichen planus several years ago. Clinical examination revealed lacy white lesions on both posterior buccal mucosae, with focal erythematous, atrophic changes on the buccal and palatal maxillary and mandibular gingivae. (*Courtesy of Ellen Eisenberg, DMD.*)

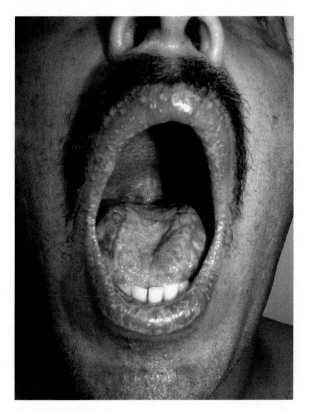

FIGURE 147-13 Lichen planus in the mouth with erosions. The lips, tongue, and palate are all involved. (*Courtesy of Eric Kraus, MD.*)

REFERENCES

1. Chuang T-Y, Stitle L. http://www.emedicine.com/derm/topic233.htm. Accessed February 14, 2007.

2. Surmond D. In: Fitzpatrick BT, Johnson RA, Wolff K, eds. *Color Atlas and Synopsis of Clinical Dermatology: Common and serious diseases.* 4th ed. New York, NY: McGraw-Hill, 2001.

3. Zakrzewska JM, Chan ES-Y, Thornhill MH. A systematic review of placebo-controlled randomized clinical trials of treatments used in oral lichen planus. *Br J Dermatol.* 2005;153:336–341.

4. Laeijendecker R, Tank B, Dekker SK, Neumann HA. A comparison of treatment of oral lichen planus with topical tacrolimus and triamcinolone acetonide ointment. *Acta Derm Venereol.* 2006;86(3): 227–229.

5. Habif TP. *Clinical Dermatology: A Color Guide to Diagnosis and Therapy.* 4th ed. Philadelphia, PA: Mosby, 2004.

6. Yoke PC, Tin GB, Kim MJ, et al. Asian Lichen Planus Study Group. A randomized controlled trial to compare steroid with cyclosporine for the topical treatment of oral lichen planus. *Oral Surg Oral Med Oral Pathol Oral Radiol Endod.* 2006;102(1):47–55.

7. Lodi G, Scully C, Carrozzo M, Griffiths M, Sugerman PB, Thongprasom K. Current controversies in oral lichen planus: Report of an international consensus meeting, Part 2. Clinical management and malignant transformation. *Oral Surg Oral Med Oral Pathol Oral Radiol Endod.* 2005;100:164–178.

8. Conrotto D, Carbone M, Carrozzo M, et al. Ciclosporine vs. clobetasol in the topical management of atrophic and erosive oral lichen planus: A double-blind, randomized controlled trial. *Br J Dermatol.* 2006;154(1):139–145.

9. Swift JC, Rees TD, Plemons JM, Hallmon WW, Wright JC. The effectiveness of 1% pimecrolimus cream in the treatment of oral erosive lichen planus. *J Periodontol.* 2005;76(4):627–635.

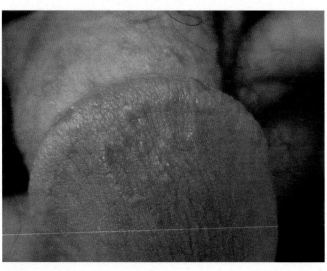

FIGURE 147-14 Lichen planus on the penis showing a lacy white pattern. (*Courtesy of Dan Stulberg, MD.*)

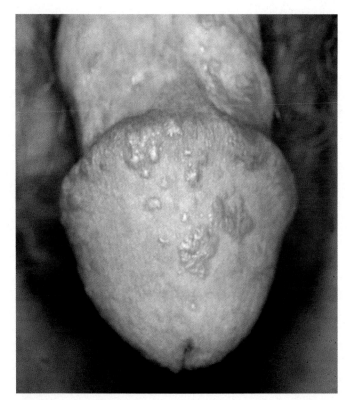

FIGURE 147-15 Lichen planus on the penis that is more similar to the pattern seen on other parts of the body. This is an example of planar, purple, polygonal papules on the penis. (*Courtesy of John Gonzales, MD.*)

148 REITER'S SYNDROME

Angela Shedd
Suraj Reddy, MD
Richard P. Usatine, MD

PATIENT STORY

A 29-year-old Hispanic man presented with concerns about an extensive rash that had developed over the previous month. The rash was reported to involve the scalp, abdomen, penis, hands, and feet (**Figures 148-1 to 148-5**). He also complained of severe joint pain, involving the back, knees, and feet. The patient described a recent history of fevers and night sweats. He denied ocular, gastrointestinal, or genitourinary complaints.

On further questioning the patient gave a history of being treated for a "sexually transmitted disease" one year ago. The patient had no other significant past medical history, and denied any illicit drugs or medications.

The patient's young age, rapid onset of symptoms, dermatological findings, arthritis, and constitutional symptoms led to the diagnosis of Reiter's syndrome. The patient's treatment was started with an NSAID and topical corticosteroids. No antibiotics were prescribed because no current infectious agent was identified. In conjunction with a dermatologist, acitretin 25 mg daily was started to treat his psoriasiform lesions.

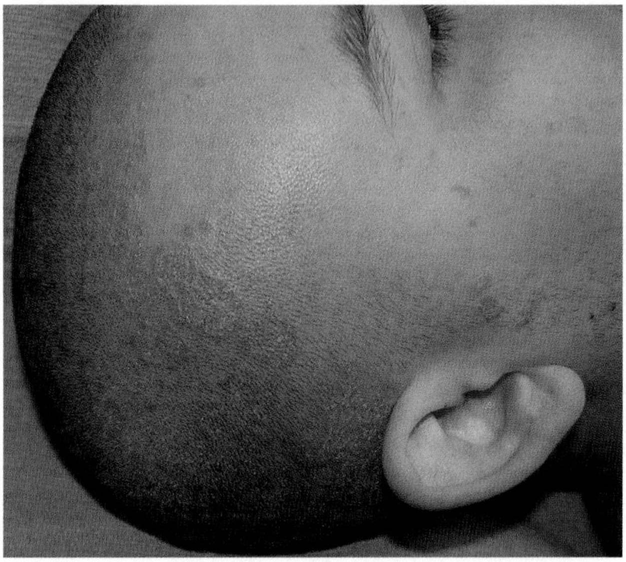

EPIDEMIOLOGY

- Reiter's syndrome (RS) may represent a reactive immune response that is usually triggered by any of several different infections.
- Major infectious associations: post-venereal (*Chlamydia* or *Ureaplasma*) and post-enteric (*Salmonella enteritidis, Yersinia enterocolitica, Campylobacter fetus, Shigella flexneri*).
- Seen most commonly in young males.
- Frequent association with HLA-B27.
- Incidence may be increased in HIV population.

ETIOLOGY AND PATHOPHYSIOLOGY

- Unknown.
- May represent a pathological CD8+ T cell response to a peptide associated with various organisms.
- Two suspected pathways: sexual transmission, which may occur 1 to 4 weeks prior to development of urethritis, conjunctivitis followed by an arthritic component; another component may involve enteric pathogens that infect the host and follow a similar time frame with the exception that diarrhea rather than urethritis may be a chief complaint.

FIGURE 148-1 Reiter's Syndrome in a young man showing annular scalp lesions (circinate plaques). (*With permission from Shedd AD, Reddy SG, Meffert JJ, Kraus EW. Acute onset of rash and oligoarthritis. J Fam Pract. 2007;56(10):811–814, Dowden Health Media.*)

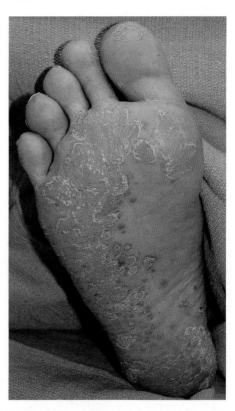

FIGURE 148-2 Keratoderma blennorrhagicum with hyperkeratotic papules, plaques, and pustules that have coalesced to form circular borders. (*With permission from Shedd AD, Reddy SG, Meffert JJ, Kraus EW. Acute onset of rash and oligoarthritis. J Fam Pract. 2007;56(10): 811–814, Dowden Health Media.*)

DIAGNOSIS

CLINICAL FEATURES

- The classic triad consists of urethritis, conjunctivitis (**Figure 148-6**), and arthritis. Few patients present with the classic triad, and thus the syndrome is often diagnosed with a peripheral arthritis >1 month and associated urethritis (or cervicitis).
- Other symptoms include malaise and fever.

TYPICAL DISTRIBUTION

Skin findings (psoriasiform) typically involve the palms, soles (keratoderma blenorrhagicum) (**Figure 148-2**), and the glans penis (balanitis circinata). Many other body surfaces may be affected including the scalp (**Figure 148-1**), intertriginous areas (**Figure 148-4**), and the oral mucosa (**Figure 148-7**). Nail dystrophy, thickening, and destruction may occur (**Figure 148-3**). Erosive lesions on the tongue and hard palate may be seen.

LABORATORY STUDIES

No specific laboratory test is used to confirm RS; however, one may see anemia, leukocytosis, thrombocytosis, and an elevated ESR. Typically a urethral swab and stool culture are performed to evaluate for an infectious source. Often an ANA, RF, and HIV are performed to rule out other disease processes. Skin biopsy if performed resembles that of psoriasis with acanthosis of the epidermis, a neutrophilic perivascular infiltrate, and spongiform pustules.

DIFFERENTIAL DIAGNOSIS

- Spondylo- and reactive-arthropathies may present with acute joint pain but often lack skin findings seen with RS (see Chapter 93, Ankylosing Spondylitis).
- Psoriatic arthritis may be easily confused especially in immunocompromised patients. Lack of constitutional symptoms and a more chronic course help differentiate from RS.
- Gonococcal arthritis is characterized by migratory polyarthralgia that settles in one or more joints. Often erythematous macules or hemorrhagic papules on acral sites help distinguish from RS.
- Rheumatoid arthritis often presents with a progressive, symmetric polyarthritis of the small joints of the hands and wrists. Females are affected more often than males (see Chapter 92, Rheumatoid Arthritis).

MANAGEMENT

- For mucosal and skin lesions, one can use topical corticosteroids.
- If infection proven, appropriate antibiotic therapy for 3 months is indicated. If chlamydial, then use tetracycline.[1] SOR **B** If infectious agent is unknown, then ciprofloxacin can serve as broad-spectrum coverage.[2] SOR **B**

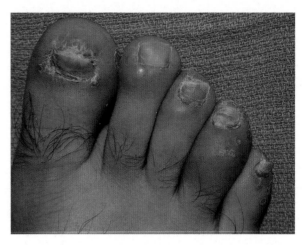

FIGURE 148-3 Erythema and scale seen on the toes of the patient in **Figure 148-1**. Note the nail involvement with subungual keratosis and onycholysis. The 4th toe is red and swollen, called dactylitis. (*With permission from Shedd AD, Reddy SG, Meffert JJ, Kraus EW. Acute onset of rash and oligoarthritis. J Fam Pract. 2007;56(10):811–814, Dowden Health Media.*)

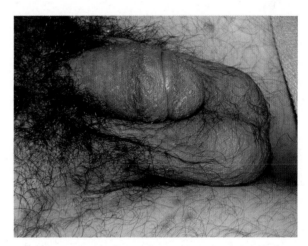

FIGURE 148-4 The patient in **Figure 148-1** with psoriasiform lesion on the corona and glans. He patient also has erythema in the inguinal area that resembles inverse psoriasis. This particular case does not exemplify classic balanitis circinata, which is characterized by annular or arcuate thin scaly plaques, as opposed to the nonspecific scaly plaques found on this patient. (*Courtesy of Suraj Reddy, MD.*)

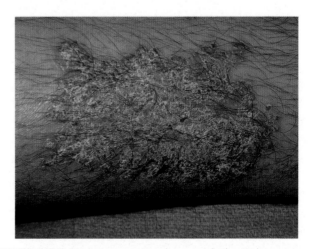

FIGURE 148-5 Psoriatic-appearing plaque on the leg in the same patient with RS in **Figure 148-1**. (*With permission from Shedd AD, Reddy SG, Meffert JJ, Kraus EW. Acute onset of rash and oligoarthritis. J Fam Pract. 2007; 56(10):811–814, Dowden Health Media.*)

- Although few studies have elucidated the long-term effects of NSAID treatment of RS, a regular schedule of high doses for several weeks is recommended for inflammation and pain management, proving most effective if given early in the disease course.[3] SOR **B**

- For refractory disease, immunosuppressive agents such as sulfasalazine at 2,000 mg/day[4] SOR **B** or subcutaneous injection of etanercept at 25 mg twice weekly[5] SOR **B** have been shown to provide therapeutic benefit.

- Psoriasiform skin lesions may be treated with some of the same medications used to treat psoriasis (including acitretin). SOR **C**

FOLLOW-UP

The majority of patients have a self-limited course, with resolution in 3 to 12 months. The disease may relapse over many years in up to a third of patients. A chronic deforming arthritis may occur in small percentage of patients.

Patient should be referred to a rheumatologist if joint problems persist.

PATIENT RESOURCES

http://healthlink.mcw.edu/article/926056398.html.

REFERENCES

1. Lauhio A, Leirisalo-Repo M, Lähdevirta J, et al. Double-blind, placebo-controlled study of three-month treatment with lymecycline in reactive arthritis, with special reference to Chlamydia arthritis. *Arthritis Rheum*. 1991;34(1): 6–14.

2. Yli-Kerttula T, Luukkainen R, Yli-Kerttula U, et al. Effect of a three month course of ciprofloxacin on the late prognosis of reactive arthritis. *Ann Rheum Dis*. 2003; 62(9):880–884.

3. Colmegna I, Cuchacovich R, Espinoza LR. HLA-B27-associated reactive arthritis: Pathogenetic and clinical considerations. *Clin Microbiol Rev*. 2004;17(2):348–369.

4. Clegg DO, Reda DJ, Weisman MH, et al. Comparison of sulfasalazine and placebo in the treatment of reactive arthritis (Reiter's syndrome). A Department of Veterans Affairs Cooperative Study. *Arthritis Rheum*. 1996; 39(12):2021–2027.

5. Flagg SD, Meador R, Hsia E, Kitumnuaypong T, Schumacher HR, Jr. Decreased pain and synovial inflammation after etanercept therapy in patients with reactive and undifferentiated arthritis: An open-label trial. *Arthritis Rheum*. 2005;53(4):613–617.

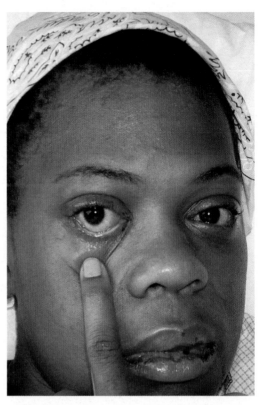

FIGURE 148-6 RS with conjunctivitis as a result of chlamydial pelvic inflammatory disease in a 42-year-old woman. She presented with fever, chills, and generalized pain in her joints, abdomen, and pelvis. (*Courtesy of Joseph Mazziotta, MD, and from Mazziotta JM, Ahmed N. Conjuctivitis and Cervicitis. J Fam Pract. 2004;53(2):121–123, Dowden Health Media.*)

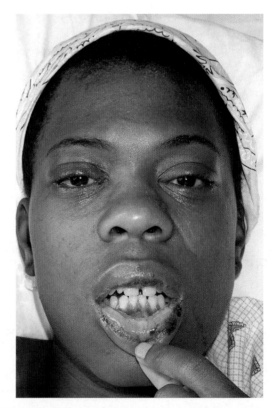

FIGURE 148-7 Oral mucosal inflammation with RS secondary to chlamydial pelvic inflammatory disease. The cervix was also inflamed on examination. (*Courtesy of Joseph Mazziotta, and from Mazziotta JM, Ahmed N. Conjuctivitis and Cervicitis. J Fam Pract. 2004;53(2): 121–123.*)

149 ERYTHRODERMA

Dave Henderson, MD

PATIENT STORY

A 56-year-old man presented with an extensive rash over his entire body (**Figures 149-1** and **149-2**). It started 2 months ago in the gluteal region and spread to cover his hands, arms, trunk, legs, feet, and most recently, his face. He had extensive pruritus and felt uncomfortable. He admitted to drinking one bottle of gin per day for the last 20 years and was not willing to stop at this time. He denied previous skin problems and had never been diagnosed with psoriasis or eczema. He denied any fevers, chills, or night sweats. Aside from his uncomfortable itchy skin, he had no other symptoms. On physical examination, he had large erythematous plaques with white scale on his hands and most of his body. In **Figure 149-1** there are individual scaling plaques on the dorsum of his left hand and extensive nail changes on the right hand. **Figure 149-2** shows the extensive erythroderma on the back gluteal region and arms. The differential diagnosis of the erythroderma included psoriasis, eczema, fungal infections, seborrheic dermatitis, and mycosis fungoides. A 4-mm punch biopsy was performed and the patient was started on topical steroids. Patient declined hospitalization for detox and dermatologic treatment. So, the patient was given a one-pound tub of 0.1% triamcinolone ointment to apply it to all affected areas twice daily. The first few days he was told to apply the triamcinolone extensively, soak cotton pajamas in warm water and put those on, wrap himself in a blanket, and remove the pajamas in 15 minutes. HIV, RPR, ANA, hepatitis B and C were negative. His TSH was normal, his liver enzymes were elevated, and his ESR was 52. Patient was told to cut back on his alcohol, drink plenty of fluids, and return the following day. Patient noted improvement and 2 days later, the pathology report came back eczematous dermatitis. With that result and knowing this was not psoriasis, we were able to give the patient a course of systemic steroids along with the topical ointment. Patient continued to improve but reached a plateau in 3 weeks. At that time, the need for stopping the alcohol for the skin to improve was emphasized more strongly and a trusting relationship had been developed. The patient went in for hospital detoxification, and after a rocky period in the intensive care unit, he came out sober with almost completely clear skin.

EPIDEMIOLOGY

Erythroderma or exfoliative dermatitis is an uncommon condition that is generally a manifestation of underlying systemic or cutaneous disorders.

- It affects all age groups from infants to the elderly people.

- In adults the average age of onset is 55 years, with a male-to-female ratio of 2.3:1.[1,2]

- It accounts for approximately 1% of all dermatologic hospital admissions.[1]

- It can be a very serious condition resulting in metabolic, infectious, cardiorespiratory, and thermoregulatory complications.[3]

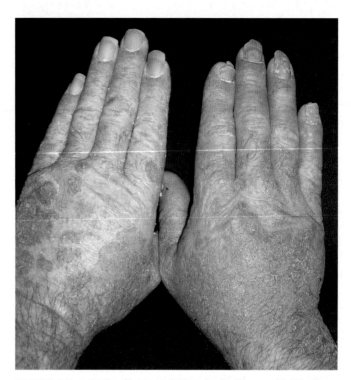

FIGURE 149-1 Erythroderma on the hands of a 56-year-old with alcoholism. The plaques and dysmorphic fingernails suggest psoriasis but the biopsy supported eczematous dermatitis. (*Courtesy of Richard P. Usatine, MD.*)

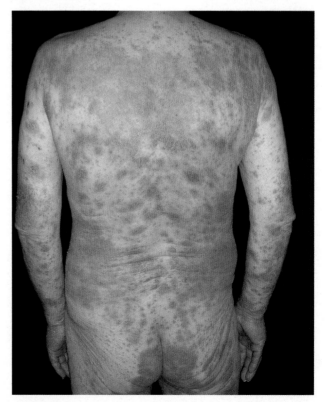

FIGURE 149-2 Erythroderma covering the back and buttocks of the patient in **Figure 149-1**. (*Courtesy of Richard P. Usatine, MD.*)

ETIOLOGY AND PATHOPHYSIOLOGY

In almost 50% of cases erythroderma occurs in the setting of a preexisting dermatosis, however it may also occur secondary to underlying systemic disease, malignancy, and drug reactions.[3] It is classified as idiopathic in 9% to 47% of cases.[3]

- The pathophysiology is not fully understood, but there is an increase in the epidermal turnover rate.
- The rapid maturation and migration of cells through the epidermal layer results in excessive scaling.
- The rapid turnover of the epidermis also results in fluid, electrolyte, and protein losses that may have severe metabolic consequences including heart failure and acute respiratory distress syndrome.
- The underlying pathogenesis may be an interaction of immunologic modulators including Interleukins 1, 2, and 8 as well as tumor necrosis factor.[1]

Dermatologic conditions most commonly associated with erythroderma include the following:

- Psoriasis-especially generalized pustular psoriasis with exfoliation (**Figure 149-3 to 149-5**).
- Pityriasis rubra pilaris.
- Seborrhea.
- Atopic and contact dermatitis.[1,3]

It may also occur secondary to a number of infectious diseases:

- HIV.
- Tuberculosis.
- Norwegian scabies.
- Hepatitis.
- Murine typhus (**Figure 149-6**).
- Histoplasmosis.[3]

Systemic diseases associated with erythroderma include the following:

- Sarcoidosis.
- Thyrotoxicosis.
- Graft versus host reaction.
- Dermatomyositis.[3]

The exact incidence of erythroderma in association with underlying malignancy is not known but reticuloendothelial neoplasms are the most common, most notably T-cell lymphomas.[1,2] It may precede or follow the diagnosis of cutaneous T-cell lymphoma, and chronic idiopathic erythroderma carries a high risk of development of cutaneous T-cell lymphoma over time (**Figure 149-7**).[4] In addition colon, lung, prostate, and thyroid malignancies account for 1% of cases of erythroderma.[1] Specifically in children it may be associated with:

- Omenn's syndrome.
- Kwashiorkor.
- Cystic fibrosis.
- Amino acid disorders.[1–5]

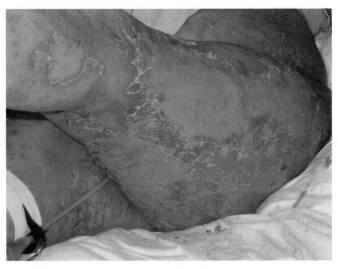

FIGURE 149-3 Erythrodermic psoriasis with sheets of exfoliation causing dehydration and life-threatening illness. This is secondary to generalized pustular psoriasis. (*Courtesy of Jack Resneck, Sr., MD.*)

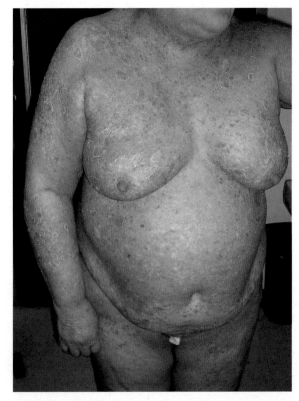

FIGURE 149-4 Generalized pustular psoriasis causing a life-threatening case of erythroderma in a 67-year-old woman. This all started 3 weeks before presentation and she had no previous history of psoriasis. Patient was hospitalized and treated with topical steroids and oral acitretin with good results. (*Courtesy of Richard P. Usatine, MD.*)

Drug reactions are a common cause of erythroderma. The list of drugs associated with erythroderma is extensive and includes both systemic and topical medications, many of which are very commonly used, including a number of herbal, homeopathic, and ayurvedic medications.[2] The list of medications includes the following:

- Penicillins.
- Sulfonamides.
- Tetracycline derivatives.
- Sulfonylureas.
- Calcium channel blockers.
- Captopril.
- Thiazides.
- NSAIDs.
- Barbiturates.
- Lithium.[1,2,3]

In children, an association with topical boric acid has been identified.[4]

The cause of erythroderma may not always be identified (**Figures 149-8** and **149-9**).

DIAGNOSIS

CLINICAL FEATURES

The clinical presentation of erythroderma may be variable depending on the underlying cause. In association with drug reactions the onset tends to be more abrupt and the resolution more rapid as well. Cutaneous manifestations begin with pruritic, erythematous patches that spread and coalesce into areas of erythema that can cover large portions of the body (**Figures 149-2, 149-4** and **149-8**). Scaling eventually develops. Large scales are seen more often in acute settings and in chronic erythroderma smaller scales predominate. Scalp involvement is very common with alopecia occurring in 25% of patients.[1] Systemic manifestations associated with compromise of the protective cutaneous barrier and loss of vasoconstriction of vessels in the dermis that occurs in erythroderma include loss of fluid and electrolytes. Protein losses can be as high as 25% to 30% in psoriatic erythroderma resulting in hypoalbuminemia and edema.[3] Increased perfusion to denuded inflamed skin may result in thermoregulatory disturbances and high output cardiac failure. In addition, there is an increased risk of Staphylococcal infection and sepsis.[1,3] Any of these complications can be life threatening.

TYPICAL DISTRIBUTION

The distribution is variable, but there is usually sparing of mucous membranes, the palms, and the soles of the feet. Sparing of the nose and nasolabial region has also been reported.[1]

LABORATORY STUDIES

Skin biopsy is often nondiagnostic. Fifty percent of individual biopsies fail to reveal a specific diagnosis and therefore multiple biopsies are recommended when evaluating patients for erythroderma. In addition to conventional histopathologic evaluation, direct immunofluorescence

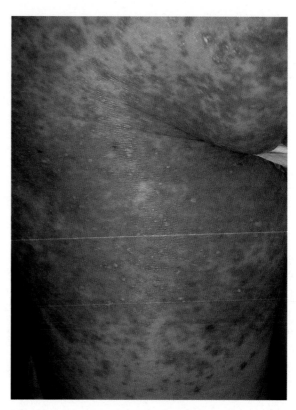

FIGURE 149-5 Close-up of posterior thigh (from patient in previous figure) showing pustules on an erythematous plaque in a new case of erythroderma from generalized pustular psoriasis. (*Courtesy of Richard P. Usatine, MD.*)

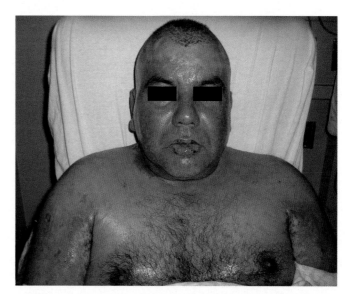

FIGURE 149-6 Murine typhus causing erythema and exfoliation in a febrile systemically-ill man in South Texas. (*Courtesy of Angela Peng, MD.*)

may be helpful in immunobullous disease (e.g., pemphigus). T-cell receptor gene rearrangement studies may aid in the diagnosis of lymphoproliferative disorders.[3] Laboratory tests are often nonspecific; however, common findings include:

- Leukocytosis.
- Lymphocytosis.
- Mild anemia.
- Eosinophilia.
- Elevated sedimentation rate.
- Polyclonal gammopathy.
- Elevated IgE levels.
- Hypoalbuminemia.
- Elevated serum creatinine.
- Elevated uric acid levels.[1–5]

HIV testing should be considered in those with risk factors.[2] In children a sweat test, zinc, amino acid, and lipid levels should be considered.[4]

DIFFERENTIAL DIAGNOSIS

Erythroderma is the dermatologic manifestation of a number of underlying disease processes, including infectious diseases, lymphoproliferative disorders, malignancies, dermatoses, acquired and inborn metabolic disorders, and drug reactions. The key to proper diagnosis and treatment is contingent on identification of the underlying cause.[1–5] (For a list of underlying conditions, see section on Pathophysiology.)

MANAGEMENT

Hospitalization and urgent dermatologic referral should be considered for patients presenting with erythroderma acutely as the metabolic, infectious, thermoregulatory, and cardiovascular complications can be life threatening (**Figures 149-1 to 149-9**).[1,4]

Therapeutic interventions:

- Topical skin care measures such as emollients, oatmeal baths and wet dressings.[1–5] SOR **C**
- Mid-potency topical steroids.[1–5] SOR **C**
- High potency steroids and immunomodulators should be avoided owing to risk of increased cutaneous absorption.[3] SOR **C**
- Systemic steroids are useful in drug reactions and eczema, but should be avoided in psoriasis.[1,3,4] SOR **C**
- Consider oral retinoids or cyclosporine for cases secondary to psoriasis (**Figures 149-3 to 149-5**).[1] SOR **C**
- Immunosuppressive agents (methotrexate, azathioprine, infliximab).[1,3] SOR **C**
- Discontinuation of all nonessential medications.[1,3] SOR **C**
- Antibiotic therapy when infection is suspected.[1,3] SOR **C**
- Close monitoring of fluid, electrolyte and nutritional status and replacement of deficits.[1,3] SOR **C**

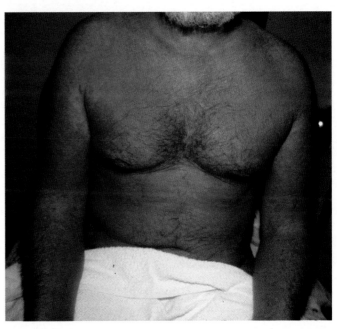

FIGURE 149-7 Erythema secondary to new onset mycosis fungoides. (*Courtesy of the University of Texas Health Sciences Center, Division of Dermatology.*)

PATIENT EDUCATION

Patients should be advised that erythroderma can be life threatening because of its infectious, thermoregulatory, metabolic, and cardiovascular complications. They should also be advised that with certain underlying etiologies, the condition may recur. This is particularly true of idiopathic erythroderma (**Figures 149-8** and **149-9**).

FOLLOW-UP

The prognosis in erythroderma is very much dependent on the underlying cause. Most deaths occur in malignancy-associated erythroderma. Drug-induced erythroderma carries the best prognosis and the lowest risk of recurrence. Relapses occur in 15% of patients with psoriatic erythroderma. Fifty percent of patients with idiopathic erythroderma experience partial remission, and one-third complete remission.[3]

REFERENCES

1. Karakayli G, Beckham G, Orengo I, Rosen T. Exfoliative Dermatitis. *Am Fam Physician*. 1990;59(3).

2. Sehgal VN, Srivastava G, Sardana K. Erythroderma/exfoliative dermatitis: A synopsis. *Int J of Dermatol*. 2004;43:39–47.

3. Rothe JH, Bernstein ML, Grant-Kels JM. Life-threatening erythroderma: Diagnosing and treating the "red man". *Clin Dermatol*. 2005;23(2):206–217.

4. Sehgal VN, Srivastava G. Erythroderma/generalized exfoliative dermatitis in pediatric practice: An overview. *Int J of Dermatol*. 2006;45:831–839.

5. Pruszkowski A, Bodemer C, Fraitag S, et al. Neonatal and Infantile Erythrodermas: A Retrospective Study of 51 Patients. *Arch Dermatol*. 2000;136:875–880.

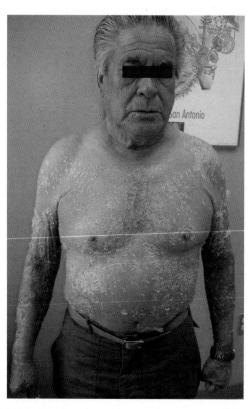

FIGURE 149-8 Complete erythroderma of unknown etiology with extreme reddening of the skin and exfoliation. (*Courtesy of Gwen Denton, MD.*)

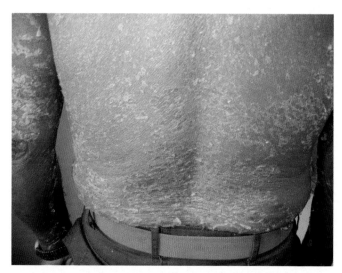

FIGURE 149-9 The back of the same patient with a closer view of the exfoliation. (*Courtesy of Gwen Denton, MD.*)

SECTION 9   BENIGN NEOPLASMS

150 SKIN TAG (ACROCHORDON)

Mindy A. Smith, MD, MS

PATIENT STORY

A 55-year-old man requests removal of multiple skin tags around his neck. He is overweight and has diabetes and acanthosis nigricans. While some of his skin tags occasionally get caught on his clothing, he just doesn't like the way they look (**Figure 150-1**).

EPIDEMIOLOGY

- Skin tags occur in 46% in the general population, particularly in patients who are obese.[1]

- Skin tags increase in frequency through the fifth decade so that as many as 59% of individuals have them by the time they are 70 years old.[1]

ETIOLOGY AND PATHOPHYSIOLOGY

- Skin tags (acrochordons; also referred to as fibroepithelial polyps) are flesh-colored, pedunculated lesions that tend to occur in areas of skin folds.

- Three types of skin tags are described:[1]
  - Small, furrowed papules of approximately 1 to 2 mm in width and height, located mostly on the neck and the axillae (**Figure 150-1**).
  - Single or multiple filiform lesions of approximately 2 mm in width and 5 mm in length occurring elsewhere on the body (**Figure 150-2**).
  - Large, pedunculated tumor or nevoid, baglike, soft fibromas that occur on the lower part of the trunk (**Figure 150-3**).

- Etiology is unknown but it is theorized that skin tags occur in local-ized areas with a paucity of elastic tissue resulting in sessile or atrophic lesions.[1] In addition, hormone imbalances appear to facili-tate their development (e.g., high levels of estrogen and progesterone seen during pregnancy) and other factors including epidermal growth factor, alpha tissue growth factor, and infection (e.g., human papillomavirus) have been implicated as cofactors.

- Acrochordons also appear to be associated with impaired carbohy-drate metabolism and diabetes mellitus (**Figure 150-1**).[2]

- Pedunculated lesions may become twisted, infarcted, and fall off spontaneously.

- Very rarely neoplasms are found at the base of skin tags. In a recent study of consecutive cutaneous pathology reports, 5 of 1335 clinically diagnosed fibroepithelial polyp specimens were malignant (i.e., four were basal cell carcinomas and one was squamous cell

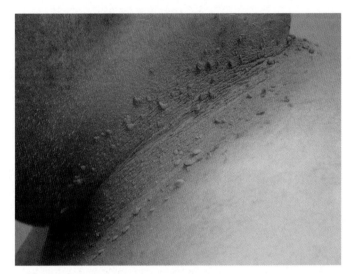

FIGURE 150-1 Many skin tags and acanthosis nigricans on the neck of a man with diabetes. (*Courtesy of Richard P. Usatine, MD.*)

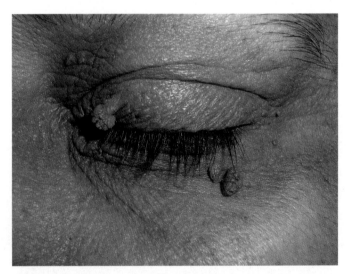

FIGURE 150-2 Filiform pedunculated skin tags on the eyelids. These were removed with a radiofrequency loop after local anesthesia with lidocaine and epinephrine to minimize bleeding. (*Courtesy of Richard P. Usatine, MD.*)

carcinoma in situ).[3] There is a selection bias here because most skin tags are not sent to the pathologist.

DIAGNOSIS

CLINICAL FEATURES

- Small, soft, usually pedunculated lesions.
- Skin colored or hyperpigmented.
- Most vary in size from 2 to 5 mm, but larger ones may be seen.
- Usually asymptomatic, but can be pruritic or become painful and inflamed by catching on clothing or jewelry.

TYPICAL DISTRIBUTION

Most typically seen on the neck and in the axillae (**Figure 150-1**), but any skin fold may be affected. They are also seen on the trunk (**Figure 150-3**), the abdomen, and the back.

BIOPSY

Not usually indicated. Skin tags, on histology, are characterized by acanthotic, flattened, or frond-like epithelium. A papillary-like dermis is composed of loosely arranged collagen fibers and dilated capillaries and lymphatic vessels.[1]

DIFFERENTIAL DIAGNOSIS

Benign lesions that can be confused with skin tags include:

- Warts—Cutaneous neoplasm caused by papilloma virus. Sessile, dome-shaped lesions about 1 cm in diameter with hyperkeratotic surface. Paring usually demonstrates central core of keratinized debris and punctate bleeding points (see Chapter 125, Common Warts).
- Neurofibromas—Benign Schwann cell tumors; cutaneous tumors tend to form multiple, soft pedunculated masses (**Figure 150-4**) (see Chapter 223, Neurofibromatosis).
- Epidermal hyperplasia in melanocytic nevi (also called keratotic melanocytic nevus)—Although most common moles are round, tan to brown, <6 mm and flat to slightly elevated, some nevi have overlying hyperplastic epidermis resembling skin tags. In a study of melanocytic nevi submitted for pathology over an 8-month period, 6% were keratotic melanocytic nevi, most often located on trunk (76%).[4] Dermal nevi can be pedunculated but they are usually larger than skin tags and may appear warty above the stalk.

MANAGEMENT

Skin tags may be removed for cosmetic reasons or because of irritation in a number of ways:

- Small lesions may be snipped with a sharp iris scissor with or without anesthesia (**Figure 150-5**).
- Larger skin tags and fibromas may be removed with shave excision after injecting with lidocaine and epinephrine (**Figure 150-3**).
- If there is any bleeding, aluminium chloride on a cotton-tipped applicator is applied for hemostasis.

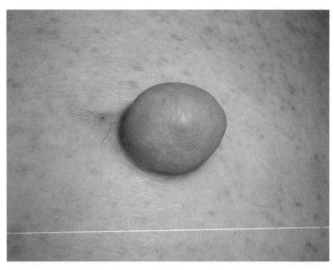

FIGURE 150-3 Large pedunculated bag-like soft fibroma on the trunk. Local anesthetic has been given prior to shave excision. (*Courtesy of Richard P. Usatine, MD.*)

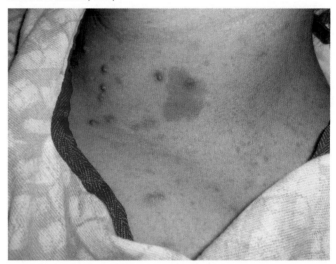

FIGURE 150-4 Multiple soft neurofibromas on the neck of a patient with neurofibromatosis. Note the coexisting café-au-lait spot. (*Courtesy of David Hiller, MD.*)

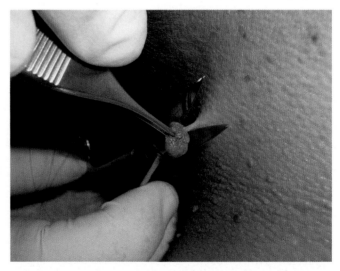

FIGURE 150-5 Snip excision of skin tag with iris scissors and no anesthesia. (*Courtesy of Richard P. Usatine, MD.*)

- Electrodesiccation with or without anesthesia works for very tiny skin tags too small to grab with the forceps.

- Skin tags on the eyelids may be removed with a radiofrequency loop after local anesthesia with lidocaine and epinephrine to minimize bleeding (the patient shown in **Figure 150-2** was treated using this technique).

- Cryotherapy can be applied directly to the skin tag with a cryogun, forceps or a cotton-tipped applicator. One preferred method involves dipping forceps into liquid nitrogen and then grasping the skin tag until it turns white. This allows you to grasp the skin tag without freezing the skin around it. This is especially helpful on the eyelids where you can pull up on the skin tag gently to remove the cold exposure from the underlying globe. CryoTweezers made by Brymill, Inc. has more metal at the end to hold the cold longer (**Figure 150-6**). This is a very efficient way to treat multiple skin tags quickly because you don't have to keep dipping the CryoTweezers back into the liquid nitrogen very often.

- Most insurance companies will not pay for the cosmetic removal of skin tags.

- To avoid large health care costs, send only suspicious-looking skin tags to the pathologist.

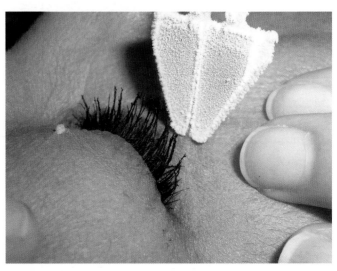

FIGURE 150-6 Cryotherapy using CryoTweezers to grasp the skin tag without freezing the skin around it. This is especially helpful on the eyelids. (*Courtesy of Richard P. Usatine, MD.*)

PATIENT EDUCATION

Advise patients that these are benign growths that can be removed if irritation occurs or for cosmetic purposes. Patients who are overweight should be encouraged to lose weight for their general health and to avoid new skin tags.

FOLLOW-UP

- Follow-up is not usually necessary.

PATIENT RESOURCES

http://www.nlm.nih.gov/medlineplus/ency/article/000848.htm.

PROVIDER RESOURCES

The CryoTweezer can be ordered from:

http://www.brymill.com/.

REFERENCES

1. Schwartz RA, Terlikowska A. http://www.emedicine.com/derm/topic606.htm. Accessed September 3, 2006.

2. Demir S, Demir Y. Acrochordon and impaired carbohydrate metabolism. *Acta Diabetol.* 2002;39(2):57–59.

3. Eads TJ, Chuang TY, Fabre VC, et al. The utility of submitting fibroepithelial polyps for histological examination. *Arch Dermatol.* 1996;132(12):1459–1462.

4. Horenstein MG, Prieto VG, Burchette JL Jr., Shea CR. Keratotic melanocytic nevus: A clinicopathologic and immunohistochemical study. *J Cutan Pathol.* 2000;27(7):344–350.

151 SEBORRHEIC KERATOSIS

Mindy A. Smith, MD, MS
Richard P. Usatine, MD

PATIENT STORY

An elderly woman noted a growth of a lesion on her chest (**Figure 151-1**). She was afraid that it might be melanoma. Her family physician recognized the typical features of a seborrheic keratosis (SK) (stuck-on with visible horn cysts) and attempted to reassure her. Dermoscopy was performed and the features were so typical of an SK; the physician was able to convince the patient to not have a biopsy (**Figure 151-2**). The white and black comedonal-like obstructions are typical of an SK and can be seen with the naked eye and magnified with a dermatoscope.

EPIDEMIOLOGY

- Most common benign tumor in older individuals; frequency increases with age.

- In an older study of individuals older than 64 years in North Carolina, 88% had at least one SK. Ten or more SKs were found in 61% of the black men and women, 38% of the white women, and 54% of the white men.[1]

- Based on international studies, between 8% and 25% of individuals younger than age 40 have at least one SK.[2]

- Familial cases of multiple SKs occur in approximately half of these patients, with an autosomal dominant mode of inheritance.[2]

ETIOLOGY AND PATHOPHYSIOLOGY

- A form of localized hyperpigmentation caused by epidermal alteration; they develop from the proliferation of epidermal cells.[2]

- In pigmented SKs, the proliferating keratinocytes secrete melanocyte-stimulating cytokines triggering the activation of neighboring melanocytes.[2]

- Reticulated SKs, usually found on sun-exposed skin, may develop from solar lentigines.[2]

- Bowen's disease (squamous cell carcinoma in situ) or malignant melanoma may rarely arise within an SK.[3]

- Multiple eruptive SKs associated with internal malignancy can be seen (the sign of Lesser-Trélat), especially with adenocarcinoma of the gastrointestinal tract (**Figure 151-3**).[2]

- An eruption of SKs may develop after an inflammatory dermatosis such as severe sunburn or eczema.[2]

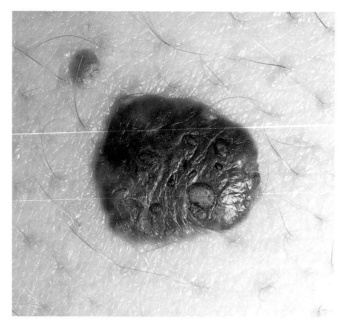

FIGURE 151-1 Seborrheic keratosis (SK) with associated horn cysts. (*Courtesy of Richard P. Usatine, MD.*)

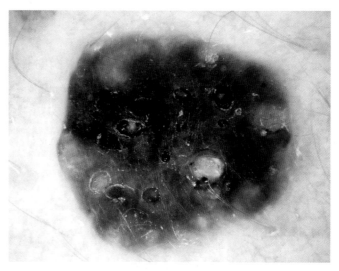

FIGURE 151-2 Dermoscopy of the SK in the previous figure showing comedo-like openings (black-like blackheads) and milia-like cysts (white-like milia). (*Courtesy of Richard P. Usatine, MD.*)

DIAGNOSIS

SKs have a variety of appearances.

CLINICAL FEATURES

- Typically oval or round brown plaques with adherent greasy scale (**Figure 151-4**).
- Color ranges from black to tan (**Figures 151-4 to 151-6**).
- Most often have a velvety to finely verrucous surface and appear to be "stuck on."
- Some are so verrucous they can appear to be warty (**Figure 151-6**).
- Lesions may be large (up to 35 × 15 cm), pigmented, and have irregular borders (**Figure 151-7**).
- SKs can also be flat.
- Many lesions show keratotic plugging of the surface (**Figures 151-1 and 151-4**).
- May have surface cracks and associated horncysts (**Figures 151-1 and 151-4**).
- Occasionally, lesions become irritated and can itch, grow, and bleed; secondary infection may occur.
- Variants of SKs:
  - Dermatosis papulosa nigra—consists of multiple brown–black dome-shaped, smooth papules found on the face in young and middle-aged persons of color—predominantly blacks (**Figures 151-8 and 151-9**).
  - Stucco keratosis—consists of large numbers of superficial gray-to-light brown flat keratotic lesions usually on the tops of the feet, the ankles, and the back of the hands and forearms (**Figure 151-10**).

TYPICAL DISTRIBUTION

- Trunk, face, back, abdomen, extremities; not present on the palms and soles or on mucous membranes. May be present on the areola and breasts (**Figures 151-11 and 151-12**).
- Dermatosis papulosa nigra is found on the face, especially the upper cheeks and lateral orbital areas (**Figures 151-8 and 151-9**).

IMAGING

- No imaging studies are needed unless there is a sudden appearance of multiple SKs as in the sign of Lesser-Trélat (**Figure 151-3**). These have been associated with adenocarcinoma of the gastrointestinal tract, lymphoma, Sézary syndrome, and acute leukemia.[2,3]

BIOPSY

- Should be performed if there is a suspicion of melanoma (**Figures 151-7 and 151-13**). Some melanomas resemble SKs and a biopsy is needed to avoid missing the diagnosis of melanoma. Do not freeze or curette a suspicious SK—these need surgical intervention to send tissue to the pathologist.

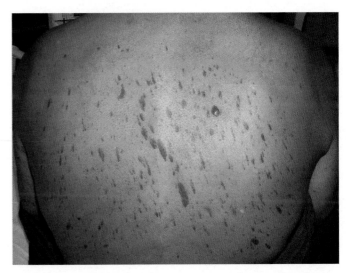

FIGURE 151-3 Multiple eruptive SKs as seen in the sign of Lesser-Trélat. In this case the malignancy workup was negative. (*Courtesy of Angela Shedd, MD.*)

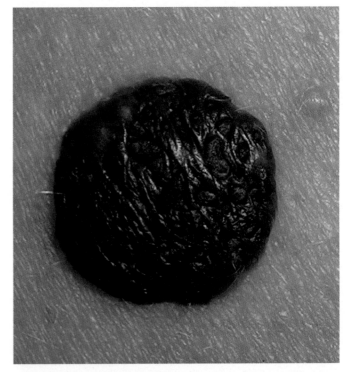

FIGURE 151-4 Round elevated SK with very visible horn cysts. (*Courtesy of Richard P. Usatine, MD.*)

DIFFERENTIAL DIAGNOSIS

- Melanoma—When keratin plugs are visible in the surface of the SK, this helps to distinguish it from a melanoma. **Figure 151-7** is an SK that has the ABCDE features of melanoma. A biopsy was performed and the lesion was definitively proven to be benign. In **Figure 151-13**, a possible SK turned out to be a melanoma in situ.

- Solar lentigo—Flat, uniformly medium, or dark brown lesion with sharp borders. These are flat and seen in sun-exposed areas, typically on the face or back of hands. Also called liver spots, these hyperpigmented areas are not palpable, whereas an SK is a palpable plaque even when the SK is thin (**Figure 151-7**) (see Chapter 165, Melanoma).

- Wart—Cutaneous neoplasm caused by papilloma virus. Sessile, dome-shaped lesions approximately 1 cm in diameter with hyperkeratotic surface. Paring usually demonstrates central core of keratinized debris and punctate bleeding points (see Chapter 125, Common Warts).

- Pigmented actinic keratosis—While most actinic keratoses are nonpigmented and do not look like an SK, occasionally a biopsy of an unknown pigmented plaque will be a pigmented actinic keratosis secondary to sun damage (see Chapter 159, Actinic Keratosis and Bowen's Disease).

- An inflamed SK may be confused with a malignant melanoma or a squamous cell carcinoma and should be biopsied to determine the diagnosis (see Chapter 164, Squamous Cell Carcinoma).

- Even a basal cell carcinoma (BCC) can have features that suggest an SK (**Figure 151-14**) (see Chapter 163, Basal Cell Carcinoma).

MANAGEMENT

- Cryosurgery with liquid nitrogen, with a 1-mm halo, is a quick and easy treatment. The risks include pigmentary changes, incomplete resolution, and scarring. Hypopigmentation is the most common complication of this treatment especially in dark-skinned individuals.

- Removal of benign lesions by curettage assures complete removal without taking the normal tissue below.

- Light electrofulguration can make the curettage so easy that it can be accomplished with a wet gauze pad.

- If the diagnosis is uncertain but there are no features suggesting a thick melanoma, suspected SK may be removed by scoop shave biopsy and the tissue sent to pathology.

- If a thick melanoma is suspected but an SK is also on the differential, perform a full-thickness biopsy by incisional or elliptical excision and send to pathology.

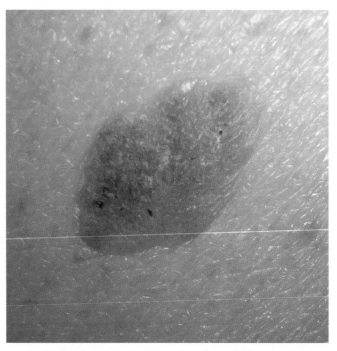

FIGURE 151-5 SK that is lightly pigmented, waxy, and appears stuck-on. (*Courtesy of Richard P. Usatine, MD.*)

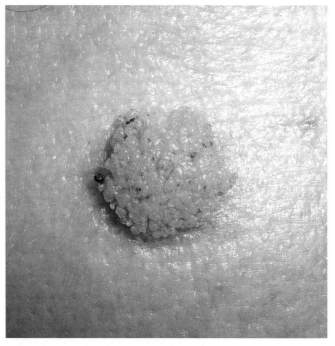

FIGURE 151-6 SK with verrucous appearance on the forehead. (*Courtesy of Richard P. Usatine, MD.*)

PATIENT EDUCATION

- Reassure patients that SKs are benign lesions that do not become cancer (except in only the most rare of circumstances). While benign SKs may grow larger and thicker with time, this is usually only a cosmetic issue.

- Unless the SK is suspicious for cancer or inflamed, removal is for cosmetic purposes only and is often not covered by insurance.

- Although SKs may resolve on occasions, spontaneous resolution does not ordinarily occur.

FOLLOW-UP

- Some experts suggest follow-up for patients with multiple SKs because malignant tumors can develop elsewhere on the body and rarely within an SK.[3] SOR **C**

PATIENT RESOURCES

http://www.nlm.nih.gov/medlineplus/ency/article/000884.htm.

http://www.aad.org/public/Publications/pamphlets/SeborrheicKeratoses.htm.

PROVIDER RESOURCES

www.emedicine.com/DERM/topic397.htm.

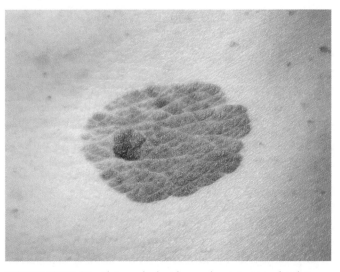

FIGURE 151-7 SK with irregular borders and variation in color that suggest a possible melanoma. (*Courtesy of Richard P. Usatine, MD.*)

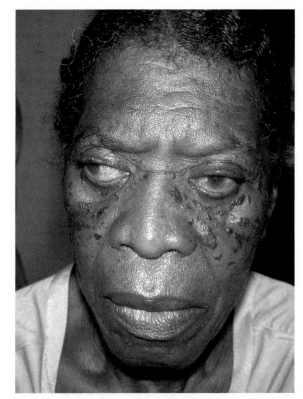

FIGURE 151-8 Dermatosis papulosa nigra with multiple SKs on the face of a Central American woman. (*Courtesy of Richard P. Usatine, MD.*)

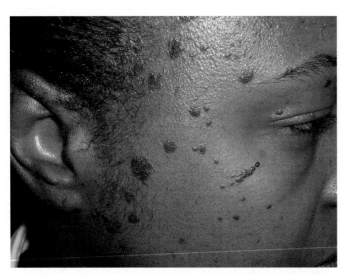

FIGURE 151-9 Dermatosis papulosa nigra on the cheeks and in the hair line. The patient was treated effectively with cryotherapy and had a great cosmetic result. (*Courtesy of Richard P. Usatine, MD.*)

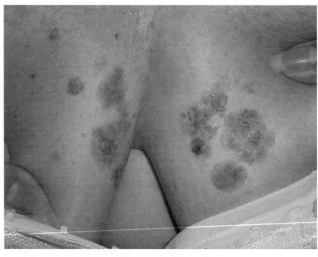

FIGURE 151-12 Waxy SKs on the breasts of this 70-year-old woman. (*Courtesy of Richard P. Usatine, MD.*)

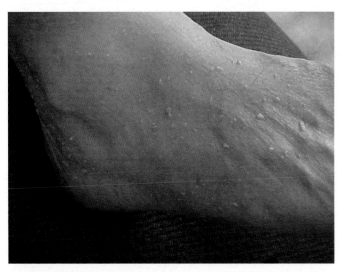

FIGURE 151-10 Stucco keratosis on the foot of an elderly man. (*Courtesy of Richard P. Usatine, MD.*)

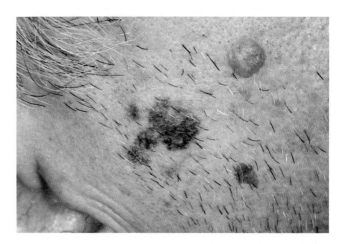

FIGURE 151-13 Melanoma in situ on the lateral face of a 48-year-old man. This resembles a SK but this large lesion also has all the ABCDE's of melanoma and needed to be biopsied. (*Courtesy of Richard P. Usatine, MD.*)

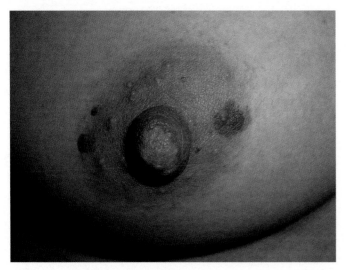

FIGURE 151-11 Multiple SKs on the areola of a 46-year-old woman. Cryotherapy cleared the SKs easily. (*Courtesy of Richard P. Usatine, MD.*)

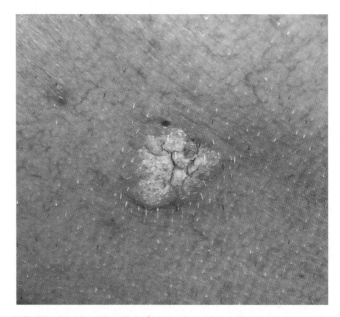

FIGURE 151-14 BCC with surface cracks and a stuck-on appearance resembling an SK. The shave biopsy demonstrated the diagnosis of BCC. (*Courtesy of Richard P. Usatine, MD.*)

REFERENCES

1. Tindall JP, Smith JG. Skin lesions of the aged and their association with internal changes. *JAMA*. 1963;186:1039–1042.

2. Balin AK. http://www.emedicine.com/derm/topic397.htm. Accessed August 21, 2006.

3. Cascajo CD, Reichel M, Sanchez JL. Malignant neoplasms associated with seborrheic keratoses. An analysis of 54 cases. *Am J Dermatopathol*. 1996;18(3):278–282.

152 SEBACEOUS HYPERPLASIA

Mindy A. Smith, MD, MS

PATIENT STORY

A 65-year-old man noted a new growth on his face for 1 year (**Figure 152-1**). On close examination, the growth was pearly with a few telangiectasias. The doughnut shape and presence of sebaceous hyperplasia scattered on other areas of the face were reassuring that this may be nothing but benign sebaceous hyperplasia. To reassure the patient and to remove the lesion a shave biopsy was performed to rule out BCC. The patient was relieved when the pathology result was in fact sebaceous hyperplasia. Additionally, he was pleased with the cosmetic result.

EPIDEMIOLOGY

- Sebaceous hyperplasia is a common, benign condition of sebaceous glands.
- It occurs in approximately 1% of the healthy population.[1]
- The prevalence of sebaceous hyperplasia is 10% to 16% in patients receiving long-term immunosuppression with cyclosporin.[2]
- Familial cases have been reported. In these cases, extensive sebaceous hyperplasia appears at puberty and tends to progress with age.[1]

ETIOLOGY AND PATHOPHYSIOLOGY

- Sebaceous glands, a component of the pilosebaceous unit, are found throughout the skin except on the palms and soles. The greatest number is found on the face, chest, back, and the upper outer arms.
- Sebaceous glands are composed of acini attached to a common excretory duct. In some areas, these ducts open directly to the epithelial surface including the lips and buccal mucosa (i.e., Fordyce spots), glans penis or clitoris (i.e., Tyson glands), areolae (i.e., Montgomery glands), and eyelids (i.e., meibomian glands).[1]
- Sebaceous glands are highly androgen sensitive (increasing in size and metabolic rate) and, along with sweat glands, account for the vast majority of androgen metabolism in the skin.[1] The glands become increasingly active at puberty and reach their maximum by the third decade of life.
- The cells that form the sebaceous gland, sebocytes, accumulate lipid material as they migrate from the basal layer of the gland to the central duct where they release the lipid content as sebum. In younger individuals, turnover of sebocytes occurs approximately every month.
- With aging, the sebocyte turnover slows, this results in crowding of primitive sebocytes within the sebaceous gland, causing a benign hamartomatous enlargement called sebaceous hyperplasia.[1]
- There is no known potential for malignant transformation.

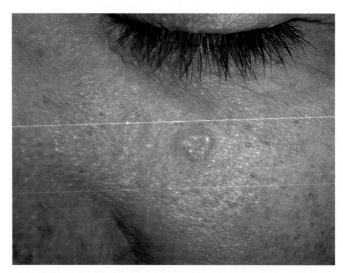

FIGURE 152-1 Large single lesion of sebaceous hyperplasia that was removed by shave biopsy to confirm that it was not a BCC. Doughnut shape visible. (*Courtesy of Richard P. Usatine, MD.*)

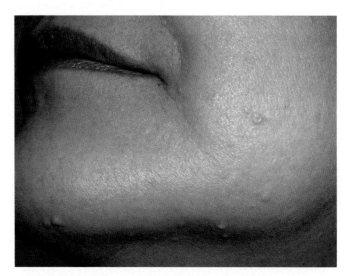

FIGURE 152-2 Multiple lesions of sebaceous hyperplasia on the cheek and chin. Simultaneous appearance of multiple lesions makes them less likely to be BCC. (*Courtesy of Richard P. Usatine, MD.*)

DIAGNOSIS

CLINICAL FEATURES

- Lesions appear as yellowish, soft, small papules ranging in size from 2 to 9 mm (**Figures 152-1** to **152-3**).[1]
- Surface varies from smooth to slightly verrucous.
- Lesions can be single or multiple.
- Increasing number of lesions with aging.
- Lesions may become red and irritated and bleed after scratching, shaving, or other trauma and may be associated with telangiectasias.
- Central umbilication (doughnut shape) from which a small amount of sebum can sometimes be expressed (**Figures 152-1** to **152-3**).

IMAGING

- Dermoscopy may aid in distinguishing between nodular basal cell carcinoma and sebaceous hyperplasia. A vascular pattern with orderly winding, scarcely branching vessels extending toward the center of the lesion is specific for hyperplastic sebaceous glands.[3] See Chapter 163 for a dermoscopic view of a BCC.

TYPICAL DISTRIBUTION

Most commonly located on the face, particularly the nose, cheeks, and forehead. May also be found on the chest, areola, mouth, and vulva.[1]

BIOPSY

Not usually necessary unless concerned about basal cell carcinoma.

DIFFERENTIAL DIAGNOSIS

- Nodular basal cell carcinoma—These lesions can appear as waxy papules with a central depression that may ulcerate, most commonly located on the head, neck, and upper back. They may have a pearly appearance, surface telangiectases, and bleed easily (**Figures 152-4** and **152-5**).
- Fibrous papule of the face is a benign, firm, papule of 1 to 5 mm that is usually dome-shaped and indurated with a shiny, skin-colored appearance. Most lesions are located on the nose and, less commonly, on the cheeks, chin, neck, and, rarely, on the lip or forehead.
- Milia are common, benign, keratin-filled cysts (histologically identical to epidermoid cysts) that occur in persons of all ages. They are 1 to 2 mm superficial, uniform, pearly white to yellowish, domed lesions usually occurring on the face (**Figure 152-6**) (see Chapter 102, Normal Skin Changes).
- Molluscum contagiosum are firm, smooth, usually 2 to 6 mm umbilicated papules that may be present in groups or widely disseminated on the skin and mucosal surfaces. The lesions can be flesh-colored, white, translucent, or even yellow in color. Lesions generally are self-limited but can persist for several years (see Chapter 124, Molluscum Contagiosum).

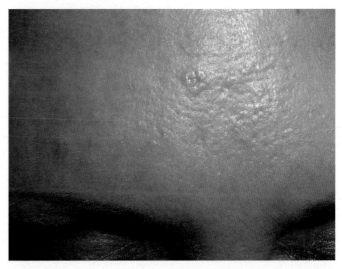

FIGURE 152-3 Large irregular sebaceous hyperplasia on the forehead with telangiectasias. Doughnut shape visible. (*Courtesy of Richard P. Usatine, MD.*)

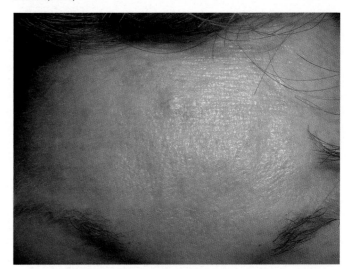

FIGURE 152-4 BCC on the forehead that could be mistaken for sebaceous hyperplasia. (*Courtesy of Richard P. Usatine, MD.*)

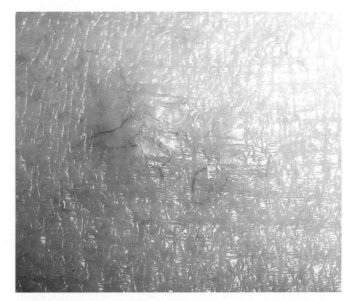

FIGURE 152-5 Close-up of same BCC on the forehead that shows irregular distribution of telangiectasias and lack of the doughnut shape. (*Courtesy of Richard P. Usatine, MD.*)

- Syringoma is a benign adnexal neoplasm formed by well-differentiated ductal elements (**Figure 152-6**). They are 1 to 3 mm skin-colored or yellowish dermal papules with a rounded or flat top arranged in clusters, and symmetrically distributed primarily on the upper parts of the cheeks and lower eyelids.

- Xanthomas are deposits of lipid in the skin or subcutaneous tissue that manifest clinically as yellowish papules, nodules or tumors. They are usually a consequence of primary or secondary hyperlipidemia and occur in patients older than age 50. The lesions are soft, velvety, yellow, flat, polygonal papules that are asymptomatic and usually bilateral and symmetric (see Chapter 215, Xanthomas).

MANAGEMENT

Sebaceous hyperplasia does not require treatment but can be removed for cosmetic purposes or if they become irritated.

- Options for removal include cryotherapy, electrodesiccation, topical chemical treatments (e.g., with bichloroacetic acid or trichloroacetic acid), laser treatment (e.g., with argon, carbon dioxide, or pulsed-dye laser), photodynamic therapy (i.e., combined use of 5-aminolevulinic acid and visible light),[4] shave excision, and punch excision. Shave excision can provide a good cosmetic result and a definitive diagnosis in a single large lesions of sebaceous hyperplasia that have suspicious features for skin cancer (**Figure 152-7**). Complications of these therapies include atrophic scarring or changes in pigmentation.

- Oral isotretinoin (10–40 mg a day for 2–6 weeks) has been used to shrink lesions, but lesions often recur within 1 month upon discontinuation. Maintenance doses (e.g., 10–40 mg every other day or 0.05% isotretinoin gel) may be indicated as suppressive treatment for widespread disfiguring sebaceous hyperplasia.[1]

PATIENT EDUCATION

- Advise patients that these are benign growths that can be removed if irritation occurs or for cosmetic purposes. These are not diet or lifestyle related and can not be prevented with special soaps or cleansers. Sebaceous hyperplasia does not become cancer and is not contagious.

FOLLOW-UP

- Follow-up is not necessary unless cosmetic treatment is being pursued.

PATIENT RESOURCES

VisualDxHealth—**http://www.visualdxhealth.com/adult/ sebaceousHyperplasia-references.htm.**

PROVIDER RESOURCES

DermNet NZ—**http://dermnetnz.org/acne/ sebaceous-hyperplasia.html** (with dermoscopic view).

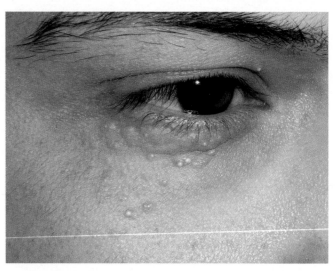

FIGURE 152-6 Syringomas and milia on the lower eyelid of a 23-year-old male. The milia are the white round epidermal cysts and the syringomas are flesh colored and larger. (*Courtesy of Richard P. Usatine, MD.*)

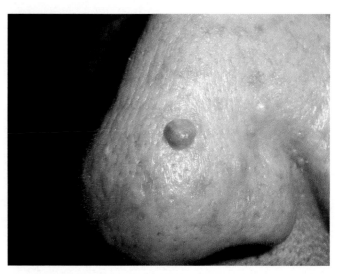

FIGURE 152-7 Single large elevated lesion of sebaceous hyperplasia on the nose of a 51 year-old man with rosacea. A shave biopsy ruled out BCC and gave the definitive diagnosis of sebaceous hyperplasia. The cosmetic result was excellent. (*Courtesy of Richard P. Usatine, MD.*)

REFERENCES

1. Hogan D, R Walker Jones, SH Mason. http://www.emedicine.com/derm/topic395.htm. Accessed September 19, 2006.

2. Boschnakow A, May T, Assaf C, et al. Ciclosporin A-induced sebaceous gland hyperplasia. *Br J Dermatol*. 2003;149(1):198–200.

3. Zaballos P, Ara M, Puig S, et al. Dermoscopy of sebaceous hyperplasia. *Arch Dermatol*. 2005;141:808.

4. Gold MH, Bradshaw WL, Boring MM, et al. Treatment of sebaceous hyperplasia by photodynamic therapy with 5-aminolevulinic acid and a blue light source or intense pulsed light source. *J Drugs Dermatol*. 2004;3(6 Suppl):S6–S9.

153 DERMATOFIBROMA

Mindy A. Smith, MD, MS
Richard P. Usatine, MD

PATIENT STORY

A 25-year-old woman reports a firm nodule on her leg that gets in the way of shaving her leg (**Figure 153-1**). Upon questioning it may have started there after she cut her leg shaving one year ago. She is worried it could be a cancer and wants it removed. Close observation showed a brown halo and a firm nodule that dimpled down when pinched. A diagnosis of a dermatofibroma (DF) was made and the choices for treatment were discussed.

EPIDEMIOLOGY

- Common, benign, scar-like nodule, most commonly found on the legs of adults.
- Occurs more often in women (female: male ratio 4:1).[1]
- Found in patients of all races.
- Approximately 20% occur in patients younger than 17 years.[1]

ETIOLOGY AND PATHOPHYSIOLOGY

- A benign fibrohistiocytic tumor, found in the mid dermis, composed of a mixture of fibroblastic and histiocytic cells (also called benign fibrous histiocytoma).
- Uncertain etiology—nodule may represent a fibrous reaction triggered by trauma, a viral infection, or insect bite; however, DFs show clonal proliferative growth seen in both neoplastic and inflammatory conditions.[1]
- Multiple DFs (i.e., >15 lesions) have been reported associated with systemic lupus erythematosus, HIV infection, or leukemia and may represent a worsening of immune function. A case of familial eruptive DFs has also been reported associated with atopic dermatitis.[2]

DIAGNOSIS

CLINICAL FEATURES

- Firm to hard nodule; skin is freely movable over the nodule, except for the area of dimpling.
- Color of the overlying skin ranges from flesh to gray, pink, red, blue, brown, or black (**Figures 153-1 to 152-5**), or a combination of hues (**Figure 153-5**).
- Dimples downward when compressed laterally because of tethering of the overlying epidermis to the underlying nodule (**Figures 153-3 and 153-4**).
- Usually asymptomatic but may be tender or pruritic.

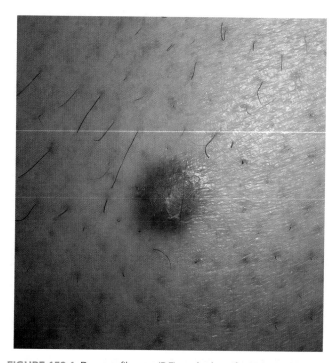

FIGURE 153-1 Dermatofibroma (DF) on the leg of a 25-year-old woman that may have begun after she cut her leg shaving 1 year ago. Note the brown halo, pink hue and raised center. (*Courtesy of Richard P. Usatine, MD.*)

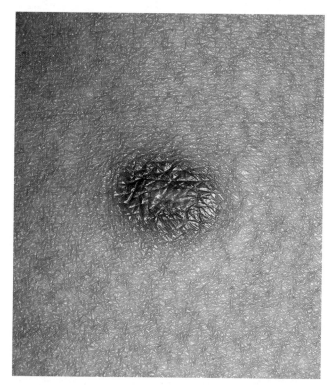

FIGURE 153-2 DF on the thigh of black woman. Note the darker brown halo around the lighter center. (*Courtesy of Richard P. Usatine, MD.*)

- Size ranges from 0.3 to 10 mm; usually <6 mm. Some DFs grow to 2 to 3 cm but these should be biopsied to rule out a malignancy called dermatofibrosarcoma protuberans (**Figure 153-6**).

- Many DFs have a hyperpigmented halo (**Figures 153-1 to 153-5**).

IMAGING

- Dermatoscopy may be a useful adjunctive diagnostic technique for DF. Three dermoscopic patterns have been seen, the most common being a peripheral pigment network with a central white area (56% of cases) (**Figure 153-7**).[3]

TYPICAL DISTRIBUTION

- May be found anywhere, but usually on the legs and arms, especially the lower legs.

BIOPSY

- A punch biopsy can be diagnostic and therapeutic if the DF is small.

DIFFERENTIAL DIAGNOSIS

DFs may be confused with the following malignant tumors; diagnosis based on histology and excision should be undertaken for enlarging or ulcerating tumors:

- Dermatofibrosarcoma protuberans—A low-grade malignant fibrotic tumor of the skin and subcutaneous tissues (**Figure 153-6**). A punch biopsy might provide adequate tissue to make the diagnosis. However, a full excisional biopsy is preferred to avoid a false negative result due to sampling error.

- Pseudosarcomatous DF—A rare connective tissue tumor arising on the trunk and limbs in young adults.

- Malignant fibrous histiocytoma—A soft tissue sarcoma occurring in the extremities. Presentation as a primary cutaneous lesion is rare and more often presents as a metastasis from another location such as the breast.

Many benign lesions have a similar appearance including:

- Pigmented seborrheic keratosis—may be macular and often larger than DF. Distinguished by surface cracks, verrucous features, stuck-on appearance, and adherent greasy scale (see Chapter 151, Seborrheic Keratosis).

- Epidermal inclusion cyst—sharply circumscribed, skin-colored nodule often with a central punctum. Most common on face, neck, or trunk. Composed of stratified epithelium surrounding a mass of keratinized material that has a foul odor when it drains.

- Hypertrophic scar—occurs within previous wounds or lacerations.

- Neurofibroma—benign Schwann cell tumors, single lesions are seen in normal individuals. Cutaneous tumors tend to form multiple, soft pedunculated masses, whereas subcutaneous nodules are skin-colored soft nodules attached to peripheral nerves. The latter show similar invagination as DF (see Chapter 223, Neurofibromatosis).

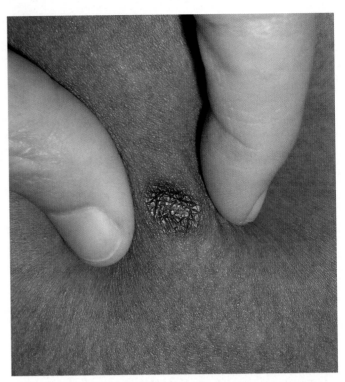

FIGURE 153-3 Dimple sign (downward skin dimpling when the DF nodule is compressed laterally). (*Courtesy of Richard P. Usatine, MD.*)

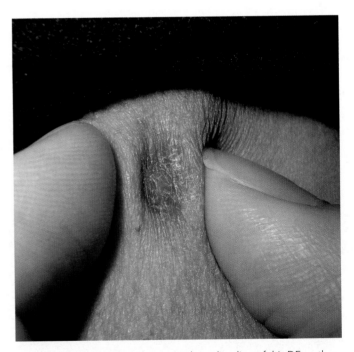

FIGURE 153-4 Pinch test showing a deep dimpling of this DF on the buttocks. (*Courtesy of Richard P. Usatine, MD.*)

MANAGEMENT

- No treatment is necessary unless the diagnosis is questioned or symptoms warrant.

- Punch excision or shave excision may be used for small lesions; the healed area may remain hard caused by the remaining fibrous tissue.

- Larger lesions may require an elliptical (fusiform) excision, down to the subcutaneous fat.

- One author noted that DFs occurring on the face often have involvement of deeper structures and an increased rate of local re-currences and, therefore, recommend excision with wider margins in comparison with DFs occurring on the extremities.[4]

- Cryotherapy has also been used, but the cure rate is low and lesions may recur.

PATIENT EDUCATION

- These are best left alone if they are relatively asymptomatic and stable. Tends to recur and so may be difficult to "cure."

PATIENT RESOURCES

www.aocd.org/skin/dermatologic_diseases/
dermatofibroma.html.

PROVIDER RESOURCES

www.emedicine.com/DERM/topic96.htm.

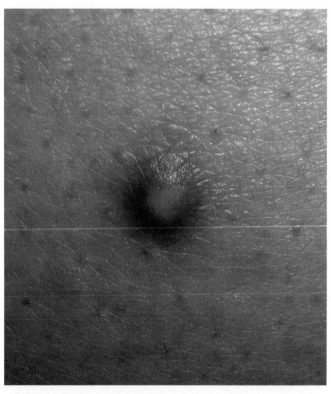

FIGURE 153-5 DF on the back. Note the brown halo around the lighter central nodule. (*Courtesy of Richard P. Usatine, MD.*)

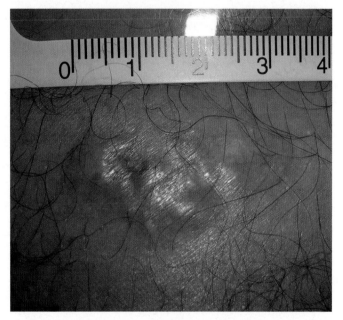

FIGURE 153-6 Large dermatofibrosarcoma protuberans growing on the thigh of this 55 year-old man. The first punch biopsy was read as a benign DF. Continued growth prompted a second biopsy that detected the malignancy. The first excision did not achieve clear margins so the final treatment consisted of Mohs surgery. Note the shiny surface and multilobular look that can be characteristic of a dermatofibrosarcoma protuberans. (*Courtesy of Richard P. Usatine, MD.*)

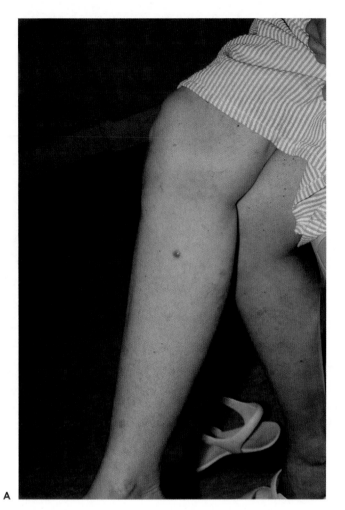

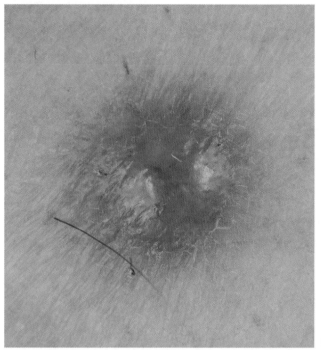

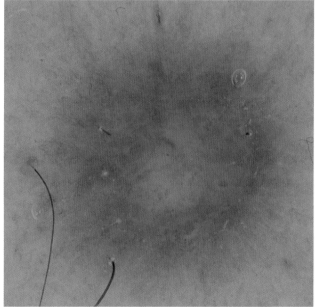

FIGURE 153-7 (A) DF on the leg that appears pink to red in color.
(B) Close-up of the DF showing the pink center and brown halo.
(C) Dermoscopic view of the DF showing the typical pattern with a
radially streaking brown halo and a pink center with little pigment.
(*Courtesy of Ashfaq Marghoob, MD.*)

REFERENCES

1. Dermatofibroma. http://www.emedicine.com/DERM/topic96.htm. Accessed July 20, 2006.

2. Yazici AC, Baz K, Ikizoglu G, et al. Familial eruptive dermatofibromas in atopic dermatitis. *J Eur Acad Dermatol Venereol.* 2006;20(1):90–92.

3. Arpaia N, Cassano N, Vena GA. Dermoscopic patterns of dermatofibroma. *Dermatol Surg.* 2005;31(10):1336–1339.

4. Mentzel T, Kutzner H, Rutten A, Hugel H. Benign fibrous histiocytoma (dermatofibroma) of the face: Clinicopathologic and immunohistochemical study of 34 cases associated with an aggressive clinical course. *Am J Dermatopathol.* 2001;23(5):419–426.

154 PYOGENIC GRANULOMA

Mindy A. Smith, MD, MS
Richard P. Usatine, MD

PATIENT STORY

A 20-year-old woman, who was being seen by her family physician for her prenatal care, presents to the office with a new growth on her lip. She stated that the growth on her lip bled very easily but was not painful. She was diagnosed with a pyogenic granuloma (PG) and preferred to wait until her pregnancy was over to have it removed. The lesion did not regress spontaneously after pregnancy and was surgically excised.

EPIDEMIOLOGY

- Common, benign, acquired, vascular neoplasm of the skin and mucous membranes.

- It is neither infections nor granulomatous, so a more accurate name has been given, lobular capillary hemangioma. Most often seen in young adults and adolescents.

- Also common during pregnancy (up to 5% of pregnancies).[1]

- PG has also been reported in the gastrointestinal tract, the larynx, and on the nasal mucosa, conjunctiva, and cornea.[1]

ETIOLOGY AND PATHOPHYSIOLOGY

- Etiology is unknown but may be the result of trauma, infection, or preceding dermatoses; a history of trauma, however, is only elicited in up to 25% of cases.

- Consists of dense proliferation of capillaries and fibroblastic stroma that is infiltrated with polymorphonuclear leukocytes.

- Multiple PGs have been reported at burn sites and following use of oral contraceptives, protease inhibitors, and topical application of tretinoin for acne.[2]

- PGs are known to regress following pregnancy. Vascular endothelial growth factor was found in one study to be high in the granulomas in pregnancy and was almost undetectable after parturition and associated with apoptosis of endothelial cells and regression of granuloma.[3]

DIAGNOSIS

CLINICAL FEATURES

- Erythematous, dome-shaped papule or nodule that bleeds easily (**Figures 154-1** to **154-6**); rarely causes anemia.

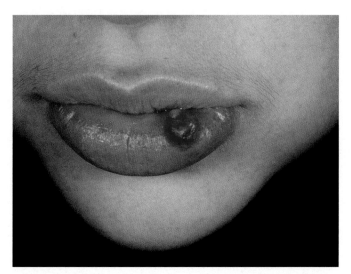

FIGURE 154-1 Pyogenic granuloma (PG) on the lower lip arising during pregnancy. (*With permission from Usatine RP, Moy RL, Tobinick EL, Siegel DM. Skin Surgery: A Practical Guide. 1998, St. Louis: Mosby.*)

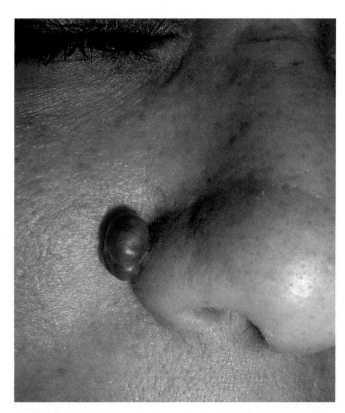

FIGURE 154-2 PG on the nose in a young adult. (*Courtesy of Richard P. Usatine, MD.*)

- Prone to ulceration, erosion, and crusting.

- Size ranges from a few millimeters to several centimeters (average size is 6.5 mm).[1]

- Rapid growth over a period of weeks to maximum size.

IMAGING

- Reddish homogeneous area surrounded by a white collarette is the most frequent dermoscopic pattern in PGs (85%).[4]

TYPICAL DISTRIBUTION

- Cutaneous PG most often found on the head and neck (specifically the gingiva, lips as in **Figure 154-1**), nose (**Figure 154-2**), and face, extremities (**Figures 154-3** to **154-6**), and upper trunk.

- Pregnancy PG occurs most commonly along the maxillary intraoral mucosal surface.

BIOPSY

- Early lesions resemble granulation tissue (numerous capillaries and venules with endothelial cells arrayed radially toward the skin surface; stroma is edematous and contains a mixed inflammatory infiltrate).[1]

- The mature PG exhibits a fibromyxoid stroma separating the lesion into lobules. Proliferation of capillaries is present, with prominent endothelial cells. Reepithelialization of the surface and a peripheral hyperplastic adnexal epithelioid collarette may be noted; less inflammatory infiltrate is present.[1] The epidermis is commonly eroded.

- A regressing PG has extensive fibrosis.

DIFFERENTIAL DIAGNOSIS

PG may be confused with a number of cutaneous malignancies including atypical fibroxanthoma, basal cell carcinoma, Kapos's sarcoma, metastatic cutaneous lesions, squamous cell carcinoma and amelanotic melanoma (**Figure 154-7**).

It is especially important to send the excised lesion that appears to be a PG for pathology to make sure that a malignancy is not missed.

Benign tumors that may be confused with PG include:

- Cherry hemangioma—Small, bright-red, dome-shaped papules that represent benign proliferation of capillaries (**Figure 154-8**) (see Chapter 194, Acquired Vascular Skin Lessions).

- Fibrous papule of the nose is a benign tumor of the nose. Most are skin colored and not confused with PG. A benign clear cell variant of a fibrous papule can closely resemble a PG as seen in **Figure 154-9**.

- Bacillary angiomatosis—A systemic infectious disease caused by two Bartonella species. Four patterns of nodules, one (globular angiomatous papules) appearing like PG (**Figure 210-5**). Nodules affect all age groups and may reach 10 cm in size. Weight loss and lymphadenopathy may occur.

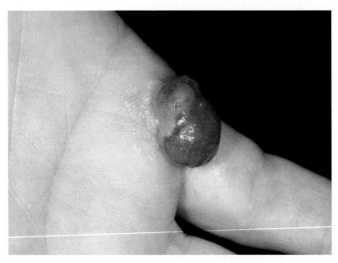

FIGURE 154-3 Large PG on the hand of a 33-year-old man present for 3 months. (*Courtesy of Richard P. Usatine, MD.*)

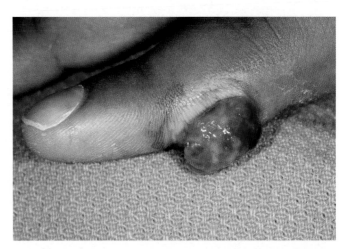

FIGURE 154-4 Large PG on the finger of a 22-year-old man present for 4 months. He was sent out of multiple clinical settings untreated until we excised this. (*Courtesy of Richard P. Usatine, MD.*)

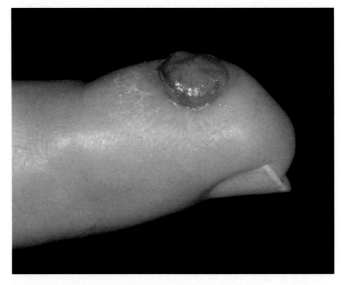

FIGURE 154-5 Small PG on the finger of a 17-year-old boy for 2 months. It started with a small injury to the finger. (*Courtesy of Richard P. Usatine, MD.*)

MANAGEMENT

- Removal of the lesion is indicated to prevent bleeding and to make sure there is no malignancy.

- Untreated PGs eventually atrophy, become fibromatous, and slowly regress, especially if the causative agent is removed.

- Removal can be accomplished with shave excision and electrodesiccation, and the latter reduces recurrence. These bleed extensively when manipulated or cut. It is important to use lidocaine with epinephrine; wait 10 minutes for the epinephrine to work and have an electrosurgery device to control bleeding. Cut the PG off with a blade and send to pathology. Curetting the base will also help stop bleeding and prevent recurrence. The base is curetted and electrodesiccated until bleeding stops. SOR **C**

- A case of successful treatment of a recurrent PG was reported using a 14-week course of twice-weekly imiquimod 5% topical application.[5] SOR **C**

- Other reported treatments include cryosurgery and laser surgery. SOR **C**.

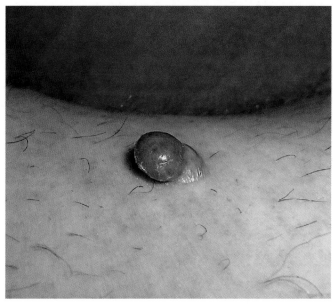

FIGURE 154-6 PG on the leg for 6 months before the patient presented for treatment. (*Courtesy of Richard P. Usatine, MD.*)

PATIENT EDUCATION

- Explain to patients that if the lesion begins to recur, they should follow-up quickly to treat the recurrence before it gets larger and harder to treat.

FOLLOW-UP

- Follow-up is only needed if the pathology does not show PG or if the lesion recurs.

PATIENT RESOURCES

VisualDxHealth **http://www.visualdxhealth.com/adult/ pyogenicGranuloma.htm.**

PROVIDER RESOURCES

http://www.emedicine.com/derm/topic368.htm and **www.emedicine.com/ped/topic1244.htm.**

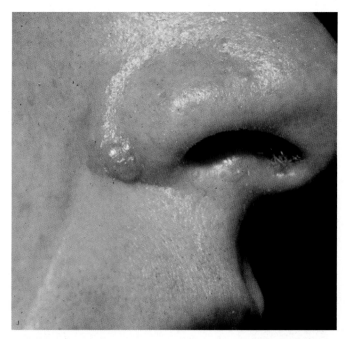

FIGURE 154-7 Amelanotic melanoma on the nose that could be confused with a PG. Always send what you suspect to be a PG to the pathologist. (*Courtesy of the University of Texas Health Sciences Center, Division of Dermatology.*)

REFERENCES

1. Pyogenic granuloma. http://www.emedicine.com/derm/topic368.htm. Accessed August 2, 2006.

2. Teknetzis A, Tonannides D, Vakali G, et al. Pyogenic granulomas following topical application of tretinoin. *J Eur Acad Dermatol Venereol.* 2004;18(3):337–339.

3. Yuan K, Lin MT. The roles of vascular endothelial growth factor and angiopoietin-2 in the regression of pregnancy pyogenic granuloma. *Oral Dis.* 2004;10(3):179–185.

4. Zaballos P, Llambrich A, Cuellar F, et al. Dermoscopic findings in pyogenic granuloma. *Br J Dermatol.* 2006;154(6):1108–1111.

5. Goldenberg G, Krowchuk DP, Jorizzo JL. Successful treatment of a therapy-resistant pyogenic granuloma with topical imiquimod 5% cream. *J Dermatolog Treat.* 2006;17(2):121–123.

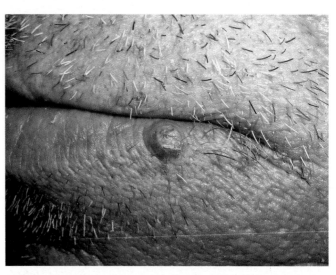

FIGURE 154-8 Hemangioma on the lip of a 67-year-old man. By appearance alone this is hard to differentiate from a pyogenic granuloma (lobular capillary hemangioma). This did not bleed extensively at time of excision and the pathology result confirmed that this was a hemangioma. (*Courtesy of Richard P. Usatine, MD.*)

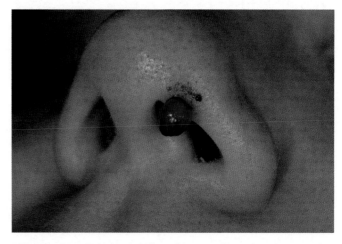

FIGURE 154-9 Vascular growth on the nose of a pregnant woman that appears to be a PG. Biopsy revealed a benign clear cell variant of a fibrous papule. (*Courtesy of Richard P. Usatine, MD.*)

SECTION 10 NEVI

155 BENIGN NEVI

Mindy A. Smith, MD, MS

PATIENT STORY

A young woman comes to the office because her husband has noted that the moles on her back are changing (**Figure 155-1**). A few have white halos around the brown pigmentation and some have lost their pigment completely, with a light area remaining (**Figure 155-2**). She has no symptoms but wants to make sure these are not skin cancers. These halo nevi are an uncommon variation of common nevi. These appear benign and the patient is reassured.

EPIDEMIOLOGY

- Acquired nevi are common lesions, forming during early childhood—few adults have none.
- Prevalence appears to be lower in dark skinned individuals.
- Present in 1% of neonates increasing through childhood and peaking at puberty; new ones may continue to appear in adulthood.
- Adults typically have 10 to 40 nevi scattered over the body. In a population study in Germany, 60.3% of 2823 adults (mean age 49 years, 50% women) exhibited 11 to 50 common nevi and 5.2% had at least one atypical nevus.[1]
- The peak incidence of melanocytic nevi (MN) is in the fourth to fifth decades of life; the incidence decreases with each successive decade.[2]

ETIOLOGY AND PATHOPHYSIOLOGY

- Benign tumors composed of nevus cells derived from melanocytes, pigment-producing cells that colonize the epidermis.
- MN represent proliferations of melanocytes that are in contact with each other, forming small collections of cells known as nests.
- Sun (ultraviolet) exposure, skin-blistering events (e.g., sunburn), and genetics play a role in the formation of new nevi.[2]
- Nevi commonly darken and/or enlarge during pregnancy. Melanocytes have receptors for estrogens and androgens and melanogenesis is responsive to these hormones.[2]
- Three broad categories of nevi (common moles) are based on location of nevus cells[1]:
  - Junctional nevi—composed of nevus cells located in the dermoepidermal junction; may change into compound nevi after childhood (except when located on the palms, soles, or genitalia) (**Figure 155-3**).

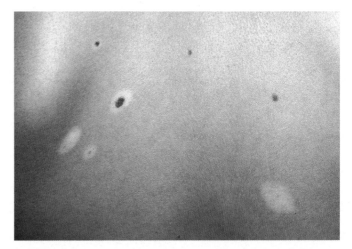

FIGURE 155-1 Multiple halo nevi on the back. (*Courtesy of Richard P. Usatine, MD.*)

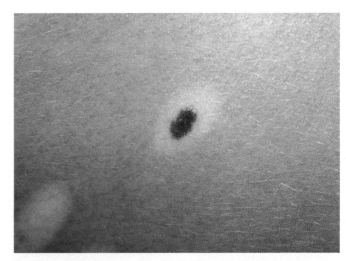

FIGURE 155-2 Close-up of halo nevi, one with remaining nevocytes and the other fully hypopigmented. (*Courtesy of Richard P. Usatine, MD.*)

- Compound nevi—a mole in which a portion of nevus cells have migrated into the dermis (**Figure 155-4**).
- Dermal nevi—composed of nevus cells located within the dermis (usually found only in adults) (**Figures 155-5 to 155-7**).

- Special categories of nevi:
  - Halo nevus—compound or dermal nevus that develops a symmetric, sharply demarcated, depigmented border (**Figures 155-1 and 155-2**). Most commonly occurs on the trunk and develops during adolescence. Repigmentation may occur.
  - Blue nevus—a dermal nevus that contains large amounts of pigment so that the brown pigment absorbs the longer wavelengths of light and scatters blue light (Tyndall effect) (**Figure 155-8**). Blue nevi are not always blue and color varies from tan to blue, black, or gray. The nodules are firm because of associated stromal sclerosis. Usually appears in childhood on the extremities, dorsum of the hands and face. A rare variant, the cellular blue nevus is large (>1 cm), frequently located on the buttocks, and may undergo malignant degeneration.
  - Nevus spilus—hairless, oval, or irregularly shaped brown lesion with darker brown to black dots containing nevus cells (**Figures 155-9 and 155-10**). May appear at any age or be present at birth; unrelated to sun exposure.
  - Becker's nevus—a brown macule, patch of hair, or both located on the shoulder, back or submammary area, most often in adolescent men (**Figures 155-11 and 155-12**). The lesion may enlarge to cover an entire shoulder or upper arm. While it is called a nevus, it does not actually have nevus cells and has no malignant potential.
  - Spitz nevus (formerly called benign juvenile melanoma because of its clinical and histologic similarity to melanoma)—hairless, red or reddish brown dome-shaped papules generally appearing suddenly in children, sometimes following trauma (**Figure 155-13**). The color is caused by increased vascularity. They may have epidermal hyperplasia and hyperkeratosis.

- Both acquired and congenital MN hold some risk for the development of melanoma; the number of MN, especially more than 100, is an important independent risk factor for cutaneous melanoma.[3]

DIAGNOSIS

CLINICAL FEATURES

Most moles are tan to brown, usually <6 mm with round shape and sharp borders.

- Junctional nevi—macular or slightly elevated mole of uniform brown to black pigmentation, smooth surface, and a round or oval border (**Figure 155-3**). Most are hairless and vary from 1 to 6 mm.

- Compound nevi—slightly elevated, symmetric, uniformly flesh colored or brown with a round or oval border, often becoming more elevated with age (**Figure 155-4**). Hair may be present and a white halo may form.

- Dermal nevi (same as intradermal nevi)—skin color or brown color that may fade with age; dome shaped is most common but shapes vary including polypoid, warty and pedunculated. Often found on the face and may have telangiectasias (**Figures 155-5 to 155-7**). Size ranges from 1 to 10 mm.

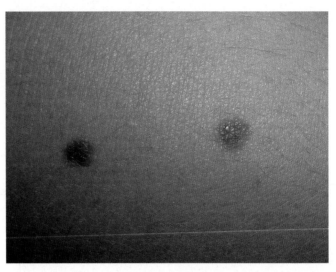

FIGURE 155-3 Two benign junctional nevi on the arm of a 19-year-old woman. Note how these are flat and macular. (*Courtesy of Richard P. Usatine, MD.*)

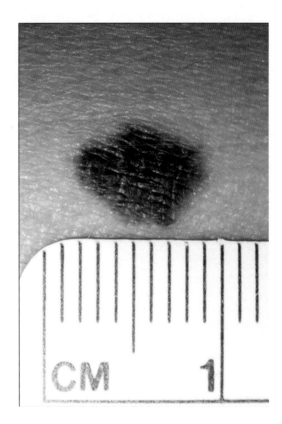

FIGURE 155-4 Benign compound nevus proven by biopsy. (*Courtesy of Richard P. Usatine, MD.*)

TYPICAL DISTRIBUTION

- Most often above the waist on sun-exposed areas but may appear anywhere on the cutaneous surface; less commonly found on the scalp, breasts, or buttocks.

- In an Australian study of white children, MN of all sizes were highest on the outer forearms, followed by the outer upper arms, neck, and face.[4] Boys had higher densities of MN of all sizes on the neck than girls ($P = 0.002$) and girls had higher densities of MN of 2 mm or greater on the lower legs ($P = 0.006$) and thighs ($P = 0.005$) than boys. Habitually sun-exposed body sites had higher densities of small MN and highest prevalence of larger MN.

BIOPSY

Biopsy is necessary if you suspect melanoma. A biopsy that cuts below the pigmented area is preferred if there is a reasonable suspicion for melanoma. This can be done with a scoop shave, a punch that gets the whole lesion or an elliptical excision. If the patient wants a raised benign appearing nevus excised for cosmetic reasons, a shave excision may be adequate. Always send all pigmented lesions to the pathologist for examination even when they appear benign to avoid missing a melanoma.

DIFFERENTIAL DIAGNOSIS

Rarely, common moles develop atypia or melanoma. This should be suspected if a lesion has atypical features including asymmetry, border irregularity, color variability, diameter greater than 6 mm, and evolving (called the ABCDE approach). Any lesion that becomes symptomatic (e.g., itchy, painful, irritated, or bleeding) or develops a loss or increase in pigmentation should be evaluated and biopsied if needed.

- Melanomas are skin cancers that may develop from a preexisting nevus. The most important skill to develop is how to distinguish a benign nevus from a nevus that might be malignant melanoma. Because clinical appearance can be misleading, a biopsy is necessary when there is a reasonable suspicion for cancer (see Chapter 165, Melanoma).

- Dysplastic or atypical nevi are variants that are relatively flat, thinly papular, and relatively broad. Often, the lesions exhibit target-like or fried egg-like morphology, with a central papular zone and a macular surrounding area with differing pigmentation (see Chapter 158, Dysplastic Nevus).[2]

- Seborrheic keratoses are benign growths that appear more with increasing age and are often hyperpigmented as seen with many nevi. These are more superficial and stuck-on in their appearance (see Chapter 151, Seborrheic Keratosis).

- Labial melanotic macules are benign dark macules on the lip that are not nevi and not melanomas (**Figure 155-14**). They can be removed for cosmetic purposes.

MANAGEMENT

MN are generally removed for cosmetic reasons or because of concern over changes in the lesion suggestive of dysplasia or

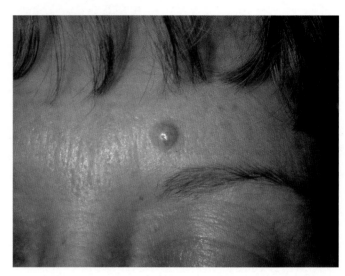

FIGURE 155-5 Dermal nevus (intradermal nevus)—dome shaped with some scattered pigmentation. (*Courtesy of Richard P. Usatine, MD.*)

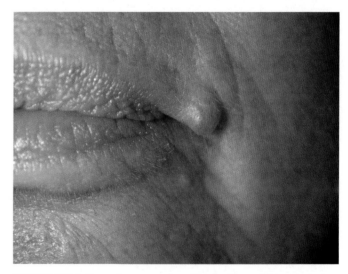

FIGURE 155-6 Dermal nevus pedunculated with small telangiectasias. (*Courtesy of Richard P. Usatine, MD.*)

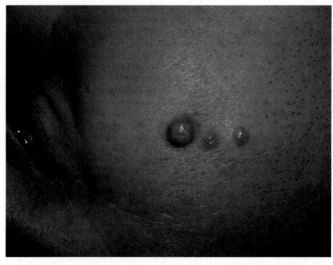

FIGURE 155-7 Three benign intradermal nevi on the face all removed using shave excisions. (*Courtesy of Richard P. Usatine, MD.*)

melanoma. Degeneration of common nevi into melanoma is very rare.

- A full excisional biopsy with a sutured closure is usually the best means to diagnose a lesion if concern exists regarding the possibility of melanoma. If the lesion is found to be benign, no further treatment is usually required.

- Punch excision can be used to excise smaller lesions.

- Scoop shave—Unfortunately, if a punch biopsy is used to sample a larger lesion it may miss the melanoma in another part of the lesion. Sometimes a broad scoop shave is better than a punch biopsy when a full elliptical excision is not possible or desirable (e.g. a large flat pigmented lesion on the face).

- Nevi removed for cosmesis are often removed by shave excision.[2]

Becker's nevi do not become melanoma because these nevi lack nevocytes. Therefore, there is no reason to excise them. Generally, these are large and the risks of excision for cosmetic reasons outweigh the benefits.

PATIENT EDUCATION

- Patients should be encouraged to use sunscreen to prevent skin cancer as well as to reduce the development of new nevi. In a trial of 209 white children, children randomized to the sunscreen group, especially those with freckles, had significantly fewer new nevi on the trunk than children in the control group at 3-year follow-up.[5]

- Patients with multiple or sizable MN appear to have an increased lifetime risk of melanoma, with the risk increasing in rough proportion to the size and/or number of lesions. Patients should be taught to look for and report asymmetry, border irregularity, new symptoms, and color and size changes.

FOLLOW-UP

- Patients with multiple or sizable MN should be followed by an experienced clinician because they appear to have an increased lifetime risk of melanoma, with the risk increasing in rough proportion to the size and/or number of lesions.

PATIENT RESOURCES

VisualDxHealth—good information with excellent photographs
http://www.visualdxhealth.com/adult/nevus.htm
http://www.visualdxhealth.com/diseaseGroups/
skinCancer_moles.htm.

American Osteopathic College of Dermatology—
www.aocd.org/skin/dermatologic_diseases/moles.html.

American Academy of Dermatology—**www.aad.org** on moles:
http://www.aad.org/public/publications/pamphlets/
common_moles.html.

PROVIDER RESOURCES

http://www.emedicine.com/derm/topic289.htm.

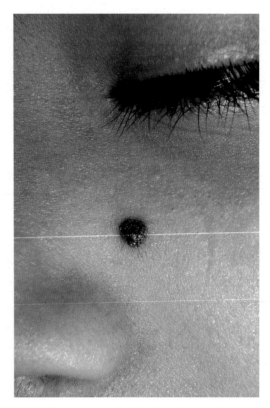

FIGURE 155-8 Blue nevus on the left cheek that could resemble a melanoma with its dark color. It was fully excised with a 5 mm punch with a good cosmetic result. (*Courtesy of Richard P. Usatine, MD.*)

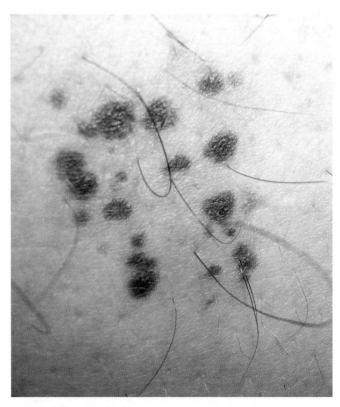

FIGURE 155-9 Speckled lentiginous nevus (nevus spilus) appearing in adolescence with large areas of absent pigment. (*Courtesy of Richard P. Usatine, MD.*)

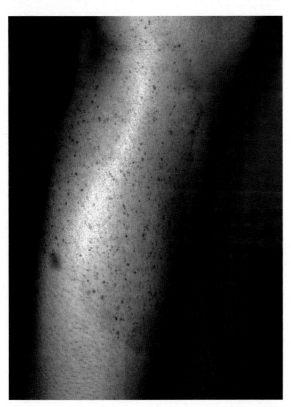

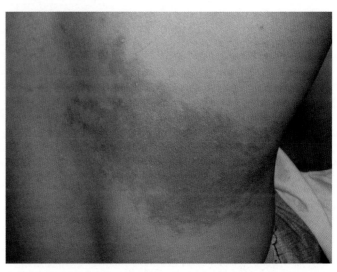

FIGURE 155-12 Becker's nevus on the back of a 16-year-old Hispanic adolescent for 2 years. While this nevus did not have hair, it did have increased acne within the area—another feature of the Becker's nevus. (*Courtesy of Richard P. Usatine, MD.*)

FIGURE 155-10 Nevus spilus on the leg of a young woman from birth. (*Courtesy of Richard P. Usatine, MD.*)

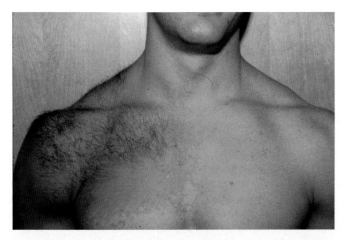

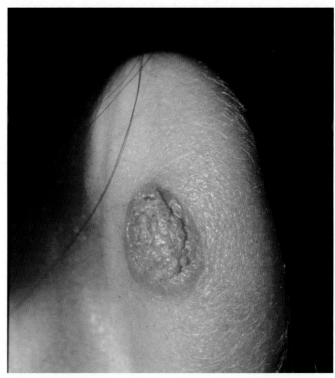

FIGURE 155-11 Becker's nevus that developed during adolescence. Hair is frequently seen on this type of nevus. There are no reported cases of Becker's nevi becoming melanoma. These nevi lack nevocytes. (*Courtesy of Jack Resneck, Sr., MD.*)

FIGURE 155-13 Spitz nevus on the right pinna of a prepubertal child. The term juvenile melanoma has been used to describe this lesion. Excision is indicated. (*Courtesy of the University of Texas Health Sciences Center, Division of Dermatology.*)

REFERENCES

1. Schafer T, Merkl J, Klemm E, et al. The Epidemiology of nevi and signs of skin aging in the adult general population: Results of the KORA-Survey 2000. *J Invest Dermatol.* 2006;126(7):1490–1496.

2. McCalmont T. http://www.emedicine.com/derm/topic289.htm. Accessed August 28, 2006.

3. Gandini S, Sera F, Cattaruzza MS, et al. Meta-analysis of risk factors for cutaneous melanoma: I. Common and atypical nevi. *Eur J Cancer.* 2005;41(1):28–44.

4. Harrison SL, Buettner PG, MacLennan R. Body-site distribution of MN in young Australian children. *Arch Dermatol.* 1999;135(1): 47–52.

5. Lee TK, Rivers JK, Gallagher RP. Site-specific protective effect of broad-spectrum sunscreen on nevus development among white schoolchildren in a randomized trial. *J Am Acad Dermatol.* 2005; 52(5):786–792.

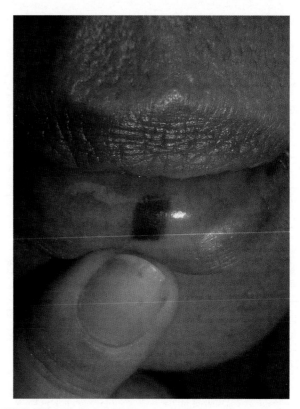

FIGURE 155-14 Labial melanotic macule. These are benign but are not nevi. (*Courtesy of Richard P. Usatine, MD.*)

156 CONGENITAL NEVI

Mindy A. Smith, MD, MS

PATIENT STORY

A small congenital nevus (**Figure 156-1**) was noted on a 6-month-old child by his new family physician during a routine examination. The parents acknowledged that it was there from birth and asked if it needed to be cut out. They were reassured that nothing needs to be done about it at this time.

EPIDEMIOLOGY

- Congenital nevi develop in 1% to 2% of newborns and are present at birth.[1]

- Nevi that are not present at birth, but are histologically identical to congenital nevi, may develop during the first 2 years of life and can be called congenital nevus tardive.[1]

- Congenital nevi are also seen in neurocutaneous melanosis, a rare syndrome characterized by the presence of congenital melanocytic nevi and melanotic neoplasms of the central nervous system.

- The development of melanoma within congenital nevi is believed to occur at a higher rate than in normal skin.
  - In a systematic review, 46 of 6571 patients with congenital melanocytic nevi (0.7%) followed for 3.4 to 23.7 years developed melanomas, representing a 465-fold increased relative risk of developing melanoma during childhood and adolescence.[2] The mean age at diagnosis of melanoma was 15.5 years (median 7). Nearly three in four melanomas appeared in large congenital nevi over 20 cm.[2]
  - Patients with giant congenital melanocytic nevi appear to be at highest risk where subsequent melanoma has been reported in 5% to 7% by age 60.[3]
  - However, in one prospective study of 230 medium-sized congenital nevi (1.5 to 19.9 cm) in 227 patients from 1955 to 1996, no melanomas occurred. The average follow-up period being 6.7 years to an average age of 25.5 years.[4]

ETIOLOGY AND PATHOPHYSIOLOGY

- The etiology of congenital nevi is unknown.

- Congenital nevi result from a proliferation of benign melanocytes in the dermis, epidermis, or both. Melanocytes of the skin originate in the neuroectoderm, although the specific cell type from which they derive remains unknown.[1]

- Congenital nevi have been stratified into 3 groups according to size[1]:
  - Small nevi—less than 1.5 cm in greatest diameter (**Figure 156-1**).

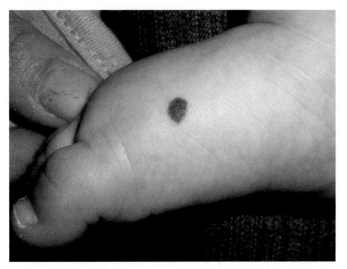

FIGURE 156-1 Small congenital nevus found on the foot of a 6-month-old child. The parents were counseled to not get it excised at this time. (*Courtesy of Richard P. Usatine, MD.*)

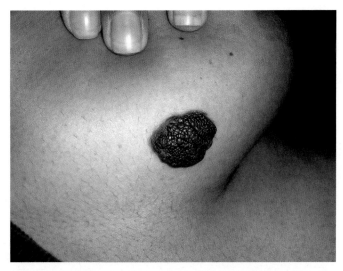

FIGURE 156-2 Congenital nevus on the breast of a 24-year-old woman. It is verrucous, but entirely benign. (*Courtesy of Richard P. Usatine, MD.*)

○ Medium nevi—1.5 to 19.9 cm in greatest diameter (**Figures 156-2** and **156-3**).

○ Large or giant nevi—greater than 20 cm in greatest diameter (**Figures 156-4** to **156-7**). Giant nevi are often surrounded by several smaller satellite nevi (**Figures 156-5** to **156-7**).

DIAGNOSIS

CLINICAL FEATURES

• Variable mixtures of color including tan, brown, black, and red within a single lesion (**Figures 156-2** to **156-7**); color usually remains constant over time.

• Irregular borders (all Figures); pigment may fade off into surrounding skin (**Figures 156-3** and **156-4**).

• Nevi may become raised over time (**Figures 156-2** and **156-3**).

• Macular portion usually found at edges.

• Usually >6 mm, may be >10 mm.

IMAGING

• Dermoscopy findings depend on the age and location. In one study, the globular pattern was most common in children younger than 11 years of age and on the trunk.[5] The majority of reticular lesions were located on the limbs and the variegated pattern was the most specific for congenital nevi.

• Magnetic resonance imaging of the central nervous system can be a useful diagnostic tool in patients suspected of having neurocutaneous melanosis.[1]

TYPICAL DISTRIBUTION

• Congenital nevi may be found anywhere on the body.

BIOPSY

Distinguishing histologic features of congenital nevi[1]:

• Involvement by nevus cells of deep dermal appendages and neurovascular structures (e.g., hair follicles, sebaceous glands, arrector pili muscles, and within walls of blood vessels).

• Extension of nevus cells to deep dermis and subcutaneous fat.

• Infiltration of nevus cells between collagen bundles.

• A nevus cell—poor subepidermal zone.

In contrast to congenital nevi, acquired nevi are usually composed of nevus cells that are limited to the papillary and upper reticular dermis and do not involve the skin appendages.[1]

DIFFERENTIAL DIAGNOSIS

Other melanocytic lesions similar to congenital nevi:

• Becker's nevus—a brown macule, patch of hair, or both on the shoulder, back, or submammary area that develops in adolescence. The border is irregular and the lesion may enlarge to cover an entire shoulder or upper arm (see Chapter 155, Benign Nevi).

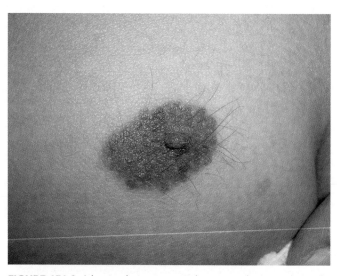

FIGURE 156-3 A benign hairy congenital nevus on the upper buttocks of a 7-year-old boy. The parents requested a consult with plastic surgery to discuss removal. (*Courtesy of Richard P. Usatine, MD.*)

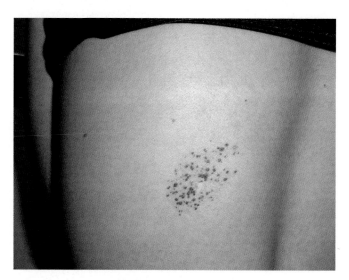

FIGURE 156-4 A speckled congenital nevus (nevus spilus) on the back of a young woman. (*Courtesy of Richard P. Usatine, MD.*)

• Nevus spilus—hairless, oval, or irregularly shaped brown lesion with darker brown to black dots containing nevus cells. May appear at birth or any age; unrelated to sun exposure (**Figure 156-4** and see Chapter 155, Benign Nevi).

MANAGEMENT

The management of congenital nevi depends on size and location of the lesion, the age of patient, the effect on cosmesis, and the potential for malignant transformation.

• For small and medium-sized congenital melanocytic nevi, the risk of malignant transformation is small and prophylactic removal is not recommended. For cosmesis, treatments include dermabrasion, curettage, laser therapy, and surgical excision.

• Larger congenital nevi can be surgically removed but may require tissue expanders, tissue grafts, and tissue flaps to close large defects. Because the melanocytes may extend deep into underlying tissues (including muscle, bone, and central nervous system), removing the cutaneous component may not eliminate the risk of malignancy.[1]

• In one case in the meta-analysis of 14 studies, a melanoma occurred underneath a previously excised congenital nevus.[2] The impact of prophylactic surgical measures on the risk of melanoma was stated as too difficult to assess from the existing data.[2] While the removal of melanocytic cells might reduce the risk of melanoma, the heterogeneity of the studies does not permit this conclusion.[2]

• Laser treatment of the lesions has been performed with a number of different types of lasers.[1,6] Because of the lack of penetrance to deeper tissue levels, long-term recurrence or malignant transformation is also an issue with these techniques.

• Careful lifelong follow-up with photographs is an acceptable approach, especially now with the affordability of digital cameras.

• Bathing trunk nevi (**Figures 156-5** to **156-7**):

  ○ 50% of the melanomas develop before age 5 in bathing trunk nevi.[7]

  ○ Melanomas can be missed by observation because they can have nonepidermal origins.[7]

  ○ Surgical excision is recommended by some experts to prevent melanoma.[7] SOR **C**

Changes to watch for that call for a biopsy:

• Partial regression (depressed white areas).

• Inflammation.

• Rapid growth or color change.

• Development of a firm nodule (**Figure 156-8**).

PATIENT EDUCATION

• All patients should be told about the importance of protection from ultraviolet light exposure. This is especially important in people with giant congenital nevi, because they are at a significantly increased risk of melanoma.

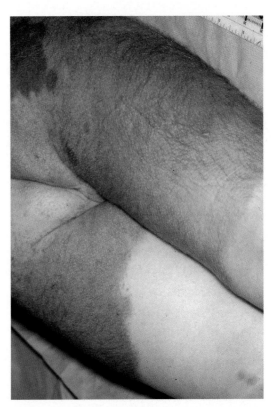

FIGURE 156-5 Large bathing trunk nevus seen on the legs of this older child. (*Courtesy of Jack Resneck, Sr., MD.*)

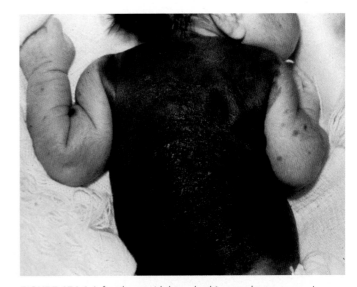

FIGURE 156-6 Infant born with large bathing trunk nevus covering most of the back and chest. (*Courtesy of the University of Texas Health Sciences Center, Division of Dermatology.*)

- Parents of children with large congenital nevi need to be given information about the known risks and benefits of prophylactic surgical removal. If a referral to a plastic surgeon is desired, it is good to know one in your community that is experienced with the removal of large congenital nevi.

FOLLOW-UP

- Patients with giant congenital nevi or multiple congenital nevi may benefit from consultation with a neurologist, pediatrician, or both because of the risk of neurocutaneous melanosis and its neurologic manifestations or obstructive hydrocephalus.

- Bathing trunk nevi can also be associated with spina bifida, meningocele, and neurofibromatosis.[7]

- Patients with all forms of congenital nevi, especially giant congenital melanocytic nevi, have an increased risk of developing melanoma. Physicians should consider baseline photography and regular follow-up with an experienced clinician for these patients.

PATIENT RESOURCES

www.nevusnetwork.org.

PROVIDER RESOURCES

http://www.emedicine.com/derm/topic903.htm and www.dermatlas.org.

REFERENCES

1. Steen CJ, Rothenberg J, Thomas I, Schwartz RA. http://www.emedicine.com/derm/topic903.htm. Accessed August 12, 2006.

2. Krengel S, Hauschild A, Schafer T. Melanoma risk in congenital melanocytic nevi: A systematic review. *Br J Dermatol.* 2006;155(1): 1–8.

3. Bett BJ. Large or multiple congenital melanocytic nevi: Occurrence of cutaneous melanoma in 1008 persons. *J Am Acad Dermatol.* 2005;52(5):793–797.

4. Sahin S, Levin L, Kopf AW, et al. Risk of melanoma in medium-sized congenital melanocytic nevi: A follow-up study. *J Am Acad Dermatol.* 1998;39:428–433.

5. Seidenari S, Pellacani G, Martella A, et al. Instrument-, age- and site-dependent variations of dermoscopic patterns of congenital melanocytic naevi: A multicentre study. *Br J Dermatol.* 2006; 155(1):56–61.

6. Ferguson RE, Jr., Vasconez HC. Laser treatment of congenital nevi. *J Craniofac Surg.* 2005;16(5):908–914.

7. Habif T. *Clinical Dermatology: A Color Guide to Diagnosis and Therapy.* 4th ed. Philadelphia: Mosby, 2003.

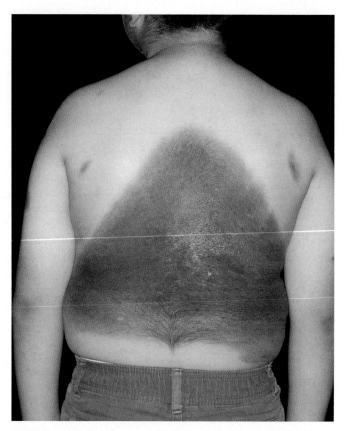

FIGURE 156-7 Giant congenital bathing trunk nevus surrounded by satellite nevi in a 7-year-old Hispanic boy. The patient was referred for staged removal of this potentially dangerous lesion. (*Courtesy of Richard P. Usatine, MD.*)

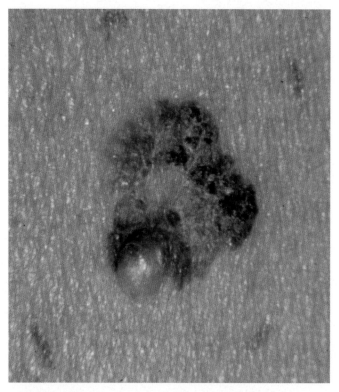

FIGURE 156-8 Melanoma arising in an acquired nevus showing features of central regression and a new elevated nodule. These are the same features that make a congenital nevus suspicious for melanoma. (*Courtesy of the University of Texas Health Sciences Center, Division of Dermatology.*)

157 EPIDERMAL NEVUS AND NEVUS SEBACEOUS

Mindy A. Smith, MD, MS

PATIENT STORY

A 15-year-old boy is brought in by his mother with a concern about the growth of his birthmark. It has become somewhat more raised and bumpy in the past year (**Figure 157-1**). The adolescent reports no symptoms and is not worried about the appearance. The boy is otherwise healthy with no neurologic symptoms. The joint decision of the family and the doctor is to not excise the epidermal nevus at this time. He may choose to have this removed by a plastic surgeon in the future.

EPIDEMIOLOGY

- Epidermal nevi (EN) are uncommon (approximately 1%–3% of newborns and children), sporadic, and usually present at birth, although they can appear in early childhood (**Figures 157-1** and **157-2**).

- EN are associated with disorders of the eye, nervous, and musculoskeletal systems in 10% to 30% of patients. In one study, 7.9% of patients with EN had a syndrome with one or more of these disorders (an estimated 1 per 11,928 pediatric patients).[1]

- Nevus sebaceus (a subtype of EN) may be present at birth or noted in early childhood and are found equally in males and females.

ETIOLOGY AND PATHOPHYSIOLOGY

- EN are congenital hamartomas of ectodermal origin classified on the basis of their main component—sebaceous, apocrine, eccrine, follicular, or keratinocytic.

- Nevus sebaceous (NS) or sebaceous nevus demonstrate three stages of evolution paralleling the histologic differentiation of normal sebaceous glands:
  - Infancy and young children—smooth to slightly papillated, waxy, hairless thickening (**Figure 157-3**).
  - Puberty—epidermal hyperplasia resulting in verrucous irregularity of the surface covered with numerous closely aggregated yellow-to-brown papules (**Figures 157-4** and **157-5**).
  - Development of secondary appendageal tumors—occurs in 20% to 30% of patients, most are benign (most commonly syringocystadenoma papilliferum (**Figure 157-6**) or trichoblastoma). Single (most commonly basal cell carcinoma) or multiple malignant tumors of both epidermal and adnexal origins may be seen, and metastases have been reported. Rarely, these malignancies are seen in childhood.

- Squamous cell carcinoma, basal cell carcinoma, and keratoacanthoma have rarely been associated with a keratinocytic EN.[2]

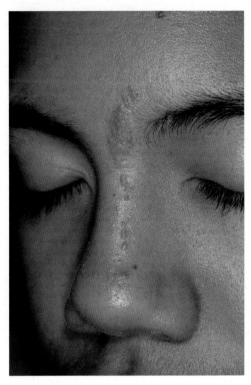

FIGURE 157-1 Epidermal nevus on the face of a teenager. This nevus has been present since birth, and the patient is otherwise healthy. (*Courtesy of Richard P. Usatine, MD.*)

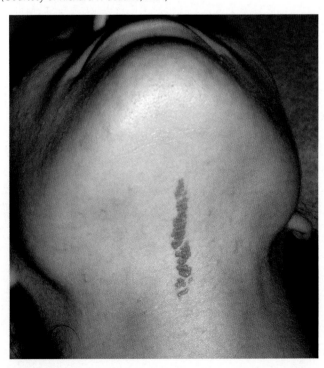

FIGURE 157-2 Linear epidermal nevus on the neck that appeared in early childhood. The patient had no neurologic, musculoskeletal, or vision problems. (*Courtesy of Richard P. Usatine, MD.*)

DIAGNOSIS

CLINICAL FEATURES OF EPIDERMAL NEVI

- EN—linear, round, or oblong, well circumscribed, elevated, and flat-topped (**Figures 157-1** and **157-2**).
- Color—yellow tan to dark brown.
- Surface is uniform velvety or warty (**Figures 157-1** and **157-2**).

CLINICAL FEATURES OF NEVUS SEBACEOUS

- NS—an oval to linear shape ranging from 0.5 to 10 cm.
- NS—usually solitary, smooth, waxy, hairless thickening noted on the scalp at birth or in early childhood (**Figures 157-4** and **157-5**).
- Early NS—may be pink, orange, yellow or tan (**Figure 157-3**); later lesions can appear verrucous and nodular (**Figures 157-4** and **157-6**).

TYPICAL DISTRIBUTION

- EN—occurs most commonly on the head and neck followed by the trunk and proximal extremities; only 13% have wide spread lesions. Lesions may spread beyond their original distribution with age.
- NS—commonly found on the scalp followed by forehead and retroauricular region and rarely involves the neck, trunk, or other areas.

Biopsy is the most definitive method for diagnosing these EN. A biopsy not needed if the clinical picture is clear and no operative intervention is planned. A shave biopsy should provide adequate tissue for diagnosis because the pathology is epidermal and in the upper dermis.

DIFFERENTIAL DIAGNOSES

- Linear lichen planus (**Figure 157-7**)—discrete, pruritic, violaceous papules are arranged in a linear fashion.
- Syringoma (**Figure 157-8**)—benign adnexal tumor derived from sweat gland ducts. Autosomal dominant transmission, soft, small, skin-colored to brown papules develop during childhood and adolescence, especially around the eyes but may be found on the face, neck, and trunk.
- Lichen striatus—discrete pink, tan, or skin-colored asymptomatic papules in a linear band that suddenly appear (**Figure 157-9**). The papules may be smooth, scaly, or flat topped. It is mostly seen in children. While it is most commonly seen on an extremity, it can appear on the trunk. It can resemble a linear epidermal nevus but lichen striatus will spontaneously regress within 1 year.
- Linear porokeratosis—Characterized by small, annular, hypertrophic verrucous plaques with a linear morphology usually limited to a single extremity. The annular morphology and dermatomal distribution should help distinguish this condition from EN and NS.

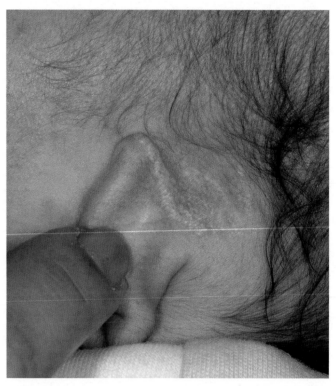

FIGURE 157-3 Nevus sebaceous behind the ear of a 2-month-old boy. He was born with this smooth to slightly papillated, waxy, and hairless thickening. (*Courtesy of Richard P. Usatine, MD.*)

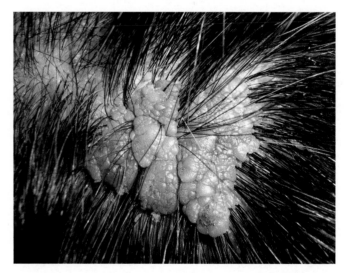

FIGURE 157-4 Nevus sebaceous on the scalp of a teen. (*Courtesy of Richard P. Usatine, MD.*)

MANAGEMENT

- There are no proven topical methods for treatment of EN.

- Surgical excision is an option that is complicated by the potential size of the scar.[3]

- Because of the potential for malignant transformation, particularly following puberty, many authors recommend early complete plastic surgical excision for NS SOR **C**—reconstructive surgery may be needed. However, in a retrospective analysis of 757 cases of NS from 1996 to 2002 in children aging 16 years and younger, investigators found no malignancies and questioned the need for prophylactic surgical removal.[4]

- Excision of large lesions may require reconstructive surgery with a rotation flap to close.[5]

FOLLOW-UP

- Patients with NS should be examined for other associated findings. Consider a consultation with a neurologist and/or ophthalmologist.
  - In a study of 196 subjects with NS examined for clinical neurologic abnormalities, only 7% had abnormalities on neurological exam by neurologists.[6] Abnormal examinations were more frequent in individuals with extensive nevi (21% vs. 5%) and a centrofacial location (21% vs. 2%). None of the patients with EN or NS had known neurologic abnormalities prior to expert evaluation. Imaging was performed in eight of the 14 with abnormalities and was abnormal in only two of the patients.[6] The cost effectiveness of such evaluations have not been established.

PROVIDER RESOURCES

Hammadi AA, Lebwohn MG. Nevus sebaceous. eMedicine.—**www.emedicine.com/DERM/topic296.htm.** Last updated August 30, 2006. Accessed September 18, 2006.

Schwartz RA, Jozwiak S. Epidermal nevus syndrome. eMedicine.—**http://www.emedicine.com/derm/topic732.htm.** Last updated July 10, 2006. Accessed September 18, 2006.

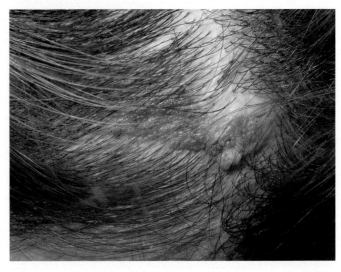

FIGURE 157-5 Nevus sebaceous on the scalp of a young woman. The patient reported a new area of elevation and bleeding. A biopsy showed no malignant transformation. (*Courtesy of Richard P. Usatine, MD.*)

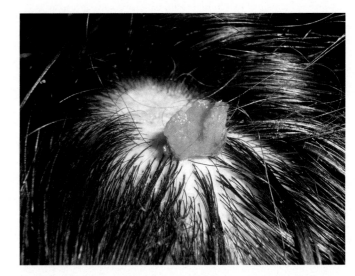

FIGURE 157-6 Nevus sebaceous with a benign tumor identified as a syringocystadenoma papilliferum by shave biopsy. Patient was referred for full removal of the NS. (*Courtesy of Richard P. Usatine, MD.*)

REFERENCES

1. Vidaurri-de la Cruz H, Tamayo-Sanchez L, Duran-McKinster C, et al. Epidermal nevus syndromes: Clinical findings in 35 patients. *Pediatr Dermatol.* 2004;21(4):432–439.

2. Happle R, Rogers M. Epidermal nevi. *Adv Dermatol.* 2002;18:175–201.

3. Schwartz RA, Jozwiak S. Epidermal nevus syndrome. eMedicine. http://www.emedicine.com/derm/topic732.htm. Last updated July 10, 2006. Accessed September 18, 2006.

4. Santibanez-Gallerani A, Marshall D, Duarte AM, et al. Should nevus sebaceus of Jadassohn in children be excised? A study of 757 cases, and literature review. *J Craniofac Surg.* 2003;14(5):658–660.

5. Davison SP, Khachemoune A, Yu D, Kauffman LC. Nevus sebaceus of Jadassohn revisited with reconstruction options. *Int J Dermatol.* 2005;44(2):145–150.

6. Davies D. Rogers M. Review of neurological manifestations in 196 patients with sebaceous naevi. *Australas J Dermatol.* 2002;43(1):20–23.

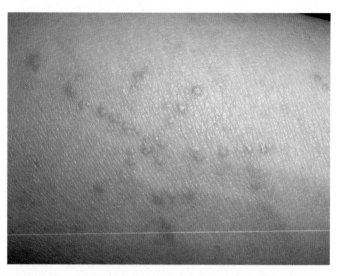

FIGURE 157-7 Lichen planus on the flexor aspect of the forearm in a linear pattern resembling a linear epidermal nevus. (*Courtesy of Richard P. Usatine, MD.*)

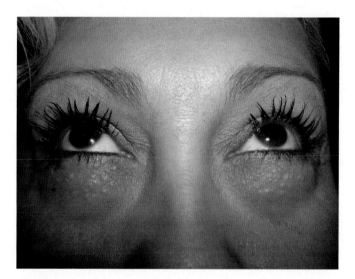

FIGURE 157-8 Syringoma on the lower eyelids. (*Courtesy of Heather Goff, MD.*)

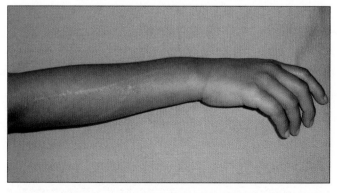

FIGURE 157-9 Lichen striatus that appeared suddenly on the arm of a young boy one year ago. This was not secondary to trauma. (*Courtesy of Richard P. Usatine, MD.*)

158 DYSPLASTIC NEVUS

Mindy A. Smith, MD, MS

PATIENT STORY

A 47-year-old man presents with concern over a mole on his back that his wife says is growing larger and more variable in color. The edges are irregular and the color almost appears to be "leaking" into the surrounding skin. He reports no symptoms related to this lesion. A shallow scoop saucerization with 2-mm margin of clinically normal skin confirmed that it was a dysplastic nevus with no signs of malignancy (**Figure 158-1**).

EPIDEMIOLOGY

- Two to nine percent of the population have dysplastic nevi (DN); also called atypical moles (AMs).[1]

- Individuals at the highest risk of DN are those of northern European background with light-colored hair and freckles. DN are rare in black, Asian, or Middle Eastern populations.[2]

- DNs appear to be dynamic throughout adulthood; in a study of the natural history of dysplastic nevi, investigators found that 51% of all evaluated nevi (297 of 593) showed clinical signs of change during an average follow-up of 89 months.[3] New nevi were common in adulthood, continuing to form in more than 20% of patients older than 50 years of age, and some nevi disappeared.

- The sudden eruption of benign and atypical melanocytic nevi has been reported and is associated with blistering skin conditions and a number of disease states, including immunosuppression. Subsets of patients with immunosuppression have increased numbers of nevi on the palms and soles.[4]

- Familial cases are seen with an autosomal dominant pattern of inheritance.

- The National Institute of Health Consensus Conference on the diagnosis and treatment of early melanoma defined a syndrome of familial atypical mole and melanoma (FAMM). The criteria of FAMM syndrome are as follows[2]:
  - The occurrence of malignant melanoma in one or more first- or second-degree relatives.
  - The presence of numerous (often >50) melanocytic nevi, some of which are clinically atypical.
  - Many of the associated nevi show certain histologic features (see below).

- The lifetime risk of developing a cutaneous melanoma in patients with FAMM is estimated to be 100% in contrast to 0.6% among whites in the United States (1 in 150 individuals).[2]

ETIOLOGY AND PATHOPHYSIOLOGY

- Dysplastic nevi (also known as Clark nevi) are acquired melanocytic lesions of the skin whose clinical and histologic definitions are controversial and still evolving.

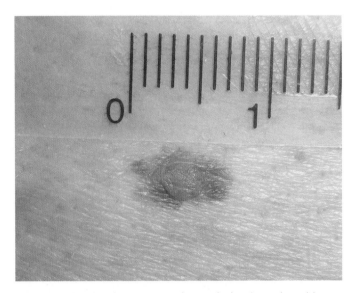

FIGURE 158-1 Dysplastic nevus with irregular border and variable pigmentation. It has the classic fried egg appearance with a raised "yoke" in the middle. (*Courtesy of Richard P. Usatine, MD.*)

- Most DN are compound nevi possessing a junctional and intradermal component (see Chapter 155, Benign Nevi).[1] The junctional component is highly cellular and consists of an irregular distribution of melanocytes arranged in nests and lentiginous patterns along the dermoepidermal junction. The dermal component, located at the center, consists of nests and strands of melanocytes with distinct sclerotic changes.[1]

- Dysplastic nevi exhibit a host response consisting of irregular rete ridge elongation, subepidermal sclerosis, proliferation of dermal capillaries, and a perivascular, lymphohistiocytic inflammatory infiltrate.[1]

- Evidence suggests that melanoma can arise directly from DNs, with a higher risk of malignant transformation among those with numerous DNs and a family history of melanoma.[2] Authors of a recent meta-analysis confirmed a substantially increased risk of melanoma associated with the number of dysplastic nevi (RR = 6.36 95%; CI: 3.80, 10.33; for 5 vs. 0).[5]

DIAGNOSIS

CLINICAL FEATURES

- Variable mixtures of color including tan, brown, black, and red within a single lesion (**Figures 158-1** to **158-3**).

- Irregular, notched borders; pigment may fade off into surrounding skin.

- Flat or slightly raised, macular portion at edge (**Figures 158-1** and **158-2**). Not verrucous or pendulous.

- Lesions frequently surrounded by a reddish hue from reactive hyperemia making them appear target-like.

- Usually >6 mm; may be >10 mm (**Figures 158-1** and **158-2**).

- Patients with FAMM syndrome may have more than 100 lesions, far greater than the average number of common moles (<50) in most individuals.

IMAGING

- Although eccentric peripheral hyperpigmented and multifocal hyper or hypopigmented types are more commonly seen in melanoma, no digital dermatoscopic criteria have been identified that can clearly distinguish dysplastic nevi from in situ melanomas.[6]

TYPICAL DISTRIBUTION

- Usually on sun-exposed areas, especially the back (**Figure 158-4**), may be found on sites where nevi are usually absent or rare such as the scalp, breasts, genital skin, buttocks, and dorsa of feet.

BIOPSY

None of the listed histologic features are diagnostic by themselves and the importance of histology is to distinguish these from melanoma. A combination of architectural and cellular features is useful in distinguishing these from nevi and melanoma and includes[1,2]:

- Melanocytes that display nuclear atypia with variability in size, shape, and staining intensity.

- Nuclear pleomorphism that is similar in different areas of the lesion in contrast to melanoma.

- A horizontal arrangement of melanocytes, which generally vary in shape from round to spindled.

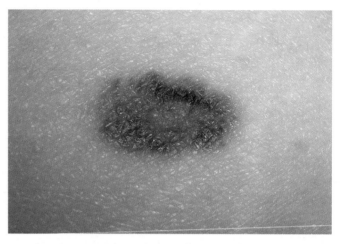

FIGURE 158-2 Dysplastic nevus in a woman with malignant melanoma in a different region of her body. The size was greater than 6 mm and there was variation in color. This was fully excised to make sure there was no melanoma present. (*Courtesy of Richard P. Usatine, MD.*)

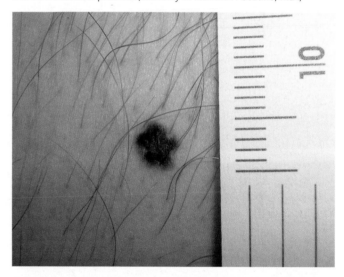

FIGURE 158-3 Dysplastic nevus on the chest of a 30-year-old man. A shave biopsy successfully removed the whole lesion and confirmed that it was not melanoma. While it was less than 6 mm, it had irregular borders and variation of color. (*Courtesy of Richard P. Usatine, MD.*)

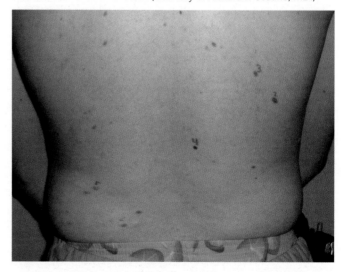

FIGURE 158-4 Multiple dysplastic nevi on the back of a young physician. Multiple biopsies have all been negative, so patient is being followed by serial digital photography with numbering of the dysplastic nevi. (*Courtesy of Richard P. Usatine, MD.*)

- A tendency for melanocytes to aggregate into variably sized nests, which fuse with adjacent rete ridges to produce bridging.

- The presence of lamellar and concentric dermal fibroplasia.

- The presence of a lymphocytic infiltrate (patchy or diffuse) in the superficial dermis.

- Extension of the junctional component many rete ridges beyond the last dermal nest to produce "shoulders."

- No pagetoid spread of atypical melanocytes at all levels of the epidermis and no atypical mitotic figures found in melanoma.

The World Health Organization Melanoma Program has proposed a similar list of characteristics/criteria for dysplastic nevi with individual lesions requiring two major and two minor criteria to be classified as a dysplastic nevus, however, these criteria are not universally accepted.[2]

DIFFERENTIAL DIAGNOSIS

- Melanocytic nevi—most common moles are tan to brown, <6 mm, round in shape, and with sharp borders (see Chapter 155, Benign Nevi).

- Melanoma—skin cancer that is often asymmetric, with irregular border and varied colors. It is usually larger than 6 mm in diameter (see Chapter 165, Melanoma).

MANAGEMENT

- Because of the low risk of any one DN developing malignant transformation, the prophylactic removal of all DNs is not recommended. SOR Ⓒ

- Removal of at least 1 lesion is reasonable to histologically confirm the diagnosis and rule out melanoma. This should be accomplished with excisional biopsy and histologic confirmation of dysplastic nevi versus melanoma. Shallow scoop saucerizations including at least a 2-mm margin of clinically normal skin surrounding the pigmented lesion is considered by some to be the best approach.[2] SOR Ⓒ

- Use the "ugly ducking" sign to find pigmented lesions that may need biopsy. Dysplastic nevi in a particular individual may all look somewhat atypical but similarly atypical. If certain lesions stand out as different than the others despite not having the typical ABCDE findings, these lesions should probably be biopsied.

- In a pilot study of five patients with dysplastic nevi treated with topical tretinoin to half of the back for 6 months, investigators found significant decreases in clinical atypia of treated lesions, with concomitant fading and even disappearance of many treated nevi concomitant with clinical and histologic improvement in a significant percentage of dysplastic nevi treated with topical tretinoin.[7] SOR Ⓒ

- Patients with FAMM syndrome should have a complete cutaneous examination performed at the first office visit and then at least every 12 months for life.[2] SOR Ⓑ

- Studies have shown that regular cutaneous examinations combined with baseline and serial color photographs of the patient's cutaneous surface decrease biopsies and lead to earlier diagnosis of melanoma.[2] SOR Ⓑ

PATIENT EDUCATION

- Patients with DNs should avoid excessive sun exposure and routinely use a broad-spectrum sunscreen with a sun protective factor of 30 or greater.

- Patients should be taught self-examination to detect changes in existing moles and to recognize clinical features of melanomas. Patients should be taught to look for and report asymmetry, border irregularity, new symptoms (e.g., pain, pruritus, bleeding, or ulceration), and color and size changes.

- In a study of 50 patients with five or more dysplastic nevi, the use of baseline digital photographs improved the diagnostic accuracy of skin self-examination on the back, chest, and abdomen and improved detection of changing and new moles.[8]

FOLLOW-UP

- Patients with numerous DNs and who have a family history of melanoma are at a higher risk of developing melanoma and should be encouraged to have regular follow-up with a provider skilled in detecting melanoma.

- Patients with FAMM should also consider a baseline ophthalmologic examination because of a possible association between uveal melanoma and FAMM syndrome.[2]

- If a patient is diagnosed with FAMM syndrome, it should be recommended that all first-degree relatives be examined.[2]

PATIENT RESOURCES

www.skincancerinfo.com/sectionf/atypicalmole.html.

Skin Cancer Foundation—**http://www.skincancer.org/ prevention/dysplastic-nevi-atypical-moles.html.**

PROVIDER RESOURCES

National Cancer Institute—**http://www.cancer.gov/ cancertopics/wyntk/moles-and-dysplastic-nevi/page8.**

REFERENCES

1. Mooi WJ. The dysplastic naevus. *J Clin Pathol.* 1997;50:711–715.

2. Wenner KA, Sloan SB, Shidham VB, Ácker SM. http://www. emedicine.com/derm/topic42.htm. Accessed August 17, 2006.

3. Trock B, Synnestvedt M, Humphreys T. Natural history of dysplastic nevi. *J Am Acad Dermatol.* 1993;29(1):51–57.

4. Woodhouse J, Maytin EV. Eruptive nevi of the palms and soles. *J Am Acad Dermatol.* 2005;52(5 Suppl 1):S96–S100.

5. Gandini S, Sera F, Cattaruzza MS, et al. Meta-analysis of risk factors for cutaneous melanoma: I. Common and atypical nevi. *Eur J Cancer.* 2005;41(1):28–44.

6. Burroni M, Sbano P, Cevenini G, et al. Dysplastic nevus vs. in situ melanoma: Digital dermoscopy analysis. *Br J Dermatol.* 2005;152(4): 679–684.

7. Halpern AC, Schuchter LM, Elder DE, et al. Effects of topical tretinoin on dysplastic nevi. *J Clin Oncol.* 1994;12(5):1028–1035.

8. Oliveria SA, Chau D, Christos PJ, et al. Diagnostic accuracy of patients in performing skin self-examination and the impact of photography. *Arch Dermatol.* 2004;140(1):57–62.

159 ACTINIC KERATOSIS AND BOWEN'S DISEASE

Richard P. Usatine, MD

PATIENT STORY

A 57-year-old woman presented with red and scaling skin on both arms (**Figure 159-1**) with a request for a prescription for 5-fluorouracil (5-FU). The patient had blue eyes and white hair and was found to have two basal cell carcinomas (BCCs) on her face and shoulder. The patient stated that 5-FU helped her arms in the past, but that the scaly lesions had returned. She avoids sun exposure now, but acknowledges receiving too much sun exposure while growing up. Another course of 5-FU was prescribed for her arms to prevent new skin cancers from forming.

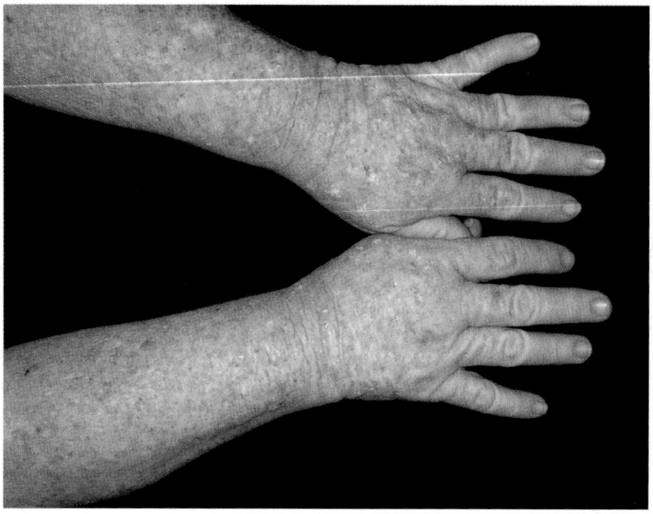

EPIDEMIOLOGY

Actinic keratoses (AKs) and Bowen's disease (BD) are seen frequently in light-skinned individuals who have had significant sun exposure. The incidence of these conditions increases with age and cumulative sun exposure.

AKs are so common that they account for over 10% of visits to dermatologists.

ETIOLOGY AND PATHOPHYSIOLOGY

Actinic keratoses and Browen's disease are both caused by cumulative sun exposure.

AKs are premalignant and have the potential to become squamous cell carcinomas (SCCs). The rate of malignant transformation has been variably estimated but is probably no greater than 6% per AK over a 10-year period.[1]

On a spectrum of malignant transformation, BD is SCC in situ before the SCC becomes invasive.

DIAGNOSIS

CLINICAL FEATURES

AKs are rough scaly spots seen on sun-exposed areas (**Figures 159-1 to 159-4**). They may be found by touch, as well as close visual inspection of the patient's skin. BD appears similar to an AK, but tends to be larger in size and thicker with a well-demarcated border (**Figures 159-5 and 159-6**).

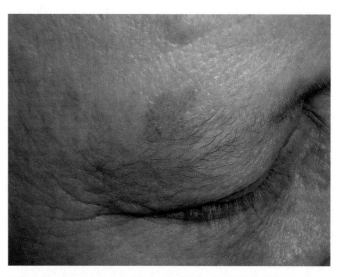

FIGURE 159-1 Actinic keratoses (AKs) covering both arms and the dorsum of both hands in a fair-skinned woman who had significant sun exposure. Note that her left arm and hand are worse due to driving a car and receiving more sun on the left arm. (*Courtesy of Richard P. Usatine, MD.*)

FIGURE 159-2 Large AK over the eyebrow of an older adult. A biopsy was performed to make sure this was not already BD or SCC. (*Courtesy of Richard P. Usatine, MD.*)

TYPICAL DISTRIBUTION

Both lesions are seen in areas with greatest sun exposure such as the face, forearms, dorsum of hands, lower legs of women, and the balding scalp (**Figure 159-3**) and tops of the ears in men.

LABORATORY STUDIES

AKs that appear premalignant may be diagnosed by observation only and treated with destructive methods (e.g., excision, electrosurgery, or cryosurgery) without biopsy. BD requires a biopsy for diagnosis. BD or SCC should be biopsied prior to treatment. A shave biopsy should produce enough tissue for histopathology.

DIFFERENTIAL DIAGNOSIS

- Nummular eczema—a type of eczema in which the scaly patches are coin-shaped. The patches are often seen in patients who have already had some eczema or atopic conditions. The patches usually respond well to topical corticosteroids and are not related to sun damage (see Chapter 139, Atopic Dermatitis).

- Seborrheic keratoses—occur in aging adults but do not have any malignant potential. Typical seborrheic keratoses are brown in color and have a stuck on appearance. Seborrheic keratoses may look greasy or verrucous and have surface cracks. Their borders tend to be more well demarcated than AKs and their color is usually more brown than pink (see Chapter 151, Seborrheic Keratosis).

- Superficial BCCs—can look like an AK or BD. Look for the pearly and thready border that may distinguish a superficial BCC from an AK or BD. Histopathology is the proven method to diagnose (see Chapter 163, Basal Cell Carcinoma).

- When in doubt, perform a shave biopsy to differentiate between an AK, BD, SCC, and superficial BCC.

MANAGEMENT

Actinic Keratoses

- No therapy or the application of an emollient is a reasonable option for mild AKs.[2] SOR **A**

- Sun screen applied twice daily for 7 months may protect against development of AKs.[2] SOR **A**

- Actinic keratoses are most often treated by cryosurgery using liquid nitrogen (**Figure 159-7**). One metaanalysis showed two months cure rate of 97.0% with 2.1% recurrences in one year.[3] SOR **A**

- Treating AKs with liquid nitrogen using a 1 mm halo freeze demonstrated complete response of 39% for freeze times of less than 5 seconds, 69% for freeze times greater than 5 seconds, and 83% for freeze times greater than 20 seconds.[4] There is considerably more hypopigmentation caused by 20 seconds of freeze time. Determine the length of the freeze time on the size and thickness of the lesion using sufficient time for clearance while attempting to avoid hypopigmentation and scarring.

- Treat multiple actinic keratoses of the face, scalp, forearms and hands topically with 5-FU, imiquimod, or diclofenac.[2] SOR **A** See **Table 159-1**.

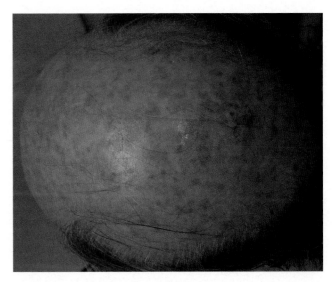

FIGURE 159-3 Actinic keratoses on the balding head of an older man. Hair loss results in less natural sun protection and is a risk factor for skin cancers on the scalp. The visible and palpable AKs were treated with cryotherapy. (*Courtesy of Richard P. Usatine, MD.*)

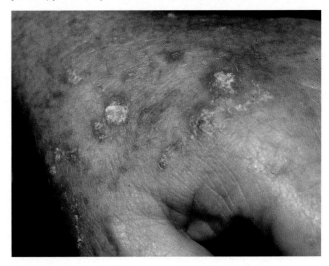

FIGURE 159-4 Actinic keratoses on the dorsum of the hand with some lesions suspicious for Bowen's disease (BD) (squamous cell carcinoma in situ). (*With permission from Usatine RP, Moy RL, Tobinick EL, Siegel DM. Skin Surgery: A Practical Guide. 1998, St. Louis: Mosby.*)

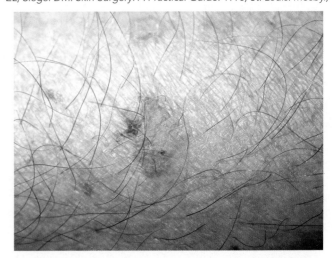

FIGURE 159-5 Lesions on the arm of an older man with BD in the central lesion and actinic keratosis on the upper lesion. (*Courtesy of Richard P. Usatine, MD.*)

- 5-Fluorouracil (5-FU) cream used twice daily for 3 to 6 weeks is effective for up to 12 months in clearance of the majority of AKs (**Figures 159-8** and **159-9**).[2] SOR **A** Due to side-effects of soreness, less aggressive regimens are often used, which may be effective, but have not been fully evaluated.[2]

- Diclofenac gel applied twice daily for 10 to 12 weeks has moderate efficacy with low morbidity in mild AKs.[2] SOR **B** There are few follow-up data to indicate the duration of benefit.[2] In one study, Diclofenac 3% gel was as effective as 5-FU cream for AK of the face and scalp and diclofenac produced less signs of inflammation.[5]

- Imiquimod 5% cream has been demonstrated to be effective over a 16-week course of treatment but studies have only measured 8 weeks of follow up.[2] SOR **B** By weight, it is 19 times the cost of 5-fluorouracil. They have similar side effects.[2]

- One metaanalysis comparing imiquimod to 5-FU showed average complete clearance of AKs for each drug was 5-FU, 52 +/− 18% and imiquimod, 70 +/− 12%.[6] SOR **A**

- Imiquimod applied topically for 12–16 weeks produced complete clearance of AKs in 50% of patients compared to 5% with vehicle (NNT = 2.2). Adverse events included erythema (27%), scabbing or crusting (21%), flaking (9%), and erosions (6%). (NNH = 3.2 to 5.9).[7]

- Topical tretinoin has some efficacy on the face, with partial clearance of AKs, but may need to be used for up to a year at a time to optimize benefit.[2] SOR **B**

- Cryosurgery is effective for up to 75% of lesions in trials comparing it with photodynamic therapy. It may be particularly superior for thicker lesions, but may leave scars.[2] SOR **A**

- Photodynamic therapy (PDT) is effective in up to 91% of AKs in trials comparing it with cryotherapy, with consistently good cosmetic result. It may be particularly good for superficial and confluent AKs, but is likely to be more expensive than most other therapies. It is of particular value where AKs are numerous or when located at sites of poor healing such as the lower leg.[2] SOR **B**

Bowen's Disease (BD)

- The main treatment options are summarized and compared in **Table 159-2**.

- The risk of progression to invasive cancer is about 3%. This risk is greater in genital BD, and particularly in perianal BD. A high risk of recurrence, including late recurrence, is a particular feature of perianal BD and prolonged follow up is recommended for this variant.[8] SOR **A**

- There is reasonable evidence to support use of 5-FU.[8] SOR **B** It is more practical than surgery for large lesions, especially at potentially poor healing sites, and has been used for 'control' rather than cure in some patients with multiple lesions.[8]

- Topical imiquimod may be used off-label for BD for larger lesions or difficult/poor healing sites.[8] SOR **B** However, it is costly and the optimum regimen has yet to be determined.[8]

- One prospective study suggests a superiority of curettage and electrodesiccation over cryotherapy in treating BD, especially for lesions on the lower leg (**Figures 159-10** and **159-11**). Curettage was associated with a significantly shorter healing time, less pain, fewer complications and a lower recurrence rate when compared with cryotherapy.

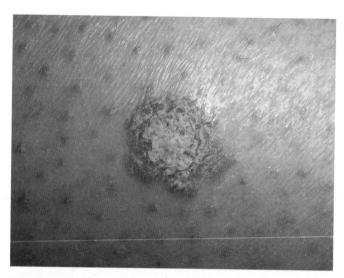

FIGURE 159-6 Bowen's disease on the leg of an older woman. (*Courtesy of Richard P. Usatine, MD.*)

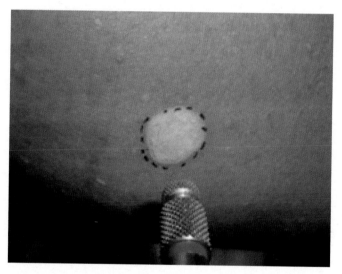

FIGURE 159-7 Cryosurgery of large actinic keratosis. The outside border was marked with a 1- to 2-mm margin. (*Courtesy of Richard P. Usatine, MD.*)

TABLE 159-1 Comparison of Topical Agents for the Treatment of AK

Topical Agent for AK	Duration of Treatment	Irritation	Cost
5-fluorouracil generic 5%	3–6 wk	High	Under $100
Diclofenac 3%	10–12 wk	Moderate	Over $130
Imiquimod	16 wk	Moderate	Over $400

PATIENT EDUCATION

Patients must understand that they acquired these conditions through cumulative sun damage, and they need to avoid further sun damage to minimize the likelihood of additional precancers and cancers. The sun damage is often from childhood and early adulthood, so the lesions are likely to form even with future sun protection. Self skin examination is recommended.

All topical treatments for AKs and BD will make the lesions look worse before they get better (**Figures 159-8** and **159-9**). The 5-FU treatments are often given with topical corticosteroid preparations to use after the treatment is over in order to minimize the symptoms of the inflammation.

FOLLOW-UP

Patients need skin examinations every 6 to 12 months to identify new precancers and cancers. SOR **C**

PATIENT RESOURCE

Skin Cancer Foundation has an excellent web site with photos and patient information—**http://www.skincancer.org/ak/index. php.** Accessed July 25, 2006.

PROVIDER RESOURCE AND GUIDELINES

Cox NH, Eedy DJ, Morton CA. Guidelines for management of Bowen's disease: 2006 update. *Br J Dermatol.* 2007;156(1):11–21.

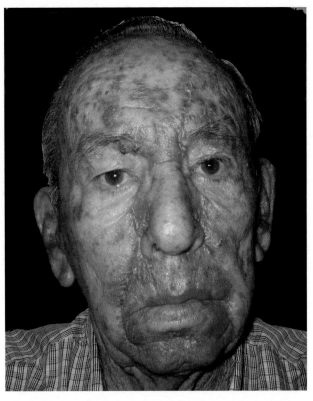

FIGURE 159-8 Actinic keratoses reddened and crusted by the application of 5-fluorouracil topically twice daily. (*Courtesy of Richard P. Usatine, MD.*)

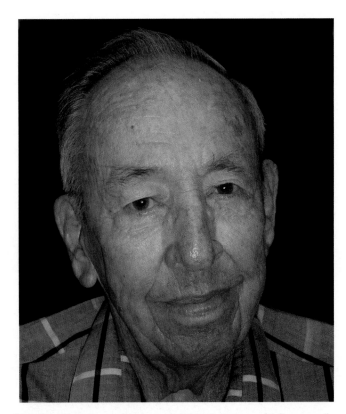

FIGURE 159-9 Face healed months after the course of 5-fluorouracil was completed. (*Courtesy of Richard P. Usatine, MD.*)

TABLE 159-2 Summary of the Main Treatment Options for Bowen's Disease[8]

Lesion Characteristics	Topical 5-FU	Topical Imiquimod*	Cryotherapy	Curettage	Excision	PDT	Radiotherapy	Laser[†]
Small, single/few, good healing site[‡]	4	3	2	1	3	3	5	4
Large, single, good healing site[‡]	3	3	3	5	5	2	4	7
Multiple, good healing site[‡]	3	4	2	3	5	3	4	4
Small, single/few, poor healing site[‡]	2	3	3	2	2	1–2	5	7
Large, single, poor healing site[‡]	3	2–3	5	4	5	1	6	7
Facial	4	7	2	2	4[§]	3	4	7
Digital	3	7	3	5	2[§]	3	3	3
Perianal	6	6	6	6	1[¶]	7	2–3	6
Penile	3	3	3	5	4[§]	3	2–3	3

*Does not have a product license for Bowen's disease.
[†]Depends on site.
[‡]Refers to the clinician's perceived potential for good or poor healing at the affected site.
[§]Consider micrographic surgery for tissue sparing or if poorly defined/recurrent.
[¶]Wide excision recommended.
5-FU, 5-fluorouracil; PDT, photodynamic therapy; 1, probably treatment of choice; 2, generally good choice; 3, generally fair choice; 4, reasonable but not usually required; 5, generally poor choice; 6, probably should not be used; 7, insufficient evidence available. The suggested scoring of the treatments listed takes into account the evidence for benefit, ease of application or time required for the procedure, wound healing, cosmetic result and current availability/costs of the method or facilities required. Evidence for interventions based on single studies or purely anecdotal cases is not included.

REFERENCES

1. Anwar J, Wrone DA, Kimyai-Asadi A, Alam M. The development of actinic keratosis into invasive squamous cell carcinoma: Evidence and evolving classification schemes. *Clin Dermatol.* 2004;22: 189–196.

2. Zouboulis CC, Rohrs H. Cryosurgical treatment of actinic keratoses and evidence-based review. *Hautarzt.* 2005;56:353–358.

3. Thai KE, Fergin P, Freeman M, et al. A prospective study of the use of cryosurgery for the treatment of actinic keratoses. *Int J Dermatol.* 2004;43:687–692.

4. Gupta AK, Davey V, McPhail H. Evaluation of the effectiveness of imiquimod and 5-fluorouracil for the treatment of actinic keratosis: Critical review and meta-analysis of efficacy studies. *J Cutan Med Surg.* 2005;9(5):209–214.

5. Hadley G, Derry S, Moore RA. Imiquimod for actinic keratosis: Systematic review and meta-analysis. *J Invest Dermatol.* 2006;126: 1251–1255.

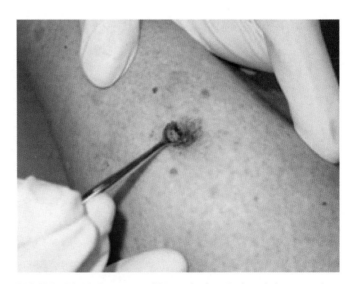

FIGURE 159-10 Curettage of BD on the leg. Each cycle begins with curettage and ends with electrodesiccation. Three cycles are performed. (*Courtesy of Richard P. Usatine, MD.*)

6. Smith SR, Morhenn VB, Piacquadio DJ. Bilateral comparison of the efficacy and tolerability of 3% diclofenac sodium gel and 5% 5-flu-orouracil cream in the treatment of actinic keratoses of the face and scalp. *J Drugs Dermatol.* 2006;5:156–159.

7. Ahmed I, Berth-Jones J, Charles-Holmes S, O'Callaghan CJ, Ilchyshyn A. Comparison of cryotherapy with curettage in the treatment of Bowen's disease: A prospective study. *Br J Dermatol.* 2000;143:759–766.

8. Cox NH, Eedy DJ, Morton CA. Guidelines for management of Bowen's disease: 2006 update. *Br J Dermatol.* 2007;156:11–21.

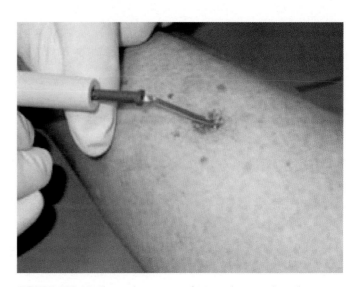

FIGURE 159-11 Electrodesiccation of BD on the same leg. Three cycles were performed to complete the procedure. (*Courtesy of Richard P. Usatine, MD.*)

160 KERATOACANTHOMAS

Richard P. Usatine, MD

PATIENT STORY

A 71-year-old woman presented with a rapidly growing lesion on her face over the past 4 months (**Figure 160-1**). The lesion had features of a basal cell carcinoma with a pearly border and telangiectasias (**Figure 160-2**). Also the central crater with keratin gave it the appearance of a keratoacanthoma (KA). A shave biopsy was performed and the pathology showed squamous cell carcinoma (SCC)—KA type. A full elliptical excision with 4 mm margins was then performed.

EPIDEMIOLOGY

- KA develops as a solitary nodule in sun-exposed areas.
- Seen more commonly later in life with a predilection for males.[1]
- Develops rapidly within 6 to 8 weeks.
- May spontaneously regresses after 3 to 6 months or may continue to grow and rarely metastasize.[2]

ETIOLOGY AND PATHOPHYSIOLOGY

- KAs share features such as infiltration and cytological atypia with SCCs.
- KAs have been reported to metastasize.
- KA is considered to be a variant of SCC, called SCC-KA type.
- Histologic criteria are not sensitive enough to discriminate reliably between KA and SCC.[3]

DIAGNOSIS

CLINICAL FEATURES

Solitary nodule in sun exposed areas. Often have a central keratin plug that resembles a volcano (**Figures 160-1** to **160-5**). Rare cases of multiple eruptive KAs have been reported.[1]

TYPICAL DISTRIBUTION

Face, arms, hands, and trunk (**Figures 160-3** and **160-5**).

LABORATORY STUDIES

Biopsy is the only reliable method to make the diagnosis. KAs are well-differentiated squamoproliferative skin lesions.

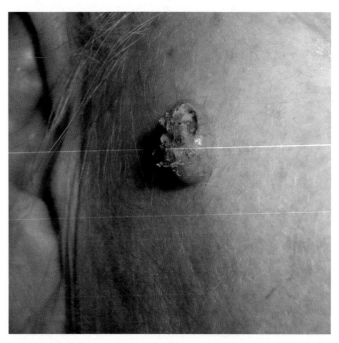

FIGURE 160-1 Pearly keratoacanthoma with telangiectasias and a central keratin core on the face of a 71-year-old woman. (*Courtesy of Richard P. Usatine, MD.*)

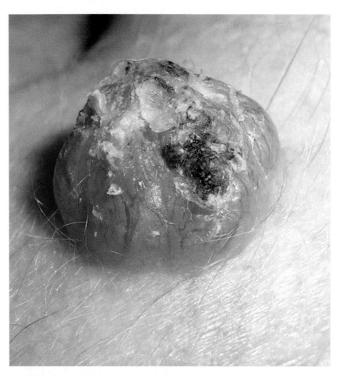

FIGURE 160-2 Close-up of the keratoacanthoma with telangiectasias and a central keratin core on the face of the same woman. (*Courtesy of Richard P. Usatine, MD.*)

DIFFERENTIAL DIAGNOSIS

- Actinic keratoses are precancerous lesions found on sun-exposed areas that may progress to SCC. Because these lesions are generally flat they are rarely confused with keratoacanthomas (see Chapter 159, Actinic Keratosis/Bowen's Disease).

- Cutaneous horn is a raised keratinaceous lesion that can arise in actinic keratoses and in all types of nonmelanoma skin cancers. It generally does not have pearly raised skin around the keratin horn and therefore does not have the crater appearance of a KA (see Chapter 162, Cutaneous Horn).

- SCCs of the skin have many forms and the keratoacanthoma is considered to be one type of SCC (see Chapter 164, Squamous Cell Carcinoma).

MANAGEMENT

- A shave biopsy may be used for diagnosis but is not an adequate final treatment. Options for definitive treatment should be discussed with patient.

- While some KAs may regress spontaneously, there is no way to distinguish between these and the ones that are variants of SCC and may go on to metastasize. Therefore, the standard of care is to remove or destroy the remaining tumor. SOR Ⓒ

- Elliptically excise a KA with margins of 3 to 5 mm as you would a SCC.[3] SOR Ⓒ

- Smaller, less aggressive KAs diagnosed with shave biopsy may be destroyed with curettage and desiccation or cryotherapy with 3 to 5 mm margins. SOR Ⓒ

- Mohs surgery may be indicated for large or recurrent KAs or KAs located in anatomic areas with cosmetic or functional considerations.[3] SOR Ⓒ

- Multiple eruptive KAs have been treated with oral retinoids, methotrexate and cyclophosphamide.[1]

PATIENT EDUCATION

KA is similar to other nonmelanoma skin cancers in that it occurs on sun exposed areas and patients that have one are at increased risk of developing new skin cancers. Therefore, sun avoidance and sun protection should be emphasized.

FOLLOW-UP

Patients should perform their own skin exams and have yearly clinical skin examinations to examine for recurrence and the development of new skin cancers.

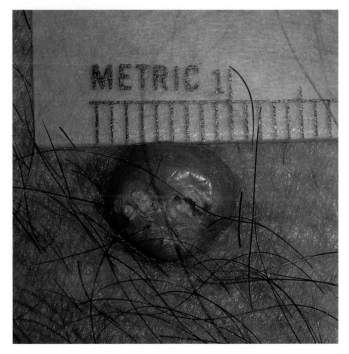

FIGURE 160-3 Keratoacanthoma on the chest of a 53-year-old man with central scaling. (*Courtesy of Richard P. Usatine, MD.*)

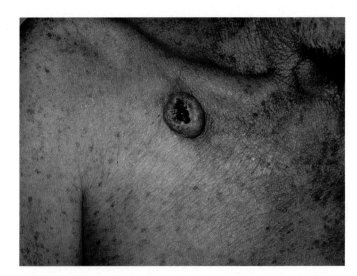

FIGURE 160-4 Giant keratoacanthoma under the clavicle. (*With permission from Usatine RP, Moy RL, Tobinick EL, Siegel DM. Skin Surgery: A Practical Guide. 1998, St. Louis: Mosby.*)

REFERENCES

1. Karaa A, Khachemoune A. Keratoacanthoma: A tumor in search of a classification. *Int J Dermatol.* 2007;46(7):671–8.

2. Clausen OP, Aass HC, Beigi M, et al. Are keratoacanthomas variants of squamous cell carcinomas? A comparison of chromosomal aberrations by comparative genomic hybridization. *J Invest Dermatol.* 2006;2308–2315.

3. Chuang, T, Brashear. Keratoacanthoma. Updated July 2005. http://www.emedicine.com/derm/topic206.htm. Accessed on May 28, 2006.

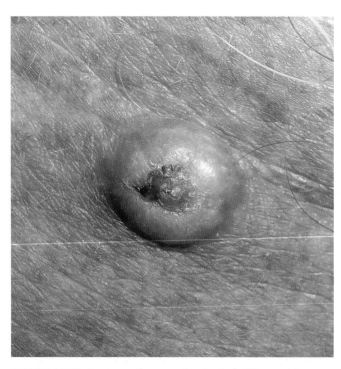

FIGURE 160-5 Keratoacanthoma on the chest of a 70-year-old man with central keratin core that resembles a volcano. (*Courtesy of Richard P. Usatine, MD.*)

161 LENTIGO MALIGNA

Richard P. Usatine, MD

PATIENT STORY

A 65-year-old woman noted that a brown spot on her face was growing larger and darker (**Figure 161-1**). A broad shave biopsy showed
lentigo maligna (LM) (melanoma in situ). The patient was referred for
Mohs surgery for definitive treatment.

EPIDEMIOLOGY

- The incidence of LM is directly related to sun exposure. In the
  United States, the incidence is greatest in Hawaii, intermediate in
  the central and southern states, and lowest in the northern states.[1]

- Generally, patients with LM are older than 40 years, with a mean
  age of 65 years.[1]

- The peak incidence occurs in the seventh to eighth decades of life.[1]

- Persons with lentigo maligna melanoma (LMM) tend to be older
  than persons with other types of melanoma.[1]

- LM and LMM have higher occupational sun exposure and lower
  recreational sun exposure.[1]

- The lesions occur more commonly on the driver's side of the head
  and neck in men in Australia.[1]

ETIOLOGY AND PATHOPHYSIOLOGY

- LM is a preinvasive pigmented lesion confined to the epidermis. It
  is one type of melanoma in situ (**Figures 161-1** to **161-3**).

- It is caused by cumulative sun exposure and, therefore, seen later in
  life.

- LMM occurs when the lesion extends into the dermis (**Figure
  161-4**).

- In melanoma the atypical melanocytes invade the rich vascular and
  lymphatic networks of the dermis, thereby establishing metastatic
  potential.[1]

- LM can be present for long periods (5–15 years) before invasion
  occurs, although rapid progression within months has been
  described.[1]

- There is a 5% estimated lifetime risk of developing LMM in
  patients diagnosed with LM at age 45.[1]

- The risk for progression to LMM appears to be proportional to the
  size of the lesion of LM.[2]

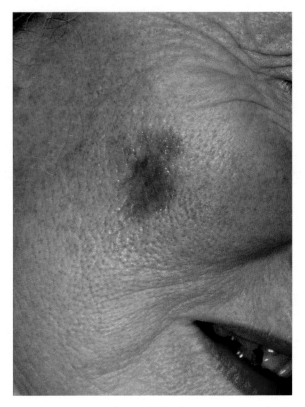

FIGURE 161-1 Lentigo maligna (LM) (melanoma in situ) on the face.
(*With permission from Usatine RP, Moy RL, Tobinick EL, Siegel DM. Skin
Surgery: A Practical Guide. 1998, St. Louis: Mosby.*)

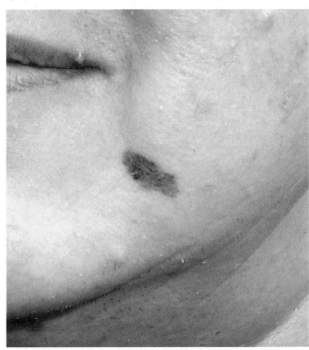

FIGURE 161-2 LM on the face, presenting as a single large evolving
pigmented lesion with changing color. (*With permission from Usatine RP,
Moy RL, Tobinick EL, Siegel DM. Skin Surgery: A Practical Guide. 1998,
St. Louis: Mosby.*)

DIAGNOSIS

CLINICAL FEATURES

- Large pigmented patch with multiple colors including brown, black, pink, and white (signifying regression) (**Figures 161-1 to 161-3**).
- May have ill-defined borders and microscopic extension that can determine the clinical borders and complete removal of the lesion difficult.

TYPICAL DISTRIBUTION

Face, head, and neck. There is a predilection for the nose and cheek (**Figures 161-1** and **161-2**).

DERMOSCOPY

- One retrospective study revealed the four most important features of LM: asymmetric pigmented follicular openings, dark rhomboidal structures, slate-gray globules, and slate-gray dots with a sensitivity of 89% and a specificity of 96%.[3] See Dermoscopy Appendix.

BIOPSY

- Complete excisional biopsy is rarely practical because these lesions are frequently large and are on the face (**Figure 161-1**). There is debate in the literature between doing broad shave biopsy, multiple punch biopsy, and incisional biopsy.[1,4] The goal is to avoid sampling error and misdiagnosing a LM or LMM as a benign lesion.
- A lesion suspicious for LM or LMM can be biopsied using a broad superficial shave biopsy approach with a Dermablade or sharp razor blade (**Figure 161-4**).[4] The goal is to sample the dermal–epidermal junction and still produce a good cosmetic result (especially if the lesion turns out to be benign).
- One option is multiple smaller biopsy samples of each morphologically distinct region of the lesion.[4]
- If an area suspicious for invasion is noted, or if there is an area of induration suspicious for associated desmoplastic melanoma, an incisional biopsy of this area should be performed.[4]
- The presence of a solar lentigo, pigmented actinic keratosis, or reticulated seborrheic keratosis (SK) could mislead the pathologist and clinician to the wrong conclusion that the incisional specimen is representative of the whole, and that no LM is present.[4]
- In a study of LM, contiguous pigmented lesions were present in 48% of the specimens obtained by broad shave biopsy or Mohs surgery. The most common lesion was a benign solar lentigo (30%), followed by pigmented actinic keratosis (24%).[4] This should be kept in mind when interpreting biopsy results to avoid false negatives.

DIFFERENTIAL DIAGNOSIS

- Solar lentigo—These hyperpigmented patches are very common on the faces and the dorsum of the hands of persons with significant sun exposure and the incidence increases with age. A possible solar lentigo is more suspicious for LM or LMM when it is larger, more

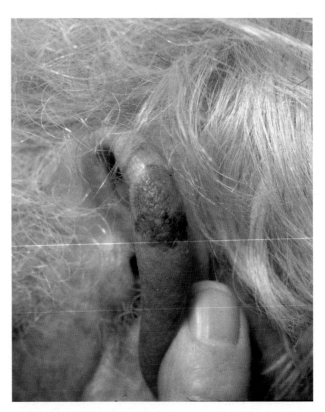

FIGURE 161-3 LM on the ear (melanoma in situ). (*With permission from Usatine RP, Moy RL, Tobinick EL, Siegel DM. Skin Surgery: A Practical Guide. 1998, St. Louis: Mosby.*)

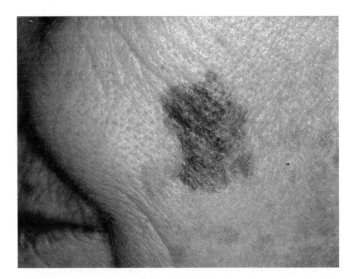

FIGURE 161-4 Lentigo maligna melanoma on the cheek. This lesion is invasive and no longer melanoma in situ. A partial broad scoop shave biopsy is a good way to make this diagnosis, since a full depth complete excisional biopsy would be prohibitively large and a punch biopsy might miss the diagnosis. (*Courtesy of the Skin Cancer Foundation.*)

asymmetric, has irregular borders and has more variation in colors. Pigmented lesions with these characteristics should be biopsied to determine the correct diagnosis. Many fair-skinned individuals have a number of solar lentigines (plural) making this a challenge. The use of dermoscopy and judicious biopsies is necessary to avoid missing LM and LMM (**Figures 161-5** and **161-6**).

- SKs are ubiquitous benign growths that occur more frequently with age. An early SK can be flat and easily resemble a solar lentigo or LM. The SKs on the back are less likely to be confused for LM, but a large flat SK on the face can easily be mistaken for an LM. More importantly, avoid missing a LM because it is assumed to be a flat early SK. When in doubt, biopsy the lesion with a quick and easy shave biopsy. Do not freeze a possible SK unless you are sure that it is truly benign (see Chapter 151, Seborrheic Keratosis).

- LMM is the feared outcome of missing an LM and not treating it properly. Any suspicious lesion requires biopsy. Don't be afraid to do a quick and easy shave biopsy rather than a full-thickness excision. If it turns out to be a LM or LMM, you can refer for definitive treatment and your biopsy technique does not change the prognosis. Early diagnosis does. LMM accounts for 4% to 15% of cutaneous melanoma (**Figure 161-4**) (see Chapter 165, Melanoma).

MANAGEMENT

- Therapy is directed toward preventing progression to invasive LMM.

- Standard therapy is margin controlled surgical excision with Mohs surgery or rush permanent sections.[5] SOR **B**

- The perimeter technique is a method of margin-controlled excision of LM with rush permanent sections. The main advantage is that all margins are examined with permanent sections. The main drawback is that multiple operative sessions are required to complete the procedure.[6]

- Recommended margins for standard excision of melanoma in situ are 0.5 cm. This margin is often inadequate for LM because of the subclinical extension that can occur. The average margin required to clear LM in 90% to 95% of cases in one study was greater than 0.5 cm.[5] Therefore, margin-controlled excision of LM is recommended.[5] SOR **B**

- Other methods reported but not as effective, include electrodestruction, topical imiquimod, radiation therapy and cryotherapy. SOR **C**

- Cryosurgery may be used in patients who are not good surgical candidates. In a study of 18 such patients with LM, the lesions resolved clinically in all cases, with no recurrence or metastasis detected during a mean follow-up of 75.5 months.[7] SOR **C** These patients were treated with two freeze-thaw cycles of liquid nitrogen under local anesthesia in a single sitting.

PATIENT EDUCATION

Patients diagnosed with LM need to minimize sun exposure and do regular self-skin examinations.

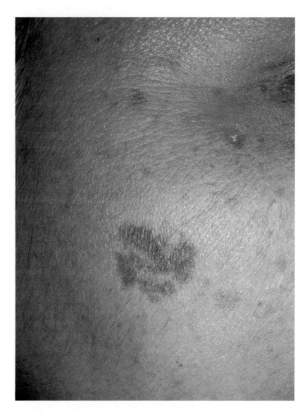

FIGURE 161-5 Solar lentigo on the face of a middle-aged Hispanic woman. (*Courtesy of Richard P. Usatine, MD.*)

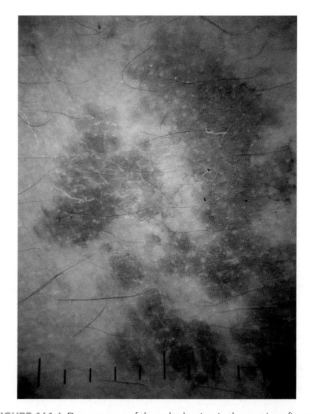

FIGURE 161-6 Dermoscopy of the solar lentigo in the previous figure. The moth-eaten appearing edges are typical of a solar lentigo. There are no suspicious patterns and a shave biopsy confirmed that it was benign. (*Courtesy of Richard P. Usatine, MD.*)

FOLLOW-UP

Patients should have regular clinical skin examinations at least yearly by their family physician or a dermatologist.

PATIENT RESOURCES

Medline Plus—**http://www.nlm.nih.gov/medlineplus/ melanoma.html.** Accessed August 14, 2007.

PROVIDER RESOURCES

The Skin Cancer Foundation—1-800-SKIN-490, or **http://www.skincancer.org.** Accessed August 14, 2007.

National Cancer Institute—**http://www.cancer.gov/ cancertopics/types/melanoma.** Accessed August 14, 2007.

Dermoscopy—**www.dermoscopy.org/** A web site on dermoscopy to learn how to improve early diagnosis of melanoma. Accessed August 14, 2007.

REFERENCES

1. Tan W Charles A. Lentigo Maligna Melanoma. http://www. emedicine.com/med/topic1278.htm. 2007. Accessed August 10, 2007.

2. Weinstock MA, Sober AJ. The risk of progression of lentigo maligna to lentigo maligna melanoma. *Br J Dermatol.* 1987;116: 303–310.

3. Schiffner R, Schiffner-Rohe J, Vogt T, et al. Improvement of early recognition of lentigo maligna using dermatoscopy. *J Am Acad Dermatol.* 2000;42:25–32.

4. Dalton SR, Gardner TL, Libow LF, Elston DM. Contiguous lesions in lentigo maligna. *J Am Acad Dermatol.* 2005;52:859–862.

5. Huang CC. New approaches to surgery of lentigo maligna. *Skin Therapy Lett.* 2004;9:7–11.

6. Mahoney MH, Joseph M, Temple CL. The perimeter technique for lentigo maligna: An alternative to Mohs micrographic surgery. *J Surg Oncol.* 2005;91:120–125.

7. de Moraes AM, Pavarin LB, Herreros F, de Aguiar MF, Velho PE, de Souza EM. Cryosurgical treatment of lentigo maligna. *J Dtsch Dermatol Ges.* 2007;5:477–480.

162 CUTANEOUS HORN

Mindy A. Smith, MD, MS

PATIENT STORY

A 74-year-old man asks about a lesion on the back of his right ear (**Figure 162-1**). It has been present for approximately 5 years. Although the lesion does not bother him, his wife is concerned because it has been slowly growing. Shave biopsy revealed that the horn was from a basal cell carcinoma.

EPIDEMIOLOGY

- Cutaneous horn (cornu cutaneum) is a morphologic (not pathologic) designation for a protuberant mass of keratin resembling the horn of an animal.
- Relatively rare lesion, most often occurring on sun-exposed areas of the skin and in elderly men.

ETIOLOGY AND PATHOPHYSIOLOGY

- Results from unusual cohesiveness of keratinized material from the superficial layers of the skin or deeply embedded in the cutis.
- Consists of marked retention of stratum corneum.
- May be benign, premalignant, or malignant at the base; in one large series, 38.9% had malignant or premalignant base pathology.[1]
- Tenderness at the base, large size, older age, and location on the penis increase the risk of underlying malignancy.[2]
- Associated with many types of skin lesions (at the base) that can retain keratin and produce horns including actinic keratosis, warts, seborrheic keratosis, keratoacanthoma, and basal or squamous cell carcinoma.
- More likely to be associated with a malignant or premalignant base in patients with a history of other malignant or premalignant lesions.[1]

DIAGNOSIS

CLINICAL FEATURES

- Horn-like protuberance (**Figures 162-1** to **162-6**).
- Lesions are usually firm; have been described as flat, keratotic, nodular, pedunculated, and ulcerated.[1]
- Size may vary from a few millimeters to several centimeters; gigantic cutaneous horns (17–25 cm length and up to 2.5 cm width) have been reported and, in one series of four cases, all were benign.[3]

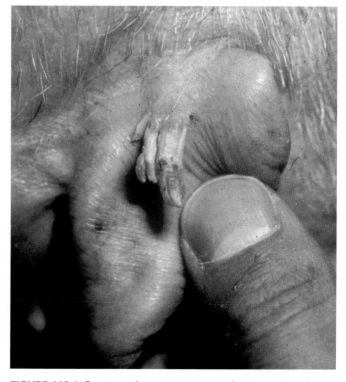

FIGURE 162-1 Cutaneous horn on posterior right pinna arising in a basal cell carcinoma. (*With permission from Usatine RP, Moy RL, Tobinick EL, Siegel DM. Skin Surgery: A Practical Guide. 1998, St. Louis: Mosby.*)

TYPICAL DISTRIBUTION

• May occur on any area of the body; approximately 30% are found on the face and scalp (**Figures 162-5** and **162-6**).

BIOPSY

• The horn itself consists of concentric layers of cornified epithelial cells (hyperkeratosis).

DIFFERENTIAL DIAGNOSIS

The differential diagnosis of lesions that can cause a cutaneous horn includes actinic keratosis, warts, seborrheic keratosis, pyogenic granuloma, keratoacanthoma, and basal or squamous cell carcinoma.

MANAGEMENT

• Shave excision, ensuring that the base of the epithelium is obtained for histologic examination, and send to pathology; if benign, may freeze any lesion that still remains.

• Excisional biopsy may also be performed, with wider margins if malignancy suspected.

See Chapter 13, sections 11 and 12 for the management of precancers and skin cancers that produce cutaneous horns.

FOLLOW-UP

• Routine follow-up is not needed provided complete removal is accomplished for malignant and premalignant lesions—in one case series of 48 eyelid cutaneous horns, there was no recurrence over a mean of 21 months.[4]

• Patients with any type of skin cancer should be seen yearly for skin examinations because one kind of cancer puts them at higher risk for all types of skin cancers. SOR **C**

PATIENT RESOURCE

VisualDxHealth **http://www.visualdxhealth.com/adult/ cutaneousHorn.htm.**

PROVIDER RESOURCES

http://www.emedicine.com/derm/topic90.htm.

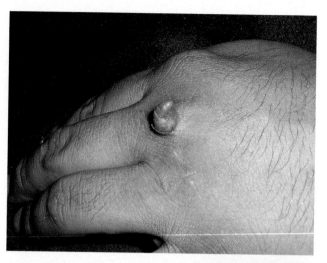

A

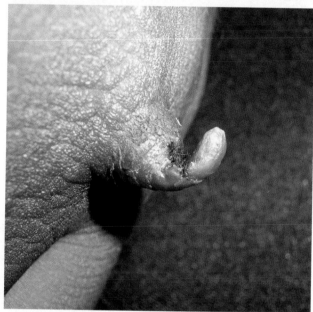

B

FIGURE 162-2 (A) Cutaneous horn on the hand of a 33-year-old man for 8 years. He clipped it with nail clippers many times but it always grew back. A shave excision successfully removed it and the pathology showed a viral wart at the base. (B) Close-up of the cutaneous horn. (*Courtesy of Richard P. Usatine, MD.*)

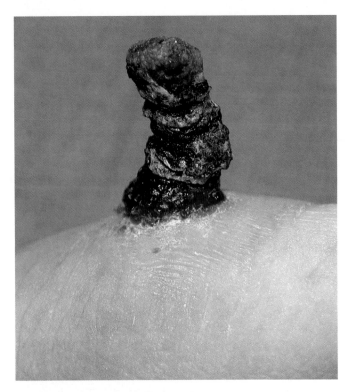

FIGURE 162-3 Cutaneous horn arising in a pyogenic granuloma. (*Courtesy of Suraj Reddy, MD.*)

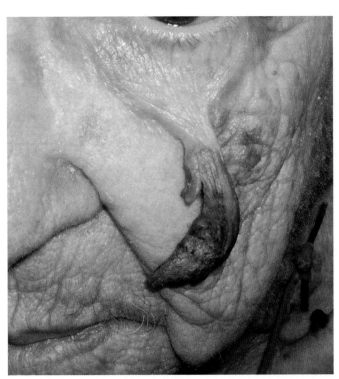

FIGURE 162-5 Large cutaneous horn on the face of an 88-year-old woman. After shave removal the pathology showed seborrheic keratosis with chronic inflammation and cutaneous horn formation. (*Courtesy of Scott Bergeaux, MD.*)

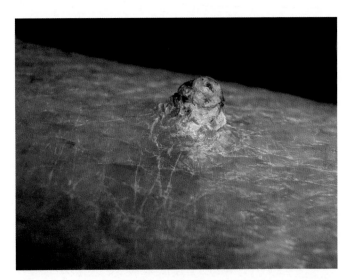

FIGURE 162-4 Cutaneous horn on the arm of a 65-year-old woman, which grew rapidly over 6 months. Biopsy revealed a squamous cell carcinoma of the keratoacanthoma type. (*Courtesy of Richard P. Usatine, MD.*)

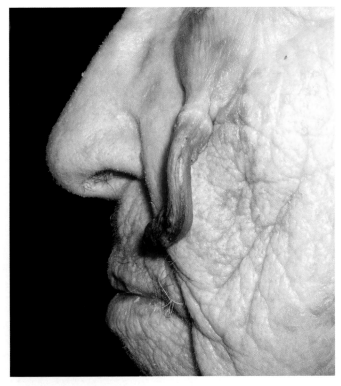

FIGURE 162-6 Another view of this amazing cutaneous horn. The patient had the lesion since her early 30s and attributed it to hot grease popping on her face. She had shown it to other physicians who declined to remove it. Patient stated it "made her feel 16 again" to have it removed. (*Courtesy of Scott Bergeaux, MD.*)

REFERENCES

1. Yu RC, Pryce DW, Macfarlane AW, Stewart TW. A histopathological study of 643 cutaneous horns. *Br J Dermatol*. 1991;124:499–452.

2. Solivan GA, Smith KJ, James WD. Cutaneous horn of the penis: Its association with squamous cell carcinoma and HPV-16 infection. *J Am Acad Dermatol*. 1990; 23(5 Pt 2):969–972.

3. Michal M, Bisceglia M, Di Mattia A, et al. Gigantic cutaneous horns of the scalp: Lesions with a gross similarity to the horns of animals: A report of four cases. *Am J Surg Pathol*. 2002;26: 789–794.

4. Mencia-Gutiérrez E, Gutiérrez-Diaz E, Redondo-Marcos I, et al. Cutaneous horns of the eyelid: Clinicopathological study of 48 cases. *J Cutan Pathol*. 2004;31:539–543.

163 BASAL CELL CARCINOMA

Richard P. Usatine, MD

PATIENT STORY

A 52-year-old woman presented to the office with a "mole" that had been increasing in size over the last year (**Figure 163-1**). This "mole" had been on her face for at least 5 years. The differential diagnosis of this lesion was a nodular basal cell carcinoma (BCC) versus an intra-dermal nevus. A shave biopsy confirmed it was a nodular BCC and the lesion was excised with an elliptical excision.

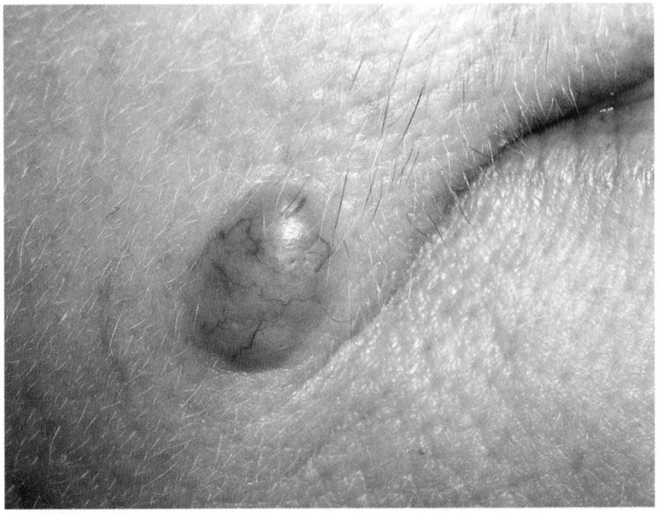

EPIDEMIOLOGY

- BCC is the most common skin cancer; 80% of skin cancers are BCCs.
- Incidence of these cancers increases with age, related to cumulative sun exposure.
- Nodular BCCs—most common type (**Figures 163-1 to 163-4**).
- Superficial BCCs—next most common type (**Figure 163-5**).
- Sclerosing BCCs—least common type (**Figures 163-6 and 163-7**).

ETIOLOGY AND PATHOPHYSIOLOGY

- Most important risk factors are sun exposure, family history, and skin type.
- BCCs spread locally and rarely metastasize.
- Basal cell nevus syndrome is a rare autosomal dominant condition in which affected individuals have multiple nevoid BCCs (**Figure 163-8**).

DIAGNOSIS

CLINICAL FEATURES

Clinical features of the three types of BCCs:

Nodular BCC

- Raised pearly white, smooth translucent surface with telangiectasias.
- Smooth surface with loss of the normal pore pattern (**Figures 163-1 to 163-4**).
- May be pigmented (**Figures 163-9 to 163-11**).

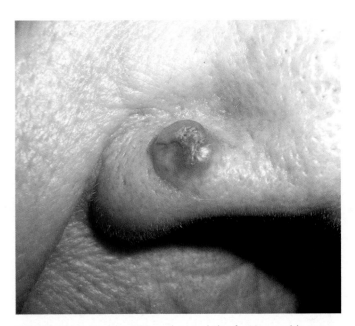

FIGURE 163-1 Pearly nodular BCC on the face of a 52-year-old woman present for 5 years. (*Courtesy of Richard P. Usatine, MD.*)

FIGURE 163-2 Nodular BCC on the nasal ala of a 82-year-old woman. The nose is a very common location for a BCC. (*Courtesy of Richard P. Usatine, MD.*)

- May ulcerate (**Figures 163-12** to **163-15**) and can leave a bloody crust.

Superficial BCC

- Red or pink scaling plaques with a thready border (slightly raised and pearly) (**Figure 163-5**).
- Found more on the trunk and upper extremities than the face.

Sclerosing BCC

- Ivory or colorless, flat or atrophic, indurated, may resemble scars, are easily overlooked (**Figures 163-6** and **163-7**).
- Called morpheaform because of their resemblance to localized scleroderma (morphea).
- Called infiltrating BCCs because the border is not well demarcated and the tumor can spread out way beyond what is visible (**Figure 163-16A** to **C**).
- These BCCs are the most dangerous and have the worst prognosis.

TYPICAL DISTRIBUTION

Ninety percent appear on face, ears, and head with some found on the trunk and upper extremities (especially the superficial type).

DERMOSCOPY

Dermoscopic characteristics of BCCs (**Figure 163-17A** to **B**) include (see Dermoscopy Appendix):

- Large gray-blue ovoid nests.
- Multiple gray-blue globules.
- Leaflike areas- that look like maple leaves.
- Spoke wheel areas.
- Arborizing "tree-like" telangiectasia.
- Ulceration.
- Shiny white areas/stellate streaks.

BIOPSY

- A shave biopsy is adequate to diagnose a nodular BCC or a thick superficial BCC.
- A scoop shave or punch biopsy is preferred for a sclerosing BCC or a very flat superficial BCC.

DIFFERENTIAL DIAGNOSIS

Nodular BCC

- Intradermal (dermal) nevi often have features in common with a BCC when present on the face. These features include being pearly and having multiple telangiectasias as seen in **Figure 163-18**. Their stable size and symmetry may be helpful in distinguishing them from a nodular BCC. A simple shave biopsy is diagnostic and produces a good cosmetic result. A large excisional biopsy with 4-mm margins for a BCC may be cosmetically deforming on the face if it turns out that the lesion was nothing more than a benign intradermal nevus. It is remarkable how similar **Figure 163-18**

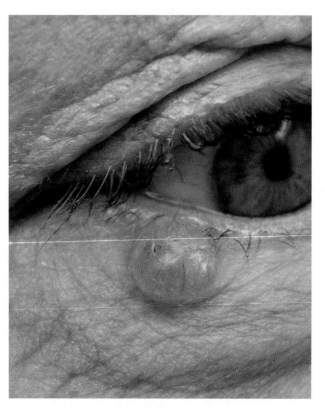

FIGURE 163-3 Nodular BCC on the lower eyelid. Patient referred for Mohs surgery. (*Courtesy of Richard P. Usatine, MD.*)

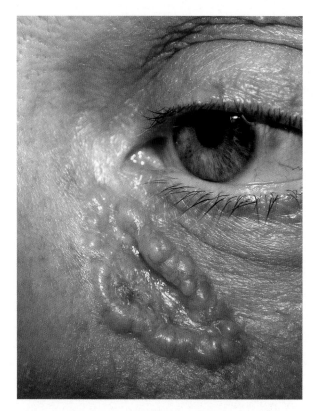

FIGURE 163-4 Large nodular BCC with an annular appearance on the face of a homeless woman. (*Courtesy of Richard P. Usatine, MD.*)

appears to **163-1** (both biopsies proven to be as labeled) (see Chapter 155, Benign Nevi).

- Sebaceous hyperplasia is a benign condition commonly seen on the face in older adults and usually occurs with more than one lesion present (**Figure 163-19**). This benign overgrowth of the sebaceous glands produces small papules that have a doughnut shape with frequent telangiectasias (see Chapter 152, Sebaceous Hyperplasia).

- Fibrous papule of the face is a benign condition with small papules that can be firm and pearly.

- Trichoepithelioma/trichoblastoma are benign tumors on the face that can appear around the nose. They may be pearly but usually do not have telangiectasias. These are best diagnosed with a shave biopsy.

- Keratoacanthoma is a type of squamous cell carcinoma that is raised, nodular and may be pearly with telangiectasias. A central keratin filled crater may help to distinguish this from a BCC (see Chapter 160, Keratoacanthoma).

Superficial BCC

- Actinic keratoses are precancers that are flat, pink and scaly. They lack the pearly and thready border of the superficial BCC (see Chapter 159, Actinic Keratosis/Bowen's Disease).

- Bowen's disease is an SCC in situ that appears like a larger thicker actinic keratosis with more distinct well-demarcated borders. It also lacks the pearly and thready border of the superficial BCC (see Chapter 159, Actinic Keratosis/Bowen's Disease).

- Nummular eczema can usually be distinguished by its multiple coin-like shapes, transient nature, and rapid response to topical steroids. These lesions are pruritic and most patients will have other signs and symptoms of atopic disease (see Chapter 139, Atopic Dermatitis).

Sclerosing BCC

- Scars may look like a sclerosing BCC. Ask about previous surgeries or trauma to the area. If the so-called scar is flat, shiny, and enlarging, a biopsy still may be needed to rule out a sclerosing BCC.

MANAGEMENT

- Mohs micrographic surgery (three studies, $n = 2,660$) is the gold standard but is not needed for all BCCs. Recurrence rate[1] is 0.8% to 1.1%. Mohs micrographic surgery is the removal of tumor by scalpel in sequential horizontal layers in which each tissue sample is frozen, stained, and microscopically examined. This is repeated until all the margins are clear (**Figure 163-16A to C**). This is the treatment of choice for BCCs with poorly defined margins involving areas of cosmetic or functional importance such as nose or eyelids.[1] SOR **A**

- Surgical excision (three studies, $n = 1303$): Recurrence rate[1] was 2% to 8%. Mean cumulative 5-year rate[1] (all 3 studies) was 5.3%. Recommended margins are 4 to 5 mm.[1] SOR **A**

- Cryosurgery (Four studies, $n = 796$): Recurrence rate was 3.0% to 4.3%. Cumulative 5-year rate (three studies) ranged from 0% to 16.5%.[1] SOR **A** Recommended freeze times are 30 to 60 seconds

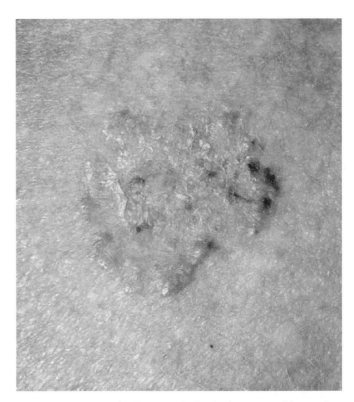

FIGURE 163-5 Superficial BCC on the back of a 45-year-old man who enjoys running in the California sun without his shirt. Note the diffuse scaling, thready border (slightly raised and pearly), and spotty hyperpigmentation. (*Courtesy of Richard P. Usatine, MD.*)

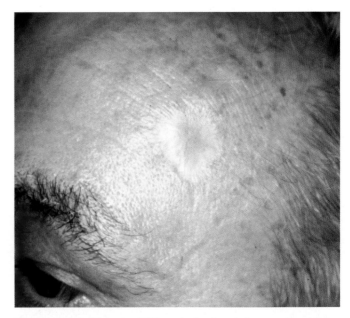

FIGURE 163-6 Sclerosing BCC on the forehead of a man resembling a scar. Note the white color with shiny atrophic skin. (*Courtesy of Skin Cancer Foundation.*)

with 5 mm halo. This can be divided up into two 30 second freezes with a thaw in between. Some patients might prefer local anesthetic if the freezing is too painful. SOR **C**

- Curettage and desiccation (six studies, $n = 4212$): Recurrence rate ranged from 4.3% to 18.1%; cumulative 5-year rate ranged from 5.7% to 18.8%.[1] Three cycles of curettage and desiccation can produce higher cure rates than one cycle.[1] SOR **A**

- Imiquimod is FDA approved for the treatment of superficial BCCs less than 2 cm in diameter.[2] SOR **B** Confirm diagnosis with biopsy and use when surgical methods are contraindicated.[2]

PATIENT EDUCATION

While most of the sun damage has been done, patients should still practice skin cancer prevention by sun-protective behaviors such as avoiding peak sun, covering up and using sunscreen.

FOLLOW-UP

Patients should be seen at least yearly after the diagnosis and treatment of a BCC. The 3-year risk of BCC recurrence after having a single BCC is 44%.[3]

PATIENT RESOURCES

The Skin Cancer Foundation has an excellent web site with photos and patient information—**http://www.skincancer.org/basal/index.php.**

PROVIDER RESOURCE

British Journal of Dermatology (1999;141:415–423) for specific guidelines for managing BCC—**http://www.bad.org.uk/healthcare/guidelines/Basal_Cell_Carcinoma.pdf.**

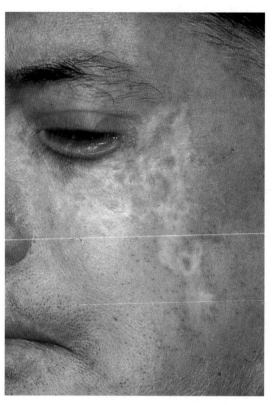

FIGURE 163-7 Advanced sclerosing BCC on the cheek of a man, causing ectropion (the eyelid is being pulled down by the sclerotic skin changes). (*With permission from Usatine RP, Moy RL, Tobinick EL, Siegel DM. Skin Surgery: A Practical Guide. 1998, St. Louis: Mosby.*)

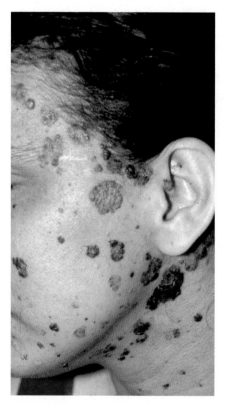

FIGURE 163-8 Basal cell nevus syndrome with multiple nevoid BCCs on the face and neck of a young woman. This is a rare autosomal dominant condition. (*Courtesy of the University of Texas Health Sciences Center, Division of Dermatology.*)

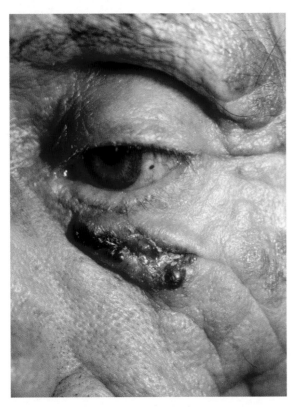

FIGURE 163-9 Large pigmented nodular BCC on the face with ulceration. (*With permission from Usatine RP, Moy RL, Tobinick EL, Siegel DM. Skin Surgery: A Practical Guide. 1998, St. Louis: Mosby.*)

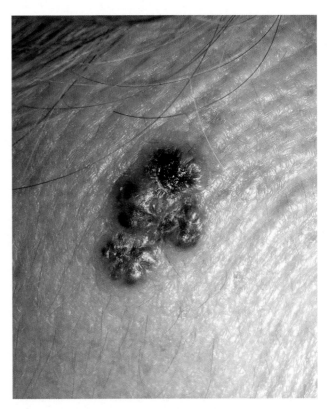

FIGURE 163-11 Darkly pigmented BCC with pearly borders and some ulceration in a 73-year-old Hispanic woman. A biopsy was performed to rule out melanoma before this was excised. (*Courtesy of Richard P. Usatine, MD.*)

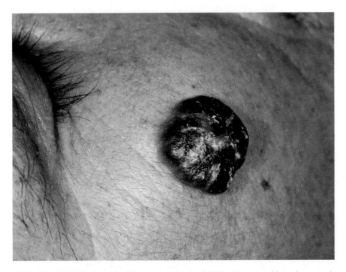

FIGURE 163-10 Darkly pigmented large BCC with raised borders and some ulceration in a 53-year-old Hispanic man. A biopsy was performed to rule out melanoma before this was excised. (*Courtesy of Richard P. Usatine, MD.*)

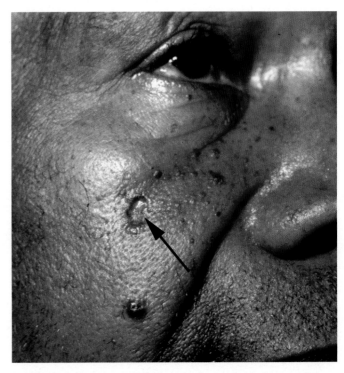

FIGURE 163-12 Ulcerated BCC on the cheek of a black man. (*With permisson from Usatine RP, Moy RL, Tobinick EL, Siegel DM. Skin Surgery: A Practical Guide. 1998, St. Louis: Mosby.*)

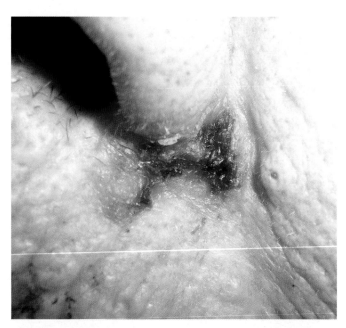

FIGURE 163-13 BCC in the nasal alar groove. There is a high risk of recurrence at this site so Mohs surgery is indicated for removal. (*Courtesy of Richard P. Usatine, MD.*)

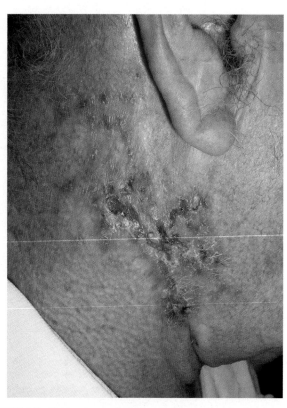

FIGURE 163-15 Very large ulcerating BCC on the neck of a 65-year-old white man, which has been growing there for 6 years. It was excised in the operating room with a large flap from his chest used to close the big defect. (*Courtesy of Richard P. Usatine, MD.*)

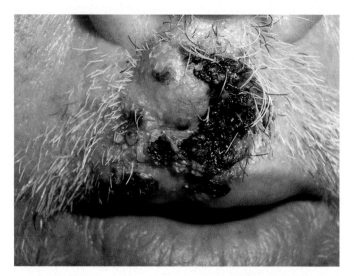

FIGURE 163-14 Large advanced BCC with ulcerations and bloody crusting infiltrating the upper lip. The patient was referred for Mohs surgery. (*Courtesy of Richard P. Usatine, MD.*)

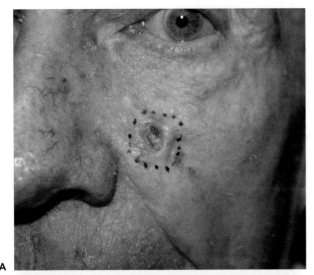

A

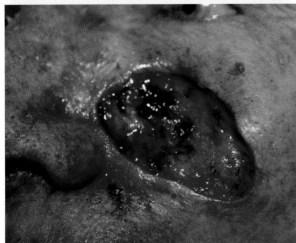

B

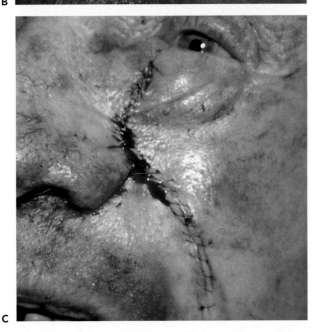

C

FIGURE 163-16 (A) Sclerosing BCC in an elderly man. The size of the BCC did not appear large by clinical examination. (B) Mohs surgery of the same sclerosing BCC. This took four shave excisions to get clean margins. Usual 4- to 5-mm margins with an elliptical excision would not have removed the full tumor. (C) Repair by Mohs surgery to close the large defect. The cure rate should be close to 99%. (*Courtesy of Ryan O'Quinn, MD.*)

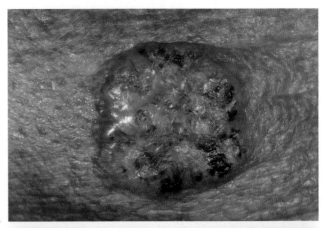

A

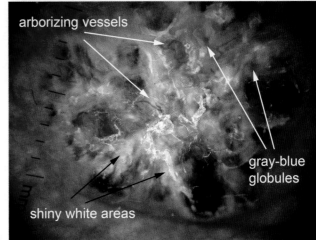

B

FIGURE 163-17 (A) Large nodular BCC on the cheek of a 52-year-old man. There is a loss of normal pore pattern, pearly appearance, telangiectasias, and some areas of dark pigmentation. (B) Dermoscopy of the previous nodular BCC. There are visible arborizing "tree-like" telangiectasias, ulcerations, shiny white areas and blue-grey globules all consistent with a BCC. (*Courtesy of Richard P. Usatine, MD.*)

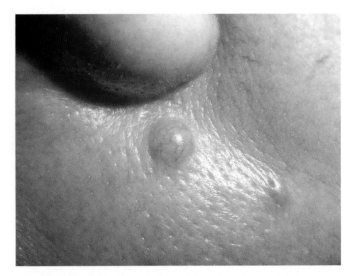

FIGURE 163-18 Pearly dome-shaped intradermal nevus near the nose with telangiectasias closely resembling a BCC. A shave biopsy proved that this was an intradermal nevus. (*Courtesy of Richard P. Usatine, MD.*)

REFERENCES

1. Thissen MR, Neumann MH, Schouten LJ. A systematic review of treatment modalities for primary basal cell carcinomas. *Arch Dermatol*. 1999;135(10):1177–1183.

2. Geisse J, Caro I, Lindholm J, Golitz L, Stampone P, Owens M. Imiquimod 5% cream for the treatment of superficial basal cell carcinoma: Results from two phase III, randomized, vehicle-controlled studies. *J Am Acad Dermatol*. 2004;50(5):722–733.

3. Marcil I, Stern RS. Risk of developing a subsequent nonmelanoma skin cancer in patients with a history of nonmelanoma skin cancer: A critical review of the literature and meta-analysis. *Arch Dermatol*. 2000;136(12):1524–1530.

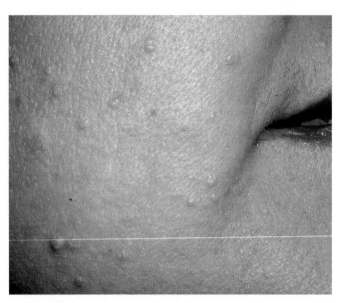

FIGURE 163-19 Extensive sebaceous hyperplasia on the cheek of a 52-year-old woman. Largest one has visible telangiectasias and could be mistaken for a BCC. (*Courtesy of Richard P. Usatine, MD.*)

164 SQUAMOUS CELL CARCINOMA

Richard P. Usatine, MD

PATIENT STORY

A 66-year-old farmer presents with new growths on his scalp (**Figure 164-1**). The patient admits to lots of sun exposure and has already had one squamous cell carcinoma (SCC) excised from the scalp 5 years ago. On close inspection there are four particularly suspicious areas. **Figure 164-1** shows four sites that have already been biopsied with shave biopsies. The final pathology demonstrated that three out of four sites were positive for SCC. **Figure 164-2** demonstrates the shave biopsy technique using a Dermablade. The patient was referred for Mohs surgery to fully excise the three positive areas.

EPIDEMIOLOGY

- SCC is the second most common skin cancer seen accounting for 16% of skin cancers.

- The most important risk factors for SCC of the skin are sun exposure and skin type.

- Less common predisposing factors include chemical exposures, HPV, and burns.

- Incidence of SCC increases with age, related to cumulative sun exposure.

- Metastasis from SCC occurs in 2% to 6% of cases.[1]

- SCCs that metastasize most often start on the mucous membranes or lips or sites of chronic inflammatory skin conditions.

- In the United States, approximately 2,500 people die from SCC every year.[1]

PATHOPHYSIOLOGY

SCC is a malignant tumor of keratinocytes. Most SCCs arise from actinic keratoses. SCCs usually spread by local extension but are capable of regional lymph node metastasis and distant metastasis. HPV-related lesions may be found on the penis, labia, or in the periungual region.[1]

DIAGNOSIS

- The only sure method of making the diagnosis is a biopsy. Biopsy suspicious lesions (thickened, indurated, ulcerated, or crusting) in areas with signs of sun exposure. Even suspicious lesions in non-sun-exposed areas need biopsy and can be SCCs.

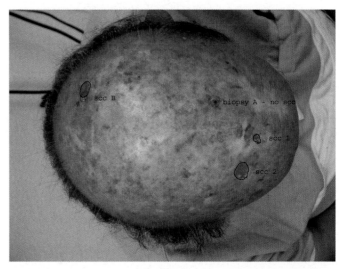

FIGURE 164-1 Three squamous cell carcinomas (SCCs) on the scalp of a farmer. The SCCs were found at the sites labeled SCC 1, SCC 2, and SCC B. (*Courtesy of Richard P. Usatine, MD.*)

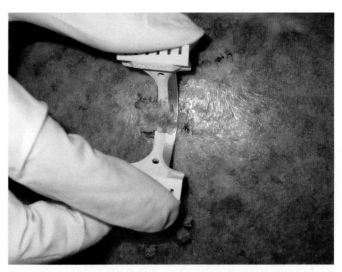

FIGURE 164-2 Shave biopsy of a new SCC on the head of the patient in **Figure 164-1** one year later. (*Courtesy of Richard P. Usatine, MD.*)

CLINICAL FEATURES

SCC often present as areas of persistent ulceration, crusting, hyperkeratosis, and erythema, especially on skin showing evidence of sun damage.

Less common types of SCC:

- Marjolin's ulcer—SCC of the extremities found in chronic skin ulcers or burn scars (**Figure 164-3**).

- Erythroplasia of Queyrat—SCC in situ on the penis or vulva related to HPV infection (**Figure 164-4**). This can progress to full invasive SCC of the penis (**Figure 164-5**).

TYPICAL DISTRIBUTION

SCC is found in all sun exposed areas and on mucus membranes. The most common sites are:

- Face (**Figures 164-6** and **164-7**).
- Lower lip (**Figures 164-8** and **164-9**).
- Ears (**Figure 164-10**).
- Scalp (**Figures 164-1** and **164-11**).
- Extremities—arm—(**Figures 164-12** and **164-13**).
- Bands (**Figure 164-14**).
- Fingers (**Figure 164-15**).
- Mucus membranes (see Chapter 42, Oral Cancer).

BIOPSY

- Deep shave biopsy is adequate to make the diagnosis of most SCCs.

- Punch biopsy is an alternative for lesions that are pigmented or appear to be deeper.

FACTORS AFFECTING METASTATIC POTENTIAL OF CUTANEOUS SCC[2]

The following factors are taken from the "Multiprofessional guidelines for the management of the patient with primary cutaneous squamous cell carcinoma."[2]

- Site.

Tumor location influences prognosis: sites are listed in order of increasing metastatic potential.[2]

1. SCC arising at sun-exposed sites excluding lip and ear.

2. SCC of the lip (**Figures 164-8** and **164-9**).

3. SCC of the ear (**Figure 164-10**).

4. Tumors arising in non-sun-exposed sites (e.g., perineum, sacrum, sole of foot) (**Figures 164-4** and **164-5**).

5. SCC arising in areas of radiation or thermal injury, chronic draining sinuses, chronic ulcers, chronic inflammation, or Bowen's disease, such as the SCC arising in a burn site (**Figure 164-3**).

- Size: diameter.

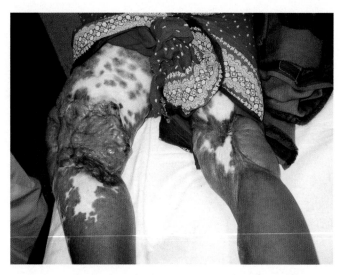

FIGURE 164-3 Marjolin's ulcer (SCC) arising in a large burn that occurred years before on the legs of a woman living in India. (*Courtesy of Colby McLaren, MD.*)

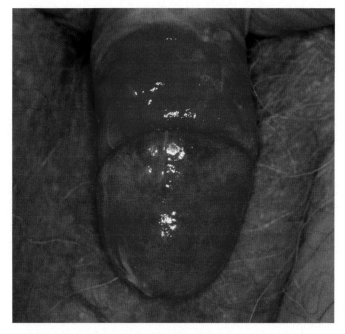

FIGURE 164-4 Erythroplasia of Queyrat (SCC in situ) under the foreskin of an uncircumcised man. This is related to HPV infection as is cervical cancer. (*Courtesy of John Pfenninger, MD.*)

Tumors larger than 2 cm in diameter are twice as likely to recur locally (15.2% vs 7.4%), and three times as likely to metastasize (30.3% vs 9.1%) as smaller tumors.

• Size: depth.

Tumors greater than 4 mm in depth (excluding surface layers of keratin) or extending down to the subcutaneous tissue (Clark level V) are more likely to recur and metastasize (metastatic rate 45.7%) compared with thinner tumors. Recurrence and metastases are less likely in tumors confined to the upper half of the dermis and less than 4 mm in depth (metastatic rate 6.7%).

• Histologic differentiation.

Poorly differentiated tumors have a poorer prognosis, with more than double the local recurrence rate and triple the metastatic rate of better differentiated SCC. Tumors with perineural involvement are more likely to recur and to metastasize.

• Host immunosuppression.

Tumors arising in patients who are immunosuppressed have a poorer prognosis. Host cellular immune response may be important both in determining the local invasiveness of SCC and the host's response to metastases. **Figures 164-16** to **164-18** are SCCs in patients that are HIV positive.

• Previous treatment and treatment modality.

The risk of local recurrence depends upon the treatment modality. Locally recurrent disease itself is a risk factor for metastatic disease. Local recurrence rates are considerably less with Mohs' micrographic surgery than with any other treatment modality.

DIFFERENTIAL DIAGNOSIS

• Actinic keratoses are precancers on sun-exposed areas, which can progress to SCC (see Chapter 159, Actinic Keratosis and Bowen's Disease).

• Bowen's disease is SCC in situ before it invades the basement membrane (see Chapter 159, Actinic Keratosis and Bowen's Disease).

• Keratoacanthoma is a lesion that can grow rapidly and often has a central keratinized crater. **Figure 164-18** resembles a keratoacanthoma but is actually a SCC. Keratoacanthomas can also be considered to be a type of SCC (see Chapter 160, Keratoacanthomas).

• Basal Cell Carcinoma cannot always be distinguished from SCC by clinical appearance alone. Both **Figures 164-16** and **164-17** could be BCCs by appearance but were proven to be SCC by biopsy (see Chapter 163, Basal Cell Carcinoma).

• Market cell carcinoma (neuroendocrine carcinoma of the skin) is a rare aggressive malignancy. It is most commonly seen on the face of white elderly persons. It can resemble a SCC and the diagnosis is made on biopsy (**Figure 164-19**).

• Nummular eczema can usually be distinguished by the multiple coin-like shapes, transient nature, and pruritus (Chapter 139, Atopic Dermatitis).

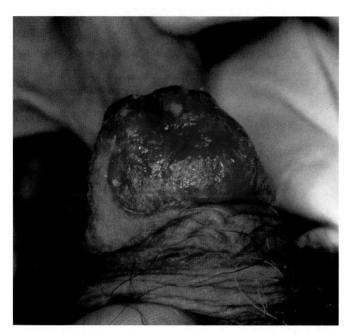

FIGURE 164-5 SCC of the penis. (*Courtesy of Jeff Meffert, MD.*)

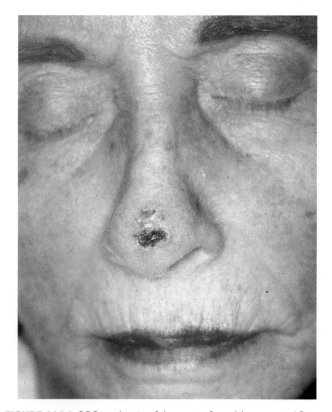

FIGURE 164-6 SCC on the tip of the nose of an older woman. (*Courtesy of the Skin Cancer Foundation.*)

MANAGEMENT

The following recommendations are derived from the "Multiprofessional guidelines for the management of the patient with primary cutaneous squamous cell carcinoma."[2] See **Table 164-1** for a summary of treatment options.

Surgical resection for definitive treatment should include margins as given below:

4-mm margin—should be adequate for well-defined, low-risk tumors less than 2 cm in diameter, such margins are expected to remove the primary tumor mass completely in 95% of cases.[2] SOR A

6-mm margin—recommended for larger tumors, high-risk tumors, tumors extending into the subcutaneous tissue and those in high-risk locations (ear, lip, scalp, eyelids, nose).[2]

MOHS' MICROGRAPHIC SURGERY

Allows precise definition and excision of primary tumor growing in continuity, thereby reducing errors in primary treatment that may arise owing to clinically invisible tumor extension. There is good evidence that the incidence of local recurrent and metastatic disease are low after Mohs' micrographic surgery and it should, therefore, be considered in the surgical treatment of high-risk SCC, particularly at difficult sites where wide surgical margins may be technically difficult to achieve without functional impairment.[2] SOR B

CURETTAGE AND ELECTRODESICCATION

Excellent cure rates have been reported in several series, and experience suggests that small (<1 cm) well-differentiated primary slow-growing tumors arising on sun-exposed sites can be removed by experienced physicians with curettage.[2]

The experienced clinician undertaking curettage can detect tumor tissue by its soft consistency and this may be of benefit in identifying invisible tumor extension and ensuring adequate treatment. Electrodesiccation is applied to the curetted wound and the curettage-cautery cycle then repeated twice. SOR C

CRYOSURGERY

Good short-term cure rates have been reported for small, histologically confirmed SCC treated by cryosurgery in experienced hands. Prior biopsy is necessary to establish the diagnosis histologically. There is great variability in the use of liquid nitrogen for cryotherapy. Start by drawing a 4- to 6-mm margin around the SCC and then use a total freeze time of 60 seconds. This can be divided up into two 30-second freezes with a thaw in between. Some patients might prefer local anesthetic if the freezing is too painful. SOR C

Cryosurgery and curettage and electrodesiccation are not appropriate for locally recurrent disease.

RADIOTHERAPY

Radiation therapy alone offers short- and long-term cure rates for SCC that are comparable with other treatments. It is recommended for lesions arising on the lip, nasal vestibule (and sometimes the outside of the nose), and ear. Certain very advanced tumors, where surgical morbidity would be unacceptably high, may also be best treated by radiotherapy. SOR C

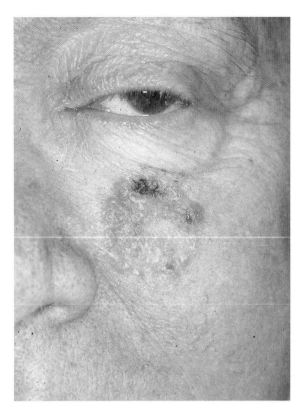

FIGURE 164-7 Large SCC on the cheek of an older man. (*Courtesy of the Skin Cancer Foundation.*)

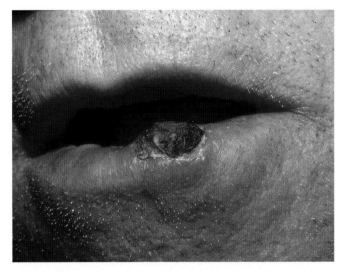

FIGURE 164-8 SCC on the lower lip. (*Courtesy of the Skin Cancer Foundation.*)

ELECTIVE PROPHYLACTIC LYMPH NODE DISSECTION

Elective prophylactic lymph node dissection has been proposed for SCC on the lip greater than 6 mm in depth and cutaneous SCC greater than 8 mm in depth, but evidence for this is weak. SOR Ⓒ

FOLLOW-UP

Patients should be seen at least yearly for skin examinations after the diagnosis and treatment of a SCC. The 3-year risk of recurrence of a new SCC after having a single SCC is 18%.[3]

PATIENT EDUCATION

Includes use of a hat and sunscreen on a regular basis with frequent follow-up for early recognition of new skin cancers.

PATIENT AND PROVIDER RESOURCE

Skin Cancer Foundation has an excellent web site with photos and patient information **http://www.skincancer.org/squamous/index.php.**

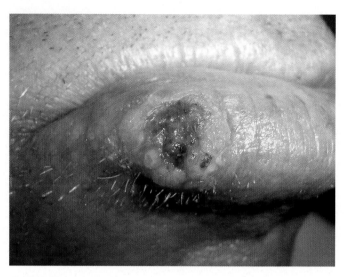

FIGURE 164-9 SCC showing ulceration on the lower lip. (*Courtesy of Richard P. Usatine, MD*)

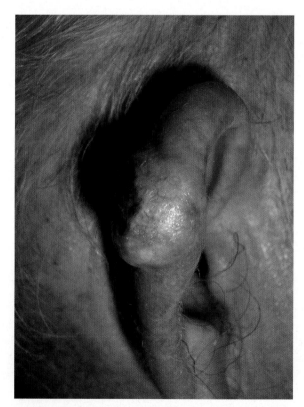

FIGURE 164-10 Large SCC on the pinna that has features suggestive of a BCC or keratoacanthoma. (*Courtesy of the Skin Cancer Foundation.*)

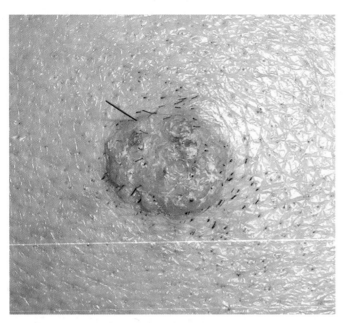

FIGURE 164-11 SCC on the shaven scalp of a 35-year-old man, which was formerly mistaken for a wart. (*Courtesy of Richard P. Usatine, MD.*)

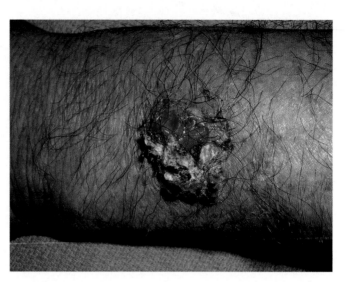

FIGURE 164-13 Large ulcerating SCC on arm. (*Courtesy of Richard P. Usatine, MD.*)

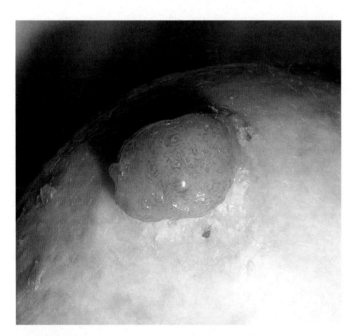

FIGURE 164-12 Large pedunculated SCC on the shoulder of a 92-year-old woman. (*Courtesy of Richard P. Usatine, MD.*)

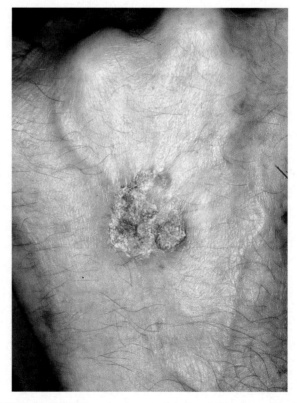

FIGURE 164-14 SCC on the dorsum of the hand. (*Courtesy of the Skin Cancer Foundation.*)

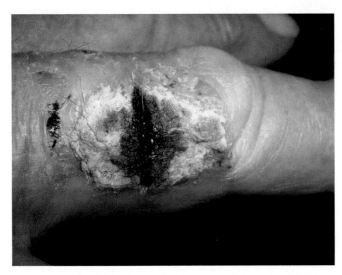

FIGURE 164-15 SCC on the finger. It took two biopsies to establish the correct diagnosis. (*Courtesy of Richard P. Usatine, MD.*)

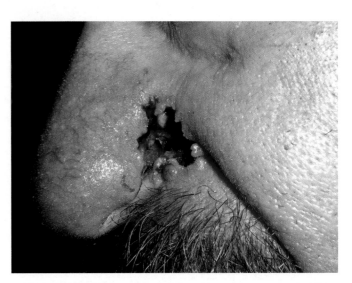

FIGURE 164-17 SCC invading the internal nasal structures in an HIV-positive man who was afraid of having a biopsy done earlier. Patient referred to ENT. (*Courtesy of Richard P. Usatine, MD.*)

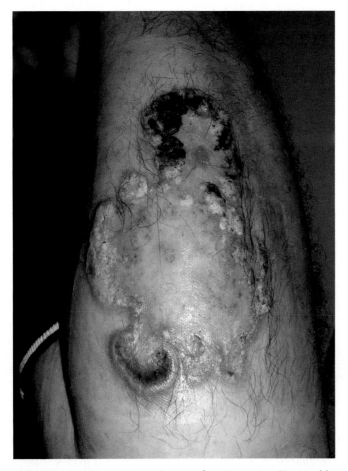

FIGURE 164-16 Large SCC on the arm of an HIV positive 51-year-old man. It grew to this size in one year and took two biopsies to get a definitive diagnosis. Differential diagnosis includes mycosis fungoides. (*Courtesy of Richard P. Usatine, MD.*)

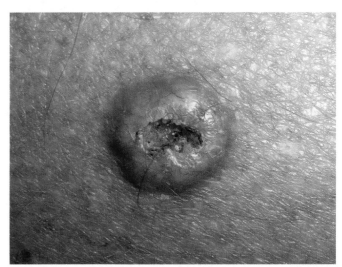

FIGURE 164-18 SCC on the shoulder of an HIV positive man. Note that the pearly borders and telangiectasias resemble a BCC and the central crater suggests that this could be a keratoacanthoma. (*Courtesy of Richard P. Usatine, MD.*)

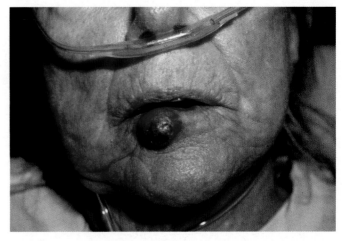

FIGURE 164-19 Merkel cell carcinoma on the lower lip of an elderly woman. This is an aggressive cancer with a high mortality rate. (*Courtesy of Jeff Meffert, MD.*)

TABLE 164-1 Summary of Treatment Options for Primary Cutaneous Squamous Cell Carcinoma[2]

Treatment	Indications	Contraindications	Notes
Surgical excision	All resectable tumors	Where surgical morbidity is likely to be unreasonably high	Generally treatment of choice for SCC High-risk tumors need wide margins or histologic margin control
Mohs' micrographic surgery/excision with histologic control	High-risk tumors, recurrent tumors	Where surgical morbidity is likely to be unreasonably high	Treatment of choice for high-risk tumors
Radiotherapy	Nonresectable tumors	Where margins are ill-defined	
Curettage and cautery	Small, well-defined, low-risk tumors	High-risk tumors	Curettage may be helpful prior to surgical excision
Cryotherapy	Small, well-defined, low-risk tumors	High-risk tumors, recurrent tumors	Only suitable for experienced practitioners

Reprinted from Motley R, Kersey P, Lawrence C. Multiprofessional guidelines for the management of the patient with primary cutaneous squamous cell carcinoma. *Br J Plast Surg.* 2003;56:85–91.

REFERENCES

1. Goldman, G. Squamous Cell Carcinoma. www.emedicine.com/DERM/topic401.htm. 2007. Accessed November 7, 2007.

2. Motley R, Kersey P, Lawrence C. Multiprofessional guidelines for the management of the patient with primary cutaneous squamous cell carcinoma. Br J Plast Surg. 2003;56:85–91.

3. Marcil I, Stern RS. Risk of developing a subsequent nonmelanoma skin cancer in patients with a history of nonmelanoma skin cancer: A critical review of the literature and meta-analysis. *Arch Dermatol.* 2000;136:1524–1530.

165 MELANOMA

Richard P. Usatine, MD

PATIENT STORIES

A 55-year-old woman noticed a new dark spot on her arm near the antecubital fossa (**Figure 165-1**). On examination the spot was 10 mm in its longest diameter, was asymmetrical, with irregular borders, and had a variation in color. A scoop biopsy demonstrated melanoma in situ. The spot was excised with 0.5 cm margins and no residual tumor was found in the excised ellipse. The prognosis is excellent for a 100% cure.

The wife of a 73-year-old man noticed that a "mole" on his back was enlarging and bleeding. (**Figure 165-2**). It had been there for years and a year ago a doctor had told him not to worry about it. His wife sent him to have it checked out again. **Figure 165-3** shows a close-up of the pigmented lesion showing ulcerations and bleeding. An elliptical excision was performed and the tissue appeared to be a nodular melanoma with dark pigment into the subcutaneous fat (**Figure 165-4**). The pathology was read as nodular melanoma with a Breslow depth of 22 mm and Clark's level V. The patient was referred to surgical and medical oncology. The next step was a wide excision with 2-cm margins and a sentinel node biopsy. Sentinel node was positive and further nodal dissection showed a total of another four axillary lymph nodes positive (one on right and three on left). The lymph nodes on left were black and enlarged. No distant mets were found. This makes him a stage IIIC because of the presence of more than two macroscopic regional nodes positive. He underwent radiation treatment to original site and both axilla. The prognosis is poor.

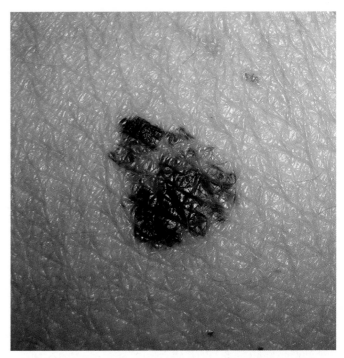

FIGURE 165-1 Melanoma in situ on the arm showing asymmetry, irregular borders, variation in color and a diameter of 10 mm. (*With permission from Leight A. Photo Rounds: A non-healing ulcerated fingertip following injury. Am Fam Phys, 2006;55(3):225–229.*)

EPIDEMIOLOGY

- Approximately 59,940 people developed invasive cutaneous melanoma in 2007 in the United States, with an additional 48,290 cases of melanoma in situ.[1]

- In 2007, approximately 8,110 people died in the United States from metastatic melanoma.[1]

- While the incidence of melanoma in the United States increased in the 1970s, it has plateaued since the 1990s.[2]

- One study showed that in a 5-year period the incidence of melanoma increased 2.4-fold, whereas the biopsy rate over the same period increased a similar 2.5 times. This suggests that the rate of melanoma may not be increasing, but the detection rate is.[3]

- The median age at melanoma diagnosis is 53 years.[4]

- Melanoma is the most common cancer in women aged 25 to 29 years.[4]

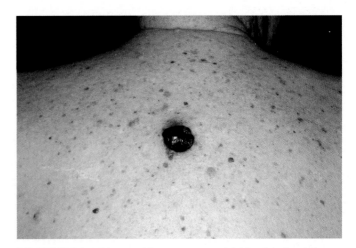

FIGURE 165-2 A 73-year-old man presents with bleeding "mole" on his back. Elliptical excision demonstrates this to be a nodular melanoma of 22 mm depth. (*From Swetter S. Malignant Melanoma. Reprinted with permission from emedicine.com, 2008. Available at: http://www.emedicine.com/derm/topic257.htm. Accessed August 18, 2008.*)

RISK FACTORS

- There is a positive association between early age sunburn and subsequent risk of melanoma.[5]
- Primary risk factors for melanoma include:[4]
  - A changing mole (most important risk factor).
  - Atypical/dysplastic nevi (particularly >5–10).
  - Large numbers of common nevi (>100).
  - Large (giant) congenital nevi (>20 cm diameter in an adult).
  - A history of melanoma.
  - Sun sensitivity/history of excessive sun exposure or sunburn.
  - Melanoma in a first-degree relative.
  - Prior nonmelanoma skin cancer (basal cell and squamous cell carcinoma).
  - Male gender.
  - Age >50 years.
  - Presence of xeroderma pigmentosum or familial atypical mole melanoma syndrome.
  - A fair-skin phenotype (blue/green eyes, blond or red hair, light complexion, sun sensitivity) and the occurrence of blistering sunburns in childhood and adolescence.[4]

DIAGNOSIS

CLINICAL FEATURES

Remember the *ABCDE* guidelines for diagnosing melanoma (**Figure 165-5**).[6]

A = Asymmetry. Most early melanomas are asymmetrical: a line through the middle will not create matching halves. Benign nevi are usually round and symmetrical.

B = Border. The borders of early melanomas are often uneven and may have scalloped or notched edges. Benign nevi have smoother, more even borders.

C = Variation in color. Benign nevi are usually in a single shade of brown. Melanomas are often in varied shades of brown, tan, or black. As melanomas progress, they may appear red, white, and blue.

D = Diameter greater than or equal to 6 mm. Early melanomas tend to grow larger than most nevi. (Note: Congenital nevi are often large).

E = Evolving. Any evolving or enlarging nevus should make you suspect melanoma. Evolving could be in size, shape, symptoms (itching, tenderness), surface (especially bleeding), and shades of color.

- A prospective controlled study compared 460 cases of melanoma with 680 cases of benign pigmented tumors and found significant differences for all individual ABCDE criteria (*p* <0.001) between melanomas and benign nevi.[6]
- Sensitivity of each criterion: A 57%, B 57%, C 65%, D 90%, E 84%; Specificity of each criterion: A 72%, B 71%, C 59%, D 63%, E 90%.[6]

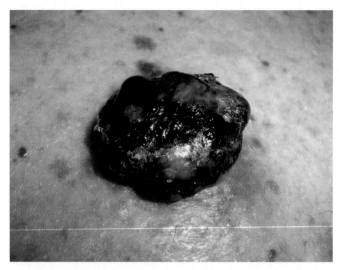

FIGURE 165-3 Close-up of the nodular melanoma showing it to be thick with ulcerations and bleeding. (*Courtesy of Richard P. Usatine, MD.*)

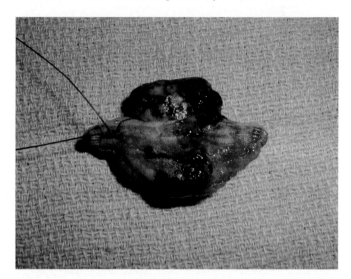

FIGURE 165-4 Nodular melanoma after initial resection showing dark pigment into the subcutaneous fat. The Breslow depth is 22 mm with Clark's level V. (*Courtesy of Richard P. Usatine, MD.*)

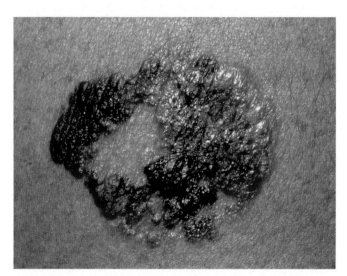

FIGURE 165-5 Superficial spreading melanoma with multiple colors and ABCDE features of melanoma. (*Courtesy of the Skin Cancer Foundation.*)

- Sensitivity of ABCDE criteria varies depending upon the number of criteria needed: using two criteria was 89.3%, with three criteria 65.5%. Specificity was 65.3% using two criteria and 81% using three.[6]

- The number of criteria present was different between benign nevi (1.24 ± 1.26) and melanomas (3.53 ± 1.53; $p < 0.001$). Unfortunately, no significant difference was found between melanomas and atypical nevi.[6]

There are four major categories of melanomas. With the exception of nodular melanoma, the growth patterns of the three other subtypes are characterized by a radial growth phase that lacks the biologic potential to metastasize and may last from months to years before dermal invasion occurs.[4] Here are the major categories of melanomas:

1. *Superficial spreading melanoma* is the most common type, representing 70% of all melanoma (**Figures 165-5** to **165-9**). This melanoma has the radial growth pattern before dermal invasion occurs. The first sign is the appearance of a flat macule or slightly raised discolored plaque that has irregular borders and is somewhat geometrical in form. The color varies, with areas of tan, brown, black, red, blue, or white. These lesions can arise in an older nevus. The melanoma can be seen almost anywhere on the body, but is most likely to occur on the trunk in men, the legs in women, and the upper back in both. Most melanomas found in the young are of the superficial spreading type.[4]

2. *Nodular melanoma* occurs in 15% to 30% of cases (**Figures 165-2** to **165-4, 165-10** and **165-11**).[4] It is usually invasive at the time it is first diagnosed, and the malignancy is recognized when it becomes a bump. The color is most often black, but occasionally is blue, gray, white, brown, tan, red, or nonpigmented. The nodule in **Figure 165-11** is multicolored.

3. *Lentigo maligna melanoma* occurs in 4% to 15% of cutaneous melanoma.[4] It is similar to the superficial spreading type and appears as a flat or mildly elevated mottled tan, brown, or dark brown discoloration. This type of melanoma is found most often in the elderly and arises on chronically sun-exposed, damaged skin on the face, ears, arms, and upper trunk. These account for most melanomas on the face. The average age of onset is 65 years and it grows slowly over 5 to 20 years. The precursor lesion, lentigo maligna, goes on to melanoma in approximately 5% of cases. The in situ precursor lesion is usually >3 cm in diameter and has existed for a minimum of 10 to 15 years (**Figures 165-12** and **165-13**) (see Chapter 161, Lentigo Maligna).[4]

4. *Acral lentiginous melanoma* is the least common subtype of melanoma (2% to 8% of melanoma cases in white people; 29% to 72% of melanoma cases in dark-skinned individuals such as African-Americans, Asians, and Hispanics.[4] It occurs under the nail plate or on the soles or palms (**Figures 165-14** to **165-17**). This subtype may be associated with a worse prognosis because of delays in diagnosis. Subungual melanoma may manifest as diffuse nail discoloration or a longitudinal pigmented band within the nail plate. When subungual pigment spreads to the proximal or lateral nail fold, it is referred to as Hutchinson's sign, and is highly suggestive of acral lentiginous melanoma (**Figure 165-16**) (see Chapter 184, Pigmented Nail Disorders).

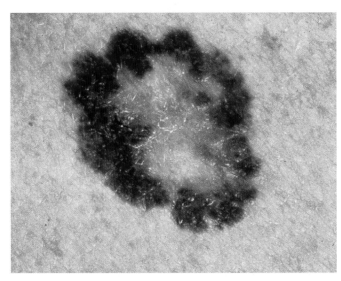

FIGURE 165-6 Superficial spreading melanoma showing area of central regression. (*Courtesy of the Skin Cancer Foundation.*)

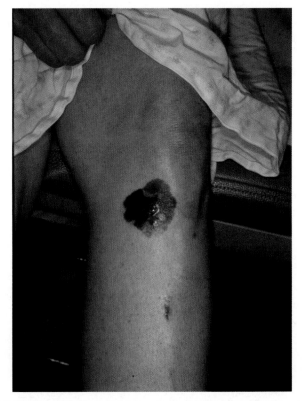

FIGURE 165-7 Large superficial spreading melanoma on the leg of a 41-year-old woman. Clark's level III, Depth 0.9 mm. (*Courtesy of Armand Cognetta, MD.*)

Less common types of melanomas include:

- *Amelanotic melanoma* (<5% of melanomas) is nonpigmented and appears pink or flesh-colored, often mimicking basal cell or squamous cell carcinoma or a ruptured hair follicle. It may be a nodular melanoma subtype or melanoma metastasis to the skin, because of the inability of these poorly differentiated cancer cells to synthesize melanin pigment (**Figures 165-18 to 165-20**).[4]

- Other rare melanoma variants include (1) desmoplastic/neurotropic melanoma, (2) mucosal (lentiginous) melanoma, (3) malignant blue nevus, and (4) melanoma arising in a giant congenital nevus.[4]

TYPICAL DISTRIBUTION

Melanoma occurs most commonly on the trunk in white males and the lower legs and back in white females. The most common site in African Americans, Hispanics, and Asians is the plantar foot, followed by the subungual, palmar, and mucosal sites.[4]

DERMOSCOPY

Dermoscopy can be used to determine if a pigmented lesion has features suspicious for a melanoma, and it can also help determine when a biopsy is needed.[7] In a prospective study of 401 lesions evaluated for melanoma by experts in dermoscopy, the sensitivity of 66.6% with ABCDE criteria improved to 80%, and specificity rose from 79.3% to 89.1% (**Figure 165-21**).[7]

In a study of dermoscopy done by 60 physicians (35 general practitioners, 10 dermatologists, and 16 dermatology trainees) on unaided photos of 40 lesions using the ABCD rule, the Menzies method, a 7-point checklist, and pattern analysis, the sensitivity rose over the unaided eye.[8] The physicians were instructed in each of the dermoscopy methods using a CD-ROM. The unaided eye using a standard photo of the lesion was 61% sensitive and 85% specific with a 73% diagnostic accuracy. The dermoscopic photo increased sensitivity (68% for pattern analysis, 77% for the ABCD rule, 81% for the 7-point checklist, and 85% for the Menzies method). The specificity did not improve. Sensitivity is more important than specificity to avoid missing melanoma. While the number of biopsies could increase with some drop in specificity, the biopsy itself is the most specific test to differentiate melanoma from benign pigmented lesions.[8]

Accepted dermoscopic local features of melanoma include:

- Atypical network (includes branched-streaks).
- Streaks: pseudopods and radial streaming.
- Atypical dots and globules.
- Negative pigment network.
- Blotch (off center).
- Blue-white veil/peppering over macular areas (regression).
- Blue-white veil over raised areas.
- Vascular structures.
- Peripheral tan/brown structureless areas.

Figure 165-21 demonstrates a number of these features. See Dermoscopy Appendix.

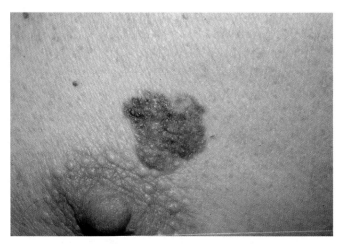

FIGURE 165-8 Superficial spreading melanoma near the areola. It is important to not mistake this for a seborrheic keratosis. Note the area of pigment regression near the top of the lesion. (*Courtesy of the University of Texas Health Sciences Center, Division of Dermatology.*)

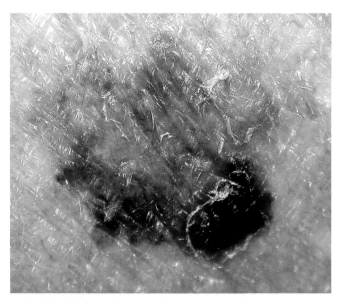

FIGURE 165-9 Superficial spreading melanoma on the arm with depth of 0.25 mm. Note the pale pink coloration along with the black area with some erosion. (*Courtesy of Eric Kraus, MD.*)

BIOPSY

A full thickness skin biopsy is the gold standard for diagnosing melanoma. A complete excisional biopsy is preferred if the lesion is small. If the lesion is too large to excise in the office, perform, an incisional biopsy, a scoop shave or a 5-mm punch biopsy, of the darkest and thickest portion. Performing a partial excision of a melanoma as the first step in the diagnosis is safe and does not increase the risk of metastasis. The initial partial excision can provide information about melanoma depth that can be used to determine the width of the margins needed to excise the full lesion (**Table 165-1**). If the pathology from a partial excision is benign and goes against your clinical impression, do a more complete biopsy or refer the patient for additional surgery.

Avoid doing a superficial shave biopsy if you suspect melanoma because important depth information can be lost. However, a broad scoop shave can often provide better tissue to the pathologist than a single punch biopsy. For suspected lentigo maligna melanoma, the risk of misdiagnosis is high if only punch biopsy specimens are taken (**Figures 165-12** and **165-13**). Some experts recommend a broad scoop shave biopsy of lentigo maligna melanoma (LMM) because a complete full thickness excision of a large suspected LMM on the face can be unnecessarily disfiguring if the ultimate diagnosis is benign.[4] SOR **C**

DIFFERENTIAL DIAGNOSIS

Nevi of all types, including congenital nevi, can mimic melanoma. Congenital nevi can be especially large and asymmetrical. Therefore, it is important to ask the patient if the pigmented area has been there from birth. Because some melanomas arise in congenital nevi, a congenital nevus that is changing needs to be biopsied to rule out melanoma.

- Dysplastic nevi, also called atypical moles, can mimic melanoma. When an atypical nevus is suspicious for melanoma, perform a full thickness biopsy or a broad scoop shave for histology. Only the less suspicious dysplastic nevi should be followed with photography or serial exams (see Chapter 158, Dysplastic/atypical Nevus).

- Seborrheic keratoses (SKs) usually look like they are stuck-on with surface cracks and a verrucous (wart-like) appearance. These are benign and not precancerous. SKs can be darkly pigmented, asymmetrical with irregular borders and have varied colors. Perform a biopsy if the diagnosis is uncertain. (Be careful to not mistake a lesion such as the one in **Figure 165-8** for a SK) (see Chapter 151, Seborrheic Keratosis).

- Solar lentigines often appear as light brown macules on the face and the dorsum of the hands. Many patients call them liver spots, but they have nothing to do with the liver. A large isolated solar lentigo on the face can mimic LMM. In this case, perform a broad scoop shave of the most suspicious area.

- Dermatofibromas are fibrotic nodules that occur most frequently on the legs and arms. They can be any color from skin color to black and often have a brown halo surrounding them. A pinch test will produce a dimpling of the skin in most cases (see Chapter 153, Dermatofibroma).

- Pigmented basal cell carcinomas (BCCs) may resemble a melanoma. However, the pigment in the BCC is often scattered

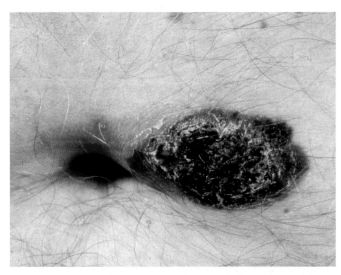

FIGURE 165-10 Nodular melanoma in the periumbilical region. This melanoma is almost entirely black. (*Courtesy of the Skin Cancer Foundation.*)

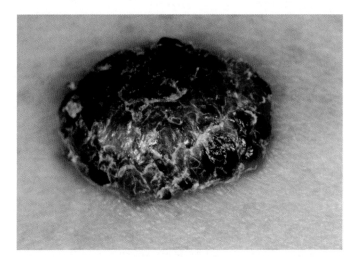

FIGURE 165-11 Raised thick nodular melanoma on the shoulder of a 37-year-old white woman with history of multiple sunburns from childhood. Note the multiple colors visible in the nodule. The Breslow depth is 8.5 mm with Clark's level V. The sentinel node was negative and the patient underwent chemotherapy after wide excision. (*Courtesy of Richard P. Usatine, MD.*)

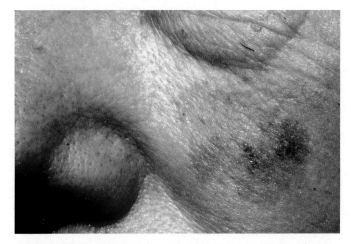

FIGURE 165-12 Lentigo malignant melanoma presenting as a large pigmented area on the face of an elderly man. (*Courtesy of the Skin Cancer Foundation.*)

throughout the lesion, and it has other features of a BCC, such as a pearly appearance with a rolled border (**Figure 165-22**) (see Chapter 163, Basal Cell Carcinoma).

MANAGEMENT

- Cutaneous melanoma is surgically treated with complete full skin depth excision using margins determined by the Breslow depth. This depth is a measure of tumor thickness from the granular layer of the epidermis to the point of deepest invasion using an ocular micrometer.

- WHO recommendations for excision margins range from 5 mm for in situ lesions to 1 to 2 cm for invasive lesions. See **Table 165-1** for a comparison of world recommendations.[9] SOR **A**

- Mohs micrographic surgery, performed by specially trained physicians, may prove useful in completely removing subclinical tumor extension in certain subtypes of melanoma in situ, such as lentigo maligna, desmoplastic melanoma, and acral lentiginous melanoma in situ.[4]

- Sentinel lymph node biopsies are recommended for tumors of greater than or equal to 1 mm in depth.[4] SOR **A** Melanomas with ulceration or areas of regression may also warrant sentinel lymph node biopsy even if the depth is less than 1 mm. A metastatic workup should be initiated if the lymph node is positive for tumor.

- Patients with advanced melanoma should be referred to a medical oncologist to consider adjuvant therapy with interferon-alpha. This may offer a small benefit in terms of recurrence-free and overall survival.[10] SOR **B**

- Little progress has been made in the medical treatment of disseminated metastasis of melanoma. Therapy with dacarbazine and a few other single agents remains the first-line treatment approach of choice. New treatment modalities, including targeted molecules and immunologic approaches with monoclonal antibodies, are under development.[10] SOR **C**

PATIENT EDUCATION

Advise patients to avoid future sun exposure and monitor their skin for new and changing moles. Recommend a complete skin examination yearly by a physician trained to detect early melanoma.

FOLLOW-UP

The need for follow-up is largely determined by the stage of the disease. The 2002 American Joint Committee on Cancer staging system is provided in **Table 165-2**. The prognosis is worsened by increasing depth, presence of ulceration, positive lymph nodes, and metastases. While Clark's levels are not used to determine surgical margins, they are used in differentiating between stage 1A and 1B disease. Patients with more advanced disease need special imaging studies and measurements of serum lactic dehydrogenase (LDH) to monitor the disease and determine medical therapies.

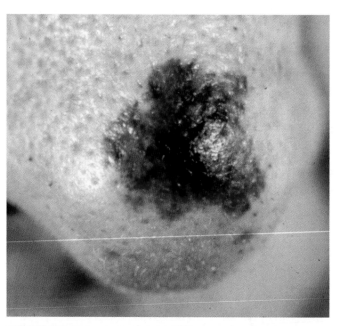

FIGURE 165-13 Lentigo maligna melanoma on the tip of the nose. (*Courtesy of the Skin Cancer Foundation.*)

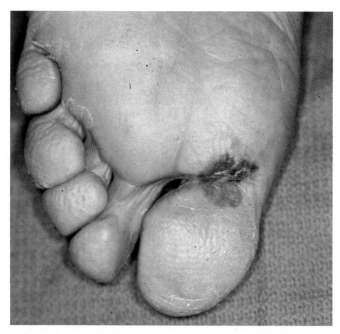

FIGURE 165-14 Acral lentiginous melanoma on the bottom of the foot where it went undetected for years. (*Courtesy of the University of Texas Health Sciences Center, Division of Dermatology.*)

The follow-up for stage 0 and 1 cutaneous melanoma is regular skin examinations by the patient and physician. The rate of subsequent cutaneous melanomas among persons with a history of melanoma was found to be more than 10 times the rate of a first cutaneous melanoma.[11]

PATIENT RESOURCES

Medline Plus—**http://www.nlm.nih.gov/medlineplus/melanoma.html** (Accessed August 14, 2007).

PROVIDER RESOURCES

The Skin Cancer Foundation—**http://www.skincancer.org** (Accessed August 14, 2007).

National Cancer Institute—**http://www.cancer.gov/cancertopics/types/melanoma** (Accessed August 14, 2007).

Dermoscopy—**www.dermoscopy.org/** A web site on dermoscopy to learn how to improve early diagnosis of melanoma. (Accessed August 14, 2007).

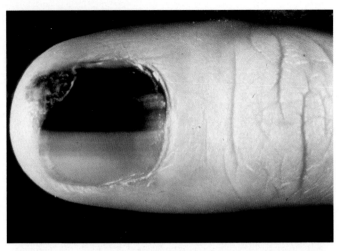

FIGURE 165-15 Subungual melanoma in a white man showing hyperpigmentation of the nail and nail bed. (*Courtesy of the Skin Cancer Foundation.*)

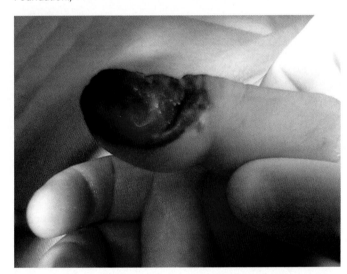

FIGURE 165-16 Acral lentiginous melanoma that started after trauma to the thumb which led to a delay in diagnosis. (*From the Journal of Family Practice, Dowden Health Media and Adam Leight, MD.*)

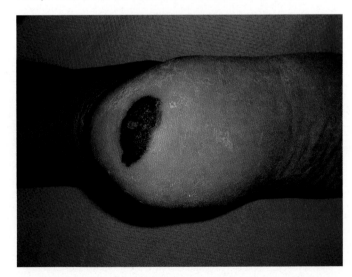

FIGURE 165-17 Nodular and acral lentiginous melanoma of the foot in a 30-year-old black woman. There is ulceration and the depth was 5.5 mm. Sentinel node biopsy was positive for 2 out of 2 nodes sampled. Clarke's level IV and Stage IIIC (pT4b N2a MO). (*Courtesy of Richard P. Usatine, MD.*)

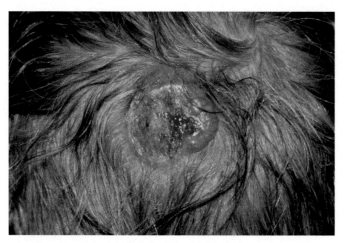

FIGURE 165-18 Amelanotic melanoma that looks like a large basal cell carcinoma (BCC) on the scalp. (*Courtesy of the University of Texas Health Sciences Center, Division of Dermatology.*)

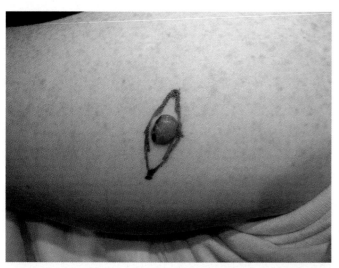

FIGURE 165-19 Amelanotic melanoma on the arm of a young woman prior to elliptical excision. The diagnosis was unexpected and shows the importance of excising suspicious lesions even when they are not pigmented. (*Courtesy of E.J. Mayeaux, Jr., MD.*)

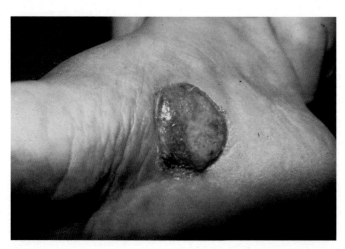

FIGURE 165-20 Amelanotic melanoma on the medial side of the foot presenting as a nonhealing lesion of unknown etiology. (*Courtesy of the University of Texas Health Sciences Center, Division of Dermatology.*)

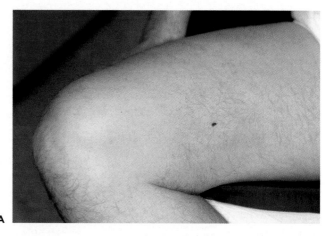

A

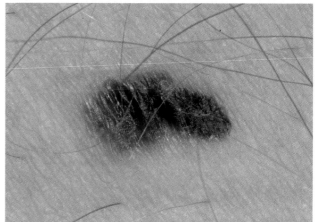

B

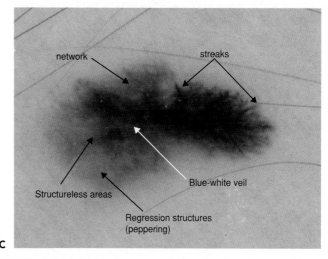

C

FIGURE 165-21 (A) A melanoma on the leg that could be missed because of its small size (7-mm long). (B) Close-up of that melanoma showing the asymmetry, irregular borders and a variation in color. (C) Dermoscopy of a melanoma showing a blue-white veil, radial streaks, pigment network, structureless areas and regression structures with peppering. This early superficial-spreading melanoma was proven to be 0.55 mm at the time of excision. (*Courtesy of Ashfaq Marghoob, MD.*)

TABLE 165-1 Currently Recommended Excision Margins for Primary Melanoma[8]

Tumor Thickness	Excision Margin			
	UK MSG	WHO	Australian	Dutch MSG
In situ	2–5 mm	5 mm	5 mm	2 mm
<1 mm	1 cm	1 cm	1 cm	1 cm
1–2 mm	1–2 cm	1 cm*	1 cm	1 cm
2.1–4 mm	2–3 cm (2 cm preferred)	2 cm	1 cm	2 cm
>4 mm	2–3 cm	2 cm	2 cm	2 cm

*For melanomas thicker than 1.5 mm, recommended excision margin is 2 cm.
MSG, Melanoma Study Group; WHO, World Health Organization.
With permission from Lens MB, et al. Excision margins in the treatment of primary cutaneous melanoma: A systematic review of randomized controlled trials comparing narrow versus wide excision. *Arch Surg.* 2002;137:1101–1105.

REFERENCES

1. Jemal A, Siegel R, Ward E, Murray T, Xu J, Thun MJ. Cancer statistics, 2007. *CA Cancer J Clin.* 2007;57:43–66.

2. Jemal A, Murray T, Ward E, et al. Cancer statistics, 2005. *CA Cancer J Clin.* 2005;55:10–30.

3. Welch HG, Woloshin S, Schwartz LM. Skin biopsy rates and incidence of melanoma: population based ecological study. *BMJ.* 2005;331:481.

4. Swetter S. Malignant Melanoma. http://www.emedicine.com/derm/topic257.htm. Updated March 18, 2006. Accessed March 29, 2007.

5. Oliveria SA, Saraiya M, Geller AC, Heneghan MK, Jorgensen C. Sun exposure and risk of melanoma. *Arch Dis Child.* 2006;91:131–138.

6. Thomas L. Semiological value of ABCDE criteria in the diagnosis of cutaneous pigmented tumors. *Dermatology.* 1998;197:11–17.

7. Benelli C. The dermoscopic versus the clinical diagnosis of melanoma. *Eur J Dermatol.* 1999;9:470–476.

8. Dolianitis C, Kelly J, Wolfe R, Simpson P. Comparative Performance of 4 Dermoscopic Algorithms by Nonexperts for the Diagnosis of Melanocytic Lesions. *Arch Dermatol.* 2005;141:1008–1014.

9. Lens MB, Dawes M, Goodacre T, Bishop JAN. Excision margins in the treatment of primary cutaneous melanoma: A systematic review of randomized controlled trials comparing narrow vs wide excision. *Arch Surg.* 2002;137:1101–1105.

10. Garbe C, Eigentler TK. Diagnosis and treatment of cutaneous melanoma: State of the art 2006. *Melanoma Res.* 2007;17:117–127.

11. Tsao H, Atkins MB, Sober AJ. Management of cutaneous melanoma. *N Engl J Med.* 2004;351:998–1012.

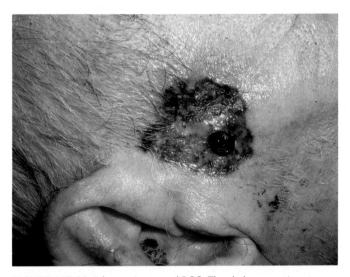

FIGURE 165-22 A large pigmented BCC. The darkest spot is an area healing from a punch biopsy. The pearly surface and spotty color tend to suggest a BCC rather than a melanoma. (*Courtesy of Richard P. Usatine, MD.*)

TABLE 165-2 Revised Melanoma Staging

Stage	TNM Classification	Histologic/Clinical Features	5-Year Survival Rate, %
0	Tis N0 M0	Intraepithelial/in situ melanoma	100
IA	T1a N0 M0	≤1 mm without ulceration and level II/III	≥95
IB	T1b N0 M0 T2a N0 M0	≤1 mm with ulceration or level IV/V 1.01–2 mm without ulceration	89–91
IIA	T2b N0 M0 T3a N0 M0	1.01–2 mm with ulceration 2.01–4 mm without ulceration	77–79
IIB	T3b N0 M0 T4a N0 M0	2.01–4 mm with ulceration >4 mm without ulceration	63–67
IIC	T4b N0 M0	>4 mm with ulceration	45
IIIA	T1–4a N1a M0 T1–4a N2a M0	Single regional nodal micrometastasis, nonulcerated primary 2–3 microscopic positive regional nodes, nonulcerated primary	63–69
IIIB	T1–4bN1a M0 T1–4bN2a M0 T1–4a N1b M0 T1–4a N2b M0 T1–4a/b N2c M0	Single regional nodal micrometastasis, ulcerated primary 2–3 microscopic regional nodes, nonulcerated primary*	46–53 30–50
IIIC	T1–4b N2a M0 T1–4b N2b M0 Any T N3 M0	Single macroscopic regional node, ulcerated primary 2–3 macroscopic metastatic regional nodes, ulcerated primary 4 or more metastatic nodes*	24–29
IV	Any T any N M1a Any T any N M1b Any T any N M1c	Distant skin, subcutaneous, or nodal metastasis with normal LDH levels Lung metastasis with normal LDH	7–19

*Shortened for space considerations
With permission from Swetter S. Malignant Melanoma. http://www.emedicine.com/derm/topic257.htm. Updated March 18, 2006. Accessed March 29, 2007.

SECTION 13 INFILTRATIVE IMMUNOLOGIC

166 GRANULOMA ANNULARE

Melissa Muszynski
Richard P. Usatine, MD

PATIENT STORY

A 39-year-old woman presents with raised rings on her right hand only. Not knowing the correct diagnosis, another physician prescribed topical steroids and antifungal medicines with no benefit. The diagnosis of granuloma annulare (GA) was made by the typical clinical appearance and the patient was offered intralesional steroids. Triamcinolone acetonide was injected as seen in **Figure 166-1**. The patient noted improvement over the subsequent weeks, but within a month new lesions began to appear on her other hand (**Figure 166-2**). Additional injections were provided and 1 month later the patient had regression of the treated lesions but had new lesions on the right arm (**Figure 166-3**). At the next visit patient had new lesions on her feet as well (**Figure 166-4**). The diagnosis of disseminated GA was made and systemic treatment was started.

EPIDEMIOLOGY

- GA affects twice as many women as men.[1]
- Four presentations of GA are localized, disseminated/generalized, perforating, and subcutaneous.
- Of the four variations, the localized form is seen most often.[1]

ETIOLOGY AND PATHOPHYSIOLOGY

- Benign cutaneous, inflammatory disorder of unknown origin.[1]
- Disease may be self-limiting, but may persist for many years.
- GA has been reported to follow trauma, malignancy, and viral infections (including human immunodeficiency).[2]
- One proposed mechanism for GA is a delayed-type hypersensitivity reaction as a result of Th-1 lymphocytic differentiation of macrophages. These macrophages become effector cells that express TNF-α and matrix metalloproteinases. The activated macrophages are responsible for dermal collagen matrix degradation.[3]
- An association between high expression of gil-1 oncogene and granulomatous lesions of the skin, including GA, has recently been established.[4]

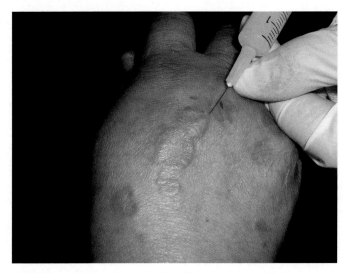

FIGURE 166-1 Granuloma annulare (GA) in a 42-year-old woman. Intralesional steroids were administered on the first visit with resolution of the injected lesions. (*Courtesy of Richard P. Usatine, MD.*)

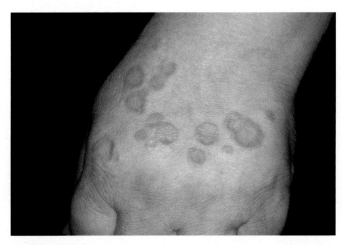

FIGURE 166-2 The patient in **Figure 116-3** 3 months later with new annular lesions on the opposite hand. She requested additional injections. (*Courtesy of Richard P. Usatine, MD.*)

DIAGNOSIS

CLINICAL FEATURES

Annular lesions have raised borders that are skin-colored to erythematous (**Figures 166-1** to **166-4**). The rings may become hyperpigmented as seen in **Figure 166-4**. There is often a central depression within the ring. These lesions range from 2 mm to 5 cm. Although the classical appearance of GA is annular, the rings may not always be complete (**Figure 166-5**). Most importantly, there should be no scaling as seen in tinea corporis (ringworm).

TYPICAL DISTRIBUTION

Each of the four types of GA has a different distribution. Localized and disseminated GA differ only in that disseminated lesions can spread to trunk and neck and may be more pronounced in sun-exposed areas.[5]

Localized—This is the most common form of GA affecting 75% of GA patients.[1] It typically presents on the dorsal surfaces of extremities, especially of hands and feet (**Figure 166-6**).

Disseminated or generalized—Adults are most affected by this form which begins in the extremities and can spread to the trunk and neck (**Figures 166-2** to **166-4**).

Perforating—Children and young adults present with one to hundreds of 1 to 4 mm annular papules that may coalesce to form a typical annular plaque. Although this form can appear anywhere on the body, it has an affinity for extremities especially the hands and fingers.[6] The papules may exude a thick and creamy or clear and viscous fluid.

Subcutaneous—These lesions present as rapidly growing, nonpainful, subcutaneous or dermal nodules on the extremities, scalp, and forehead. Subcutaneous GA mainly affects children with a mean age of 3.9 years (**Figures 166-7** and **166-8**).[5] The lesions are deeper so more swelling is seen with less surface definition.

LABORATORY STUDIES

Often a diagnosis of GA is made on clinical presentation alone, without the need for biopsy. Subcutaneous GA may be an exception because of its unusual appearance. Histologic examination reveals localized degeneration of collagen in the dermis surrounded by granulomatous inflammation. There are no signs of epidermal damage.[1,2]

DIFFERENTIAL DIAGNOSIS

- Tinea corporis has a raised, scaling border and can present on any body surface. KOH preparation reveals hyphae with multiple branches (see Chapter 132, Tinea Corporis).

- Erythema annulare centrifugum has an affinity for thighs and legs. The diameter of these lesions can expand at a rate of 2 to 5 mm/d and may present with a trailing scale inside the advancing border.[2] Biopsy is helpful to differentiate this condition from GA (see Chapter 199, Erythema Annulare Centrifugum).

- Nummular eczema presents commonly on extremities, but is almost always associated with scaling plaques and intense itching (see Chapter 141, Hand Eczema).

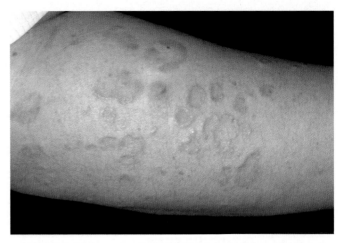

FIGURE 166-3 The patient in **Figure 166-1** 1 month later with new crops of lesions on the arms and feet. She has disseminated GA. Note the central area of hypopigmentation secondary to a previous steroid intralesional steroid injection. (*Courtesy of Richard P. Usatine, MD.*)

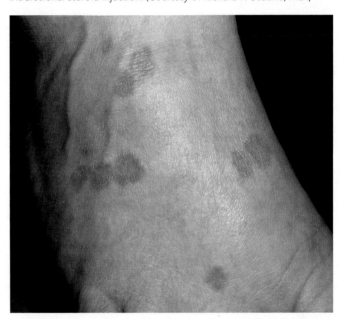

FIGURE 166-4 Disseminated GA on the foot of the patient in **Figure 166-1**. The rings are flatter and many are conjoined. (*Courtesy of Richard P. Usatine, MD.*)

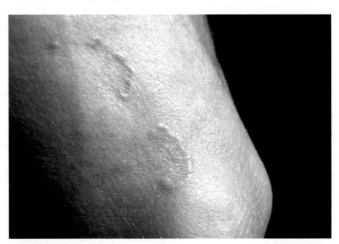

FIGURE 166-5 GA on the elbow showing how the rings may not be complete. This patient is in her fifties and has had new crops of lesions over the past 10 years. (*Courtesy of Richard P. Usatine, MD.*)

- Pityriasis rosea often has annular lesions with collarette scale. The lesions are flatter and have scale that is absent in GA (see Chapter 146, Pityriasis Rosea).

- Rheumatoid nodules may mimic appearance of subcutaneous GA. These nodules are often seen over the elbows, fingers, and other joints in a patient with joint pains and other clinical signs of arthritis (see Chapter 92, Rheumatoid Arthritis).

MANAGEMENT

The evidence for various treatments is at best small series of cases that are not randomized controlled trials. This disease is asymptomatic, and treatments only improve cosmetic appearance. Often the best solution may be letting the lesions resolve without intervention. Although several treatments below have shown promise, these treatments may appear to work when in fact the resolution was natural.

Localized GA:

- In a retrospective study of children with localized GA (mean age 8.6 years), 39 of 42 presented with complete clearance within 2 years. The average duration was 1 year. Researchers of this study consider most treatments unnecessary because of the self-limiting nature of this variation.[7] One treatment option is watchful waiting.[7] SOR **B**

- Intralesional corticosteroids can be injected into GA lesions with resolution of the area injected (**Figure 163-1**). Inject directly into the ring itself with 3 to 5 mg/cc triamcinolone acetonide (Kenalog) using a 27-gauge needle. SOR **C** A completed ring may take four injections to reach 360 degrees of the circle. The major complications include hypopigmentation (**Figure 166-3**) and skin atrophy at the injected sites.

- Cryotherapy was studied using nitrous oxide for nine patients and liquid nitrogen for 22 patients. The results showed 80% clearing after a single freeze; however, 4 of 19 patients treated with liquid nitrogen developed atrophic scars when lesions were larger than 4 cm. All patients developed blisters.[8] Cryoatrophy may possibly be prevented by avoiding freeze thaw cycles greater than 10 seconds and not overlapping treatment areas.[9] SOR **C**

Generalized/disseminated GA:

- This variant is more difficult to treat, and often has a longer duration than localized GA. Many treatments have been claimed to be effective, but the studies touting these treatments have small sample sizes and were not randomized.

- Successful treatment of six patients with GA was achieved with 100 mg of Dapsone, once a day. Complete clearance in all patients took between 4 weeks and 3 months.[10] SOR **C**

- UVA1 phototherapy provided good or excellent results in half of 20 patients with disseminated GA. In patients with only a satisfactory treatment response, the disease reappeared soon after phototherapy was discontinued.[11] SOR **C**

- In a study of four patients, topical 5% imiquimod cream was effective when used once daily for an average of 2 months. After discontinuing treatment, three patients went an average of 12 months

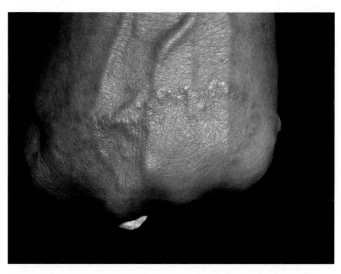

FIGURE 166-6 One single large irregular annular lesion of GA. This ring is also not complete. (*Courtesy of Richard P. Usatine, MD.*)

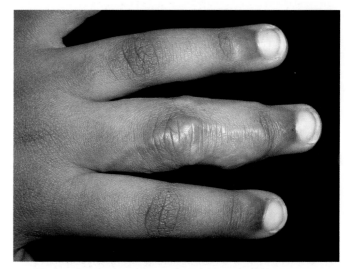

FIGURE 166-7 Subcutaneous GA in a 7-year-old girl showing one large ring on the dorsum of the finger with soft tissue infiltration. (*Courtesy of Richard P. Usatine, MD.*)

without recurrence; the fourth patient had remission 10 days after treatment stopped, but after an additional 6 weeks of applying cream once daily, he was lesion-free for 18 months.[12] SOR Ⓒ

- Four patients were treated with twice daily topical application of 0.1% tacrolimus ointment for 6 weeks; all reported improvement after 10 to 21 days. At treatment conclusion, two patients had complete clearance and the other two had marked improvement.[13] SOR Ⓒ

- Treatment with 0.5 to 1 mg/kg of isotretinoin daily has produced some positive results across multiple small studies; however because of the potential for adverse effects, this option should be reserved for very severe, nonresponsive cases.[14] SOR Ⓒ

- Three patients were treated with vitamin E 400 IU daily and zileuton 2400 mg daily. All responded within 3 months with complete clinical clearing.[15] SOR Ⓒ

Perforating, Subcutaneous:

- While we could find no specific data to inform the treatment of these less common types of GA, treatments for both localized and disseminated GA could be applied based on clinical judgement along with patient's severity and preferences.

PATIENT EDUCATION

It is important to reassure patients that this disease is self-limiting. Despite a displeasing appearance, the best treatment may be to let lesions resolve naturally. Numerous individual case studies and treatments have been attempted without consistent success. Treatments may produce side effects that are equally as unwanted, but more permanent, than the GA.

FOLLOW-UP

Follow-up visits should be offered to patients who want active treatment.

PATIENT RESOURCES

VisualDxHealth—**http://www.visualdxhealth.com/adult/granulomaAnnulare.htm.**

PROVIDER RESOURCES

http://www.emedicine.com/DERM/topic169.htm.

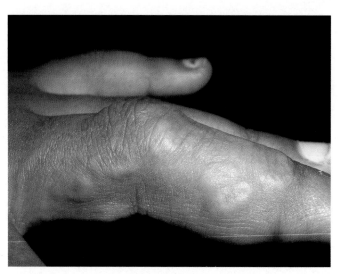

FIGURE 166-8 Subcutaneous GA in a 7-year-old girl showing thickening of the involved finger along with the small annular patterns. Note the soft tissue infiltration that has distorted the finger anatomy. (*Courtesy of Richard P. Usatine, MD.*)

REFERENCES

1. Cyr PR. Diagnosis and management of granuloma annulare. *Am Fam Physician*. 2006;74(10):1729–1734.

2. Ghadially R, Garg A. Granuloma annulare. http://www.emedicine.com/DERM/topic169.htm. Accessed June 28, 2007.

3. Fayyazi A, Schweyer S, Eichmeyer B, et al. Expression of IFNgamma, coexpression of TNF-alpha and matrix metalloproteinases and apoptosis of T lymphocytes and macrophages in granuloma annulare. *Arch Dermatol Res*. 2000;292:384–390.

4. Macaron NC, Cohen C, Chen SC, Arbiser JL. gli-1 Oncogene is highly expressed in granulomatous skin disorders, including sarcoidosis, granuloma annulare, and necrobiosis lipoidica diabeticorum. *Arch Dermatol*. 2005;141:259–262.

5. Habif TP. *Clinical Dermatology*. 4th ed. St Louis: Mosby, 2004.

6. Smith MD, Downie JB, DiCostanzo D. Granuloma annulare. *Int J Dermatol*. 1997;36:326–333.

7. Martinón-Torres F, Martinón-Sánchez JM, Martinón-Sánchez F. Localized granuloma annulare in children: A review of 42 cases. *Eur J Pediatr*. 1999;158(10):866

8. Blume-Peytavi U, Zouboulis CC, Jacobi H, et al. Successful outcome of cryosurgery in patients with granuloma annulare. *Br J Dermatol*. 1994;130(4):494–497.

9. Lebwohl MG, Berth-Jones M, Coulson I. *Treatment of Skin Disease, Comprehensive Theraperutic Strategies*, 2nd ed. St. Louis: Mosby, 2006: 251.

10. Czarnecki DB, Gin D. The response of generalized granuloma annulare to Dapsone. *Acta Derm Venereol (stockh)*. 1986;66:82–84.

11. Schnopp C, Tzaneva S, Mempel M, Schulmeister K, Abeck D, Tanew A. UVA1 phototherapy for disseminated granuloma annulare. *Photodermatol Photoimmunol Photomed*. 2005;:21(2):68–71.

12. Badavanis G, Monastirli A, Pasmatzi E, Tsambaos D. Successful treatment of granuloma annulare with imiquimod cream 5%: A report of four cases. *Acta Derm Venereol*. 2005;85(6):547–548

13. Jain S, Stephens. Successful treatment of disseminated granuloma annulare with topical tacrolimus. *Br J Dermatol*. 2004;150:1042–1043

14. Looney M. Isotretinoin in the treatment of granuloma annulare. *Ann Pharmacother*. 2004;38(3):494–497.

15. Smith KJ, Norwood C, Skelton H. Treatment of disseminated granuloma annulare with a 5-lipoxygenase inhibitor and vitamin E. *Br J Dermatol*. 2002;146(4):667–670.

167 PYODERMA GANGRENOSUM

Damian Flowers, MD
Richard P. Usatine, MD

PATIENT STORY

A 35-year-old woman was diagnosed with Crohn's disease 10 years prior to her visit for this nonhealing leg ulcer. The patient experienced minor trauma to her leg 2 years ago and this ulcer developed (pathergy). Multiple treatments have been tried and the ulcer persists (**Figures 167-1** and **167-2**).

EPIDEMIOLOGY

- Pyoderma gangrenosum (PG) occurs in about 1 person per 100,000 people each year.[1]
- No racial predilection is apparent.
- A slight female predominance may exist.
- Predominately occurs in fourth and fifth decade, but all ages may be affected.

ETIOLOGY AND PATHOPHYSIOLOGY

- Etiology is poorly understood.
- Pathergy (initiation at the site of trauma or injury) is a common process and it is estimated that 30% of patients with PG experienced pathergy.[1]
- Up to 50% of cases are idiopathic.[2]
- At least 50% of cases are associated with systemic diseases such as inflammatory bowel disease, hematologic malignancy, and arthritis.[2]
- Biopsies usually show a polymorphonuclear cell infiltrate with features of ulceration, infarction, and abscess formation.

DIAGNOSIS

CLINICAL FEATURES

Typically PG presents with deep painful ulcer with a well-defined border, which is usually violet or blue. The ulcer edge is often undermined and the surrounding skin is erythematous and indurated. Usually starts as small papules which coalesce and the central area then undergoes necrosis to form a single ulcer.[3]

The lesions are painful and the pain can be severe.[2] Patients may have malaise, arthralgia, and myalgia.

- Two main variants of PG exist: classic and atypical.[2]
  - Classic PG is characterized by a deep ulceration with a violaceous border that overhangs the ulcer bed.[2] These lesions of PG most

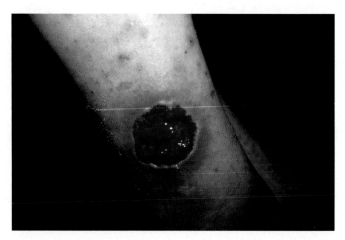

FIGURE 167-1 Classic Pyoderma gangrenosum (PG) on the leg of a 35-year-old woman with Crohn's disease. This ulcer started with minor trauma (pathergy) and has been there for 2 years. (*Courtesy of Richard P. Usatine, MD.*)

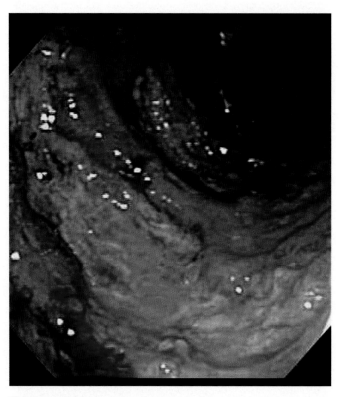

FIGURE 167-2 Friable inflamed mucosa of the colon in Crohn's disease. (*Courtesy of Shashi Mittal, MD.*)

commonly occur on the legs[2] (**Figures 167-1** and **167-3** to **167-5**).

 ○ Atypical PG has a vesiculopustular "juicy" component (**Figures 167-6** to **167-8**). This is usually only at the border, is erosive or superficially ulcerated, and most often occurs on the dorsal surface of the hands, the extensor parts of the forearms, or the face.[2]

• Other variants:

 ○ Peristomal PG may occur around stoma sites. This form is often mistaken for a wound infection or irritation from the appliance.[2]

 ○ Vulvar or penile PG occurs on the genitalia and must be differentiated from ulcerative sexually transmitted diseases (STDs) such as chancroid and syphilis.[2]

 ○ Intraoral PG is known as pyostomatitis vegetans. Occurs primarily in patients with inflammatory bowel disease.[2]

TYPICAL DISTRIBUTION

Most commonly seen on the legs and hands, but can occur on any skin surface including the genitalia, and around a stoma.

LABORATORY STUDIES

CBC, UA, and LFTs should be obtained. Order a hepatitis profile to rule out hepatitis.[2] Systemic disease markers may be elevated if associated conditions exist i.e., ESR and rheumatoid factor. Obtain RPR, protein electrophoresis, and skin cultures as indicated. Consider culturing the ulcer/erosion for bacteria, fungi, atypical mycobacteria, and viruses.[2]

 Biopsy an active area of disease along with the border. A punch biopsy is preferred. While there are not specific pathological signs of PG, the biopsy can be used to rule out other causes of ulcerative skin lesions. The pathologist may be able to confirm your clinical impression.

 If GI symptoms exist, perform or refer for colonoscopy to look for inflammatory bowel disease.

DIFFERENTIAL DIAGNOSIS

PG is sometimes a diagnosis of exclusion diagnosed with successful wound healing following immunosuppressant therapy.[4] When misdiagnosed it is often confused for vascular occlusive or venous disease, vasculitis, cancer, primary infection, drug-induced or exogenous tissue injury, and other inflammatory disorders.[5] Biopsy of a questionable lesion may be the only way to ultimately distinguish PG as the cause of ulcerative skin lesions.

• Ulcerative STDs such as chancroid and syphilis can resemble vulvar or penile PG. These STDs are more common than PG and should be diagnosed with appropriate tests including RPR and bacterial culture for *hemophilus ducreyi*. If these tests are negative, then PG should be considered. RPR should also be repeated in 2 weeks if it is initially negative at the start of a chancre—it takes some weeks to become positive and syphilis is so easily treatable (see Chapter 209, Syphilis).

• Acute febrile neutrophilic dermatosis (Sweet's syndrome) is a neutrophilic dermatosis like PG but the patients are generally febrile

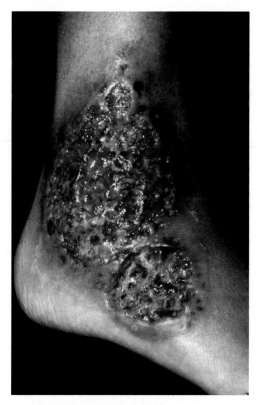

FIGURE 167-3 PG showing dusky red border with undermined edges. The surface appears purulent and necrotic. (*Courtesy of Jack Resneck, Sr., MD.*)

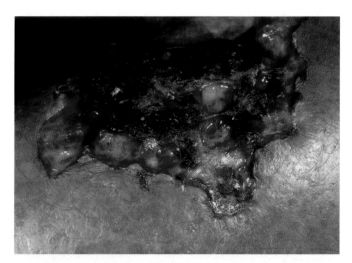

FIGURE 167-4 PG ulcer on the leg with purulent undermined edges and black eschar. (*Courtesy of Jeff Meffert, MD.*)

with systemic symptoms (**Figure 167-9**). The diagnosis of Sweet's syndrome is made when the patient fulfills two of two major criteria and two of four minor criteria. The two major criteria are (a) an abrupt onset of tender or painful erythematous plaques or nodules occasionally with vesicles, pustules, or bullae and (b) predominantly neutrophilic infiltration in the dermis without leukocytoclastic vasculitis. Minor criteria include specific preceding or concurrent medical conditions, fever, abnormal lab values including leukocytosis and an elevated sedimentation rate and a rapid response to systemic steroids.

- Systemic vasculitis is perhaps the most difficult to differentiate, but history of minor trauma in the area preceding lesion formation (pathergy) and undermining of the violaceous border should lead one toward the diagnosis of PG.[5]

- Ecthyma is a type of impetigo in which ulcers form. Bacterial cultures will be positive and this disease should respond to cephalexin or other oral antibiotics (see Chapter 110, Impetigo).

- Spider bites from the black recluse spider can easily resemble PG when they ulcerate. The history of a spider bite can help differentiate this from PG.

- Sporotrichosis is a fungal infection that often starts from an injury while gardening with roses. It is usually on the arm or hand and can resemble PG. Use fungal culture to diagnose this when the history suggests this as the diagnosis. Oral antifungal medications can treat this (**Figure 167-10**).

- Squamous cell carcinoma with ulcerations may look like PG. Its diagnosis requires a biopsy. If the ulcer is on sun-exposed area, squamous cell carcinoma should be considered. A shave or punch biopsy can be used to diagnose this malignancy (see Chapter 164, Squamous Cell Carcinoma).

- Venous insufficiency ulcers are typically seen around the medial malleolus and the most severe of these ulcers resembles PG. The presence of signs and symptoms of venous insufficiency should help differentiate this from PG (see Chapter 50, Venous Insufficiency).

- Mycosis fungoides is a cutaneous T-cell lymphoma that can ulcerate and resemble PG. Use tissue biopsy to differentiate these two conditions (see Chapter 169, Mycosis Fungoides).

MANAGEMENT

Patients frequently are in pain from the lesions and so treatment is aimed at pain relief as well as healing the skin lesions.

- Topical medications are first-line therapy in cases of localized PG that is not severe: Start with potent corticosteroid ointments or tacrolimus ointment.[6] SOR **B**

- Small ulcers can be managed with topical steroid creams, silver sulfadiazine, or potassium iodide solution. SOR **C**

- Intralesional injections with corticosteroids are one option.[6] SOR **B**

- Systemic treatment with oral corticosteroids (e.g., methylprednisolone or prednisone 0.5–1 mg/kg/d) or oral cyclosporine (e.g., 5 mg/kg/d) alone or together appears to be effective (in the absence of controlled trials) in many cases and should be considered first-line therapy.[6] SOR **B** Response is usually rapid, with stabilization of the PG within 24 hours.[7]

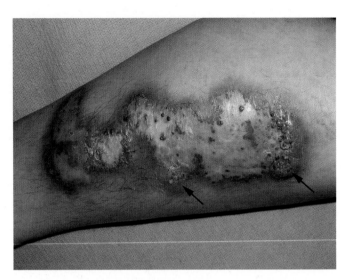

FIGURE 167-5 Partially healed PG on the leg of a 29-year-old Hispanic woman. Note the areas of healed ulcerations and the dusky elevated borders. There remain two areas of active disease (arrows) with pain, erythema, swelling, and purulent discharge. The patient improved with dapsone. (*Courtesy of Richard P. Usatine, MD.*)

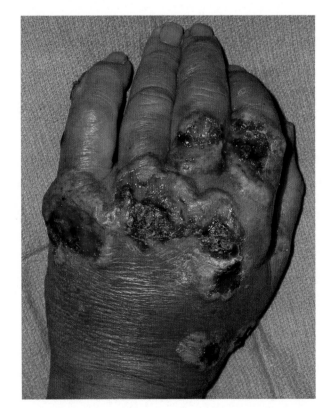

FIGURE 167-6 Atypical PG with a vesiculopustular "juicy" component on the dorsal surface of the hand. Bulla were previously present before the ulcerations developed. (*Courtesy of Eric Kraus, MD.*)

- Systemic treatment with corticosteroids in pulsed doses (e.g., methylprednisolone 1 g/d for 1–5 days) can be used as an alternate regimen to induce remission.[7] SOR **B**

- In steroid-refractory PG associated with inflammatory bowel disease, immunomodulatory therapy and biological response modifiers are promising.[6] SOR **C**

- To date, case reports have been published that show therapeutic efficacy of mycophenolate mofetil, oral tacrolimus, dapsone, azathioprine, and infliximab.[6] SOR **C**

- Surgical debridement is contraindicated since pathergy occurs in 25% to 50% of cases and surgery will make the lesions worse. SOR **B**

PATIENT EDUCATION

- PG is a rare ulcerative skin condition that is poorly understood.

- A skin biopsy is needed to rule out other diagnoses.

- Most treatments are empirical and based on small studies.

- The risks and benefits of steroids and/or other immunosuppressive medications needs to be explained.

FOLLOW-UP

All patients suspected of having PG need close and frequent follow-up to obtain a definitive diagnosis and treat this challenging condition. In many cases referral to a dermatologist will be needed.

PATIENT RESOURCES

American Autoimmune Related Diseases Association, Inc. Tel: (800)598–4668—**http://www.aarda.org/.**

Crohn's and Colitis Foundation of America Tel: 8009322423—**http://www.ccfa.org.**

PROVIDER RESOURCES

eMedicine—**http://www.emedicine.com/ DERM/topic367.htm.**

NIH/National Arthritis and Musculoskeletal and Skin Diseases Information Clearinghouse—**http://www.niams.nih.gov.**

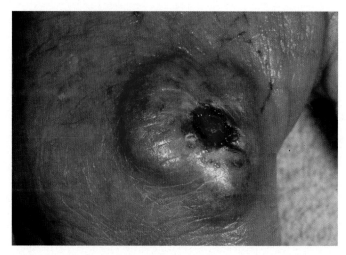

FIGURE 167-7 PG rapidly progressing with suppurative border and central ulceration over the first MCP joint following minor trauma. (*Courtesy of Jeff Meffert, MD.*)

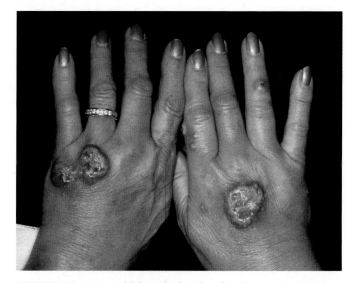

FIGURE 167-8 Atypical PG on the hands with violaceous borders that match the fingernail color. The lesions are "juicy" and resemble those seen in Sweet's syndrome and have occurred at sites of minor (pathergy). (*Courtesy of Jeff Meffert, MD.*)

REFERENCES

1. Brooklyn T, Brooklyn T, Dunnill G, Probert C. Diagnosis and treatment of pyoderma gangrenosum. *BMJ*. 2006;333(7560): 181–184.

2. Jackson JM, Callen JP. eMedicine. Pyoderma gangrenosum. http://www.emedicine.com/DERM/topic367.htm. Accessed on June 30, 2007.

3. Habif T. *Clinical dermatology*. 4th ed. Philadelphia: Mosby, 2004: 653–654.

4. Banga F, Schuitemaker N, Meijer P. Pyoderma gangrenosum after caesarean section: A case report. *Reprod Health*. 2006;3:9.

5. Weenig RH, Davis MD, Dahl PR, Su WP. Skin ulcers misdiagnoised as pyoderma gangrenosum. *N Engl J Med*. 2002;347(18):1412–1418.

6. Reichrath J, Bens G, Bonowitz A, Tilgen W. Treatment recommendations for pyoderma gangrenosum: An evidence-based review of the literature based on more than 350 patients. *J Am Acad Dermatol*. 2005;53(2):273–283.

7. Chow RK, Ho VC. Treatment of pyoderma gangrenosum. *J Am Acad Dermatol*. 1996;34:1047–1060.

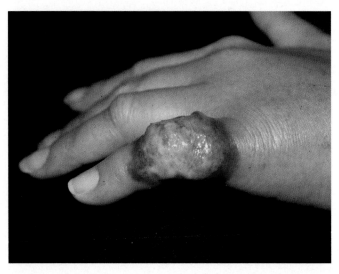

FIGURE 167-9 Sweet's syndrome is the eponym for acute febrile neutrophilic dermatosis. The lesion looks like PG and occurs at sites of minor trauma (pathergy). However, this patient has a fever and is systemically ill. (*Courtesy of John Gonzalez, MD.*)

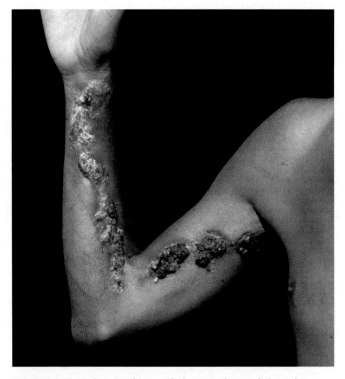

FIGURE 167-10 Sporotrichosis with the typical spread along the arm. (*Courtesy of Eric Kraus, MD.*)

168 SARCOIDOSIS

Khashayar Sarabi, MD
Amor Khachemoune, MD

PATIENT STORY

A 42-year-old man presents with "multiple bumps" that had been growing on his scalp, the back of the neck, and on area of previous scars (**Figure 168-1**). These lesions started developing slowly over a period of 1 year. The differential diagnosis of these lesions included cutaneous sarcoidosis, acne keloidalis nuchae and pseudofolliculitis barbae. A punch biopsy was performed and the diagnosis of sarcoidosis was made.

EPIDEMIOLOGY

- Cutaneous manifestations occur in approximately 25% of systemic sarcoidosis patients.

- Patients with sarcoid-like lesions in the skin, without systemic disease, are in ratio of one to three compared to patients with multisystem involvement.

- Specific cutaneous involvement is seen most commonly in older, female patients of African descent (**Figures 168-2 to 168-3**).

- Common types are maculopapular, lupus pernio, cutaneous, or subcutaneous nodules, and infiltrative scars.

- Nonspecific—most common lesion is erythema nodosum (EN) occurring in 3% to 34% of patients (see Chapter 171, Erythema Nodosum).

- Sarcoidosis related EN is more prevalent in whites, especially Scandinavians. Irish and Puerto Rican females are also affected more often.

- EN occurs between second and fourth decades of life with more occurrences in women than in men.

- Nonspecific lesions of sarcoidosis reported, besides EN, include erythema multiforme, pruritus, calcinosis cutis, prurigo, and lymphedema. Nail changes can include clubbing, onycholysis, subungual keratosis, and dystrophy, with or without underlying changes in the bone (cysts).

ETIOLOGY AND PATHOPHYSIOLOGY

- Sarcoidosis is a granulomatous disease with involvement of multiple organ systems with an unknown etiology.

- The typical findings in sarcoid lesions are characterized by the presence of circumscribed granulomas of epithelioid cells with little or no caseating necrosis, although fibrinoid necrosis is not uncommon.

- Granulomas are usually in the superficial dermis but may involve the thickness of dermis and extend to the subcutaneous tissue. These granulomas are referred to as "naked" because they only have a sparse lymphocytic infiltrate at their margins.

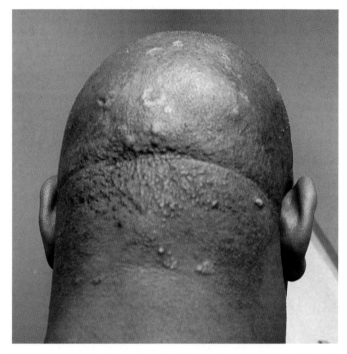

FIGURE 168-1 Papular and annular lesions of sarcoid on the scalp and neck of a 42-year-old black man. (*Courtesy of Amor Khachemoune, MD.*)

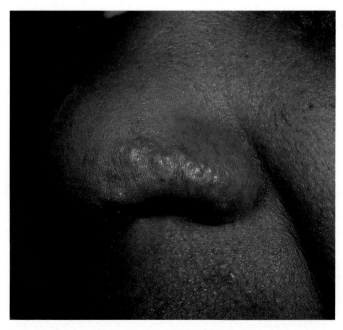

FIGURE 168-2 Lupus pernio in a 45-year-old black woman with sarcoid involving the nasal rim. (*Courtesy of Richard P. Usatine, MD.*)

DIAGNOSIS

CLINICAL FORMS OF DISEASE

Cutaneous involvement is either *specific* or *nonspecific*.

- Specific
  - Typical noncaseating granulomas, no evidence of infection, foreign body, or other causes.
  - May be disfiguring, but almost always nontender and rarely ulcerate.
  - Maculopapular type is most common, red–brown, or purplish and usually smaller than 1 cm and found mostly on face, neck, upper back, and limbs (**Figure 168-4**).
  - Lupus pernio type are most distinctive lesions and present as purplish lesions resembling frostbites with shiny skin covering them, typically affecting nose, cheeks, ears, and lips and distal extremities (**Figures 168-2, 168-3** and **168-5**).
  - Lupus pernio may occur as a syndrome involving upper respiratory tract with pulmonary fibrosis, or be associated with chronic uveitis and bone cysts.
  - Annular or circinate type appear ribbon-like, with mild scaling and yellowish red in color, with centrifugal progression and central healing and depigmentation (**Figure 168-1**).
  - Plaque sarcoidosis is typically chronic but may heal without scarring, and occur over bone, forehead, arms, legs, and shoulders (**Figure 168-6**).
  - Nodular cutaneous and subcutaneous that are skin-colored or violaceous without epidermal involvement typically seen in advanced systemic sarcoidosis (**Figure 168-7**).
  - Areas of old scars that are damaged by trauma, radiation, surgery, or tattoo may also be infiltrated with sarcoid granulomas (**Figures 168-8** and **168-9**). Appearance is red or purple discoloration and induration and lesions and may be tender.

- Nonspecific
  - EN lesions usually are not disfiguring, but tender to touch especially when they occur along with symptoms of fever, polyarthralgias, and sometimes arthritis and acute iritis.
  - EN appears abruptly with warm, tender, reddish nodules on lower extremity, most commonly anterior tibial surfaces, ankles, and knees.
  - The EN nodules are 1 to 5 cm and usually bilateral and evolve through color stages: first bright red, then purplish, and lastly a bruise-like yellow or green appearance.
  - EN bouts occur with fatigue, fever, symmetrical polyarthritis, and skin eruptions that typically last 3 to 6 weeks with more than 80% of cases resolving within 2 years.[4]
  - EN is seen in the setting of Löfgren syndrome appearing in conjunction with hilar lymphadenopathy (bilateral most often), and occasionally anterior uveitis and/or polyarthritis.
  - Löfgren syndrome is associated with right paratracheal lymph node involvement seen on x-ray.
  - Ulceration is typically not observed in EN and plaques and nodules heal without scarring.
  - Other nonspecific lesions of sarcoidosis include lymphedema, calcinosis cutis, prurigo, and erythema multiforme.
  - Nail changes seen in sarcoidosis may appear as clubbing, onycholysis, and subungual keratosis.

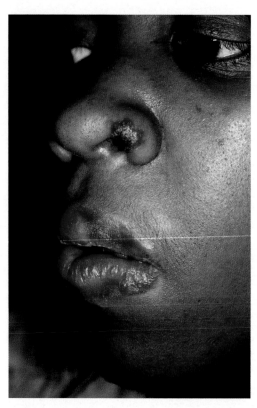

FIGURE 168-3 Lupus pernio with red to violaceous sarcoid papules and plaques on the nose and lips. (*Courtesy of Amor Khachemoune, MD.*)

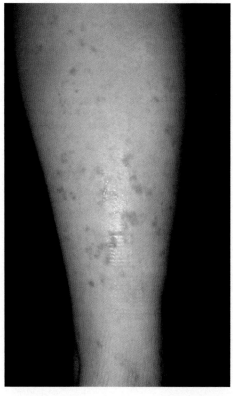

FIGURE 168-4 Maculopapular sarcoidosis on the leg of a 46-year-old white woman. (*Courtesy of Amor Khachemoune, MD.*)

LABORATORY STUDIES

- CBC count with differential and platelets
  - Leukopenia (5%–10%) and/or thrombocytopenia may be seen.
  - Eosinophilia occurs in 24% of patients, and anemia occurs in 5% of patients.
  - Hypergammaglobulinemia (30%–80%), positive rheumatoid factor and decreased skin test reactivity.
  - Autoimmune hemolytic anemia and hypersplenism can occur in some patients, although rare.
  - Hypocapnia and hypoxemia maybe present in certain patient populations, and these symptoms are worsened by exercise.

- Serum calcium and 24-hour urine calcium levels
  - Hypercalciuria has been found in 49% of patients in some studies, whereas 13% of patients had hypercalcemia.
  - Hypercalcemia occurs in sarcoidosis because of increased intestinal absorption of calcium that results from overproduction of a metabolite of vitamin D by pulmonary macrophages.

- Serum angiotensin-converting enzyme (ACE) level
  - Serum ACE level is elevated in 60% of patients.
  - Serum ACE levels are helpful in monitoring disease activity and treatment response. ACE is derived from epithelioid cells of the granulomas, therefore, it reflects granuloma load in the patient.

- Serum chemistries, such as alanine aminotransferase, aspartate aminotransferase, alkaline phosphatase, BUN, and creatinine levels. These levels may be elevated with hepatic and renal involvement.

- Other: Elevated erythrocyte sedimentation rate, elevated antinuclear antibodies (30%), diabetes insipidus, and renal failure may be noted.

IMAGING STUDIES

- Chest radiography
  - Radiographic involvement is seen in almost 90% of patients. Chest radiography is used in staging the disease.
  - Stage I disease shows bilateral hilar lymphadenopathy (BHL). Stage II disease shows BHL plus pulmonary infiltrates. Stage III disease shows pulmonary infiltrates without BHL. Stage IV disease shows pulmonary fibrosis.

- CT of the thorax
  - CT of the thorax may demonstrate lymphadenopathy or granulomatous infiltration.
  - Other findings may include small nodules with a bronchovascular and subpleural distribution, thickened interlobular septae, honeycombing, bronchiectasis, and alveolar consolidation.

- Pulmonary function tests
  - Evidence of both restrictive abnormalities and obstructive abnormalities may be found.

BIOPSY

- Punch biopsy is adequate to obtain a sample of skin that includes dermis.

- If EN nodules are deep, a biopsy should also include subcutaneous tissue.

- Biopsy specimens are sent for histologic examination, as well as stains and cultures to rule out infectious causes.

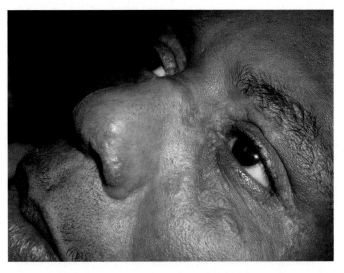

FIGURE 168-5 Lupus pernio in a 48-year-old black man with sarcoid lesions on the nose and around the eyes. (*Courtesy of Richard P. Usatine, MD.*)

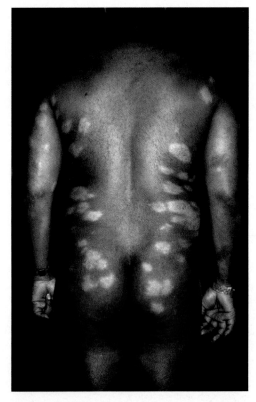

FIGURE 168-6 Hypopigmented widespread cutaneous plaque sarcoidosis predominantly on the back of a black man. (*Courtesy of Eric Kraus, MD.*)

DIFFERENTIAL DIAGNOSIS

- Granulomatous skin disease
  - Granuloma annulare (GA) is also a granulomatous skin disease, which appears in single or multiple rings in adults and children (see Chapter 166, Granuloma Annulare).
  - Rheumatoid nodules: These usually appear in the context of a diagnosed rheumatoid arthritis with joint disease present (see Chapter 92, Rheumatoid Arthritis).
  - Granulomatous mycosis fungoides. This is a type of cutaneous lymphoma with many clinical forms including granuloma formation (see Chapter 169, Mycosis Fungoides).

- Maculopapular type
  - Lupus vulgaris: This is a type of cutaneous involvement with mycobacterium tuberculosis.
  - Syringoma: These are small firm adnexal benign tumors usually appearing around the upper cheeks and lower eyelids.
  - Xanthelasma: These are the most common type of xanthomas. They are benign yellow macules, papules, or plaques often appearing on the eyelids. Approximately one half of the patients with xanthelasma have a lipid disorder (see Chapter 215, Xanthomas).
  - Lichen planus: This is a very pruritic skin involvement with pink to violaceous papules and plaques. It may present in different body locations but the most common areas are the writs and ankles (see Chapter147, Lichen Planus).
  - Granulomatous rosacea: This is a variant of rosacea made of uniform papules involving the face.
  - Acne keloidalis nuchae: This is commonly seen in dark-skinned patients. It presents with multiple perifollicular papules and nodules. The most common location is the back of the neck at the hairline (see Chapter 108, Pseudofolliculitis and Acne Keloidalis Nuchae).
  - Pseudofolliculitis barbae: This is most commonly seen in patients with darker skin color. The triggering factor is often ingrown hair at the beard area (see Chapter, 108 Pseudofolliculitis and Acne Keloidalis Nuchae).

- Annular or circinate type
  - GA: Annular type of previously described GA (see Chapter 166, Granuloma Annulare).
  - Annular form of necrobiosis lipoidica: A granulomatous disease with area of necrobiosis. This is usually seen on the pretibial areas of patients with diabetes. But not all patients have diabetes (see Chapter 214, Necrobiosis Lipoidica).
  - These two entities maybe differentiated histologically.

- Nodular cutaneous and subcutaneous type:
  - Morphea: It is also known as localized scleroderma. It is caused by excessive collagen deposition in the dermis or subcutaneous tissue leading to the formation of nodules (see Chapter 175, Scleroderma and Morphea).
  - Epidermal inclusion cyst: This is an encapsulated keratin filled nodule of different sizes and is often found in the subcutaneous tissue. A central pore or punctum is often noted on examination of the overlying epidermis.
  - Lipoma: These are soft nodules of different sizes. They are composed of mature fat cells and often found in the subcutaneous tissue.

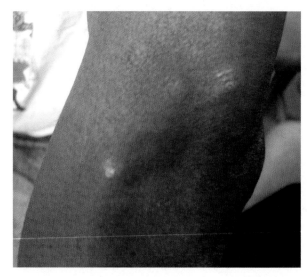

FIGURE 168-7 Subcutaneous sarcoid (Darier–Roussy syndrome) in a patient with advanced systemic sarcoidosis. (*Courtesy of Amor Khachemoune, MD.*)

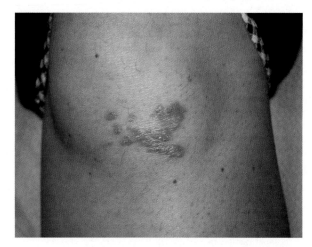

FIGURE 168-8 Sarcoidal plaque of the knee, which appeared after a trauma to the knee. (*Courtesy of Amor Khachemoune, MD.*)

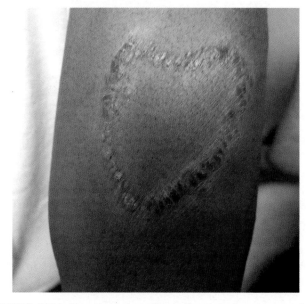

FIGURE 168-9 Sarcoid on a heart-shaped homemade tattoo over the knee. (*Courtesy of Amor Khachemoune, MD.*)

○ Metastatic carcinoma: These nodular lesions often present in the context of a diagnosed primary carcinoma of other internal organs.

○ Foreign body granuloma: This is usually localized to the area of introduction of the foreign body into the skin.

MANAGEMENT

- Cutaneous involvement of sarcoidosis is typically not life-threatening and, therefore, the major rationale for treatment is to prevent or minimize disfigurement. Cosmetic issues are particularly important on the face. Also, the lesions can be painful.

- Corticosteroids are the mainstay of treatment.[1–5] SOR Ⓑ

- Limited cutaneous disease responds to very high potency topical corticosteroids, or intralesional triamcinolone repeated monthly.[3,4] SOR Ⓑ

- Photochemotherapy (PUVA) is successful in erythrodermic and hypopigmented lesions. SOR Ⓒ

- Lupus pernio patient may benefit from pulsed-dye or carbon dioxide laser treatments. SOR Ⓒ

- Resistant lesions to topical therapy or large and diffuse lesions require prednisone.[2,5] SOR Ⓑ

- To prevent complications from long-term treatment by steroids, hydroxychloroquine or chloroquine are used as steroid-sparing agents.[6] SOR Ⓒ

- Other combinations that have been successful in chronic cutaneous disease and lung disease are methotrexate or azathioprine with low-dose prednisone.[5] SOR Ⓒ

- Agents such as cyclophosphamide and cyclosporin are also used but with caution because of severe drug toxicity.[7] SOR Ⓒ

- Future treatments look toward the use of antihuman TNF-alpha monoclonal antibody and infliximab.[8] SOR Ⓒ

PATIENT EDUCATION

Inform patients about the risk that systemic sarcoidosis can occur even if the skin is the only area currently involved.

FOLLOW-UP

Patient with cutaneous sarcoidosis should be worked up for systemic sarcoidosis. Regular follow up is necessary.

PATIENT RESOURCES

http://www.nhlbi.nih.gov/health/dci/Diseases/sarc/sar_whatis.html.

PROVIDER RESOURCE

http://www.emedicine.com/DERM/topic381.htm.

REFERENCES

1. Grutters JC, van den Bosch JM. Corticosteroid treatment in sarcoidosis. *Eur Respir J.* 2006;28(3):627–636.

2. English JC, 3rd, Patel PJ, Greer KE. Sarcoidosis. *J Am Acad Dermatol.* 2001;44(5):725–743; quiz 744–746.

3. Khatri KA, Chotzen VA, Burrall BA. Lupus pernio: Successful treatment with a potent topical corticosteroid. *Arch Dermatol.* 1995;131:617–618.

4. Yeager H, Sina B, Khachemoune A. Dermatologic disease. In: Baughman RP ed. *Sarcoidosis.* New York: *Taylor & Francis*, 2006:593–604.

5. Mosam A, Morar N. Recalcitrant cutaneous sarcoidosis: An evidence-based sequential approach. *J Dermatol Treat.* 2004;15(6):353–359.

6. Baughman RP. Infliximab for refractory sarcoidosis. *Sarcoidosis Vasc Diffuse Lung Dis* 2001;18:70–74; erratum in: *Sarcoidosis Vasc Diffuse Lung Dis* 2001;18:310.

7. Kouba DJ, Mimouni D, Rencic A, Nousari HC. Mycophenolate mofetil may serve as a steroid-sparing agent for sarcoidosis. *Br J Dermatol.* 2003;148:147–148.

8. Baughman RP, Judson MA, Teirstein AS, Moller DR, Lower EE. Thalidomide for chronic sarcoidosis. *Chest.* 2002;122:227–232.

169 MYCOSIS FUNGOIDES

Anjeli Nayar, MD
Richard P. Usatine, MD

PATIENT STORY

A 52-year-old black woman presented with a 7-month history of a hypopigmented rash in a symmetric distribution on her upper thighs and arms (**Figures 169-1** and **169-2**). She had been from evacuated New Orleans following Hurricane Katrina. She had waded through polluted waters for hours before being rescued by a boat.[1] Four days passed before she had access to a shower at which time she noticed a single erythematous spot the size of a silver dollar on her left thigh. Over the next several weeks, it faded to hypopigmented macules and plaques and eventually spread to both thighs and arms. The physical examination revealed no lymphadenopathy. A hematoxylin and eosin stain of a full thickness punch biopsy revealed "cerebriform" lymphocytes at the dermal-epidermal junction characteristic of mycosis fungoides (MF), a type of cutaneous T-cell lymphoma (CTCL). Her blood tests were essentially normal, and she was HIV negative. The patient reported no improvement with topical high-potency generic steroid to affected areas and is currently receiving narrow-band UVB treatment twice weekly.

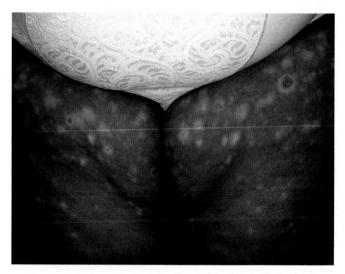

FIGURE 169-1 The hypopigmented patches of MF on the thighs of a 52-year-old black woman. This is the patch stage of the disease. This mimics vitiligo but the distribution and appearance warranted a biopsy that provided a definitive diagnosis of MF. (*Courtesy of Richard P. Usatine, MD.*)

EPIDEMIOLOGY

- CTCL is a rare disease with 1000 new cases per year in the United States, comprising approximately 0.5% of all non-Hodgkin's lymphoma cases.[1,2]

- MF is the most common CTCL, and Sézary syndrome (SS) is a variant of MF comprising 5% of cases.

- It is more common in African Americans than in white individuals with an incidence ratio of 6:1.[1]

- It is more common in males, with a male-to-female ratio of 2:1, and most commonly presents at 50 to 60 years. However, children and adolescents can be affected and have similar clinical outcomes.

ETIOLOGY AND PATHOPHYSIOLOGY

- The exact etiology of CTCL is unknown, but environmental, infectious and genetic causes have been suggested. CTCL is a malignant lymphoma of helper T cells that usually remain confined to skin and lymph nodes (LN). MF is a specific type of CTCL named for the mushroom-like skin tumors seen in severe cases.[1]

- Human T-lymphocytic virus (HTLV) types 1 and 2, HIV-1, CMV, EBV and Borrelia burgdorferi have been suggested but unproven infectious causes of MF.[2,3] Environmental exposure to Agent Orange may be responsible for some cases.[1] There is one case report of possible conjugal transmission of MF between a heterosexual couple who developed advanced MF within 14 months of one another.[3]

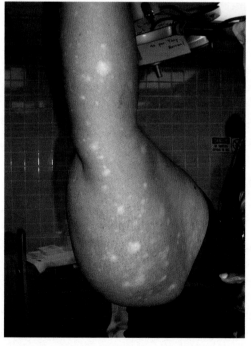

FIGURE 169-2 Hypopigmented patches on the arm of the woman in **Figure 169-2** with MF. (*Courtesy of Richard P. Usatine, MD.*)

- MF and SS have been associated with specific HLA types (Aw31, Aw32, B8, Bw38, and DR5).[2] Genetic predisposition is also suggested by detection of HLA class II alleles DRB1*11 and DQB1*03 in association with sporadic and familial malignancy and familial clustering among Israeli Jews.[2,4]

- Metastasis, to the liver, spleen, lungs, gastrointestinal tract, bone marrow, and the CNS may occur via T-cell spread through the lymphatic system.[1,2]

- The reduction of T-cell receptor complexity contributes to immunosuppression in advanced MF and SS, and may manifest clinically as herpes simplex or zoster.[5] Death is usually secondary to systemic infection, especially from *Staphylococcus aureus* and *Pseudomonas aeruginosa*.

- Host antitumor immunity also deteriorates, and patients have an increased risk for secondary malignancies, including higher-grade non-Hodgkin's lymphoma, Hodgkin disease, secondary melanoma, and colon cancer in addition to cardiopulmonary complications.[5]

DIAGNOSIS

CLINICAL FEATURES

- The most common initial presentation involves patches or scaly plaques with a persistent rash that is often pruritic and usually erythematous (**Figures 169-1** to **169-4**).[1] Patches may evolve to generalized, infiltrated plaques or to ulcerated, exophytic tumors (**Figures 169-5** and **169-6**).[2,6]

- Hypo- or hyperpigmented lesions, petechiae, poikiloderma (skin atrophy with telangectasia), and alopecia with or without mucinosis are other findings.

- A "premycotic" phase may precede definitive diagnosis for months to decades, which involves nonspecific, slightly scaling skin lesions that intermittently appear and may eventually resolve with topical steroids.

- SS is characterized by generalized exfoliative erythroderma, lymphadenopathy, and atypical Sézary cells in the peripheral blood. Diffuse infiltration of malignant T cells in SS may exaggerate facial lines, creating a leonine facies.[6]

- "Invisible MF" describes pruritus without visible lesions but the skin biopsy is positive for monoclonal T-cell infiltrates.[2]

TYPICAL DISTRIBUTION

- Lesions may affect any skin surface, but typically develop on non-sun-exposed areas initially such as the trunk below the waistline, flanks, breasts, inner thighs and arms, and the periaxillary areas.[7]

- If there is follicular involvement, lesions may be found on the face or scalp.

- MF occasionally presents as a refractory dermatosis of the palms or soles.

BIOPSY AND LABORATORY STUDIES

- Biopsies: A full-thickness punch biopsy of the lesion is the most important diagnostic tool. If the initial biopsy is negative but the rash persists, the biopsy should be repeated.[1] Topical treatments and

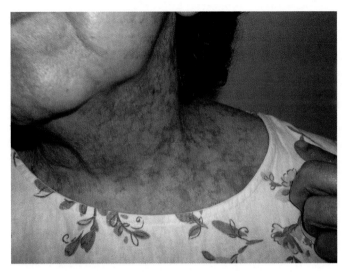

FIGURE 169-3 Reticulated MF. This netlike pattern of MF is also called parapsoriasis variegata. (*Courtesy of Heather Goff, MD.*)

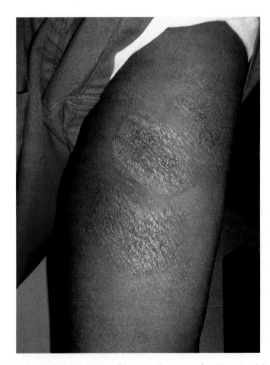

FIGURE 169-4 Plaque stage of MF on the arm of a 57-year-old nurse. She has had MF for 8 years and has intermittantly been on chemotherapy. Recently her MF has worsened and she was started on nitrogen mustard. (*Courtesy of E.J. Mayeaux, Jr., MD.*)

systemic immunosuppressants should be discontinued 2 to 4 weeks before the biopsy.[8]

- If the lymph nodes (LN) are palpable or lymphadenopathy is suspected, also known as "dermatopathic lymphadenitis," biopsies should be performed.[2]

- A bone marrow biopsy should be performed if there is proven nodal or blood involvement.

- Histology: The skin biopsy may reveal Pautrier microabscesses or an inflammatory cell bandlike infiltrate lining the basal layer or in the upper dermis ("mononuclear epidermotropism"). Malignant lymphocytes have hyperchromatic and convoluted or "cerebriform" nuclei. Capillary dermal fibrosis may also be observed.[8]

- Radiography: A chest radiography and CT scan of the abdomen and pelvis are recommended for advanced stages IIB to IIIB, or, if visceral disease is suspected.[7] A combination of CT and PET scans offers more sensitive detection of LN involvement than either imaging study alone.[2]

- Blood tests for infectious etiology: HIV test, human T-cell lymphocyte virus type 1, EBV, CMV, as indicated by clinical history.

- Serology and blood tests: A complete blood cell count with differential, a buffy coat smear to screen for Sézary cells, lactic dehydrogenase and uric acid as markers for bulky or aggressive disease, and liver function tests to detect hepatic involvement should be measured. Progression of MF is associated with increased serum concentrations of immunoglobin E (IgE) and IgA.[2] Peripheral eosinophilia is an independent marker for poor prognosis and disease progression.[2,9]

- Flow cytometry: This test may be used to detect malignant clones and to quantify CD8+ lymphocytes to assess immunocompetence.

- Immunophenotyping may be used to support histology results.

- PCR and Southern blot testing are recommended to detect T-cell rearrangements, if histology and immunophenotyping results are equivocal and to detect abnormal cells in LN.[2]

- The International Society for Cutaneous Lymphoma proposed criteria for diagnosing early "classic" MF by incorporating clinical, histopathologic, molecular biologic and immunopathologic features including the presence of persistent or progressive patches or thin plaques in unexposed areas and/or poikiloderma, superficial lymphoid infiltrate, epidermotropism with spongiosis, lymphocytes with hyperchromatic and cerebriform nuclei, epidermal/dermal discordance between CD2, CD3, CD5, or CD7, and clonal T-cell receptor rearrangement.[8] The International Society for Cutaneous Lymphoma also proposed criteria for diagnosing SS with leukemic blood involvement including an absolute Sézary cell count of >1000/mm^3, a CD4:CD8 ratio of ≥10, T-cell chromosomal abnormalities detected by Southern blot or PCR, increased circulation of T cells and aberrant expression of pan T-cell markers as assessed by flow cytometry.[6]

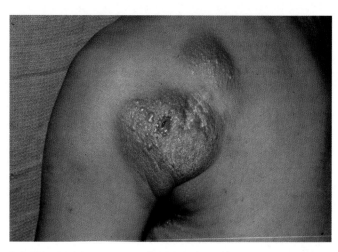

FIGURE 169-5 Tumor stage of MF. (*Courtesy of the University of Texas Health Sciences Center, Division of Dermatology.*)

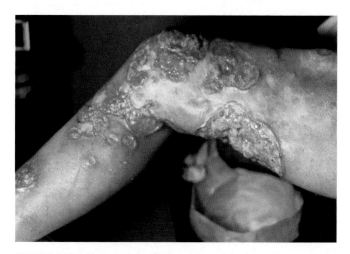

FIGURE 169-6 Tumor stage of MF with large leg ulcers. (*Courtesy of the University of Texas Health Sciences Center, Division of Dermatology.*)

DIFFERENTIAL DIAGNOSIS

- "Premycotic" period preceding diagnosis of MF may resemble parapsoriasis en plaque or nonspecific dermatitis.[2,8]

- MF with erythroderma must be distinguished from generalized atopic dermatitis, contact dermatitis, photodermatitis, drug eruptions, erythrodermic psoriasis, and idiopathic hyper-eosinophilic syndrome (see Chapter 149, Erythroderma).[2,6]

- Unilesional MF may resemble nummular eczema, lichen simplex chronicus, erythema chronicum migrans, tinea corporis, or digitate dermatosis (a variant of small plaque parapsoriasis).[8]

- Vitiligo typically involves discrete, hypopigmented macules on the hands and face that coalesce into larger areas.[1] However, some MF may mimic vitiligo as seen in (**Figures 169-1** and **169-2**). The distribution of the hypopigmented macules in this case is atypical for vitiligo and this prompted a biopsy that led to the diagnosis of MF (see Chapter 191, Vitiligo).

- Idiopathic guttate hypomelanosis is a benign condition involving smaller hypopigmented macules than those seen in MF.[1]

- In patients with HIV, histopathology; resembling MF may represent a reactive inflammatory condition instead. Nonepidermotrophic large T-cell cutaneous lymphoma and B-cell diffuse cutaneous lymphoma are more frequent complications than MF in these patients.[10]

MANAGEMENT

- The rarity of MF precludes data supporting evidence-based treatment, and well designed, prospective controlled clinical studies comparing various therapies are lacking.[1,2]

- For stage I disease localized to the skin, symptomatic treatment with emollients, antipruritics (Doxepin cream 5%) and topical high-potency steroids (Clobestol cream 0.05% twice daily) on an outpatient basis are recommended.[7] SOR ⓒ. Topical retinoids (bexarotene 300 mg/m[2] per day PO once daily) or topical chemotherapy (nitrogen mustard, bischloroethylnitrosourea, or carmustine) are treatment alternatives for localized disease and effective adjuvants in generalized disease.[1,7,11,12] SOR ⓑ

- Bexarotene 1% topical gel may be used if disease persists despite treatment or if other medication is not tolerated.[12] When used in combination with psoralen-enhanced ultraviolet light (PUVA), bexarotene decreases the total UVA dosage needed and if used as maintenance therapy increases the duration of remission.[12] SOR ⓒ

- Alternatively, PUVA may also be used concurrently with interferon (IFN), three times weekly, or retinoids until skin lesions clear, then continued as maintenance therapy at a reduced frequency.[12] SOR ⓒ

- For a plaque recalcitrant to PUVA and retinoid combination therapy, one case study showed that Imiquimod 5% topical cream effectively cleared the lesion.[5] SOR ⓒ

- UVA may also be enhanced with methoxsalen or oxsoralen instead of psoralen.[7] SOR ⓒ

- Narrowband UVB light has proven effective in early MF and prolonging remission, although an optimal maintenance protocol still needs to be established.[13] SOR ⓒ

- Photodynamic therapy with 5-aminolevulinic acid (PDT-ALA) was found to effectively eradicate localized infiltrates better than topical steroids, but more studies are needed before it becomes standard-

ized treatment.[11] SOR ⓒ In general, photodynamic therapy works via direct cytotoxicity, vascular damage and immune host response.[6,14]

- Stage II disease involves the regional LN and may be treated the same as for stage I. For stage IIB, total skin electron beam therapy (EBT) followed by nitrogen mustard treatment for ≥6 months is most recommended.[12] SOR ⓒ For disease relapse after EBT, PUVA may be used in combination with IFN or a systemic retinoid.[12] SOR ⓒ Other systemic therapies include fusion toxins, monoclonal antibody treatment, and single-agent chemotherapy.[7] For recalcitrant tumors, there is no evidence that combination systemic chemotherapy regimens offer superior survival outcome than single agents.[7,12] SOR ⓒ

- Stage III, or erythrodermic disease without extracutaneous disease or with limited LN involvement, should be treated with chemotherapy or photophoresis for 4 weeks.[12] SOR ⓒ Extracorporeal photochemotherapy involves irradiation of white blood cells with PUVA after leukophoresis before reinfusing the blood cells intravenously.[7] If the response is delayed, photophoresis may be combined with IFN or systemic retinoids.

- Stage IV extracutaneous disease should be treated with systemic chemotherapy. Although response rates are improved with combination chemotherapy, the response duration is less than 1 year. Regimens include cyclophosphamide, vincristine, and prednisone (CVP), CVP plus adriamycin, CVP plus methotrexate, or cyclophosphamide, vincristine, adriamycin, and etoposide. Adjuvants treatments may include IFN, systemic retinoids, and photophoresis. Single agent chemotherapy includes methotrexate, liposomal doxorubicin, gemcitabine, etoposide, cyclophosphamide, and purine analogs.[12] SOR ⓒ The patient should be referred to a dermatologist, and medical and radiation oncologists.[1]

- The patient should be monitored for development of secondary malignancies.

PATIENT EDUCATION

- Patients should avoid sun exposure, stay in a cool environment, and keep their skin lubricated.

FOLLOW-UP AND PROGNOSIS

- Patients have a normal life expectancy, if diagnosed early during stage IA in which the patch or plaque is limited to <10% of the skin surface area.[1]

- MF and SS are otherwise difficult to cure and have a prognosis of 3.2 years for stage IIB cutaneous tumors, 4 to 6 years for stage III generalized erythroderma, and <1.5 years for stage IVA and stage IVB with LN and visceral involvement, respectively.[7]

PATIENT AND PROVIDER RESOURCES

http://www.emedicine.com/MED/topic1541.htm.

REFERENCES

1. Mahan RD, Usatine RP. Hurricane Katrina evacuee develops a persistent rash. *J Fam Pract.* 2007;56(6):454–457.

2. Hoppe RT, Kim YH. Clinical features, diagnosis, and staging of mycosis fungoides and Sezary syndrome. http://www.utdol.com/utd/content/topic.do?topicKey=lymphoma/7439&type=A&selectedTitle=1~10. Updated December 15, 2006. Accessed June 19, 2007.

3. Adriana N, Schmidt AN, Jason B, Robbins JB, Greer JP, Zic JA. Conjugal transformed mycosis fungoides: The unknown role of viral infection and environmental exposures in the development of cutaneous T-cell lymphoma. *J Am Acad Dermatol.* 2006;54(5): S202–S205.

4. Hodak E, et al. Familial mycosis fungoides: Report of 6 kindreds and a study of the HLA system. *J Am Acad Dermatol.* 2005;52(3): 393–402.

5. Navi D, Huntley A. Imiquimod 5 percent cream and the treatment of cutaneous malignancy. *Dermatol Online J.* 2004; 10(1):4. Available at http://www.mdconsult.com/das/citation/body/73715997-14/jorg=journal&source=MI&sp=15008885&sid=598240728/N/15008885/1.html. Accessed June 19, 2007.

6. Girardi M, et al. The pathogenesis of mycosis fungoides. *N Engl J Med.* 2004;350(19):1978–1988.

7. Pinter-Brown LC. Mycosis fungoides. Updated September 8, 2006. http://www.emedicine.com/MED/topic1541.htm. Accessed June 19, 2007.

8. Pimpinelli N, et al. Defining early mycosis fungoides. *J Am Acad Dermatol.* 2005;53(6):1053–1063.

9. Querfeld C, et al. Phase II trial of subcutaneous injections of human recombinant interleukin-2 for the treatment of mycosis fungoides and Sezary syndrome. *J Am Acad Dermatol.* 2007;56(4): 580–583.

10. Honda KS. HIV and skin cancer. *Dermatol Clin.* 2006;24(4): 521–530.

11. Blume JE, Oseroff AR. Aminolevulinic acid photodynamic therapy for skin cancers. *Dermatol Clin.* 2007;25(1):5–14.

12. Hoppe RT, Kim YH. Treatment of mycosis fungoides and Sezary syndrome. Updated December 14, 2006. http://www.utdol.com/utd/content/topic.do?topicKey=lymphoma/6747&type=A&selectedTitle=2~10. Accessed June 19, 2007.

13. Boztepe G, et al. Narrowband ultraviolet B phototherapy to clear and maintain clearance in patients with mycosis fungoides. *J Am Acad Dermatol.* 2005;53(2):242–246.

14. Nayak CS. Photodynamic therapy in dermatology. *Indian J Dermatol Venereol Leprol.* 2005;71(3):155–160. http://www.ijdvl.com. Accessed June 19, 2007.

170 ERYTHEMA MULTIFORME, STEVENS-JOHNSON SYNDROME AND TOXIC EPIDERMAL NECROLYSIS

Carolyn Milana, MD
Mindy A. Smith, MD, MS

PATIENT STORY

A 2-year-old Hispanic girl developed typical target lesions of erythema multiforme (EM) after starting a sulfa-containing antibiotic 1 week prior for an otitis media (**Figure 170-1**). In this mild version of EM, the target lesions were on the extensor surface of the arm and face. The antibiotic was stopped and the EM cleared.

EPIDEMIOLOGY

- EM has been estimated to range from 1 in 1000 persons to 1 in 10,000 persons.[1] The true incidence of the disease is not known.[1]

- Stevens-Johnson syndrome (SJS) and toxic epidermal necrolysis (TEN) are severe cutaneous reactions often caused by drugs—both are believed to be the same disorder as EM but are more severe; the incidence is rare.

- EM most commonly occurs between the ages of 10 and 30 years, with 20% of cases occurring in children and adolescents.[2]

- With respect to EM, men are affected slightly more often than women.[2]

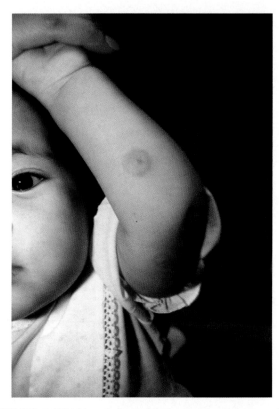

FIGURE 170-1 EM with typical target lesions on the extensor surface of the arm and face from a drug reaction. The center of each target lesion has a vesicle. (*Courtesy of Richard P. Usatine, MD.*)

ETIOLOGY AND PATHOPHYSIOLOGY

- Numerous factors have been identified as causative agents for EM:
  - Erythema multiforme
    - Herpes simplex virus (HSV) I and II are the most common causative agents and have been implicated in at least 60% of the cases.[3,4]
    - The virus has been found in circulating blood,[5] as well as on skin biopsy of patients with EM minor.[3]
  - Stevens-Johnson syndrome and toxic epidermal necrolysis
    - 50% of cases have no identifiable cause.
    - Mycoplasma pneumoniae has been identified as the most common infectious cause for SJS.[4]

- Drugs most commonly known to cause SJS and TEN are sulfonamide antibiotics, allopurinol, nonsteroidal anti-inflammatory agents, amine antiepileptic drugs (phenytoin and carbamazepine), and lamotrigine.[6]
- Other less common causative agents for EM, SJS, and TEN include:
  - Infectious agents such as mycobacterium tuberculosis, group A streptococci, hepatitis B, Epstein Barr virus, Francisella tularensis, yersinia, enteroviruses, histoplasma, coccidioides.[1,4]
  - Neoplastic processes such as leukemia and lymphoma.[1,4]
  - Antibiotics such as penicillin, isoniazid, tetracyclines, cephalosporins, and quinolones.
  - Anticonvulsants such as phenobarbital and valproic acid.[1,4]
  - Other drugs including captopril, etoposide, aspirin, and allopurinol.
  - Immunizations such as Calmette-Guérin bacillus, diphtheria-tetanus toxoid, hepatitis B, measles-mumps-rubella, and poliomyelitis.[3]
  - Other agents or triggers including radiation therapy, sunlight, pregnancy, connective tissue disease, and menstruation.[1,4]
- The pathogenesis of EM, SJS, and TEN remains unknown, however, recent studies have shown that it may be as a result of a host specific cell mediated immune response to an antigenic stimulus that activates cytotoxic T-cells and results in damage to keratinocytes.[3,6]
  - The epidermal detachment (skin peeling) seen in SJS and TEN appears to result from epidermal necrosis in the absence of substantial dermal inflammation.

DIAGNOSIS

CLINICAL FEATURES

- In all of these conditions, there is a rapid onset of skin lesions.
- EM is a disease in which patients present with the following lesions:
  - Classic lesions begin as red macules and expand centrifugally to become target-like papules or plaques with an erythematous outer border and central clearing (iris or bull's eye lesions) (**Figures 170-1 to 170-3**). Iris lesions, although characteristic, are not necessary to make the diagnosis. The center of the lesion may have vesicles or erosions (**Figure 170-4**).
  - Lesions can coalesce and form larger lesions up to 2 cm in diameter with centers that can become dusky purple to necrotic at this time (**Figures 170-4 and 170-5**).
  - Unlike urticarial lesions, the lesions of EM do not appear and fade; once they appear they remain fixed in place.
  - Patients are usually asymptomatic although a burning sensation or pruritus may be present.
  - Lesions typically resolve without any permanent sequelae within 2 weeks.
  - Recurrent outbreaks have been reported to occur and are thought to be associated with HSV infection.[3,4]
- In both SJS and TEN, patients may have blisters that develop on dusky or purpuric macules. SJS is diagnosed when less than 10% of the body surface area is involved; SJS/TEN when 10% to 30% is involved; and TEN, when >30% is involved.
  - Lesions may become more widespread and rapidly progress to form areas of central necrosis, bullae and areas of denudation (**Figure 170-6**).

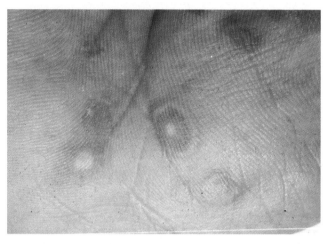

FIGURE 170-2 EM on the palm with target lesions that have a dusky red center. (*Courtesy of the University of Texas Health Sciences Center, Division of Dermatology.*)

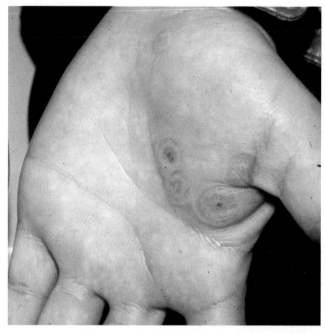

FIGURE 170-3 EM on the hands secondary to an outbreak of oral herpes. (*Courtesy of the University of Texas Health Sciences Center, Division of Dermatology.*)

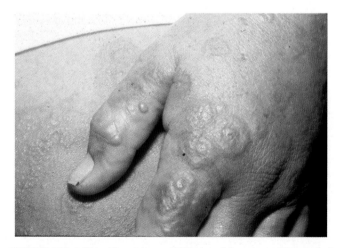

FIGURE 170-4 EM with vesicles and blistering of the targets. (*Courtesy of the University of Texas Health Sciences Center, Division of Dermatology.*)

○ Fever >39°C is often present.

○ In addition to skin involvement, there is involvement of at least two mucosal surfaces such as the eyes, oral cavity, upper airway, esophagus, gastrointestinal tract, or the anogenital mucosa (**Figures 170-7 to 170-9**).

○ New lesions occur in crops and may take 4 to 6 weeks to heal.

○ Large areas of epidermal detachment occur (**Figures 170-10 and 170-11**).

○ Severe pain can occur from mucosal ulcerations but skin tenderness is minimal.

○ Skin erosions lead to increased insensible blood and fluid losses, as well as an increased risk of bacterial superinfection and sepsis.

○ These patients are at high risk for ocular complications that may lead to blindness. Additional risks include bronchitis, pneumonitis, myocarditis, hepatitis, enterocolitis, polyarthritis, hematuria, and acute tubular necrosis.

○ For patients with SJS mortality rates have been reported of 5% to 10% and up to 30% for TEN.[6,7]

TYPICAL DISTRIBUTION

• The distribution of the rash in EM can be widespread.

○ The distal extremities, including the palms and soles, are most commonly involved.

○ Extensor surfaces are favored.

○ Oral lesions may be present.

• More severe lesions and more extensive mucosal lesions occur in SJS and TEN.

LABORATORY AND IMAGING

• There are no consistent laboratory findings with these conditions. The diagnosis is usually made based on clinical findings.

• Routine blood work may show leukocytosis, elevated liver transaminases, and an elevated erythrocyte sedimentation rate.

• In TEN, leukopenia may occur.

BIOPSY

• A cutaneous punch biopsy can be performed to confirm the diagnosis or to rule out other diseases.

• Histologic findings of EM will show a lymphocytic infiltrate at the dermal-epidermal junction. There is a characteristic vacuolization of the epidermal cells and necrotic keratinocytes within the epidermis.[1]

DIFFERENTIAL DIAGNOSIS

• Bullous pemphigoid—can be either subacute or acute with tense widespread blisters that can occur after persistent urticaria; mucosal involvement is rare. Significant pruritus can be present. As with EM, SJS, and TEN, bullous pemphigoid can occur after certain exposures such as ultraviolet radiation, or certain drugs (Chapter 177, Bullous Pemphigoid).

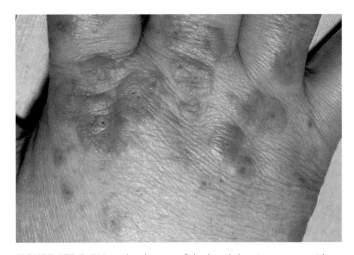

FIGURE 170-5 EM on the dorsum of the hand showing targets with small, eroded centers. There should be some epidermal erosion to diagnose EM. (*Courtesy of the University of Texas Health Sciences Center, Division of Dermatology.*)

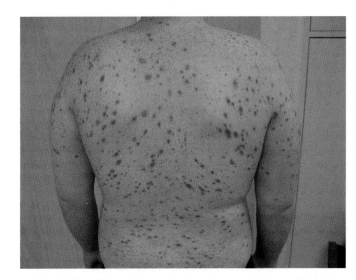

FIGURE 170-6 SJS in a 14-year-old boy who received penicillin for pneumonia. (*Courtesy of Dan Stulberg, MD.*)

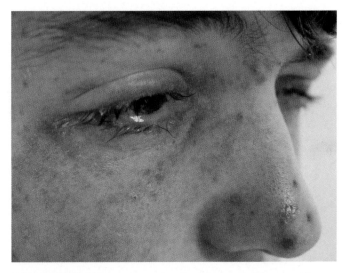

FIGURE 170-7 SJS showing mucosal involvement of the eye with a purulent appearing discharge. (*Courtesy of Dan Stulberg, MD.*)

- Urticaria—a skin reaction characterized by red wheals that are usually pruritic (**Figure 170-12**). Unlike EM, individual lesions rarely last more than 24 hours (Chapter 143, Urticaria and Angioedema).

- Kawasaki disease—fever persists at least 5 days and there must at least four of the following features[8]:
  - Changes in extremities—Acute: Erythema of palms, soles; edema of hands and feet or Subacute: Periungual peeling of fingers, and toes in weeks 2 and 3.
  - Polymorphous exanthem.
  - Bilateral bulbar conjunctival injection without exudate.
  - Changes in lips and oral cavity—erythema, lips cracking, strawberry tongue (see Chapter 33, Scarlet Fever and Strawberry Tongue), diffuse injection of oral and pharyngeal mucosae.
  - Cervical lymphadenopathy (>1.5 cm diameter), usually unilateral.

- Cutaneous vasculitis—also caused by a hypersensitivity reaction, lesions are palpable papules or purpura. Blisters, hives, and necrotic ulcers can occur on the skin. Lesions are usually located on the legs, trunk and buttocks (see Chapter 172, Cutaneous Vasculitis).

- Erythema annulare centrifugum—a hypersensitivity reaction caused by a variety of agents. Lesions look similar with erythematous papules of a few to several centimeters that enlarge and clear centrally and may be vesicular. Lesions tend to appear on the legs and thighs, but may occur on upper extremities, trunk and face; palms and soles are spared (see Chapter 199, Erythema Annulare Centrifugum).

- Staphylococcal scalded skin syndrome—rash may also follow a prodrome of malaise and fever but is macular, brightly erythematous, and initially involves the face, neck, axilla, and groin. Skin is markedly tender. Like SJS and TEN, large areas of the epidermis peel away. Unlike TEN, the site of the staphylococcal infection is usually extracutaneous (e.g., otitis media, pharyngitis) and not the skin lesions themselves (see Chapter 110, Impetigo).

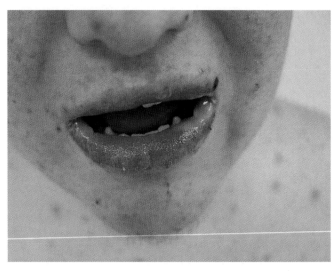

FIGURE 170-8 Same patient with SJS and mucosal mouth involvement. (*Courtesy of Dan Stulberg, MD.*)

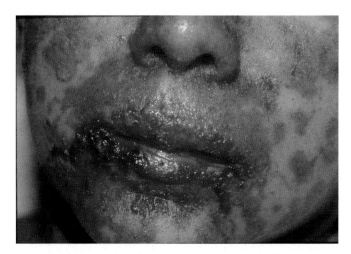

FIGURE 170-9 TEN on the face. (*Courtesy of the University of Texas Health Sciences Center, Division of Dermatology.*)

MANAGEMENT

- Erythema multiforme
  - The treatment is mainly supportive. Symptomatic relief may be provided with topical emollients, systemic anti-histamines, and acetaminophen. These do not, however, alter the course of the illness.
  - The use of corticosteroids has not been well studied, but is thought to prolong the course or increase the frequency of recurrences in HSV-associated cases.[4]
  - Prophylactic acyclovir has been used to control recurrent HSV-associated EM with some success.[4]

- Stevens-Johnson syndrome and toxic epidermal necrolysis
  - Treatment again, is mainly supportive and may require intensive care or placement in a burn unit. Early diagnosis is imperative so that triggering agents can be discontinued.
    - Oral lesions can be managed with mouthwashes and glycerin swabs.
    - Skin lesions should be cleansed with saline or Burow's solution (aluminum acetate in water).
    - IV fluids should be given to replace insensible losses.

- Daily examinations for secondary infections should occur and systemic antibiotics should be started as needed.
  ○ Consultation with an ophthalmologist is important because of the high risk of ocular sequelae.
  ○ Thus far treatments aimed at the immune response and cytokines have been ineffective in controlled trials; however, there has been some success with intravenous immunoglobulin.[6]

PATIENT EDUCATION

- If an offending drug is found to be the cause, it should be discontinued immediately.
- Patients with HSV-associated EM should be made aware of the risk of recurrence.

FOLLOW-UP

- For uncomplicated cases, no specific follow-up is needed.
- For patients with EM major and any of the complications listed above, follow-up should be arranged with the appropriate specialist.
- Prognosis is poorer for patients with SJS and TEN, if they are older, have a large percentage of body surface area involved or intestinal or pulmonary involvement.

PATIENT RESOURCES

- http://www.nlm.nih.gov/medlineplus/ency/article/000851.html.
- http://dermnetnz.org/reactions/erythema-multiforme.html.

PROVIDER RESOURCES

- http://www.emedicine.com/derm/topic137.htm.
- http://www.merck.com/mmhe/sec18/ch203/ch203f.html.

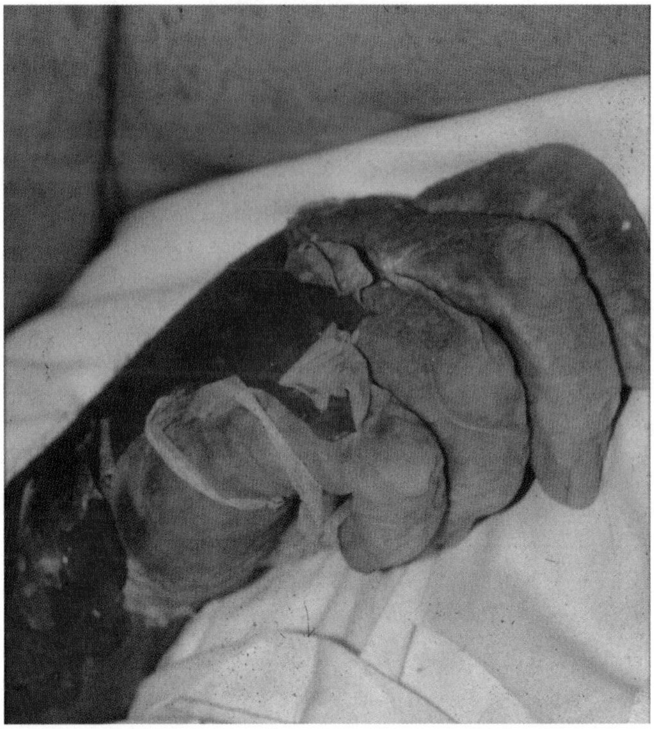

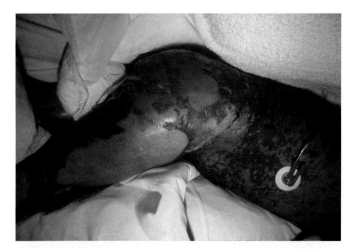

FIGURE 170-10 TEN with desquamation of skin on the hand. (*Courtesy of the University of Texas Health Sciences Center, Division of Dermatology.*)

FIGURE 170-11 TEN with large areas of desquamation on the leg. (*Courtesy of the University of Texas Health Sciences Center, Division of Dermatology.*)

REFERENCES

1. Shaw JC. Erythema multiforme. In: Noble J, Green H, Levinson W, et al., eds. *Textbook of Primary Care Medicine*. 3rd ed. St. Louis, MO: Mosby, 2001:815–816.

2. Pruksachatkunakorn C, Schachner LA. Erythema Multiforme. http://www.emedicine.com/derm/topic137.htm Accessed March 7, 2007.

3. Darmstadt GL. Erythema multiforme. In: Long S, Pickering L, Prober C, eds. *Principles and Practice of Pediatric Infectious Diseases*. 2nd ed. New York, NY: Churchill Livingstone, 2003:442–444.

4. Vesiculobullous disorders. In: Behrman R, Kliegman RM, Jenson HB, eds. *Nelson Textbook of Pediatrics*. 17th ed. Philadelphia, Saunders, 2004:2182–2184.

5. Weston WL. Herpes associated erythema multiforme. *J Invest Dermatol*. 2005;124(6):xv–xvi.

6. Chosidow OM, Stern RS, Wintroub BU. Cutaneous drug reactions. In: Kasper DL, Fauci AS, Longo DL, Braunwald EB, Hauser SL, Jameson JL, eds. *Harrison's Principles of Internal Medicine*. 16th ed. New York, NY: McGraw-Hill, 2005:318–324.

7. Habif T: *Clinical Dermatology*. 4th ed. Philadelphia: Mosby, 2004:627–631.

8. Newburger JW, Takahashi M, Gerber MA, et al. Diagnosis, treatment, and long-term management of Kawasaki disease: A statement for health professionals from the Committee on Rheumatic Fever, Endocarditis and Kawasaki Disease, Council on Cardiovascular Disease in the Young, American Heart Association. *Circulation*. 2004;110(17):2747–2771.

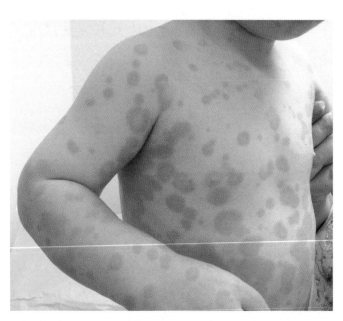

FIGURE 170-12 Urticarial drug reaction with annular lesions that are often mistaken for EM. Note there is no epidermal disruption as seen with the vesicles, bulla, or crusts in the other cases. (*Courtesy of Linda Maidment, MD.*)

171 ERYTHEMA NODOSUM

Richard Paulis, MD

PATIENT STORY

A young woman presented to the office with several days of overall malaise, fever, and sore throat. At the time of presentation she noted some painful bumps on her lower legs, and denied trauma (**Figure 171-1**). No history of recent cough or change in bowel habits has been reported. Patient was otherwise healthy and took no medications and had no known drug allergies. Her temperature was slightly elevated, but other vitals were normal. On examination, her oropharynx revealed tonsillar erythema and exudates. Bilateral lower extremities were spotted with slightly-raised, tender, erythematous nodules that varied in size from 2 to 6 cm. Rapid strep test was positive and she was diagnosed with erythema nodosum (EN) secondary to group A β-hemolytic strep. Patient was treated with penicillin and NSAIDs and was advised bedrest. She experienced complete resolution of the EN within 4 weeks.

EPIDEMIOLOGY

- EN is the most frequent septal panniculitis (inflammation of the septa of fat lobules in the subcutaneous tissue).[1]
- EN tends to occur more often in women in the adult population, generally during second and fourth decade of life (**Figures 171-1 to 171-3**).
- In one study, an overall incidence of 54 million people worldwide was cited in patients older than 14 years.[2]
- In the childhood form, the female predilection is not seen.

ETIOLOGY

Most EN is idiopathic (**Figures 171-3** and **171-4**). While the exact percentage is unknown, one study estimated that 55% of EN is idiopathic.[3] This may be influenced by the fact that EN may precede the underlying illness by more than 2 years.[4] The distribution of etiologic causes may be seasonal.[5] Identifiable causes can be infectious, reactive, pharmacologic, or neoplastic.

- Group A β-hemolytic streptococcal pharyngitis has been linked to EN (**Figure 171-1**).
  - A retrospective study of 129 cases of EN over several decades reports 28% had streptococcal infection.[3]
  - Nonstreptococcal upper respiratory tract infections may also play a role.[4]
- Historically, tuberculosis (TB) was a common underlying illness with EN, but TB is now a rare cause of EN.
  - There are reports of EN occurring in patients receiving the bacille Calmette–Guérin vaccination.[6]

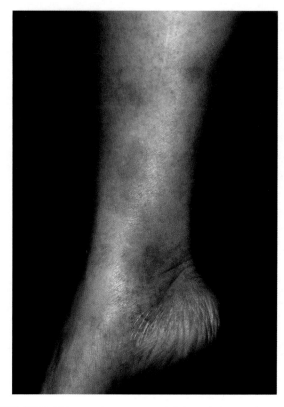

FIGURE 171-1 EN secondary to group A β-hemolytic strep in a young woman. (*Courtesy of Richard P. Usatine, MD.*)

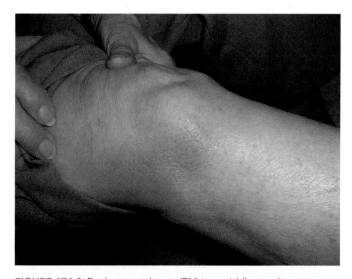

FIGURE 171-2 Erythema nodosum (EN) in a middle-aged woman around the knee secondary to sarcoidosis. (*Courtesy of Richard P. Usatine, MD.*)

- EN occurs in 3% of all patients with coccidiomycosis.[4]

- EN is less frequently associated with toxoplasmosis, syphilis, amebiasis, giardiasis, brucellosis, leprosy, and bartonella.[2]

- On of the most common noninfectious causes of EN is sarcoidosis. One study estimates sarcoidosis as being the cause of 11% of EN cases (**Figure 171-2**).[3]

- When the EN rash occurs with hilar adenopathy, the entity is called Lofgren's syndrome.
  - Lofgren's syndrome in TB represents primary infection.
  - A more common cause of Lofgren's syndrome is sarcoidosis.[7]

- The literature reports that EN is seen in patients with inflammatory bowel diseases.
  - Usually prominent around the time of gastrointestinal flare-ups, but may occur before a flare.
  - Most sources report a greater association between Crohn's disease and EN than ulcerative colitis and EN.

- Some debate exists over causality from pregnancy and oral contraceptives in the occurrence of EN.
  - The major known epidemiologic grouping for EN may have one or both of the preceding causes.

- Besides oral contraceptives, medications implicated as causing EN are antibiotics including sulfonamides and bromides. However, these may have been prescribed for the underlying infection that had caused EN.[4]

- Lymphomas are associated with EN.

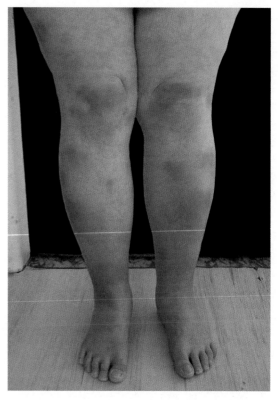

FIGURE 171-3 EN in a middle-aged woman with no known cause. These lesions are bright red, warm and painful. (*Courtesy of Dr. Hanuš Rozsypal.*)

PATHOPHYSIOLOGY

From the aforementioned diversity in etiology, EN is likely a cutaneous reactive process for which the skin has limited expressions.

- Histologic examination is most useful in defining EN.
  - Defining characteristics of EN are a septal panniculitis without presence of vasculitis.
  - That this pattern develops in certain areas of skin may be linked to local variations in temperature and efficient blood drainage.
  - Septal panniculitis begins with polymorphonuclear cells infiltrating the septa of fat lobules in the subcutaneous tissue.
  - It is thought that this is in response to existing immune complex deposition in these areas.[7]
  - This inflammatory change consists of edema and hemorrhage which is responsible for the nodularity, warmth, and erythema.
  - The infiltrate progresses from predominantly polymorphonuclear cells, to lymphocytes, and then histiocytes where fibrosis occurs around the lobules.
  - There may be some necrosis though minimal as complete resolution without scarring is the typical course.

- The histopathologic hallmark of EN is the Miescher's radial granuloma. This is a small, well-defined nodular aggregate of small histiocytes around a central stellate or banana-shaped cleft.

CLINICAL FEATURES

- The lesions of EN are deep-seated nodules that may be more easily palpated than visualized.

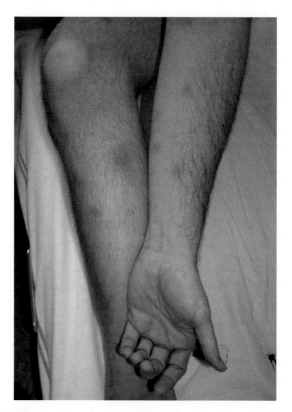

FIGURE 171-4 EN on the arms and legs of unknown cause in a young man. (*Courtesy of Dr. Hanuš Rozsypal.*)

- Lesions are initially firm, round or oval, and are poorly demarcated.
- Lesions may be bright red, warm, and painful (**Figure 171-3**).
- Lesions number from one to greater than 10.[5]
- Lesions vary in size from 1 to 15 cm.
- Over their course, the lesions begin to flatten and change to a purplish color before eventually taking on the yellowish hue of a bruise.
- A characteristic of EN is the complete resolution of lesions with no ulceration or scarring.
- A generally accepted feature of EN is systemic occurrence of fever, malaise, and polyarthralgia sometime near eruption.

LOCATION

- Lesions appear on the anterior/lateral aspect of both lower extremities (**Figures 171-1** to **171-3**).
- Although lesions may appear in other regions such as the arms, absence in the lower legs is unusual (**Figure 171-4**).[4]
- Sarcoid, in particular, may present with lesions on the ankles and knees (**Figure 171-2**).
- Lesions may appear in dependent areas in bedridden patients.

LABORATORY STUDIES

- The diagnosis of EN is mostly made on physical examination. When the diagnosis is uncertain, a biopsy that includes subcutaneous fat is performed. This can be a deep punch biopsy or a deep incisional biopsy sent for standard histology. If a biopsy is needed, this can be done by choosing a lesion not over a joint or vital structure and burying a 4 mm punch biopsy to the hilt.
- Blood tests may help to identify the underlying cause. Typical tests include complete blood count, chemistries, liver function tests, and erythrocyte sedimentation rate. Erythrocyte sedimentation rate may be elevated.
- For suspected strep cases, rapid strep test or throat cultures are best during acute illness while antistreptolysin O titers may be used in the convalescent phase.[2]
- In sarcoid, angiotensin converting enzyme levels may be helpful but are not 100% sensitive.[1] A chest x-ray and/or skin biopsy of a suspected sarcoid lesion can help make this diagnosis (see Chapter 168, Sarcoidosis).

DIFFERENTIAL DIAGNOSIS

- Cellulitis should be considered and not missed. These patients tend to be sicker and have more fever and systemic symptoms. EN tends to appear in multiple locations while cellulitis is usually is one localized area (see Chapter 114, Cellulitis).
- Nodular cutaneous and subcutaneous sarcoid is skin-colored or violaceous without epidermal involvement. The lack of surface involvement makes this resemble EN. Subcutaneous sarcoid may be

seen in advanced systemic sarcoidosis that can also be the cause of EN. Skin biopsy is the best method to distinguish between these two conditions. Either way, treatment is directed toward the sarcoidosis (see Chapter 168, Sarcoidosis).

- Erythema induratum of Bazin is a lobular panniculitis that occurs on the posterior lower extremity of women with tendency of lesions to ulcerate with residual scarring.[7] This condition is typically caused by TB and is more chronic in nature than EN.[1]
- Cutaneous polyarteritis nodosa may present with tender calf lesions, but these, like erythema induratum of Bazin, tend to ulcerate. EN does not ulcerate.

MANAGEMENT

- Look for and treat the underlying cause. There is limited evidence to guide treatment unless an underlying cause is found.
- Treat the pain and discomfort of the nodules with NSAIDs and/or other analgesics. SOR **C**
- Cool wet compresses, elevation of the involved extremities, and bedrest may help alleviate the pain. SOR **C**
- The value of oral prednisone is controversial and should be avoided unless it is being used to treat the underlying cause (such as sarcoidosis). SOR **C**
- Potassium iodide, which is contraindicated in pregnancy, has shown success.[5,7] SOR **C**
- Colchicine, hydroxychloroquine, and dapsone have been used as well.[1,7] SOR **C**

PATIENT EDUCATION

Reassure the patient that there is complete resolution in most cases within 3 to 6 weeks. Inform the patient that some EN outbreaks may persist for up to 12 weeks, and some cases are recurrent.[5]

FOLLOW-UP

Follow-up is needed to complete the work-up for an underlying cause and to make sure that the patient is responding to symptomatic treatment.

PATIENT RESOURCE

http://health.groups.yahoo.com/group/erythema_nodosum_G/.

PROVIDER RESOURCE

http://www.emedicine.com/derm/topic138.htm.

REFERENCES

1. Atzeni F, Carrabba M, Davin JC, et al. Skin manifestations in vasculitis and erythema nodosum. *Clin Exp Rheumatol*. 2006;24(1 Suppl 40):S60–S66.

2. Gonzalez-Gay MA, Garcia-Porrua C, Pujol RM, Salvarani C. Erythema nodosum: A clinical approach. *Clin Exp Rheumatol*. 2001; 19(4):365–368.

3. Cribier B, Caille A, Heid E, Grosshans E. Erythema nodosum and associated diseases. A study of 129 cases. *Int J Dermatol*. 1998; 37(9):667–672.

4. Shojania KG. Erythema nodosum. http://www.uptodate.com. 2007. Accessed March, 2007.

5. Hannuksela M. Erythema nodosum. *Clin Dermatol*. 1986;4(4): 88–95.

6. Fox MD, Schwartz RA. Erythema nodosum. *Am Fam Physician*. 1992;46(3):818–822.

7. Requena L, Requena C. Erythema nodosum. *Dermatol Online J*. 2002;8(1):4.

172 CUTANEOUS VASCULITIS

E.J. Mayeaux, Jr., MD
Richard P. Usatine, MD

PATIENT STORY

A 21-year-old woman presented with a 3-day history of a painful purpuric rash on her lower extremities (**Figures 172-1** and **172-2**). The lesions had appeared suddenly, and the patient had experienced no prior similar episodes. The patient had been diagnosed with a case of pharyngitis earlier that week and was given a course of clindamycin. She had not experienced any nausea or vomiting, fever, abdominal cramping, or gross hematuria. Urine dipstick revealed blood in her urine, but no protein. The typical palpable purpura on the legs is consistent with Henoch–Schönlein purpura (HSP).

EPIDEMIOLOGY

- Cutaneous vasculitic diseases are classified according to the size (small versus medium to large vessel) and type of blood vessel involved (venule, arteriole, artery, or vein).

- Small- and medium-sized vessels are found in the dermis and deep reticular dermis, respectively. The clinical presentation varies with the intensity of the inflammation, and the size and type of blood vessel involved.[1]

- HSP (**Figures 172-1** and **172-2**) occurs mainly in children and results from IgA-containing immune complexes in blood vessel walls in the skin, kidney, and gastrointestinal tract. HSP is usually benign and self-limiting, and tends to occur in the springtime. A streptococcal or viral upper respiratory infection often precedes the disease by 1 to 3 weeks. Prodromal symptoms include anorexia and fever. In half of the cases, there are recurrences, typically in the first 3 months. Recurrences are more common in patients with nephritis and are milder than the original episode.

- Some patients with systemic lupus erythematosus (SLE) (**Figures 172-3** and **172-4**), rheumatoid arthritis (RA), relapsing polychondritis, and other connective tissue disorders develop an associated vasculitis. It most frequently involves the small muscular arteries, arterioles, and venules. The propensity for involvement of internal organs varies with the underlying disorder.

- Leukocytoclastic vasculitis (**Figures 172-5** to **172-8**) is the most commonly seen form of small vessel vasculitis. Prodromal symptoms include fever, malaise, myalgia, and joint pain. The palpable purpura begins as asymptomatic localized areas of cutaneous hemorrhage that become palpable. Few or many discrete lesions are most commonly seen on the lower extremities but may occur on any dependent area. Small lesions itch and are painful, but nodules, ulcers, and bullae may be very painful. Lesions appear in crops, last for 1 to 4 weeks, and may heal with residual scarring and hyperpigmentation. Patients may experience one episode (drug reaction or

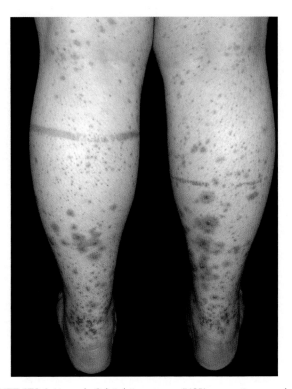

FIGURE 172-1 Henoch–Schönlein purpura (HSP) presenting as palpable purpura on the lower extremity. The visible sock lines are from lesions that formed where the socks exerted pressure on the legs. (*Courtesy of Richard P. Usatine, MD.*)

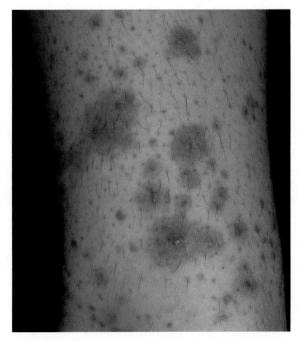

FIGURE 172-2 Closeup of palpable purpura from the patient in **Figure 172-1**. Some lesions look like target lesions but this is HSP and not erythema multiforme. (*Courtesy of Richard P. Usatine, MD.*)

viral infection) or multiple episodes (RA or SLE). The disease is usually self-limited and confined to the skin.

  ○ Systemic manifestations of leukocytoclastic vasculitis may include kidney disease, heart, nervous system, gastrointestinal tract, lungs, and joint involvement.

ETIOLOGY AND PATHOPHYSIOLOGY

• Vasculitis is defined as inflammation of the blood vessel wall. All forms of vasculitis are either autoimmune or allergic (immune-complex) phenomenon.

• Vasculitis induced injury to blood vessels may lead to increased vascular permeability, vessel weakening, causing aneurysm formation or hemorrhage, and intimal proliferation and thrombosis that result in obstruction and local ischemia.[2]

• Small vessel vasculitis is initiated by hypersensitivity to various antigens (drugs, chemicals, microorganisms, and endogenous antigens), with formation of circulating immune complexes that are deposited in walls of postcapillary venules. The vessel-bound immune complexes activate complement, which attracts polymorphonuclear leukocytes. They damage the walls of small veins by release of lysosomal enzymes. This causes vessel necrosis and local hemorrhage.

• Small-vessel vasculitis most commonly affects the skin and rarely causes serious internal organ dysfunction, except when the kidney is involved. Small vessel vasculitis is associated with leukocytoclastic vasculitis, HSP, essential mixed cryoglobulinemia, connective tissue diseases or malignancies, serum sickness and serum sickness-like reactions, chronic urticaria, and acute hepatitis B or C infection.

• Leukocytoclastic (hypersensitivity) vasculitis causes acute inflammation and necrosis of venules in the dermis. The term leukocytoclastic vasculitis describes the histologic pattern produced when leukocytes fragment.

DIAGNOSIS

• Initially, determining the extent of visceral organ involvement is more important than identifying the type of vasculitis, so that organs at risk of damage are not jeopardized by delayed or inadequate treatment. It is critical to distinguish vasculitis occurring as a primary autoimmune disorder from vasculitis secondary to infection, drugs, malignancy, or connective tissue disease such as SLE or RA.[2]

CLINICAL FEATURES

Small vessel vasculitis is characterized by necrotizing inflammation of small blood vessels, and may be identified by the finding of "palpable purpura." The lower extremities typically demonstrate "palpable purpura," varying in size from a few millimeters to several centimeters

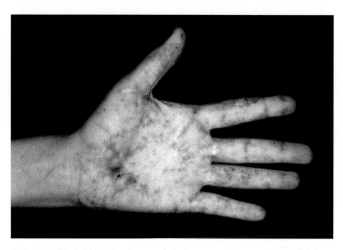

FIGURE 172-3 Necrotizing vasculitis in a young Asian woman with systemic lupus erythematosus (SLE). The circulation to the fingertips was compromised and the woman was treated with high-dose intravenous steroids and intravenous immunoglobulins to prevent tissue loss. (*Courtesy of Richard P. Usatine, MD.*)

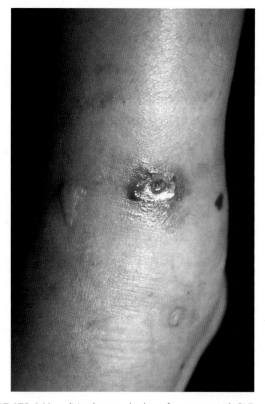

FIGURE 172-4 Vasculitis ulcer on the leg of a woman with SLE. (*Courtesy of Everett Allen, MD.*)

(**Figures 172-2, 172-6,** and **172-7**). In its early stages leukocytoclastic vasculitis may not be palpable (**Figure 172-5**).

The clinical features of HSP include nonthrombocytopenic palpable purpura mainly on the lower extremities and buttocks (**Figures 172-1** and **172-2**), gastrointestinal symptoms, arthralgia, and nephritis.

TYPICAL DISTRIBUTION

Cutaneous vasculitis is found most commonly on the legs, but may be seen on the hands and abdomen (**Figures 172-3** and **172-8**).

LABORATORY STUDIES

Laboratory evaluation is geared to finding the antigenic source of the immunologic reaction. Consider throat culture, antistreptolysin-O titer, erythrocyte sedimentation rate, platelets, CBC, serum creatinine, urinalysis, antinuclear antibody, serum protein electrophoresis, circulating immune complexes, hepatitis B surface antigen, hepatitis C antibody, cryoglobulins, and rheumatoid factor. The erythrocyte sedimentation rate is almost always elevated during active vasculitis. Immunofluorescent studies are best done within the first 24 hours after a lesion forms. The most common immunoreactants present in and around blood vessels are IgM, C3, and fibrin. The presence of IgA in blood vessels of a child with vasculitis suggests the diagnosis of HSP.

Basic laboratory analysis to assess the degree and types of organs affected should include serum creatinine, creatanine kinase, liver function studies, hepatitis serologies, urinalysis, and possibly chest x-ray and electrocardiogram.

BIOPSY

The clinical presentation is so characteristic that a biopsy is generally unnecessary. In doubtful cases, a punch biopsy should be taken from an early active (nonulcerated) lesion or, if necessary, from the edge of an ulcer (**Figure 172-4**).

DIFFERENTIAL DIAGNOSIS

- Schamberg's disease (**Figure 172-9**) is a capillaritis characterized by extravasation of erythrocytes in the skin with marked hemosiderin deposition.
- Meningococcemia that presents with purpura in severely ill patients with central nervous system symptoms (**Figures 172-10** and **172-11**).
- Rocky mountain spotted fever is a rickettsial infection that presents with pink to bright red, discrete 1 to 5 mm macules that blanch with pressure and may be pruritic. The lesions start distally and spread to the soles and palms (**Figure 172-12**).
- Malignancies, such as cutaneous T-cell lymphoma (mycosis fungoides) (see Chapter 169, Mycosis Fungoides).
- Stevens–Johnson syndrome and toxic epidermal necrolysis (see Chapter 170, Hypersensitivity Syndromes).
- Idiopathic thrombocytopenia purpura can be easily distinguished from vasculitis by measuring the platelet count.

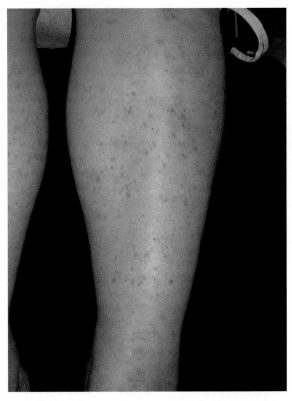

FIGURE 172-5 Mild leukocytoclastic vasculitis in a middle-aged woman. The patient was asymptomatic but was worried about the new rash on her legs. (*Courtesy of Richard P. Usatine, MD.*)

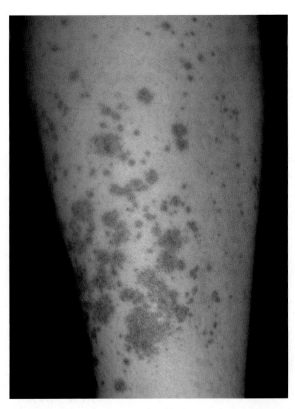

FIGURE 172-6 More severe episode of leukocytoclastic vasculitis in the woman in **Figure 172-5** months later. (*Courtesy of Richard P. Usatine, MD.*)

- Wegener granulomatosis is an unusual multisystem disease characterized by necrotizing granulomatous inflammation and vasculitis of the respiratory tract, kidneys, and skin.
- Churg–Strauss syndrome (Allergic granulomatosis) that presents with a systemic vasculitis associated with asthma, transient pulmonary infiltrates, and hypereosinophilia.
- Cutaneous manifestations of cholesterol embolism which are leg pain, livedo reticularis (blue–red mottling of the skin in a netlike pattern,) and/or blue toes in the presence of good peripheral pulses.

MANAGEMENT

- An antihistamine might be used for itching associated with urticaria. The offending antigen should be identified and removed whenever possible. No other treatment may be necessary. SOR ⓒ
- In leukocytoclastic (hypersensitivity) vasculitis, the cutaneous lesions usually resolve without sequelae. Visceral involvement (such as kidney and lung) most commonly occurs in HSP, cryoglobulinemia and vasculitis associated with SLE.[2] Extensive internal organ involvement should prompt an investigation for coexistent medium-sized vessel disease and referral to a rheumatologist.
  - Oral prednisone is used to treat visceral involvement and more severe cases of vasculitis of the skin. Short courses of prednisone (60–80 mg/d)[3] are effective and should be tapered slowly.[4,5] SOR ⓑ
  - Colchicine (0.6 mg twice daily for 7–10 days) and Dapsone (100–150 mg/d) may be used to inhibit neutrophil chemotaxis. SOR ⓑ They are tapered and discontinued when lesions resolve. Azathioprine, cyclophosphamide, and methotrexate have also been studied. SOR ⓒ
- In HSP, treatment with nonsteroidal anti-inflammatory drugs is usually preferred. Treatment with corticosteroids may be of more benefit in patients with more severe disease such as more pronounced abdominal pain and renal involvement.[6] SOR ⓑ Adding cyclophosphamide to the steroids may also be effective. SOR ⓒ Azathioprine also may be used.[7]

FOLLOW-UP

Relapses may occur, especially when the precipitating factor is an autoimmune disease. Regular monitoring is necessary.

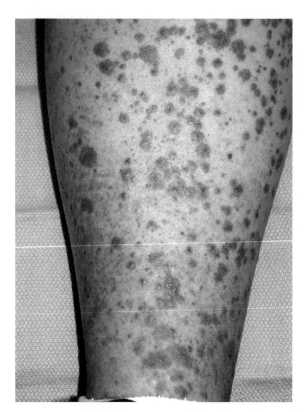

FIGURE 172-7 Very palpable purpura on the leg of a middle-aged woman with leukocytoclastic vasculitis. (*Courtesy of Eric Kraus, MD.*)

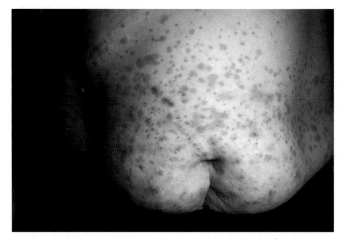

FIGURE 172-8 Vasculitis on the abdomen of a middle-aged woman who also has the vasculitis on her legs. (*Courtesy of Everett Allen, MD.*)

PATIENT RESOURCES

MedicineNet Patient education handout—
http://www.medicinenet.com/vasculitis/article.htm.

MedlinePlus: Vasculitis Multimedia tutorial—**http://www.nlm.nih.gov/medlineplus/tutorials/vasculitis/htm/index.htm.**

National Heart Blood and Lung Institute patent information—
http://www.nhlbi.nih.gov/health/dci/Diseases/vas/vas_whatis.html.

National Kidney and Urologic Diseases Information Clearinghouse patent information—**http://kidney.niddk.nih.gov/kudiseases/pubs/HSP/.**

PROVIDER RESOURCES

Fpnotebook on Vasculitis—**http://www.fpnotebook.com/RHE13.htm.**

AFP. An approach to diagnosis and initial management of systemic vasculitis. (*Am Fam Physician* 1999:60:1421–30)—
http://www.aafp.org/afp/991001ap/1421.html.

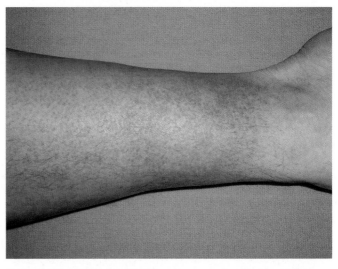

FIGURE 172-9 Schamberg's disease in a man showing hemosiderin deposits and a cayenne pepper small vessel vasculitis. (*Courtesy of Richard P. Usatine, MD.*)

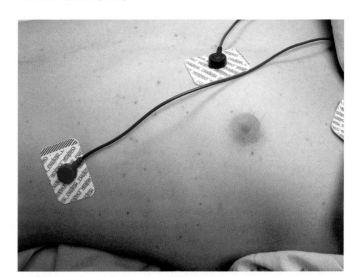

FIGURE 172-10 Petechiae of meningococcemia on the trunk of a hospitalized adolescent. (*Courtesy of Tom Moore, MD.*)

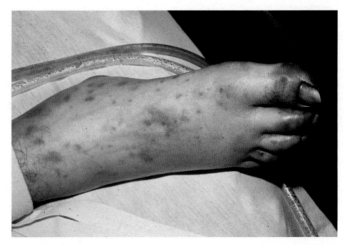

FIGURE 172-11 Petechiae, purpura and acrocyanosis in a severely ill patient with meningococcemia. (*Courtesy of the University of Texas Health Sciences Center Division of Dermatology.*)

REFERENCES

1. Stone JH, Nousari HC. "Essential" cutaneous vasculitis: What every rheumatologist should know about vasculitis of the skin. *Curr Opin Rheumatol.* 2001;13(1):23–34.

2. Roane DW, Griger DR. An approach to diagnosis and initial management of systemic vasculitis. *Am Fam Physician.* 1999;60: 1421–1430.

3. Nurnberg W, Grabbe J, Czarnetzki BM. Urticarial vasculitis syndrome effectively treated with dapsone and pentoxifylline. *Acta Derm Venereol.* 1995;75:54–56.

4. Martinez-Taboada VM, Blanco R, Garcia-Fuentes M, Rodriguez-Valverde V. Clinical features and outcome of 95 patients with hypersensitivity vasculitis. *Am J Med.* 1997;102:186–191.

5. Sais G, Vidaller A, Jucgla A, et al. Colchicine in the treatment of cutaneous leukocytoclastic vasculitis. Results of a prospective, randomized controlled trial. *Arch Dermatol.* 1995;131:1399–1402.

6. Weiss PF, Feinstein JA, Luan X, et al. Effects of corticosteroid on Henoch-Schonlein purpura: A systematic review. *Pediatrics* 2007; 120:1079–1087.

7. Saulsbury FT. Henoch-Schönlein purpura. *Curr Opin Rheumatol.* 2001;13:35–40.

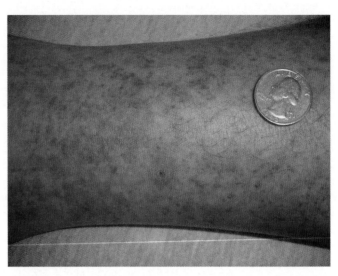

FIGURE 172-12 Rocky mountain spotted fever with many petechiae visible around the original tick bite. This rickettsial disease looks similar to vasculitis. (*Courtesy of Tom Moore, MD.*)

SECTION 15   CONNECTIVE TISSUE DISEASE

173 LUPUS ERYTHEMATOSUS (SYSTEMIC AND CUTANEOUS)

E.J. Mayeaux, Jr., MD

PATIENT STORY

A 39-year-old black woman presented to the clinic with 2 months of swelling of her upper lip and cheeks with new dark spots on her face (**Figure 173-1**). An antinuclear antibody (ANA) was positive at a 1:80 dilution. A homogeneous nuclear pattern was present as commonly seen in systemic lupus erythematosus (SLE) and drug-induced lupus. The punch biopsy of a facial lesion was consistent with chronic cutaneous lupus erythematosus. The remainder of her laboratory tests were normal. The patient's facial lesions did not respond to topical steroids and hence she was started on a short course of systemic steroids. The improvement was seen 3 weeks later (**Figure 173-2**). Hyperpigmentation remained but erythema, swelling, and pruritus were gone.

EPIDEMIOLOGY

- In the United States, the prevalence of SLE plus incomplete SLE (disease only partially meeting diagnostic requirements for SLE) is 40 to 50 cases per 100,000 persons.[1] It is more common in women and patients with African ancestry.[1]

- Discoid lupus (DL) develops in up to 25% of patients with SLE, but may also occur in the absence of any other clinical feature of SLE.[2] Patients with only cutaneous DL have a 5% to 10% risk of eventually developing SLE, which tends to follow a mild course.[3] DL lesions usually slowly expand with active inflammation at the periphery, and then to heal, leaving depressed central scars, atrophy, telangiectasias, and hypopigmentation.[4] The female–male ratio of discoid lupus erythematosus (DLE) is 2:1.

ETIOLOGY AND PATHOPHYSIOLOGY

- Many of the signs and symptoms of LE are caused by circulating immune complexes or by the direct effects of antibodies to cells.

- A genetic predisposition for SLE exists. The concordance rate in monozygotic twins is between 25% and 70%. If a mother has SLE, her daughter's risk of developing the disease is 1:40 and her son's risk is 1:250.

- The course of SLE is one of intermittent remissions punctuated by disease flares. Organ damage often progresses over time.

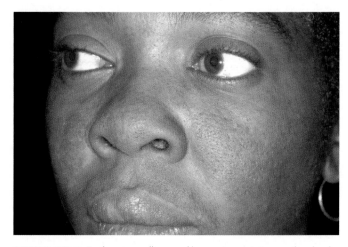

FIGURE 173-1 Erythema, swelling, and hyperpigmentation on the cheeks and lips of a 39-year-old black woman as the initial presentation of chronic cutaneous lupus erythematosus. (*From Hochberg MD. Cupdating the American College of Rheumatology revised criteria for the classification of SLE [letter]. Arthritis Rheum. 1997;40:1725.*)

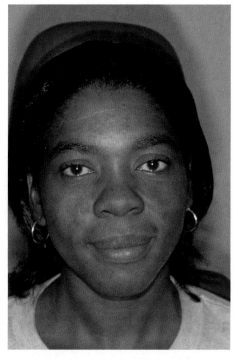

FIGURE 173-2 Hyperpigmented malar rash 3 weeks later; the patient was treated with oral and topical steroids. The erythema and swelling are now gone and patient is feeling better. (*Courtesy of Richard P. Usatine, MD.*)

- Rarely, neonates may develop a lupus rush from acquired antibodies through transplacental transmission from mother if she has active SLE (**Figure 173-3**).

DIAGNOSIS

CLINICAL FEATURES

- SLE is a chronic, recurrent, potentially fatal inflammatory disorder that can be difficult to diagnose. It is an autoimmune disease involving multiple organ systems that is defined clinically with associated autoantibodies directed against cell nuclei. The disease has no single diagnostic sign or marker. Accurate diagnosis is important because treatment can reduce morbidity and mortality.[5]

- SLE most often presents with a mixture of constitutional symptoms. The mean length of time between onset of symptoms and diagnosis is 5 years.

- The disease is characterized by exacerbations and remissions as well as symptoms. The diagnosis of SLE is made if four or more of the manifestations mentioned below are either present, serially or simultaneously, in the patient at the time of presentation or were present in the past. If two to three manifestations are present, some clinicians refer to the syndrome as "incomplete lupus."[6]

  ○ Systemic symptoms such as low-grade fever, fatigue, malaise, anorexia, nausea, and weight loss.

  ○ Arthralgias, which are often the initial complaint, are usually out of proportion to physical findings. The polyarthritis is symmetric, nonerosive, and usually nondeforming. In longstanding disease, rheumatoid-like deformities with swan-neck fingers are commonly seen.

  ○ A malar or butterfly rash is fixed erythema over the cheeks and bridge of the nose sparing the nasolabial folds (**Figures 173-2, 173-4,** and **173-5**). It may also involve the chin and ears. More severe malar rashes may cause severe atrophy, scarring, and hypopigmentation (**Figure 173-5**).

  ○ Rash associated with photosensitivity to ultraviolet (UV) light.

  ○ A discoid rash consisting of erythematosus raised patches with adherent keratotic scaling and follicular plugging. Atrophic scarring may occur in older lesions.

  ○ Ulcers (usually painless) in the nose, mouth, or vagina are frequent complaints.

  ○ Pleurities as evidenced by a convincing history of pleuritic pain or rub or evidence of pleural effusion.

  ○ Pericarditis as documented by EKG, rub, or evidence of pericardial effusion.

  ○ Renal disorder such as cellular casts or persistent proteinuria >0.5 g/d or $>3+$ if quantitation not performed.

  ○ Central nervous system (CNS) symptoms ranging from mild cognitive dysfunction to psychosis or seizures. Any region of CNS can be involved. Intractable headaches and difficulties with memory and reasoning are the most common features of neurologic disease in lupus patients.

  ○ Hematologic disorders such as hemolytic anemia, leukopenia ($<4000/mm^3$ total on two or more occasions), lymphopenia ($<1500/mm^3$ on two or more occasions), or thrombocytopenia ($<100,000/mm^3$ in the absence of precipitating drugs).

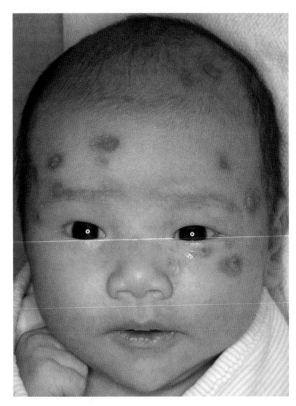

FIGURE 173-3 Neonatal lupus from acquired antibodies through transplacental transmission from the mother with active SLE. (*From Warner AM, Frey KA, Connolly S. Photo Rounds: Annular rash on a newborn. J Fam Pract 2006;55(2):128–129, Dowden Health Media.*)

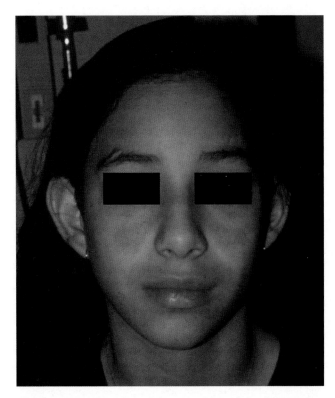

FIGURE 173-4 Malar rash in adolescent Hispanic girl with SLE. Note the relative sparing of the nasolabial fold. (*Courtesy of the University of Texas Health Sciences Center, Division of Dermatology*).

○ GI symptoms may include abdominal pain, diarrhea, and vomiting. Intestinal perforation and vasculitis are important diagnoses to exclude.

○ Vasculitis (**Figures 173-6** and **173-7**) can be severe and can include retinal vasculitis.

○ Immunologic disorders such as a positive antiphospholipid antibody, anti-DNA, anti-SM, or a false positive serologic test for syphilis (known to be positive for at least 6 months and confirmed by a negative treponema specific test).

○ An abnormal titer of antinuclear antibody at any point in time and in the absence of durgs associated with "drug-induced lupus."

• DL lesions are characterized by discrete, erythematous, slightly infiltrated papule or plaques covered by a well-formed adherent scale (**Figures 173-8** to **173-11**). As the lesion progresses, the scale often thickens and becomes adherent. Hypopigmentation develops in the central area and hyperpigmentation develops at the active border. Resolution of the active lesion results in atrophy and scarring. When they occur in the scalp, scarring alopecia often results (**Figure 173-11**). If the scale on the scalp is removed, it may leave a "carpet tack sign" from follicular plugging.

TYPICAL DISTRIBUTION

• Discoid lesions are most often seen on the face, neck, and scalp, but also occur on the ears, and infrequently on the upper torso.

○ DLE lesions may be localized or widespread. Localized DLE occurs only in the head and neck area, while widespread DLE occurs anywhere. Patients with widespread involvement are more likely to develop SLE.

LABORATORY STUDIES

• The American College of Rheumatology recommends ANA testing in patients who have two or more unexplained signs or symptoms that could be lupus. Elevation of the ANA titer to or above 1:80 is the most sensitive of the American College of Rheumatology diagnostic criteria. Although many patients may have a negative ANA titer early in the disease, more than 99% of SLE patients will eventually have an elevated ANA titer.[7] The ANA test is not specific for lupus, and the most common reason for a positive ANA test without SLE (usually at titers <1:80) is the presence of another connective tissue disease.

• Patients with only cutaneous DL generally have negative or low-titer ANA titers, and rarely have low titers of anti-Ro antibodies.[8]

DIFFERENTIAL DIAGNOSIS

• Drug-induced lupus is a lupus-like syndrome most strongly associated with procainamide, hydralazine, isoniazid, chlorpromazine, methyldopa, and quinidine.

• Scleroderma presents with thickening of the skin and multi-system sclerosis (see Chapter 175, Scleroderma and Morphea).

• Actinic keratosis on the face may become confluent but lack the systemic symptoms of lupus (see Chapter 159, Actinic Keratosis and Bowen's Disease).

• Dermatomyositis presents with facial swelling, "heliotrope" rash around the eyes, Gottron's papules and periungual erythema in the

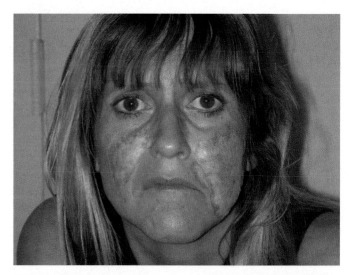

FIGURE 173-5 Malar rash with severe atrophy, scarring, and hypopigmentation in a young woman with arthritis and other signs of more severe systemic lupus. (*Courtesy of Richard P. Usatine, MD.*)

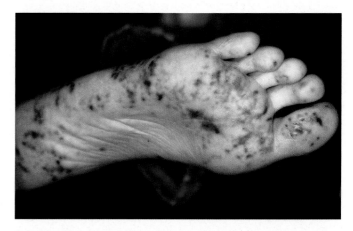

FIGURE 173-6 Necrotizing angiitis in a 28-year-old Japanese American woman with a severe lupus flare. Palpable purpura was evident on both feet and hands. (*Courtesy of Richard P. Usatine, MD.*)

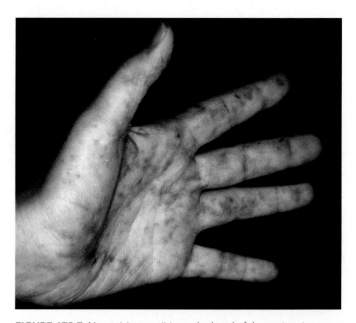

FIGURE 173-7 Necrotizing angiitis on the hand of the patient in **Figure 173-6** with lupus. (*Courtesy of Richard P. Usatine, MD.*)

hands, and proximal muscular limb girdle weakness. It is often associated with internal malignancy (see Chapter 174, Dermatomyositis).

- Lichen planus produces a polygonal pruritic purple papular rash (see Chapter 147, Lichen Planus).

- Psoriasis demonstrates silver-white plaques that cover the elbows, knees, scalp, back, or vulva. There may also be nail and scalp involvement (see Chapter 145, Psoriasis).

- Rosacea is associated with mid-facial skin erythema, papules, and pustules without the systemic symptoms of LE, and usually involves the nasolabial folds (see Chapter 107, Rosacea).

- Sarcoidosis may produce skin plaques but without the central clearing and atrophy of LE (see Chapter 168, Sarcoidosis).

- Syphilis may produce a plaque like rash that can be confused with DLE. The short course of the disease and serologic testing can distinguish the diseases. However, lupus autoantibodies may produce a false-positive screening test for syphilis (see Chapter 209, Syphilis).

MANAGEMENT

SYSTEMIC LUPUS ERYTHEMATOSUS

- Conservative management with nonsteroidal anti-inflammatory drugs or cyclooxygenase-2 selective inhibitors is recommended for arthritis, arthralgias, and myalgias. SOR Ⓒ

- Antimalarial drugs (hydroxychloroquine (Plaquenil) 200 mg bid, maximum 6.5 mg/kg/d) most commonly for skin manifestations and for musculoskeletal complaints that do not adequately respond to nonsteroidal anti-inflammatory drugs. They may also prevent major damage to the kidneys and CNS and reduce the risk of disease flares.[9] SOR Ⓑ

- Systemic glucocorticoids (1–2 mg/kg/d of prednisone or equivalent) alone or with immunosuppressive agents for patients with significant renal and CNS disease or any other organ threatening manifestation.[10] SOR Ⓑ Lower doses of glucocorticoids (prednisone 10–20 mg/d) for symptomatic relief of severe or unresponsive musculoskeletal symptoms. In severe, life-threatening situations, methylprednisolone bolus (1 gm IV/d) can be given for 3 consecutive days.

- Immunosuppressive medications (e.g., methotrexate, cyclophosphamide, azathioprine, mycophenolate, or rituximab) are generally reserved for patients with significant organ involvement, or who have had an inadequate response to glucocorticoids. SOR Ⓒ

- Patients with thrombosis, usually associated to the presence of antiphospholipid antibodies, require anticoagulation with warfarin for a target international normalized ratio of 3:3.5 for arterial thrombosis and 2:3 for venous thrombosis.[11]

DISCOID LUPUS ERYTHEMATOSUS

- DLE therapy includes corticosteroids (topical or intralesional) and antimalarials. SOR Ⓒ Alternative therapies include auranofin, oral or topical retinoids, and immunosuppressive agents.

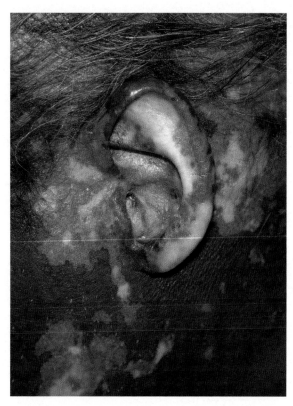

FIGURE 173-8 Discoid lupus in a middle-aged black man with hypopigmentation and scarring of the pinna. (*Courtesy of Richard P. Usatine, MD.*)

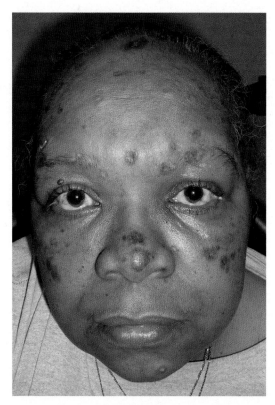

FIGURE 173-9 Discoid lupus on the face and scalp of a 56-year-old woman with hyperpigmented lesions that are indurated and atrophic. She also has similar lesions on the back and has scarring alopecia. (*Courtesy of Richard P. Usatine, MD.*)

PATIENT EDUCATION

- Educate the patient on the necessity of protection from the sun, since UV exposure can cause lupus flares. They should use sun screens, preferably those that block both UV-A and UV-B, with a minimum skin protection factor of 30.

- Since cigarette smoking may increase the risk of developing LE and smokers generally have more active disease, smokers with LE should be counseled to quit smoking.

- Have patients report any signs of superinfection in their rash, since this requires antibiotic therapy (**Figure 173-12**).

- If possible, avoid sulfa drugs, which have been related to lupus flares.

FOLLOW-UP

- The patient should have regular follow-up appointments to monitor for and attempt to prevent end organ damage. Regular follow-up visits are needed to monitor medication benefits and side-effects and to coordinate care of the whole person.

PATIENT RESOURCES

- The National Women's Health Information Center lupus page—**http://www.4 woman.gov/faq/lupus.htm.**
- SLE Foundation Information—**http://www.4 woman.gov/faq/lupus.htm.**
- Lupus foundation of America—**http://www.lupus.org/newsite/index.html.**

PROVIDER RESOURCES

- MedlinePlus lupus information links—**http://www.nlm.nih.gov/medlineplus/lupus.html.**
- Emedicine systemic lupus erythematosus—**http://www.emedicine.com/emerg/topic564.htm.**

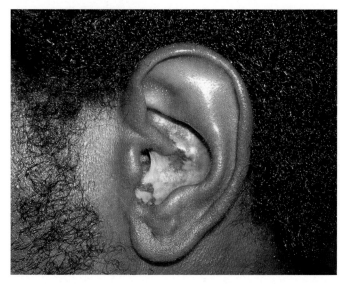

FIGURE 173-10 Discoid lupus with hypopigmentation and scarring inside the pinna. (*Courtesy of E.J. Mayeaux, Jr., MD.*)

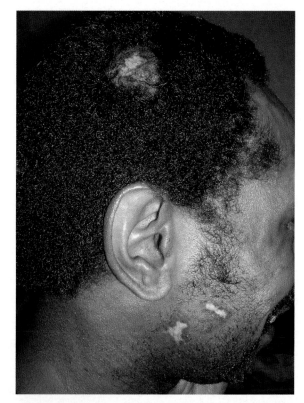

FIGURE 173-11 Discoid lupus with scarring alopecia and hypopigmentation on the scalp and face. (*Courtesy of E.J. Mayeaux, Jr., MD.*)

REFERENCES

1. Lawrence RC, Helmick CG, et al. Estimates of the prevalence of arthritis and selected musculoskeletal disorders in the United States. *Arthritis Rheum*. 1998;41:778–799.

2. Pistiner M, Wallace DJ, Nessim S, et al. Lupus erythematosus in the 1980s: A survey of 570 patients. *Semin Arthritis Rheum*. 1991;21:55.

3. Healy E, Kieran E, Rogers S. Cutaneous lupus erythematosu—a study of clinical and laboratory prognostic factors in 65 patients. *Ir J Med Sci*. 1995;164:113.

4. Rowell NR. Laboratory abnormalities in the diagnosis and management of lupus erythematosus. *Br J Dermatol*. 1971;84:210.

5. Gill JM, Quisel AM, Rocca PV, Walters DT. Diagnosis of systemic lupus erythematosus. *Am Fam Physician*. 2003;68:2179–2186.

6. Hochberg MC. Updating the American College of Rheumatology revised criteria for the classification of SLE [letter]. *Arthritis Rheum*. 1997;40:1725.

7. Tan EM, Cohen AS, Fries JF, et al. The 1982 revised criteria for the classification of systemic lupus erythematosus. *Arthritis Rheum*. 1982;25:1271–1277.

8. Provost TT. The relationship between discoid and systemic lupus erythematosus. *Arch Dermatol*. 1994;130:1308.

9. Fessler BJ, Alarcon GS, McGwin G Jr., et al. Systemic lupus erythematosus in three ethnic groups: XVI. Association of hydroxychloroquine use with reduced risk of damage accrual. *Arthritis Rheum*. 2005;52:1473–1480.

10. Parker BJ, Bruce IN. High dose methylprednisolone therapy for the treatment of severe systemic lupus erythematosus. *Lupus* 2007;16:387–393.

11. Erkan D, Lockshin MD. New treatments for antiphospholipid syndrome. *Rheum Dis Clin N Am*. 2006;32:129–148.

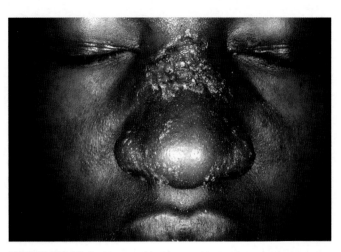

FIGURE 173-12 An 18-year-old girl presenting with crusted sores on her nose and malar rash. This was impetigo over malar rash from new onset SLE. Months later she developed a severe lupus cerebritis. (*Courtesy of Richard P. Usatine, MD.*)

174 DERMATOMYOSITIS

Anna Allred, MD
Richard P. Usatine, MD

PATIENT STORY

A 55-year-old Hispanic woman presented with a widespread rash and increasing muscle weakness. The initial rash 2 months prior was thought to be a photosensitivity reaction to her new hydrochlorothiazide prescription. She stopped the hydrochlorothiazide and the rash initially improved with some topical corticosteroids. At the time of her presentation (**Figures 174-1 to 174-4**), she had trouble getting up from a chair, walking, and lifting her arms over her head. She had the pathognomonic heliotrope rash of dermatomyositis along with Gottron's papules on the fingers (**Figure 174-4**). She also had periungual erythema and a scaly red scalp. Her neurologic examination was consistent with proximal myopathy. She also had some trouble swallowing bread. Muscle enzymes were only slightly raised. The patient was started on 60 mg of prednisone daily and topical steroids for the affected areas. The patient responded well to prednisone and 2 weeks later was (**Figure 174-5**) feeling stronger and the rash was fading. After 6 weeks of 60 mg of prednisone daily she was started on 10 mg of methotrexate weekly in order to eventually taper her steroids. The patient continued to do well but the rash recurred when her steroids were being tapered. The patient was sent for physical therapy and started on calcium supplementation to protect her from steroid-induced osteoporosis. She was also given 1 mg of folic acid a day to minimize the adverse effects of methotrexate. Six months later she was feeling great on 7.5 mg of methotrexate weekly and 20 mg prednisone daily.

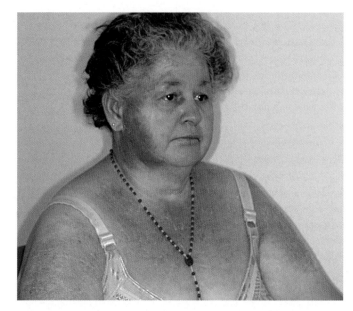

FIGURE 174-1 Initial presentation of dermatomyositis in a 55-year-old Hispanic woman. Prominent violaceous erythema with scale is visible on the chest, face, and arms. Deep red erythema is especially visible on the side of the face. The scalp is red and scaling. (*Courtesy of Richard P. Usatine, MD.*)

EPIDEMIOLOGY

- Rare idiopathic inflammatory disease involving the striated muscles and skin.
  - Progressive symmetrical proximal muscle weakness.
  - Characteristic heliotrope rash (**Figures 174-2, 174-3, 174-5, and 174-6**).
- Annual incidence of 5.5 per million.[1]
- Seen more commonly in women, with a female-to-male ratio of 2:1.[1]
- Affect any age; however, it is more common in children and adults >40 years.[1]
  - Has been linked to malignancy in 15% to 25%, suspect in adults >50 years.[1]
  - Cancers most commonly associated are breast, ovary, lung, and gastrointestinal tract. Ovarian cancer is overrepresented in those patients with dermatomyositis and cancer. Cancer is not typically seen in children with dermatomyositis.

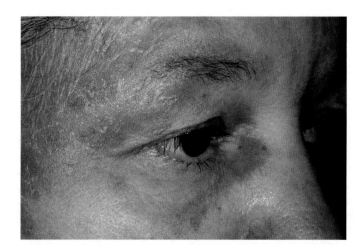

FIGURE 174-2 Close-up of the heliotrope (violaceous) rash around the eyes of the patient in **Figure 174-1**. (*Courtesy of Richard P. Usatine, MD.*)

ETIOLOGY AND PATHOPHYSIOLOGY

- Dermatomyositis is considered an autoimmune disease of unknown etiology. Environmental exposure and infectious agents may play a role in disease pathogenesis.

- Dermatomyositis has been shown to be a microangiopathy that affects the skin and muscle. The muscle weakness and skin manifestations may be a result of activation and deposition of complement, which cause lysis of endomysial capillaries and muscle ischemia.

DIAGNOSIS

CLINICAL FEATURES

- Bilateral periorbital heliotrope erythema (pathognomonic (**Figures 174-2, 174-3, 174-5** and **174-6**)) and scaling violaceous papular dermatitis in a patient complaining of proximal muscle weakness points to dermatomyositis.

- The patient may classically complain of difficulty climbing stairs, rising from a seat, or combing their hair. Notably the skin manifestations may precede, follow, or present simultaneously with muscle involvement; a patient may even have skin manifestations for greater than a year prior to developing muscle weakness.

- Hand involvement includes abnormal nail folds and Gottron's papules. "Moth-eaten" cuticles, also called the Samitz sign, evidenced by periungual erythema and telangiectasias (**Figures 174-7** to **174-9**).

- Gottron's papules, smooth, purple to red papules and plaques are classically located over the knuckles and on the sides of fingers (**Figures 174-4, 174-7** and **174-8**). Plaques may be present over the knuckles instead of or in addition to papules. The papules are much more evident upon presentation of juvenile-onset dermatomyositis (**Figure 174-8**).

TYPICAL DISTRIBUTION

- Face—the characteristic heliotrope rash occurs around the eyes. The color "heliotrope" is a pink-purple tint named after the color of the heliotrope flower. This color is best seen in **Figure 174-6**. The heliotrope rash can also be a dusky-red color as seen in the **Figures 174-1** to **174-5**. This heliotrope rash is bilaterally symmetrical.

- Hands—There is usually hand involvement with Gottron's papules (and plaques) and abnormal nail folds and cuticles (**Figures 174-4** and **174-7** to **174-9**).

- Neck and upper trunk—a red or poikiloderma-type rash can be seen in a V-neck (**Figure 174-10**) or in a shawl distribution. Poikiloderma refers to hyperpigmentation of the skin demonstrating a variety of shades and associated with telangiectasias. The rash here can be scaling and look psoriasiform.

- Extremities may have erythematous plaques and papules with scale.

- Scalp is often involved with erythema and scale and appears similar to seborrhea or psoriasis.

- Sun exposed areas are often involved and worsen with sun exposure. This is why so many of the skin findings are on the face and upper chest. However, patients rarely complain of sun sensitivity.

LABORATORY STUDIES AND DIAGNOSTIC TESTS

- Elevated muscle enzymes, evidence of inflammation on EMG and inflammatory infiltrates on muscle biopsy confirm the diagnosis of dermatomyositis. The following serum muscle enzymes can be drawn during the acute active phase and may be found to be elevated: creatine kinase, lactate dehydrogenase, alanine aminotransferase, aspartate aminotransferase, and aldolase. Of

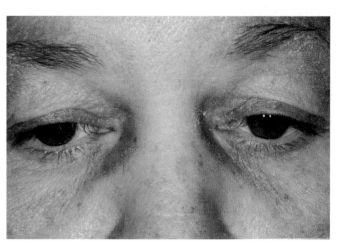

FIGURE 174-3 View showing the bilateral heliotrope rash of the patient in **Figure 174-1**. A pathognomonic sign of dermatomyositis. (*Courtesy of Richard P. Usatine, MD.*)

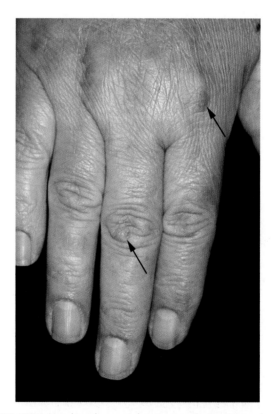

FIGURE 174-4 Hand involvement showing two Gottron's papules over the knuckles (*arrows*) end erythematous nail folds (periungual erythema) in the patient in **Figure 174-1**. (*Courtesy of Richard P. Usatine, MD.*)

note, it is necessary to measure all of the aforementioned enzymes as only one of them may be elevated.

- The diagnosis may be made with confidence in a patient with characteristic skin findings and elevated muscle enzymes. If the presentation is not straightforward, then electromyography and muscle biopsy should be performed.

- The diagnosis can be supported with positive antibodies such as ANA, anti-Mi-2 and anti-Jo-1. It is not necessary to order these antibodies to make the diagnosis of dermatomyositis. In fact these myositis-specific antibodies are only positive in 30% of patients with dermatomyositis. Patients with anti-Mi-2 generally have a better overall prognosis.

- Other papulosquamous diseases such as lichen planus and psoriasis may be differentiated from dermatomyositis with a punch biopsy, but the histology of dermatomyositis is indistinguishable from cutaneous lupus erythematosus.

DIFFERENTIAL DIAGNOSIS

- Polymyositis is another form of inflammatory myopathy. It is distinguished from dermatomyositis by its lack of cutaneous involvement. Dermatomyositis can also occur without muscle involvement. This is called dermatomyositis sine myositis or amyopathic dermatomyositis.

- Polymorphous light eruption or other photosensitivity reactions may be mistaken for the dermatologic findings of dermatomyositis. As in the case of our patient, her cutaneous findings preceded her muscle weakness and the cutaneous findings were only in light-exposed areas. Therefore, it is essential in the management and follow-up with patients with suspected photosensitivity reactions to inquire about muscle weakness and to look for other signs of dermatomyositis. Examination of the hands and tests for muscle enzyme elevations might help to distinguish dermatomyositis from photosensitivity reactions (see Chapter 192, Photosensitivity).

- Hypothyroidism can cause a proximal myopathy just like polymyositis and dermatomyositis. While hypothyroidism can cause a dermopathy, it does not resemble the skin findings of dermatomyositis. All patients with proximal muscle weakness should have a screening TSH to rule out hypothyroidism regardless of their skin findings (see Chapter 216, Goitrous Hypothyroidism).

- Rosacea causes an erythematous rash on the face as is often seen in dermatomyositis. Of course rosacea does not cause muscle weakness and the erythema of rosacea is generally confined to the face only (see Chapter 107, Rosacea).

- Steroid myopathy may develop as a side effect of systemic steroid therapy. The symptoms develop 4 to 6 weeks after starting oral steroids for dermatomyositis and other autoimmune diseases. Therefore if muscle weakness recurs after improving it could be from the steroids not the disease.

- Dermatomyositis-like reaction rarely may present with similar skin findings with initiation of the following medications and improvement with their discontinuation: penicillamine, nonsteroidal anti-inflammatory drugs, and carbamazepine.

- Overlap syndrome. The term "overlap" denotes that certain signs are seen in both dermatomyositis and other connective tissue

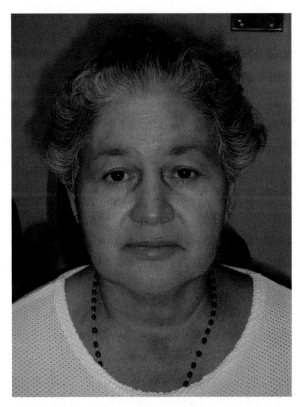

FIGURE 174-5 Patient improving after 2 weeks of oral prednisone. The heliotrope rash is still visible around the eyes and upper chest. The hair line erythema is from scalp involvement. (*Courtesy of Richard P. Usatine, MD.*)

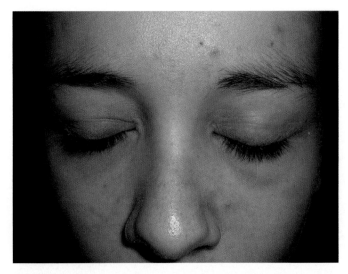

FIGURE 174-6 Classic heliotrope rash around the eyes of this 19-year-old woman newly diagnosed with dermatomyositis. The color "heliotrope" is a pink-purple tint named after the color of the heliotrope flower. As expected, her heliotrope rash is bilaterally symmetrical. This rash has resolved on prednisone and hydroxychloroquine. (*Courtesy of Richard P. Usatine, MD and from Goodall J, Usatine RP. Skin rash and muscle weakness. J Fam Pract. 2005;54(10):864–868, Dowden Health Media.*)

diseases such as scleroderma, rheumatoid arthritis, and lupus erythematosus. Scleroderma and dermatomyositis are the most commonly associated conditions and have been termed sclerodermatomyositis or mixed connective disease. In mixed connective tissue disease, features of SLE, scleroderma, and polymyositis are evident such as malar rash, alopecia, Raynaud's phenomenon, waxy-appearing skin, and proximal muscle weakness.

MANAGEMENT

Treatment is geared toward the proximal muscle weakness and the skin changes. Cutaneous manifestations do not always parallel muscle disease in response to therapy. Effective therapies for the myopathy are oral corticosteroids, immunosuppresant, biologic agents, and/or immunoglobin. Effective therapies for the skin disease are sun protection, topical corticosteroids, antimalarials, methotrexate, and/or immunoglobulin. These treatments are used individually and in combination in routine clinical practice; however, the optimal therapeutic regimen remains unclear because of a lack of high quality randomized controlled trials.[2]

TOPICAL

- Therapy of the skin disease begins with high potency topical corticosteroids.[3–5] SOR **B** Triamcinolone ointment may be used for less severe areas or on the face at first. Consider a short course of a very-high potency steroid such as clobetasol for more severe involvement not on the face.[5]

- Topical tacrolimus 0.1% has been shown to be a useful adjunct in the treatment of refractory skin manifestations.[6] SOR **B**

ORAL TREATMENT

- Therapy for the muscle disease begins with systemic corticosteroids with or without an immunosuppressive agent—Methotrexate, Cyclosporin A, or Azathioprine.

- First line therapy is Prednisone 0.5 to 1.0 mg/kg body weight per day (or 60 mg/d) until muscle enzyme levels trend toward normal limits after which a steroid taper should be initiated.[2,5,7,8] SOR **B**

- Methotrexate has been shown to be effective in childhood and adult refractory dermatomyositis and in patients needing a steroid-sparing agent, secondary to steroid side effects.[9] SOR **B**
  - Recent studies have shown that methotrexate use early in the disease course allows for faster recovery, less medication use and less disease sequelae.[8]
  - Combinations therapy with Prednisone and methotrexate is becoming common, allowing the reduction in corticosteroid dose to < or = 5 mg/d.[7–9]
  - Suggested Methotrexate dosing starts at 7.5 to 10 mg/wk. The dose is then increased 2.5 mg/wk until a total dose of 15 to 25 mg/wk is reached.[5] The total dose of methotrexate will also be determined by how well that patient can tolerate this medication.
  - As the methotrexate dose is increased the dose of Prednisone should be tapered.

- Cyclosporin A plus methotrexate has shown some benefit in the treatment of refractory juvenile dermatomyositis.[7] SOR **B**

- Azathioprine is commonly used in chronic inflammatory diseases as a steroid-sparing agent; however, studies of azathioprine 2 mg/kg

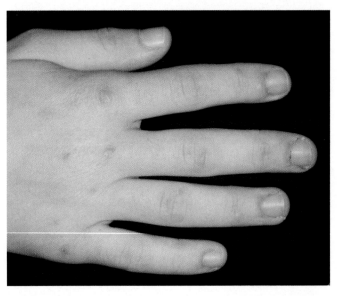

FIGURE 174-7 Hand involvement in the 19-year-old woman in **Figure 174-6** with Gottron's papules over the finger joints. She has nail fold erythema and ragged cuticles (Samitz sign). (*Courtesy of Richard P. Usatine, MD and from Goodall J, Usatine RP. Skin rash and muscle weakness. J Fam Pract. 2005;54(10):864–868, Dowden Health Media.*)

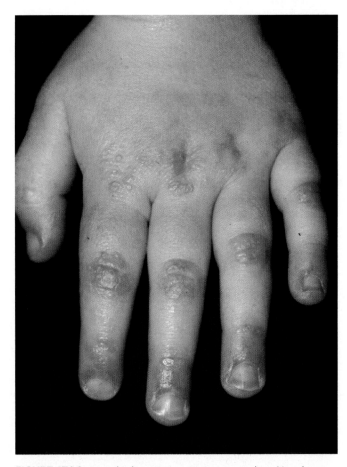

FIGURE 174-8 Juvenile dermatomyositis in a young boy. Note how the erythematous papules and plaques are most prominent over the finger joints and spares the space between joints. This is a good example of Gottron's papules being very visible in juvenile dermatomyositis. (*Courtesy of Richard P. Usatine, MD and from Goodall J, Usatine RP. Skin rash and muscle weakness. J Fam Pract. 2005;54(10):864–868, Dowden Health Media.*)

per day versus placebo showed no significant improvement in muscle strength compared to placebo.[7] SOR Ⓒ

- Hydroxychloroquine is one option for a steroid-sparing agent to be considered for young women with mild disease. SOR Ⓒ

- Various combination therapies with two of the following agents have been studied, but are still empirical–Azathioprine, cyclosporine A, intramuscular Methotrexate and oral Methotrexate.[2,5,7] SOR Ⓒ

- It is important to look at these medications' side-effect profile and monitor the patient accordingly during treatment. Patients must not get pregnant while on these medications and various labs need to be followed. A liver biopsy may be needed for patients taking methotrexate after 1.5-g cumulative dose.

INTRAVENOUS

- Pulsed intravenous methylprednisolone has been advocated for severe disease and in refractory cases of myositis.[7,8,10] SOR Ⓒ

- A number of patients have been found to be resistant or only partially responsive to steroids or immunosuppressive drugs. Recent studies have found intravenous immunoglobulin to be an effective second-line therapy.[7,8,11] SOR Ⓒ
  - Intravenous immunoglobulin therapy in patients with dermatomyositis has shown a statistically significant improvement in muscle strength score and even reported improvement in cutaneous disease.[7,11]
  - Patients were treated with 1 g/kg/d of immunoglobulin for 2 days every 4 weeks.[7]

OTHER

- Physical and/or occupational therapy to regain strength is highly recommended.[7]

- Photoprotection consisting of a broad-spectrum sunscreen, protective outerwear and limiting sun exposure.[3,4,7] SOR Ⓑ

- New agents termed biologics, including TNF-alpha inhibitors, are currently being tested for use in juvenile and adult dermatomyositis.[8] SOR Ⓒ

MALIGNANCY WORK-UP

- In patients older than 50 years, the physician should look for evidence of malignancy after initiating treatment.

- For women without risk factors, a complete annual physical examination is generally sufficient, including pelvic, breast, and rectal examination.[5,9]

- After considering the patient's age and family history, a mammogram and/or colonoscopy may be indicated. Some experts recommend total body scanning for persons just diagnosed with dermatomyositis after age 50. SOR Ⓒ

- Searching for malignancy, more than 2 years after the diagnosis, is unnecessary. A sixfold increase in diagnosing a primary malignancy is present during the first year. The risk normalized to that of the general population after the first year.[5]

PATIENT EDUCATION

Discuss the importance of sun protection. Counseling about the serious nature of the disease and prognosis is important since many

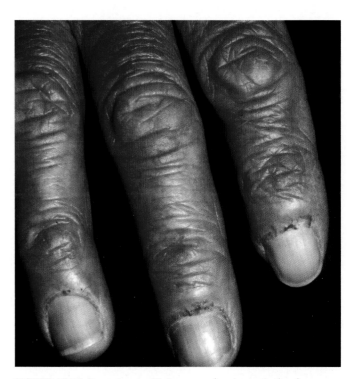

FIGURE 174-9 Dermatomyositis in a man showing cuticular changes that are thick, rough, and hyperkeratotic with telangiectasias. This moth-eaten appearance of the cuticles is called Samitz sign. (*Courtesy of the University of Texas Health Sciences Center, Division of Dermatology.*)

patients are left with residual weakness even after good disease control is obtained. Patients need to understand that the medications being used have many risks along with their benefits and need to report side effects to their physicians. Pregnancy prevention is needed for women of child-bearing potential while on a number of the medications used to treat this disease.

FOLLOW-UP

The patients need very close and frequent follow-up to manage their medications and overall care. This is because high doses of steroids and steroid sparing agents, such as methotrexate, have numerous potential side effects. The patients need to be closely followed with laboratory tests and careful titration of the toxic medicines used for treatment. Also the patients need physical therapy and specific supplements including calcium and folic acid to prevent some of the side effects of the strong medications being prescribed.

PATIENT RESOURCES

www.myositis.org.

www.ninds.nih.gov/disorders/dermatomyositis/dermatomyositis.htm.

PROVIDER RESOURCES

http://www.emedicine.com/med/topic2608.htm.

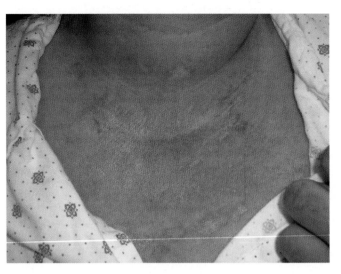

FIGURE 174-10 A 35-year-old Hispanic woman dermatomyositis and erythema and poikiloderma of the neck area. This is related to sun exposure. (*Courtesy of Richard P. Usatine, MD, and from Goodall J, Usatine RP. Skin rash and muscle weakness. J Fam Pract. 2005;54(10)864–868.*)

REFERENCES

1. Callen J. Dermatomyositis. eMedicine. www.emedicine.com/med/topic2608.htm. Accessed February 15, 2008.

2. Choy EH, Hoogendijk JE, Lecky B, Winer JB. Immunosuppressant and immunomodulatory treatment for dermatomyositis and polymyositis. *Cochrane Database Syst Rev.* 200520;(3):CD003643.

3. Callen JP. Dermatomyositis: Diagnosis, evaluation and management. *Minerva Med.* 2002;93(3):157–167.

4. Callen JP, Wortmann RL. Dermatomyositis. *Clin Dermatol.* 2006; 24(5):363–373.

5. Habif T. *A Color Guide to Diagnosis and Therapy, Clinical Dermatology*. 4th ed. St Louis, MO: Mosby, 2004.

6. Hollar CB, Jorizzo JL. Topical tacrolimus 0.1% ointment for refractory skin disease in dermatomyositis: A pilot study. *J Dermatolog Treat.* 2004;15(1):35–39.

7. Choy EH, Isenberg DA. Treatment of dermatomyositis and polymyositis. *Rheumatology (Oxford).* 2002;41(1):7–13.

8. Reed AM, Lopez M. Juvenile dermatomyositis: Recognition and treatment. *Paediatr Drugs.* 2002;4(5):315–321.

9. Dalakas MC, Hohlfeld R. Polymyositis and dermatomyositis. *Lancet.* 200320;362(9388):971–982.

10. Sontheimer RD. The management of dermatomyositis: Current treatment options. *Expert Opin Pharmacother.* 2004;5(5): 1083–1099.

11. Dalakas MC. The role of high-dose immune globulin intravenous in the treatment of dermatomyositis. *Int Immunopharmacol.* 2006;6(4):550–556. Epub 2005.

175 SCLERODERMA AND MORPHEA

E.J. Mayeaux, Jr., MD

PATIENT STORY

A 35-year-old woman presented with areas of shiny tough skin in patches over her abdomen (**Figure 175-1**). The patient was otherwise in good health and was puzzled by this new condition. She feared that all her skin would become this way. The skin was slightly uncomfortable but not painful. A 3-mm punch biopsy confirmed the clinical suspicion of morphea or localized scleroderma. The patient was treated with topical clobetasol and calcipotriol with some improvement in skin quality and symptoms. An anti-nuclear antibody (ANA) test was positive but she has not developed progressive systemic sclerosis.

EPIDEMIOLOGY

- The prevalence rates of diseases that share scleroderma as a clinical feature are reported ranging from 4 to 253 cases per 1,000,000 individuals.[1]

- Systemic sclerosis has an annual incidence of 1 to 2 per 100,000 individuals in the United States.[1] The peak onset is between the ages of 30 and 50 years.[1]

- In the United States, the incidence of morphea has been estimated at 25 cases per million per year.[1]

ETIOLOGY AND PATHOPHYSIOLOGY

- The scleroderma disorders can be subdivided into three groups: localized scleroderma (morphea, **Figures 175-1** to **175-3**), systemic sclerosis (**Figures 175-4** to **175-9**), and other scleroderma-like disorders that are marked by the presence of thickened, sclerotic skin lesions.

- The most common vascular dysfunction associated with scleroderma is Raynaud's phenomenon (**Figure 175-10**). Raynaud's phenomenon is produced by arterial constriction in the digits. The characteristic color changes progress from white pallor, to blue (acrocyanosis), to finally red (reperfusion hyperemia). Raynaud's phenomenon generally precedes other disease manifestations, sometimes by years. Many patients develop progressive structural changes in their small blood vessels, which permanently impair blood flow, and can result in digital ulceration or infarction. Other forms of vascular injury include pulmonary artery hypertension, renal crisis, and gastric antral vascular ectasia.

- Systemic sclerosis is used to describe a systemic disease characterized by skin induration and thickening accompanied by variable tissue fibrosis and inflammatory infiltration in numerous visceral organs. Systemic sclerosis can be diffuse (DcSSc) or limited to the skin and adjacent tissues (limited cutaneous systemic sclerosis [LcSSc]).

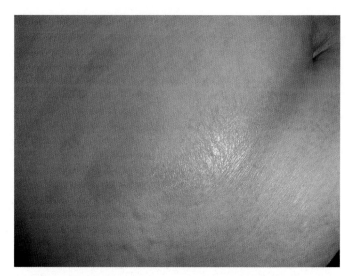

FIGURE 175-1 Morphea on the abdomen in a 35-year-old woman. (*Courtesy of Richard P. Usatine, MD.*)

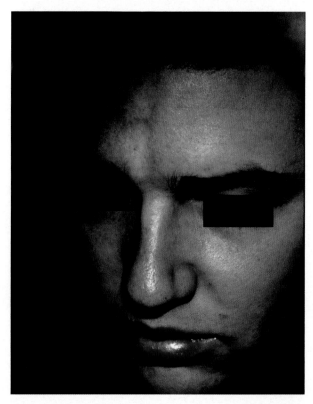

FIGURE 175-2 Linear morphea on the forehead called "En coup de sabre" meaning the blow of a sword. (*Courtesy of John Gonzalez, MD.*)

- Patients with LcSSc usually have skin sclerosis restricted to the hands, and to a lesser extent, the face and neck. With time, some patients develop scleroderma of the distal forearm. They often display the CREST syndrome, which presents with Raynaud's phenomenon (**Figure 175-10**), esophageal dysmotility, sclerodactyly (**Figures 175-4** to **175-7**), and telangiectasias (**Figures 175-8** and **175-9**), and calcinosis cutis (**Figure 175-11**).

- Patients with DcSSc often present with sclerotic skin on the chest, abdomen, or upper arms and shoulders. The skin may take on a "salt-and-pepper" look (**Figure 175-12**). They are more likely to develop internal organ damage caused by ischemic injury and fibrosis than those with LcSSc or morphea.

- Almost 90% of patients with systemic sclerosis have some gastrointestinal involvement,[2] although half of these patients may be asymptomatic. Any part of the gastrointestinal tract may be involved. Potential signs and symptoms include dysphagia, choking, heartburn, cough after swallowing, bloating, constipation and/or diarrhea, pseudo-obstruction, malabsorption, and fecal incontinency. Chronic gastroesophageal reflux and recurrent episodes of aspiration may contribute to the development of interstitial lung disease. Vascular ectasia in the stomach (often referred to as "watermelon stomach" on endoscopy) is common, and may lead to gastrointestinal bleeding and anemia.

- Pulmonary involvement is seen in more than 70% of patients, usually presenting as dyspnea on exertion and a nonproductive cough. Fine "Velcro" rales may be heard at the lung bases with lung auscultation. Pulmonary vascular disease occurs in 10% to 40% of patients with systemic sclerosis, and is more common in patients with limited cutaneous disease. The risk of lung cancer is increased approximately fivefold in patients with scleroderma.

- Autopsy data suggest that 60% to 80% of patients with DcSSc have evidence of kidney damage.[3] Some degree of proteinuria, a mild elevation in the plasma creatinine concentration, and/or hypertension are observed in as many as 50% of patients.[4] Severe renal disease develops in 10% to 15% of patients, most commonly in patients with DcSSc.

- Symptomatic pericarditis occurs in 7% to 20% of patients, which has a 5 year's mortality rate of 75%.[5] Primary cardiac involvement includes pericarditis, pericardial effusion, myocardial fibrosis, heart failure, myocarditis associated with myositis, conduction disturbances, and arrhythmias.[6] Patchy myocardial fibrosis is characteristic of systemic sclerosis, and is thought to result from recurrent vasospasm of small vessels. Arrhythmias are common and are most caused by fibrosis of the conduction system.

- Pulmonary vascular disease occurs in 10% to 40% of patients with scleroderma, and is more common in patients with limited cutaneous disease. It may occur in the absence of significant interstitial lung disease, generally a late complication, and is usually progressive. Severe pulmonary arterial hypertension, sometimes with pulmonale and right-sided heart failure or thrombosis of the pulmonary vessels may develop.

- Joint pain, immobility and contractures may develop, with contractures of the fingers being most common (**Figure 175-6**). Neuropathies and central nervous system involvement, including headache, seizures, stroke, vascular disease, radiculopathy, and myelopathy, occur.

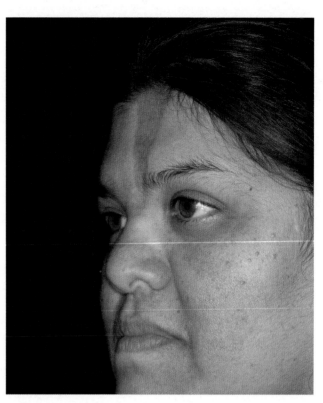

FIGURE 175-3 Linear morphea that started 3 years before on the forehead of a 41-year-old Hispanic woman. Another example of "En coup de Sabre" meaning the blow of a sword. (*Courtesy of Richard P. Usatine, MD.*)

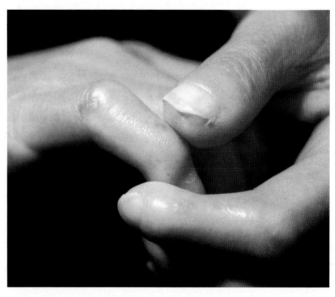

FIGURE 175-4 Scleroderma showing sclerodactyly with tight shiny skin over the fingers. (*Courtesy of Everett Allen, MD.*)

• Scleroderma produces sexual dysfunction in men and women. In men, it is very frequently associated with erectile dysfunction.

DIAGNOSIS

CLINICAL FEATURES

The diagnosis of systemic sclerosis and related disorders is based primarily upon the presence of characteristic clinical findings. Skin involvement is characterized by variable thickening and hardening of the skin. Skin pigmentary changes may occur, especially a salt-and-pepper appearance from spotty hypopigmentation (**Figure 175-12**). Other prominent skin manifestations:

• Pruritus and edema in the early stages.
• Sclerodactyly (**Figures 175-4** to **175-6**).
• Digital ulcers and pitting at the fingertips (**Figures 175-8** and **175-10**).
• Telangiectasia (**Figures 175-8** and **175-9**).
• Calcinosis cutis (**Figure 175-11**).

The diagnosis of localized scleroderma (morphea) is suggested by the presence of typical skin thickening and hardening confined to one area (**Figures 175-1** to **175-3**). The diagnosis of systemic sclerosis is suggested by the presence of typical skin thickening and hardening (sclerosis) that is not confined to one area (i.e., not localized scleroderma). The combination of skin signs plus one or more of the typical systemic features supports the diagnosis of systemic sclerosis.

The American College of Rheumatology criteria[7] for the diagnosis of systemic sclerosis requires one major criterion or two minor criteria:

• The major criterion is typical sclerodermatous skin changes: tightness, thickening, and nonpitting induration, excluding the localized forms of scleroderma including:
  ◦ Sclerodactyly: above-indicated changes limited to fingers and toes.
  ◦ Proximal scleroderma: above-indicated changes proximal to the metacarpophalangeal or metatarsophalangeal joints, affecting other parts of the extremities, face, neck, or trunk (thorax or abdomen) almost always including sclerodactyly.
• Minor criteria:
  ◦ Digital pitting scars or a loss of substance from the finger pad.
  ◦ Bilateral finger or hand pitting edema.
  ◦ Abnormal skin pigmentation: hyperpigmentation often with areas of punctate or patchy hypopigmentation.
  ◦ Raynaud's phenomenon.
  ◦ Bibasilar pulmonary fibrosis.
  ◦ Lower (distal) esophageal dysmotility.
  ◦ Colonic sacculations: wide-mouthed diverticula of colon located along the antimesenteric border.

LABORATORY STUDIES

A positive ANA with a speckled, homogenous, or nucleolar staining pattern is common in scleroderma. Anti-centromere antibodies are often associated with LcSSc. Anti-DNA topoisomerase I (Scl-70) antibodies are highly specific for both systemic sclerosis, and related

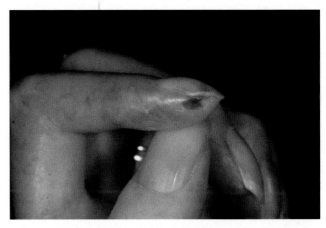

FIGURE 175-5 Sclerodactyly with tapering of the fingers and mottled hyperpigmentation. (*Courtesy of Jeffrey Meffert, MD.*)

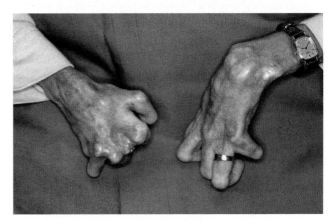

FIGURE 175-6 Severe scleroderma with deformity of hands as a result of sclerodactyly leading to severe flexion contractures. (*Courtesy of Jeffrey Meffert, MD.*)

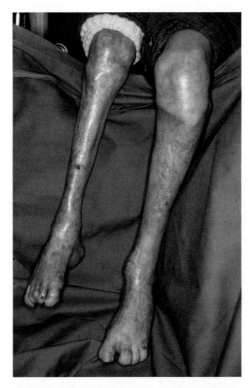

FIGURE 175-7 Scleroderma in the patient in **Figure 175-6** showing leg involvement with muscle atrophy. (*Courtesy of Jeffrey Meffert, MD.*)

interstitial lung and renal disease.[8] Although not very sensitive, anti-RNA polymerase I and III antibodies are specific for systemic sclerosis. Other testing for specific organ dysfunction is routinely done.

- The presence of characteristic autoantibodies, such as anti-centromere, anti-topoisomerase-I (Scl-70), anti-RNA polymerase, or U3-RNP antibodies, is supportive of the diagnosis of systemic sclerosis.

BIOPSY

A punch biopsy can be used to diagnose morphea and scleroderma.

DIFFERENTIAL DIAGNOSIS

- Idiopathic occurrence of systemic sclerosis associated diseases such as Raynaud's phenomenon, renal failure, and gastroesophageal reflux disease.

- SLE presents with systemic symptoms and a typical rash that may be scaring. Antinuclear antibody testing usually helps establish the diagnosis (see Chapter 173, Lupus Erythematosus).

- DLE presents as localized plaque lesion that eventually scar. Biopsy usually makes the diagnosis (see Chapter 173, Lupus Erythematosus).

- Myxedema is associated with hypothyroidism and is characterized by thickening and coarseness of the skin. Thyroid testing usually makes the diagnosis (see Chapter 216, Goiter and Hypothyroidism).

- Amyloidosis of the skin may result in thickening and stiffness of the skin. Skin biopsy reveals amyloid infiltration. Biopsy usually makes the diagnosis.

- Mycosis Fungoides presents with purplish macules and plaques throughout the body. Biopsy usually makes the diagnosis (see Chapter 169, Mycosis Fungoides).

MANAGEMENT

- Localized scleroderma, including morphea, appears to soften with ultraviolet-A light therapy.[9] SOR **B** Other options include highly potent topical glucocorticoids and topical calcipotriol.[10] SOR **B** Methotrexate can be started at 7.5 mg PO weekly and titrated up as needed. The combination of high-dose systemic glucocorticoids and low dose methotrexate has also been used successfully.[11] SOR **B**

- For symptomatic therapy, skin lubrication, histamine 1 (H1) and histamine 2 (H2) blockers, oral doxepin and low dose oral glucocorticoids may be used to treat pruritus. SOR **C**

- Telangiectasias may be covered with foundation make-up or treated with laser therapy.

- Calcium channel blockers, prazosin, prostaglandin derivatives, dipyridamole, aspirin, and topical nitrates may help symptoms of Raynaud's phenomenon.[12,13] SOR **B** Sildenafil (20 mg PO tid) has also been shown to be effective in patients with primary Raynaud's.[14] SOR **B** Patients should be advised to avoid cold, stress, nicotine, caffeine, and sympathomimetic decongestant medications. Acid reducing agents may be used empirically for gastroesophageal reflux disease. Prokinetic agents such as erythromycin may be useful for patients with esophageal hypomotility. SOR **C**

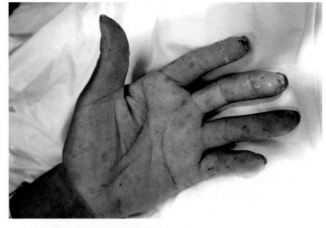

FIGURE 175-8 Scleroderma with telangiectasias and digital necrosis of the hands. (*Courtesy of Everett Allen, MD.*)

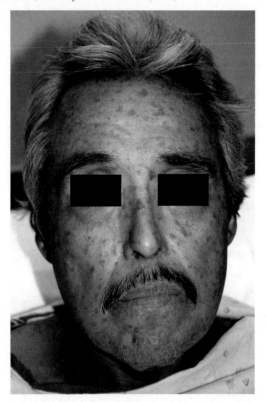

FIGURE 175-9 Telangiectasias on the face of the patient in **Figure 175-8**. (*Courtesy of Everett Allen, MD.*)

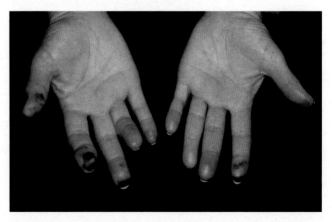

FIGURE 175-10 Raynaud's phenomenon with severe ischemia leading to the necrosis of the fingertips. (*Courtesy of L. Ricardo Zuniga-Montes, MD.*)

- Some localized lesions can be removed surgically.

- Unapproved therapies for skin disease include interferon-gamma, mycophenolate mofetil (1–1.5 g PO bid), and cyclophosphamide (50–150 mg/d PO in a single am dose). Extensive skin disease is being experimentally treated with D-penicillamine (250–1500 mg/d PO bid/tid on empty stomach divided.)[15] SOR Ⓑ

- The mainstay of treatment of renal disease is control of blood pressure, with angiotensin converting enzyme (ACE) inhibitors being the first-line agent. SOR Ⓒ Hemodialysis or peritoneal dialysis may be used as needed.

- Treatments of pulmonary hypertension associated with SSc being tested include the endothelin receptor antagonist bosentan (62.5 mg PO bid for 4 wk, then increase to 125 mg PO bid), the phosphodiesterase-5 inhibitor sildenafil and various prostacyclin analogs (e.g., epoprostenol, treprostinil, and iloprost). Pulmonary fibrosing alveolitis may be treated with cyclophosphamide.[16] SOR Ⓑ

- Myositis may be treated with steroids, methotrexate, and azathioprine (50–150 mg/d PO qam). Doses of prednisone greater than 40 mg/d are associated with a higher incidence of sclerodermal renal crisis.[17] SOR Ⓑ Arthralgias can be treated with acetaminophen and nonsteroidal anti-inflammatory drugs. SOR Ⓒ

PATIENT EDUCATION

Instruct the patient to avoid skin trauma (especially in the finger) cold exposure, and smoking. Make the patients aware of potential complications and have them watch for signs of systemic disease occurrence or progression.

FOLLOW-UP

The patient with systemic sclerosis needs to be evaluated at least every 3 to 6 months to monitor disease activity and progression.

PATIENT RESOURCES

- American College of Rheumatology Scleroderma Page— **http://www.rheumatology.org/public/factsheets/ scler_new.asp.**

- Scleroderma Foundation—**http://www.scleroderma.org/.**

- International Scleroderma Network—**http://www.sclero. org.**

PROVIDER RESOURCES

- The Arthritis Foundation—**http://www.arthritis.org.**

- National Institute of Arthritis and Musculoskeletal and Skin Diseases Information Clearinghouse—**http://www.niams.nih. gov.**

- eMedicine: Scleroderma—**http://www.emedicine.com/ med/topic2076.htm.**

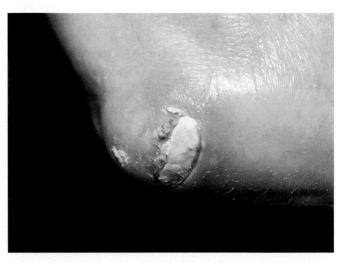

FIGURE 175-11 Calcinosis over the elbow in a patient with CREST syndrome. (*Courtesy of Everett Allen, MD.*)

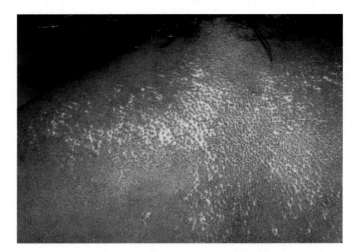

FIGURE 175-12 Scleroderma with mottled hypopigmentation. The skin may have a salt-and-pepper appearance as shown here. (*Courtesy of Jeffrey Meffert, MD.*)

REFERENCES

1. Lawrence RC, Helmick CG, Arnett FC, et al. Estimates of the prevalence of arthritis and selected musculoskeletal disorders in the United States. *Arthritis Rheum*. 1998;41:778.

2. Akesson A, Wollheim FA. Organ manifestations in 100 patients with progressive systemic sclerosis: A comparison between the CREST syndrome and diffuse scleroderma. *Br J Rheumatol*. 1989;28:281.

3. Medsger TA, Jr., Masi AT. Survival with scleroderma. II. A life-table analysis of clinical and demographic factors in 358 male U.S. veteran patients. *J Chronic Dis*. 1973;26:647.

4. Tuffanelli DL, Winklemann RK. Systemic scleroderma, A clinical study of 727 cases. *Arch Dermatol*. 1961;84:359.

5. Janosik DL, Osborn TG, Moore TL, et al. Heart disease in systemic sclerosis. *Semin Arthritis Rheum*. 1989;19:191.

6. Byers RJ, Marshall DA, Freemont AJ. Pericardial involvement in systemic sclerosis. *Ann Rheum Dis*. 1997;56:393.

7. American Rheumatism Association Diagnostic and Therapeutic Criteria Committee. Preliminary criteria for the classification of systemic sclerosis (scleroderma). Subcommittee for scleroderma criteria of the American Rheumatism Association Diagnostic and Therapeutic Criteria Committee. *Arthritis Rheum*. 1980;23(5): 581–590.

8. Reveille JD, Solomon DH. Evidence-based guidelines for the use of immunologic tests: Anticentromere, Scl-70, and nucleolar antibodies. *Arthritis Rheum*. 2003;49:399.

9. Kreuter A, Breuckmann F, Uhle A, et al. Low-dose UVA1 phototherapy in systemic sclerosis: Effects on acrosclerosis. *J Am Acad Dermatol*. 2004;50:740.

10. Seyger MM, van den Hoogen FH, de Boo T, de Jong EM. Low-dose methotrexate in the treatment of widespread morphea. *J Am Acad Dermatol*. 1998;39:220.

11. Kreuter A, Gambichler T, Breuckmann F, et al. Pulsed high-dose corticosteroids combined with low-dose methotrexate in severe localized scleroderma. *Arch Dermatol*. 2005;141:847.

12. Thompson AE, Shea B, Welch V, Fenlon D, Pope JE. Calcium-channel blockers for Raynaud's phenomenon in systemic sclerosis. *Arthritis Rheum*. 2001;44:1841.

13. Clifford PC, Martin MF, Sheddon EJ, Kirby JD, Baird RN, Dieppe PA. Treatment of vasospastic disease with prostaglandin E1. *Br Med J*. 1980;281:1031.

14. Fries R, Shariat K, von Wilmowsky H, Bohm M. Sildenafil in the treatment of Raynaud's phenomenon resistant to vasodilatory therapy. Circulation. 2005;112:2980.

15. Falanga V, Medsger TA, Jr. D-penicillamine in the treatment of localized scleroderma. *Arch Dermatol*. 1990;126(5):609–612.

16. Tashkin DP, Elashoff R, Clements PJ, et al. Cyclophosphamide versus placebo in scleroderma lung disease. *N Engl J Med*. 2006; 354:2655.

17. Steen VD, Medsger TA, Jr. Case-control study of corticosteroids and other drugs that either precipitate or protect from the development of scleroderma renal crisis. Arthritis Rheum. 1998;41:1613.

176 BULLOUS DISEASES— OVERVIEW

Ana Treviño Sauceda, MD
Richard P. Usatine, MD

PATIENT STORY

A 100-year-old black woman with diabetes was brought to the office by her family concerned about the large blister on her leg that started earlier that day (**Figure 176-1**). This large bulla appeared spontaneously without trauma and there was no surrounding erythema. The bulla contained clear fluid and there were no signs of infection. The bulla was drained with a sterile needle and no further bullae developed. The diagnosis is bullosis diabeticorum, a benign self-limited condition.

APPROACH TO THE DIAGNOSIS

The approach to a patient with a blistering disorder begins with a complete history and physical examination. To make the final diagnosis, laboratory investigations or tissue biopsies may be needed.

DIAGNOSIS

HISTORY

- How did the eruption present?
- Has it changed in morphology or location?
- Has it responded to any therapies?
- Are there any associated symptoms or aggravating factors?
- How has it impacted the patient's life?
- Does the patient have any chronic medical conditions?
- Does the patient take any medications?
- Does the patient have any significant family history?

PHYSICAL EXAMINATION

- Note the location of the eruption.
- Are the bullae flaccid or tense?
- Are there other lesions present (erosions, excoriations, papules, wheals)?
- Is Nikolsky sign positive or negative? (Does the skin shear off when lateral pressure in applied to unblistered skin?).
- Is Asboe-Hansen sign positive or negative? (**Figure 176-2**) (Do the bullae extend to surrounding skin when vertical pressure is

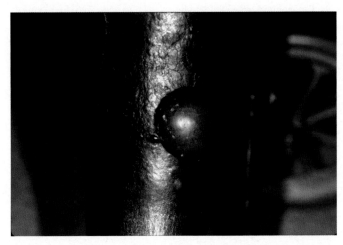

FIGURE 176-1 Bullosis diabeticorum on the lower leg of an older black woman with diabetes. This large bulla appeared spontaneously without trauma and there is no surrounding erythema. The bulla contained clear fluid and there was no infection. (*Courtesy of Richard P. Usatine, MD.*)

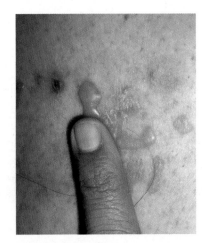

FIGURE 176-2 Testing for Asboe-Hanson sign on the back of a patient with bullous pemphigoid. The bulla did not extend with vertical pressure so the sign was negative. (*Courtesy of Richard P. Usatine, MD.*)

applied?) Sometimes the Asboe-Hansen sign is also attributed to Nikolsky and called a Nikolsky sign too.

- Is Darier's sign positive or negative? (Do wheals form with rubbing of the skin?).
- Note the skin background (sun-exposed skin, postinflammatory hyperpigmentation, lichenification and scarring).
- Does the patient have lymphadenopathy or hepatosplenomegaly?

CLINICAL FEATURES

- Autoimmune.
  - In bullous pemphigoid, patients have large, tense bullae that primarily involve the trunk, groin, axilla, proximal extremities, and flexor surfaces[1] (**Figure 176-2**).
  - Pemphigus vulgaris is characterized by erosions and flaccid bullae that frequently involve the mouth. In fact, mucosal membrane involvement may be the initial presentation. If the skin is involved, then Nikolsky and Asboe-Hansen signs are positive[1] (**Figures 176-3** and **178-1** to **178-4**).
  - Pemphigus foliaceus presents with cutaneous erosions and never involves the mucosal membranes. Nikolsky and Asboe-Hansen signs are positive[1] (**Figures 178-7** to **178-10**).
  - Pemphigus vegetans is characterized by verrucous plaques that involve the body folds, particularly the axillary region and the groin[1] (**Figures 178-5** and **178-6**).
  - Pemphigus erythematosus clinically resembles the malar rash of lupus with lesions localized to the nose, cheeks, and ears[1] (**Figure 178-11**).
  - Pemphigoid gestationis is a condition during pregnancy or during the postpartum period that can have a bullous component. The patient usually presents with urticarial papules and plaques with bullae developing around the umbilicus and extremities. The eruption eventually generalizes and involves the palms and soles. There usually is sparing of the face, scalp, and oral mucosa[1] (**Figure 176-4**).
  - Cicatricial pemphigoid involves the oral mucosa in 90% of cases and the conjunctiva in 66% of cases. Patients frequently present with a desquamative gingivitis. Cutaneous lesions are seen in 25% of patients.[1] (**Figures 177-4** to **177-6**).
  - Epidermolysis bullosa acquisita presents with trauma-induced blistering and erosions usually on the distal extremities. The patient should have background scarring, milia, and nail dystrophy. Patients have an increased risk of solid cancers, particularly adenocarcinomas.[1]
  - Dermatitis herpetiformis classically is a symmetrical, pruritic eruption that involves the extensor surfaces, scalp, and buttocks. The patient presents with pruritic vesicles and crusted papules with overlying excoriations[1] (**Figures 179-9** and **179-10**).
  - Linear IgA bullous dermatosis may produce a ring-like pattern of distribution and can occur in childhood (**Figure 176-5**). Patients may have mucous membrane involvement in up to 50% of cases.[1]
- Traumatic/Physical Stress.
  - Friction blisters form at sites of pressure and friction, frequently on the distal lower extremities.[1]
  - Bullous diabeticorum is trauma-induced, painless blistering, frequently in an acral distribution, in individuals with diabetes mellitus[1] (**Figure 176-1**).

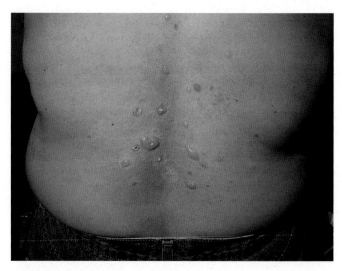

FIGURE 176-3 Pemphigus vulgaris with intact bullae. (*Courtesy of E. J. Mayeaux, Jr., MD.*)

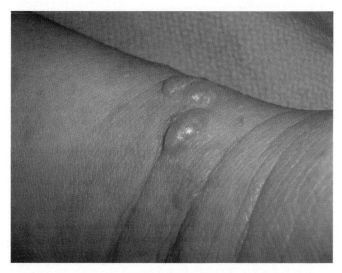

FIGURE 176-4 Pemphigoid gestationis with bullae on the wrist. (*Courtesy of Richard P. Usatine, MD.*)

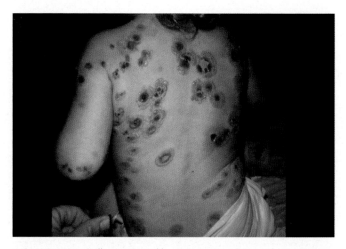

FIGURE 176-5 Bullae in a ring-like pattern in a young girl with IgA bullous dermatosis of childhood. (*Courtesy of Jack Resneck, Sr., MD.*)

○ Postburn blistering occurs in the hours after the insult, such as is seen in severe second degree sunburns.[1]

○ Miliaria is caused by keratinous obstruction of the eccrine ducts in response to heat. Small superficial vesicles may involve the face, trunk, or extremities.[1]

• Metabolic.

○ Porphyria cutanea tarda (PCT) involves sun-exposed skin, particularly the dorsal hands, forearms, ears, and face. The patient will have associated milia, scarring, and background dyspigmentation. PCT has been associated with hepatitis C infection[1] (**Figure 176-6**).

• Immunologic.

○ Pityriasis lichenoides et varioliformis acuta usually presents as a papulonecrotic eruption but may have vesicles resembling varicella (**Figure 176-7**). It usually involves the anterior trunk, flexor surfaces of the upper extremities, and the axilla. The general health of the patient is unaffected, although most have lymphadenopathy. CD8 T-cells are the predominant cell-type in lesional skin.[1] It is seen more frequently in young men and can go on to become chronic.

○ Allergic-contact and irritant-contact dermatitis, if severe, can cause blistering. Special attention should be placed on the location and pattern of involvement. For example, linear vesicles and bullae would suggest a plant-induced dermatitis such as poison ivy, poison oak, or poison sumac (**Figure 176-8**). Blistering in the periumbilical area is consistent with nickel dermatitis. Involvement of the dorsal feet is frequently seen with footwear dermatitis; likewise, involvement of the dorsal hands is consistent with glove dermatitis[2] (see Chapter 140, Contact Dermatitis).

• Drug.

○ Bullous drug eruptions may be localized to two mucosal surfaces with minimal cutaneous involvement or may be generalized involving all mucosal surfaces and a majority of the skin surface area. Nikolsky and Asboe-Hansen signs are positive on affected skin[1] (see Chapter 170, Hypersensitivity syndromes and Chapter 196, Cutaneous Drug Reactions).

• Infections and Bites.

○ Bullous arthropod reaction can occur after an insect bite (**Figure 176-9**).[1]

○ Bacterial infections should be considered when evaluating a localized blistering eruption. Amongst these infections is bullous impetigo (**Figure 176-10**). When evaluating the extremities, vesiculation overlying cellulitis may be associated with the more severe staphylococcal and streptococcal infections, and a thorough evaluation should be conducted to rule-out necrotizing fasciitis. As with most bacterial infections, the patient typically presents with fever and has an elevated white blood cell count.[2]

○ Herpes simplex viruses should always be considered when blistering of the mucosal surfaces is observed. Generalized blistering in the adult could be because of disseminated herpes and should prompt an evaluation for immunosuppression. Blistering in a dermatomal distribution is characteristic of herpes zoster (**Figure 176-11**).[2]

○ Scabies, tinea, and candida can also have bullous or pustular presentations in the classic sites of involvement.[2]

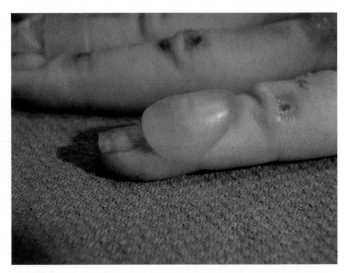

FIGURE 176-6 PCT with large bulla on the finger. (*Courtesy of Lewis Rose, MD.*)

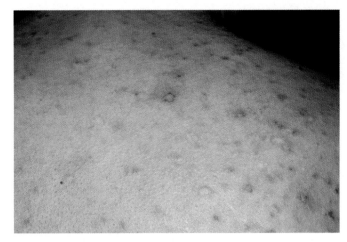

FIGURE 176-7 Pityriasis lichenoides et varioliformis acuta in a young man showing erosions where vesicles and bullae had been previously. (*Courtesy of Richard P. Usatine, MD.*)

- Hydrostatic.
  - Edema blisters form from the osmotic pressure experienced during the third spacing of fluid. As such, patients usually have a diagnosis of heart failure, cirrhosis, or kidney failure.[1]
- Congenital.
  - Erythema toxicum neonatorum are asymptomatic pink macules, papules, pustules, or wheals on the face, trunk, proximal arms, or buttocks, usually sparing the palms and soles, that occur from birth to 2 weeks of age and spontaneously resolve. Affects approximately 10% of term neonates[3] (**Figures 102-5** and **102-6**).[3]
  - Miliaria is a disorder caused by obstruction of the eccrine ducts. Clinically, noninflammatory vesicles may involve the face, trunk, or extremities. It affects 15% of neonates, and is more common in warm climates[3] (**Figure 102-7**).
  - Transient Neonatal Pustular Melanosis are pustules or vesicles without associated erythema located in clusters on the forehead, posterior ears, chin, neck, upper chest, back, buttocks, abdomen, and thighs, that spontaneously heal leaving behind pigmented macules. TNPM affects up to 4% of term infants and is more commonly seen in the African American population[3] (**Figures 104-4** and **104-5**) (see Chapter 104, Pustular Diseases of Childhood).
  - Acropustulosis of infancy develops during the first few weeks to months of life and spontaneously remits at 2 to 3 years of age. In this condition, crops of vesicles and pustules involve palms and soles, causing pruritus[3] (see Chapter 104, Pustular diseases of Childhood) (**Figures 104-1** to **104-3**).
  - Eosinophilic pustular folliculitis is a rare condition where yellowish pustules involve the face, scalp, trunk, and extremities usually causing pruritus and irritability. Work-up for bacterial, viral, and fungal infections is negative.[3] It can be seen in patients who are HIV positive (see Chapter 111, Folliculitis).
  - Neonatal herpes gestationis is associated with maternal disease. The neonate clinically has erythematous macules, papules, vesicles, and bullae involving the trunk, head, and extremities. There is spontaneous resolution by 1 month of age, but lesions may persist for up to 2 years after delivery.[3]
  - Neonatal pemphigus occurs in neonates whose mothers have active pemphigus vulgaris (not pemphigus foliaceus). The patient is born with bullae that spontaneously resolve within 1 to 2 weeks.[3]
  - The epidermolysis bullosa diseases are hereditary conditions in which minimal friction or trauma causes vesicles, bullae, and erosions. The distal extremities are frequently involved[4] (**Figures 179-3** to **179-6**).
  - Congenital infections with herpes simplex virus usually present with vesicles. In addition, a vesicular eruption in the neonate could be caused by neonatal syphilis, which is the only form of syphilis with a vesicular presentation.[2]
- Hematologic.
  - Bullous mastocytosis is caused by mast cell accumulation in the skin. The bullous presentation is very rare, but may involve any area of the body (**Figure 176-12**). On examination, Darier's sign should be positive and dermatographism should be present. Care should be taken to not irritate the patient as generalized degranulation of mast cells may ensue. Work-up should be conducted to determine the presence of systemic involvement, which may

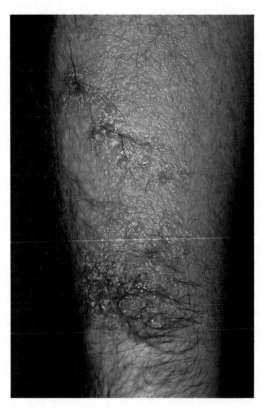

FIGURE 176-8 Bullae and vesicles on the extremity of a patient with poison ivy. Acute contact dermatitis can present with bulla and vesicles. (*Courtesy of Richard P. Usatine, MD.*)

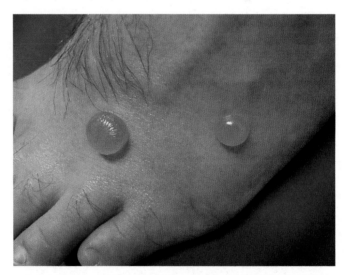

FIGURE 176-9 Bullous arthropod bites secondary to fire ants. (*With permission from Lane K, Lumbang W. Photo Rounds: Pruritic blisters on legs and feet. From J Fam Pract 2008;57(3):177–180, Dowden Health Media.*)

include a mast cell leukemia. A good lymph node and abdominal examination is recommended to evaluate for lymphadenopathy and hepatosplenomegaly.[3]

LABORATORY STUDIES AND WORK-UP

If the clinical picture is not clear, various laboratory studies may assist the clinician in making the diagnosis. Some diagnoses should be confirmed by histology even if the diagnosis appears clear. For example, all cases of suspected pemphigus should be biopsied because the management will involve long-term use of potentially toxic medications and it is crucial to know exactly what you are treating. The information in Chapter 177, Bullous Pemphigoid, and Chapter 178, Pemphigus, will help you to decide which tests to use in some of the autoimmune blistering diseases. Consulting a dermatologist is very appropriate for many of the more rare and lethal conditions.

POSSIBLE LABORATORY STUDIES

- Direct fluorescent antibody test can be done on a scraping of a lesion if herpes simplex or varicella zoster is suspected. In many laboratories, a result can be obtained within 24 hours.
- Mineral oil scraping for scabies (see Chapter 137, Scabies).
- KOH scraping for possible blistering tinea infections (such as bullous tinea pedis). See Fungal section.
- Genetic studies for suspected genetic defects—consider referral to geneticist.

POSSIBLE BIOPSIES

- One 4-mm punch biopsy for pathologic evaluation—biopsy an established lesion including the edge of the blister. A shave biopsy is an alternative as long as the epidermis of the blister stays attached to the specimen.
- 4-mm punch biopsy for immunofluorescence—biopsy the perilesional skin and send the specimen in special media. One exception occurs if you suspect dermatitis herpetiformis then a biopsy for immunofluorescence should be of non-involved skin.
- Consider two 4-mm punch biopsy for bacterial, fungal, and viral cultures and stains if infections are suspected and cultures and other less invasive studies are not providing the diagnosis. Send the specimens in a sterile urine cup on top of a sterile gauze soaked with sterile saline. Preservative-free anesthetic and saline should be used when performing a biopsy for culture.

FURTHER EVALUATIONS

Patients with cicatricial pemphigoid and toxic epidermal necrolysis need an ophthalmologic evaluation. Patients with several of the epidermolysis bullosa diseases and dermatitis herpetiformis need a gastroenterologic evaluation.

For possible paraneoplastic conditions, such as in epidermolysis bullosa acquisita and cicatricial pemphigoid, thorough cancer screening and studies targeting the patient's symptomatology are indicated.

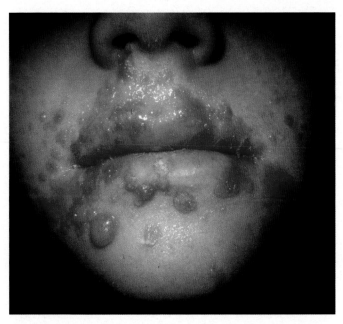

FIGURE 176-10 Bullous impetigo on the face of a child. Note the honey crusts. (*Courtesy of Jack Resneck, Sr., MD.*)

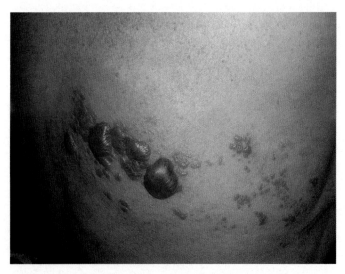

FIGURE 176-11 Herpes zoster with large bulla in a dermatomal pattern. (*Courtesy of Rose Walczak, MD.*)

REFERENCES

1. Bolognia JL, Jorizzo JL, Rapini RP. *Dermatology*. London: Elsevier Health Sciences, 2003.

2. James WD, Berger TG, Elston DM. *Andrews' Diseases of the Skin: Clinical Dermatology*. 10th ed. Philadelphia: Elsevier Health Sciences, 2005.

3. Schachner LA, Hansen RC. *Pediatric Dermatology*. 3rd ed. New York: Mosby, 2003.

4. Spitz JL. *Genodermatoses: A Clinical Guide to Genetic Skin Disorders*. Philadelphia: Lippincott Williams & Wilkins, 2004.

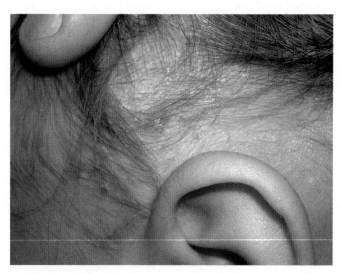

FIGURE 176-12 Bullous mastocytosis on the scalp of a 9-month-old child. (*Courtesy of Richard P. Usatine, MD.*)

177 BULLOUS PEMPHIGOID

Asad K. Mohmand, MD

PATIENT STORY

A native of Panama was seen for extensive bullous disease that is classic for bullous pemphigoid (BP) (**Figures 177-1** and **177-2**). The presence of so many intact bullae would make pemphigus very unlikely. The patient was treated with oral prednisone and began to respond quickly with a good outcome.

EPIDEMIOLOGY

- BP is an uncommon condition of the elderly.
- Average age of onset is approximately 65 years.[1]
- There is no racial or gender predilection.

ETIOLOGY AND PATHOPHYSIOLOGY

- BP is a chronic autoimmune disorder of the skin.
  - IgG autoantibodies against BP180 antigen of the basement membrane protein are considered pathognomonic and can be found in up to 65% of patients.[2]
  - Anti-BP230 antibodies are present in virtually all patients but are not considered pathognomonic.[3]
- The binding of antibodies to the basement membrane activates complement leading to chemotaxis of inflammatory cells (eosinophils and mast cells) that release proteases. The subsequent degradation of hemidesmosomal proteins leads to blister formation.
- There are several morphologically distinct clinical presentations:
  - Generalized bullous form is the most common (**Figures 177-1** to **177-3**). Tense bullae occurring on both erythematous (**Figure 177-3**) and normal appearing skin surfaces, which usually heal without scarring.
  - Vesicular form characterized by clusters of small tense blisters with an urticarial or erythematous base.
  - Other forms are very uncommon and include vegetative (intertriginous vegetating plaques), generalized erythroderma (exfoliative lesions with or without vesicles/bullae), urticarial (without any bullae), nodular (resembling prurigo nodularis), and acral forms (bullae on palms, soles, and face in children associated with vaccination).
- Pemphigoid gestationis is a variant of BP occurring during or after pregnancy. Lesions resolve after delivery, but may recur with subsequent pregnancies or in the nonpregnant state (see Chapter 72, Pemphigoid Gestationis).[4]
- Drug-induced BP has been reported with drugs containing sulfhydryl groups including penicillamine, furosemide, captopril, and sulfasalazine.

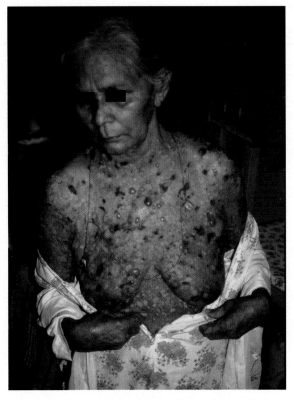

FIGURE 177-1 Extensive untreated bullous pemphigoid (BP) in a Panamanian woman. (*Courtesy of Eric Kraus, MD.*)

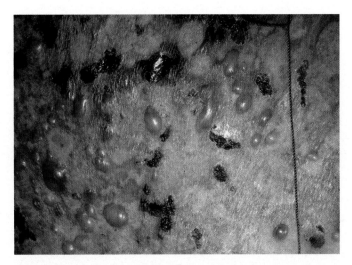

FIGURE 177-2 Close-up of intact bulla and dark crusts in the Panamanian woman in **Figure 177-1**. (*Courtesy of Eric Kraus, MD.*)

DIAGNOSIS

CLINICAL FEATURES

- Tense blisters involving normal or inflamed skin or mucus membranes (**Figures 177-1 to 177-3**).

- Intense pruritus is a common feature and may precede blistering by months.[5]

- Nikolsky's sign (wrinkling and sheet-like peeling of the skin when lateral pressure is applied to unblistered skin) is usually negative.[6]

TYPICAL DISTRIBUTION

- Flexure surfaces of the arms and legs.

- Lower abdomen and groin.

- Mucus membranes are involved in 10% to 25% of cases.

BIOPSY

Biopsy is required for establishing diagnosis and to differentiate it from other conditions that can have a similar clinical presentation:

- 4-mm punch biopsy from edge of an early blister including part of the normal-appearing skin for histopathologic review shows a subepidermal blister and an eosinophil-rich mixed dermal inflammatory infiltrate. (A scoop shave biopsy under a small intact blister is also a good method of making a diagnosis of BP or other bullous diseases.) Start with this standard biopsy and perform another biopsy for direct immunofluorescence (DIF) if needed.

- A second 4-mm punch biopsy from perilesional skin, transported in Michel's solution for DIF. DIF demonstrates linear IgG and complement C3 deposits at the dermal–epidermal junction.
  - If DIF is positive, indirect immunofluorescence (IDIF) can be performed on patient's serum using salt-split normal human skin substrate, which will reveal IgG on the epidermal side of split skin (blister roof). This is rarely needed.

DIFFERENTIAL DIAGNOSIS

- Cicatricial pemphigoid (**Figures 177-4 to 177-6**)—predominant mucosal involvement and lesions heal with prominent scarring; IgG localizes to blister floor on IDIF.

- Dermatitis herpetiformis—grouped vesicles, extensor distribution (see Chapter 179, Other Bullous Diseases).

- Epidermolysis bullosa acquisita—IgG localizes to blister floor on IDIF (see Chapter 179, Other Bullous Diseases).

- Erythema multiforme—targetoid lesions; linear IgG immunofluorescence is negative (see Chapter 170, Erythema Multiforme).

- Linear IgA dermatosis—usually drug-induced (e.g., vancomycin[7]); DIF demonstrates IgA deposits. Also called chronic bullous dermatosis of childhood (see Chapter 176, Bullous Diseases—Overview including **Figure 176-5**).

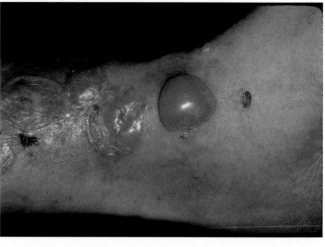

FIGURE 177-3 Localized BP with large bulla on the ankle. (*Courtesy of Eric Kraus, MD.*)

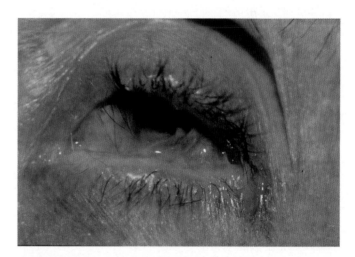

FIGURE 177-4 Cicatricial BP of the eye, causing scarring and blindness. (*Courtesy of Eric Kraus, MD.*)

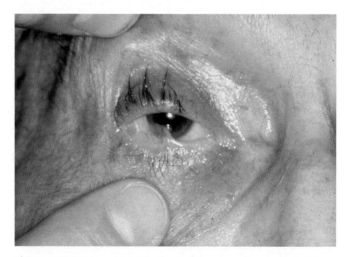

FIGURE 177-5 Cicatricial BP with scarring connecting the lower lid to the cornea. (*Courtesy of Eric Kraus, MD.*)

MANAGEMENT

- High potency topical corticosteroids are considered first-line treatment for moderate to severe generalized disease (e.g., clobetasol).[8] SOR **A**

- Oral corticosteroids.[8] SOR **A**
  - Prednisone 0.5 to 1 mg/kg/d.
  - Increase dose until new blisters cease to develop.
  - Reduce dose at ~10% every 2 to 3 weeks to reach dose of 15 to 20 mg/d.

- Adjuvant antibiotic treatment should be considered for all patients:
  - Tetracycline (1.5–2 g/d) with or without niacinomide (1.5–2 g/d).[9] SOR **B** Both tetracycline and niacinomide come in 500 mg capsules and may be taken three to four times daily. Niacinomide contains niacin (Vitamin B$_3$) and is available over the counter.

- Steroid-sparing drugs and adjuvant for patients whose disease is not controlled with steroids and tetracycline:
  - Azathioprine 50 to 200 mg divided bid or tid (first-line adjuvant).[8] SOR **B**
  - Mycophenolate mofetil 0.5 to 2 g/d divided bid or tid (less hepatotoxic than azathioprine).[10] SOR **C**
  - Cyclophosphamide 1 to 5 mg/kg/d. SOR **C**

- Disease resistant to combination of corticosteroids and steroid-sparing agents:
  - Intravenous immunoglobulin (IVIG) can produce a rapid and dramatic but very transient response; requires multiple cycles of IVIG. SOR **C**

- Consultations
  - Dermatology consultation for recommending therapy based on extent of disease and for changes in therapy when required.
  - Nutrition consultation if patient is having difficulty maintaining weight.

PATIENT EDUCATION

- Avoid mechanical irritation, direct sun-exposure, dental prostheses, extremes of temperature.

- Recommend high-protein, low-carbohydrate and low-fat diet; calcium and vitamin D supplementation for patients on corticosteroids.

- Provide information on wound care, stress-reduction, appropriate exercise, and side effects of medications.

FOLLOW-UP SOR **C**

- Ask patient about recurrent lesions, pruritus, and side effects from treatment.

- Perform periodic skin examinations looking for new lesions to adjust dose of prednisone and to monitor for lymphadenopathy and skin cancer in patients using immunosuppressive medications.

- Monitor for drug-specific laboratory abnormalities (e.g., glucose and triglycerides with steroid use; CBC, renal function, and liver function tests for azathioprine).

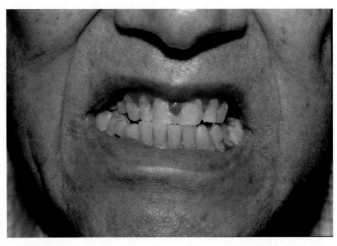

FIGURE 177-6 Cicatricial BP of the mouth showing gingivitis. Over 50% of cases of BP have oral involvement. (*Courtesy of Eric Kraus, MD.*)

- Make sure patients do not run out of their medications because this can result in recurrent lesions (**Figure 177-7**).

- Adjust treatment if patient relapses (e.g., increase steroid dose or add an immunosuppressive agent).

- Taper steroids slowly (as above) after dissipation of disease flare.

PATIENT RESOURCES

http://www.patient.co.uk/showdoc/23069059/.

PROVIDER RESOURCES

- ACP Pier—**http://pier.acponline.org/physicians/diseases/d1023/d1023.html.**

- eMedicine—**http://www.emedicine.com/DERM/topic64.htm.**

REFERENCES

1. Chan L. Bullous Pemphigoid. eMedicine: http://www.emedicine.com/DERM/topic64.htm. Accessed March 23, 2008.

2. Zillikens D, Rose PA, Balding SD, et al. Tight clustering of extra-cellular BP180 epitopes recognized by bullous pemphigoid autoantibodies. *J Invest Dermatol*. 1997;109:573–579.

3. Yancey KB, Egan CA. Pemphigoid: Clinical, histologic, immunopathologic, and therapeutic considerations. *JAMA*. 2000;284:350–356.

4. Kroumpouzos G, Cohen LM. Specific dermatoses of pregnancy: An evidence-based systematic review. *Am J Obstet Gynecol*. 2003;188(4):1083–1092.

5. Bingham EA, Burrows D, Sandford JC. Prolonged pruritus and bullous pemphigoid. *Clin Exp Dermatol*. 1984;9:564–570.

6. Habif TP. *Clinical Dermatology: A Color Guide to Diagnosis and Therapy*. 4th ed. Mosby: St Louis, 2004.

7. Kuechle MK, Stegemeir E, Maynard B, Gibson LE. Drug-induced linear IgA bullous dermatosis: Report of six cases and review of the literature. *J Am Acad Dermatol*. 1994;30:187–192.

8. Khumalo N, Kirtschig G, Middleton P, et al. Interventions for bullous pemphigoid. *Cochrane Database Syst Rev*. 2003;(3): CD002292.

9. Fivenson DP, Breneman DL, Rosen GB, et al. Nicotinamide and tetracycline therapy of bullous pemphigoid. *Arch Dermatol*. 1994;130(6):753–758.

10. Böhm M, Beissert S, Schwarz T, et al. Bullous pemphigoid treated with mycophenolate mofetil. *Lancet*. 1997;349(9051):541.

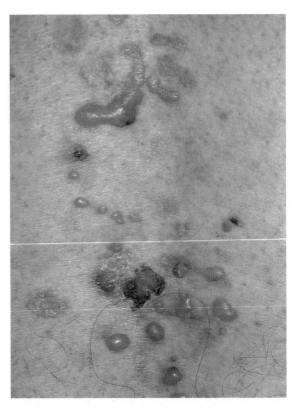

FIGURE 177-7 Recurrent bullous pemphigoid on the back of a 57-year-old man who ran out of his prednisone for a few days. (*Courtesy of Richard P. Usatine, MD.*)

178 PEMPHIGUS

Shashi Mittal, MD

PATIENT STORY

A young man presented with painful blisters on his face and mouth (**Figure 178-1**). The patient was referred to dermatology that day. The dermatologist recognized likely pemphigus vulgaris (PV) and did shave biopsies for histopathology and direct immunofluorescence of facial vesicles/bullae to confirm the presumed diagnosis. The patient was started on 60 mg of prednisone daily until the pathology confirmed PV. Steroid sparing therapy was then discussed with the patient.

EPIDEMIOLOGY

- Pemphigus is a rare but serious autoimmune disease that is marked by vesiculobullous lesions of the skin and mucus membranes.
- There are three major types of pemphigus:
  - Pemphigus Vulgaris (PV) (**Figures 178-1 to 178-4**):
    - Most common form of pemphigus in the United States.
    - Annual incidence is 0.75 to 5 cases per million.[1]
    - Usually occurs between 30 to 50 years of age.[2]
    - Increased incidence in Ashkenazi Jews and Mediterraneans.[2]
    - Pemphigus vegetans is a variant form of PV (**Figures 178-5 and 178-6**).
  - Pemphigus foliaceus (PF) (**Figures 178-7 to 178-10**): Superficial form of pemphigus.
    - More prevalent in Africa.[1]
    - Variant forms include pemphigus erythematosus (**Figure 178-11**) and fogo selvagem.
    - Fogo selvagem is an endemic form of PF seen in Brazil and affects teenagers and individuals in their twenties.[1]
  - Paraneoplastic pemphigus (PNP): Onset 60 years and older.
    - Associated with occult neoplasms commonly lymphoreticular.
    - Malignancies like non-Hodgkin's lymphoma and chronic lymphocytic leukemia.
    - Leukemia; also associated with benign neoplasms such as thymoma and Castleman's disease.[2]

ETIOLOGY AND PATHOPHYSIOLOGY

- The basic abnormality in all three types of pemphigus is acantholysis, a process of separation of keratinocytes from one another. This occurs as a result of autoantibody formation against desmoglein (the adhesive molecule that holds epidermal cells together). Separation of epidermal cells leads to formation of intraepidermal clefts, which enlarge to form bullae.[1]
- The mechanism that induces the production of these autoantibodies in most individuals is unknown. Yet PF may be triggered by drugs,

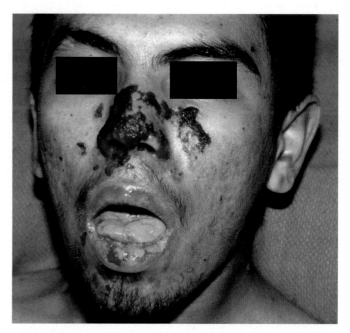

FIGURE 178-1 Pemphigus vulgaris (PV) on the face of a young man with mouth involvement. (*Courtesy of Eric Kraus, MD.*)

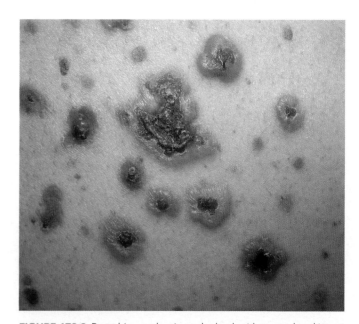

FIGURE 178-2 Pemphigus vulgaris on the back with crusted and intact bullae. Downward pressure on a bulla demonstrates a positive Asboe-Hansen sign with lateral spread of a fresh bullae. (*Courtesy of Eric Kraus, MD.*)

most commonly thiol compounds like penicillamine, captopril, piroxicam, and others like penicillin and imiquimod.[3] An environmental trigger in the presence of susceptible HLA gene is suggested to induce autoantibodies in fogo selvagum.[1]

- The autoantibodies in pemphigus are usually directed against desmoglein 1 and 3 molecules (Dsg1 and Dsg3). Dsg1 is present predominantly in the superficial layers of the epidermis whereas Dsg3 is expressed in deeper epidermal layers and in mucus membranes. As a result, clinical presentation depends on the antibody profile. In PV, a limited mucosal disease occurs when only Anti-Dsg3 antibody is present but extensive mucosal and cutaneous disease occurs when both Anti-Dsg1 and Dsg3 antibodies are present. In PF, mucosal lesions are absent and the cutaneous lesions are superficial because of isolated Anti-Dsg1 antibody.[2]

- Patients with PNP demonstrate both anti-Dsg1 and Dsg3 antibodies. However, unlike PV, autoantibodies against plakin proteins (another adhesive molecule) are also observed in patients with PNP and these autoantibodies form a reliable marker for this type of pemphigus.[3]

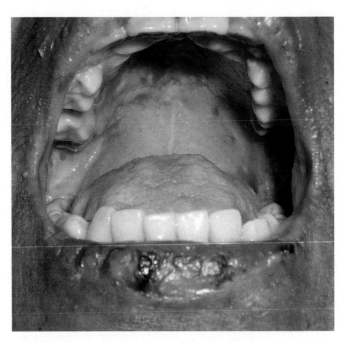

FIGURE 178-3 PV involving the lips and palate of a 55-year-old woman. (*Courtesy of Dan Shaked, MD.*)

DIAGNOSIS

CLINICAL FEATURES

- PV (**Figures 178-1** to **178-4**): Classical lesions are flaccid bullae that rupture easily creating erosions. Since bullae are short-lived, erosions are the more common presenting physical finding. Lesions are typically tender and heal with postinflammatory hyperpigmentation that resolves without scarring. A positive Asboe-Hansen or Nikolsky sign may be present, but these not diagnostic. A positive Asboe-Hansen sign occurs when a bulla extends to surrounding skin while pressure is applied directly to the bulla. The Nikolsky sign is positive when skin shears off while lateral pressure is applied to unblistered skin during active disease. Sometimes the Asboe-Hansen sign is also attributed to Nikolsky and called a Nikolsky sign too.

- Pemphigus vegetans is a variant of PV where healing is associated with vegetating proliferation of the epidermis (**Figures 178-5** and **178-6**).

- Pemphigus foliaceous: multiple red, scaling, crusted, and pruritic lesions described as "corn flakes" are seen. Shallow erosions arise when crusts are removed but intact blisters are rare as the disease is superficial (**Figures 178-7** to **178-10**).

- PNP (**Figure 178-11**): Lesions are similar to PV though lichen planus, morbilliform or erythema multiforme-like lesions may also be seen in addition to blisters and erosions. Another distinctive feature is the presence of epithelial necrosis and lichenoid changes in the lesions. Pulmonary involvement secondary to acantholysis of bronchial mucosa is seen in 30% to 40% of cases of PNP.

TYPICAL DISTRIBUTION

- PV: Common mucosal site is oral mucosa, though any stratified squamous epithelium may be involved. Mucosal lesions may be followed by skin lesions after weeks to months usually on scalp, face, and upper torso. PV should be suspected if an oral ulcer persists beyond a month (**Figures 178-1** to **178-4**).

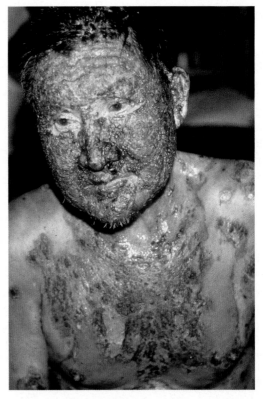

FIGURE 178-4 Severe fatal PV. (*Courtesy of Eric Kraus, MD.*)

- Pemphigus vegetans: usually seen in intertriginous areas like the axilla, groin, and genital region (**Figures 178-5** and **178-6**).

- Pemphigus foliaceous: initially affects face and scalp though may progress to involve chest and back (**Figures 178-7** to **178-10**). When the facial involvement in PF is in a lupus-like pattern, this is called pemphigus erythematosus (**Figure 178-11**).

- PNP: common sites include oral mucosa and conjunctiva. Columnar and transitional epithelia may also be involved besides stratified squamous epithelium (**Figure 178-11**).

LABORATORY STUDIES AND BIOPSY

- Skin biopsy is essential for accurate diagnosis. The depth of acantholysis and site of deposition of antibody complexes help differentiate pemphigus from other bullous diseases. Two biopsies are preferred. The first is sent in formalin for routine histopathology. This biopsy should be of the freshest lesion with an intact bulla, if possible. Perform a shave or punch of the edge of the bulla to include the epidermis. The second, a 4-mm perilesional punch from adjacent normal skin, is sent on a gauze soaked in normal saline or Michel's solution for DIF.[2] Routine histopathology demonstrates suprabasal acantholysis and DIF shows antibody deposition in the intercellular spaces of the epidermis.

- A blood test may be ordered to measure circulating desmoglein antibodies levels using indirect immunofluorescence. It may be helpful in monitoring disease activity and evaluating therapy.

DIFFERENTIAL DIAGNOSIS

- Bullous pemphigoid—Bullae are tense because they occur in the deeper subepidermal layer. Mucus membrane involvement is rare. Biopsy illustrates subepidermal acantholysis and immunoglobulin deposition along the basement membrane[4] (see Chapter 177, Bullous Pemphigoid).

- Cicatricial pemphigoid—Also known as mucus membrane pemphigoid. Usually affects oral mucosa and conjunctiva. Lesions heal with scarring, which results in irreversible sequelae such as blindness, subglottic stenosis, and esophageal strictures.[4] Histology demonstrates antibody complexes in the basement membrane with submucosal infiltrate and prominent fibroblast proliferation[3] (see Chapter 177, Bullous Pemphigoid).

- Dermatitis herpetiformis—Herpes like lesions in form of grouped vesicles, papules, urticaria, and rarely bullae are seen. It is associated with gluten enteropathy. Biopsy reveals neutrophilic microabscesses at the tips of dermal papillae with deposition of IgA antibody complexes. Furthermore, antireticulin and endomysial antibodies are found in the patient's sera[4] (see Chapter 179, Other Bullous Diseases).

- Linear IgA dermatosis—Typical lesions are described as "string of pearls," which is an urticarial plaque surrounded by vesicles. Histologically, IgA antibodies are deposited in a linear fashion along the basement membrane[5] (see Chapter 176, Overview of Bullous Diseases).

- Porphyria cutanea tarda—Bullae are seen on sun-exposed areas. Histology shows antibody deposition in the capillary walls and

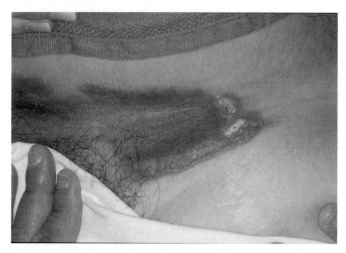

FIGURE 178-5 Pemphigus vegetans in the groin of a middle-aged woman. (*Courtesy of Eric Kraus, MD.*)

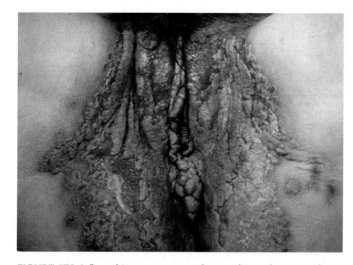

FIGURE 178-6 Pemphigus vegetans widespread over the external genitalia and buttocks. (*Courtesy of Eric Kraus, MD.*)

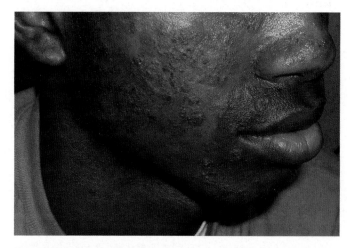

FIGURE 178-7 Pemphigus foliaceous on the face of a black man. (*Courtesy of Jack Resneck, Sr., MD.*)

dermoepidermal junction. Serum iron, ferritin, and transaminase levels are elevated as well as 24-hour urine porphyrins.[5] Elevations in urine porphyrins are diagnostic (see Chapter 179, Other Bullous Disease).

MANAGEMENT

Treatment of pemphigus should be undertaken in consultation with a dermatologist. Treatment is directed initially at disease control and remission followed by disease suppression. The goal is to eventually discontinue all medications and achieve complete remission.

SYSTEMIC THERAPY

- Corticosteroids are the mainstay of treatment.[6] SOR Ⓐ Mild disease may be controlled with prednisone 20 to 40 mg/d but for rapidly progressive and extensive disease, a higher dose prednisone 70 to 90 mg/d is initiated.[1] The dose may be increased by 50% every 1 to 2 weeks until disease activity is controlled. However, some experts will not go beyond 1 mg/kg/d.[7] Once remission is induced, the dose is tapered by 25% every 1 to 2 weeks to the lowest dose needed to suppress recurrence of new lesions.[1]

- Pulse therapy with intravenous methylprednisolone 1 g/d for 5 days may be tried in severe cases in an attempt to decrease the cumulative dose of steroids, especially when high dose oral steroids are ineffective.[6] SOR Ⓒ

- High dose and prolonged treatment with steroids can have serious side effects. Therefore, it is advisable to start adjuvant steroid-sparing therapy within 2 to 4 weeks of treatment. Adjuvant agents have a lag period of 4 to 6 weeks before they become effective, so starting them sooner allows for earlier steroid taper.[1] They may be used alone to maintain remission after steroid withdrawal.

- Adjuvant agents include azathioprine, cyclophosphamide, mycophenolate, gold, and methotrexate.[6] SOR Ⓑ Dapsone is the preferred adjuvant for PF.[6] SOR Ⓒ

- Mycophenolate (CellCept) has become the preferred adjuvant for PV.[6] SOR Ⓒ

- IVIG could be considered as an adjuvant therapy in refractory cases in combination with cytotoxic drugs.[6] SOR Ⓑ

- Rituximab (chimeric monoclonal antibody used in the treatment of non-Hodgkin's lymphoma) has been shown in small case series to be effective in pemphigus.[6] SOR Ⓒ

LOCAL THERAPY

- Solitary lesions may be treated with topical high-potency steroids, such as clobetasol or with intralesional steroid injections e.g., 20 mg/ml triamcinolone acetonide. Isolated oral lesions may be treated with steroid paste, sprays, or lozenges.

- Normal saline compresses or bacteriostatic solutions such as potassium permanganate are useful in keeping lesions clean. Oral hygiene is crucial. Mouthwashes such as chlorhexidine 0.2% or 1:4 hydrogen peroxide may be used. Topical anesthetics may be used for pain.[6]

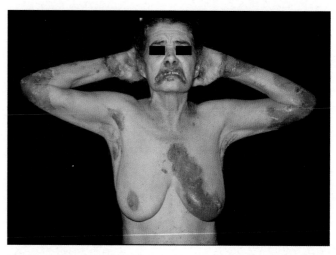

FIGURE 178-8 Pemphigus foliaceous on the face, chest, and arms. (*Courtesy of Eric Kraus, MD.*)

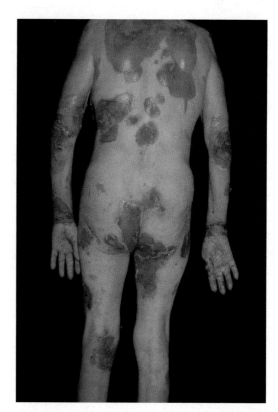

FIGURE 178-9 Pemphigus foliaceous widespread on the back of the patient in **Figure 178-1**. (*Courtesy of Eric Kraus, MD.*)

PATIENT EDUCATION

- Educate patients regarding disease, complications, and side effects of medications.

- Advise patients on avoiding trauma to skin such as with contact sports. Similarly, oral lesions may be aggravated by nuts, spicy foods, chips, and dental plates and bridges.

- Instruct patients on wound care to prevent infections and relieve local discomfort.

- Provide information on support groups such as the International Pemphigus Foundation.

FOLLOW-UP

- Prolonged follow-up is needed for medication adjustment, monitoring disease activity and side effects of drugs.

PATIENT RESOURCES

http://www.mayoclinic.com/health/pemphigus/DS00749.

PROVIDER RESOURCES

http://www.emedicine.com/DERM/topic319.htm.

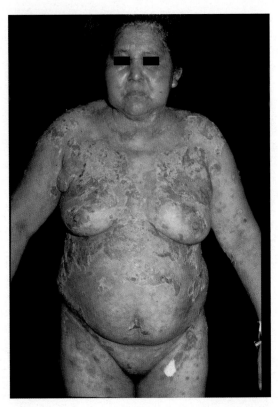

FIGURE 178-10 Widespread pemphigus foliaceous. (*Courtesy of Eric Kraus, MD.*)

REFERENCES

1. Bystryn J, Rudolph JL. Pemphigus. *Lancet*. 2005;366:61–73.

2. Ettlin DA. Pemphigus. *Dent Clin N Am*. 2005;49:107–125.

3. Goldstein BG, Goldstein AO. Pemphigus and bullous pemphigoid. http://www.uptodate.com. Accessed July 16, 2007.

4. Bickle KM, Roark TR. Autoimmune bullous dermatosis: A review. http://www.aafp.org/afp/20020501/1861.html. Accessed July 16, 2007.

5. Yeh SW, Ahmed B, Sami N, Razzaque Ahmed A. Blistering disorders: diagnosis and treatment. *Dermatol Ther*. 2003;16(3): 214–223.

6. Harman KE, Albert S, Black MM. Guidelines for the management of pemphigus vulgaris. *Br J Dermatol*. 2003;149:926–937.

7. Zeina B, Ali M, Mansoor S. Pemphigus Vulgaris. http://www.emedicine.com/DERM/topic319.htm. Accessed July 16, 2007.

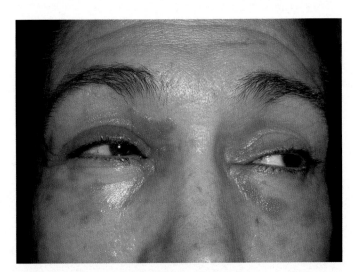

FIGURE 178-11 Pemphigus erythematosus on the face of a 55-year-old woman. (*Courtesy of Richard P. Usatine, MD.*)

179 OTHER BULLOUS DISEASES

Jimmy Hara, MD
Richard P. Usatine, MD

PORPHYRIA CUTANEA TARDA

PATIENT STORY

A middle-aged woman presented with tense blisters on the dorsum of her hand (**Figure 179-1**). One bulla was intact and the others had ruptured showing erosions. Work-up showed elevated porphyrins in the urine (which fluoresced orange-red under a Wood's lamp) and the patient was diagnosed with porphyria cutanea tarda.

EPIDEMIOLOGY

- Porphyria cutanea tarda (PCT) occurs mostly in middle-aged adults (typically 30 to 50 years of age) and is rare in children.
- It is especially likely to occur in women on oral contraceptives and in men on estrogen therapy for prostate cancer.[1]
- Alcohol, pesticides, and chloroquine have been implicated as chemicals that induce porphyria cutanea tarda.[1]
- Porphyria cutanea tarda is equally common in both genders.
- There is an increased incidence of PCT in persons with hepatitis C (**Figure 179-2**).

ETIOLOGY AND PATHOPHYSIOLOGY

- The porphyrias are a family of illnesses caused by various metabolic derangements in the metabolism of porphyrin, the chemical backbone of hemoglobin. Whereas the other porphyrias (acute intermittent porphyria and variegate porphyria) are associated with well-known systemic manifestations (abdominal pain, peripheral neuropathy, and pulmonary complications), porphyria cutanea tarda has no extracutaneous manifestations. Photosensitivity is seen (as with variegate porphyria). Porphyria cutanea tarda is associated with a reduction in hepatic uroporphyrin decarboxylase.

DIAGNOSIS

CLINICAL FEATURES

The classic presentation is that of blistering (vesicles and tense bullae) on photosensitive "fragile skin" (similar to epidermolysis bullosa). Scleroderma-like heliotrope suffusion of the eyelids and face may be seen. As the blisters heal, the skin takes on an atrophic appearance. Hypertrichosis (especially on the cheeks and temples) is also common and may be the presenting feature.

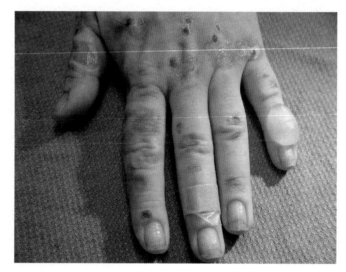

FIGURE 179-1 Porphyria cutanea tarda in a middle-aged woman. (*Courtesy of Lewis Rose, MD.*)

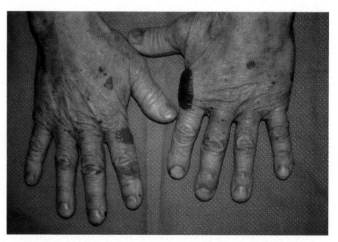

FIGURE 179-2 Porphyria cutanea tarda in a man with hepatitis C. (*Courtesy of the University of Texas Health Sciences Center, Division of Dermatology.*)

TYPICAL DISTRIBUTION

Classically, the dorsa of the hands are affected. Facial suffusion (heliotrope) may be seen along with hypertrichosis of the cheeks and temples.

LABORATORY STUDIES

The diagnosis can be confirmed by the orange-red fluorescence of the urine when examined under a Wood's lamp. Increased plasma iron may be seen (associated with increased hepatic iron in the Kupffer cells). Diabetes is said to occur in 25% of individuals.

- 24 hour urine collection for porphyrins—these will be elevated in PCT.
- Skin biopsy may help confirm PCT if the other information is not clear.
- Once the diagnosis is made, secondary causes of PCT should be investigated:
  - Serum for ferritin, iron and iron binding capacity to look for hemochromatosis.
  - Order liver function tests and if abnormal order tests for hepatitis B and C.
  - Consider alpha-fetoprotein and liver ultrasound if considering cirrhosis and/or hepatocellular carcinoma.
  - Order an HIV test if risk factors are present.

DIFFERENTIAL DIAGNOSIS

- The acral vesiculobullous lesions may suggest nummular or dyshidrotic eczema. In younger individuals, the acral blistering may suggest epidermolysis bullosa. The lesions may also suggest erythema multiforme bullosum. The heliotrope suffusion may suggest dermatomyositis and the atrophic changes may suggest systemic sclerosis.

MANAGEMENT

- If the onset is associated with alcohol ingestion, estrogen therapy, or exposure to pesticides, reducing exposure is warranted.[1]
- Phlebotomy of 500 mL of blood weekly until the hemoglobin is decreased to 10 g is associated with biochemical and clinical remission within a year.[2]
- Low-dose chloroquine can help maintain remissions, whereas high-dose chloroquine can exacerbate the illness.

PATIENT EDUCATION

- Avoidance of potential precipitants (alcohol, estrogens, pesticides) and avoidance of excess sunlight exposure (to avoid hypersensitivity) are important. Avoidance of trauma and careful wound care is also necessary.

FOLLOW-UP

- Periodic clinical follow-up until remission is achieved is necessary along with constant education and reinforcement of the need to avoid precipitants.

DYSTROPHIC EPIDERMOLYSIS BULLOSA

PATIENT STORY

A 34-year-old pregnant woman presents with active blistering in her axilla and no fingernails (**Figure 179-3**). Past history revealed that she lost her fingernails and toenails as a young child. She was diagnosed as a child with recessive dystrophic epidermolysis bullosa. None of her children had been affected since her husband was neither affected nor a carrier (**Figure 179-4**). A topical steroid ointment helped relieve the pain and calm the blistering in her axilla.

EPIDEMIOLOGY

- Dystrophic epidermolysis bullosa belongs to a family of inherited diseases characterized by skin fragility and blister formation caused by minor skin trauma.[3] There are autosomal recessive and autosomal dominant types. The severity of this disease may vary widely. Onset is in childhood and in later years severe dystrophic deformities of hands and feet are characteristic (**Figures 179-5** and **179-6**). Malignant degeneration is common, especially squamous cell carcinoma, in sun-exposed areas.

ETIOLOGY AND PATHOPHYSIOLOGY

- Dystrophic epidermolysis bullosa has vesiculobullous skin separation occurring at the sub-basal lamina level, as opposed to junctional epidermolysis bullosa which blisters at the intralamina lucida layer, and epidermolysis bullosa simplex which blisters at the intraepidermal layer.[4,5]

DIAGNOSIS

CLINICAL FEATURES

Acral skin fragility and blistering are the hallmark in childhood. Minor trauma can induce severe blistering. As the disease progresses initially, painful and ultimately debilitating dystrophic deformities are typical. Repeated blistering of the hands can lead to fusion of the fingers and the so-called mitten deformity (**Figure 179-5**).

TYPICAL DISTRIBUTION

The typical distribution is acral although blistering may extend proximally secondary to trauma (**Figures 179-3** to **179-6**).

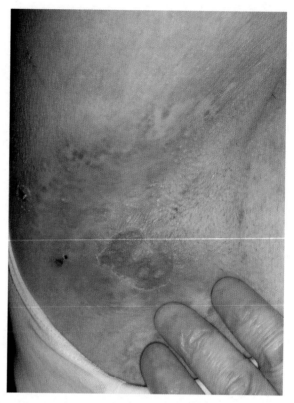

FIGURE 179-3 Recessive dystrophic epidermolysis bullosa in a 34-year-old pregnant woman with active blistering in her axilla and previous loss of all her finger and toe nails as a young child. (*Courtesy of Richard P. Usatine, MD.*)

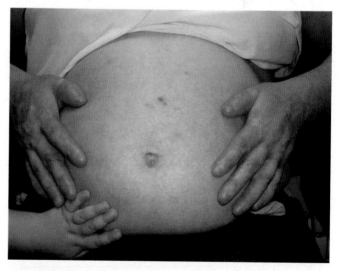

FIGURE 179-4 The pregnant woman in **Figure 179-3** with recessive dystrophic epidermolysis bullosa showing complete loss of her fingernails. Note that her daughter does not have the disease and, therefore, has normal fingers. (*Courtesy of Richard P. Usatine, MD.*)

LABORATORY STUDIES AND BIOPSY

There are no laboratory tests to confirm the diagnosis. A punch biopsy can provide adequate tissue for the dermatopathologist to differentiate between the different forms of epidermolysis bullosa: simplex, junctional, and dystrophic.

DIFFERENTIAL DIAGNOSIS

- Erythema multiforme bullosum may have a similar appearance, but the distribution is less apt to be limited to the distal extremities. The appearance of an acral blistering on fragile skin is also characteristic of porphyria cutanea tarda, but the age of onset of porphyria cutanea tarda is typically in middle age and not in childhood. The first appearance of the condition may be confused with staphylococcal scalded skin syndrome (see Chapter 110, Impetigo).[6]

MANAGEMENT

- Management is primarily prevention of trauma, careful wound care, and treatment of complicating infections. Other supportive measures such as pain management and nutritional support are often necessary. Screening the skin for squamous cell carcinoma is important in the dystrophic form.

PATIENT EDUCATION

Avoid trauma and come in early if there are any signs of infection or malignancy.

FOLLOW-UP

Periodic skin examinations should be done to help manage symptoms and screen for malignancy.

PLEVA (PITYRIASIS LICHENOIDES ET VARIOLIFORMIS ACUTA)

PATIENT STORY

A 22-year-old man presented with a varicelliform eruption that he has had for 6 weeks (**Figure 179-7**). Initially he was diagnosed with varicella and given a course of acyclovir. Then he was misdiagnosed with scabies and treated with permethrin. A correct diagnosis was made of pityriasis lichenoides et varioliformis acuta (PLEVA) by clinical appearance and confirmed with biopsy. His skin lesions cleared with oral tetracycline.

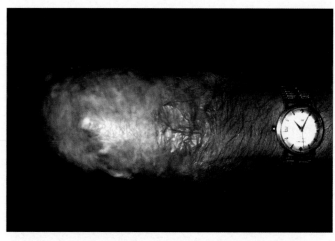

FIGURE 179-5 Severe recessive dystrophic epidermolysis bullosa in a 53-year-old Asian man with complete loss of fingers from the disease on his hands. This is the so-called mitten deformity. He has also had multiple squamous cell carcinomas excised from his hands. (*Courtesy of Richard P. Usatine, MD.*)

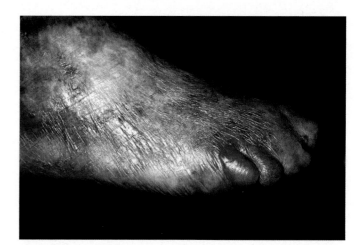

FIGURE 179-6 Severe recessive dystrophic epidermolysis bullosa in the man in **Figure 179-5** showing foot deformities with loss of normal toes. (*Courtesy of Richard P. Usatine, MD.*)

EPIDEMIOLOGY

- PLEVA or Mucha–Habermann disease and pityriasis lichenoides chronica are maculopapular erythematous eruptions that can occur in crops of vesicles that can become hemorrhagic over a course of weeks to months (**Figures 179-7** and **179-8**).[7]
- There is a predilection for males in the second and third decades.
- PLEVA occurs in preschool and preadolescent children as well.[8]

ETIOLOGY AND PATHOPHYSIOLOGY

- PLEVA has traditionally been classified as a benign papulosquamous disease. However there is increasing evidence that suggests that PLEVA should be considered a form of cutaneous lymphoid dyscrasia.[9] It may even represent an indolent form of mycosis fungoides.

DIAGNOSIS

CLINICAL FEATURES

PLEVA occurs with crops of maculopapular and papulosquamous lesions that can vesiculate and form hemorrhagic vesicles (**Figures 179-7** and **179-8**). It resembles varicella, however new crops of lesions continue to appear over weeks and months. It can be thought of as "chickenpox that lasts for weeks to months."

TYPICAL DISTRIBUTION

Lesions typically occur over the anterior trunk and flexural aspects of the proximal extremities. The face is spared.

LABORATORY STUDIES

There are no specific laboratory tests for PLEVA except biopsy.

BIOPSY

A punch biopsy is helpful in making the diagnosis. It may be necessary to differentiate PLEVA from lymphomatoid papulosis (see differential diagnosis below).

DIFFERENTIAL DIAGNOSIS

- Varicella—A varicella direct fluorescent antibody test can confirm acute varicella. If no viral testing was done and what appeared to be varicella persists, PLEVA should be considered (see Chapter 117, Chickenpox).
- Erythema multiforme is a hypersensitivity syndrome in which target lesions are seen. The target lesions have epidermal disruption in the center with vesicles and/or erosions. Look for the target lesions to help differentiate this from PLEVA (see Chapter 170, Hypersensitivity Syndromes).
- Lymphomatoid papulosis presents in a manner similar to PLEVA with recurrent crops of pruritic papules at different stages of development that appear on the trunk and extremities. While it has histologic features that suggest lymphoma, lymphomatoid papulosis

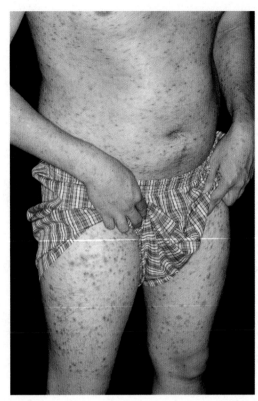

FIGURE 179-7 A 22-year-old man with pityriasis lichenoides et varioliformis acuta (PLEVA). His skin lesions cleared with oral tetracycline. (*Courtesy of Richard P, Usatine, MD.*)

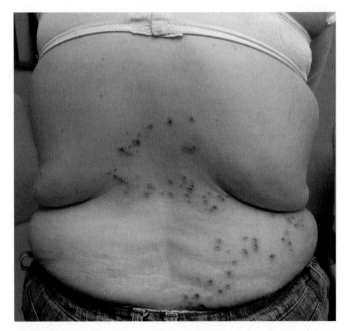

FIGURE 179-8 A young woman with PLEVA. (*Courtesy of David Anderson, MD.*)

alone is not fatal. It is important to differentiate this from PLEVA because these patients need to be worked up for coexisting malignancy. These patients tend to be older and a punch biopsy can make the diagnosis.

- Gianotti–Crosti syndrome (papular acrodermatitis of childhood) may resemble PLEVA but the lesions are usually acral in distribution.[5] The erythematous papules and vesicles are found on the extremities and sometimes on the face. It is a benign syndrome associated with many childhood viruses that may last 2 to 8 weeks.

MANAGEMENT

- Ultraviolet A1 phototherapy has been deployed with some success.[10] Various reports suggest the efficacy of macrolides and tetracyclines, probably more for their antiinflammatory properties than for their antibacterial effects.

PATIENT EDUCATION

This is usually a temporary disease but if it becomes chronic there are treatments that could help such as oral macrolides or tetracycline.

FOLLOW-UP

Needed only if the disease does not resolve.

DERMATITIS HERPETIFORMIS

PATIENT STORY

A young man with a past history of diarrhea and malabsorption carries a past diagnosis of gluten-induced enteropathy. He indicates that he periodically develops a vesicular eruption over the extensor aspects of his extremities (**Figure 179-9**). A punch biopsy confirms dermatitis herpetiformis.

EPIDEMIOLOGY

- Dermatitis herpetiformis is a chronic recurrent symmetric vesicular eruption that is usually associated with diet-related enteropathy.[11] It most commonly occurs in the 20 to 40 years age group. Men are affected more often than women.

ETIOLOGY AND PATHOPHYSIOLOGY

- The disease is related to gluten and other diet-related antigens that cause the development of circulating immune complexes and their subsequent deposition in the skin. The term herpetiformis refers to the grouped vesicles that appear on extensor aspects of the extremities

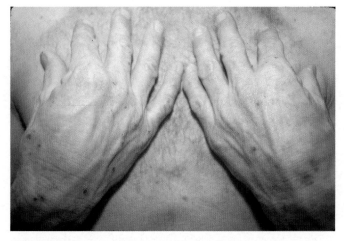

FIGURE 179-9 A man with dermatitis herpetiformis and gluten-induced enteropathy. (*Courtesy of Richard P. Usatine, MD.*)

and trunk and is not a viral infection or related to the herpes viruses. The disease is characterized by the deposition of IgA along the tips of the dermal papillae. The majority of patients will also have blunting and flattening of jejunal villi, which leads to diarrhea even to the point of steatorrhea and malabsorption.

DIAGNOSIS

CLINICAL FEATURES

The clinical eruption is characterized by severe itching, burning, or stinging in the characteristic extensor distribution. Herpetiform vesicles and urticarial plaques may be seen. Because of the intense pruritus, characteristic lesions may be excoriated beyond recognition (**Figures 179-9** and **179-10**).

TYPICAL DISTRIBUTION

Classically, the lesions (or excoriations) are seen in the extensor aspects of the extremities (**Figure 179-10**), shoulders, lower back, and sacrum.

LABORATORY STUDIES

If the patient has gluten-induced enteropathy, antigliadin and antiendomysial antibodies may be present. A blood test for antigliadin antibody is a sensitive test for gluten-induced enteropathy.

BIOPSY

Diagnosis is confirmed by a punch biopsy. It is best to biopsy new crops of lesions. A standard histologic examination will show eosinophils and microabscesses of neutrophils in the dermal papillae and subepidermal vesicles. Direct immunofluorescence reveals deposits of IgA and complement within the dermal papillae.

DIFFERENTIAL DIAGNOSIS

• Scabies may have a similar appearance with pruritus, papules, and vesicles. If the lesions and distribution suggest scabies, it should be ruled out with skin scraping looking for the mite, feces, and eggs. If the scraping is negative, but the clinical appearance suggests scabies, empiric treatment with permethrin should be considered as well. If the lesions persist, consider a punch biopsy to look for dermatitis herpetiformis (see Chapter 137, Scabies).

• Nummular and dyshidrotic eczema may also be diagnostic considerations, but response to steroids in eczema may be helpful in differentiation (see Chapters 139, Atopic Dermatitis and 141, Hand Eczema).

• The classic differential for PCT is pseudoporphyria (caused by NSAIDS like naprosyn), epidermolysis bullosa acquisita and variegate porphyria.

MANAGEMENT

• With a gluten-free diet, 80% of patients will show improvement in the skin lesions. The degree of benefit is dependent upon the strictness of the diet.[11]

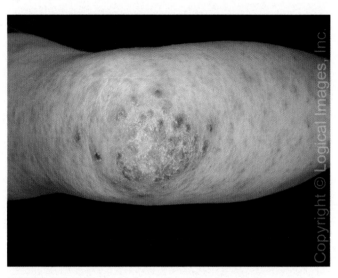

FIGURE 179-10 Dermatitis herpetiformis on the extensor aspect of the arm with excoriations on the elbow. (*Courtesy of Logical Images, Inc.*)

- A gluten-free diet may help the enteropathy and decrease the subsequent development of small bowel lymphoma.
- Dapsone at an initial dose of 100 to 200 mg daily with gradual reduction to a 25- to 50-mg maintenance level may be necessary indefinitely.[12]

PATIENT EDUCATION

Nutritional counseling is important for all patients with gluten-induced enteropathy. Persons with dermatitis herpetiformis and gluten-induced enteropathy should not eat wheat and barley but can eat rice, oats and corn.

FOLLOW-UP

Follow-up is needed to control the disease and monitor nutritional status.

PATIENT AND PROVIDER RESOURCES

Medline Plus article on porphyria for patients—**http://www.nlm.nih.gov/medlineplus/ency/article/001208.htm.**

Genetics Home Reference: Epidermolysis bullosa simplex (National Library of Medicine)—**http://ghr.nlm.nih.gov/condition=epidermolysisbullosasimplex.**

Epidermolysis Bullosa (National Institute of Arthritis and Musculoskeletal and Skin Diseases)—**http://www.niams.nih.gov/Health_Info/Epidermolysis_Bullosa/default.asp.**

Dermatitis Herpetiformis (Gluten Intolerance Group)—**http://www.gluten.net/dh.htm.**

Mayo Clinic on PLEVA—**http://www.mayoclinic.com/health/pleva/AN00709.**

PROVIDER RESOURCES

Dermnet Skin Disease Image Atlas module on bullous disease—**http://www.dermnet.com/moduleIndex.cfm?moduleID=5.**

PatientPlus from the UK on Bullous Dermatoses—**http://www.patient.co.uk/showdoc/40001035/.**

REFERENCES

1. Gonzalez E, Gonzales S. Drug photosensitivity, idiopathic photodermatoses, and sunscreens. *J Am Acad Dermatol.* 1996;35:871.

2. Kauppinen R, Timonen K, Mustajoki P. Treatment of the porphyrias. *Ann Med.* 1994;26:31.

3. Horn HM, Tidman MJ. The clinical spectrum of epidermolysis bullosa. *Brit J Dermatol.* 2002;146:267.

4. Margileth AM. Dermatologic conditions. In: Avery GB, Fletcher MA, McDonald MG eds. *Neonatology.* 5th ed. Philadelphia: Lippincott Williams and Wilkins, 1999:1323.

5. Paller AS, Mancini AJ. Bullous diseases in children. In: Paller AS, Mancini AJ eds. *Hurwitz's Clinical Pediatric Dermatology.* 3rd ed. Philadeplphia: Elsevier, 2006:345.

6. Patel GK, Finlay AY. Staphylococcal scalded skin syndrome: Diagnosis and management. *Am J Clin Dermatol.* 2003;4:165.

7. Bowers S, Warshaw EM. Pityriasis lichenoides and its subtypes. *J Am Acad Dermatol.* 2006;55:557.

8. Ersoy-Evans S, Greco MF, Mancini AJ, Subasi N, Paller AS. Pityriasis lichenoides in childhood: A retrospective review of 124 patients. *J Am Acad Dermatol.* 2007;56:205.

9. Magro C, Crowson AN, Kovatich A, Burns. Pityriasis lichenoides: A clonal T-cell lymphoproliferative disorder. *Human Pathol.* 2002;33:788.

10. Pinton PC, Capezzera R, Zane C, De Panfilis G. Medium dose ultraviolet A1 therapy for pityriasis lichenoides et varioliformis acuta and pityriasis lichenoides chronica. *J Am Acad Dermatol.* 2002;47:410.

11. Dermatitis herpetiformis. PatientPlus. http://www.patient.co.uk/showdoc/40001007/. Accessed October 7, 2007.

12. Fine JD. Management of acquired bullous skin diseases. *N Engl J Med.* 1995;333:1475.

180 ALOPECIA AREATA

James W. Haynes, MD

PATIENT STORY

An 8-year-old Hispanic girl was brought to her physician by her mother, who noticed two bald spots on the back of her daughter's scalp while brushing her hair. The child had no itching or pain. The mother was more worried that her beautiful girl would become bald. The girl was pleased that the bald spots could be completely covered with her long hair, but she did not want anyone to see them. The child was otherwise healthy. When the mother lifted the hair in the back, two round areas of hair loss were evident (**Figure 180-1**). On close inspection, there was no scaling or scarring. The mother and child were reassured that alopecia areata (AA) is a condition in which the hair is likely to regrow without treatment. Neither of them wanted intralesional injections or topical therapies. During a well-child examination 1 year later, it was noted that the girl's hair had fully regrown.[1]

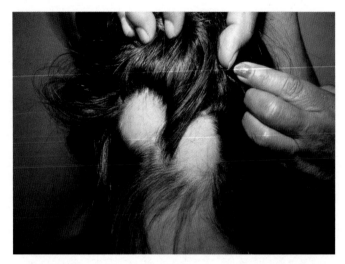

FIGURE 180-1 Alopecia areata (AA) in an 8-year-old girl.[1] (*With permission from Usatine RP. Bald spots on a young girl. J Fam Pract. 2004;53:33–36, Dowden Health Media.*)

EPIDEMIOLOGY

- Alopecia areata is a common, chronic skin disorder manifested as a sudden loss of hair without accompanying inflammation or scarring. It affects about 0.2% of the population at any given time with ~1.7% of the population experiencing an episode during their lifetime.[2,3]

- Alopecia areata may extend to involve the whole scalp, alopecia totalis (AT) (**Figures 180-2 and 180-3**), or the whole body, alopecia universalis (AU).

- Men and women are equally affected.

- Most patients are younger than 40 years at disease onset with the average age being 25 to 27 years.[2,4]

ETIOLOGY AND PATHOPHYSIOLOGY

- The etiology is unknown but experts presume that the AA spectrum of disorders is secondary to an autoimmune phenomenon involving antibodies, T cells, and cytokines.[5]

DIAGNOSIS

CLINICAL FEATURES

- Sudden onset of one or more 1 to 4 cm areas of hair loss on the scalp (**Figures 180-1 and 180-4**).

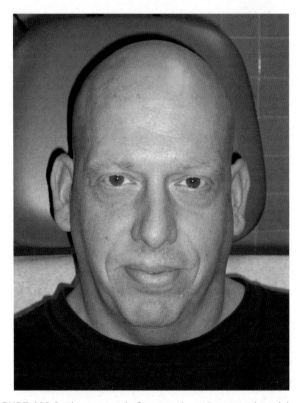

FIGURE 180-2 Alopecia totalis for more than 10 years in this adult man. (*Courtesy of Richard P. Usatine, MD.*)

- The affected skin is smooth and white and may have short stubble hair growth.
- When hair begins to regrow, it often comes in as fine white hair (**Figure 180-5**).

TYPICAL DISTRIBUTION

- Scalp, but can progress to involve total body hair loss.

LABORATORY STUDIES

- Typically, the diagnosis can be made with history and physical examination alone.
- Microscopic evaluation of the hair from the periphery of the involved skin reveals "exclamation point" hairs, which are characterized by proximal thinning while the distal portion remains of normal caliber.
- Thyroid abnormalities, vitiligo, and pernicious anemia often accompany AA and hence screening laboratory tests (e.g., thyroid stimulating hormone, CBC) may be helpful to look for thyroid disorders and anemia.

BIOPSY

Not needed. Histology examination shows peribulbar lymphocytic infiltration, frequently including eosinophils and the above mentioned "exclamation point" hairs.

DIFFERENTIAL DIAGNOSIS

- Trichotillomania—history of hair pulling; short, "broken" hairs are seen (see Chapter 181, Traction Alopecia and Trichotillomania).
- Telogen effluvium—even distribution of hair loss; may be drug-induced (e.g., warfarin, beta blockers, lithium) or occur after pregnancy (see Chapter 70, Normal Skin Findings in Pregnancy).
- Anagen effluvium—history of drug use (e.g., antimitotic agents); even distribution of hair loss.
- Tinea Capitis—skin scaling and inflammation; KOH prep or fungal culture, if necessary (see Chapter 131, Tinea Capitis).
- Secondary syphilis—"moth-eaten" appearance in beard or scalp; risk factors and RPR will help distinguish (see Chapter 209, Syphilis).
- Lupus erythematosus—skin scarring; antinuclear antibody (ANA) if clinical presentation compatible with this diagnosis (see Chapter 173, Lupus-Systemic and Cutaneous).

MANAGEMENT

- Many patients with AA will have significant comorbid anxiety and depression, so the management of psychological implications is paramount to successful management.
- Treatment for alopecia includes immune-modulating agents (e.g., corticosteroids, anthralin, psoralen plus ultraviolet A [PUVA]),

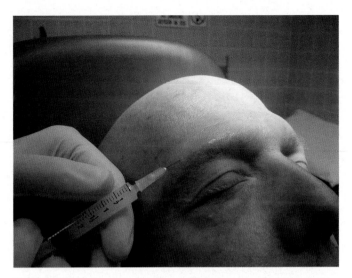

FIGURE 180-3 The patient in **Figure 180-2** receiving steroid injection to encourage regrowth of his eyebrows. This therapy has worked before and patient is requesting it again. (*Courtesy of Richard P. Usatine, MD.*)

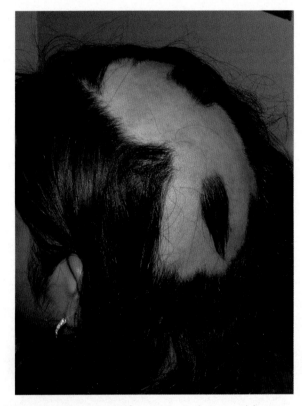

FIGURE 180-4 Extensive AA for over 6 months in an adult woman. (*Courtesy of Richard P. Usatine, MD.*)

contact sensitizers (e.g., dinitrochlorobenzene, squaric acid dibutyl ester, diphenylcyclopropenone), and biologic response modifiers (e.g., minoxidil).[5,6] SOR Ⓒ

○ A commonly used treatment in patients older than 10 years of age with less than 50% scalp involvement is intralesional steroids (**Figure 180-3**). SOR Ⓒ

■ Triamcinolone acetonide (Kenalog)—dilute with sterile saline to 5 mg per mL. Inject with a 3-mL or 5-mL syringe and a 27 or 30-gauge needle. Inject into the dermis of the involved areas but not to exceed 4 mL per visit. Use 2.5 mg per mL for involved areas of the eyebrows or beard. SOR Ⓒ

■ Skin atrophy can be reduced by injecting intradermally and limiting both the volume per site and the frequency of injections (>4–6 wk between injections). Do not reinject areas that show atrophy and in most cases, the artophy will resolve spontaneously. SOR Ⓒ

■ Because spontaneous regrowth can occur, steroid injections should be discontinued after 6 months if there is no response.

○ For patients younger than 10 years, 5% minoxidil, mid-potency topical steroids, and/or anthralin can be used. The combination of anthralin with topical steroids and/or minoxidil is a good choice for children and for those with extensive disease caused by its easy use and effectiveness without skin irritation. SOR Ⓒ

○ For patients with more than 50% of scalp involvement, topical immunotherapy with contact sensitizers may be an effective treatment.

■ Topical diphenylcyclopropenone (DPCP) is a contact immunotherapy that has some proven benefit with extensive alopecia areata. In one study, 56 patients with chronic, extensive alopecia areata (duration ranging from 1 to 10 years, involving 30% to 100% of the scalp) were treated with progressively higher concentrations of DPCP in a randomized crossover trial. Twenty-five of 56 patients had total hair regrowth at 6 months, and no relapse occurred in 60% of patients.[7] SOR Ⓑ

■ These contact sensitizers have potential severe side effects including mutagenesis, blistering, hyperpigmentation, and scarring and hence should be used by clinicians with significant experience with these agents or in consultation with a dermatologic specialist.

■ Minoxidil, PUVA, and anthralin have been used with varying effectiveness and can be considered.

• Hairpieces and transplants may be used for those patients with unresponsive, recalcitrant disease.

• One randomized controlled trial showed aromatherapy with topical essential oils to be a safe and effective treatment for AA.[8] SOR Ⓑ

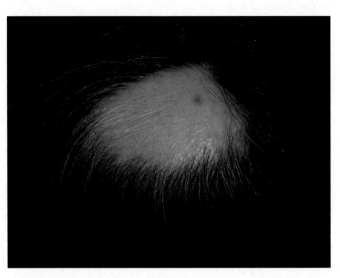

FIGURE 180-5 New growth of white hair after 7 months of AA in this middle-aged woman. (*Courtesy of Richard P. Usatine, MD.*)

PATIENT EDUCATION

• Although spontaneous recovery usually occurs, the course of AA is unpredictable and often characterized by recurrent periods of hair loss and regrowth.

• Spontaneous long-term regrowth in AT and AU is poor.

• Prognosis is worse if the alopecia persists longer than 1 year.

FOLLOW-UP

- Spontaneous recovery usually occurs within 6 to 12 months and the prognosis for total permanent regrowth with limited involvement (AA) is excellent.

- The regrown hair is usually of the same texture and color but may be fine and white at first (**Figure 180-5**).

- Ten percent of patients' never regrow hair and advance to chronic disease. Clinicians should provide contact information to the National Alopecia Areata Foundation and offer follow-up in the office as necessary.

- Patients with a family history of AA, younger age at onset, coexisting immune disorders, nail dystrophy, atopy, and widespread hair loss have a poorer prognosis.[5]

PATIENT RESOURCES

The National Alopecia Areata Foundation (**http://www.naaf.org/**) publishes a newsletter and can provide information regarding these support groups as well as hairpiece information.

http://www.niams.nih.gov/hi/topics/alopecia/ ff_alopecia_areata.htm.

PROVIDER RESOURCES

- **www.emedicine.com/derm/topic14.htm.**

REFERENCES

1. Usatine RP. Bald spots on a young girl. *J Fam Pract*. 2004;53:33–36.

2. Firooz A, Firoozabadi MR, Ghazisaidi B, Dowlati Y. Concepts of patients with alopecia about their disease. *BMC Dermatol*. 2005;12(5):1.

3. Springer K, Brown M, Stulberg DL. Common hair loss disorders. *Am Fam Physician*. 2003;68:93–102,107–108.

4. Choi HJ, Ihm CW. Acute alopecia totalis. *Acta Dermatoven Alp Panonica Adriat*. 2006;15:27–34.

5. Habif TP. Hair diseases. In: Habif TP ed. *Clinical Dermatology: A Color Guide to Diagnosis and Therapy*. 4th ed. Mosby: St Louis, 2004.

6. Price VH. Treatment of hair loss. *N Engl J Med*. 1999;341(13): 964–973.

7. Cotellessa C, Peris K, Caracciolo E, Mordenti C, Chimenti S. The use of topical diphenylcyclopropenone for the treatment of extensive alopecia areata. *J Am Acad Dermatol*. 2001;44:73–76.

8. Hay IC, Jamieson M, Ormerod AD. Randomized trial of aromatherapy. Successful treatment for alopecia areata. *Arch Dermatol*. 1998;134:1349–1352.

181 TRACTION HAIR LOSS AND TRICHOTILLOMANIA

E.J. Mayeaux, Jr., MD
Zoe Draelos, MD

PATIENT STORY

A 38-year-old woman was found to have hair thinning on the anterior scalp. She had long thick heavy hair that she always styled in a bun on the top of her head. She was concerned about the slow, steady loss of hair that she was experiencing. **Figure 181-1** shows the appearance of the thinned hair as a result of chronic traction. A 4-mm punch biopsy was performed to confirm the clinical impression and the histology was supportive of this diagnosis.

EPIDEMIOLOGY

*   The prevalence of traction alopecia (**Figure 181-1**) is unknown and varies by cultural hair style practices. It is most commonly seen in females and children.[1]

*   The prevalence of trichotillomania (**Figures 181-2 to 181-5**) is also difficult to determine, but is estimated to be about 1.5% of males and 3.4% of females in the United States. The mean age of onset of trichotillomania is 8 years in boys and 12 years in girls, and it is the most common cause of childhood alopecia.[2]

ETIOLOGY AND PATHOPHYSIOLOGY

*   Traction alopecia is seen in individuals who place chronic tension on the hair shafts with tight braids, heavy natural hair, use of hair prostheses, or chronic pulling (**Figure 181-1**).[1] It also occurs commonly in female athletes who pull their hair into tight ponytails.

*   Chronic tension on the hair shaft seems to create inflammation within the hair follicle that eventually leads to cessation of hair growth. Hair loss from traction alopecia may become permanent, thus prevention and early treatment are important.

*   It is seen most frequently in black women who tightly braid or pull the hair into a hair style during youth and on into adulthood. May also be seen in individuals who wear hair prostheses or extensions for a prolonged period of time.

*   Trichotillomania is a subtype of traction alopecia manifested by chronic hair pulling (**Figures 181-2 to 181-4**) and sometimes hair eating (trichophagy), which can lead to a trichobezoar. It is classified as a psychiatric impulse-control disorder.[3]

*   Trichotillomania may be a manifestation of the inability to cope with stress rather than more severe mental disorders.

*   Children who exhibit trichotillomania may discontinue the hair pulling with parental support and maturity. Adults who exhibit trichotillomania, even though they are aware of the problem, may

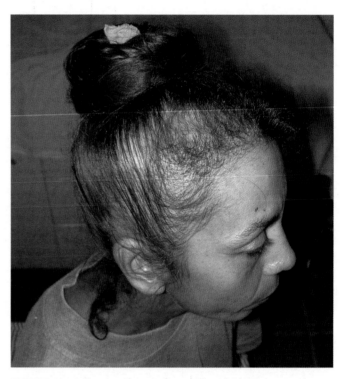

FIGURE 181-1 Traction alopecia from pulling the hair up in a tight bun. (*Courtesy of Richard P. Usatine, MD.*)

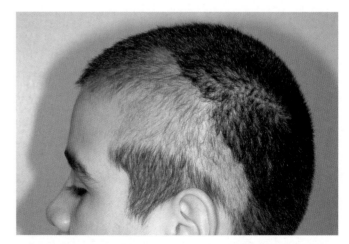

FIGURE 181-2 Trichotillomania in an 11-year-old boy. Note the incomplete hair loss and unusual geometric pattern. He was receiving help and the hair is now growing in. (*Courtesy of Richard P. Usatine, MD.*)

require psychiatric intervention to limit the behavior. The hair loss is initially reversible but may become permanent if the habits persist.

DIAGNOSIS

CLINICAL FEATURES

In patients with traction alopecia, there are decreased follicular ostia in the affected area coupled with decreased hair density. The hair loss usually occurs in the frontal and temporal areas but depends on the precipitating hairstyle (**Figure 181-1**). No scalp inflammation or scaling is typically visible. No pain or other discomfort is associated with the condition. Patients with trichotillomania often demonstrate short broken hairs (**Figure 181-5**) without the presence of inflammation or skin scale early in the disease. The affected areas are not bald, but rather possess hairs of varying length. There may be a telltale stubble of hairs too short to pull. The hair loss often follows bizarre patterns with incomplete areas of clearing. The scalp may appear normal or have areas of erythema and pustule formation. With chronic pulling, the hair loss becomes permanent (**Figures 181-3** and **181-4**). The patient may be observed pulling or twisting the hair by friends or family members.

TYPICAL DISTRIBUTION

Trichotillomania most commonly occurs on the scalp and can involve any area of the body that can be reached by the patient.[1] Traction alopecia can occur anywhere on the scalp, but is most commonly seen at the anterior hairline. This is the site where the hair is pulled back from the face into braids or a bun.

LABORATORY STUDIES

Laboratory tests are not needed to make the diagnosis. A hand lens can be used to examine the affected scalp for decreased follicular ostia, if desired. A scalp biopsy (4-mm punch biopsy) may be necessary to make the diagnosis and rule out other etiologies, especially in trichotillomania, because patients may not acknowledge the habit.

Hypothyroidism or hyperthyroidism may be associated with telogen effluvium or alopecia areata. It may be worth ordering a TSH if the history and physical exam are not completely convincing for self-induced hair loss.

DIFFERENTIAL DIAGNOSIS[1]

- Alopecia areata is characterized by the total absence of hair in an area and the presence of exclamation point hairs. These hairs are thinner in diameter closer to the scalp and thicker in diameter away from the scalp creating the appearance of an exclamation point. Hairs are often white when they start to regrow (see Chapter 180, Alopecia Areata).

- Tinea capitis exhibits hairs broken off at the skin surface and the presence of scale and/or inflammation. Some varieties fluoresce when examined with a Wood's light (UV light). Microscopy of a KOH preparation may detect the dermatophyte. Sometimes it is

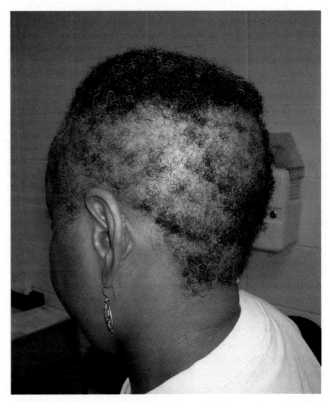

FIGURE 181-3 Chronic hair loss in a 39-year-old woman with trichotillomania. (*Courtesy of E.J. Mayeaux, Jr., MD.*)

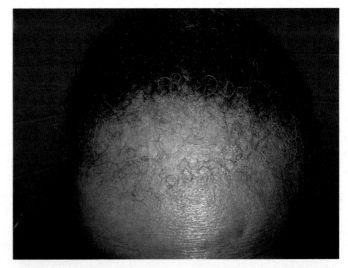

FIGURE 181-4 Forehead of the same patient as shown in **Figure 181-3**. The hair loss has become permanent as a result of chronic injury. (*Courtesy of E.J. Mayeaux, MD.*)

necessary to culture some hairs and scale to make this diagnosis (see Chapter 131, Tinea Capitis).

- Scarring alopecia (lichen planopilaris, folliculitis decalvans) is observed as loss of the follicular ostia and the absence of hairs. The scalp may appear scarred with changes in pigmentation (see Chapter 182, Scarring Alopecia).

- Telogen effluvium (postpregnancy hair loss) is associated with hair loss during the postpartum period and can happen after other stressful events such as surgery or severe illness (see Chapter 70, Normal Skin Findings in Pregnancy). The hair loss is evenly distributed across the head and the hair is thinned all over rather than in patches as in traction alopecia.

- Androgenetic alopecia produces central thinning in women and temple and crown thinning in males. It should be considered in women with symptoms of hormonal abnormalities such as hirsutism, amenorrhea, or infertility.

MANAGEMENT

- Stop hair styling practices that led to the traction alopecia. No tight braiding or buns should be worn.[1]

- Topical corticosteroids can be used to decrease scalp inflammation if erythema is present. SOR **C**

- Topical minoxidil is sometimes used to speed hair regrowth in the area. SOR **C**

- The principal treatments for trichotillomania are counseling and behavior modification techniques.[1] SOR **C**

- Cognitive behavioral therapy usually is successful if the patient is recalcitrant to simple education.[4] SOR **C**

- Fluoxetine hydrochloride (Prozac) 20 to 40 mg a day in adults or clomipramine (Anafranil) 25 to 250 mg/d in adults or a maximum of 3 mg/kg/d in children has had some success for alleviating compulsive hair pulling.[3–5] SOR **B**

- Open discussions with the patient, and the family, if appropriate, are important to understand the reason for the behavior. Many times there are secondary social or emotional issues that must be resolved before the trichotillomania ceases.

- No topical medication is effective in stopping either type of alopecia. However, scalp itching can be treated with topical liquid corticosteroid preparations.

PATIENT EDUCATION

Explain that in traction alopecia, current grooming practices are responsible for the hair loss and a new hair style must be selected. It is important to tell the patient that some of the hair loss may be permanent and no guarantee can be given regarding the amount of expected hair regrowth. Similar hair grooming practices should be avoided in the patient's children to prevent traction alopecia from occurring. Prevention is definitely the best treatment.

Explain that trichotillomania is a self-induced disease that can often resolve if the hair pulling or twisting is discontinued. Patients may exhibit hair pulling or twisting unconsciously when stressed or use it as

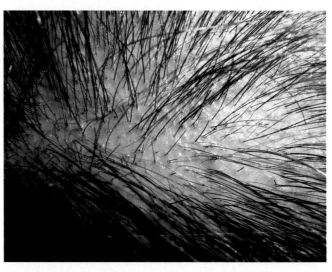

FIGURE 181-5 Close-up of broken hairs on the scalp of a 16-year-old athletic girl with trichotillomania. At first she denied manipulating her hair but a 4-mm punch biopsy was highly suggestive of trichotillomania. She then admitted to ironing her hair daily and sometimes pulling on it to make it straight. (*Courtesy of Richard P. Usatine, MD.*)

a calming activity when relaxing or going to sleep. The underlying reasons for the behavior should be explored and discussed. Sometimes trichotillomania can be substituted with another behavior, such as playing with beads or rubbing a stone.

FOLLOW-UP

Specific follow-up is not required for traction alopecia but psychiatric/behavioral counseling follow-up is indicated for trichotillomania.

PATIENT RESOURCES

- Trichotillomania Support and Therapy Site. Emphasis on Growth: **http://www.trichotillomania.co.uk/**.
- Trichotillomania—Quest Diagnostics Patient Health Library: **http://www.bioportfolio.co.uk/**.
- Traction Alopecia: Causes and Treatment Options: **http://www.traction-alopecia.com/**.

PROVIDER RESOURCES

- eMedicine—Trichotillomania: **http://www.emedicine. com/DERM/topic433.htm**.
- eMedicine—Traction Alopecia: **http://www.emedicine. com/derm/topic895.htm**.

REFERENCES

1. Springer K, Brown M, Stulberg DL. Common hair loss disorders. *Am Fam Physician*. 2003;68:93–102,107–108.

2. Messinger ML, Cheng TL. Trichotillomania. *Pediatr Rev*. 1999;20: 249–250.

3. Christenson GA, Crow SJ. The characterization and treatment of trichotillomania. *J Clin Psychiat*. 1996;57(Suppl 8):42–27.

4. Streichenwein, SM, Thornby, JI. A long-term, double-blind, placebo-controlled crossover trial of the efficacy of fluoxetine for trichotillomania. *Am J Psychiat*. 1995;152:1192.

5. Ninan, PT, Rothbaum, BO, Marsteller, FA, et al. A placebo-controlled trial of cognitive-behavioral therapy and clomipramine in trichotillomania. *J Clin Psychiat*. 2000;61:47, 10.

182 SCARRING ALOPECIA

Richard P. Usatine, MD

PATIENT STORY

A 32-year-old woman presents with severe hair loss along with chronic pustular eruptions of her scalp. Previous biopsy has shown folliculitis decalvans. She has had many courses of antibiotics, but the hair loss continues to progress. The active pustular lesions are cultured and grow out methicillin-resistant *Staphylococcus aureus*. The patient was treated with trimethoprim sulfamethoxazole twice daily and mupirocin on the affected areas and nasal mucosa twice daily. Two weeks later, the pustular lesions are less prominent although the alopecia is permanent (**Figures 182-1** and **182-2**).

EPIDEMIOLOGY

- Scarring alopecias (primary cicatricial alopecias) are all rare, except acne keloidalis nuchae.

ETIOLOGY

Scarring alopecia is caused by a wide variety of conditions including various immunologic diseases such as discoid lupus erythematosus (DLE) and lichen planus. It can also be caused by rare pustular diseases such as folliculitis decalvans and more common acneiform conditions such as acne keloidalis nuchae (see Chapter 108, Pseudofolliculitis and Acne Keloidalis Nuchae).

PATHOPHYSIOLOGY

Scarring alopecia occurs when there is inflammation and destruction of the hair follicles leading to fibrous tissue formation.[1] While there can be secondary infections as seen in folliculitis decalvans, the actual process is more inflammatory than infectious.

The type of inflammatory infiltrates can vary and are used to classify the scarring alopecias (primary cicatricial alopecias):

- Lymphocytic: DLE, lichen planopilaris (LPP), and central centrifugal scarring alopecia.
- Neutrophilic: folliculitis decalvans and dissecting folliculitis.
- Mixed: acne keloidalis nuchae.[1]

DIAGNOSIS

Scarring alopecias can vary by distribution and appearance. Most patients will need a biopsy to confirm the clinical impression and determine the specific type of alopecia.

- Folliculitis decalvans is a chronic painful neutrophilic bacterial folliculitis characterized by bogginess or induration of the scalp with pustules, erosions, crusts, and scale.[1] It is postulated that this

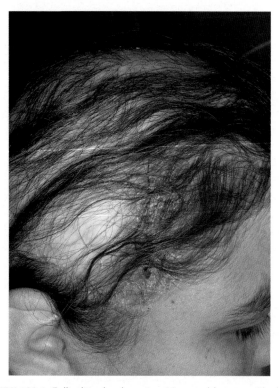

FIGURE 182-1 Folliculitis decalvans in a 32-year-old woman. She has an active area of pustular lesions on the periphery with wide areas of scarring and hair loss. (*Courtesy of Richard P. Usatine, MD.*)

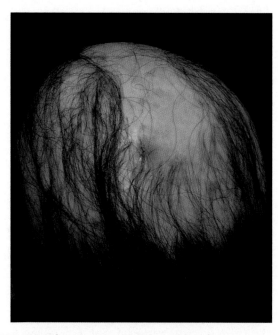

FIGURE 182-2 Same patient (see **Figure 182-1**) showing permanent hair loss on the top of the head with some small active pustular lesions. (*Courtesy of Richard P. Usatine, MD.*)

results from an abnormal host response to *S. aureus*, which is often cultured from the lesions (**Figures 182-1** and **182-2**). In one case series, the disease ran a protracted course with temporary improvement while on antibiotic and flare up of disease when antibiotics were stopped.[2]

- Tufted folliculitis is a term for a clinical picture in which multiple hairs are growing from the same follicle. While this is frequently seen in folliculitis decalvans (**Figure 182-3**), these hair tufts can be seen in other types of scarring alopecias.

- DLE presents with lesions that can be erythematous, atrophic, and/or hypopigmented. Scarring alopecia may be accompanied by follicular plugging on the scalp. Hypopigmentation may develop in the central area of the inflammatory lesions and hyperpigmentation may develop at the active border. The external ear and ear canal are often involved (**Figure 182-4**) (see Chapter 173, Lupus—Systemic and Cutaneous).

- LPP most commonly affects middle-aged women; it mostly occurs on the frontal and parietal scalp and causes follicular hyperkeratosis, pruritus, perifollicular erythema, violaceous color of scalp, and scalp pain (**Figure 182-5**).[1] It may also affect other hair-bearing sites such as the groin and axilla.[1]

- Postmenopausal frontal fibrosing alopecia presents with a progressive recession of the frontal hairline affecting particularly postmenopausal women. It is considered to be a variant of LPP on the basis of its clinical, histological, and immunohistochemical features.[3]

- Dissecting folliculitis presents with deep inflammatory nodules, primarily over the occiput, that progress to coalescing regions of boggy scalp.[1] Sinus tracts may form and *S. aureus* is frequently cultured from the inflamed lesions. When dissecting folliculitis occurs with acne conglobata and hidradenitis suppurativa, the syndrome is referred to as the follicular occlusion triad (**Figures 182-6** and **182-7**).

- Central centrifugal scarring alopecia is a slowly progressive alopecia that begins in the vertex and advances to surrounding areas. It may be related to chemicals used on the hair, heat from hot combs, or chronic tension on the hair.[1]

- Erosive pustular dermatosis of the scalp is characterized by chronic, sterile, pustular erosions leading to scarring alopecia. It appears to be associated with ultraviolet light exposure and trauma.[4]

- Acne keloidalis nuchae (folliculitis keloidalis) presents with a chronic papular and pustular eruption at the nape of the neck. This can lead to scarring alopecia with large keloidal scarring. It is seen most commonly in men of color but can be seen in women as well. It is often made worse by shaving the hair (see Chapter 108, Pseudofolliculitis and Acne Keloidalis Nuchae).

- Pseudopelade of Brocq is not a distinct primary form of scarring alopecia, but is a pattern of cicatricial alopecia that resembles alopecia areata (*pelade* is the French term for alopecia areata.) It can be caused by DLE or LPP. The term pseudopelade should be abandoned and a primary pathophysiologic diagnosis should be sought.

LABORATORY STUDIES

If there is purulence, perform a bacterial culture. *S. aureus* and methicillin-resistant *S. aureus* are now frequently seen in the neutrophilic alopecias. Consider obtaining various tests such as TSH, CBC, and RPR to rule out treatable causes of alopecia. Do a KOH smear and/or culture if tinea capitis is suspected.

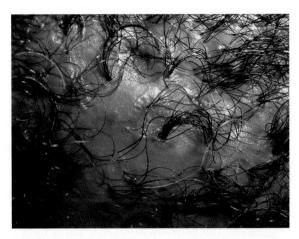

FIGURE 182-3 Tufted folliculitis showing multiple hairs growing from the same follicle along with purulence and hair loss. (*Courtesy of Richard P. Usatine, MD.*)

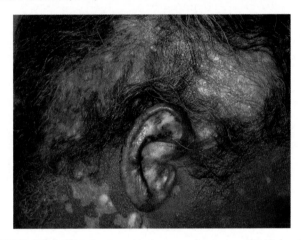

FIGURE 182-4 Chronic cutaneous lupus erythematosus (DLE) showing scarring alopecia. Prominent hypopigmentation and skin atrophy are visible on the scalp and ear. (*Courtesy of Richard P. Usatine, MD.*)

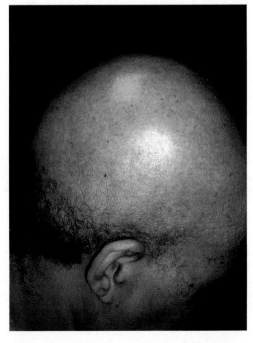

FIGURE 182-5 Lichen planopilaris in a 65-year-old woman, causing severe hair loss with visible dark dots representing follicular hyperkeratosis (plugging). (*Courtesy of Richard P. Usatine, MD.*)

BIOPSY

- Biopsy is almost always needed to diagnose the rare forms of scarring alopecia. Usually a single 4-mm punch biopsy for histology is adequate.
- A second 4-mm punch biopsy for direct immunofluorescence may be considered if pemphigus or bullous pemphigoid are suspected (uncommon).

DIFFERENTIAL DIAGNOSIS

- Alopecia areata presents with hair loss and a very smooth scalp. The hair loss is usually in round punched-out patterns and the scalp otherwise appears normal.
- Sarcoidosis of the scalp can resemble DLE but treatment will be different. Hence the importance of a biopsy diagnosis.[5]
- Secondary syphilis with moth-eaten alopecia is rare but should be considered. A highly positive RPR can easily make this diagnosis.
- Tinea capitis presents with scale and hair loss. It is diagnosed by a positive KOH and/or fungal culture. Do not miss this diagnosis because it is much easier to treat than any of the scarring alopecias.
- Trichotillomania is defined as self-induced hair loss caused by pulling at the hairs. The pattern of hair loss may be distinctive and the behavior may be discovered on history. The scalp appears normal and there is a distinctive pattern seen on biopsy.
- Traction alopecia occurs when the hair is pulled too tight for braids or ponytails.
- Androgenetic alopecia is the standard hair loss that males experience with aging. There are a number of male pattern types of hair loss. Women can also get androgenic alopecia, but the pattern tends to be more diffuse and frontal. Both are treatable with topical minoxidil and oral finasteride.
- Drug-induced alopecia is from chemotherapy and other toxic drugs.
- Seborrheic dermatitis may cause some hair loss. The presence of scale on the scalp with minimal to no hair loss helps to differentiate this from scarring alopecia.
- Telogen effluvium is a type of nonscarring alopecia that occurs after childbirth or other traumatic events. The scalp is normal.
- Various metabolic and nutritional problems can lead to alopecia. It is worth doing a CBC and TSH to rule out iron-deficiency and hyper- or hypothyroidism.
- Pemphigus or bullous pemphigoid can cause lesions on the scalp but the presence of bulla should differentiate this from the primary cicatricial alopecias. If not, then biopsy is helpful.

MANAGEMENT

- Cicatricial (scarring) alopecias are such rare conditions that there are no randomized controlled trials available to guide therapy.
- In one case report, a young man with folliculitis decalvans was successfully treated with a combination of isotretinoin, corticosteroids, and clindamycin.[6] SOR **C**
- There have been four case reports of successful treatment of erosive pustular dermatosis of the scalp with topical tacrolimus. Tacrolimus 0.1% ointment was used after intralesional steroids and oral

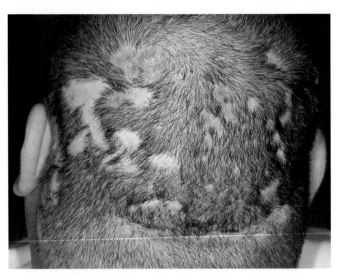

FIGURE 182-6 Dissecting folliculitis of the scalp causing painful purulent nodules and sinus tracts leading to scarring alopecia. The patient also has severe hidradenitis suppurativa and therefore has two of three elements of the follicular occlusion triad (he does not have acne conglobata). (*Courtesy of Richard P. Usatine, MD.*)

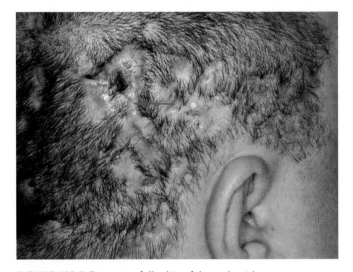

FIGURE 182-7 Dissecting folliculitis of the scalp with arrow on one sinus tract. (*Courtesy of Richard P. Usatine, MD.*)

antibiotics and it helped to resolve the atrophy and prevented relapse of inflammation.[4] SOR **C**

- Imiquimod cream 5% was reported to cause regression of discoid lupus of the scalp and face in a single patient when applied to the lesions once a day three times a week. After 20 applications, Gul et al. reported that the lesions had regressed significantly.[7] SOR **C**

- Dapsone at 75 to 100 mg per day for 4 to 6 months was well tolerated and rapidly effective in treating two cases of folliculitis decalvans. Long-term low-dose (25 mg daily) maintenance treatment avoided disease relapses. Paquet and Pierard chose dapsone because of its antimicrobial activity and its anti-inflammatory action directed to the neutrophil metabolism.[8] SOR **C**

- Surgical excision of cicatricial alopecias includes excision and tissue expansion. Unfortunately, the outcomes have been disappointing to the patients and surgeons.[9] SOR **C**

- In one review article, Price suggests that scarring alopecias with predominantly lymphocytic infiltrates should be treated with immunomodulating agents and those with predominantly neutrophilic infiltrates should be treated with antimicrobial agents.[10] SOR **C** This makes sense pathophysiologically.
  ○ Lymphocytic infiltrate predominates (discoid lupus and LPP)—Price suggests high potency corticosteroids or topical tacrolimus to the involved areas; intralesional injections of triamcinolone acetonide, 10 mg/mL; and hydroxychloroquine if oral therapy is needed.[10] SOR **C** If severe symptoms and signs of activity persist after 3 to 6 months of hydroxychloroquine, then mycophenolate mofetil is considered (especially in LPP).[10] SOR **C** Both oral agents have specific toxicity that requires careful monitoring. Consider referral to a specialist with experience using these oral agents.
  ○ Neutrophilic infiltrate predominates (folliculitis decalvans and dissecting folliculitis)—The purulent scalp lesions are cultured and the treatment is directed to the predominant pathogen (most commonly *S. aureus*). Both oral rifampin 300 mg twice daily and oral clindamycin 300 mg twice daily for 10 weeks are suggested.[10] SOR **C** Sustained remission is achieved in many patients after one course, although a second or third course may be needed for such a remission. For patients who cannot take clindamycin, oral ciprofloxacin 750 mg twice daily, or cephalexin 500 mg 4 times daily, or doxycycline 100 mg twice daily is given along with rifampin. The nostrils and perineum are cultured, and if the patient is found to be a staph carrier, topical mupirocin ointment is applied daily for 1 week and then once a month.[10] SOR **C** In patients with dissecting cellulitis, isotretinoin may be effective in inducing a prolonged remission. Price suggests starting with a 20 mg daily, to avoid a flare, and then slowly increase to 1 mg/kg per day for many months.[10] SOR **C**

- See Chapter 108, Pseudofolliculitis and Acne Keloidalis Nuchae, for treatment of acne keloidalis nuchae.

PATIENT EDUCATION

The following points are based upon information from the Cicatricial Alopecia Research Foundation—**http://www.carfintl.org/faq.html**

- The goal of treatment is to control scalp inflammation and stop the progression of the disease. While hair regrowth is desirable, it should not be expected.

- Scarring alopecias often reactivate after a quiet period of one or more years. Patients should be encouraged to self-monitor for recurrence and to seek care early to prevent hair loss.

- It is safe to wash the hair with gentle hair products, if desired even daily.

- When severe hair loss occurs, hats, scarves, hairpieces, and wigs may be used safely for cosmetic purposes.

FOLLOW-UP

Close follow-up is needed for patients put on oral agents. Monitoring for side effects will be agent specific.

PATIENT RESOURCES

Cicatricial Alopecia Research Foundation—**http://www.carfintl.org/faq.html.**

PROVIDER RESOURCES

Good review article on all types of hair loss with helpful algorithms: Springer K, Brown M, Stulberg, D. Common hair loss disorders. *Am Fam Physician*. 2003;68:93–102,107–108. Full text and photos—**http://www.aafp.org/afp/20030701/93.html.**

REFERENCES

1. Wolff K, Johnson RA, Suurmond D. *Fitzpatrick's Color Atlas & Synopsis of Clinical Dermatology*. 5th ed. New York, NY: McGraw-Hill; 2005:968–973.

2. Chandrawansa PH, Giam YC. Folliculitis decalvans—a retrospective study in a tertiary referred centre, over five years. *Singapore Med J*. 2003;44:84–87.

3. Moreno-Ramirez D, Camacho MF. Frontal fibrosing alopecia: a survey in 16 patients. *J Eur Acad Dermatol Venereol*. 2005;19:700–705.

4. Cenkowski MJ, Silver S. Topical tacrolimus in the treatment of erosive pustular dermatosis of the scalp. *J Cutan Med Surg*. 2007;11:222–225.

5. Henderson CL, Lafleur L, Sontheimer RD. Sarcoidal alopecia as a mimic of discoid lupus erythematosus. *J Am Acad Dermatol*. 2008;59:143–145.

6. Gemmeke A, Wollina U. Folliculitis decalvans of the scalp: response to triple therapy with isotretinoin, clindamycin, and prednisolone. *Acta Dermatovenerol Alp Panonica Adriat*. 2006;15:184–186.

7. Gul U, Gonul M, Cakmak SK, Kilic A, Demiriz M. A case of generalized discoid lupus erythematosus: successful treatment with imiquimod cream 5%. *Adv Ther*. 2006;23:787–792.

8. Paquet P, Pierard GE. Dapsone treatment of folliculitis decalvans. *Ann Dermatol Venereol*. 2004;131:195–197.

9. Duteille F, Le FB, Hepner LD, Pannier M. The limitation of primary excision of cicatricial alopecia: a report of 63 patients. *Ann Plast Surg*. 2000;45:145–149.

10. Price VH. The medical treatment of cicatricial alopecia. *Semin Cutan Med Surg*. 2006;25:56–59.

183 NORMAL NAIL VARIANTS

E.J. Mayeaux, Jr., MD

PATIENT STORY

A 28-year-old man is in the office for a work physical and asks about the white streaks on his fingernail (**Figure 183-1**). He has had them on and off all of his adult life, but recently developed more of them and was concerned he may have a vitamin deficiency. He was reassured that this is a normal nail finding often associated with minor trauma.

ETIOLOGY AND PATHOPHYSIOLOGY

- *Leukonychia* represents benign, single or multiple, white spots or lines in the nails. Patchy patterns of partial, transverse white streaks (transverse striate leukonychia, **Figure 183-1**) or spots (leukonychia punctata, **Figure 183-2**) are the most common patterns of leukonychia.[1] Leukonychia is common in children and becomes less frequent with age. Parents may fear that it represents a dietary deficiency, in particular a lack of calcium, but this concern is almost always unfounded.
  - Most commonly, no specific cause for leukonychia can be found. It is usually the result of minor trauma to the nail cuticle or matrix and is the most commonly found nail condition in children.[2] When the lesions are caused by overly aggressive manicuring or nervous habit, behavior modification often is helpful. Leukonychia can also be an indirect manifestation of autoimmunity, including alopecia areata or thyroid disease. Histologically, the nail plate contains a greater number of nucleated cells that are associated with lack of cohesion between the corneocytes, producing reflective properties of the nail.
- *Longitudinal melanonychia* (LM, **Figure 183-3**) represents a longitudinal pigmented band in the nail plate. LM may involve of one or several digits, vary in color from light brown to black, vary in width (most range from 2 to 4 mm), and have sharp or blurred borders. They must be differentiated from subungual melanoma (see Chapter 184, Pigmented Nail Disorders).
- *Nail hypertrophy and onychogryphosis* (ram's horn nail—lateral nail hypertrophy, **Figure 183-4**) is the development of opaque thickened nails with exaggerated upward or lateral growth. It may be associated with age, fungal infections and trauma. It can cause pain with pressure.
- *Habit-tic deformity* (**Figure 183-5**) is caused by habitual picking of the proximal nail fold. The resulting inflammation induces the nail plate to be wavy and ridged, while its substance remains intact and hard.
- *Beau's lines* are transverse linear depressions in the nail plate (**Figure 183-6**). They are thought to result from suppressed nail growth secondary to local trauma or severe illness.[3] They most commonly appear symmetrically in several or all nails and may have associated

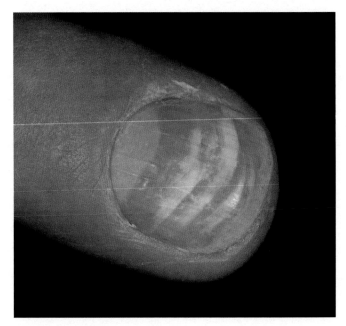

FIGURE 183-1 Transverse striate leukonychia (transverse white streaks) in a healthy patient. Note that the lines do not extend all of the way to the lateral folds, which indicates a probable benign process. (*Courtesy of Richard P. Usatine, MD.*)

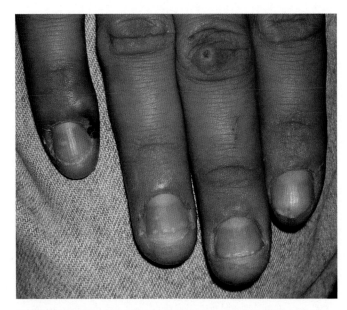

FIGURE 183-2 Leukonychia punctata in a patient who bites his nails. Note he also has an acute paronychia of the fifth digit. (*Courtesy of E.J. Mayeaux, Jr., MD.*)

white lines. They usually grow out over several months. One may estimate the time since onset of systemic illness by measuring the distance from the Beau's line to the proximal nail fold and applying the conversion factor of 6 to 10 days per millimeter of growth.[2]

DIAGNOSIS

Biopsy—definitive diagnosis of a nail discoloration may be made with a biopsy of the nail or matrix. Patients with darker skin tones and multiple digits with translucent LM often need only be observed. A new dark line in a single nail should be biopsied. A 3-mm punch biopsy can be performed at the origin of the darkest part of a dark band. This usually involves reflecting the skin of the proximal nail fold back while performing a punch biopsy of the distal matrix. Histologic diagnosis of atypical melanocytic hyperplasia necessitates the complete removal of the lesion.

DIFFERENTIAL DIAGNOSIS

- Pigmented lesions in the nail bed do not cause LM only nail matrix lesions do. Nail bed lesions make spots under the nails but do not grow out as stripes. These are viewed through the nail as a grayish to brown or black spot.[4]

- The diagnosis of subungual melanoma must always be considered in patients with longitudinal melanonychia. A biopsy should be performed in an adult if the cause of longitudinal melanonychia is not apparent. Extension of pigmentation to the skin adjacent to the nail plate involving the nail folds or the fingertip is called Hutchinson sign, which is an important indicator of nail melanoma (see Chapter 184, Pigmented Nail Disorders).

- Hematoma may be confused with LM, but the color grows out with the nail plate, exhibiting a proximal border that reproduces the shape of the lunula. A hole punched in the nail plate allows for the visualization of the underlying nail bed and confirmation of the nature of the coloration.

- Mees' and Muehrcke's lines may be confused with leukonychia or Beau's lines. Mees' lines are multiple white transverse lines that begin in the nail matrix and extend completely across the nail plate (**Figure 183-7**). They are due to heavy metal poisoning or severe systemic insults. Muehrcke's lines are double white transverse lines that represent an abnormality of the nail vascular bed and may occur with chronic hypoalbuminemia. **Table 183-1** shows clinical signs that help differentiate local trauma-induced lesions from those associated with systemic disease.

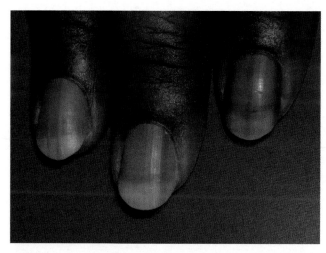

FIGURE 183-3 Longitudinal melanonychia (LM) in multiple fingers— bands of translucent nail pigment in multiple fingers. (*Courtesy of E.J. Mayeaux, Jr., MD.*)

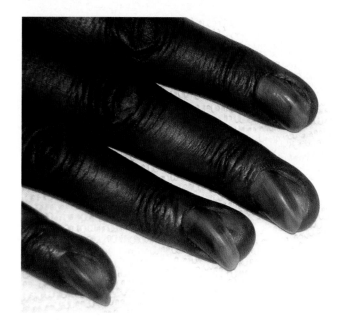

FIGURE 183-4 Onychogryphosis (ram's horn nail) is a type of lateral nail hypertrophy. (*Courtesy of E.J. Mayeaux, Jr., MD.*)

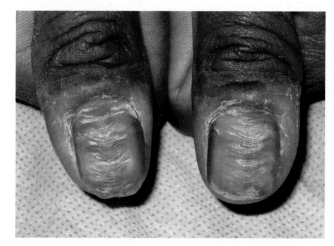

FIGURE 183-5 Habit-tic deformity caused by a conscious or unconscious rubbing or picking of the proximal nails and nail folds. Horizontal grooves are formed proximally and move distally with fingernail growth. The thumbnails are most often affected. (*Courtesy of Edwin A. Farnell, MD.*)

TABLE 183-1 Signs that Help Differentiate Local Trauma-Induced Lesions from Those Associated with Systemic Disease

Mees' and Muehrcke's Lines	Leukonychia and Trauma-induced Lesions
Tend to occur on several nails at once	Usually on one or two nails
Spread across the entire breadth of the nail bed or plate and tend to be more homogeneous	Often do not span the entire breadth of the nail plate.
Tend to have contour similar to the distal lunula, with a rounded distal edge	More linear and resemble the contour of the proximal nail fold
History of a systemic insult is correlated with the onset of the lines	History of sufficient physical trauma to the cuticle area

PROVIDER RESOURCES

- Emedicine Nail Surgery—**http://www.emedicine.com/ derm/topic818.htm.**
- Color pictures at Dermatlas.org—**http://www.dermatlas. com/derm/.**
- Medscape nail disorders—**http://www.medscape.com/ viewarticle/470942_19.**

REFERENCES

1. Grossman M, Scher RK. Leukonychia. Review and classification. *Int J Dermatol*. 1990;29:535–541.

2. Baran R, Kechijian P. Diagnosis and management. *J Am Acad Dermatol*. 1989;21:1165–1175.

3. Daniel CR, Zaias N. Pigmentary abnormalities of the nails with emphasis on systemic diseases. *Dermatol Clin*. 1988;6:305–313.

4. Noronha PA, Zubkov B. Nails and nail disorders in children and adults. *Am Fam Phys*. 1997;55:2129–2140.

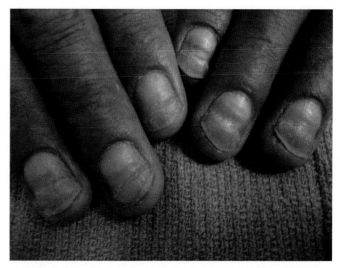

FIGURE 183-6 Beau's lines most likely secondary to an acute cholecystitis episode a couple of months prior. (*Courtesy of Suraj Reddy, MD.*)

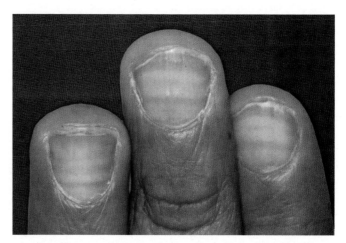

FIGURE 183-7 Mee's lines that spread transversely across the entire breadth of the nail and are somewhat rounded with a contour similar to the distal lunula. (*Courtesy of Jeffrey Meffert, MD.*)

184 PIGMENTED NAIL DISORDERS

E.J. Mayeaux, Jr., MD

PATIENT STORY

An African American medical student presented with a new dark band on her index finger for 1 year (**Figure 184-1**). The dark color and the lack of melanonychia in other fingers made this concerning. A biopsy of the nail matrix was performed and the result showed a benign nevus.

EPIDEMIOLOGY

Longitudinal melanonychia (LM) is more common in more darkly pigmented persons. It occurs in 77% of African Americans older than 20 years and in almost 100% of those older than 50 years.[1] It also occurs in 10% to 20% of persons of Japanese descent. LM is common in Hispanic and other dark-skinned groups. LM is unusual in Caucasians occurring in only about 1% of the population.[1]

Melanoma is the seventh most common cause of cancer in patients in the United States. Subungual melanoma is a relatively rare tumor with reported incidences between 0.7% and 3.5% of all melanoma cases in the general population.[2]

ETIOLOGY AND PATHOPHYSIOLOGY

- Longitudinal melanonychia (LM) represents a longitudinal pigmented band in the nail plate (**Figures 184-1** and **184-2**). It may involve of one or several digits, vary in color from light brown to black, vary in width (most range from 2 to 4 mm), and have sharp or blurred borders.

- LM originates in the nail matrix and results from increased deposition of melanin within the nail plate. This deposition may result from greater melanin synthesis or from an increase in the total number of melanocytes. Pigment clinically localized within the dorsal half of the nail plate indicates a proximal matrix origin, and pigment localized within the ventral nail plate indicates a distal matrix origin. Look at the distal edge of the nail in cross section view to see whether the pigment is dorsal or ventral.

- LM may also be caused by chronic trauma, especially in the great toes.

- Inflammatory changes accompanying skin diseases located in the nail unit, such as psoriasis, lichen planus, amyloidosis, and localized scleroderma may rarely result in LM.

- Benign melanocytic hyperplasia (lentigo) is observed in 9% of the adult cases and 30% of the pediatric cases of single-biopsied LM.[3]

- Nevi represent 12% of LM in adults but almost 50% of cases in children. A brown-black coloration is observed in two-thirds of the

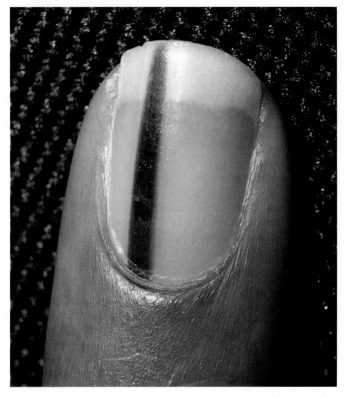

FIGURE 184-1 Longitudinal melanonychia—single dark band of nail pigment appearing in the matrix region and extended to the tip of the nail. This is concerning for melanoma. This young woman had a biopsy that showed a benign nevus. (*Courtesy of Richard P. Usatine, MD.*)

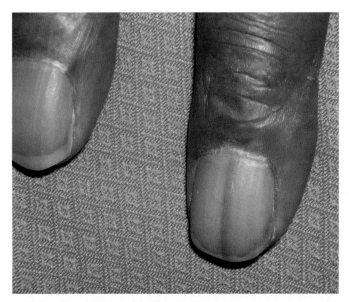

FIGURE 184-2 Close up of longitudinal melanonychia in a single finger. Note the color band is translucent. (*Courtesy of E.J. Mayeaux, Jr., MD.*)

cases and periungual pigmentation (benign pseudo-Hutchinson's sign) in one third.

- Certain drugs may also cause LM, especially chemotherapeutic agents (**Figure 184-3**), and antimalarial drugs (mepacrine, amodiaquine, and chloroquine).

- Endocrine disorders, such as Addison disease, Cushing syndrome, hyperthyroidism, and acromegaly can be responsible for LM.

- The diagnosis of subungual melanoma must always be considered in patients with longitudinal melanonychia (**Figures 184-4** and **184-5**). Separating benign from malignant lesions is often difficult. Both arise most often in the thumb or index fingers, and both are more common in dark-skinned persons.[4] A biopsy should be performed in an adult if the cause of longitudinal melanonychia is uncertain. Diagnostic clues for subungual melanomas are shown in **Table 184-1**. Extension of pigmentation to the skin adjacent to the nail plate involving the nail folds or the fingertip is called Hutchinson's sign, which is an important indicator for nail melanoma (**Figures 184-4** and **184-5**).[5]

- Pseudo-Hutchinson's sign is the presence of dark pigment around the proximal nail fold secondary to benign conditions such as racial melanosis and not melanoma (**Figure 184-6**). Another cause of Pseudo-Hutchinson's sign is a translucent cuticle below which the pigment of LM is visible. Trauma and drug-induced pigmentation can also produce a Pseudo-Hutchinson's sign.

- Subungual melanoma arises on the hand in 45% to 60% of cases, and most of those occur in the thumb[4] (**Figures 184-5** and **184-6**). On the foot, subungual melanoma usually occurs in the great toe.[4] The median age at which subungual melanoma is usually diagnosed is in the sixth and seventh decades. It appears with equal frequency in males and females.[4]

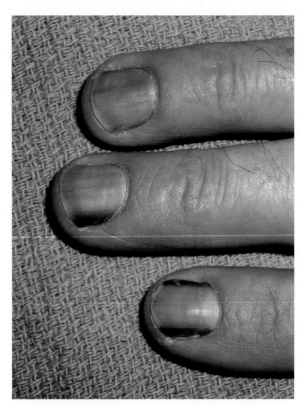

FIGURE 184-3 Melanonychia secondary to chemotherapy for metastatic penile cancer. (*Courtesy of Richard P. Usatine, MD.*)

TABLE 184-1 Diagnostic Clues That Indicate Longitudinal Melanonychia Is Subungual Melanoma

Hutchinson's sign (melanoma until proven otherwise)

In a single digit

Sixth decade of life or later

Develops abruptly in a previously normal nail plate

Suddenly darkens or widens (change in the LM morphology)

Occurs in either the thumb, index finger, or great toe

History of digital trauma

Dark-skinned patient, particularly if the thumb or great toe is affected

Blurred, rather than sharp, lateral borders

History of malignant melanoma

Increased risk for melanoma (e.g., FAM-M syndrome)

Nail dystrophy, such as partial nail destruction or disappearance

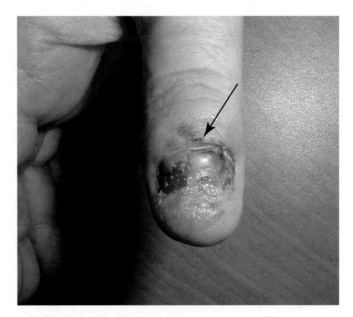

FIGURE 184-4 Advanced acrolentiginous melanoma of the thumb. Note the hyperpigmentation in the center of the ventral fold (Hutchinson's sign) which is strongly indicative of melanoma. (*Courtesy of Dr. Dubin at http://www.skinatlas.com.*)

MAKING THE DIAGNOSIS

- Distribution—the digits used for grasping (thumb, index finger, and middle finger) are the most commonly involved in longitudinal melanonychia and melanoma, but either may be found in any finger or toe.
- There is an ABCDEF mnemonic system that applies to subungual melanoma:
  - In this system "A" stands for age (peak incidence being between the fifth to seventh decades) and African Americans, Asians, and native Americans in whom subungual melanoma accounts for one third of melanoma cases.
  - "B" stands for "brown to black" and with "breadth" of 3 mm or more.
  - "C" stands for change in the nail band coloration or lack of change after adequate treatment.
  - "D" stands for the digit most commonly involved.
  - "E" stands for extension of the pigment onto the proximal and/or lateral nailfold (Hutchinson's sign).
  - "F" stands for family or personal history of dysplastic nevus or melanoma.
- Biopsy—definitive diagnosis of a nail discoloration may be made with a biopsy of the nail matrix. Patients with darker skin color and multiple digits with translucent LM often need only be observed. Single dark lines in whites should always be biopsied. A 3-mm punch biopsy can be performed at the origin of the darkest part of a dark band within the nail matrix (**Figure 184-7**). Histologic diagnosis of atypical melanocytic hyperplasia necessitates the complete removal of the lesion.

DIFFERENTIAL DIAGNOSIS

- Pigmented lesions in the nail bed usually do not cause LM and are viewed through the nail as a grayish to brown or black spot.[6]
- Subungual hematoma may be confused with LM, but the color grows out with the nail plate, exhibiting a proximal border that reproduces the shape of the lunula. A hole punched in the nail plate allows for the visualization of the underlying nail bed and confirmation of the nature of the coloration.

TREATMENT

- No treatment is required for benign LM.
- Treatment of primary subungual melanomas includes amputation at the level of the interphalangeal joint for thumb lesions SOR B, the distal interphalangeal joint for fingers SOR C, and the metatarsophalangeal joint for toes.[7] For melanoma in situ, it may be possible to remove the full nail apparatus and save the digit. Regional lymph node dissection can help with establishment of disease stage. Chemotherapy is recommended for nodal or visceral metastases. The 5-year survival is approximately 74% for patients with stage I and 40% for patients with stage II disease. Prognostic variables negatively affecting survival include stage at diagnosis, deeper Clark's level of invasion, African American race, and ulceration.[8]

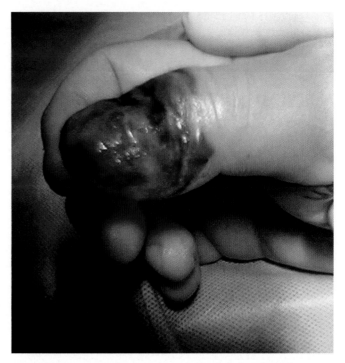

FIGURE 184-5 Acral lentiginous melanoma that started after trauma to the thumb, which led to a delay in diagnosis. (*Reproduced with permission from Photo Rounds: A non-healing ulcerated fingertip following injury. The Journal of Family Practice, March 2006;55(3):225, Dowden Health Media*)

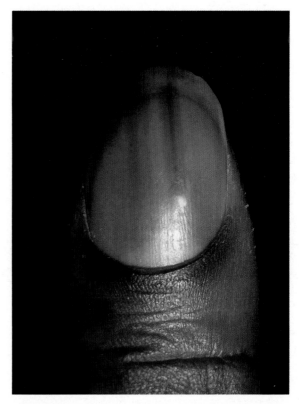

FIGURE 184-6 Benign LM in a black person demonstrating pseudo-Hutchinson's sign (dark pigment around the proximal nail fold secondary to racial melanosis and not melanoma). (*Courtesy of Richard P. Usatine, MD.*)

FOLLOW-UP

Because LM may indicate an undiagnosed melanoma of the nail unit, regular monitoring is extremely important. Have the patient report any rapid changes in pigmentation of the nail plate or nail folds, and strongly consider biopsy in these individuals.

PATIENT RESOURCES

- Nail Diseases & Disorders—**http://www.hooked-on-nails.com/naildisorders.html.**

PROVIDER RESOURCES

- EMedicine Nail Surgery—**http://www.emedicine.com/derm/topic818.htm.**
- Color pictures at Dermatlas.org—**http://www.dermatlas.com/derm/.**
- Medscape nail disorders—**http://www.medscape.com/viewarticle/470942_19.**
- Braun RP, Baran R, Le Gal FA, et al. Diagnosis and management of nail pigmentation. *J Am Acad Dermatol.* 2007;56(5): 835–847.
- Jellinek N. Nail matrix biopsy of longitudinal melanonychia: diagnostic algorithm including the matrix shave biopsy. *J Am Acad Dermatol.* 2007;56(5): 803–810.

REFERENCES

1. Baran R, Kechjijian P. Longitudinal melanonychia (melanonychia striata): Diagnosis and management. *J Am Acad Dermatol.* 1989;21:1165–1175.

2. Finley RK, Driscoll DL, Blumenson LE, Karakousis CP. Subungual melanoma: An eighteen year review. *Surgery.* 1994;116:96–100.

3. Goettmann-Bonvallot S, André J, Belaich S, Longitudinal melanonychia in children: A clinical and histopathologic study of 40 cases. *J Am Acad Dermatol.* 1999;41:17–22.

4. Papachristou DN, Fortner, JG. Melanoma arising under the nail. *J Surg Oncol.* 1982;21:219–22.

5. Mikhail GR. Hutchinson's sign. *J Dermatol Surg Oncol.* 1986;12: 519–21.

6. Baran R, Perrin C. Linear melanonychia due to subungual keratosis of the nail bed: Report of two cases. *Br J Dermatol.* 1999;140:730–733.

7. Moehrle M, Metzger S, Schippert W, Garbe C, Rassner G, Breuninger H. "Functional" surgery in subungual melanoma. *Dermatol Surg.* 2003; 29(4):366–374.

8. O'Leary JA, Berend KR, Johnson JL, Levin LS, Seigler HF. Subungual melanoma: A review of 93 cases with identification of prognostic variables. *Clin Orthop Relat Res.* 2000;378:206–212.

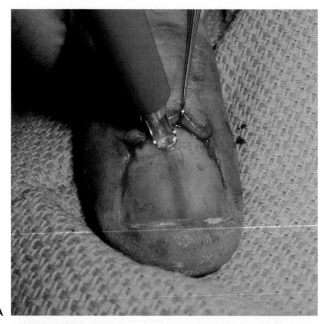

A

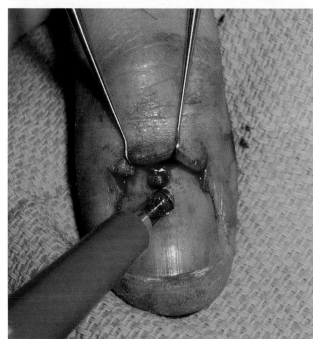

B

FIGURE 184-7 (A) The proximal nail fold is reflected back to perform a nail matrix biopsy in a young man with new onset of LM. The 3-mm punch is placed over the origin of the dark band at the distal matrix. (B) The 3 mm punch now contains the specimen for pathology. The LM was caused by melanocytic hyperplasia. (*Courtesy of Richard P. Usatine, MD.*)

185 ONYCHOCRYPTOSIS (INGROWN TOENAIL)

E.J. Mayeaux, Jr., MD

PATIENT STORY

A 24-year-old woman presents with a history of multiple ingrown nails of both great toes. She has a 2-week history of pain, redness, and swelling of the medial nail fold of the right great toe. Soaking the toe in Epsom salts has not helped. A partial nail removal after a digital block was successful.

INTRODUCTION

Onychocryptosis (ingrown toenails) is a common childhood and adult problem. The prevalence of onychocryptosis is unknown since many patients do not seek medical care and it is not a reportable disease.

ETIOLOGY AND PATHOPHYSIOLOGY

- Onychocryptosis occurs when the lateral nail plate damages the lateral nail fold. It is a common affliction that can result from a variety of conditions that cause improper fit of the nail plate in the lateral nail grove (**Figure 185-1**).
- Ingrown toenails at birth and in early childhood do occur, but are very rare.
- Patients often seek treatment because of the significant levels of discomfort and disability associated with the condition.
- Predisposing factors include poor-fitting footwear, excessive trimming of the lateral nail plate, pincer nail deformity (**Figure 185-2**), trauma, sports in which kicking or running is important, sweaty feet, and anatomic features such as nail fold width.

DIAGNOSIS

- Clinical features—characteristic signs and symptoms include pain, edema, exudate, and granulation tissue (**Figure 185-1**).
- Typical distribution—the great toe is most commonly affected and fingers are rarely involved except when nail biting is present.
- The diagnosis is based upon clinical appearance and rarely is difficult.

DIFFERENTIAL DIAGNOSIS

- Cellulitis—presents with redness, pain, and swelling beyond the nail fold (see Chapter 114, Cellulitis).

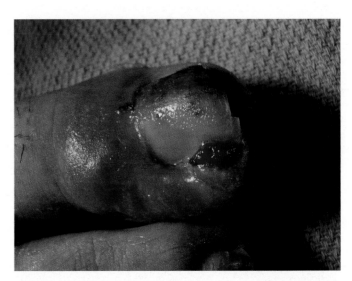

FIGURE 185-1 Ingrown toenail of the lateral aspect of the right great toe showing inflammation and granulation tissue. (*Courtesy of Richard P. Usatine, MD.*)

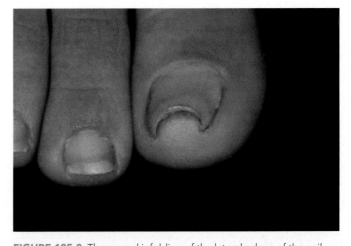

FIGURE 185-2 The curved infolding of the lateral edges of the nail-plate indicates this patient has a pincer nail, which predisposes to onychocryptosis. (*Courtesy of Richard P. Usatine, MD.*)

- Paronychia—presents with redness and abscess formation (pus) in a nail fold (see Chapter 187, Paronychia).

MANAGEMENT

- The treatment of ingrown toenails depends upon the age of the patient and the severity of the lesion.

- Lesions characterized by minimal to moderate pain, little erythema, and no discharge can be treated conservatively with soaking the affected foot in warm water for 20 minutes, three times per day, and pushing the lateral nailfold away from the nail plate.[1,2] SOR **C** Other palliative measures include cotton wedging underneath the lateral nail plate and trimming the lateral part of the nail plate below the area of nail fold irritation.

- Nonresponders to conservative therapy and patients with more severe lesions (substantial erythema, granulation tissue and pus) need surgical therapy. SOR **C**

- Surgical intervention involves partial or full nail plate avulsion.

- Although many elect to treat apparent infections with oral antibiotics, studies show the use of antibiotics does not decrease healing time or postprocedure morbidity in otherwise normal patients.[3] SOR **A**

- Patients who develop recurrent ingrown toenails benefit from permanent nail ablation of the lateral nail matrix. This may be achieved with the combination of surgical excision plus phenol or electrosurgical ablation, which can cut recurrence rates by 90%.[4–6] SOR **A** Electrosurgical ablation can be performed with electrosurgery units on the fulguration setting or using a special matrixectomy electrode with a high-frequency electrosurgical unit (**Figures 185-3** and **185-4**). There is a higher rate of postoperative secondary infections with ablation techniques.

PATIENT EDUCATION

- Patients should be educated about proper nail trimming in order to minimize trauma to the lateral nail fold. The lateral nail plate should be allowed to grow well beyond the lateral nail fold before trimming horizontally.

- Patients should also be educated about the importance of avoiding shoes that are too tight over the toes to help minimize recurrences.

FOLLOW-UP

After surgical intervention, consider follow-up in 3 to 4 days to assess treatment and exclude cellulitis.

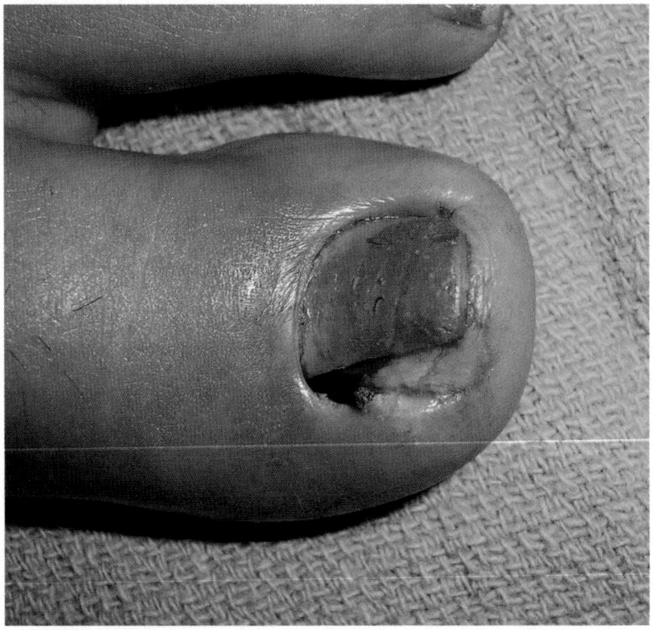

FIGURE 185-3 Status post partial nail avulsion procedure for an ingrown toenail. Note the char where the corner of the matrix was destroyed with electrosurgery to prevent recurrence. (*Courtesy of Richard P. Usatine, MD.*)

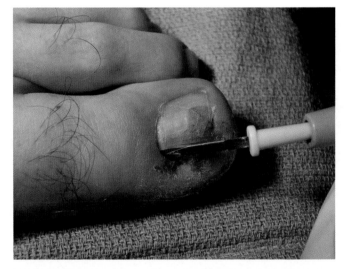

FIGURE 185-4 Use of electrosurgery to ablate the lateral nail matrix. This results in a narrower nail and a decreased likelihood of onychocryptosis recurrence. (*Courtesy of Richard P. Usatine, MD.*)

PATIENT RESOURCES

- American Academy of Orthopaedic Surgeons Information—**http://orthoinfo.aaos.org/fact/thr_report.cfm?Thread_ID=197.**

- FamilyDoc.org patient information—**http://familydoctor.org/208.xml.**

- FootPhysicans.com—**http://www.footphysicians.com/footankleinfo/ingrown-toenail.htm.**

PROVIDER RESOURCES

- Ingrown Toenail Removal by AFP—**http://www.aafp.org/afp/20020615/2547.html.**

- EMedicine.com—**http://www.emedicine.com/ped/topic942.htm.**

REFERENCES

1. Connolly B, Fitzgerald RJ. Pledgets in ingrowing toenails. *Arch Dis Child*. 1988;63:71.

2. Senapati A. Conservative outpatient management of ingrowing toenails. *J R Soc Med*. 1986;79:339.

3. Reyzelman AM, Trombello KA, Vayser DJ, et al. Are antibiotics necessary in the treatment of locally infected ingrown toenails? *Arch Fam Med*. 2000;9:930.

4. Grieg JD, Anderson JH, Ireland AJ, Anderson JR. The surgical treatment of ingrowing toenails. *J Bone Joint Surg [Br]*. 1991;73:131.

5. Rounding C, Bloomfield S. Surgical treatments for ingrowing toenails. *Cochrane Database Syst Rev*. 2003;1:CD001541, doi:10.1002/14651858.CD001541.pub2.

6. Rounding C, Bloomfield S. Surgical treatments for ingrowing toenails. *Cochrane Database Syst Rev*. 2005;2:CD001541.

186 ONYCHOMYCOSIS

E.J. Mayeaux, Jr., MD

PATIENT STORY

A 29-year-old woman presents with thickened and discolored toenails for 1 year (**Figure 186-1**). She is embarrassed to wear sandals and wants treatment. The entire nail plates are involved and there is subungual keratosis. She did not realize that she had tinea pedis but a fine scale was seen on the soles and sides of the feet indicative of tinea pedis in a moccasin distribution. A KOH scraping from the subungual debris was positive for hyphae. She has no history of liver disease or risk factors for liver disease. An oral antifungal was prescribed for 3 months.

EPIDEMIOLOGY

- Onychomycosis is a fungal infection of the nail plate and other parts of the nail unit including the nail matrix.

- Most patients (7.6%) only have toenail involvement and only 0.15% have fingernail involvement alone.[1] The prevalence of onychomycosis varies from 4% to 18%.[2, 3]

- The disease is very common in adults, but may also occur in children.

ETIOLOGY AND PATHOPHYSIOLOGY

- Dermatophytes are responsible for most finger and toenail infections.

- Nonpathogenic fungi and Candida (in the rare syndrome of chronic mucocutaneous candidiasis) also can infect the nail plate (**Figure 186-2**).

- Dermatophytic onychomycosis (tinea unguium) occurs in three distinct forms: distal subungual, proximal subungual, and white superficial.

- The vast majority of distal and proximal subungual onychomycosis results from *Trichophyton rubrum* (**Figure 186-3**).

- White superficial onychomycosis is usually caused by *T. mentagrophytes*, although cases caused by *T. rubrum* have also been reported (**Figure 186-4**).

- Yeast onychomycosis is most common in the fingers caused by *Candida albicans*.

- Trauma predisposes to infection but can also cause a dysmorphic nail that can be confused for onychomycosis.

- Extensive disease may be a sign of deteriorating immune status in AIDS patients (**Figures 186-5** and **186-6**).[4]

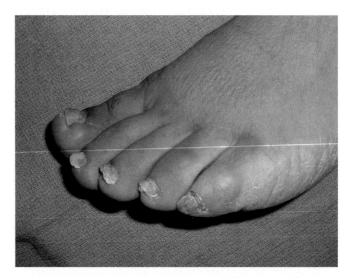

FIGURE 186-1 Onychomycosis in all toenails of this 29-year-old woman. Note the nail plate thickening and discoloration along with the subungual keratosis. She also has tinea pedis in a moccasin distribution. (*Courtesy of Richard P. Usatine, MD.*)

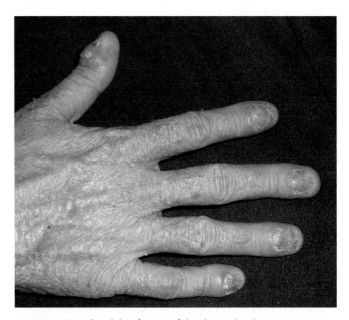

FIGURE 186-2 Candida infection of the skin and nails in an immunosuppressed patient with chronic mucocutaneous candidiasis. (*Courtesy of Richard P. Usatine, MD.*)

DIAGNOSIS

- Clinical features—distal subungual onychomycosis is the most common presentation.
  - Distal subungual onychomycosis begins with a whitish, yellowish, or brownish discoloration of a distal corner of the nail, which gradually spreads to involve the entire width of the nail plate and extends slowly toward the cuticle. Keratinous debris collecting between the nail plate and its bed is the cause of the discoloration (**Figures 186-1**, **186-3** and **186-7**).
  - Proximal subungual onychomycosis progresses in a manner similar to distal subungual onychomycosis but affects the nail in the vicinity of the cuticle first and extends distally. It usually occurs in individuals with a severely compromised immune system (**Figure 186-5**).
  - White superficial onychomycosis appears as dull white spots on the surface of the nail plate (**Figure 186-4**). Eventually the whole nail plate may be involved. The white areas may be soft and can be lightly scraped to yield a chalky scale that may be examined or cultured.

- Typical distribution—nail infection may occur in a single digit but most often occurs simultaneously in multiple digits of the foot. Toenails and fingernails may be affected at the same time especially in patients that are immunocompromised (**Figures 186-5** and **186-6**).

- KOH and culture—clippings of nail plate and scrapings of subungual keratosis can be examined with KOH and microscopy and/or sent to the laboratory in a sterile container to be inoculated onto Sabouraud's medium to culture.

- Clippings—nail clippings may be sent to pathology in formalin to be examined with periodic acid-Schiff (PAS) stain for fungal elements. This can be more, sensitive than KOH and culture.

- Comparison of diagnostic methods:
  - In a 2003 study by Weinberg et al., the sensitivities for onychomycosis detection were KOH 80%, Bx/PAS 92%, and culture 59%. The specificities were KOH 72%, Bx/PAS 72%, and culture 82%. The positive predictive values were KOH 88%, Bx/PAS 89.7%, and culture 90%. The negative predictive values were KOH 58%, Bx/PAS 77%, and culture 43%.[5]
  - In a 2007 study of the diagnosis of onychomycosis by Hsiao et al, the sensitivities of KOH, PAS and culture were 87%, 81%, and 67%, and the negative predictive values of KOH, PAS, and culture were 50%, 40%, and 28%, respectively. One reason that the KOH may have done so well is that the nail specimen was immersed in 20% KOH in a test tube for 30 min or longer before looking under the microscope.[6]

- KOH may be equivalent to PAS if done and read properly. Consider it as the first line test since it is less expensive and the results are available while the patient is in the office. PAS is a good second line if the KOH is negative and the suspicion for onychomycosis is still present.

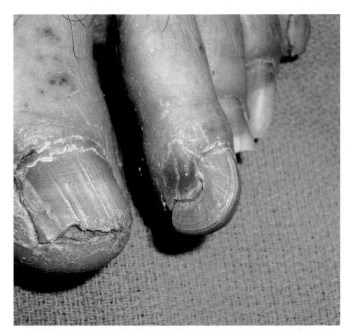

FIGURE 186-3 Severe toenail onychomycosis demonstrating subungual keratosis in the first nail and onychogryphosis (ram's horn nail) in the second nail because of the fungal infection. The culture grew Trichophyton rubrum. (*Courtesy of Richard P. Usatine, MD.*)

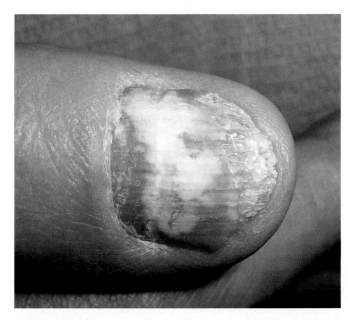

FIGURE 186-4 White superficial onychomycosis of the thumb nail. The culture was positive for Trichophyton mentagrophytes. (*Courtesy of Richard P. Usatine, MD.*)

DIFFERENTIAL DIAGNOSIS

- Nail trauma can cause a dysmorphic nail that is discolored and thickened. It is especially seen in the big toenail in runners. Ask about nail trauma before diagnosing onychomycosis. While onychomycosis often starts in the big toenail, it usually spreads to other nails. Traumatic changes often present with only one nail involved.

- Psoriatic nail changes may easily be confused with onychomycosis, especially when the psoriasis causes nail thickening and discoloration. Pitting of the nail plate surface, which is common in psoriasis, is not a feature of fungal infection. It is possible for a patient with psoriasis to get onychomycosis. Fungal studies can help determine if the changes are truly secondary to onychomycosis (see Chapter 188, Psoriatic Nails).

- Pseudomonal nail infection—produces a blue-green tint to the nail plate (**Figure 186-8**).

- Leukonychia—white spots or bands that appear proximally and proceed out with the nail may be confused with white superficial onychomycosis (see Chapter 183, Normal Nail Variants).

- Habitual picking of the proximal nail fold—induces the nail plate to be wavy and ridged, while its substance remains intact and hard (see Chapter 183, Normal Nail Variants).

MANAGEMENT

- Treating onychomycosis can be discouraging. Topical creams and lotion do not penetrate the nail plate and are of little value except in controlling inflammation at the nail folds.

- Oral therapy (**Table 186-1**) is expensive and may be followed by recurrence or reinfection when the medication is discontinued; however, it has the highest success rate.

- A Cochrane review found that the evidence suggests that terbinafine is more effective than griseofulvin and that terbinafine and itraconazole are more effective than no treatment.[7] SOR **A**

- Another Cochrane review found two trials of nail infections that did not provide any evidence of benefit for topical treatments (ciclopirox not included) compared with placebo.[8] SOR **A**

- Terbinafine has a preferable drug interaction profile, may have better long-term cure rates, and daily dosing may be the most effective treatment.[4,7] SOR **A**

- Itraconazole (Sporanox) has more drug interactions. Pulse dosing is as effective as daily dosing.

- Fluconazole (Diflucan) is not currently FDA approved for nail therapy and is not as effective as other oral therapies.[4,9] SOR **B**

- Ciclopirox 8% nail lacquer (Penlac) used daily (with weekly nail cleaning and filing) is a FDA approved topical treatment for mild to moderate onychomycosis. A meta-analysis of two randomized controlled trials showed a clinical cure rate of 8% vs 1% for vehicle alone.[10] Such a low cure rate is disappointing but a larger group of patients had some improvement without cure. This is one option for persons able to afford this topical treatment and not able to take oral antifungals.

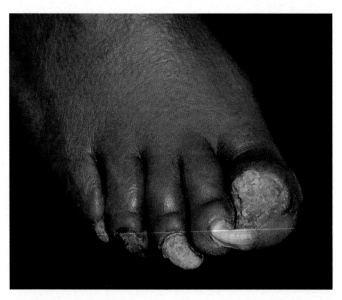

FIGURE 186-5 Extensive onychomycosis involving all toenails in an HIV positive man. His second toenail shows onychogryphosis (ram's horn nail) secondary to the fungal infection. (*Courtesy of Richard P. Usatine, MD.*)

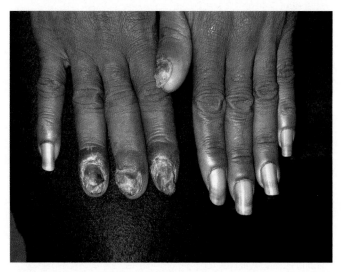

FIGURE 186-6 Fungal infection involving 4 out of 10 nails on the hands of the same HIV positive man. (*Courtesy of Richard P. Usatine, MD.*)

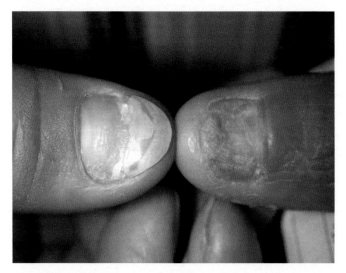

FIGURE 186-7 Onychomycosis involving both thumbnails. (*Courtesy of Richard P. Usatine, MD.*)

PATIENT EDUCATION

Patients should be advised that with treatment, nails may not appear normal for up to 1 year. The normal nail must grow out as treatment progresses.

PATIENT RESOURCES

• Fungal Infections of Fingernails and Toenails from family doctor.org.—**Available at http://www.familydoctor. org/663.xml.** Accessed October 15, 2007.

• EMedicineHealth on onychomycosis. Available at: **http:// www.emedicinehealth.com/onychomycosis/article_ em.htm.** Accessed October 15, 2007.

PROVIDER RESOURCES

• Onychomycosis on doctorfungus. Available at: **http://www. doctorfungus.org/mycoses/human/other/ onychomycosis_general.htm.** Accessed October 15, 2007.

• Blumberg M, Kantor GR. Onychomycosis—**http://www. emedicine.com/derm/topic300.htm.** Accessed October 15, 2007.

• Roger P, Bassler, M. American Family Physician Treating Onychomycosis—**http://www.aafp.org/afp/20010215/ 663.html.** Accessed October 15, 2007.

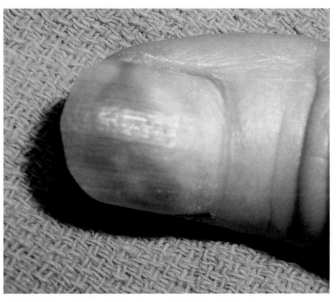

FIGURE 186-8 Pseudomonas of the nail showing a blue-green discoloration. (*Courtesy of Richard P. Usatine, MD.*)

TABLE 186-1 Common Treatments for Onychomycosis[4,7,8]

Drug	Pediatric Dose	Adult Dose	Course	Toenail Cure Rate*
Griseofulvin (Grifulvin V)	Microsize 15–20 mg/kg/d	500 mg po qd	4–9 months (f), 6–12 months (t)	60% ± 6%
Terbinafine (Lamisil)	10–20 kg: 62.5 mg/d 20–40 kg: 125 mg/d	250 mg po qd	6 weeks (f), 12 weeks (t)	76% ± 3%
Terbinafine (Lamisil) pulse†	—	250 mg bid 1 wk/mo	2 months (f), 3 months (t)	NR
Itraconazole (Sporanox)	—	200 mg daily	6 weeks (f), 12 weeks (t)	59% ± 5%
Itraconazole (Sporanox) pulse	<20 kg: 5 mg/kg/d for 1 wk/mo 20–40 kg: 100 mg daily for 1 wk/mo	200 mg bid or 5 mg/kg/d capsules for 1 wk/mo	2 months (f), 3 months (t)	63% ± 7%
Fluconazole (Diflucan)*	3–6 mk/kg once a wk	150 mg once a wk	12–16 weeks (f), 18–26 weeks (t)	48% ± 5%
Ciclopirox 8% nail lacquer (Penlac)	—	Apply daily to nail and surrounding 5-mm skin	Up to 48 weeks	~7%

*In a randomized trial meta-analysis. 10 NR = Not recorded.
†Not indicated for treating onychomycosis by the FDA.

REFERENCES

1. Gupta AK. Prevalence and epidemiology of onychomycosis in patients visiting physicians' offices: A multicenter Canadian survey of 15,000 patients. *J Am Acad Dermatol.* 2000;43:244.

2. Erbagci Z, Tuncel A, Zer Y, Balci I. A prospective epidemiologic survey on the prevalence of onychomycosis and dermatophytosis in male boarding school residents. *Mycopathologia.* 2005;159:347.

3. Sahin I, Kaya D, Parlak AH, et al. Dermatophytoses in forestry workers and farmers. *Mycoses.* 2005;48:260.

4. Harrell TK, Necomb WW, Replogle WH, King DS, Noble SL. Onychomycosis: Improved cure rates with Itraconazole and Terbinafine. *J Am Board Fam Pract.* 2000;13(4):268–273.

5. Weinberg JM, Koestenblatt EK, Tutrone WD, Tishler HR, Najarian L. Comparison of diagnostic methods in the evaluation of onychomycosis. *J Am Acad Dermatol.* 2003;49(2):193–197.

6. Hsiao YP, Lin HS, Wu TW, et al. A comparative study of KOH test, PAS staining and fungal culture in diagnosis of onychomycosis in Taiwan. *J Dermatol Sci.* 2007;45(2):138–140.

7. Bell-Syer S, Porthouse J, Bigby M. Oral treatments for toenail onychomycosis. *Cochrane Data Syst Rev.* 2004;(2): Art. No.: CD004766. DOI: 10.1002/14651858.CD004766. Accessed April 12, 2006.

8. Crawford F, Hart R, Bell-Syer S, Torgerson D, Young P, Russell I. Topical treatments for fungal infections of the skin and nails of the foot. *Cochrane Data Syst Rev.* 1999;(3): Art. No.: CD001434. DOI: 10.1002/14651858.CD001434. Accessed April 12, 2006.

9. Havu V, Heikkila H, Kuokkanen K, et al. A double-blind, randomized study to compare the efficacy and safety of terbinafine (Lamisil) with fluconazole (Diflucan) in the treatment of onychomycosis. *Br J Dermatol.* 2000;142(1):97–102.

10. Gupta AK, Joseph WS. Ciclopirox 8% nail lacquer in the treatment of onychomycosis of the toenails in the United States. *J Am Podiatr Med Assoc.* 2000;90(10):495–501.

187 PARONYCHIA

E.J. Mayeaux Jr., MD

PATIENT STORY

A 41-year-old woman presented with a 3-day history of localized pain, redness, and tenderness of the lateral nail fold of the index finger. A small abscess had developed in the last 24 hours at the nail margin (**Figure 187-1**). After informed consent was given, a digital block was performed. This acute paronychia was treated with incision and drainage using a #11 scalpel (**Figure 187-2**). A significant amount of pus was drained. She soaked her finger four times daily as directed. Two days later the patient's finger was much better and the culture grew out *Staphylococcus aureus*. Draining the abscess was sufficient treatment.

DEFINITIONS

- Paronychia is a localized, superficial infection or abscess of the nail folds. It is one of the most common infections of the hand.

- Paronychia can be acute or chronic. Chronic paronychia is defined as being present for longer than 6 weeks duration.

- Acute paronychia usually presents as an acutely painful abscess in the nail fold.

- Chronic paronychia is a red, tender, swelling of the proximal or lateral nail folds. It is usually nonsuppurative and is more difficult to treat.

EPIDEMIOLOGY

Paronychia is a relatively common problem in adults. The prevalence is unknown since many patients do not seek medical care.

ETIOLOGY AND PATHOPHYSIOLOGY

- Paronychial infections develop when a disruption occurs between the seal of the nail fold and the nail plate or the skin of a nail fold is disrupted and allows a portal of entry for invading organisms.

- Acute paronychia commonly results from nail biting (**Figure 187-3**), finger sucking, aggressive manicuring (**Figure 187-4**), hang nails (**Figure 187-5**), trauma, and artificial nails.[1]

- Acute paronychia is most commonly caused by *Staphylococcus aureus*, followed by streptococci and pseudomonas.

- Children are prone to acute paronychia through direct infection of fingers with mouth flora from finger sucking and nail biting.

- Chronic paronychia more likely results from chronic *Candida albicans* (95%) (**Figures 187-6** and **187-7**). Other rare causes include atypical mycobacteria and gram-negative rods. There is some evidence that chronic paronychia is at least partially an

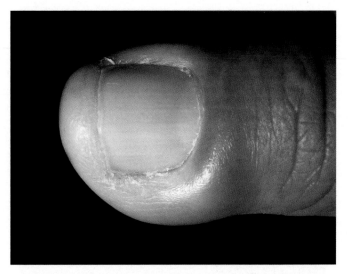

FIGURE 187-1 Painful acute paronychia around the fingernail of a 41-year-old woman. Note the swelling and erythema with a small white-yellow area suggesting underlying purulence. (*Courtesy of Richard P. Usatine, MD.*)

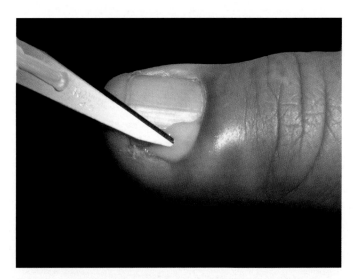

FIGURE 187-2 Incision and drainage of the acute paronychia in the previous figure with a #11 scalpel. Note the exuberant pus draining from the incision. (*Courtesy of Richard P. Usatine, MD.*)

eczematous process and that Candida infection is a secondary phenomenon.[2]

- People at risk of developing chronic paronychia include those who are repeatedly exposed to liquid irritants or alkali, and those whose hands are chronically wet. People with occupations such as baker, bartender, housekeepers, and dishwashers are predisposed to developing chronic paronychia.

- Untreated persistent chronic paronychia may cause horizontal ridging, undulations and other changes to the nail plate (**Figures 187-6** and **187-7**).

- Patients with diabetes mellitus, compromised immune systems, or a history of oral steroid use are at increased risk for paronychia. Retroviral therapy use, especially indinavir and lamivudine, may be associated with an increased incidence of paronychia.[3]

DIAGNOSIS

CLINICAL FEATURES

- Acute paronychia presents with localized pain and tenderness. The nail fold appears erythematous and inflamed, and a collection of pus usually develops (**Figures 187-1** through **187-4**). Granulation tissue may develop along the nail fold, and cellulitis may develop (**Figure 187-5**).

- Chronic paronychia is a red, tender, painful swelling of the proximal or lateral nail folds. A small collection of pus or abscess may form but typically only redness and swelling are present. Eventually, the nail plates may become thickened and discolored, with pronounced horizontal ridges[4] (**Figures 187-6** and **187-7**). *Candida albicans* may be cultured.

DIFFERENTIAL DIAGNOSIS

- Mucus cyst, which presents as a painless swelling lateral and proximal to the nail plate (**Figure 187-8**). This can also cause changes in the nail morphology.

- Glomus tumor, which presents with constant severe pain, nail plate elevation, bluish-discoloration of the nail plate, and blurring of the lunula.

- Proximal onychomycosis—involves the nail plate and not the nail folds (see Chapter 186, Onychomycosis).

- Herpetic whitlow, which results from herpes simplex virus (HSV) infection presents with acute onset of vesicles or pustules, severe edema, erythema, and pain. Tzanck staining of vesicles will demonstrate multinucleated giant cells and viral culture will grow HSV (see Chapter 123, Herpes Simplex).

- Felon—Paronychia must be distinguished from a felon, which is an infection of the digital pulp. It is characterized by severe pain, swelling, and erythema in the pad of the fingertip.

- Benign and malignant neoplasms, which may present early with redness and swelling should always be ruled out when chronic paronychia does not respond to conventional treatment.

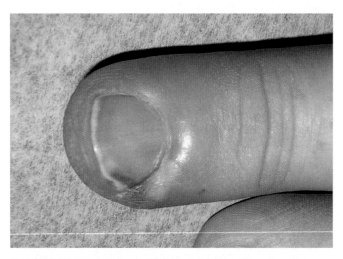

FIGURE 187-3 Acute paronychia from nail biting. Note abscess formation in the lateral nail fold that is extending into the proximal fold. (*Courtesy of E.J. Mayeaux, Jr., MD.*)

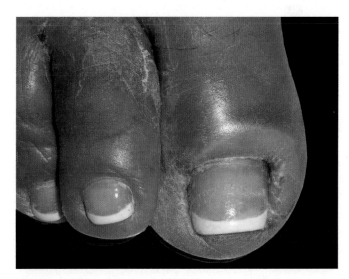

FIGURE 187-4 Acute paronychia of the great toe. Note extensive manicure of the nails, which may predispose to paronychia if the cuticle or nail folds are disrupted. (*Courtesy of Jennifer P. Pierce, MD.*)

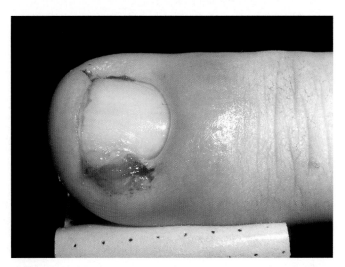

FIGURE 187-5 Paronychia with cellulitis of the skin of the fingertip and granulation tissue formation. This all started when the patient began manipulating a hang nail. (*Courtesy of Richard P. Usatine, MD.*)

MANAGEMENT

- Acute paronychia:
  - Milder cases of acute paronychia without abscess formation may be treated with warm soaks for 20 minutes three to four times a day.[1] SOR **C**
  - Addition of an oral antistaphylococcal agent (dicloxacillin 500 mg three times daily, cephalexin 500 mg two to three times daily for 7 to 10 days, erythromycin 333–500 mg three times daily or azithromycin 500 mg on day one followed by 250 mg daily for 4 days) may be added for more severe or unresponsive cases. SOR **C** Children who suck their fingers and patients who bite their nails should be covered against anaerobes. Clindamycin and amoxicillin-clavulanate potassium are effective against most pathogens isolated from infections originating in the mouth.[5]
  - When abscess or fluctuance is present, drainage is necessary.[6] SOR **C** It is performed with digital block anesthesia. The affected nail fold is incised with a scalpel with the blade parallel to the edge of the nail plate and the pus expressed (**Figure 187-2**). Warm soaks four times a day are initiated to keep the incision from sealing until all of the pus is gone.[7] Between soakings, an adhesive bandage can protect the nail fold. Antibiotic therapy is usually not necessary unless there is accompanying cellulitis.
- Chronic paronychia:
  - Long-term treatment of chronic paronychia primarily involves avoiding predisposing factors such as prolonged exposure to water, nail trauma and finger sucking. Treatment with a combination of topical steroids and an antifungal agent has been shown to be successful.[1,2] SOR **B** Oral antifungal therapy is usually not necessary.[1]

PATIENT EDUCATION

Measures that may prevent or improve paronychia:

- Keep the hands dry as much as possible.
- Avoid work that keeps the hands wet, or dry them off as soon as possible.
- Use cotton glove liners under waterproof gloves to keep hands dry from sweat and condensation.
- Keep fingernails clean.
- After dirty work, wash thoroughly with soap and water, rinse off, and dry carefully.
- Moisturize the skin, don't let it become chafed and cracked.

PATIENT RESOURCES

- Paronychia—Infection Around the Nails @ About.com— **http://dermatology.about.com/cs/paronychia/a/paronychia.htm.**
- Paronychia (nail fold infection) @ DermNet NZ— **http://dermnetnz.org/fungal/paronychia.html.**

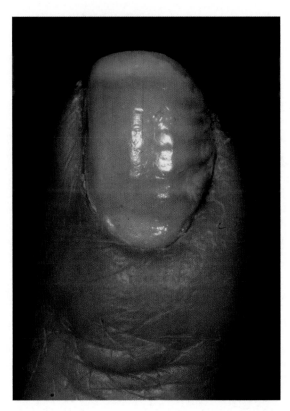

FIGURE 187-6 Chronic paronychia. Note horizontal ridges on one side of the nail plate as a result of chronic inflammation. (*Courtesy of Richard P. Usatine, MD.*)

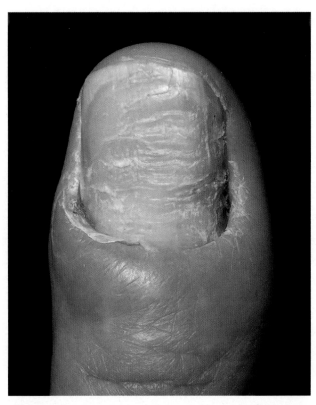

FIGURE 187-7 Chronic candida paronychia causing a dysmorphic fingernail with horizontal ridging. (*Courtesy of Richard P. Usatine, MD.*)

PROVIDER RESOURCES

• eMedicine Paronychia—**http://www.emedicine.com/ emerg/topic357.htm.**

• Acute and Chronic Paronychia—American Family Physician (*Am Fam Physician* 2001;63:1113–1116)—**http://www.aafp.org/ afp/20010315/1113.html.**

REFERENCES

1. Hochman LG. Paronychia: More than just an abscess. *Int J Dermatol*. 1995;34:385–386.

2. Tosti, A, Piraccini, BM, Ghetti, E, Colombo, MD. Topical steroids versus systemic antifungals in the treatment of chronic paronychia: An open, randomized double-blind and double dummy study. *J Am Acad Dermatol*. 2002; 47:73.

3. Tosti A, Piraccini BM, D'Antuono A, Marzaduri S, Bettoli V. Paronychia associated with antiretroviral therapy. *Br J Dermatol*. 1999;140(6):1165–1168.

4. Canales FL, Newmeyer WL 3d, Kilgore ES. The treatment of felons and paronychias. *Hand Clin*. 1989;5:515–523.

5. Brook I. Aerobic and anaerobic microbiology of paronychia. *Ann Emerg Med*. 1990;19:994–996.

6. Keyser JJ, Littler JW, Eaton RG. Surgical treatment of infections and lesions of the perionychium. *Hand Clin*. 1990;6(1):137–153.

7. Zuber T, Mayeaux EJ, Jr. *Atlas of Primary Care Procedures*. Philadelphia: Lippincott, Williams, & Wilkins, 2003:233–238.

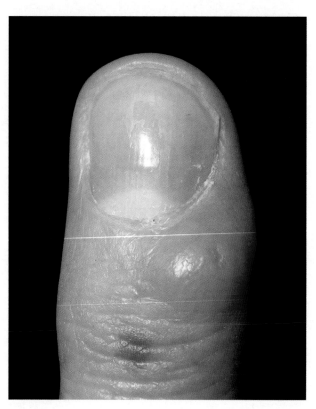

FIGURE 187-8 Digital mucus cyst presenting as a painless swelling of the nail fold in a young woman. (*Courtesy of Richard P. Usatine, MD.*)

188 PSORIATIC NAILS

E.J. Mayeaux, Jr., MD

PATIENT STORY

A 19-year-old man with a 4-year history of plaque psoriasis presents with nail abnormalities in several fingers (**Figure 188-1**). He is particularly concerned about the recently acquired greenish discoloration of his fifth digit.

EPIDEMIOLOGY

- Psoriasis is a hereditary disorder of skin with numerous clinical expressions. It affects millions of people throughout the world.[1] The prevalence increases with age.

- Nails are involved in up to 50% of persons with psoriasis.[1] In most cases, nail involvement coexists with cutaneous psoriasis, although the skin surrounding the affected nails need not be involved. Psoriatic nail disease without overt cutaneous disease occurs in 1% to 5% of psoriasis. Patients with nail involvement are thought to have a higher incidence of associated arthritis.[2]

- The most common nail change seen with psoriasis is nail plate pitting (**Figures 188-1** and **188-2**).

ETIOLOGY AND PATHOPHYSIOLOGY

- The proximal nail matrix forms the superficial portion of the nail plate, so that involvement in this part of the matrix results in pitting of the nail plate (**Figures 188-1** and **188-2**.) The pits may range in size from pinpoint depressions to large punched out lesions. People without psoriasis can have nail pitting.

- Longitudinal matrix involvement produces longitudinal nail ridging or splitting (**Figure 188-2**). When transverse matrix involvement occurs, solitary or multiple "growth arrest" lines (Beau's lines) may occur (see Chapter 183, Normal Nail Variants). Psoriatic involvement of the intermediate portion of the nail matrix leads to leukonychia and diminished nail plate integrity.

DIAGNOSIS

- The diagnosis of nail psoriasis is usually straightforward when characteristic nail findings coexist with cutaneous psoriasis. Nail psoriasis and onychomycosis are often indistinguishable by clinical examination alone. Potassium hydroxide (KOH) preparation and fungal culture will usually provide an answer. However, it may be necessary to clip a portion of the nail plate and send it for fungal staining (periodic acid-Schiff [PAS] stain) if the first test results are not consistent with the clinical picture.[3] Psoriasis and onychomycosis can occur concomitantly.

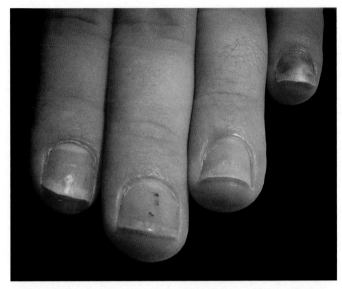

FIGURE 188-1 Patient with nail psoriasis demonstrating the oil drop sign (second digit), nail pitting (second and third digit), onycholysis (second, fourth and fifth digit), and secondary pseudomonas infection (fifth digit). (*Courtesy of E.J. Mayeaux, Jr., MD.*)

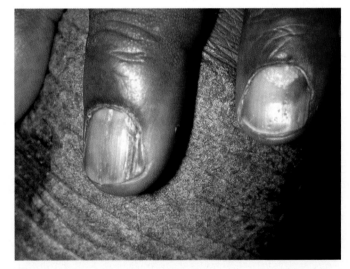

FIGURE 188-2 Nail psoriasis demonstrating nail pitting, onycholysis, oil drop sign and longitudinal ridging. Nails held over the silvery plaque on the knee. (*Courtesy of Richard P. Usatine, MD.*)

- Psoriasis at the hyponychium produces subungual hyperkeratosis and distal onycholysis (**Figures 188-1, 188-3,** and **188-4**). Trauma may accentuate this process. Secondary microbial colonization by Candida or Pseudomonas organisms may occur (**Figure 188-1**, digit 5).

- Nail bed psoriasis produces localized onycholysis which often appears like a drop of oil on a piece of paper (oil drop sign) (**Figures 188-2, 188-3,** and **188-5**). This same condition is also called the salmon patch sign.

- Extensive germinal matrix involvement may result in loss of nail integrity and transverse (horizontal) ridging (**Figure 188-4**).

- Psoriasis causes dermal vascular dilatation and tortuosity, and in the nails is associated with splinter hemorrhages of the nail bed caused by foci of capillary bleeding. Extravasated blood becomes trapped between the longitudinal troughs of the nail bed and the overlying nail plate grows out distally along with the plate (**Figure 188-6**). The splinter hemorrhages of the psoriatic nail are analogous to the cutaneous Auspitz sign.

DIFFERENTIAL DIAGNOSIS

- Onychomycosis produces distal onycholysis and hyperkeratosis that appear identical to psoriasis and may coexist with it (see Chapter 182, Onychomycosis).

- Darier disease (keratosis follicularis) is an autosomal dominant disorder that results in abnormal keratinization and loss of adhesion between epidermal cells. It typically presents in the second decade of life with hyperkeratotic, yellow-brown, greasy-appearing papules that coalesce into verrucous-like plaques in a seborrheic distribution. Nails may demonstrate red/white longitudinal stripes, subungual hyperkeratosis, and notching of the distal nail margins (**Figure 188-7**). The course of the illness is chronic and persistent.

- Alopecia areata also can produce pitting of the nails. As a general rule, pitting in psoriasis is more irregular and broader based; pitting in alopecia areata is more regular, shallow, and geometric and produces fine pits (see Chapter 180, Alopecia Areata).

- Neoplastic and dysplastic diseases may produce psoriasiform nail changes in a single nail. Bowen's disease, squamous cell carcinoma, and verruca vulgaris may appear as an isolated subungual or periungual plaque, possibly with accompanying nail plate destruction. A biopsy can establish a definitive diagnosis.

MANAGEMENT

- Psoriatic nail disease is often persistent and refractory to treatment. There is insufficient evidence to recommend a standard treatment.

- Psoriatic nail changes may be reversible because scarring typically does not occur. An exception to this may develop in severe cases of generalized pustular psoriasis. Systemic retinoid therapy is often effective for pustular psoriasis, and early intervention is most likely to prevent chronic nail-associated scarring.

- One treatment option for nail psoriasis, especially with matrix involvement, is intralesional corticosteroid injection. Triamcinolone acetonide (0.4 mL, 10 mg/mL) into the nail bed and matrix

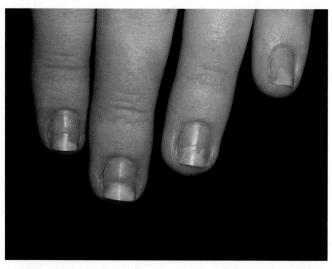

FIGURE 188-3 Nail psoriasis with onycholysis and oil drop sign in a young woman. Note that end of the nail plates are no longer attached to the nail bed and there is a light brown discoloration where the nail loses its attachment. (*Courtesy of Richard P. Usatine, MD.*)

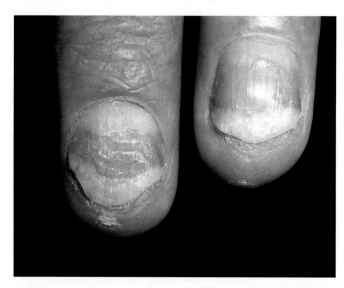

FIGURE 188-4 Nail psoriasis demonstrating onycholysis, pits, and transverse (horizontal) ridging. (*Courtesy of Richard P. Usatine, MD.*)

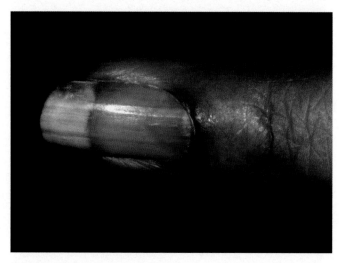

FIGURE 188-5 Nail psoriasis with the oil drop (or salmon patch) sign. (*Courtesy of Richard P. Usatine, MD.*)

following digital block, and then at 3-month intervals (**Figure 188-6**).[4] SOR Ⓑ Subungual hyperkeratosis, ridging, and thickening respond better than pitting and onycholysis, with benefit sustained for at least 9 months.[4]

- Nail bed disease, including subungual hyperkeratosis, distal onycholysis, and "oil drop" changes may also need the lateral nail folds injected close to the nail bed. Direct injection into the nail bed is prevented by the nail plate and extreme pain sensitivity of the hyponychial region. Atrophy and subungual hematoma formation are potential complications.

- Other topical therapies that have shown effectiveness include topical 1% 5-fluorouracil solution or 5% cream applied twice daily to the matrix area for 6 months, topical calcipotriol, topical anthralin, topical tazarotene, and topical cyclosporine. Systemic therapies for psoriasis may improve nail manifestations. Oral and topical Psoralen plus long-wave ultraviolet light (PUVA) for 3 to 6 months, acitretin, methotrexate, and cyclosporine have been found to be helpful for nail psoriasis.[5] SOR Ⓑ In a single-blinded study, Feliciani et al. found that combination therapy (oral cyclosporine and topical calcipotriol) was more effective than monotherapy (cyclosporine alone) on nail psoriasis.[6]

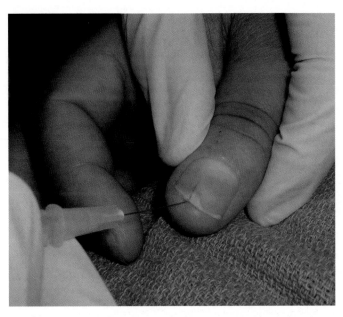

FIGURE 188-6 Injecting a psoriatic nail with triamcinolone after doing a digital block.[4] The nail matrix was injected prior to injecting the distal nail bed. This 23-year-old woman wanted treatment to normalize nail appearance, which currently has onycholysis and splinter hemorrhages. (*Courtesy of Richard P. Usatine, MD.*)

PATIENT EDUCATION

Nail psoriasis is mainly a cosmetic problem. Nail polish or artificial nails can be used in some patients to conceal psoriatic pitting and onycholysis. When subungal hyperkeratosis becomes uncomfortable because of pressure exerted by footwear, the nail can be pared down to relieve the pressure.

Patients should be instructed to trim nails back to the point of firm attachment with the nail bed to minimize further nail-bed and nail-plate disassociation. Wearing gloves while working may minimize trauma to the nails. Tell patients to avoid vigorous cleaning and scraping under the nails since this may break the skin where the nail is attached and lead to an infection.

FOLLOW-UP

Follow-up can be combined with regular follow-ups for cutaneous psoriasis.

PATIENT RESOURCES

- Psoriasis and Psoriatic Arthritis information site—Nail Psoriasis—**http://www.paalliance.org/nail_psoriasis. htm.**
- DermNet Nail Psoriasis—**http://dermnetnz.org/scaly/ nail-psoriasis.html.**

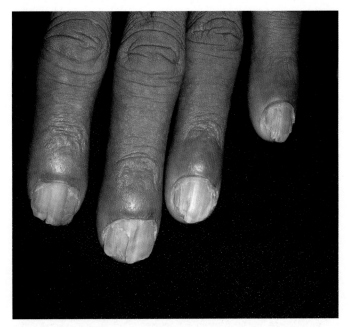

FIGURE 188-7 A woman with Darier's disease (keratosis follicularis) demonstrating brittle nails with brown/white longitudinal stripes and notching of the distal nail plate. (*Courtesy of Richard P. Usatine, MD.*)

PROVIDER RESOURCES

- E medicine Nail Psoriasis—**http://www.emedicine.com/ derm/topic363.htm.**
- National Psoriasis Foundation Psoriasis of the nails— **http://www.psoriasis.org/about/psoriasis/sites/nails. php.**
- Dermatology Online Journal Psoriasis confined to the nails— **http://dermatology.cdlib.org/94/NYU/Nov2001/ 8.html.**
- Comprehensive review—Jiaravuthisan MM, Sasseville D, Vender RB, Murphy F, Muhn CY. Psoriasis of the nail. Anatomy, pathology, clinical presentation, and a review of the literature on therapy. *J Am Acad Dermatol.* 2007;57(1):1–27.

REFERENCES

1. Jiaravuthisan MM, Sasseville D, Vender RB, Murphy F, Muhn CY. Psoriasis of the nail. Anatomy, pathology, clinical presentation, and a review of the literature on thereapy. *J Am Acad Dermatol.* 2007;57(1):1–27.

2. Noronha PA, Zubkov B. Nails and nail disorders in children and adults. *Am Fam Phys.* 1997;55:2129–2140.

3. Grammer-West NY, Corvette DM, Giandoni MB, Fitzpatric JE. Clinical Pearl: Nail plate biopsy for the diagnosis of psoriatic nails. *J Am Acad Dermatol.* 1998;38:260–262.

4. de Berker DA, Lawrence CM. A simplified protocol of steroid injection for psoriatic nail dystrophy. *Br J Dermatol.* 1998;138(1): 90–95.

5. Cassell, S, Kavanaugh, AF. Therapies for psoriatic nail disease. A systematic review. *J Rheumatol.* 2006;33:1452.

6. Feliciani C, Zampetti A, Forleo P, et al. Nail psoriasis: combined therapy with systemic cyclosporine and topical calcipotriol. *J Cutan Med Surg.* 2004;8:122–125.

189 SUBUNGUAL HEMATOMA (NAIL TRAUMA)

E.J. Mayeaux, Jr., MD

PATIENT STORY

A 22-year-old woman dropped an iron on her toe the day before she visited our free clinic. Her toe was painful at rest and worse when walking (**Figure 189-1**). This subungual hematoma needed to be drained and we did not have an electrocautery unit. A paperclip was bent open and held in a hemostat and heated with a torch. With some pressure it pierced the patient's nail plate and the blood spontaneously drained (**Figures 189-2** and **189-3**). This relieved the pressure and gave the patient immediate pain relief. The remaining old blood was drained with a little pressure on the proximal nail fold (**Figure 189-4**). While we were concerned about a possible underlying fracture the patient did not have health insurance and chose to postpone an x-ray. Her toe healed well and no radiographs were ever taken. (*Story by Richard P. Usatine, MD.*)

EPIDEMIOLOGY

Subungual hematoma is a common childhood and adult injury.

ETIOLOGY AND PATHOPHYSIOLOGY

- Subungual hematomas may be simple (i.e., the nail and nail margin are intact) or accompanied by injuries to the nail bed and possibly associated underlying fractures.[1]
- Subungual hematoma is usually caused by a blow to the distal phalanx (i.e., stubbing a toe or crush injury).
- The patient may not be aware of the precipitating trauma, because it may have been minor and/or chronic (e.g., rubbing in a tight shoe).
- The injury causes bleeding of the nail matrix and nail bed which results in subungual hematoma formation (**Figures 189-1 to 189-5**).
- In most cases it grows out with the nail plate, exhibiting a proximal border that reproduces the shape of the lunula. Occasionally, a hematoma does not migrate because of repeated daily trauma. An extended, nonmigrating hematoma should be considered suspicious. Nail plate punch biopsy will often reveal the dark streak to be a subungual hematoma since the color lifts off with nail plate (**Figure 189-5**).
- Potential complications of subungual hematoma include onycholysis, nail deformity (usually splitting as in **Figure 189-6**), and infection. Complications are more likely to occur when presentation is delayed or there is an underlying fracture.[2]

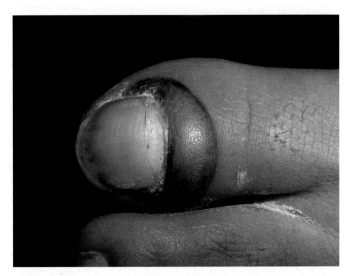

FIGURE 189-1 Acute subungual hematoma 1 day after dropping an iron on her toe. It was painful at rest and worse when walking. (*Courtesy of Richard P. Usatine, MD.*)

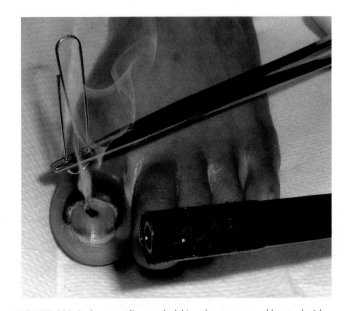

FIGURE 189-2 A paperclip was held in a hemostat and heated with a torch to pierce the patient's nail plate in order to relieve the subungual hematoma. (*Courtesy of Richard P. Usatine, MD.*)

DIAGNOSIS

- Patients complain of throbbing pain and blue-black discoloration under the nail as the hematoma progresses. Pain is relieved immediately in most patients with simple nail trephination (**Figure 189-3**).
- If the mechanism of injury and clinical picture suggest a possible distal phalanx or DIP fracture, obtain a radiograph. SOR ©

DIFFERENTIAL DIAGNOSIS

- Nail bed nevus—appears as a stable or slowly growing painless dark spot in the nail bed or matrix.
- Longitudinal melanonychia—appears as painless pigmented bands that start in the matrix and extend the length of the nail (see Chapter 184, Pigmented Nail Disorders).
- Subungual melanoma—may start as a painless darkly pigmented band in the matrix and extend the length of the nail. It may be associated with pigment deposition in the proximal nail fold (Hutchinson's sign) (see Chapter 184, Pigmented Nail Disorders).
- Splinter hemorrhages—appears as reddish streaks in the nail bed and are seen in psoriasis more commonly than endocarditis (see Chapter 188, Psoriatic Nails).
- The diagnosis of child abuse must be considered in cases of chronic or frequently recurrent subungual hematomas in children.[3]

MANAGEMENT

- Subungual hematomas are treated with nail trephination, which removes the extravasated blood and relieves the pressure and resulting pain. SOR ©
- Nail trephination is a painless procedure because there are no nerve endings in the nail plate that is perforated. The nail is perforated with a hot metal wire or steel paper clip (**Figures 189-2 to 189-4**), an electrocautery device, or by spinning a large-bore needle against the nail plate like a mechanical spade bit. This allows the collected blood to drain out (**Figures 189-3 and 189-4**). The hole must be large enough for continued drainage, which can continue for 24 to 36 hours. The puncture site should be kept covered with sterile gauze dressing while the wound drains and the gauze is changed daily.
- Some authors recommend removal of the nail with inspection instead of nail trephination when the hematoma involves more than 25% to 50% of the nail because of the increased likelihood of significant nail bed injury and fracture of the distal phalanx.[4,5]
- When deeper injuries are involved, nail plate removal after a digital block will allow for nail bed repair.[6] SOR ©

PATIENT EDUCATION

- Potential complications of subungual hematoma and nail trephination should be discussed with the patient and/or his or her parents or guardian.

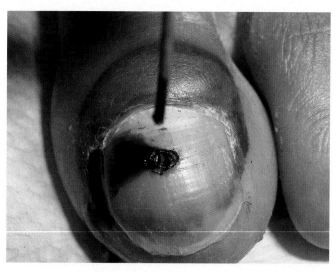

FIGURE 189-3 The hot paper-clip formed a nice hole in the nail plate and the blood drained out spontaneously. This relieved the pressure and gave the patient immediate pain relief. (*Courtesy of Richard P. Usatine, MD.*)

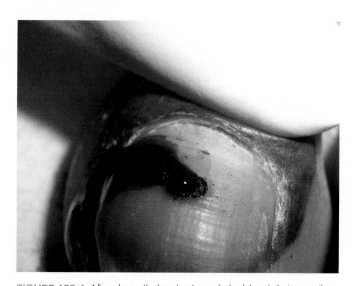

FIGURE 189-4 After the nail plate is pierced, the blood drains easily with a little pressure on the proximal nail fold. (*Courtesy of Richard P. Usatine, MD.*)

• Inform the patient that residual discoloration usually slowly grows out with the nail.

FOLLOW-UP

Follow-up in about a week to assess for reaccumulation of blood or infection.

PATIENT RESOURCES

• Emedicinehealth subungual hematoma—**http://www.emedicinehealth.com/subungual_hematoma_bleeding_under_nail/article_em.htm.**

• HealthSquare subungual hematoma—**http://www.healthsquare.com/mc/fgmc0728.htm.**

PROVIDER RESOURCES

• American Family Physician Fingertip Injuries—**http://www.aafp.org/afp/20010515/1961.html.**

• InteliHealth Nail Trauma—**http://www.intelihealth.com/IH/ihtIH/WSIHW000/9339/25971.html.**

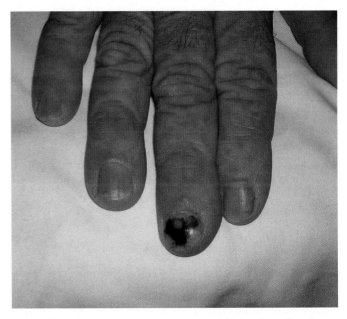

FIGURE 189-5 This persistent discoloration of the nail was found to be a subungual hematoma by nail plate biopsy using a punch biopsy instrument. (*Courtesy of E.J. Mayeaux, Jr., MD.*)

REFERENCES

1. Roser, SE, Gellman, H. Comparison of nail bed repair versus nail trephination for subungual hematomas in children. *J Hand Surg [Am]*. 1999;24:1166.

2. Meek, S, White, M. Subungual haematomas: Is simple trephining enough? *J Accid Emerg Med*. 1998;15:269.

3. Gavin, LA, Lanz, MJ, Leung, DY, Roesler, TA. Chronic subungual hematomas: A presumed immunologic puzzle resolved with a diagnosis of child abuse. *Arch Pediatr Adolesc Med*. 1997;151:103.

4. Zook, EG, Guy, RJ, Russell, RC. A study of nail bed injuries: Causes, treatment, and prognosis. *J Hand Surg [Am]*. 1984;9:247.

5. Zacher, JB. Management of injuries of the distal phalanx. *Surg Clin North Am*. 1984;64:747.

6. Hart, RG, Kleinert, HE. Fingertip and nail bed injuries. *Emerg Med Clin North Am*. 1993;11:755.

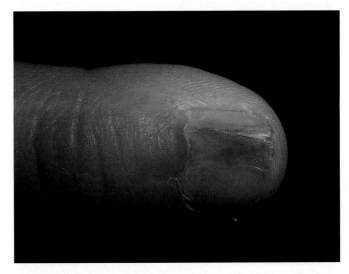

FIGURE 189-6 Split nail deformity in a 6-year-old girl 1 year after her finger was closed in a car door and sutured in the ER. The matrix did not come together well and the nail will remain split (onychoschizia). (*Courtesy of Richard P. Usatine, MD.*)

190 MELASMA

E.J. Mayeaux, Jr., MD

PATIENT STORY

A young hispanic woman delivers a healthy baby boy. On the first postpartum day, she is sitting in the rocking chair after breast-feeding her
son. Her doctor notes that she has melasma and asks her about it. She
states that the hyperpigmented areas on her face have become darker
during this pregnancy (**Figure 190-1**). She noted the dark spots
started with her first pregnancy but they are worse this time. On physical examination, hyperpigmented patches are noted on the cheeks and
upper lip (**Figure 190-2**). While the patient hopes the pigment will
fade, she does not want to treat the melasma at this time.

EPIDEMIOLOGY

- It is a relatively common disorder that affects sun-exposed areas of
  skin, most commonly the face. It is believed to affect up to 75% of
  pregnant women.[1]

- It usually affects women (**Figures 190-1** to **190-3**) and is particularly
  prevalent in women with darker complexions (especially Hispanics)
  and who live in areas of intense ultraviolet radiation exposure.

ETIOLOGY AND PATHOPHYSIOLOGY

- Melasma (mask of pregnancy) is a localized facial
  hyperpigmentation, most commonly caused by pregnancy or the
  use of sex steroid hormones such as oral contraceptive pills.

- Melasma caused by pregnancy usually regresses within a year, but
  areas of hyperpigmentation may never completely resolve.[2] It may
  increase with each subsequent pregnancy becoming more obvious.

- The precise cause of melasma has not been determined. Multiple
  factors have been implicated, including pregnancy, oral contraceptives, genetics, sun exposure, cosmetic use, thyroid dysfunction,
  and antiepileptic medications.[3,4]

- Women with melasma not related to pregnancy or oral contraceptive use may have hormonal alterations that are consistent with
  mild ovarian dysfunction.[5]

- Melasma in men (**Figure 190-4**) shares the same clinical features as
  in women, but it is not known if hormonal factors play a role.[6]

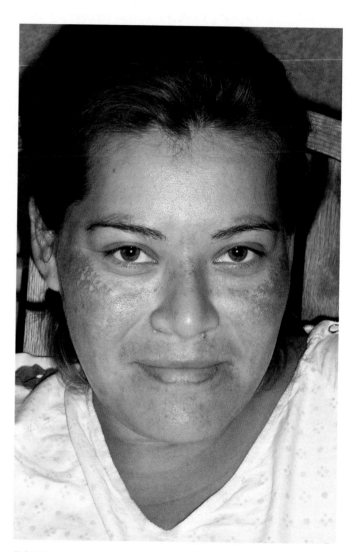

FIGURE 190-1 Melasma (chloasma) in the typical distribution in a
woman that just gave birth to her second child. This is sometimes
called the mask of pregnancy. (*Courtesy of Richard P. Usatine, MD.*)

DIAGNOSIS

CLINICAL FEATURES

The diagnosis of melasma is based upon clinical appearance. Affected patients exhibit splotchy areas of hyperpigmented macules on the face (**Figures 190-1** to **190-4**). In natural light, epidermal melasma appears light to dark brown, and the dermal pattern is blue or gray.

TYPICAL DISTRIBUTION

The lesion is found typically on sun-exposed areas. The three typical patterns of involvement are: 1 centrofacial involving the cheeks, forehead, upper lip, nose, and chin; 2 malar involving the cheeks and nose; 3 and mandibular involving the ramus of the mandible.

BIOPSY

Histologically, there is an increased number of melanocytes, with the deposition of additional melanin and a background of solar elastosis. There are two main histologic patterns that are epidermal and dermal, depending on the skin layers involved.

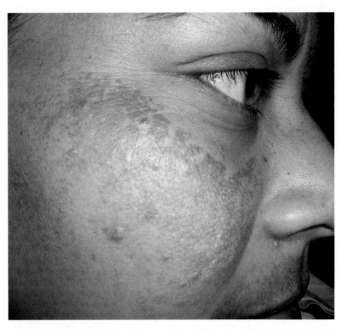

FIGURE 190-2 Closeup of the melasma showing the hyperpigmented patches on cheeks and upper lip. (*Courtesy of Richard P. Usatine, MD.*)

DIFFERENTIAL DIAGNOSIS

- The facial rash of systemic lupus may be confused with melasma as they both can have a butterfly pattern. Melasma is hyperpigmented, while the lupus facial rash is usually inflammatory. An antinuclear antibody (ANA) test should be positive in SLE and negative in melasma. False positive antinuclear antibodies are usually low titer and the patient does not have other criteria for lupus (see Chapter 173, Lupus Erythematosus).

- Discoid lupus or cutaneous lupus can occur across the face but is usually seen with scarring. In this condition, the ANA is often negative (see Chapter 173, Lupus Erythematosus).

- Contact dermatitis on the face may be confused with melasma but usually appears much more inflammatory (see Chapter 140, Contact Dermatitis).

MANAGEMENT

- Melasma treatment is started only when the patient is disturbed by the hyperpigmentation. All patients can benefit from sun protection and this is always a good place to start.

- It is important to give the patient realistic treatment goals. The treatments that follow may lighten the hyperpigmentation but do not generally remove all the hyperpigmentation.

- Tretinoin 0.1% (Retin-A) cream applied once daily at bedtime or hydroquinone (over-the-counter: 2%, by prescription: 4%), a bleaching agent, are the main topical treatments. SOR Ⓑ Combining tretinoin and hydroquinone can potentiate their effects. SOR Ⓒ

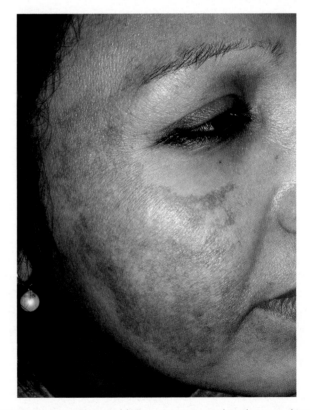

FIGURE 190-3 A 39-year-old Hispanic woman with melasma seeking treatment. She is disturbed by this dark color on her face. Note the hyperpigmentation reaches the eyebrows but does not cover the upper lip. She has not been pregnant for years and is not taking hormonal contraceptives. (*Courtesy of Richard P. Usatine, MD.*)

- Bleaching agents are best tried only after patch testing elsewhere on the body. Bleaching agents should be avoided on inflamed skin to prevent more to postinflammatory changes and further hyperpigmentation. It is applied twice daily for up to three months with subsequent tapering.

- A new medication that contains tretinoin, 0.05%; hydroquinone, 4.0%; and fluocinolone acetonide, 0.01% (Tri-Luma) has been effective in the treatment of melasma.[7] SOR Ⓑ

- Azelaic acid (20%), kojic acid formulations, and alpha-hydroxy acids (such as glycolic acid) also have been useful in the treatment of melasma. SOR Ⓒ

- Side effects of all topical treatments include allergic and contact dermatitis, depigmentation of surrounding normal skin, and postinflammatory hyperpigmentation. Tretinoin should never be used during pregnancy.

- Chemical peels are one option for in patients with moderate to severe melasma that has not responded to bleaching agents and are seeking further treatment.

PATIENT EDUCATION

Strict avoidance of sun exposure is important to control the disease. SOR Ⓒ Broad-spectrum sunscreens (with ultraviolet B and ultraviolet A protection), such as titanium dioxide, micronized zinc oxide, or avobenzone/Parsol are essential.[8]

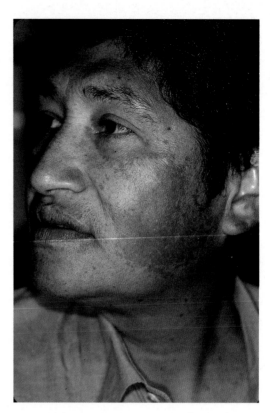

FIGURE 190-4 Melasma in a man. (*Courtesy of Richard P. Usatine, MD.*)

FOLLOW-UP

Follow-up is advisable when using bleaching agents. Long-term follow-up and reinforcement of limiting sun exposure can be accomplished during routine prevention visits.

PATIENT RESOURCES

WebMD: Skin Problems of Pregnancy—**http://www.webmd. com/content/Article/67/79983.htm?printing=true.**

American Pregnancy Association: Skin Changes During Pregnancy—**http://www.americanpregnancy.org/ pregnancyhealth/skinchanges.html. http://www.aafp.org/afp/20031115/1963.html.**

PROVIDER RESOURCES

AAFP: Common Hyperpigmentation Disorders in Adults: Part II—**http://www.aafp.org/afp/20031115/1955.html.**

Habif T, ed. *Clinical Dermatology*. 4th ed. New York, NY: Mosby, 2004:692–693.

REFERENCES

1. Goldstein BG, Goldstein AO Melasma. http://www.uptodate. com/. Accessed April 30, 2008.

2. Elling SV, Powell FC. Physiological changes in the skin during pregnancy. *Clin Dermatol.* 1997;15:35.

3. Grimes PE. Chloasma. Etiologic and therapeutic considerations. *Arch Dermatol.* 1995;131:1453.

4. Wong RC. Physiologic skin changes in pregnancy. In: Skin changes and diseases in pregnancy. Harahap M, Wallach RC eds. New York, NY: Marcel Dekker, Inc., 1996:37.

5. Hassan I, Kaur I, Sialy R, Dash RJ. Hormonal milieu in the maintenance of chloasma in fertile women. *J Dermatol.* 1998;25:510.

6. Vazquez M, Maldonado H, Benmaman C, Sanchez JL. Chloasma in men. A clinical and histologic study. *Int J Dermatol.* 1988;27:25.

7. Taylor SC, Torok H, Jones T, et al. Efficacy and safety of a new triple-combination agent for Cutis. 2003;72(1):67–72.

8. Vazquez M, Sanchez JL. The efficacy of a broad-spectrum sunscreen in the treatment of chloasma. *Cutis.* 1983;32:92.

191 VITILIGO

Karen A. Hughes, MD
Richard P. Usatine, MD

PATIENT STORY

An 8-year-old Hispanic boy is brought in to the clinic by his mother, who is concerned about his pigment loss (**Figure 191-1**). He is starting to develop this vitiligo around the eyes, and his mother wants him to be treated. The child was started on a topical steroid, and the use of narrow band UVB was discussed if the steroid does not prove helpful. Realistic expectations of the treatments were provided to the mother and her son.

EPIDEMIOLOGY

- Vitiligo is an acquired, progressive loss of pigmentation of the epidermis.
- It occurs in approximately 0.5% of the worldwide population.[1]
- It can occur at any age but typically develops between the ages of 10 and 30 years.[1]
- Vitiligo has equal rates in men and women.[1]
- It occurs in all races but is more prominent in those with darker skin.

ETIOLOGY AND PATHOPHYSIOLOGY

- Autoimmune disease with destruction of melanocytes.
- Genetic component in approximately 30% of cases.
- Can trigger or worsen with illness, emotional stress, and/or skin trauma (Koebner phenomenon).

DIAGNOSIS

CLINICAL FEATURES

- Macular regions of depigmentation with scalloped, well-defined borders (**Figures 191-1** to **191-3**).
- Depigmented areas often coalesce over time to form larger areas (**Figures 191-4** and **191-5**).
- Depigmented areas are more susceptible to sunburn. Tanning of the normal surrounding skin makes the depigmented areas more obvious.

TYPICAL DISTRIBUTION

- Widespread, but generally seen first on the face, hands, arms, and genitalia (**Figure 191-6**).
- Depigmentation around body openings such as eyes, mouth, umbilicus, and anus is common.

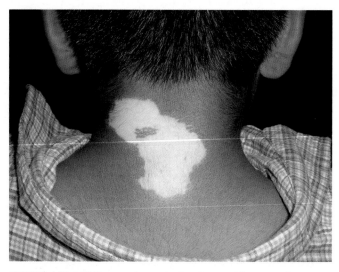

FIGURE 191-1 Vitiligo on the neck of an 8-year-old Hispanic boy. (*Courtesy of Richard P. Usatine, MD.*)

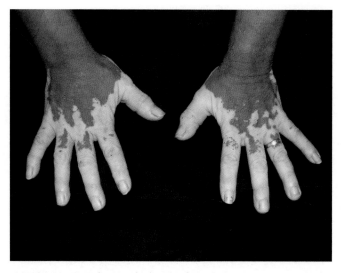

FIGURE 191-2 Vitiligo on the hands of a Hispanic man. (*Courtesy of Richard P. Usatine, MD.*)

LABORATORY AND IMAGING

- Evaluation for endocrine disorders such as hyper- or hypothyroidism (e.g., TSH) and diabetes mellitus (e.g., fasting blood sugar) is indicated, as vitiligo can be associated with these disorders.[2]

- Pernicious anemia and lupus erythematosus should be considered; obtain CBC with indices and an antinuclear antibody (ANA).

BIOPSY

Not indicated unless the diagnosis is not clear and then a 3–4 mm punch biopsy will suffice.

DIFFERENTIAL DIAGNOSIS

- Pityriasis alba—areas of decreased pigmentation with scaling and mild itching. Seen in young children and usually associated with eczema and improves with age (see Chapter 139, Atopic Dermatitis).

- Ash leaf spots—lance-shaped macules of hypopigmentation, which remain stable in size and shape over time. Often the earliest sign of tuberous sclerosis.

- Halo nevus—hypopigmentation confined to areas surrounding pigmented nevi that typically appear in adolescents and young adults (see Chapter 155, Nevus).

- Idiopathic guttate hypomelanosis—confetti-like 2 to 5 mm areas of depigmentation predominantly on sun-exposed areas (**Figure 191-7**).

- Nevus anemicus—a congenital hypopigmented macule or patch that is stable in relative size and distribution. It occurs as a result of localized hypersensitivity to catecholamines and not a decrease in melanocytes. On diascopy (pressure with a glass slide) the skin is indistinguishable from the surrounding skin. Its presence from birth helps distinguish it from vitiligo (**Figure 191-8**).

- Nevus depigmentus is usually present at birth or starts in early childhood. There is a decrease number of melanosomes within a normal number of melanocytes. It typically has a serrated or jagged edge. Its presence at birth or early in childhood help to differentiate it from vitiligo (**Figure 191-9**).

MANAGEMENT

- Addressing the psychological distress that this disfiguring skin disorder causes should be a primary focus as little can be done to modify the condition itself.

- According to one retrospective study of 101 children with vitiligo, moderate- to high-potency topical corticosteroids are efficacious in children with vitiligo.[3] SOR **B** of these 101 children 64% (45 of 70) had repigmentation of the lesions, 24% (17 of 70) showed no change, and 11% (8 of 70) were worse than at the initial presentation. Local steroid side effects were noted in 26% of patients at 81.7 +/− 44 days of follow-up. Cortisol levels were abnormal in 29% of patients (21 of 73). Two children with low-cortisol levels were given the diagnosis of steroid-induced adrenal suppression.

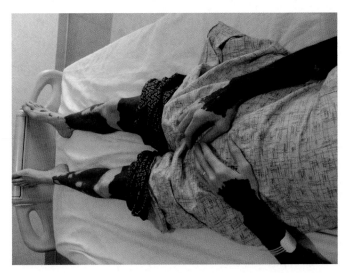

FIGURE 191-3 Vitiligo on the hands knees and feet of a black woman. (*Courtesy of Dan Stulberg, MD.*)

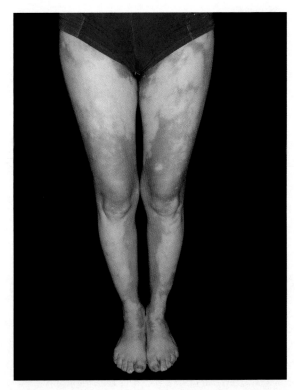

FIGURE 191-4 Vitiligo covering more than 50% of this young Hispanic woman's body. The patient is starting topical monobenzone to attempt to bleach the unaffected skin so that she has one matching skin color. (*Courtesy of Richard P. Usatine, MD.*)

Children with head and/or neck affected areas were 8.36 times more likely to have an abnormal cortisol level compared with children who affected in other body areas.[3] Therefore, a trial of topical steroids may be valuable in vitiligo that is not widespread and does not predominantly involve the head and neck. SOR **C**

- The 308-nm excimer laser is being used in the treatment of vitiligo with some success. In one prospective study of 14 patients, repigmentation rates for 1×, 2× and 3× weekly treatment approached each other (60%, 79% and 82%, respectively) at 12 weeks. Although repigmentation occurred fastest with 3× weekly treatment, the final repigmentation depends on the total number of treatments, not their frequency.[4] SOR **B**

- In a recent evidence-based analysis of the literature, the available studies were largely case studies, pilot studies, and clinical studies with only few patients and often-poor control. Only a few RCTs exist with high levels of evidence.[5] The major conclusions of this evidence-based analysis are as follows:
  - The face and neck were found to respond best to all therapeutic approaches, while the acral areas are least responsive.[5] SOR **B**
  - For generalized vitiligo, phototherapy with UVB radiation is most effective with the fewest side effects (**Figure 191-10**); PUVA is the second best choice.[5] SOR **B**
  - Excimer laser is an alternative to UVB therapy achieving good responses especially in localized vitiligo of the face; here the excimer laser may even be superior to UVB therapy. By combining with topical immunomodulators, treatment response can be accelerated.[5] SOR **B**
  - Topical corticosteroids are the preferred drugs for localized vitiligo.[5] SOR **A** Topical immunomodulators (tacrolimus, pimecrolimus) are an alternative for localized vitiligo and display comparable effectiveness with fewer side effects.[5] SOR **B**
  - No single therapy for vitiligo can be regarded as the most effective as the success of each treatment modality depends on the type and location of vitiligo.[5] SOR **B**

- Management of inciting factors such as illness, stress, and skin trauma. SOR **C**

- Use of sunscreen to prevent burns to the depigmented areas and further trauma to unaffected skin, and to minimize contrast between these areas.

- Bleaching of the unaffected skin in patients with widespread depigmentation to reduce contrast with depigmented areas can improve cosmetic appearance. A monobenzylether of hydroquinone 20% cream (Benoquin) is available by prescription to produce a permanent bleaching of the skin around the vitiligo. It is irreversible and makes the skin higher risk for sunburn.

PATIENT EDUCATION

- Reassurance that this is a benign condition while acknowledging any psychological distress.

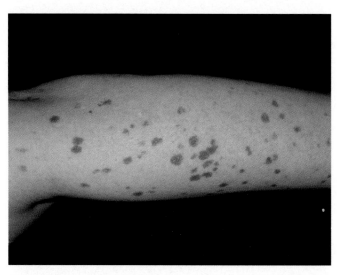

FIGURE 191-5 This previously dark-skinned woman has only a few spots of pigment remaining on her arm because of the extensive vitiligo. Her father has the same condition. (*Courtesy of Richard P. Usatine, MD.*)

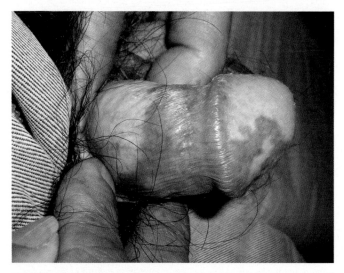

FIGURE 191-6 Vitiligo on the penis of a 72-year-old man. (*Courtesy of Richard P. Usatine, MD.*)

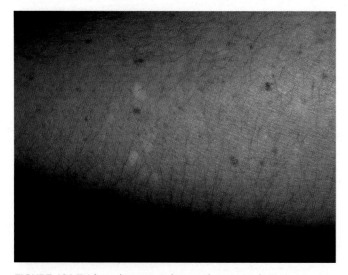

FIGURE 191-7 Idiopathic guttate hypomelanosis on the arm. (*Courtesy of Richard P. Usatine, MD.*)

FOLLOW-UP

- Counseling and emotional support are the mainstay of follow-up treatment.

REFERENCES

1. Njoo MD, Westerhof W. Vitiligo: Pathogenesis and treatment. *Am J Clin Dermatol.* 2001;2(3):167–181.

2. Hacker SM. Common disorders of pigmentation: When are more than cosmetic cover-ups required? *Postgrad Med.* 1996;99(6): 177–186.

3. Kwinter J, Pelletier J, Khambalia A, Pope E. High-potency steroid use in children with vitiligo: a retrospective study. *J Am Acad Dermatol.* 2007;56(2):236–241.

4. Hofer A, Hassan AS, Legat FJ, Kerl H, Wolf P. Optimal weekly frequency of 308-nm excimer laser treatment in vitiligo patients. *Br J Dermatol.* 2005;152(5):981–985.

5. Tobias, Stefan, Eggert S. Current state of vitiligo therapy—evidence-based analysis of the literature *J Dtsch Dermatol Ges.* 2007;5(6):467–475. DOI:10.1111/j.1610-0387.2007.06280.x

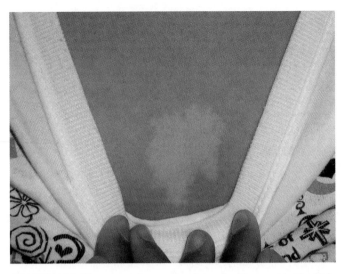

FIGURE 191-8 Nevus anemicus on the chest of a 12-year-old girl, which was there since birth. This is a congenital hypersensitivity to localized catecholamines. On diascopy the skin was indistinguishable from the surrounding skin. The irregular broken-up outline is seen in nevus anemicus and nevus depigmentus. (*Courtesy of Richard P. Usatine, MD.*)

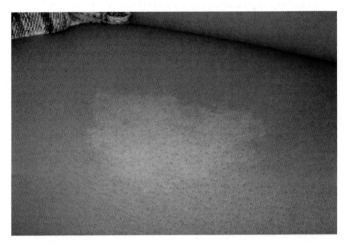

FIGURE 191-9 Nevus depigmentus present, since birth, on the thigh of an 11-year-old girl. Note the serrated or jagged edge. Vitiligo is not present at birth. (*Courtesy of Richard P. Usatine, MD.*)

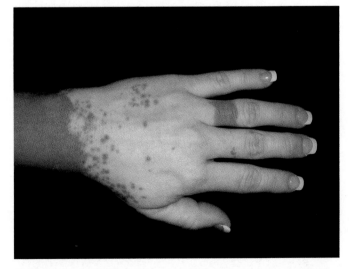

FIGURE 191-10 Vitiligo, which spared the area under a ring; the patient has spotty return of pigment on hand with narrow band UVB treatment. (*Courtesy of Richard P. Usatine, MD.*)

192 PHOTODERMATITIS

E.J. Mayeaux, Jr., MD
Chris Wenner, MD

PATIENT STORY

A 50-year-old woman presented to the clinic with an abrupt onset of an intensely pruritic rash that extended over the dorsal aspect of both arms (**Figure 192-1**). The patient notes no new medicines and no recent exposures to any new chemicals. She acknowledged recent time spent outside in the sun. The plaques were photodistributed, with sparing of her watch area. A clinical diagnosis of polymorphous light eruption (PMLE) was made, and the patient was started on oral antihistamines and topical steroids. She was told to minimize her sun exposure.

EPIDEMIOLOGY

- PMLE (**Figures 192-1** and **192-2**) may affect up to 10% of the population, with a predilection for females.[1] The prevalence increases in northern latitudes. It may appear spontaneously at any age.

- The incidence of drug-induced photosensitivity in the United States is unknown. Phototoxic reactions are much more common than photoallergic reactions.

ETIOLOGY AND PATHOPHYSIOLOGY

- There are three common types of photodermatitis:
  - PMLE (**Figures 192-1** and **192-2**).
  - Phototoxic eruptions (**Figures 192-3** to **192-7**).
  - Photoallergic eruptions (**Figure 192-8**).

- *PMLE* is an idiopathic, delayed-type hypersensitivity reaction to UVA light and, to a lesser extent, UVB light (**Figures 192-1** and **192-2**). PMLE is the most common photoeruption encountered in clinical practice. The reaction will remit spontaneously with time and absence of sun exposure, but occasionally it will last as long as sun exposure occurs.
  - PMLE usually begins in the first three decades of life and occurs more commonly in women.
  - The rash develops within hours to days after exposure to sunlight and lasts for several days to a week.
  - There is a broad range of degrees of photosensitivity with PMLE. Extremely sensitive individuals can tolerate only minutes of exposure, whereas many people have a low sensitivity and require prolonged exposure to sunlight before developing a reaction.
  - PMLE is a recurrent condition that persists for many years in most patients.[2]

- *Phototoxic reactions* are the most common drug-induced photoeruptions (**Figures 192-3** to **192-7**). They are caused by absorption of ultraviolet rays by the causative drug, which releases energy and damages cell membranes, or, in the case of psoralens, DNA.

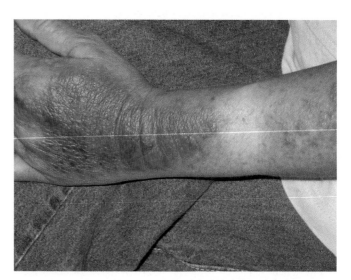

FIGURE 192-1 Polymorphous light eruption noted over dorsum of left forearm. Note absence of the lesion where the patient had been wearing her watch. (*Reproduced with permission from Photo Rounds: A bright red pruritic rash on the forearms. The Journal of Family Practice, August 2007;56(8):627, Dowden Health Media*)

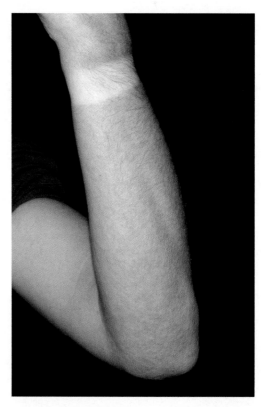

FIGURE 192-2 Polymorphous light eruption on the arm of a young man. Note the sparing of the skin under his watchband. (*Courtesy of Richard P. Usatine, MD.*)

- The drugs that most frequently cause phototoxic reactions are NSAIDs, quinolones, tetracyclines, amiodarone, and the phenothiazines[3] (see **Table 192-1**).
- Most have at least one resonating double bond or an aromatic ring that can absorb radiant energy. Most compounds are activated by wavelengths within the UVA (320–400 nm) range, although some compounds have a peak absorption within the UVB or visible range.
- Phytophotodermatitis are phototoxic reactions to psoralens, which are plant compounds found in limes, celery, figs, and certain drugs. They can cause dramatic inflammation and bullae where the psoralen comes into contact with the skin (**Figures 192-5 to 192-7**). The inflammation is frequently followed by hyperpigmentation.

- *Photoallergic eruptions* are a lymphocyte-mediated reaction. Photoactivation of a drug or agent results in the development of a metabolite that can bind to proteins in the skin to form a complete antigen. The antigen is presented to lymphocytes by Langerhans cells, causing an inflammatory response and a spongiotic dermatitis (eczema). The eruption is characterized by widespread eczema in the photodistribution areas such as the face, upper chest, arms, and back of hands (**Figure 192-8**).
- Most photoallergic reactions are caused by topical agents such as antibiotics and halogenated phenolic compounds added to soaps and fragrances.[4] Systemic photoallergens such as the phenothiazines, chlorpromazine, sulfa products, and NSAIDs can produce photoallergic reactions, although most of their photosensitive reactions are phototoxic (see **Table 192-2**).

DIAGNOSIS

CLINICAL FEATURES

- The appearance of the PMLE varies from person to person but is consistent in a given patient. Erythematous pruritic papules, sometimes with vesicles, are most common (**Figures 192-1 and 192-2**). Lesions may coalesce to form plaques. The rash typically involves the V of the neck and the arms, legs, or both. The face, which is exposed to sunlight in both summer and winter, tends to be spared. It tends to present in spring/summer, with the first significant UV exposure of the year. The rash typically develops 1 to 4 days after sun exposure.
- Phototoxic reaction occurs 2 to 6 hours after exposure to sunlight. The eruption typically appears as an exaggerated sunburn, with mild cases causing slight erythema and severe cases causing vesicles or bullae (**Figures 192-3 to 192-7**).
- Phytophotodermatitis reactions are asymmetric and localized to the area in which the plant psoralen was in contact with the skin. Accompanying hyperpigmentation is a good clue to a phytophotodermatitis reaction (**Figures 192-5 to 192-7**). Ask the patient if he or she had any contact with limes, celery, or figs. Squeezing lime juice into drinks is a particularly common cause of this reaction.
- Photo-onycholysis phototoxicity reactions (sun-induced separation of the nail plate from the nail bed) have been reported with the use of tetracycline, psoralen, chloramphenicol, fluoroquinolones,

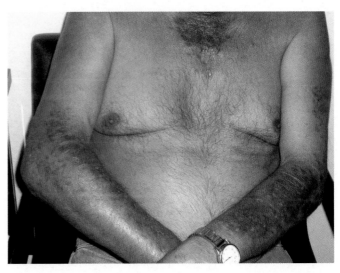

FIGURE 192-3 Severe phototoxic drug reaction secondary to HCTZ use. (*Courtesy of Richard P. Usatine, MD.*)

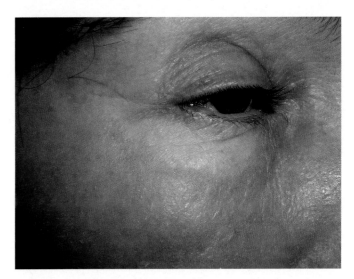

FIGURE 192-4 Phototoxic drug reaction secondary to ibuprofen. (*Courtesy of Richard P. Usatine, MD.*)

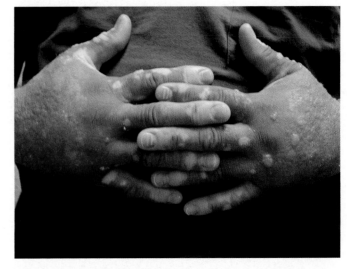

FIGURE 192-5 Phototoxic drug reaction secondary to treatment of vitiligo with oral psoralen and UV light (phytophotodermatitis). Note the bullae. (*Courtesy of Richard P. Usatine, MD.*)

oral contraceptives, quinine, and mercaptopurine. Photo-onycholysis may be the only manifestation of phototoxicity in individuals with heavily pigmented skin.

- Photoallergic eruptions are characterized by widespread eczema in the photodistribution areas such as the face, upper chest, arms, and back of hands. They resemble allergic contact dermatitis, but the distribution is mostly limited to sun-exposed areas of the body (**Figure 192-8**).

TYPICAL DISTRIBUTION

All photodermatitis reactions occur in sun-exposed areas.

LABORATORY STUDIES

Most cases of photodermatitis can be diagnosed on the basis of the patient's history. Punch biopsy of PMLE demonstrates extensive spongiosis and edema of the dermis with a deep lymphohistiocytic infiltrate. In acute phototoxic reactions, necrotic keratinocytes are observed. Photopatch testing may be applied for the diagnosis of photoallergic dermatitis.

DIFFERENTIAL DIAGNOSIS

- Systemic lupus erythematosus (SLE)—sunlight can precipitate a lupus rash. Serum antinuclear antibody (ANA) is usually positive (see Chapter 173, Lupus-Systemic and Cutaneous).

- Porphyria cutanea tarda reactions can also be precipitated by sunlight. It tends to present with vesicles or bullae in sun-exposed areas such as the back of the hands. The bullae generally do not have any surrounding erythema, and urine for porphyrins should be positive (see Chapter 179, Other Bullous Disease).

- Dermatomyositis may cause an erythematous or violaceous eruption in sun-exposed areas. If these cutaneous findings precede the muscle weakness it can appear to be a photosensitivity reaction such as PMLE or a phototoxic drug reaction. Therefore, it is essential in the management and follow-up of patients with suspected PMLE or other photosensitivity to inquire about muscle weakness and to look for other signs of dermatomyositis on the hands and/or through laboratory tests for muscle enzyme elevations (see Chapter 174, Dermatomyositis). The dermatomyositis patient story in Chapter 174 is one in which the initial rash was thought to be a photosensitivity reaction to a new hydrochlorothiazide (HCTZ) prescription.

- Contact dermatitis appears the same as photoallergic dermatitis but is usually not limited to sun-exposed areas (see Chapter 140, Contact Dermatitis).

MANAGEMENT

- The management of PMLE is aimed mainly at prevention. Patients who have mild disease should adopt a program of sun avoidance that consists of avoiding sun exposure, wearing tightly woven clothing and hats, and using broad-spectrum sunscreens with a sun-protection factor of 50 or higher. SOR **C**

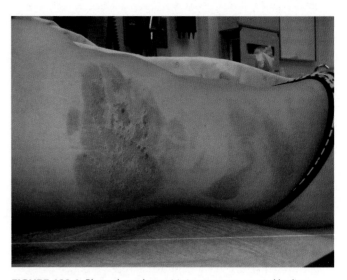

FIGURE 192-6 Phytophotodermatitis in a woman, caused by lime juice and sun exposure on the beach. Note the hand print of her fiancé who had been squeezing limes into their tropical drinks. This contact occurred when they posed for a photograph. (*Reproduced with permission from Photo Rounds: Hyperpigmentation and vesicles after beach vacation. The Journal of Family Practice, December 2006;55(12):1050, Dowden Health Media.*)

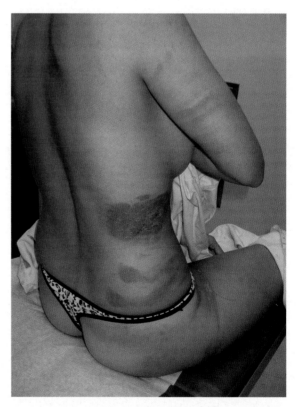

FIGURE 192-7 Phytophotodermatitis visible on the arm, trunk, and leg caused by lime juice and sun exposure on the beach. Note the hyperpigmentation that occurs in conjunction with the erythema. (*With permission from Photo Rounds. Hyperpigmentation and vesicles after beach vacation. J Fam Pract. 2006;55(12):1050, Dowden Health Media and Andrea Darby-Stewart, MD.*)

- Patients with severe PMLE can be desensitized in the spring with the use of phototherapy and maintained in the nonreactive state with weekly 1 hour unprotected exposure to sunlight. SOR **C** A course of psoralen and UVA radiation, or a course of narrowband UVB, three times a week for 4 weeks provides protection.[5] SOR **B** These treatments may induce a typical rash or erythema but otherwise have no major adverse effects.

- Acute episodes of photodermatitis respond rapidly to topical and/or oral corticosteroids. Topical steroids should provide symptomatic relief and decrease the inflammation. For more severe reactions, a course of 30 mg of prednisone daily for 5 to 7 days may be used.[6] SOR **B**

- Patients with acute drug-induced photodermatitis need to practice sun avoidance until well after the drug is discontinued. Topical and oral corticosteroids may be used, especially with photoallergic reactions, but their efficacy is unproven. SOR **C**

PATIENT EDUCATION

- Patients with any type of photodermatitis should apply strong broad-spectrum sunscreens daily and use protective clothing (hats and shirts that cover the arms and v-neck). The sunscreen should be water resistant and applied to exposed areas before sun exposure.[7] Sunscreens should be reapplied every 2 hours if there is continued sun exposure. Some of the most effective sunscreens contain avobenzone (Parsol 1789), Mexoryl, and/or titanium dioxide or zinc oxide to block UVA and UVB.

- Tell your patients that if they develop an allergy to one sunscreen, they should find another with different ingredients.

- It is important to avoid sunlight during the mid-day whenever possible.

- Explain to patients that phototoxic reactions may cause hyperpigmentation, which can take weeks to months to resolve. There is no guarantee that all the hyperpigmentation will go away.

- Avoid repeated rubbing and scratching, which can lead to skin thickening and chronic lichenification. Use the topical medications prescribed to treat the itching and to avoid lichenification.

FOLLOW-UP

- Follow-up is needed if the photosensitivity persists.

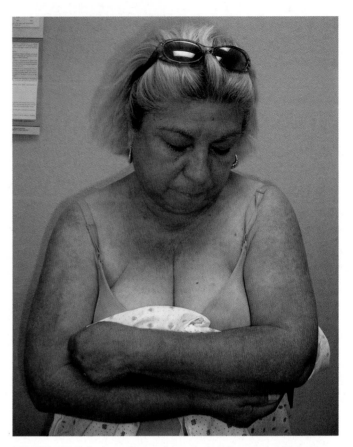

FIGURE 192-8 A photoallergic drug reaction characterized by widespread eczema in the photodistribution areas such as the face, upper chest, arms, and back of hands. A punch biopsy showed a spongiotic dermatitis (eczema). The exact photoallergen was not found. (*Courtesy of Richard P. Usatine, MD.*)

REFERENCES

1. Morison WL, Stern RS. Polymorphous light eruption: A common reaction uncommonly recognized. *Acta Derm Venereol*. 1982;62: 237–240.

2. Hasan T, Ranki A, Jansen CT, Karvonen J. Disease associations in polymorphous light eruption: A long-term follow-up study of 94 patients. *Arch Dermatol*. 1998;134:1081–1085.

3. Stern RS, Shear NH. Cutaneous reactions to drugs and biological modifiers. In: Arndt KA, LeBoit PE, Robinson JK, Wintroub BU eds. *Cutaneous Medicine and Surgery*. Vol. 1. Philadelphia: W.B. Saunders, 1996:412.

4. Gonzalez, E, Gonzalez, S. Drug photosensitivity, idiopathic photodermatoses, and sunscreens. *J Am Acad Dermatol*. 1996;35:871.

5. Bilsland D, George SA, Gibbs NK, Aitchison T, Johnson BE, Ferguson J. A comparison of narrow band phototherapy (TL-01) and photochemotherapy (PUVA) in the management of polymorphic light eruption. *Br J Dermatol*. 1993;129:708–712.

6. Patel DC, Bellaney GJ, Seed PT, McGregor JM, Hawk JLM. Efficacy of short-course oral prednisolone in polymorphic light eruption: A randomized controlled trial. *Br J Dermatol*. 2000;143: 828–831.

7. Morison WL. Photosensitivity. *N Engl J Med*. 2004;350: 1111–1117.

TABLE 192-1 Common Medications That Cause **Phototoxic** Reactions*

Class	Medication
Antibiotics	Tetracyclines
	Fluoroquinolones
	Sulfonamides
	Ibuprofen
Nonsteroidal anti-inflammatory drugs (NSAIDs)	Ketoprofen
	Naproxen
	Diuretics
	Furosemide
	Hydrochlorothiazide
Retinoid	Isotretinoin
	Acitretin
PDT pro-photosensitizers	5-Aminolevulinic acid
	Methyl-5-aminolevulinic acid
	Verteporfin
	Photofrin
Neuroleptic drugs	Phenothiazines
	Thioxanthenes (chlorprothixene and thiothixene)
	Other drugs
	Itraconazole
	5-FU
	Amiodarone
	Diltiazem
	Quinidine
	Coal tar
Sunscreens	Para-aminobenzoic acid (PABA)

*Data for table comes from eMedicine—Drug-induced photosensitivity: **http://www.emedicine.com/derm/topic108.htm**

TABLE 192-2 Common Medications That Cause **Photoallergic** Reactions*

5-FU

6-Methylcoumarin

Benzophenones

Celecoxib

Cinnamates

Dapsone

Hormonal contraceptives

Hydrochlorothiazide

Itraconazole

Musk ambrette

Para-aminobenzoic acid (PABA)

Phenothiazines

Salicylates

Sulfonylureas (glipizide and glyburide)

Quinidine

*Data for table comes from eMedicine—Drug-induced photosensitivity: **http://www.emedicine.com/derm/topic108.htm**

193 ERYTHEMA AB IGNE

Amor Khachemoune, MD, CWS
Khashayar Sarabi, MD

PATIENT STORY

A 50-year-old woman presented to the office with bilateral erythematous lesions on the inner aspects of both of her lower extremities (**Figures 193-1** and **193-2**). The lesions started developing for the past 6 months. They became progressively more noticeable but stayed localized in the inner aspects of the lower extremities. She mentioned that she was using a hot water bottle in the area involved to keep her warm at night when she was sleeping in bed. Although our working clinical diagnosis was erythema ab igne, clinical entities such as livedo reticularis, poikiloderma atrophicans vasculare, and acanthosis nigricans were also considered in the differential diagnosis. A skin biopsy was performed and confirmed the diagnosis of erythema ab igne. The patient was advised to abandon the hot water bottle application to the skin. Over the course of 4 months her skin lesions started to clear with no further intervention.

EPIDEMIOLOGY

- Rare disease.
- Women, in particular those who are overweight, are affected more often than men.

ETIOLOGY AND PATHOPHYSIOLOGY

- The skin findings form as a result of multiple exposures to an intense source of heat.
- Erythema ab igne has been noted for many years, and the sources of heat have changed over time. It used to be reported in women who stay for long periods of time in front of open fires, fireplaces, or furnaces to cook.[1-4] Most of the lesions were appearing on the medial side of the thigh and the lower leg in general.
- Currently, erythema ab igne is seen on different parts of the body, depending on what source of heat initiated the pathology, the angle of the heat radiation, the morphology of the skin, and the layers of clothing. Some of the modern-day examples are repeated application of hot water bottles or heating pads to treat chronic pain, exposure to car heaters and furniture with internal heaters, the use of a laptop computer for long periods, and cooks and chefs who stand for long periods in the range of heat. Ultrasound physiotherapy was also reported as a cause of erythema ab igne. Recently, there was a reported case of frequent prolonged hot baths that caused the disease.[5]

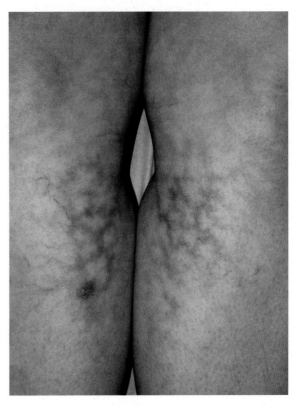

FIGURE 193-1 Mottled or mesh-like pigmentary changes on the legs of a 50-year-old woman who slept with a hot water bottle between her legs. (*Reproduced with permission from Photo Rounds: Bilateral lesions on the legs. The Journal of Family Practice, January 2007;56(1):37, Dowden Health Media.*)

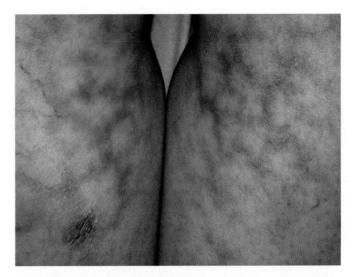

FIGURE 193-2 Close up of previous figure. (*Reproduced with permission from Photo Rounds: Bilateral lesions on the legs. The Journal of Family Practice, January 2007;56(1):37, Dowden Health Media.*)

DIAGNOSIS

CLINICAL FEATURES

- Some patients have mild pruritus or burning sensation but the majority of patients are asymptomatic.

- Skin lesions may not appear immediately after the exposure; it might take a period of 1 month to show up. Skin changes start as a reddish-brown pigmentation distributed as a mottled rash and are followed by skin atrophy (**Figures 193-1 to 193-3**).

- Telangiectasias with diffuse hyperpigmentation and subepidermal bullae may also develop.

- The rash appears mesh-like or like a net in the area exposed to the heat. The heat can be from fire places, heating pads, laptop computers and hot water bottles (**Figures 193-1 to 193-3**).

- In some rare cases, Merkel cell carcinoma has developed in areas of erythema ab igne.[6]

TYPICAL DISTRIBUTION

At the area of heat exposure which is most often the legs or back.

LABORATORY STUDIES

None recommended.

SKIN BIOPSY

- In most all cases, the diagnosis is based on the history and physical exam.

- If clinically warranted, a biopsy is performed to exclude the possibility of malignant transformation. Histopathology shows epidermal atrophy, subepidermal separation, and haziness of the dermoepidermal junction. Dilatation of capillaries and connective tissue disintegration, elastosis, hemosiderin deposition, melanocytosis, and abundance of inflammatory cells are all seen in the dermis. Some of these lesions might progress to actinic keratosis, which could be a precursor for squamous cell carcinoma of the skin.

- In some rate cases, Market cell carcinoma has developed in areas of erythema ab igne.[6]

DIFFERENTIAL DIAGNOSIS

Erythema ab igne should be differentiated from other diseases with skin changes that mimic its presentation.

LIVEDO RETICULARIS (FIGURE 193-4)

- Reticular cyanotic cutaneous discoloration surrounding pale central areas caused by dilation of capillary blood vessels and stagnation of blood.

- Occurs mostly on the legs, arms, and trunk and appears to be a purplish mottling of the skin.

- More pronounced in cold weather.

- Idiopathic condition that may be associated with systemic diseases such as SLE (**Figure 193-4**).

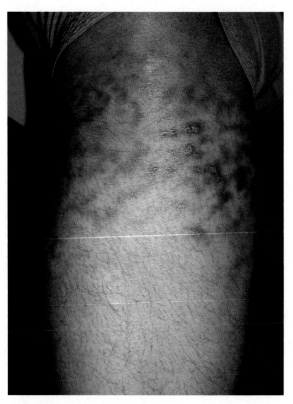

FIGURE 193-3 Mottled hyperpigmentation and hint of blistering and crusting on the anterior leg area in a 23-year-old woman who spent significant time close to a fire place. (*Courtesy of Amor Khachemoune, MD.*)

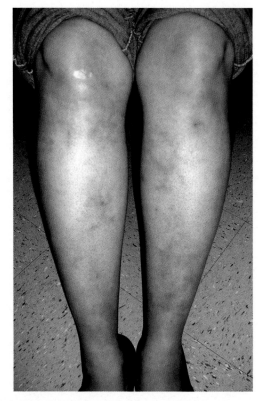

FIGURE 193-4 Livedo reticularis in a 27-year-old woman with lupus. The mottled purple color gets worse when she is exposed to colder temperature. (*Courtesy of Richard P. Usatine, MD.*)

POIKILODERMA ATROPHICANS VASCULARE

- A variant of mycosis fungoides (cutaneous t-cell lymphoma) (see Chapter 169, Mycosis Fungoides).

- Circumscribed violaceous erythema.

- Occurs mostly in posterior shoulders, back, buttocks, V-shaped area of anterior neck and chest.

- May be asymptomatic or mildly pruritic.

- May remain stable in size or gradually increase.

- Numerous atypical lymphocytes are observed around dermal blood vessels, and some epidermotropism is observed.

ACANTHOSIS NIGRICANS

- Velvety, light-brown-to-black markings usually on the neck, under the arms, or in the groin (see Chapter 212, Acanthosis Nigricans).

- Most often associated with being overweight.

- More common in people with darker skin pigmentation.

- A disorder that may begin at any age may be inherited as a primary condition or associated with various underlying syndromes.

- Should be able to distinguish from erythema ab igne by the typical location around the neck and in the axilla.

MANAGEMENT

- The first goal of treatment is to identify the source of heat radiation to avoid further exposure. For mild lesions, no intervention is needed after the heat source is removed and the probability of full resolution is good.

- Topical retinoids, vitamin A derivatives, hydroquinone, and 5-fluorouracil have been prescribed to treat the abnormal skin pigmentation.[7] Laser therapy has been used to even out the skin color.[4,7] SOR **C**

PATIENT EDUCATION

Patients should avoid excessive and prolonged localized heat exposures (i.e., fire places, heating pads, laptop computers, and hot water bottle applications).

FOLLOW-UP

Follow-up visits are recommended if there are new changes to the skin after removing the source of heat. This is to diagnose and manage any malignant transformation.

PATIENT RESOURCES

http://tray.dermatology.uiowa.edu/EryAbIgne01.htm.

PROVIDER RESOURCES

http://www.emedicine.com/derm/topic130.htm.

http://dermnetnz.org/vascular/erythema-ab-igne.html.

REFERENCES

1. Meffert JJ, Davis BM. Furniture-induced erythema ab igne. *J Am Acad Dermatol*. 1996;34(3):516–517.

2. Helm TN, Spigel GT, Helm KF. Erythema ab igne caused by a car heater. *Cutis*. 1997;59(2):81–82.

3. Bilic M, Adams BB. Erythema ab igne induced by a laptop computer. *J Am Acad Dermatol*. 2004;50(6):973–974.

4. El-Ghandour A, Selim A, Khachemoune A. Bilateral lesions on the legs. *J Fam Pract*. 2007;56(1):37–39.

5. Weber MB, Ponzio HA, Costa FB, Camini L. Erythema ab igne: A case report. *An Bras Dermatol*. 2005;80(2):187–188.

6. Hewitt JB, Sherif A, Kerr KM, Stankler L. Merkel cell and squamous cell carcinomas arising in erythema ab igne. *Br J Dermatol*. 1993;128(5):591–592.

7. Sahl WJ Jr, Taira JW. Erythema ab igne: Treatment with 5-fluorouracil cream. *J Am Acad Dermatol*. 1992;27(1):109–110.

194 ACQUIRED VASCULAR LESIONS IN ADULTS

Nathan Hitzeman, MD

PATIENT STORY

A 31-year-old woman presented with a new swelling on her lower lip. This was clinically recognized as a venous lake (**Figure 194-1**). The patient was bothered by its appearance and wanted it removed. She chose to have cryotherapy, which eradicated the venous lake. A closed-probe was used on a Cryo-Gun to get some compression while the freeze was applied using liquid nitrogen.

EPIDEMIOLOGY

- Venous lakes are acquired vascular lesions of the face and ears.[1]

- Cherry angiomas are common vascular malformations that occur in many adults after the age of 30 years (**Figure 194-2**). Cherry angiomas may be more common during pregnancy.[1]

- Angiokeratomas, the most common form being angiokeratomas of the scrotum (Fordyce), develop during adult years (**Figure 194-3**).[1] Angiokeratomas can also occur on the vulva (**Figure 194-4**).

- Glomangiomas, also known as glomuvenous malformations or glomus tumors, are a type of rare venous malformation (**Figure 194-5**). Approximately two-thirds of patients with glomangiomas have a family history of similar lesions.[2]

- Cutaneous angiosarcomas are malignant vascular tumors most commonly found on the head and neck areas of elderly men. These are very rare (**Figure 194-6**).[3]

ETIOLOGY AND PATHOPHYSIOLOGY

- Venous lakes are benign dilated vascular channels (**Figure 194-1**).

- Cherry angiomas are common benign vascular malformations (**Figure 194-2**). They may occur during pregnancy. Several case reports have cited increased cherry angiomas after exposure to toxins.[4]

- Angiokeratomas are dilated superficial blood vessels that may be associated with increased venous pressure (such as in pregnant patients and patients with hemorrhoids)[1] (**Figures 194-3** and **193-4**).

- Glomangiomas are a distinct type of venous malformation caused by abnormal synthesis of the protein glomulin[2] (**Figure 194-5**).

- Cutaneous angiosarcomas are rare malignant vascular tumors thought to arise from vascular endothelium. Elevation of several

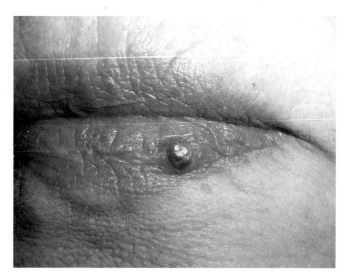

FIGURE 194-1 Venous lake on the lip of a young woman. This was eradicated with cryotherapy. (*Courtesy of Richard P. Usatine, MD.*)

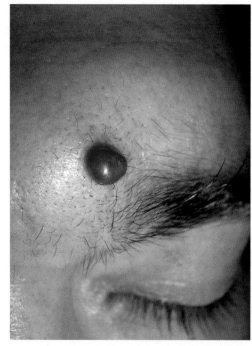

FIGURE 194-2 Large cherry angioma treated with shave excision and electrodesiccation of the base. (*Courtesy of Richard P. Usatine, MD.*)

growth factors and cytokines has been associated with this malignancy[3] (**Figure 194-6**).

DIAGNOSIS

CLINICAL FEATURES

- Venous lakes are dark blue, slightly raised, and less than a centimeter in size. The lesions empty with firm compression. They may bleed with trauma.
- Cherry angiomas are deep red papules with a distinct cherry color.
- Angiokeratomas are multiple red-to-purple papules with associated hyperkeratosis. They may bleed easily with trauma.
- Glomangiomas are blue-purple, partially compressible nodules with a cobblestone appearance. Lesions are tender to the touch.
- Cutaneous angiosarcomas present as progressively enlarging erythematous plaques.

TYPICAL DISTRIBUTION

- Venous lakes are found on the face and ears, particularly the vermilion border of the lips (**Figure 194-1**).
- Cherry angiomas favor the trunk but may occur on other parts of the body. Number of lesions ranges from several to hundreds.
- Angiokeratomas typically occur on the scrotum or vulva (**Figures 194-3** and **193-4**).
- Glomangiomas tend to occur on the extremities (**Figure 194-5**). Solitary glomangiomas often occur in the nail bed.
- Cutaneous angiosarcomas often present on the head and neck areas (**Figure 194-6**).

LABORATORY STUDIES AND BIOPSY

- Diagnosis of venous lakes, cherry angiomas, and angiokeratomas is usually by history and physical examination alone. If these are removed surgically, it is still best to send them to pathology for confirmation of diagnosis. If the diagnosis is not clear clinically, a biopsy is warranted to rule out malignancy.
- Diascopy is a technique in which a microscope slide is used to compress a vascular lesion, allowing the clinician the ability to see the red or purple color of a vascular lesion blanch under pressure (**Figure 194-7**).
- Skin biopsy of glomangioma reveals distinct rows of glomus cells that surround distorted vascular channels.[2]
- Skin biopsy of cutaneous angiosarcoma reveals irregular vascular channels and atypical endothelial cells.[3]

DIFFERENTIAL DIAGNOSIS

- Melanoma lesions are irregularly shaped, usually pigmented lesions identified by the ABCDE guidelines discussed in Chapter 165, Melanoma. Unlike venous lakes, they do not change consistency with firm compression.
- Angiokeratomas typically occur on the scrotum or vulva. They may bleed easily with trauma.

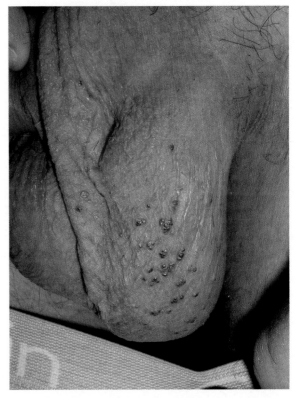

FIGURE 194-3 Angiokeratosis on the scrotum. Fordyce spots. (*Courtesy of Lewis Rose, MD.*)

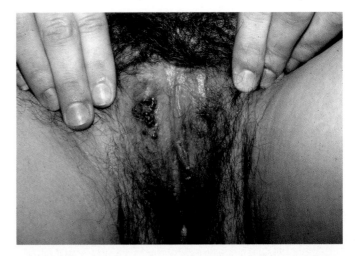

FIGURE 194-4 Angiokeratosis on the vulva. This might be mistaken for a melanoma. (*Courtesy of Eric Kraus, MD.*)

- Glomangiomas have a cobblestone appearance and are tender. Unlike venous lakes, these anomalies do not empty with compression.
- Cutaneous angiosarcomas present as progressively enlarging erythematous plaques that may resemble cellulitis, rosacea, or erysipelas. Recently, the head-tilt maneuver has been described to aid in its detection.[5] Having a patient lower his or her head below the level of the heart for 5 to 10 seconds will make the lesion more engorged and violaceous, thus confirming its vascular nature.

MANAGEMENT

OBSERVATION

- Patients can be reassured that venous lakes and most other acquired vascular lesions (with the exception of angiosarcomas) are benign lesions that develop during adult years.

SURGICAL

- Venous lakes, cherry angiomas, and other acquired vascular lesions can be eradicated by cryotherapy, electrodesiccation, sclerotherapy, intense pulsed light, and other laser modalities.[1,6,7] SOR **C** Compared with intense pulsed light, the Nd:YAG laser system may yield superior results in the treatment of benign vascular lesions.[8] SOR **B** Hyperpigmentation is the most common complication of treatment.
- When using cryotherapy to treat vascular lesions, it helps to compress the lesion at the same time as it is frozen. This can be done with a cryogun that has a solid probe for compression. SOR **C**
- Cherry angiomas can be treated with light electrodesiccation using an electrosurgical instrument on a low setting without anesthesia. SOR **C**
- Larger cherry angiomas can be removed with a shave excision after injecting with lidocaine and epinephrine. The base can be treated with electrodesiccation if needed. SOR **C**
- Isolated glomangiomas may be surgically excised. Sclerotherapy may be useful for multiple lesions or large segmental lesions.[9] SOR **C**
- Cutaneous angiosarcoma is best treated with excision and wide surgical margins, as the primary tumor is often more extensive than appears on examination. Postoperative radiotherapy is then used at the primary site and regional lymphatics. If inoperable, palliative chemotherapy may be considered.[3] SOR **C**

PATIENT EDUCATION

- When discussing any new lesions in sun-exposed areas, the clinician should take the opportunity to counsel patients on sunscreen use, avoiding direct sun during peak hours and performing periodic skin examination.
- Patients should be fully informed about the risk of pigmentary changes and chance of recurrence if they elect for cosmetic removal of benign lesions.

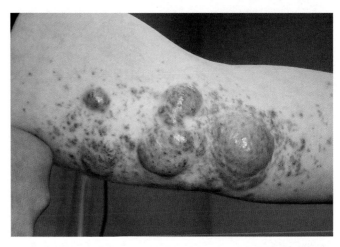

FIGURE 194-5 Large glomangiomas of the arm. (*Courtesy of Jack Resneck, Sr., MD.*)

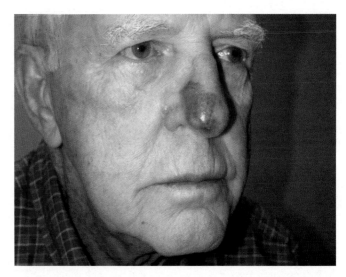

FIGURE 194-6 Angiosarcoma on the nose. A lesion like this requires an urgent biopsy. (*Courtesy of Amor Khachemoune, MD.*)

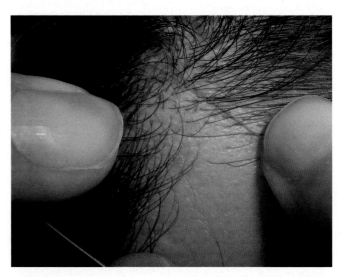

FIGURE 194-7 Diascopy in which a microscope slide is being used to compress a vascular lesion. The red color of this vascular hemangioma is blanching under pressure. (*Courtesy of Richard P. Usatine, MD.*)

FOLLOW-UP

None typically needed for benign lesions unless lesions recur or the patient is concerned about growth or changes to the lesions.

PATIENT RESOURCES

Cherry Angioma. Medline Plus. **http://www.nlm.nih.gov/medlineplus/ency/article/001441.htm.**

PROVIDER RESOURCES

Laser Treatment of Acquired and Congenital Vascular Lesions. eMedicine. **http://www.emedicine.com/derm/topic518.htm.**

REFERENCES

1. Habif TP. Acquired vascular lesions. In: *Clinical Dermatology: A Color Guide to Diagnosis and Therapy*. 4th ed. Philadelphia: Mosby, 2004:824–825. http:www.clinderm.com. Accessed on June 6, 2007.

2. Boon LM, Mulliken JB, Enjolras O, Vikkula M. Glomuvenous malformation (glomangioma) and venous malformation: Distinct clinicopathologic and genetic entities. *Arch Dermatol*. 2004;140(8): 971–976.

3. Mendenhall WM, Mendenhall CM, Werning JW, et al. Cutaneous angiosarcoma. *Am J Clin Oncol*. 2006;29(5):524–528.

4. Hefazi M, Maleki M, Mahmoudi M, et al. Delayed complications of sulfur mustard poisoning in the skin and the immune system of Iranian veterans 16–20 years after exposure. *Int J Dermatol*. 2006;45(9):1025–1031.

5. Asgari MM, Cockerell CJ, Weitzul S. The head-tilt maneuver. *Arch Dermatol*. 2007;143:75–77.

6. Suhonen R, Kuflik EG. Venous lakes treated by liquid nitrogen cryosurgery. *Br J Dermatol*. 1997;137:1018–1019.

7. Bekhor PS. Long-pulsed Nd:YAG laser treatment of venous lakes: Report of a series of 34 cases. *Dermatol Surg*. 2006;32:1151–1154.

8. Fodor L, Ramon Y, Fodor A, et al. A side-by-side prospective study of intense pulsed light and Nd:YAG laser treatment for vascular lesions. *Ann Plastic Surg*. 2006;56:164–170.

9. Parsi K, Kossard S. Multiple hereditary glomangiomas: Successful treatment with sclerotherapy. *Australes J Dermatol*. 2002;43:43.

195 HEREDITARY AND CONGENITAL VASCULAR LESIONS IN ADULTS

Nathan Hitzeman, MD

PATIENT STORY

A 56-year-old woman has had recurrent nosebleeds starting in childhood and has visible telangiectasias on her lips and tongue (**Figure 195-1**). In early adulthood, she was diagnosed with hereditary hemorrhagic telangiectasias (HHT) (Osler–Weber–Rendu syndrome) and was found to have an arteriovenous malformation (AVM) in the lung requiring surgical resection. She has led a normal productive life and has two children who have not inherited this condition. Her mom had recurrent epistaxis but never had an AVM.

EPIDEMIOLOGY

- Hereditary hemorrhagic telangiectasias is an autosomal-dominant vascular disease with a minimum estimated prevalence of one in 10,000 (**Figure 195-1**). Certain populations in northern Japan, Europe, and the United States have a higher prevalence of this disease.[1]

- Nevus flammeus, or port-wine stains, are congenital vascular malformations that occur in 0.1% to 0.3% of infants as developmental anomalies (**Figure 195-2**).[2] They may be associated with rare syndromes such as Klippel–Trenaunay and Sturge–Weber syndromes (**Figure 195-3**).

- Maffucci's syndrome is a rare nonhereditary condition characterized by hemangiomas and enchondromas involving the hands and feet and long bones (**Figure 195-4**).[3]

ETIOLOGY AND PATHOPHYSIOLOGY

- Hereditary hemorrhagic telangiectasias is associated with mutations in genes that regulate transforming growth factor beta in endothelial cells. Arterioles become dilated and connect directly with venules without a capillary in between. Although manifestations are not present at birth, telangiectasias later develop on the skin, mucus membranes, and gastrointestinal tract. In addition, AVMs often develop in the hepatic (30%–40% of patients), pulmonary (30%–50%), and cerebral circulations (10%–20%). Any of these lesions may become fragile and prone to bleeding.[4,5]

- Port-wine stains are vascular ectasias or dilatations thought to arise from a deficiency of sympathetic nervous innervation to the blood vessels. Dilated capillaries are present throughout the dermis layer of the skin.

- The bone and vascular lesions of Maffucci's syndrome exist at birth or develop during childhood. Progression usually does not occur after completion of puberty.

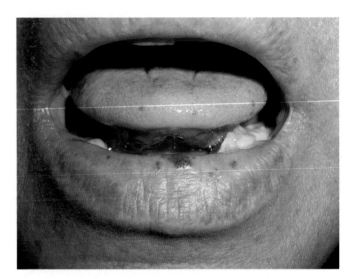

FIGURE 195-1 Hereditary hemorrhagic telangiectasias (Osler–Weber–Rendu syndrome) in a 56-year-old woman with recurrent nosebleeds and an arteriovenous malformation in the lung. (*Courtesy of Richard P. Usatine, MD.*)

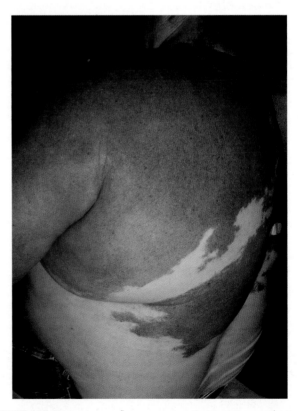

FIGURE 195-2 Large nevus flammeus or port-wine stain over the trunk of a 55-year-old man since birth. (*Courtesy of Casey Pollard, MD.*)

DIAGNOSIS

CLINICAL FEATURES

- Hereditary hemorrhagic telangiectasias is diagnosed if three of the following four criteria are met: recurrent spontaneous nosebleeds (the presenting sign in more than 90% of patients, often during childhood), mucocutaneous telangiectasia (typically develops in the third decade of life), visceral involvement (lungs, brain, liver, and colon), and/or an affected first-degree relative.[6]

- Port-wine stains are irregular red-to-purple patches that start out smooth in infancy but may hypertrophy and develop a cobblestone texture with age. Nuchal port-wine stains are associated with alopecia areata.[7] Klippel–Trenaunay syndrome is characterized by vascular malformations, venous varicosities, and soft-tissue hyperplasia. Patients with Sturge–Weber syndrome often have mental retardation, epilepsy, and eye problems.[2]

- The cobblestone deformity of the hands and feet in Maffucci's syndrome is striking (**Figure 195-4**).

TYPICAL DISTRIBUTION:

- Hereditary hemorrhagic telangiectasias skin manifestations are few to numerous lesions on the tongue, lips, nasal mucosa, hands, and feet. However, any skin area or internal organ may be involved.

- Port-wine stains tend to affect the face and neck, although lesions may affect any body surface, including mucous membranes. Lesions of Klippel–Trenaunay syndrome tend to affect the lower extremities. A diagnosis of Sturge–Weber syndrome requires that a port-wine stain be present in the V1 trigeminal nerve distribution. Patients with port-wine stains of the eyelids, bilateral trigeminal lesions (40% of patients with Sturge–Weber syndrome), and unilateral lesions involving all three divisions of the trigeminal nerve are particularly at risk of Sturge–Weber syndrome.[2]

LABORATORY STUDIES

- Check a CBC and iron studies in patients with HHT. They are at higher risk for iron-deficiency anemia because of recurrent nosebleeds and/or gastrointestinal bleeding.

- Patients with benign-appearing port-wine stains, who lack other concerning symptoms, do not require laboratory testing (**Figure 195-5**).

- If Sturge–Weber syndrome is suspected, perform neuroimaging and glaucoma testing. Neuroimaging may reveal leptomeningeal malformations ipsilateral to the port-wine stain. An electroencephalogram may reveal epilepsy. Elevated ocular pressures or visual field deficits may indicate glaucoma.

- Investigate the musculoskeletal system with Maffucci's syndrome. It is associated with various benign and malignant tumors of the bone and cartilage.[3]

DIFFERENTIAL DIAGNOSIS

- CREST (calcinosis, Raynaud's phenomenon, esophageal involvement, sclerodactyly, and telangiectasia) syndrome and scleroderma

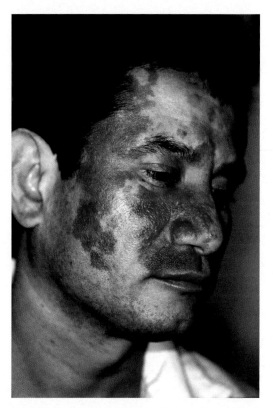

FIGURE 195-3 Port-wine stain, since birth, on the face of a man. Its distribution puts this patient at risk of Sturge-Weber syndrome. (*Courtesy of Richard P. Usatine, MD.*)

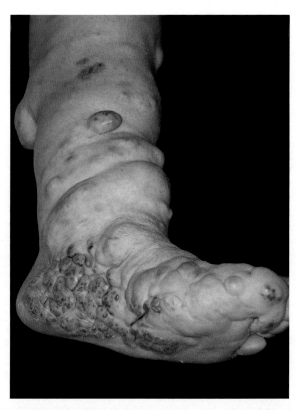

FIGURE 195-4 Hereditary hemangiomatosis, also called Maffucci's syndrome. Note the cobblestone deformity of the foot. (*Courtesy of Tran Shellenberger, MD.*)

usually have multiple telangiectasias as in HHT. Other clinical features and laboratory tests such as the ANA and skin biopsies can differentiate between these rheumatologic conditions and HHT (see Chapter 175, Sclerodema and Morphea).

- Port-wine stains are often isolated findings but may indicate underlying Klippel–Trenaunay or Sturge–Weber syndrome. Further investigations may be necessary when these syndromes are suspected.

- Glomangiomas are blue-purple, partially compressible nodules with a cobblestone appearance. These glomuvenous malformations may appear similar to Maffucci's syndrome but lack the rheumatologic component (see Chapter 194, Acquired Vascular Skin Lesions).

- Salmon patches, also known as "stork bites" or "angel kisses" (present in 40%–70% of newborns), are a type of nevus flammeus or port-wine stain. Salmon patches are more pink than purple but are true congenital vascular malformations, not hemangiomas. The angel kisses over the face tend to fade with time but the stork bites on the nape of the neck often persist as seen in **Figure 195-6** (see Chapter 103, Childhood Hemangiomas).[2]

MANAGEMENT

- Hereditary hemorrhagic telangiectasias has no cure. Oral iron supplementation and transfusions are sometimes needed as a result of bleeding. Few randomized controlled trials exist regarding treatment of bleeding. Estrogen/progesterone supplementation for heavily transfusion-dependent patients decreases recurrent bleeding.[8] SOR **B** Case reports and uncontrolled studies regarding epistaxis treatment show some benefit from laser treatment, surgery, embolization, and topical therapy. SOR **C** Cauterization is not recommended because of complications from local tissue damage. Embolization procedures have been described for AVMs in the liver, lungs, and brain. Surgical resection of AVMs is sometimes done as a last resort when other measures fail. In short, it is often best to do as little intervention as possible with HHT and, if so, with input from specialists experienced with this disease, as complications and recurrence are frequently encountered.[5]

- Port-wine stains may be treated with makeup (see patient resources). Pulsed-dye laser treatment is another option, albeit expensive. Laser treatments blanch most port-wine lesions to some degree, but complete resolution is difficult to achieve and the recurrence rate is high.[9] SOR **C**

- Patients with Maffucci's syndrome often require multiple orthopedic surgeries for their enchondromatous deformities and for cosmetic purposes.[3,10]

PATIENT EDUCATION

- Whatever the vascular condition is, patients can benefit from reliable information about the current and future outlook for their condition.

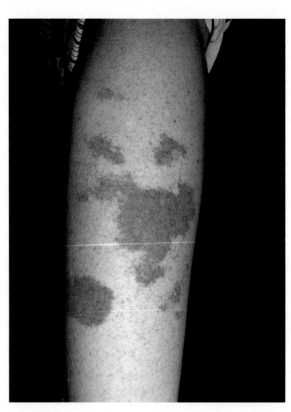

FIGURE 195-5 Nevus flammeus or port-wine stain, since birth, on the arm of a 34-year-old woman. She has had no problems with this benign capillary malformation. (*Courtesy of Richard P. Usatine, MD.*)

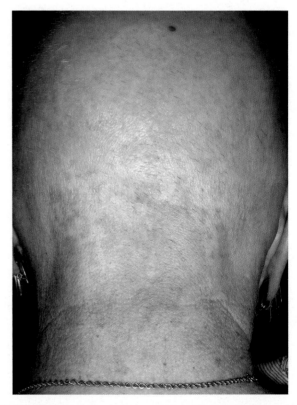

FIGURE 195-6 Stork bite (salmon patch) that has persisted since birth in this 72-year-old woman. This benign capillary malformation is more visible now, caused by the hair loss from chemotherapy. (*Courtesy of Richard P. Usatine, MD.*)

FOLLOW-UP

- Patients with port-wine stains should have periodic skin checks, as other lesions may develop within the port-wine stains. Several case reports of basal cell cancers developing within port-wine stains have been described.[11]

- Patients with Sturge-Weber syndrome should have yearly eye examinations, which include intraocular pressures. SOR Ⓒ

- Patients with Maffucci's syndrome should be monitored closely for both skeletal and nonskeletal tumors, particularly of the brain and abdomen.[10] SOR Ⓒ

PATIENT RESOURCES

- Excellent patient information on HHT can be found through the HHT Foundation International at **www.hht.org.**

- Port-wine stains are often psychologically detrimental. Cosmetic makeup may be purchased through Covermark at www.covermark.com. Dermablend is another effective product available at **www.dermablend.com.**[2]

PROVIDER RESOURCES

Laser treatment of acquired and congenital vascular lesions. eMedicine. **http://www.emedicine.com/derm/topic518.htm.**

REFERENCES

1. Guttmacher AE, Marchuk DA, White RI. Hereditary hemorrhagic telangiectasia. *N Engl J Med*. 1995;333:918–924.

2. Habif TP. Vascular tumors and malformations. In: *Clinical Dermatology: A Color Guide to Diagnosis and Therapy*. 4th ed. Philadelphia: Mosby, 2004:814–833.

3. Jermann M, Eid K, Pfammatter T, Stahel R. Maffucci's syndrome. *Circulation*. 2001;104:1693.

4. Abdalla SA, Letarte M. Hereditary haemorrhagic telangiectasia: Current views on genetics and mechanisms of disease. *J Med Genet*. 2006;43(2):97–110.

5. Begbie ME, Wallace GM, Shovlin CL. Hereditary haemorrhagic telangiectasia (Osler–Weber–Rendu syndrome): A view from the 21st century. *Postgrad Med J*. 2003;79(927):18–24.

6. Shovlin CL, Guttmacher AE, Buscarini E, et al. Diagnostic criteria for hereditary haemorrhagic telangiectasia (Rendu–Osler–Weber syndrome). *Am J Med Genet*. 2000;91: 66–67.

7. Akhyani M, Farnaghi F, Seirafi H, Nazari R, Mansoori P, Taheri A. The association between nuchal nevus flammeus and alopecia areata: A case-control study. *Dermatology*. 2005;211(4):334–337.

8. Van Cutsem E, Rutgeerts P, Vantrappen G. Treatment of bleeding gastrointestinal vascular malformations with oestrogen-progesterone. *Lancet*. 1990;335:953–955.

9. Lanigan SW, Taibjee SM. Recent advances in laser treatment of port-wine stains. *Br J Dermatol*. 2004;151(3):527–533.

10. Gupta N, Kabra M. Maffucci syndrome. *Indian Pediatr*. 2007;44(2):149–150.

11. Silapunt S, Goldberg LH, Thurber M, Friedman PM. Basal cell carcinoma arising in a port-wine stain. *Dermatol Surg*. 2004;30(9):1241–1245.

SECTION 20 OTHER SKIN DISORDERS

196 CUTANEOUS DRUG REACTIONS

Anna Allred, MD
Richard P. Usatine, MD

PATIENT STORY

A 20-year-old college student was seen for fatigue and an upper respiratory infection and started on amoxicillin for a sore throat. Six days later she broke out with a red rash all over her body (**Figure 196-1**). She then went to see her family physician back home with the rash and lymphadenopathy. A monospot was then drawn and found to be positive. This morbilliform rash (like measles) is typical of an amoxicillin drug eruption in a person with mononucleosis. Amoxicillin was stopped, and diphenhydramine was used for the itching.

EPIDEMIOLOGY

- Cutaneous drug reactions are common complications of drug therapy occurring in 2% to 3% of hospitalized patients.[1]

- One study found that 45% of all adverse drug reactions were manifested in the skin.[1]

- Maculopapular eruptions, also known as exanthematous drug eruptions, are the most frequent of all cutaneous drug reactions, representing 95% of skin reactions.[2] They are often confused with viral exanthems. This occurs most commonly with beta-lactams such as amoxicillin but also with barbiturates, gentamicin, isoniazid, phenytoin, sulfonamides, thiazides, and trimethoprim–sulfamethoxazole (**Figures 196-1** and **196-2**).

- Urticarial drug reactions are the second most common skin eruptions, representing approximately 5% of cutaneous drug reactions.[2] This reaction can result from any drug but commonly occurs with aspirin, penicillin, sulfa, ACE inhibitors, aminoglycosides, and blood products. Urticaria results from IgE reactions within minutes to hours of drug administration (**Figures 196-3** and **196-4**).

- Drug-induced hyperpigmentation, as occurs with antiarrhythmics (amiodarone), antibiotics (minocycline), NSAIDs, and chemotherapy agents (Adriamycin) (**Figures 196-5** and **196-6**).

- Warfarin-induced skin necrosis (WISN) is a rare but serious side effect predominantly seen in obese women and presents between days 3 and 6 of warfarin treatment. WISN is more common in those with thrombophilic abnormalities, given large loading doses (**Figure 196-7**).

- Fixed drug eruptions (FDEs) occur with phenolphthalein, tetracycline, ibuprofen, sulfonamide antibiotics, and barbiturates. FDEs are more commonly found in males (**Figures 196-8** to **196-11**).

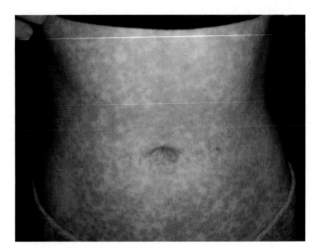

FIGURE 196-1 Amoxicillin rash in a young woman with mononucleosis. (*Courtesy of Richard P. Usatine, MD.*)

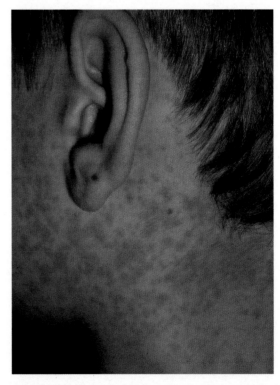

FIGURE 196-2 Maculopapular drug eruption in a 5-year-old boy with an upper respiratory infection started on amoxicillin for a questionable otitis media. Four days later he broke out with a red rash all over his face and body. This morbilliform rash (like measles) is typical of an amoxicillin drug eruption. (*Courtesy of Robert Tunks, MD.*)

- Erythema multiforme (EM) and Stevens–Johnson syndrome (SJS) can occur secondary to drug reactions (**Figures 196-12** and **196-13**). Incidence of SJS is estimated at 1.2 per 6 million. SJS has 5% mortality, and toxic epidermis necrolysis (TEN) has a mortality of 30%.[1]

- **Tables 196-1** and **196-2** list the most common medications associated with allergic cutaneous drug reactions and the rates of reactions found.[3]

- **Table 196-3** lists the medications that have not been found to cause allergic cutaneous drug reactions.[3]

ETIOLOGY AND PATHOPHYSIOLOGY

- Two mechanisms are responsible for cutaneous drug reactions: immunologic including all four types of hypersensitivity reactions and more commonly nonimmunologic.

- Warfarin-induced skin necrosis (WISN) develops during the hypercoagulable state as a result of a more rapid fall in concentration of protein C compared to the other vitamin-K-dependent procoagulant factors. Thrombophilic abnormalities such as familial or acquired deficiency of protein C or S and antiphospholipid antibodies have been implicated in WISN.

- SJS/TEN is most commonly associated with penicillins and sulfonamide antibiotics but can also occur with anticonvulsants, NSAIDS, allopurinol, and corticosteroids.

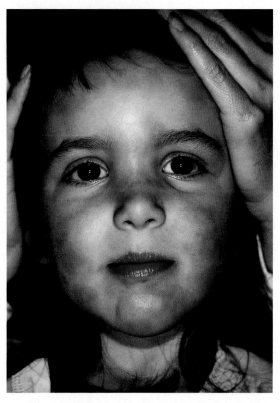

FIGURE 196-3 Urticarial drug eruption secondary to trimethoprim/sulfamethoxazole. (*Courtesy of Richard P. Usatine, MD.*)

DIAGNOSIS

CLINICAL FEATURES AND TYPICAL DISTRIBUTION OF THE MOST COMMON AND IMPORTANT DRUG ERUPTIONS

Maculopapular—These eruptions, red macules with papules, can occur anytime after drug therapy is initiated (often 7–10 days) and last 1 to 2 weeks. The reaction usually starts on the upper trunk or head and neck then spreads symmetrically downward to limbs. The eruptions may become confluent in a symmetric, generalized distribution that spares the face (**Figure 196-1**). Mild desquamation is normal as the exanthematous eruption resolves.

Urticaria and angioedema—Urticaria reactions present as circumscribed areas of blanching-raised erythema and edema of the superficial dermis (**Figures 196-3** and **196-4**). They may occur on any skin area and are usually transient, migratory, and pruritic. Angioedema represents a deeper reaction with swelling usually around the lips and eyes (see Chapter 143, Urticaria and Angioedema).

Hyperpigmentation—Drug-induced hyperpigmentation presents in many ways. Amiodarone causes a dusky red coloration that turns blue-gray with time in photoexposed areas. Minocycline can cause a blue-gray color in acne lesions, on the gingiva and on the teeth. Phenytoin (Dilantin) and other hydantoins may cause melasma-like brown pigmentation on the face. Bleomycin can cause a streaking hyperpigmentation on the trunk and extremities. Adriamycin, as evident in the case above, can cause hyperpigmentation of the face and nails (**Figure 196-5**).

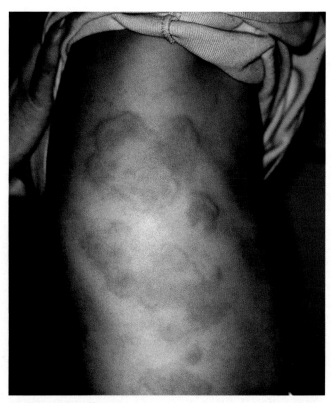

FIGURE 196-4 Giant urticarial eruption in the patient in **Figure 196-3** with drug reaction to sulfa. (*Courtesy of Richard P. Usatine, MD.*)

WISN—It presents with sudden onset of painful localized skin lesion that is initially erythematous and/or hemorrhagic that becomes bullous, culminating in gangrenous necrosis (**Figure 196-7**). It develops more often in obese women in their 50s in areas with high subcutaneous fat content such as breasts, thighs, and buttocks. This is different from a warfarin bleed secondary to too much anticoagulation (**Figure 196-14**).

Fixed or bullous drug eruption—An FDE presents with single or multiple sharply demarcated circular, violaceous, edematous plaques that may include central blister (**Figures 196-9** to **196-11**). The lesion(s) appear after drug exposure and reappear exactly at the same site each time the drug is taken. The site resolves, leaving an area of macular hyperpigmentation (**Figure 196-8**). Lesions can occur anywhere including the hands and feet but are found most commonly on the glans penis (**Figure 196-11**). The eruption presents 30 minutes to 8 hours after drug administration. Bullous FDEs occur when the lesion blisters and erodes, followed by desquamation and crusting.

EM—It presents with typical target or raised edematous papules distributed acrally. Most importantly, there should be some type of epidermal disruption with bullae or erosions within the target lesions (**Figure 196-12**). Severe EM becomes and more widespread epidermal detachment may occur involving less than 10% of total body surface area (see Chapter 170, Erythema Multiforme).

SJS—It presents with erythematous or pruritic macules, widespread blisters on the trunk and face, and erosions of one or more mucous membranes (**Figure 196-13**). Epidermal detachment occurs and involves less than 30% of total body surface area.

TEN—It is on the most severe side of the SJS spectrum. EM is diagnosed when less than 10% of the body surface area is involved, SJS/TEN when 10% to 30% is involved, and TEN when more 30% is involved.

• Drugs most commonly known to cause SJS and TEN are sulfonamide antibiotics, allopurinol, nonsteroidal anti-inflammatory agents, amine antiepileptic drugs (phenytoin and carbamazepine), and lamotrigine (see Chapter 170, Erythema Multiforme).[4] Fifty percent of SJS/TEN cases have no identifiable cause.

LABORATORY STUDIES

The diagnosis of drug eruptions is usually made based on history and physical examination.

• An FDE may be diagnosed by "provoking" the appearance of the lesion with an oral rechallenge with the suspected drug; however, this can be dangerous in bullous cases.

• Severe reactions may need a CBC with differential and comprehensive serum chemistry panel to look for systemic involvement and check hydration status.

• In more challenging cases, a skin biopsy may be helpful to confirm the diagnosis.

• Intradermal skin testing may be hazardous to patients, and patch tests are not useful.

• Skin biopsies are usually not required for diagnosis of WISN, but may aid in the diagnosis.

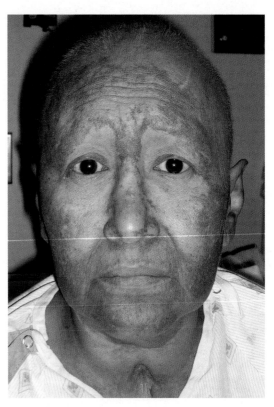

FIGURE 196-5 Facial hyperpigmentation secondary to Adriamycin. (*Courtesy of Richard P. Usatine, MD.*)

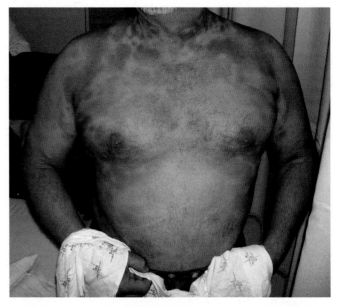

FIGURE 196-6 Hyperpigmentation with a drug reaction to an NSAID. (*Courtesy of Heather Goff, MD.*)

- Testing for thrombophilia (high platelet count) may also be done in WISN.

DIFFERENTIAL DIAGNOSIS

- Viral exanthems look just like generalized maculopapular drug eruptions. Sometimes when a patient is given an antibiotic for an upper respiratory infection, the rash that ensues may be the viral exanthem rather than a drug eruption. The best way to avoid this confusion is only to use antibiotics when the evidence for bacterial infection is sufficient to justify the risks of a drug reaction. See "Viral Infection" chapters for more information on viral exanthems.

- Urticarial reactions present as transient migratory circumscribed areas of blanching-raised erythema and edema of the superficial dermis. Patients experience itching. Identifying urticaria is easy compared with finding the precipitating factors. If there is a temporal association with starting a new drug, it is best to stop the drug (in most cases) and see if the urticaria resolves. See Chapter 143 for more strategies in diagnosis and treatment.

- EM presents with sudden onset of rapidly progressive, symmetrical, and cutaneus lesions with centripetal spread. The patient may have a burning sensation in affected areas but usually have no pruritus. EM is most often caused by a reaction to an infection such as HSV or mycoplasma but may be caused by a drug reaction. Careful history and physical examination can help differentiate between the possible causes (see Chapter 170, Erythema Multiforme, Stevens-Johnson Syndrome and Toxic Epidermal Necrolysis).

- SJS and TEN present with generalized cutaneous lesion with blisters, fever, malaise, arthralgias, headache, sore throat, nausea, vomiting, and diarrhea. The patient may also have difficulty in eating, drinking, or opening their mouth secondary to erosion of oral mucous membranes (**Figure 196-13**). Not all SJS or TEN is secondary to drug exposure, but it is the job of the clinician to investigate this cause and stop any suspicious medications. SJS and TEN can be life threatening (see Chapter 170, Erythema Multiforme, Stevens-Johnson Syndrome and Toxic Epidermal Necrolysis).

- Pityriasis rosea (PR) is a mysterious eruption of unknown etiology, which could easily mimic a maculopapular drug eruption. Look and ask for the herald patch to help make the diagnosis of PR. In PR, look for the collarette scale and observe whether the eruption follows the skin lines (causing a Christmas tree pattern on the back). These features should help positively identify PR because there are no laboratory tests that are specific to PR or most drug eruptions (see Chapter 146, Pityriasis Rosea).

- Syphilis is the great imitator. Any generalized rash without a known etiology may be due to secondary syphilis. An RPR will always be positive in secondary syphilis and is easy to run (see Chapter 209, Syphilis).

- Bullous pemphigoid and pemphigus vulgaris can resemble a bullous drug eruption. Biopsies are the best way to diagnose these bullous diseases. Their clinical pictures are described in detail in Chapters 177, Bullous Pemphigoid, and Chapter 178, Pemphigus.

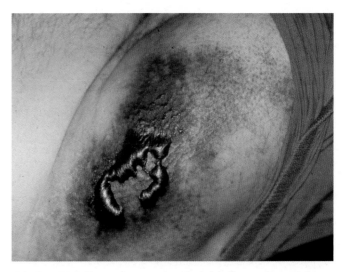

FIGURE 196-7 Coumadin necrosis with dark bullae on the arm of a woman just started on coumadin. (*Courtesy of Eric Kraus, MD.*)

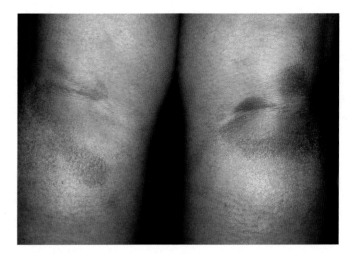

FIGURE 196-8 Hyperpigmented fixed drug eruption. (*Courtesy of Jeffrey Meffert, MD.*)

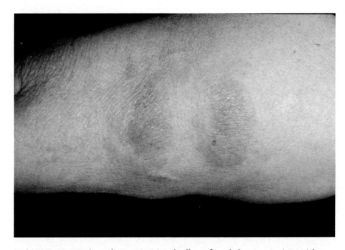

FIGURE 196-9 Annular appearing bullous fixed drug eruption with dusky center. (*Courtesy of Jeffrey Meffert, MD.*)

- Hematoma is a much more common complication of warfarin therapy and must be distinguished from WISN early to decrease permanent tissue damage; a high index of suspicion is needed and an very elevated INR will confirm that bleeding is due to over coagulation (**Figure 196-14**).

MANAGEMENT

- Discontinue the offending medication for all types of drug reactions whenever possible. Older patients with drug eruptions may be on multiple medications and may be very ill; however, efforts should be made to discontinue all nonessential medications.[2] SOR **C**
  - Patients with maculopapular reactions may continue to be treated with the offending agent if it is essential for treating a serious underlying condition.[2]
  - Maculopapular drug eruptions are not a precursor to severe reactions such as TEN.[2]
- Maculopapular- and urticarial/angioedema-type drug reactions are treated with antihistamines. If the angioedema is causing airway compromise, epinephrine and other treatments will be necessary.[2] SOR **C** Usually an H1 blocker is started. In some cases of urticaria/angioedema, an H2 blocker is added on for broader antihistamine effects (see Chapter 143, Urticaria and Angioedema).
  - Diphenhydramine (Benadryl)—adult dosing is 25 to 50 mg orally every 4 to 6 hours (OTC).
  - Hydroxyzine (Atarax)—adults receive 25 mg orally every 6 hours. Pediatric dose 0.5 to 1.0 mg/kg/d orally four times daily.[2]
  - Loratadine (Claritin)—10 to 20 mg orally one time daily[2] (OTC).
  - Any H2 blocker can be used by prescription or OTC.
- Topical steroids such as triamcinolone or desonide may be used for symptomatic relief of pruritus.[2] SOR **C**
- Oral steroids have been used, but little benefit has been shown.[2] SOR **C**
- Hyperpigmentation—stop the drug if possible. In the case of Adriamycin-induced skin hyperpigmentation, the Adriamycin may be continued if it is the best chemotherapy for a life-threatening malignancy (**Figure 196-5**).
- WISN treatment is generally supportive including discontinuing the warfarin, admission to the hospital, and administration of vitamin K and fresh-frozen plasma.[5,6]
  - Many clinicians recommend resuming heparin therapy if needed for the patients underlying pathology that prompted the use of initial anticoagulation therapy.[5,6]
  - Local wound care, debridements, and skin grafting may need to be performed to repair resultant disfigurement from necrosis.[5,6]
- FDEs are treated by discontinuing the drug and applying topical corticosteroids to the affected area.[1] SOR **C**
- EM—stop the medication if that is believed to be the cause.
- SJS and TEN—start with early diagnosis, rapid discontinuing of offending agent, intravenous fluid replacement, and placement in an ICU or burn unit[1,2] (see Chapter 170, Erythema Multiforme, Steven-Johnson Syndrome and Toxic Epidermal Necrolysis).

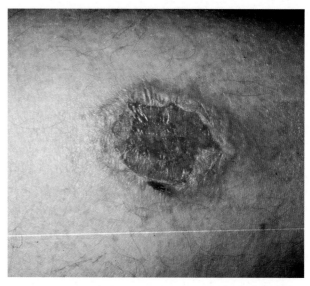

FIGURE 196-10 Bullous fixed drug eruption in which the bulla has opened. (*Courtesy of Jeffrey Meffert, MD.*)

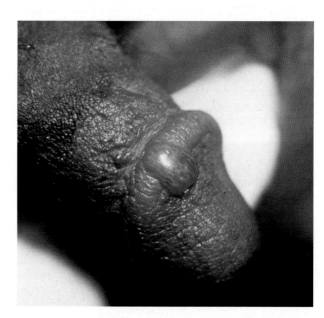

FIGURE 196-11 Bullous fixed drug eruption on the glans penis—a common location for this fixed drug eruptions. (*Courtesy of Jeffrey Meffert, MD.*)

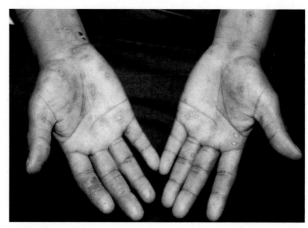

FIGURE 196-12 Erythema multiforme showing target lesions on the palms. (*Courtesy of the University of Texas Health Sciences Center, Division of Dermatology.*)

- Most experts and studies now agree that systemic corticosteroids should not be used.[1] SOR Ⓑ
- Nutritional support, careful wound care, temperature control, and anticoagulation are recommended.[1] SOR Ⓒ
- Daily skin samples should be sent for bacterial gram stain and culture to monitor for developing infection.[1] SOR Ⓒ

PATIENT EDUCATION

Most patients with drug eruptions recover fully without any complications. Patient should be warned even after the responsible medication is stopped the eruptions may clear slowly or even worsen first; the patient should be advised that the reaction may not resolve for 1 to 2 weeks. The patient should also be counseled that mild desquamation is normal as the exanthematous eruption resolves. Confirming the diagnosis of an FDE, especially lesions presenting on the glans, with a drug challenge may allay the patient anxiety about the venereal origin of the disease. The family should be counseled as to the genetic predisposition of some drug-induced eruptions. The patient should be advised to enroll in a medic alert program and to wear a bracelet detailing the allergy.

FOLLOW-UP

Follow-up is most important when the case is severe or the diagnosis is uncertain. Clear-cut mild drug reactions may not need scheduled follow-up.

PATIENT RESOURCES

From familydoctor.org and the AAFP: **http://familydoctor. org/online/famdocen/home/seniors/seniors-meds/ 231.html.**

PROVIDER RESOURCES

http://www.emedicine.com/derm/topic104.htm.

If the skin eruption is rare, serious, or unexpected, the drug reaction should be reported to manufacturer and FDA.

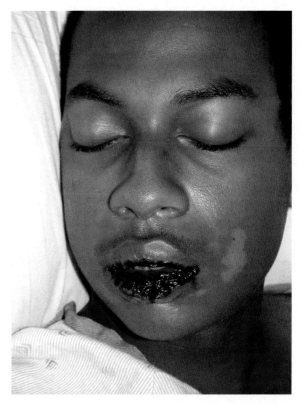

FIGURE 196-13 Stevens-Johnson syndrome secondary to a sulfa antibiotic. (*Courtesy of Eric Kraus, MD.*)

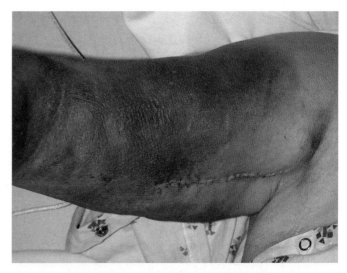

FIGURE 196-14 Large bleed in the arm secondary to overcoagulation with Coumadin. The large hematoma was surgically evacuated to prevent neurovascular compromise to the arm. (*Courtesy of Richard P. Usatine, MD.*)

TABLE 196-1 Allergic Cutaneous Reactions to Drugs Received by at Least 1000 Patients (BCDSP)*

Drug	Reactions, No.	Recipients, No.	Rate, %	95% Confidence Interval
Amoxicillin	63	1225	5.1	3.9–6.4
Ampicillin	215	4763	4.5	3.9–5.1
Co-trimoxazole (TMP/ sulfamethoxazole)	46	1235	3.7	2.7–4.8
Semisynthetic penicillins	41	1436	2.9	2.0–3.7
Red blood cells	67	3386	2.0	1.5–2.4
Penicillin G	68	4204	1.6	1.2–2.0
Cephalosporins	27	1781	1.5	0.9–2.1
Gentamicin	13	1277	1.0	0.5–1.6

*BCDSP indicates Boston Collaborative Drug Surveillance Program.
Represented with permission from Bigby M. Rates of cutaneous reactions to drugs. *Arch Dermatol.* 2001;137(6):765–770.

TABLE 196-2 Allergic Cutaneous Reactions to Drugs Received by at Least 1000 Patients (van der Linden et al[2])

Drug	Reactions, No.	Recipients, No.	Rate, %	95% Confidence Interval
Floroquinolones	16	1015	1.6	0.8–2.3
Amoxicillin	4o	3233	1.2	0.9–1.6
Augmentin	12	1000	1.2	0.5–1.9
Penicillins	63	5914	1.1	0.8–1.3
Nitrofurantoin	7	1085	0.6	0.2–1.1
Tetracycline	23	4981	0.5	0.3–0.7
Macrolides	5	1435	0.3	0.0–0.7

Represented with permission from Bigby M. Rates of cutaneous reactions to drugs. *Arch Dermatol.* 2001;137(6):765–770.

TABLE 196-3 Drugs Received by at Least 1000 Patients With No Allergic Cutaneous Reactions Reported (BCDSP)*

Drug	Recipients, No.	Upper 95% Confidence Limit, %
Digoxin	9399	0.04
Milk of magnesia	5436	0.07
Acetaminophen	4507	0.08
Meperidine	4080	0.09
Dioctyl sodium sulfosuccinate	3506	0.11
Maalox (Rhone-Poulenc Rorer, Antony, France)	3390	0.11
Multivitamins	3016	0.12
Aminophylline	2988	0.12
Aspirin	2926	0.13
Diphenhydramine	2681	0.14
Bisacodyl	2478	0.15
Prochlorperazine	2472	0.15
Spironolactone	2325	0.16
Prednisone	2312	0.16
Gelusil (Parke-Davis, Morris Plains, NJ)	2277	0.16
Ferrous sulfate	2189	0.17
Nitroglycerin	2165	0.17
Codeine	2045	0.18
Methyldopa	2043	0.18
Insulin, regular	1936	0.19
Thiamine	1889	0.19
Phosphate enema	1684	0.22
Propranolol	1653	0.22
Castor oil	1610	0.23
Morphine	1576	0.23
Hydrochlorothiazide	1489	0.25
Vitamin B complex	1462	0.25
Tetracycline	1428	0.26
Potassium iodide	1404	0.26
Warfarin	1371	0.27
Hydrocortisone	1279	0.29
Magnesium citrate	1202	0.31
Folic acid	1179	0.31
Isosorbide	1173	0.31
Lidocaine	1130	0.33
Prednisolone	1126	0.33
Magaldrate	1032	0.36

*BCDSP indicates Boston Collaborative Drug Surveillance Program.

REFERENCES

1. Nigen S, Knowles SR, Shear NH. Drug eruptions: approaching the diagnosis of drug-induced skin diseases. *J Drugs Dermatol*. 2003;3: 278–299.

2. Habif T. *Skin Disease Diagnosis and Treatment*. 2nd ed. Philadelphia: Mosby, 2005.

3. Bigby M. Rates of cutaneous reactions to drugs. *Arch Dermatol*. 2001;137(6):765–770.

4. Chosidow OM, Stern RS, Wintroub BU. Cutaneous drug reactions. In: Kasper DL, Fauci AS, Longo DL, Braunwald EB, Hauser SL, Jameson JL eds. *Harrison's Principles of Internal Medicine*. 16th ed. New York: McGraw-Hill, 2005:318–324.

5. Alves DW, Chen IA. Warfarin-induced skin necrosis. *Hosp Physician*. 2002;38(8):39–42.

6. Stewart AJ, Penman ID, Cook MK, Ludlam CA. Warfarin-induced skin necrosis. *Postgrad Med J*. 1999;75:233–235.

197 KELOIDS

Alejandra Varela, MD
Richard P. Usatine, MD

PATIENT STORY

A 64-year-old black woman comes to the office because the keloids on her chest are itching (**Figure 197-1**). The horizontal keloid started during childhood when she was scratched by a branch of a tree. The vertical keloid is the result of bypass surgery 1 year ago. The lower portion of this area could be called a hypertrophic scar because it does not advance beyond the borders of the original surgery. The patient did not want surgical treatment for the keloid/hypertrophic scar and was happy to receive intralesional steroids to decrease her symptoms.

EPIDEMIOLOGY

- Individuals with darker pigmentation are more likely to develop keloids. Sixteen percent of black persons reported having keloids in a random sampling.[1]

- Men and women are generally affected equally except that keloids are more common in young adult women—probably secondary to a higher rate of piercing the ears (**Figure 197-2**).[1]

- Highest incidence is in individuals aged 10 to 20 years.[1]

ETIOLOGY AND PATHOPHYSIOLOGY

- Keloids are dermal fibrotic lesions that are a variation of the normal wound healing process in the spectrum of fibroproliferative disorders.

- Keloids are more likely to develop in areas of the body that are subjected to high skin tension such as over the sternum (**Figures 197-1 and 197-3**).

- These can occur even up to a year after the injury and will enlarge beyond the scar margin. Burns and other injuries can heal with a keloid in just one portion of the area injured (**Figure 197-4**).

- Wounds subjected to prolonged inflammation (acne cysts) are more likely to develop keloids.

DIAGNOSIS

CLINICAL FEATURES

- Some keloids present with pruritic pain or a burning sensation around the scar.

- Initially manifest as erythematous lesions devoid of hair follicles or other glandular tissue.

- Papules to nodules to large tuberous lesions (**Figure 197-5**).

- Range in consistency; can be soft and doughy to rubbery and hard.[1]

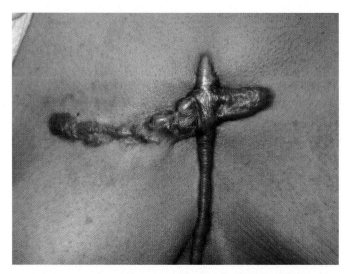

FIGURE 197-1 Two keloids that cross the chest of a 64-year-old black woman. The horizontal keloid came from a scratch during childhood, and the vertical keloid is a result of open heart surgery. (*Courtesy of Richard P. Usatine, MD.*)

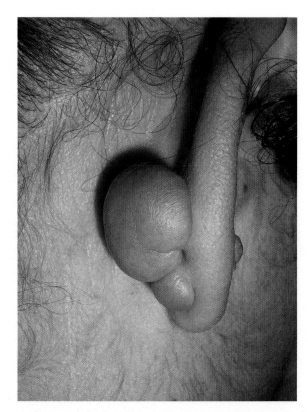

FIGURE 197-2 A keloid on the earlobe that started from piercing the ear. (*Courtesy of Richard P. Usatine, MD.*)

- Most often, the lesions are the color of normal skin but can become brownish red or bluish and then pale as they age.[1]
- May extend in a claw-like fashion far beyond any slight injury.
- Lesions on neck, ears, and abdomen tend to become pedunculated.[1]

TYPICAL DISTRIBUTION

- Anterior chest, shoulders, flexor surfaces of extremities, anterior neck, earlobes, and wounds that cross skin tension lines.

LABORATORY STUDIES

Biopsy is rarely needed to make a diagnosis because the clinical appearance is usually distinctive and clear.

DIFFERENTIAL DIAGNOSIS

- Hypertrophic scars can appear similar to keloids but are confined to the site of original injury.
- Dermatofibromas are common button-like dermal nodules usually found on the legs or arms. They may umbilicate when the surrounding skin is pinched. These often have a hyperpigmented halo around them and are less elevated than keloids (see Chapter 153, Dermatofibroma).
- Dermatofibrosarcoma protuberans is a malignant version of the dermatofibroma. Usually presents as an atrophic, scar-like lesion developing into an enlarging firm and irregular nodular mass. If this is suspected, a biopsy is needed (see Chapter 153, Dermatofibroma).

MANAGEMENT

Patients frequently want keloids treated because of symptoms (pain and pruritus) and concerns about appearance.

- Cryosurgery and intralesional triamcinolone have been used to treat keloids secondary to acne with similar success.[2] SOR **B**
- Silicon gel sheeting as a treatment for hypertrophic and keloid scarring is supported by poor-quality trials susceptible to bias. There is only weak evidence of a benefit of silicon gel sheeting as a prevention for abnormal scarring in high-risk individuals.[3] SOR **B**
- Intralesional steroid injections—intralesional injection of triamcinolone acetonide (10–40 mg/mL) may decrease pruritus, as well as decrease keloid size (**Figure 197-6**). SOR **C** This may be repeated monthly as needed.
- Combined cryosurgery and intralesional triamcinolone—the lesion is initially frozen with liquid nitrogen spray and allowed to thaw for 10–15 minutes. Then it is injected with triamcinolone acetate (10–40 mg/mL). SOR **C**
- Earlobe keloids can be treated with imiquimod 5% cream following tangential shave excision on both sides of the earlobe.[4,5] SOR **B** Patients were instructed to administer imiquimod 5% cream to the excision sites the night of the surgery and daily for 6 to 8 weeks postsurgery. Imiquimod 5% cream only temporarily prevented the recurrence of presternal keloids after excision.[6]

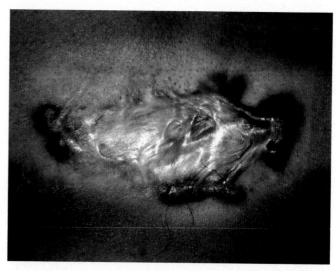

FIGURE 197-3 A keloid over the sternum of an Asian man. The hypopigmented area around it is the result of using steroid-impregnated tape as a treatment. (*Courtesy of Richard P. Usatine, MD.*)

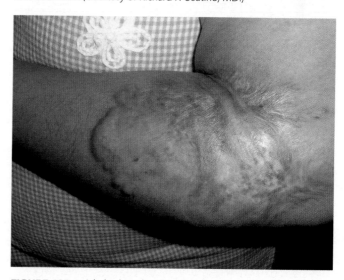

FIGURE 197-4 A keloid on the arm of a Hispanic woman burned accidentally by a hot iron at the age of 1 year. Most of the burn scar is not a keloid. The keloid is at the distal edge where the skin is raised nodular and pink. She has pruritus in that area. (*Courtesy of Richard P. Usatine, MD.*)

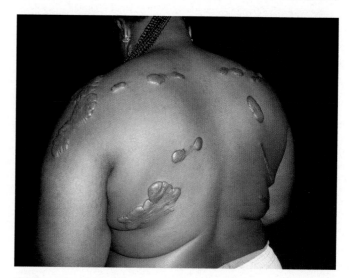

FIGURE 197-5 Many keloids in a woman, who develops keloids with even the most minor skin injuries. (*Courtesy of Richard P. Usatine, MD.*)

- Earlobe keloids can be surgically excised with a shave technique and then injected with triamcinolone acetate (10–40 mg/mL) after hemostasis is obtained. The triamcinolone injection can be repeated in one month to decrease the chance of recurrence. SOR **C**

- New combination methods with intralesional triamcinolone and 5-fluorouracil along with pulsed-dye laser have been reported for treatment of keloid and hypertrophic scars.[7]

PATIENT EDUCATION

Advise patients to avoid local skin trauma, for example, ear piercing, body piercing, and tattoos, and to control inflammatory acne.

FOLLOW-UP

Follow-up is based on the chosen treatment. Follow-up for intralesional steroid injections is usually in one month.

PATIENT RESOURCES

VisualDxHealth—**http://www.visualdxhealth.com/adult/keloid.htm.**

PROVIDER RESOURCES

http://www.emedicine.com/derm/topic205.htm.

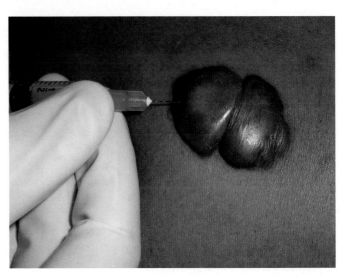

FIGURE 197-6 Performing a steroid injection into a keloid on the back of a young black woman. The patient understood that this injection would not remove the keloid, but it did succeed in taking away the pruritus at that site. (*Courtesy of Richard P. Usatine, MD.*)

REFERENCES

1. Berman B, Perez OA. Keloid and hypertrophic scar. http://www.emedicine.com/derm/topic205.htm. 2007. 8-25-0007. Ref Type: electronic citation.

2. Layton AM, Yip J, Cunliffe WJ. A comparison of intralesional triamcinolone and cryosurgery in the treatment of acne keloids. *Br J Dermatol.* 1994;130:498–501.

3. O'Brien L, Pandit A. Silicon gel sheeting for preventing and treating hypertrophic and keloid scars. *Cochrane Database Syst Rev.* 2006;(1):CD003826. Doi:10.1002/14651858.CD003826.pub2.

4. Patel PJ, Skinner RB, Jr. Experience with keloids after excision and application of 5% imiquimod cream. *Dermatol Surg.* 2006;32:462.

5. Stashower ME. Successful treatment of earlobe keloids with imiquimod after tangential shave excision. *Dermatol Surg.* 2006;32:380–386.

6. Malhotra AK, Gupta S, Khaitan BK, Sharma VK. Imiquimod 5% cream for the prevention of recurrence after excision of presternal keloids. *Dermatology.* 2007;215:63–65.

7. Asilian A, Darougheh A, Shariati F. New combination of triamcinolone, 5-fluorouracil, and pulsed-dye laser for treatment of keloid and hypertrophic scars. *Dermatol Surg.* 2006;32:907–915.

198 GENODERMATOSES

Michael Babcock, MD
Richard P. Usatine, MD

INTRODUCTION

There are more than a hundred genetic syndromes with cutaneous manifestations that are referred to as genodermatoses. For example, there are disorders of pigmentation (albinism), cornification (the ichthyoses and Darier's disease), vascularization (Sturge–Weber syndrome), connective tissue (Ehlers–Danlos syndrome), porphyrin metabolism, other errors of metabolism (phenylketonuria), and the immune system (Wiskott–Aldrich syndrome) to name a few. Some textbooks are dedicated to the topic of genodermatoses alone. The purpose of this chapter is to introduce the topic and illustrate a couple of genodermatoses. We have chosen two problems of cornification for the remainder of the chapter—Darier's disease and ichthyoses.

PATIENT STORY

A 45-year-old black man presents with greasy scale over his face and large parts of his chest and back (**Figures 198-1** and **198-2**). A previous biopsy was diagnostic for Darier's disease. His mother had a milder version of the same condition. His sister has the full blown disease. His brother has similar nail findings, but his skin is affected only behind the ears. The patient has suffered with this condition for whole life and feels that he has been ostracized from normal social life because of his appearance and bad body odor. He suffers from depression and has used various substances to treat his pain. Topical steroids provide some help for the itching and scaling, but the patient is looking for a more effective treatment. The cost of oral retinoids is currently prohibitive, but an application has been put in for patient assistance to receive acitretin.

EPIDEMIOLOGY

- Darier's disease (keratosis follicularis)—1:30,000 to 1:100,000. Males and females are equally affected. Clinically becomes apparent near puberty.
- X-linked ichthyosis—1:2,000 to 1:6,000 males. Clinical lesions present typically during the first 1 to 2 months of life.

ETIOLOGY AND PATHOPHYSIOLOGY

- Darier's disease—An abnormal calcium pump in the sarco/endoplasmic reticulum, SERCA2, results from a gene mutation in the ATP2A2 gene. It is inherited in an autosomal-dominant fashion and results in abnormal epidermal differentiation.

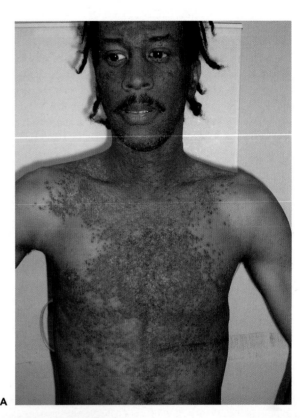

A

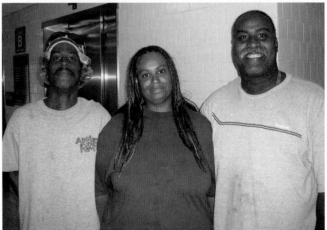

B

FIGURE 198-1 (A) Greasy, hyperkeratotic, and hyperpigmented papule and plaques with scale in a seborrheic distribution involving the face, neck, and chest of a man with Darier's disease. (B) Three siblings with Darier's disease. The brother on the left and the sister have the full blown disease. The sister's face cleared after 3 months of acitretin. The brother on the right has similar nail findings, but his skin is affected only behind the ears. As a family doctor, I take care of this whole family. (*Courtesy of Richard P. Usatine, MD.*)

- X-linked ichthyosis—A deletion of the steroid sulfatase gene results in keratinocyte retention by inhibiting degradation of the desmosome. It is inherited in an X-linked recessive manner.

DIAGNOSIS

- Darier's disease
  - ○ Clinical features—Greasy, hyperkeratotic, yellowish-brown papules in a seborrheic distribution (**Figures 198-1** to **198-4**). The feet can be covered with hyperkeratotic plaques (**Figure 198-5**). The palms may have pits or keratotic papules, and the nails can have V-shaped nicking (**Figures 198-6** and **198-7**) and alternating longitudinal red and white bands. The keratotic papules can be intensely malodorous such that it can interfere with normal social situations.
  - ○ Typical distribution—The clinical lesions involve skin in the seborrheic distribution (face, ears, scalp, upper chest, upper back, and groin) (**Figures 198-1** to **198-4**). In early, mild, or partially treated disease, only the ears may be affected. The nails are characteristically involved.
  - ○ Laboratories—Skin biopsy reveals the characteristic histopathology. A test for the ATP2A2 gene mutation can be performed.
- X-linked ichthyosis
  - ○ Clinical features—Firm, adherent, brown scale in a typical distribution as noted below (**Figures 198-8** and **198-9**). These patients can have corneal opacities on Descemet's membrane of the posterior capsule, which does not affect their vision. They have an increased incidence of cryptorchidism and are at an increased risk of testicular cancer, independent of the risk from cryptorchidism alone. Often they are delivered by cesarian section because a placental sulfatase deficiency results in failure of labor progression.
  - ○ Tight skin over the fingers can be as a manifestation of X-linked ichthyosis (**Figure 198-10**).
  - ○ Typical distribution—Most of the body is involved, except for the typical sparing of the flexures, face, palms, and soles. There is an accentuation noted on the neck, giving these patients a characteristic "dirty neck" appearance.
  - ○ Laboratories—Increased levels of serum cholesterol sulfate levels (steroid sulfatase hydrolyses cholesterol sulfate). Steroid sulfatase activity can also be measured directly.

DIFFERENTIAL DIAGNOSIS

- Darier's disease
  - ○ Hailey–Hailey disease—Another genodermatosis with crusted erosions and flaccid vesicles distributed in the intertriginous areas as opposed to the greasy keratotic papules in the seborrheic distribution.
  - ○ Grover's disease—This presents sporadically as many small, pruritic, erythematous to reddish-brown hyperkeratotic papules on the trunk of older adults. These typically result from conditions that cause sweating or occlusion (like lying in a hospital bed) (see Chapter 111, Folliculitis).

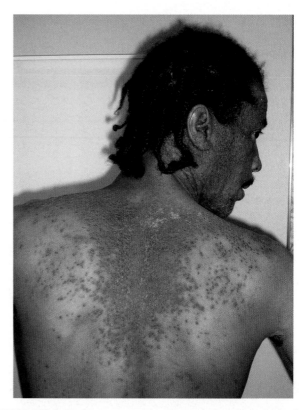

FIGURE 198-2 Similar-appearing papules and plaques on the back, neck, ears, and scalp of the patient in **Figure 198-1** with Darier's disease. Sunlight and heat make his disease worse. (*Courtesy of Richard P. Usatine, MD.*)

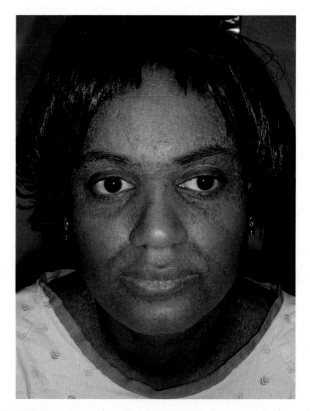

FIGURE 198-3 Greasy, hyperkeratotic scaling plaques on the face of the 44-year-old woman (sister of the patient in **Figure 198-1**) with Darier's disease prior to her use of acitretin. She is wearing a wig to cover the alopecia and plaques on her scalp. (*Courtesy of Richard P. Usatine, MD.*)

- Seborrheic dermatitis—Erythematous patches and thin plaques with yellow greasy scale on the scalp, central face, and chest. This is rarely as severe as Darier's disease (see Chapter 144, Seborrheic Dermatitis).

- X-linked ichthyosis
  - Ichthyosis vulgaris—A relatively common condition (approximately one in 250 people affected) that usually presents with a fine adherent scale in similar distribution to X-linked ichthyosis, but the scale is typically lighter in color. These patients frequently have hyperlinear palms, keratosis pilaris, and atopic dermatitis, which are not commonly associated with X-linked ichthyosis.
  - Lamellar ichthyosis—A more severe and rare disorder that has a plate-like scale, which involves most of the body, including the face and flexures. These patients are typically born as a collodion baby (they have a thin translucent membrane that surrounds the baby at birth).
  - Asteatotic eczema—Dry skin that has a "dried riverbed" or "cracked porcelain" appearance, which usually involves the lower extremities. There may be erythema and serous exudate associated with the cracks. It typically presents in the winter, improves during the rest of the year, and is also known as winter itch or eczema craquelé (see Chapter 139, Atopic Dermatitis).
  - Xerosis—Dry scaly skin most notably on legs without significant inflammation. This is very common compared with any ichthyosis.

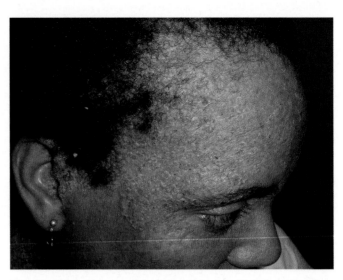

FIGURE 198-4 Close-up of the hyperkeratotic scaling plaques on the forehead, scalp, and ears of the 44-year-old woman (sister of the patient in **Figure 198-1**) with Darier's disease prior to her use of acitretin. With the wig off, the alopecia and plaques on the scalp are visible. Note how the keratosis follicularis follows a seborrheic distribution. (*Courtesy of Richard P. Usatine, MD.*)

MANAGEMENT

- Darier's disease is so rare that there are no randomized controlled trials to guide treatment.

- The intense malodor that accompanies the disease, as well as the facial involvement, often adversely affects the patient's quality of life; thus, treatment is often warranted. Mild-to-moderate disease can be treated by avoiding exacerbating factors (sunlight, heat, and occlusion) and with topical medications, SOR **C** but severe disease is best treated with oral retinoids. SOR **C**
  - Topical retinoids (adapalene, tretinoin, or tazarotene) are effective in some patients, but their main limitation is irritation. Adapalene use may be effective in localized variants. SOR **C** All retinoids are contraindicated in pregnancy.
  - Topical corticosteroids may be of some help. Lower-potency topical corticosteroids should be used on the face, groin, and axillae to minimize side effects in these areas. SOR **C**
  - Systemic retinoids (acitretin or isotretinoin) are the most potent treatment. SOR **C** They should only be prescribed by physicians who have experience with these medications. Patients on systemic retinoids require close monitoring and careful selection, as they are teratogenic (category X) and can cause hyperlipidemia, hypertriglyceridemia, mucous membrane dryness, alopecia, hepatotoxicity, and possible mood disturbances. Females must not get pregnant for at least 1 month after stopping isotretinoin and at least 3 years after stopping acitretin.
  - Cyclosporine can be used for acute flares but should also only be prescribed by a physician who has experience with this medication. It should only be used temporarily and requires close follow-up for monitoring hypertension and nephrotoxicity. It is

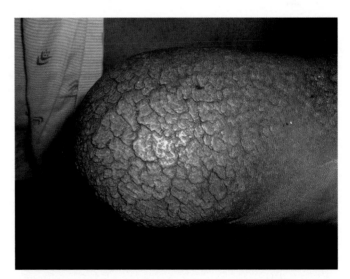

FIGURE 198-5 Thick hyperkeratotic plaque on the heel of the woman in **Figure 198-4** with Darier's disease. (*Courtesy of Richard P. Usatine, MD.*)

metabolized by the common cytochrome P450 3A4 system and has many medication interactions.

- Laser, radiation, photodynamic therapy, and gene therapy are newer treatment modalities that are being investigated.

• X-linked ichthyosis is rare and treatments are based on the clinical experience of experts rather than large studies.

- Frequent application of emollients, humectants, and keratinolytics are the mainstay of therapy. SOR **C** There are many effective over-the-counter and prescription products that contain propylene glycol, urea, or lactic acid. Salicylic acid products should be used only on a limited body surface area, as systemic absorption has led to salicylate toxicity in some patients.

- Topical retinoids can be used, SOR **C** but systemic retinoids are rarely used.

- Refer to an urologist or ophthalmologist if testicular abnormality or corneal opacities are detected. SOR **C**

- Gene therapy has also been studied but has not yet become a viable treatment option.

PATIENT EDUCATION

• Darier's disease
  - Avoid direct sunlight, heat, occlusion, and people acutely infected with HSV or varicella-zoster virus.
  - Watch for signs of secondary cutaneous bacterial or viral infections.

• X-linked ichthyosis
  - Use daily moisturizers, especially in dry climates and in the winter.

FOLLOW-UP

• Darier's disease—Follow-up is needed if patients are on oral retinoids to monitor patients' lipid panel and liver function tests approximately every 3 months. They should also be monitored for signs of secondary bacterial infection.

• X-linked ichthyosis—Monitoring for corneal opacities and for testicular cancer in men should be performed at follow-up visits.

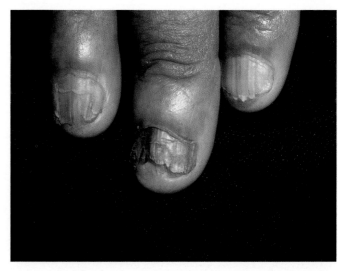

FIGURE 198-6 Typical nail findings in Darier's disease showing longitudinal bands, longitudinal splitting. (*Courtesy of Richard P. Usatine, MD.*)

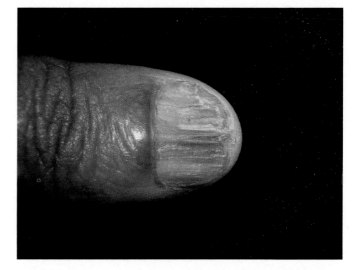

FIGURE 198-7 V-shaped nick at the free margin of the fingernail—the most pathognomonic nail finding in Darier's disease. (*Courtesy of Richard P. Usatine, MD.*)

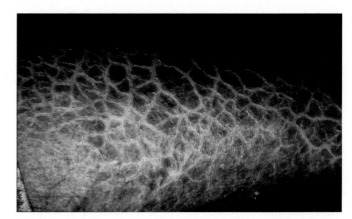

FIGURE 198-8 Heavy fish scale of X-linked ichthyosis. (*Courtesy of the University of Texas Health Sciences Center, Division of Dermatology.*)

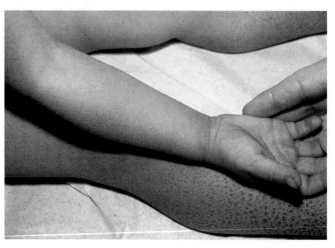

FIGURE 198-9 Ichthyosis in a young boy showing sparing of flexural regions of the arm. (*Courtesy of the University of Texas Health Sciences Center, Division of Dermatology.*)

REFERENCES

1. Bolognia J, Jorizzo J, Rapini R. *Dermatology*. London: Mosby, 2003.

2. James W, Berger T, Elston D. *Andrews' Diseases of the Skin: Clinical Dermatology*. 10th ed. Amsterdam: Elsevier, 2006.

3. Spitz J. *Genodermatoses: A Clinical Guide to Genetic Skin Disorders*. 2nd ed. Philadelphia: Lippincott Williams and Wilkins, 2005.

4. Sehgal V, Srivastava G. Darier's (Darier-White) disease/keratosis follicularis. *Int J Dermatol*. 2005;44(3):184–192.

5. Khachemoune A, Lockshin B. Chronic papules on the back and extremities. *J Fam Pract*. 2004;53(5):361–363.

6. Hazan C, Orlow S, Schagger J. X-linked recessive ichthyosis. *Dermatol Online J*. 2005;11(4):12.

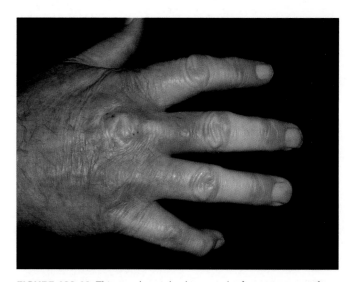

FIGURE 198-10 This man has tight skin over the fingers as a manifestation of his X-linked ichthyosis. (*Courtesy of Richard P. Usatine, MD.*)

199 ERYTHEMA ANNULARE CENTRIFUGUM

Shehnaz A. Zaman, MD
Richard P. Usatine, MD

PATIENT STORY

A 57-year-old farm worker presents with itchy red rings on his body that have come and gone for over 13 years (**Figures 199-1** and **199-2**). The erythematous annular eruption was visible on his abdomen, legs, and arms. **Figure 199-2** shows the typical "trailing scale" of erythema annular centrifugum (EAC). A KOH preparation was negative for fungal elements and the patient was given the diagnosis of EAC. He recently began using paint thinner to "dry out the rash" and decrease the itching. Since topical steroids did not provide any relief for him in the past, we offered the option of using calcipotriol ointment. He chose to try the calcipotriol and stop using paint thinner.

EPIDEMIOLOGY

- Uncommon inflammatory skin disease characterized by slowly migrating annular or configurate erythematous lesions.
- It may begin at any age with a mean age of onset of 39.7 years, with no predilection for either sex.[1]
- The mean duration of skin condition is 2.8 years but may last between 4 weeks and 34 years.[2]

ETIOLOGY AND PATHOPHYSIOLOGY

- Unknown etiology and pathogenesis, but erythema annulare centrifugum has been associated with other medical conditions such as fungal infections in 72% of cases,[1] malignancy, and other systemic illness. Few case reports have reported the diagnosis of cancer 2 years after presentation of erythema annulare centrifugum.[2]
- Other infections identified as triggers for erythema annulare centrifugum include bacterial infections such as cystitis, appendicitis, and TB; viral infections such as EBV, molluscum contagiosum, and herpes zoster; and parasites such as ascaris.[2]
- Certain drugs such as chloroquine, hydroxychloroquine, estrogen, cimetidine, penicillin, salicylates, piroxicam, hydrochlorathiazide, amytriptyline, and etizolam can also trigger erythema annulare centrifugum.[2–4]
- Systemic diseases involving the liver, dysproteinemias, autoimmune disorders, HIV, and pregnancy have been shown to be associated with erythema annulare centrifugum by various case reports.[2,5,6]
- Since injections of *Trichophyton, Candida,* tuberculin, and tumor extracts have been reported to induce erythema annulare centrifugum, a type IV hypersensitivity reaction is thought to be one possible mechanism for its development.[7]

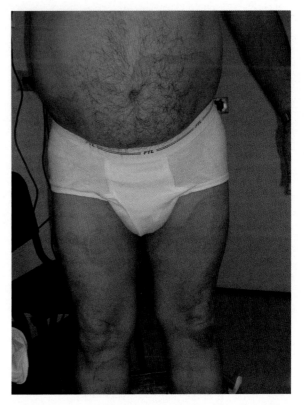

FIGURE 199-1 Erythema annulare centrifugum with large erythematous rings on the trunk and legs of a 57-year-old man. (*Reproduced with permission from Photo Rounds: Persistent itchy pink rings. The Journal of Family Practice, February 2005;54(2):131, Dowden Health Media.*)

DIAGNOSIS

CLINICAL FEATURES

- Large, scaly, erythematous plaques, which begin as papules and spread peripherally with a central clearing forming a "trailing" scale. The margins are indurated and may vary in width from 4 to 6 mm[1,2] (**Figures 199-1** to **199-4**).

- Pruritis is common but not always present.[2]

- Slowly progressing but may enlarge up to 2 to 5 mm/d.[2]

- Evaluation of a skin biopsy specimen by light microscopy reveals parakeratosis and spongiosis within the epidermis and a tightly cuffed lymphohistiocytic perivascular infiltrate with focal extravasation of erythrocytes in the papillary dermis.[8]

TYPICAL DISTRIBUTION

- Lesions typically found in lower extremities, particularly the thighs, but can be found on trunk and face as well.[1,2]

LABORATORY STUDIES

- No specific laboratory tests are necessary to diagnose erythema annulare centrifugum, but laboratory tests may be obtained to rule out other common conditions. Consider a KOH prep to search for tinea corporis or cutaneous candidiasis. If the patient has been in an area with Lyme disease, consider *Borrelia* titers to rule out Lyme disease.[2,5]

- Biopsy: If the diagnosis is uncertain, a punch biopsy can be performed to look for the typical histology of EAC, and a PAS stain can be performed on the specimen to look for fungal elements. Other diseases on the differential diagnosis such as psoriasis, cutaneous lupus, and sarcoidosis can be diagnosed with a punch biopsy.

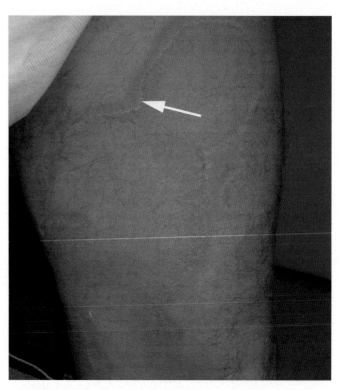

FIGURE 199-2 Erythema annulare centrifugum with conjoined rings on the thigh. Arrow pointing to "trailing scale," which appears as a white scaling line within the erythematous border. (*Reproduced with permission from Photo Rounds: Persistent itchy pink rings. The Journal of Family Practice, February 2005;54(2):131, Dowden Health Media.*)

DIFFERENTIAL DIAGNOSIS

- Pityriasis rosea has erythematous patch distributed on trunk and lower extremities, but these patches have distinctive colarette border and typically have a "herald patch" that appears first. Classically, the patches have a "Christmas tree" pattern in the back and, unlike erythema annulare centrifugum, lasts only 6 to 8 weeks[2] (see Chapter 146, Pityriasis Rosea).

- Tinea corporis (ring worm) presents with one or multiple areas of annular plaques caused by fungal infection. Tinea corporis often produces red scaling rings that resemble erythema annulare centrifugum. However, the scale in tinea corporis tends to lead with the erythema inside the ring and the scale on the outside. This is the opposite of the trailing scale seen with EAC. KOH prep shows branched hyphae with septae. Tinea corporis responds to antifungal treatment.[2] **Figure 199-4** shows a case of EAC that was mistaken for tinea corporis by a number of physicians (see Chapter 132, Tinea Corporis).

- Psoriatic plaques can be annular but do not have the trailing scale that is characteristic of erythema annulare centrifugum. Psoriasis will respond to steroid therapy[2] (see Chapter 145, Psoriasis).

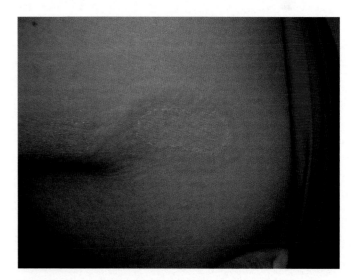

FIGURE 199-3 A single ring of erythema annulare centrifugum in a 35-year-old Hispanic woman with obvious trailing scale. She has had EAC on and off since the age of 20 years without any cause ever identified. (*Courtesy of Christopher Patton, MD.*)

- Erythema migrans seen in Lyme disease is a large annular rash with central clearing. The red ring in erythema migrans is usually smooth without the scale seen in EAC. Patients usually have other signs of infection, positive antibodies, and may have a history of tick bite (see Chapter 211, Lyme Disease).

- Cutaneous lupus could present with annular or papulosquamous plaques, with or without scales on sun-exposed areas. Patients with lupus generally have other systemic symptoms and positive antinuclear antibodies[9] (see Chapter 173, Lupus—Systemic and Cutaneous).

- Sarcoidosis may present with annular indurated papules and plaques, but are more commonly found on the face. Patients may have other systemic manifestations of sarcoidosis. Sarcoidosis can effectively be treated with systemic corticosteroids[9] (see Chapter 168, Sarcoidosis).

MANAGEMENT

- There is no proven treatment for EAC. Identifying and treating underlying medical conditions may help resolve the skin condition. Since EAC is seen in association with certain drugs, discontinuing the offending medication may resolve the problem.

- Topical corticosteroids have been traditionally used but there is little evidence to support their use. SOR C

- Case reports have reported benefits of using calcipotriol (Dovonex) daily for EAC.[10] Another case report described a good outcome for a patient with EAC being treated with calcipotriol and narrow-band UVB phototherapy.[11]

PATIENT EDUCATION

- EAC is not contagious or malignant.

- While the treatment might not work and the condition may recur, it is not dangerous and is confined to the skin only.

FOLLOW-UP

- Follow-up depends on the type of treatment provided and patient's preferences.

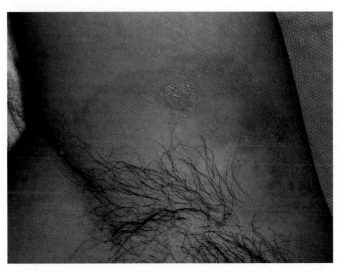

FIGURE 199-4 EAC in the axilla of a 28-year-old man, which had repeatedly been mistaken for tinea corporis. The trailing scale is visible and a punch biopsy confirmed the diagnosis of EAC. (*Courtesy of Richard P. Usatine, MD.*)

REFERENCES

1. Kim KJ, Chang SE, Choi JH, Sung KJ, Moon KC, Koh JK. Clinicopathologic analysis of 66 cases of erythema annulare centrifugum. *J Dermatol*. 2002;29(2):61–67.

2. Brand ME, Usatine RP. Persistent itchy pink rings. *J Fam Pract*. 2005;54(2):131–133.

3. Garcia-Doval I, Pereiro C, Toribio J. Amitriptyline-induced erythema annulare centrifugum. *Cutis*. 1999;63(1):35–36.

4. Kuroda K, Yabunami H, Hisanaga Y. Etizolam-induced superficial erythema annulare centrifugum. *Clin Exp Dermatol*. 2002;27(1): 34–36.

5. Rosina P, Francesco S, Barba A. Erythema annulare centrifugum and pregnancy. *Int J Dermatol*. 2002;41(8):516–517.

6. Gonzalez-Vela MC, Gonzalez-Lopez MA, Val-Bernal JF, Echevarria S, Arce FP, Fernandez-Llaca H. Erythema annulare centrifugum in a HIV-positive patient. *Int J Dermatol*. 2006;45(12):1432–1435.

7. White JW. Gyrate erythema. *Dermatol Clin*. 1985;3:129–139.

8. Weyers W, Diaz-Cascajo C, Weyers I. Erythema annulare centrifugum: Results of a clinicopathologic study of 73 patients. *Am J Dermatopathol*. 2003;25(6):451–462.

9. Hsu S, Le FH, Khoshevis MR. Differential diagnosis of annular lesions. *Am Fam Physician*. 2001;64(2):289–296.

10. Gniadecki R. Case report: Calcipotriol for erythema annulare centrifugum. British Association of Dermatologists. *Br J Dermatol*. 2002;146:317–319.

11. Reuter J, Braun-Falco M, Termeer C, Bruckner-Tuderman L. Erythema annulare centrifugum Darier: Successful therapy with topical calcitriol and 311 nm-ultraviolet B narrow band phototherapy. *Hautarzt*. 2007;58(2):146–148.

PART 14

PODIATRY

200 CALLUSES AND CORNS

Naohiro Shibuya, DPM
Javier La Fontaine, DPM

PATIENT STORY

A 52-year-old man with diabetes and mild sensory neuropathy presented with callus under "the ball of his foot" for at least 5 years. He recently noticed that the callus had grown thicker as he gained weight.

Sharp debridement of the callus was performed, and an offloading pad was placed (**Figure 200-1**). The patient walked out of the office with less pain and discomfort. He was encouraged to use a pumice stone gently after bathing. One important goal is to avoid an ulcer (**Figure 200-2**).

EPIDEMIOLOGY

Corns and callus are two very common problems of the feet that can lead to pain and ulcerations.

ETIOLOGY AND PATHOPHYSIOLOGY

Calluses and corns in the foot are caused by multiple factors. These factors include the following:

- Mechanical pressure from abnormal biomechanics, underlying spur/exostosis, ill-fitting shoes, physiologic repetitive activities, and foot surgery or amputation that result in increased focal pressure at the distance site.[1]

- Shearing force from ill-fitting shoes, foot deformities (e.g., hammer toe and bunion), and physiologic repetitive activities.

- A foreign body.

- Smoking.

DIAGNOSIS

The diagnosis of callus or corn formation is made clinically. Radiographic examination is helpful in identifying the cause of the lesion.

CLINICAL FEATURES

- Common signs include a hard hyperkeratotic (nucleated/non-nucleated) lesion or hard callus seen on the weight-bearing surface commonly under the metatarsal heads, plantar-medial hallux interphalangeal joint, distal tip of the digits, plantar heel, fifth metatarsal base, dorsolateral fifth digit, and nail folds.

- Corns can be seen in a non-weight-bearing surface, such as:
  - Dorsal proximal interphalangeal joints in patients with hammertoe deformity. It is often referred to as a hard corn in that location (**Figure 200-3**).

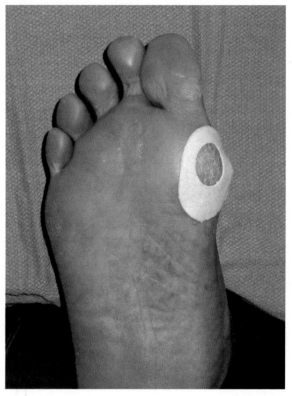

FIGURE 200-1 Typical callus under the first metatarsal head. An offloading device can alleviate pain caused by the callus. (*Courtesy of Naohiro Shibuya, DPM.*)

○ Interdigital spaces (commonly in the fourth space) often referred to as a soft corn (**Figure 200-4**).

- The lesion is often slightly hyperpigmented or normal colored and usually well demarcated.

- The lesion may have a hard or soft nucleus upon debridement.

- Common associated signs: Prominent underlying bony structure, gross deformity of the foot (e.g., cavus [high-arch] foot deformity, flatfoot deformity, bunion deformity, or lesser digital deformity), decreased ankle dorsiflexion, and an overall decrease in pedal joint range of motion.

IMAGING

- Weight-bearing plain radiographs are obtained in dorsoplantar, lateral, and medial oblique views, with a metal marker placed on the lesion.

- An exostosis (or spur) may be detected in the area of the marker.

- Underlying deformities can also be assessed with plain radiographs.

DIFFERENTIAL DIAGNOSIS

Other painful hyperkeratotic lesions in the foot can be caused by the following:

- Plantar warts are common painful HPV skin infections found on the sole of the foot. These can be small and single or large and multifocal as seen in mosaic warts. Look for evidence of black dots (thrombosed capillaries) and disruption of skin lines to differentiate these warts from callus or corns (see Chapter 128, Planter Warts).

- Acrolentiginous melanoma can occur on the foot and become painful over time. These are usually pigmented with irregular borders and variations in color. If these are amelanotic they may be harder to diagnose. Any unusual growth on the foot should be biopsied (see Chapter 165, Melanoma).

- Nonmelanoma skin cancers can rarely occur on the foot and are more likely to be on the dorsum of the foot where there is more sun exposure. These cancers are hyperkeratotic and may ulcerate. If suspicious, a shave biopsy should be adequate for diagnosis (see Chapter 163, Basal Cell Carcinoma, and Chapter 164, Squamous Cell Carcinoma).

- Porokeratosis is a deep, seeded callus that has been described as a "plugged sweat duct" and is not necessarily located in a weight-bearing area.

- Surgical physiologic/hypertrophic scar can be easily identified by the surgical orientation of the incision and patient history.

MANAGEMENT

First, consider the following conservative measures:

- Suggest that the patient change shoes to something that puts less pressure on the area involved.

- Pad the foot to limit shearing force from shoes (**Figure 200-1**).

- Use interdigital spacers to relieve pressure (**Figure 200-5**).

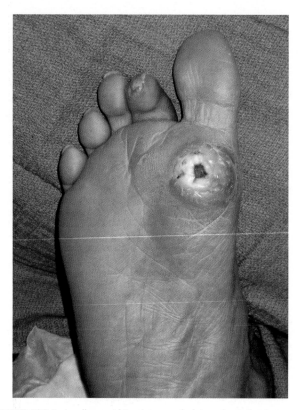

FIGURE 200-2 A callus resulting in an underlying ulceration in a person with diabetes. A neglected callus in a high-risk patient can result in infection. (*Courtesy of Naohiro Shibuya, DPM.*)

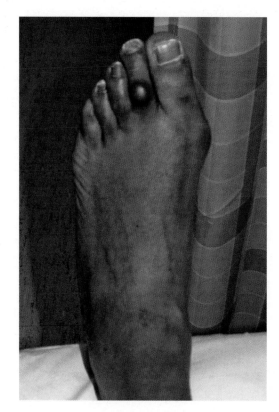

FIGURE 200-3 A dorsal hard corn formed secondary to a hammer-toe deformity. (*Courtesy of Naohiro Shibuya, DPM.*)

- Incorporate offloading devices or "cut-offs" in custom-made orthoses to realign an underlying deformity to minimize abnormal biomechanics.
- Suggest the patient reduce activity level on the feet.
- Encourage the patient to stop smoking and offer assistance.

If conservative measures fail to work, consider these surgical options:

- Sharp debridement of the lesion provides instant temporary relief from pain and discomfort. Infiltration of a local anesthetic may be necessary before debridement of an extremely painful lesion, but most calluses and corns can be debrided without anesthesia. Perform sharp debridement with a No. 10 or 15 surgical blade. The No. 10 blade is especially good for large callus. Debride the lesion down to soft, nonkeratotic tissue and remove the hard nucleus.
- In a patient with recurring lesions, consider a surgical referral to a foot specialist to correct an underlying deformity.
- Exostectomy of the prominent underlying bone can be done with a minimal incision technique.
- Consider prophylactic correction of the deformity and/or removal of exostosis in a high-risk patient (e.g., patients with diabetes who are immunocompromised and neuropathic) to reduce the risk of future ulceration and infection.
- Plastic procedures (e.g., excisional biopsy with primary closure or local flap) may be necessary in patients with a chronic lesion of idiopathic origin.

PATIENT EDUCATION

Conservative measures are effective in mild lesions. If conservative measures fail, surgical management is indicated to correct the underlying cause of the problem. Surgical correction can result in a "transferred lesion" by shifting the pressure point away from the original site.[2] Tell patients with neuropathy and/or their caregivers to examine the patient's feet daily for potential ulceration. An overlying hyperkeratotic lesion can mask an underlying ulcer. Drainage, maceration, and malodor are signs of underlying ulceration and infection.

FOLLOW-UP

A healthy patient can be seen in an "as-needed" basis. However, in a high-risk patient, periodic follow-up and sharp debridement of the lesion are necessary to prevent development of a neurotrophic ulcer. Use the University of Texas Diabetic Foot and Diabetic Wound Classification System to assess the risk of the diabetic patients.[3] (http://www.medicalcriteria.com/criteria/dbt_foot.htm. Accessed April 28, 2008.) If the patient develops an open lesion, obtain plain radiographs to rule out osteomyelitis and gas gangrene. An irregular, hyperpigmented, fast-growing lesion needs to be biopsied.

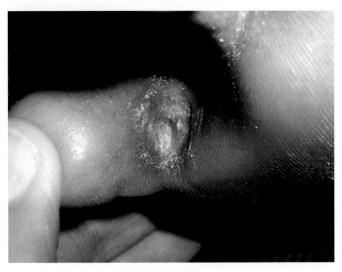

FIGURE 200-4 A soft corn at the base of the fifth digit. (*Courtesy of Richard P. Usatine, MD.*)

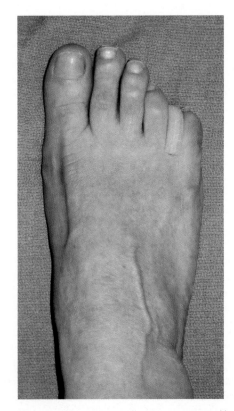

FIGURE 200-5 A simple spacer can alleviate pain caused by the corn in the fourth interdigital space. (*Courtesy of Naohiro Shibuya, DPM.*)

REFERENCES

1. Freeman DB. Corns and calluses resulting from mechanical hyperkeratosis. *Am Fam Physician*. 2002;65(11):2277–2280.

2. McGlamry ED, Banks AS. *McGlamry's Comprehensive Textbook of Foot and Ankle Surgery*. 3rd ed, Vol. 1, Chapter 9. Philadelphia, PA: Lippincott Williams & Wilkins, 2001:253–372.

3. Armstrong DG, Lavery LA, Harkless LB. Who is at risk for diabetic foot ulceration? *Clin Podiatr Med Surg*. 1998;15(1):11–19.

201 BUNION DEFORMITY

Naohiro Shibuya, DPM
Javier La Fontaine, DPM

PATIENT HISTORY

A healthy 34-year-old woman has had "bunion pain" for 5 years (**Figure 201-1**). The patient claimed that the medial prominence at the big toe joint was there ever since she could remember and it had been getting larger over the years. She had been given custom-made orthoses, but it alleviated only 50% of the pain. The patient was concerned about progression of the bunion since her mother had a severe bunion too. On examination, the patient had a very flexible foot with severe lateral deviation of the hallux. The second digit is mildly dorsiflexed. There is no pain on range of motion at the first metatarsophalangeal (MTP) joint; however, there is severe tenderness at the medial prominence. The lateral deviation of the hallux was reducible. A biomechanical hyperkeratotic lesion was found under the second metatarsal head region. **Figure 201-2** shows medial angulation of the first metatarsal and lateral deviation of the hallux. On the lateral view, the first metatarsal was slightly elevated and showed mild sign of flatfoot deformity.

The patient was referred to podiatry for surgical correction of the bunion deformity. First metatarsal–cuneiform joint fusion was chosen to correct the medial angulation and dorsal elevation of the first metatarsal, and lateral soft tissue release at the first MTP joint was done to correct the lateral deviation of the hallux. The medial aspect of the first metatarsal head was also resected.

The patient was placed in a short-leg cast for 6 weeks and slowly progressed to a regular shoe over the next month. The patient was encouraged to use the custom-made orthoses for her flatfoot to prevent recurrence of the bunion.

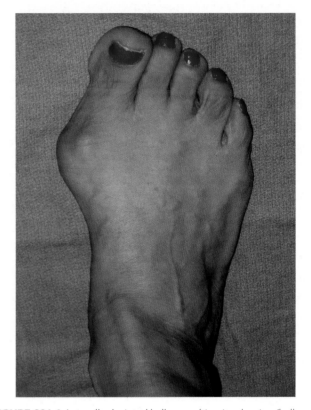

FIGURE 201-1 Laterally deviated hallux resulting in a bunion (hallux abducto valgus deformity). (*Courtesy of Naohiro Shibuya, DPM.*)

EPIDEMIOLOGY

The prevalence of bunions (hallux abducto valgus deformity) ranges from 2% to 50%.[1] It is far more common in women.

ETIOLOGY AND PATHOPHYSIOLOGY

Hallux abducto valgus deformities (bunions) are caused by multiple factors:

- Genetic and hereditary factors.
- Abnormal biomechanics (limb length discrepancy, hypermobility/ligament laxity, flatfoot deformity, malaligned skeletal structures, and ankle equinus).[2]
- Neuromuscular diseases.
- Ill-fitting shoes.
- Trauma.
- Iatrogenic causes.

DIAGNOSIS

The diagnosis of hallux abducto valgus deformity is made clinically and radiographically.

CLINICAL FEATURES

• Common signs include laterally deviated hallux, erythema, edema, tenderness on the medial eminence at the first MTP joint, and pain through the first MTP joint range of motion.

• Commonly associated signs: hypermobility, flatfoot deformity, second MTP joint pain, pain under the second metatarsal head, overlapped second digit, decreased ankle dorsiflexion, concurrent gout, decreased first MTP joint range of motion, sesamoiditis, hyperkeratosis, and hammertoe deformity. A unilateral bunion deformity is often a result of limb length discrepancy (**Figure 201-3**).

IMAGING

• Weight-bearing plain radiographs are obtained in dorsoplantar, lateral, and medial oblique views (**Figure 201-2**).

• Lateral deviation of the hallux and medial deviation of the first metatarsal bone are noted in the dorsoplantar view.

• The first MTP joint narrowing, osteophyte formation, subchondral cysts, and sclerosis are indicative of osteoarthritis.

• The lateral view is useful in assessing elevation of the first metatarsal, dorsal spur formation at the first MTP joint, and hammertoe deformity.

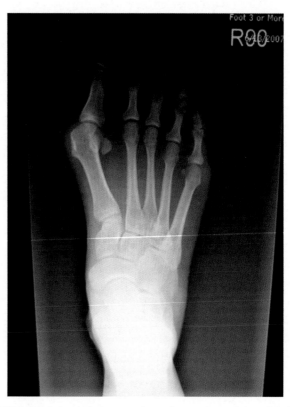

FIGURE 201-2 A weight-bearing dorsoplantar plain radiograph helps in assessing severity of the deformity and determining treatment plan. (*Courtesy of Naohiro Shibuya, DPM.*)

DIFFERENTIAL DIAGNOSIS

Pain and swelling around the first MTP joint may be caused by the following:

• Gout or pseudogout presents with acute pain with signs of inflammation and prior history of gout/pseudogout. Joint aspiration may be performed to rule out septic joint (see Chapter 94, Gout).

• Rheumatoid arthritis presents with pain, inflammation, and loss of range of motion and is often symmetrical. Radiographic evidence of other small pedal joints involvement is usually evident (see Chapter 92, Rheumatoid Arthritis).

• Septic joint presents with acute pain, loss of range of motion, and systemic signs and symptoms of infectious process.

MANAGEMENT

Conservative measures and surgical treatments are described below.

CONSERVATIVE MEASURES

• Change in shoes.

• Placing a toe spacer in the first interdigital space straightens the hallux and decreases the irritation caused by rubbing of the first and second digits.

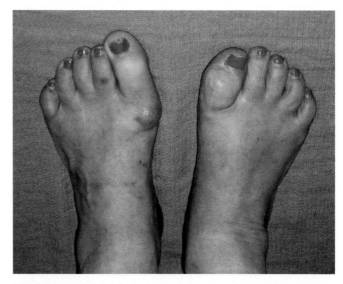

FIGURE 201-3 A unilateral bunion deformity is often a result of limb length discrepancy. Note the prominent erythema around the first MTP joint of the left foot only. (*Courtesy of Naohiro Shibuya, DPM.*)

- Padding to limit shearing force from shoes (**Figure 201-4**).

- Water-soluble cortisone injection into the first MTP joint may help a patient who complains of joint pain secondary to early-stage osteoarthritis.

- Custom-made orthoses help slow progression of the deformity caused by biomechanical factors.

- Resting, NSAIDs, and ice may help an inflamed joint and/or shoe irritation.

- Physical therapy may help improve joint range of motion, reduce edema, or decrease nerve pain.

SURGICAL TREATMENT

- Consider surgical referral to a foot specialist for correction of the deformity.

- The tendon and ligament balancing procedure is used for minor, flexible deformities.

- Exostectomy may help patients who have no joint pain, but complain about extra-articular "bump pain."

- Osteotomy to realign the bony structure is indicated for moderate to severe deformities (**Figure 201-5**).

- Arthrodesis of the first MTP or metatarsocuneiform joint is indicated in a severe deformity.

- Adjunctive procedures (e.g., correction of hammertoe deformities, flatfoot deformity, ankle equinus, and resection of the sesamoid bone) may be required for a positive long-term outcome.

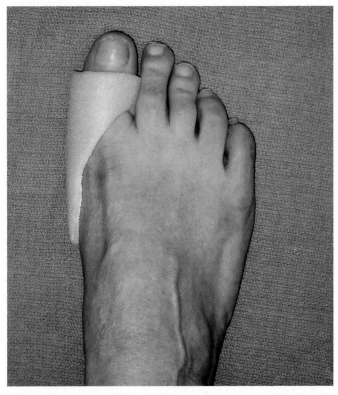

FIGURE 201-4 Simple padding can alleviate shoe irritation from the bunion deformity. (*Courtesy of Naohiro Shibuya, DPM.*)

PATIENT EDUCATION

Conservative measures may or may not provide temporary relief and prevent progression of the deformity. Surgical management is necessary to correct the deformity. Surgical treatment will typically require 2 to 6 weeks of non-weight-bearing status postoperatively, depending on the procedure performed. More severe deformities will require a more extensive surgical approach and longer recovery period.

FOLLOW-UP

The patient may be seen on an as-needed basis. Serial plain radiographs can be obtained to follow the progression of the deformity and arthritic changes in the first MTP joint. Follow-up for surgery will be arranged by the surgeon.

PATIENT RESOURCES

Penn State Milton S. Hershey Medical Center. Bunion. Available at: **http://www.hmc.psu.edu/healthinfo/b/bunion.htm.** (Accessed August 18, 2007).

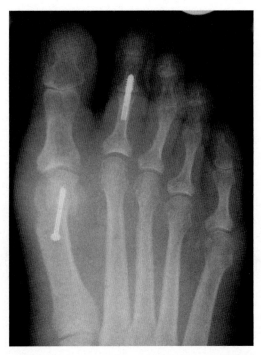

FIGURE 201-5 Surgical correction is indicated if conservative measures fail. (*Courtesy of Naohiro Shibuya, DPM.*)

PROVIDER RESOURCES

American College of Foot and Ankle Surgeons. Bunions. Available at: **http://www.footphysicians.com/footankleinfo/bunions.htm.** (Accessed August 18, 2007).

Shiel WC, Jr. Bunions. MedicineNet.com. Available at: **http://www.medicinenet.com/bunions/article.htm.** (Accessed August 18, 2007).

REFERENCES

1. McGlamry ED, Banks AS. *McGlamry's Comprehensive Textbook of Foot and Ankle Surgery*. 3rd ed. 2 v. xxiv, 2117. Philadelphia: Lippincott Williams & Wilkins, 2001:66.

2. Chang TJ. *Master Techniques in Podiatric Surgery: The Foot and Ankle*. Vol. xvii. Philadelphia: Lippincott Williams & Wilkins, 2005:560.

202 HAMMERTOE DEFORMITIES

Naohiro Shibuya, DPM
Javier La Fontaine, DPM

PATIENT HISTORY

A 44-year-old woman presented with pain in the ball of her left foot on weight-bearing. She works as a nurse and does a lot of walking all day long. Two months ago she noticed a new deformity of the second digit of her left foot (**Figure 202-1**). She denied any injury. She had a rupture of the plantar plate from overuse, which resulted in a hammertoe deformity of her second digit. The digit was contracted with a nonreducible proximal interphalangeal joint and reducible metatarsophalangeal (MTP) joint. Her x-ray is seen in **Figure 202-2**.

She was referred to a podiatrist who fused her proximal interphalangeal joint and released her extensor tendon and dorsal capsule at the MTP joint to reduce the deformity. The plantar plate was also repaired. The patient started protective ambulation with a surgical shoe on the postoperative day 3. An internal fixation wire, which was utilized to fixate the fusion site, was removed in 4 weeks. She returned to work and her regular activities within 6 weeks of the operation.

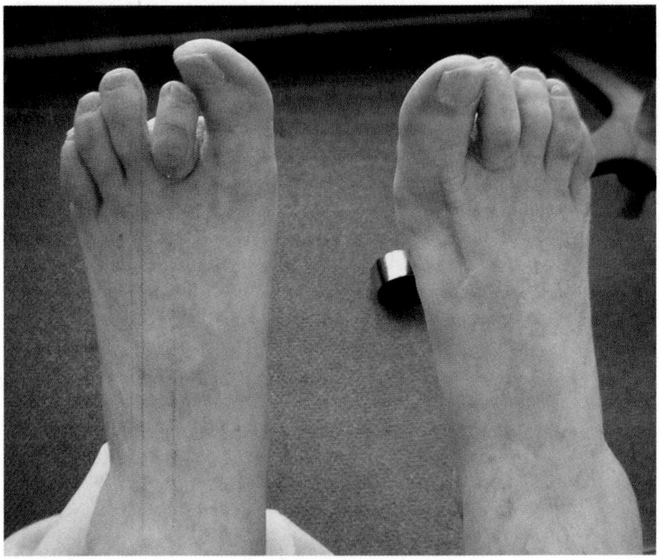

EPIDEMIOLOGY

Hammertoe deformity is the most common digital deformity, and it can affect up to 60% of adults. The second digit is most commonly affected.[1]

ETIOLOGY AND PATHOPHYSIOLOGY

A hammertoe is caused by multiple factors:

- Genetic and hereditary factors.
- Abnormal biomechanics (cavus or high-arch foot, flatfoot deformity, loss of intrinsic muscle function, and hypermobile first ray).
- Long metatarsal and/or digit.
- Systemic arthridities.
- Neuromuscular diseases such as Charcot-Marie-Tooth disease (**Figure 202-3**).
- Ill-fitted shoes.
- Trauma.
- Iatrogenic causes.

DIAGNOSIS

The diagnosis of hammertoe deformity is made clinically and radiographically.

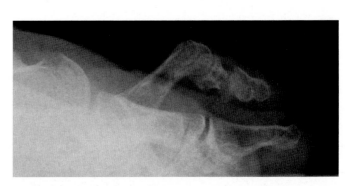

FIGURE 202-1 A plantar plate rupture at the MTP joint from overuse often causes an acute isolated hammertoe deformity. (*Courtesy of Naohiro Shibuya, DPM.*)

FIGURE 202-2 This lateral plain film shows dorsiflexion of the proximal phalanx at the MTP joint and plantarflexion of the middle phalanx at the proximal interphalangeal joint of the second digit. (*Courtesy of Naohiro Shibuya, DPM.*)

CLINICAL FEATURES

- In a hammertoe deformity the proximal phalanx is dorsiflexed at the MTP joint and the middle phalanx is plantarflexed at the proximal interphalangeal joint of the lesser digit. Transverse and frontal plane deformities can coexist with the main, sagittal plane deformity.

- Common signs include contracted digit(s), callus formation at the dorsal aspect of the proximal interphalangeal joint and/or distal aspect of the digit, edema, and tenderness on the plantar aspect of the lesser MTP joint(s).

- Commonly associated signs include cavus foot deformity, flatfoot deformity, bunion deformity, transverse deformity of the digits, decreased ankle dorsiflexion, and bowstringing of the extensor and/or flexor tendons.

- Evaluation of the digit in weight-bearing and non-weight-bearing conditions helps assess reducibility and rigidity of the deformity. In the case of predislocation syndrome (acute rupture or tear of the MTP joint capsule or plantar plate), the deformity may not be appreciated unless the foot is evaluated in the weight-bearing position.[2]

IMAGING

- Weight-bearing plain radiographs are obtained in dorsoplantar, lateral, and medial oblique views (**Figure 202-2**).

- Dorsal angulation and/or translation of the proximal phalanx on the metatarsal head with plantar angulation of the middle phalanx are noted in the lateral view. Degenerative changes in the digital joints and dislocation in the MTP joint may be evident.

- Transverse deformity can be assessed in the dorsoplantar view. Abnormal metatarsal length can also be assessed in this view.

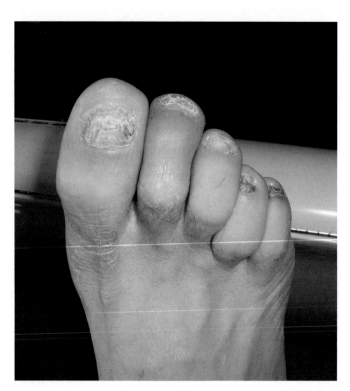

FIGURE 202-3 Severe hammertoe deformity caused by Charcot-Marie-Tooth disease, an autosomal-dominant neuromuscular disease. (*Courtesy of Richard P. Usatine, MD.*)

DIFFERENTIAL DIAGNOSIS

Pain and swelling in the digit may be caused by the following:

- Gout or pseudogout presents with acute pain with signs of inflammation, and prior history of gout/pseudogout. Joint aspiration may be performed to rule out septic joint (see Chapter 94, Gout).

- Rheumatoid arthritis presents with pain, inflammation, and loss of range of motion and is often symmetrical. Radiographic evidence of other small foot joint involvement usually is evident (see Chapter 92, Rheumatoid Arthritis).

- Septic joint presents with acute pain, loss of range of motion, and systemic signs and symptoms of infectious process.

- Fractured toe caused by sudden trauma.

- Neuroma in the intermetatarsal space (Morton's neuroma) with compression of the intermetatarsal nerves – numbness and cramping of the innervated toes are the most common symptoms.

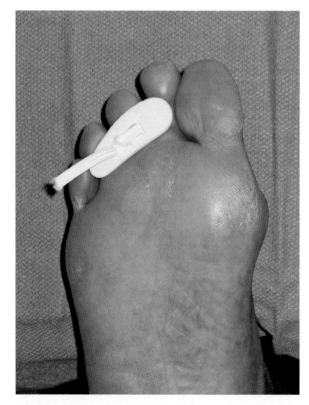

FIGURE 202-4 A crest pad prevents painful callus formation at the distal tip of the digit. (*Courtesy of Naohiro Shibuya, DPM.*)

MANAGEMENT

Conservative measures and surgical treatment may be used to correct this condition. Note that a neglected hammertoe deformity could result in ulceration in a patient with diabetes.

CONSERVATIVE MEASURES

- Change in shoes.
- Padding to limit shearing force from shoes. A crest pad can be used to prevent painful callus formation at the distal tip of the digit (**Figure 202-4**).
- Splinting can be used in an early flexible hammertoe.
- Water-soluble steroid injection into the MTP joint may help a patient who complains of joint pain secondary to early-stage osteoarthritis or capsulitis. Avoid excessive steroid injections, as these can result in further damage of the capsule and worsening of the deformity.
- Custom-made orthoses are helpful to slow down progression of the deformity if it is caused by biomechanical factors.
- Resting, NSAIDs, and ice help an inflamed joint and/or shoe irritation.

SURGICAL TREATMENT

- Consider surgical referral to a foot specialist to correct the deformity.
- Percutaneous tenotomy and/or capsulotomy are used for mild, flexible deformities.
- Resectional arthroplasty at the proximal interphalangeal joint may be beneficial for a more rigid deformity.
- Shortening osteotomy of the metatarsal is indicated in the deformities resulting from the long metatarsal.
- Arthrodesis (fusion) of the proximal interphalangeal joint and/or flexor tendon transfer is indicated for a severe deformity (**Figure 202-5**).
- Adjunctive procedures (e.g., correction of bunion, cavus foot, flatfoot deformities, and ankle equinus) may be necessary for a good long-term outcome.

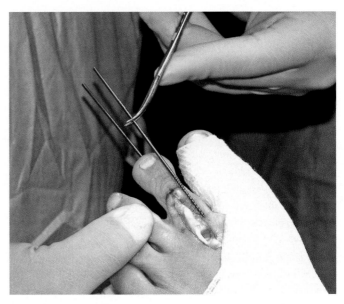

FIGURE 202-5 Proximal interphalangeal joint arthrodesis (fusion) is often used to correct hammertoe deformity. (*Courtesy of Naohiro Shibuya, DPM.*)

PATIENT EDUCATION

Explain to patients that conservative measures may prevent progression of the deformity and provide temporary relief, but that surgical management is necessary to correct the deformity. Surgical treatment can require up to 4 to 6 weeks of non-weight-bearing status postoperatively in severe deformities. A less involved surgical approach in correction of a mild deformity can allow a patient to walk on the same day of the surgery. In many cases, fixation with a pin, small screw, or implant may be necessary to correct the deformity.

FOLLOW-UP

Periodic debridement of the calluses developed from the deformity may be sufficient in many of the patients if the deformity is not progressive. Serial plain radiographs can be obtained to follow the progression of the deformity and arthritic changes in the first MTP joint. In a high-risk, immunocompromised, neuropathic patient, prophylactic surgical correction of the deformity may be indicated.

PATIENT RESOURCES

Cluett J. About.com:orthopedics. Available at: **http://orthopedics.about.com/cs/toeproblems/a/toeproblems_2.htm.** (Accessed August 19, 2007).

PROVIDER RESOURCES

Watson A. *Hammertoe Deformity.* eMedicine. Available at: **http://www.emedicine.com/orthoped/topic457.htm.** Accessed April 28, 2008.

REFERENCES

1. McGlamry ED, Banks AS. *McGlamry's Comprehensive Textbook of Foot and Ankle Surgery.* 3rd ed. 2 v. xxiv, 2117. Philadelphia: Lippincott Williams & Wilkins, 2001:66.

2. Yu GV, et al. Predislocation syndrome. Progressive subluxation/dislocation of the lesser metatarsophalangeal joint. *J Am Podiatr Med Assoc.* 2002;92(4):182–199.

203 ISCHEMIC ULCER

Javier La Fontaine, DPM
Naohiro Shibuya, DPM

PATIENT STORY

A 38-year-old woman with type 2 diabetes and hypercholesterolemia presented with a 2-month history of a nonhealing ulceration on her left foot (**Figure 203-1**). She remembered stepping on a tack, but she continued walking. Her physician referred her to a wound-care center. She reported smoking one pack of cigarettes daily for 20 years and had not been taking her diabetes medication. She presented with loss of protective sensation and a nonpalpable posterior tibial pulse. The patient had limited joint mobility at the first metatarsophalangeal joint, which led to increased pressure under the joint. Arterial noninvasive studies showed severe vascular disease; therefore, she was a candidate for revascularization. While in the hospital, she quit smoking and began taking her diabetes medication again. She underwent revascularization and appropriate off-loading therapy. Her ulcer healed and she continues to take her diabetes medications and does not smoke.

EPIDEMIOLOGY

The incidence of ischemic ulcers among all diabetic ulcers is unknown.[1] These ulcers are very difficult to heal with basic wound care and commonly require advanced therapy (e.g., hyperbaric oxygen treatment or bioengineered skin substitutes). If not aggressively treated, these ulcers will become infected and may have to be amputated.

ETIOLOGY AND PATHOPHYSIOLOGY

Microvascular dysfunction is an important component of the disease processes that occur in diabetic foot disease. The abnormalities observed in the endothelium in patients with diabetes are not well understood and evidence suggests that endothelial dysfunction could be involved in the pathogenesis of diabetic macroangiopathy and microangiopathy.[2] Microangiopathy is a functional disease where neuropathy and autoregulation of capillaries lead to poor perfusion of the tissues, especially at the wound base.

DIAGNOSIS

CLINICAL FEATURES

- Gray/yellow fibrotic base (**Figures 203-1** and **203-2**).
- Undermining skin margins.
- Punched-out appearance.
- Pain.
- Most common location: distal aspect of the toes.

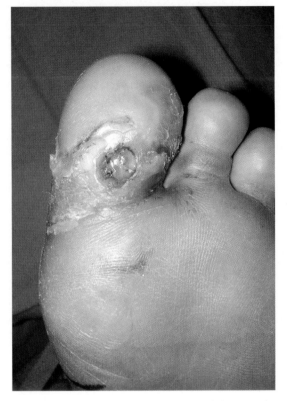

FIGURE 203-1 A 38-year-old woman with type 2 diabetes and an ischemic ulcer on the first digit of the left foot. The base of the wound is grey in color with pink surrounding wound margins. (*Courtesy of Javier La Fontaine, DPM.*)

- Nonpalpable pulses.
- Associated trophic skin changes (e.g., absent pedal hair and thin shiny skin).

IMAGING

- Noninvasive studies (e.g., arterial Doppler and pulse volume recordings) are important for baseline assessment of the patient's blood flow.[3]
- Radiographs may be necessary to rule out osteomyelitis.

DIFFERENTIAL DIAGNOSIS

- Neuropathic ulcer usually presents with beefy red wound base and hyperkeratosis at the skin margins (see Chapter 204, Neuropathic Ulcer).
- Infected wound presents with localized redness, edema, drainage, and warmness in any of the diabetic-type wounds with lack of systemic symptoms of infection.
- Gangrene usually well-demarcated, black eschar in the dysvascular foot (see Chapter 206, Gangrene).

MANAGEMENT

- Consider vascular surgery to evaluate the possibility of revascularization.
- It is important to rule out a concomitant infection. Antibiotics are not indicated unless infection is present.
- Avoid aggressive debridement until optimization of blood flow occurs.
- Change dressings twice daily to evaluate the wound and keep a low bacterial load. Many advanced therapies can be added to accomplish the same goals.
- If the wound is plantar, offloading is important to prevent the wound from increasing in size.

PATIENT EDUCATION

- Prevention measures such as smoking cessation are important to aid wound healing.[4]
- Promote successful treatment by encouraging adherence with use of offloading devices.
- Strive for normal glycemic control to optimize outcome for healing and surgical intervention.

FOLLOW-UP

- Schedule weekly to biweekly visits to monitor the ulcer.
- Obtain serial radiographs every 4 weeks to monitor for the development of osteomyelitis.

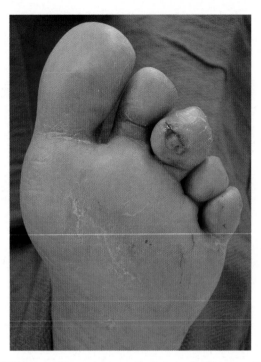

FIGURE 203-2 A 57-year-old man with diabetes for 25 years with an ischemic ulcer of the third toe. A grayish base is a common finding in this type of ulcer. (*Courtesy of Javier La Fontaine, DPM.*)

- Closely monitor the patient every 3 to 4 months once healing has occurred. Patients who have had history of ulcerations are 36 times more likely to develop another ulcer.[5]

PATIENT RESOURCES

Frykberg RG. Diabetic foot problems. Available at: **http://www.footdokter.com/treatments/diabetes.htm.** (Accessed May 14, 2007).

PROVIDER RESOURCES

Frykberg RG. Diabetic foot ulcers: Pathogenesis and management. 2002 Nov 1;66(9):1655–1662. Available at: **http://www.aafp.org/afp/20021101/1655.html.** (Accessed May 14, 2007).

Kruse I, Edelman S. Evaluation and treatment of diabetic foot ulcers. *Clin Diabetes.* 2006;24:91–93.

REFERENCES

1. Tooke JE. A pathophysiological framework for the pathogenesis of diabetic microangiopathy. In: Tooke JE ed. *Diabetic Angiopathy.* New York: Oxford University Press Inc, 1999:187.

2. La Fontaine J, Allen M, Davis C, Harkless LB, Shireman PK. Current concepts in diabetic microvascular dysfunction. *JAPMA.* 2006;96(3):245–252.

3. Sykes MT, Godsey JB. Vascular evaluation of the problem diabetic foot. *Clin Podiatr Med Surg.* 1998;15(1):49–82.

4. American Diabetes Association Guidelines. Preventive foot care in people with diabetes. *Diabetes Care.* 2000;23(Suppl 1):S55–S56.

5. Armstrong DG, Lavery LA, Harkless LB. Validation of a diabetic wound classification system. The contribution of depth, infection, and ischemia to risk of amputation. *Diabetes Care.* 1998;21(5):855–859.

204 NEUROPATHIC ULCER

Javier La Fontaine, DPM
Naohiro Shibuya, DPM

PATIENT STORY

A 57-year-old man with type 2 diabetes presented with history of a neuropathic ulceration to the right foot for 2 weeks (**Figure 204-1**). The patient recalled having a callus for several months. He noticed blood on his sock 3 days ago. He denied fever or chills, but his glucose has been running higher than normal. The patient demonstrated loss of protective sensation, but vascular status was intact. He was referred to a podiatrist who immediately off-loaded his foot with a to-tal contact cast. His ulcer healed in 1 month, and he was subsequently fitted with orthopedic shoes.

EPIDEMIOLOGY

Overall 15% of people with diabetes will experience a foot ulcer dur-ing their lifetime, and 15% of these will have osteomyelitis.[1] Foot ulcers can develop in any location of the foot but are more common under the metatarsal heads, hallux, heel, or other weight-bearing areas. Foot ulcers may also result from poorly fitting footwear, which creates excessive pressure, friction, or irritation. The mechanism of injury is moderate pressure with repetitive trauma.

ETIOLOGY AND PATHOPHYSIOLOGY

Neuropathy causes approximately 50% of diabetic foot ulcers.[2] Hav-ing diabetic neuropathy alone makes a patient 1.7 times more likely to develop foot ulceration. Patients with diabetic neuropathy combined with pedal deformity are 12.1 times more likely to develop ulceration.[3] The mechanism of injury is commonly described as mod-erate pressure with repetitive trauma. Offloading is the key for heal-ing the neuropathic ulceration. Therefore, once ulceration occurs reducing pressure promotes healing.

DIAGNOSIS

The diagnosis of neuropathic ulceration is made clinically.

CLINICAL FEATURES

- A red, granular base (**Figures 204-1** and **204-2**).
- Surrounding hyperkeratosis with white, macerated margins (**Figures 204-1** and **204-2**).
- The ulcer is most commonly found under the metatarsal heads, but it can also be present in the distal and plantar aspects of the toes (**Figures 204-1** and **204-2**).

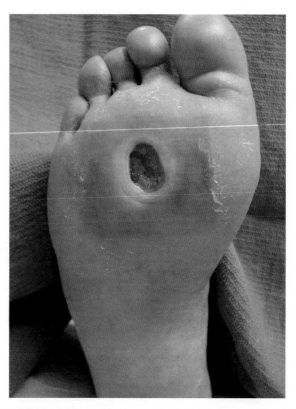

FIGURE 204-1 Neuropathic ulcer under the third metatarsal head of the right foot in a patient with diabetes. Note the red base with a white rim of hyperkeratotic tissue, a classical finding of this type of ulcer. (*Courtesy of Javier La Fontaine, DPM.*)

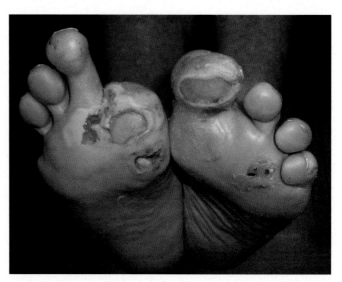

FIGURE 204-2 Neuropathic ulcers in the plantar aspect of both feet. Multiple amputations in this patient caused an increased pressure in different areas of the feet, which, in combination with neuropathy, led to new ulcerations. (*Courtesy of Richard P. Usatine, MD.*)

LABORATORY STUDIES

- Cultures are only indicated if infection is suspected. Swab cultures are not reliable. Curettage of the base of the wound may be more reliable.

IMAGING

- Radiographs may identify a foreign body, or underlying osteomyelitis.
- A biopsy may be necessary to rule out a suspected malignancy.

DIFFERENTIAL DIAGNOSIS

- Ischemic ulcer presents in the dysvascular foot and may have black eschar at the wound base. Usually presents with pink to grey wound base (see Chapter 203, Ischemic Ulcer).
- Puncture wounds may become neuropathic ulcers in the presence of neuropathy.

MANAGEMENT

Refer to Podiatry for the following management options:

- Offloading pressure from the foot is the standard of care.
- Multiple devices (e.g., removable cast boot, surgical shoes, and wedge shoes) are used for offloading; however, a total contact cast is the gold standard.[4,5]
- Diabetic shoes should not be used as offloading devices for ulcerations.
- Serial tissue debridement should be performed weekly to biweekly to maintain minimal bacterial load, low pressure surrounding the ulcer, and a metabolically active wound base.
- If no improvement in the ulcer is noticed in 4 weeks, the ulcer should be considered a chronic wound, and, therefore, adjunctive therapy (e.g., growth factors) must be considered.
- Oral antibiotics are not indicated unless infection is suspected.

PATIENT EDUCATION

- Tell patients that adherence with offloading devices is essential.
- Inform patients that control of blood sugar and blood pressure promotes healing.

FOLLOW-UP

- Weekly to biweekly visits to the podiatrist are needed to monitor and treat the ulcer.

- Serial radiographs every 4 weeks may be necessary to monitor for the development of osteomyelitis.
- Closely monitor the patient every 3 to 4 months once healing is accomplished. Patients who have had history of ulcerations are 36 times more likely to develop another ulcer.[3]

PATIENT RESOURCES

DermNet NZ. Diabetic foot ulcers. Available at: **http:// www.dermnetnz.org/systemic/diabetic-foot.html.** (Accessed May 15, 2007).

Vancouver Island Health Authority. Chapter 7: Neuropathic Ulcers. Wound and Skin Care Clinical Guidelines, April 2007. Available at: **http://www.viha.ca/NR/rdonlyres/ 7C47A7F9-1133-4D75-955C-7A4CBBD49A6E/8471/ Chapter7NeuropathicUlcers.pdf.** (Accessed April 28, 2008).

PROVIDER RESOURCES

Boulton AJM, Kirsner RS, Vileikyte L. Neuropathic diabetic foot ulcers. *N Engl J Med*. 2004;351:48–55.

Karlock L. Wound Care Q&A: Inside insights for offloading diabetic neuropathic ulcers. Podiatry Today. Available at: **http://www.podiatrytoday.com/article/2781.** (Accessed May 15, 2007).

REFERENCES

1. Levin ME. Pathogenesis and general management of foot lesions in the diabetic patient. In: Bowker JH, Pfeifer MA eds. *Levin and O'Neal's the Diabetic Foot*. 6th ed. St. Louis, MO: CV Mosby, 2001:219–260.

2. Reiber GE, Smith DG, Wallace C, et al. Effect of therapeutic footwear on foot reulceration in patients with diabetes: A randomized controlled trial. *JAMA*. 2002;287:2552–2558.

3. Armstrong DG, Lavery LA, Harkless LB. Validation of a diabetic wound classification system. The contribution of depth, infection, and ischemia to risk of amputation. *Diabetes Care*. 1998;21(5): 855–859.

4. Lavery LA, Vela SA, Lavery DC, Quebedeaux TL. Reducing dynamic foot pressures in high-risk diabetic subjects with foot ulcerations. A comparison of treatments. *Diabetes Care*. 1996;19(8): 818–821.

5. Fleischli JG, Lavery LA, Vela SA, Ashry H, Lavery DC. Comparison of strategies for reducing pressure at the site of neuropathic ulcers. *JAPMA*. 1997;87(10):466–472.

205 CHARCOT ARTHROPATHY

Javier La Fontaine, DPM
Naohiro Shibuya, DPM

PATIENT STORY

A 62-year-old man with type 2 diabetes for 15 years presents with history of erythematous, hot, swollen right foot for 2 weeks (**Figure 205-1**). He is on multiple medications for management of his diabetes, but it is not successfully controlled. The patient does not recall any trauma to the foot. Three days ago, he noticed his foot began to pain. He denies fever or chills. The radiograph of his foot (**Figure 205-2**) shows midfoot osteopenia—an early sign of acute Charcot arthropathy (also called neuroarthropathy).

EPIDEMIOLOGY

The incidence of Charcot arthropathy in diabetes ranges from 0.1% to 5%.[1] The lack of knowledge about this entity may lead to an unnecessary amputation. Untreated Charcot foot may lead to a rockerbottom foot, which in turn leads to increased plantar pressure in the neuropathic foot. This cascade will lead to an ulceration and possible amputation.[2]

ETIOLOGY AND PATHOPHYSIOLOGY

Charcot arthropathy is a gradual destruction of the joint in patients with neurosensory loss. Its most common presentation is in diabetic neuropathic patient.[3] The pathogenesis is unknown. A number of theories have been proposed to explain the etiology of Charcot arthropathy, including the following:

- Neurotraumatic theory: Following sensory-motor neuropathy, the resulting sensory loss and muscle imbalance induces abnormal stress in the bones and joints of the affected limb, leading to bone destruction.

- Neurovascular theory: Following the development of autonomic neuropathy there is an increased blood flow to the extremity, resulting in osteopenia from a mismatch in bone reabsorption and synthesis.

- Stretching of the ligaments because of joint effusion may lead to joint subluxation.

- It is most likely that Charcot arthropathy involves all of the above mechanisms together.

DIAGNOSIS

The diagnosis of Charcot arthropathy is made clinically.

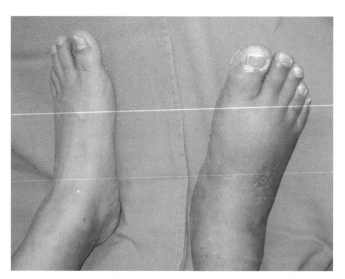

FIGURE 205-1 Charcot arthropathy in the right foot. Notice the swelling and discoloration compared to the contralateral side. (*Courtesy of Javier La Fontaine, DPM.*)

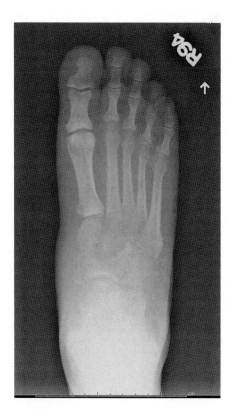

FIGURE 205-2 Anterior–posterior view of same foot demonstrating midfoot osteopenia, an early sign of acute Charcot arthropathy. (*Courtesy of Javier La Fontaine, DPM.*)

CLINICAL FEATURES

- Red, hot, swollen foot (**Figure 205-1**).
- Even with neurosensory loss, 71% of patients present with the chief complaint of pain.[2]
- Rockerbottom foot deformity is a classic finding of this entity (**Figure 205-3**).
- Patients may present with an open wound in the plantar aspect of the foot, which may complicate the diagnosis between Charcot arthropathy and infection.

IMAGING

- Radiographs are imperative for diagnosis. Usually, radiographs show arch collapse within the joints of the midfoot (tarsometatarsal joints) (**Figure 205-4**). Radiographs can also show erosions and cystic degeneration of the tarsometatarsal joints in Charcot arthropathy (**Figure 205-5**).
- When infection is suspected, other imaging modalities such as bone scan and magnetic resonance imaging may be ordered, but are often inconclusive because of the difficulty differentiating cellulitis, osteomyelitis, and Charcot arthropathy.

CULTURE AND BIOPSY

- If osteomyelitis is suspected, bone cultures and bone biopsy are recommended. Cultures need to be taken during the bone biopsy so that the suspected infected bone can be visualized for accurate sampling. Send cultures for aerobic and anaerobic cultures as well as for acid-fast bacilli.

DIFFERENTIAL DIAGNOSIS

- Infections, including cellulitis and osteomyelitis, should be considered and treated if present (see Chapter 114, Cellulitis).
- Gouty arthropathy of the foot or ankle can resemble a Charcot foot (see Chapter 94, Gout).
- Acute trauma to the foot can cause swelling and erythema, but should be easy to distinguish by the history.
- Deep venous thrombosis in the leg will generally cause swelling that extends above the ankle.

MANAGEMENT

- Offloading of pressure from the foot is the standard of care. The total contact cast is most effective, and it covers the toes for protection. Other methods that are used include the removable cast boot, crutches, and the wheelchair.
- Diabetic shoes should not be used as offloading devices for Charcot arthropathy.
- Skin temperature assessment with infrared thermometry has been demonstrated to be successful in monitoring improvement.
- Prevention of rockerbottom deformities, plantar ulcers, and amputations is the major goal of the treatment. If foot care is not optimized, a plantar ulcer can form under the Charcot's joints as seen in **Figure 205-6**.

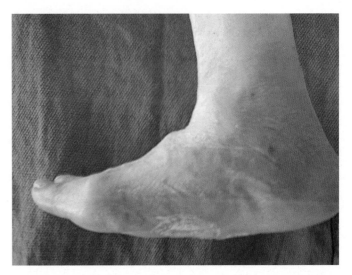

FIGURE 205-3 Lateral view of the right foot demonstrating the classic rockerbottom deformity. (*Courtesy of Javier La Fontaine, DPM.*)

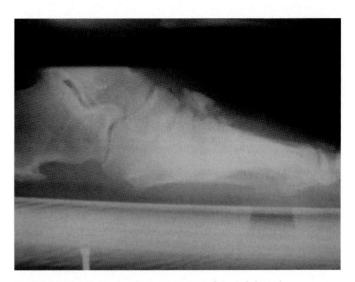

FIGURE 205-4 Lateral radiographic view of the left foot demonstrating the classic rockerbottom deformity in Charcot arthropathy with the arch collapsed at the tarsometatarsal joints. (*Courtesy of Javier La Fontaine, DPM.*)

- The bones will take approximately 4 to 5 months to heal in presence of neuropathy.
- Oral antibiotics are not indicated unless infection is suspected.
- If deformity develops, custom-molded shoes and insoles must be ordered to prevent plantar ulcers that can lead to amputation.
- If the foot develops instability at the fracture sites, surgical reconstruction may be required.

PATIENT EDUCATION

- Ensure that patients understand that adherence with offloading devices is essential.
- Tell the patient that all efforts should be made to control blood sugar and blood pressure to promote healing.

FOLLOW-UP

- Weekly to biweekly visits to the podiatrist are needed.
- Serial radiographs every 4 weeks are required to monitor bone healing and deformity.
- Once healing is accomplished, it is imperative to continue monitoring the patient every 3 to 4 months. Patients who have had history of Charcot arthropathy are 36 times more likely to develop another ulcer and are at risk of amputation.[4]

PATIENT RESOURCES

ePodiatry.com. Charcot's foot (Charcot's arthropathy or arthropathy). Available at: **http://www.epodiatry.com/ charcot-foot.htm.** (Accessed August 18, 2007).

PROVIDER RESOURCES

ePodiatry.com. Charcot's foot (Charcot's arthropathy or arthropathy). Available at: **http://www.epodiatry.com/ charcot-foot.htm** (Accessed August 18, 2007).

Sommer TC, Lee TH. Charcot foot: The diagnostic dilemma. *Am Fam Physician*. 2001;64:1591–1598. Available at: **http://www.aafp. org/afp/20011101/1591.html.** (Accessed August 18, 2007).

REFERENCES

1. Brodsky J, Rouse AM. Exostectomy for symptomatic bony prominences in diabetic Charcot feet. *Clin Orthop Relat Res*. 1993;296: 21–26.

2. Armstrong DG, Todd WF, Lavery LA, Harkless LB, Bushman TR. The natural history of acute Charcot's arthropathy in a diabetic foot specialty clinic. *JAPMA*. 1997;87(6):272–278.

3. Fryksberg R. Osteoarthropathy. *Clin Podiatr Med Surg*. 1987;4(2): 351–359.

4. Levin ME. Pathogenesis and general management of foot lesions in the diabetic patient. In: Bowker JH, Pfeifer MA eds. *Levin and O'Neal's the Diabetic Foot*. 6th ed. St. Louis: CV Mosby, 2001:219–260.

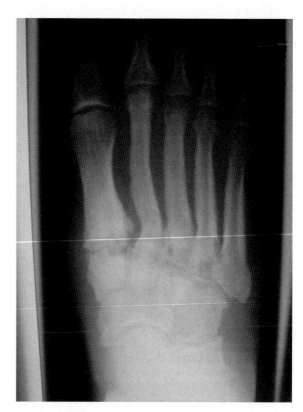

FIGURE 205-5 Anterior–posterior radiograph of the right foot demonstrating erosion and cystic degeneration at the tarsometatarsal joints in Charcot arthropathy. (*Courtesy of Javier La Fontaine, DPM.*)

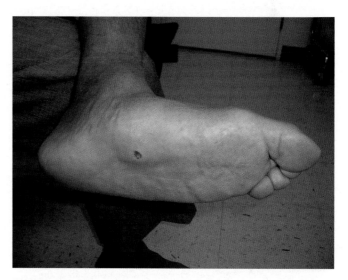

FIGURE 205-6 Foot ulcer as a result of diabetic neuropathy and a Charcot foot. Note the collapse of the arch. (*Courtesy of Richard P. Usatine, MD.*)

206 DRY GANGRENE

Javier La Fontaine, DPM
Naohiro Shibuya, DPM

PATIENT STORY

A 36-year-old woman with type 1 diabetes presented with a 4-week history of a dry, black great toe and third toe on the right foot. She said that she noticed severe maceration between the first and second interspace approximately 6 weeks ago. Subsequently, the toes changed color and became very painful. Two days ago, she noticed a foul odor from both toes. The patient reported smoking since she was 13 years old. On physical examination, there were no palpable pulses in the right foot. The patient was admitted for IV antibiotics and revascularization was performed. Subsequently, the toes were partially amputated and the wounds healed without any complications. Her physicians attempted to help her to quit smoking without success.

EPIDEMIOLOGY

Peripheral arterial disease (PAD) is a common finding in patients with diabetes. PAD is an important factor leading to lower extremity amputation in patients with diabetes.[1] Thirty percent of diabetic patients with an absent pedal pulse will have some degree of coronary artery disease.[1]

ETIOLOGY AND PATHOPHYSIOLOGY

PAD manifests in the lower extremity in two ways: macro- and microvascular diseases. The pattern of occlusion in the macrovascular tree is distal and multisegmental.[2] In other words, multiple occlusions occur below the trifurcation of the popliteal artery into the anterior tibial artery, posterior tibial artery, and peroneal artery. Risk factors such as hypercholesteremia, hyperlipidemia, and hypertension are often associated with patients with PAD and, therefore, poor wound healing.[3,4]

DIAGNOSIS

CLINICAL FEATURES (DRY GANGRENE)

- Dry, black eschar, which most commonly begins distally at the extremities (**Figures 206-1** and **206-2**).
- There is a clear demarcation between healthy tissue and necrotic tissue (**Figures 206-1** and **206-2**).
- Foul odor.
- Pain may be present.
- Trauma is the most common etiology.
- Nonpalpable pulses.
- Smoking is commonly associated with this problem.

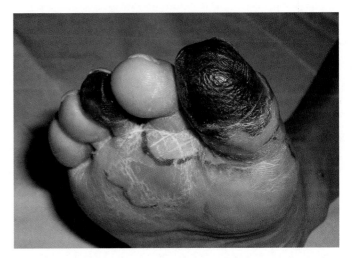

FIGURE 206-1 Dry gangrene of the first and third toes in a 36-year-old woman with poorly controlled diabetes demonstrating the typical demarcation of the necrotic eschar from the normal tissue. (*Courtesy of Richard P. Usatine, MD.*)

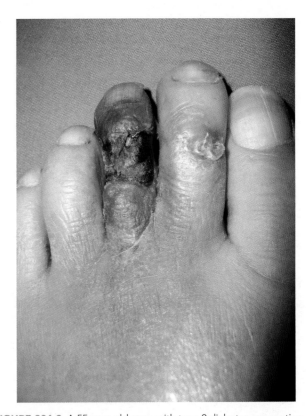

FIGURE 206-2 A 55-year-old man, with type 2 diabetes, presenting with dry gangrene of the third toe. Note a visible line of demarcation between the gangrene and normal tissue. The dry, black eschar is more distal than proximal. (*Courtesy of Javier La Fontaine, DPM.*)

- Associated trophic skin changes (e.g., absent pedal hair and thin shiny skin).

IMAGING

- Even in the presence of a palpable pulse, noninvasive studies (e.g., arterial Doppler and pulse volume recordings) are important for baseline assessment of the patient's blood flow.
- Angiogram is required to evaluate the possibility of revascularization.
- Radiographs may be necessary to rule out osteomyelitis.

DIFFERENTIAL DIAGNOSIS

- Wet Gangrene is an acute, urgent problem that is a caused by a severe infection in the dysvascular foot (**Figure 206-3**). Wet gangrene usually presents with cyanosis, purulence, foul odor, and systemic signs and symptoms of infection.
- Ischemic ulcer is an actual foot ulcer that usually presents with a pink to grey wound base (see Chapter 203, Ischemic Ulcer).

MANAGEMENT

- Vascular surgery consult is imperative.
- It is important to rule out wet gangrene. Wet gangrene is an emergent infectious process in combination with severe ischemia. Therefore, immediate debridement of infected tissue is required with antibiotics.
- Avoid amputation or debridement until optimization of blood flow occurs. This may require a vascular bypass procedure and/or interventional radiology for percutaneous angioplasty and STENT placement.
- Antibiotics are not indicated for dry gangrene unless infection is suspected.

PATIENT EDUCATION

- Avoid trauma to the amputated site.
- Advise and assist patients to stop smoking to help the wound heal and prolong the survival of the revascularization procedure.

FOLLOW-UP

- Closely monitor the patient for new gangrene or ulcers every 3 to 4 months once healing is accomplished.

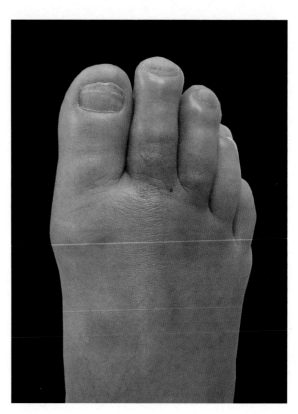

FIGURE 206-3 A 53-year-old diabetic man with wet gangrene of the second and third toes of the right foot. This diagnosis should always be considered when evaluating the ischemic limb. Wet gangrene is an emergency caused by an infectious process with severe ischemia. (*Courtesy of Javier La Fontaine, DPM.*)

REFERENCES

1. American Diabetes Association Guidelines. Preventive foot care in people with diabetes. *Diabetes Care*. 2000;23(Suppl 1):S55–S56.

2. Sykes MT, Godsey JB. Vascular evaluation of the problem diabetic foot. *Clin Podiatr Med Surg*. 1998;15(1):49–82.

3. La Fontaine J, Allen M, Davis C, Harkless LB, Shireman PK. Current concepts in diabetic microvascular dysfunction. *JAPMA*. 2006;96(3):245–252.

4. Tooke JE. A pathophysiological framework for the pathogenesis of diabetic microangiopathy. In: Tooke JE ed. *Diabetic Angiopathy*. New York: Oxford University Press, 1999:187.

PART 15

INFECTIOUS DISEASES

207 INTESTINAL WORMS AND PARASITES

Heidi Chumley, MD

PATIENT STORY

A parent brings in a 4-year-old boy suffering with anal itching. On examination the physician finds several excoriations around the anus and suspects pinworms. The physician then applies scotch tape to the perianal area and places the tape on a glass slide. Review of the slide demonstrates adult worms and ova of *Enterobius vermicularis* (pinworms) (**Figure 207-1**). The boy is treated with a single dose of chewable mebendazole and his symptoms resolve. The parent is told to repeat the mebendazole dose in 2 weeks to increase the long-term cure rate. If the scotch tape test were negative, the physician could choose to treat empirically since mebendazole is a very safe medication. Another option is to test again having the parent apply the scotch tape to the boy's perianal area first in the morning and bring that back to the office (the yield is higher in the morning).

EPIDEMIOLOGY

- Nematoda is the phylum that contains pinworms, hookworms, *Ascaris*, *Strongyloides*, and whipworms.
  - *E. vermicularis* (pinworm) is the most prevalent nematode in the United States. Two hundred and nine million persons and more than 30% of children in the world are infected[1] (**Figure 207-1**).
  - *Necator americanus* (hookworm) is found in the Americas and Caribbean and is the second most common nematode identified in stool studies in the United States[2] (**Figures 207-2** and **207-3**). *A. duodenale* (hookworm) is found mostly in Europe, Africa, China, Japan, India, and the Pacific islands.
  - *Ascaris lumbricoides* is the largest and most common human roundworm in the world, although less common in the United States, seen mostly in the rural southeast. It is found in tropical and subtropical areas including the southeastern rural United States (**Figures 207-4** and **207-5**).
  - *Strongyloides stercoralis* is seen mostly in tropical and subtropical areas, but cases also occur in temperate areas (including the south of the United States) (**Figure 207-6**). It is more frequently found in rural areas, institutional settings, and lower socioeconomic groups.
  - *Trichuris trichiura* (whipworm) is the third most common roundworm of humans, worldwide, with infections more frequent in areas with tropical weather and poor sanitation practices, and among children (**Figure 207-7**). It is estimated that 800 million people are infected worldwide. Trichuriasis occurs in the southern United States.[3]
- Cestodes (tapeworm) is a class in the phylum Platyhelminthes that contains *Taenia solium* (pork tapeworm).
  - *T. solium* is found worldwide.
  - It requires an environment where pigs and humans live in close proximity.

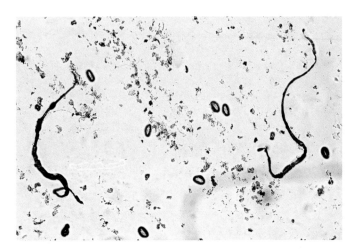

FIGURE 207-1 *Enterobius vermicularis* (pinworms and ova) seen under the microscope from a scotch tape specimen taken of the perianal region of a 4-year-old boy with anal itching. (*Courtesy of James L. Fishback, MD.*)

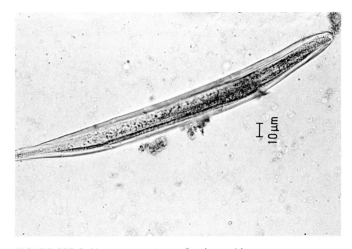

FIGURE 207-2 *Necator americanus* (hookworm) larvae can penetrate the skin, travel through veins to the heart then lungs, climb the bronchial tree to the pharynx, are swallowed, and attach to intestine walls. (*Courtesy of James L. Fishback, MD.*)

- Protozoa is the kingdom of one-celled organisms that includes *Giardia lamblia* and *E. histolytica.*
  - *G. lamblia* is the most common parasite infection worldwide and the second most common in the United States (after pinworm), causing 2.5 million infections annually (**Figure 207-8**).[4]
  - *E. histolytica* is seen worldwide, with higher incidence in developing countries. In the United States, risk groups include gay men travelers and recent immigrants, and institutionalized populations.

ETIOLOGY AND PATHOPHYSIOLOGY

- Nematodes (roundworms).
  - *E. vermicularis* (pinworm) (**Figure 207-1**) are acquired through an oral route when hands that have contacted contaminated objects are placed in the mouth. This can happen when kids play together in a sand box.
  - *N. americanus* (hookworm) (**Figure 207-2**) larvae penetrate the skin, travel through veins to the heart and then to the lungs, climb the bronchial tree to the pharynx, and then are swallowed and attach to intestine walls (**Figure 207-3**).
  - When fertilized eggs of *A. lumbricoides'* (**Figure 207-4**) are ingested, these enter the circulation through intestinal mucosa, travel to the lungs, climb to the pharynx, then are swallowed, and finally live in the small intestine.
  - *S. stercoralis* larvae penetrate the skin, travel through the circulation to the lungs and are swallowed, and travel to the small intestine (**Figure 207-6**).
  - *T. trichiura* (whipworm) (**Figure 207-7**) eggs are ingested and hatch in the small intestine; worms live in the cecum or colon.
- Cestodes (tapeworms): *T. solium* is acquired by ingesting undercooked contaminated pork. *Diphyllobothrium latum* is the fish tapeworm that is acquired by ingesting uncooked contaminated fresh-water fish.
- Protozoa.
  - *G. lamblia* cysts are ingested from contaminated water, food, or fomites and travel to the small intestine (**Figure 207-8**).
  - *E. histolytica* cysts or trophozoites are ingested from fecally contaminated food, water, or hands or from fecal contact during sexual practices; these then travel to the large intestine, where these either remain or travel through the bloodstream to the brain, liver, or lungs.

DIAGNOSIS

CLINICAL FEATURES

- Nematodes.
  - *E. vermicularis* (pinworm)—perianal pruritus, irritability (in infants) but can be asymptomatic.
  - *N. americanus* (hookworm)—can present with iron-deficiency anemia.
  - *T. trichiura* (whipworm)—frequently asymptomatic; high number of worms can cause abdominal pain or intestinal obstruction, cough, shortness of breath, or hemoptysis when in the lungs.
  - *S. stercoralis*—frequently asymptomatic; eosinophilia; may cause abdominal pain or diarrhea, cough, shortness of breath, or hemoptysis when in the lungs; can disseminate in immunocompromised

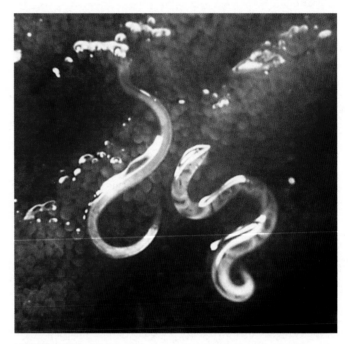

FIGURE 207-3 Adult hookworm attached to the intestinal wall. (*Courtesy of CDC.*)

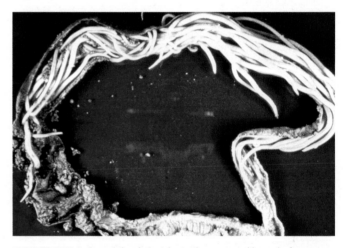

FIGURE 207-4 *Ascaris lumbricoides* in the resected bowel of a patient with bowel obstruction. (*Courtesy of James L. Fishback, MD.*)

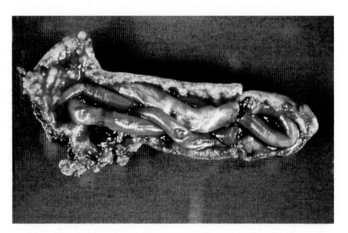

FIGURE 207-5 *Ascaris lumbricoides* in the appendix after being removed from a young adult with acute appendicitis. (*Courtesy of James L. Fishback, MD.*)

causing abdominal pain, distention, septicemia, shock, or death.

◦ *T. trichiura* (whipworm)—frequently asymptomatic; large infections can cause abdominal pain, diarrhea, or rectal prolapse.

• Cestodes: *T. solium*—frequently asymptomatic; risk of developing cysticercosis with symptoms based on location of cysts in brain (e.g. seizures, focal neurological signs, and death), eyes, heart, or spine.

• Protozoa.

◦ *G. lamblia*—diarrhea, nausea, emesis, abdominal bloating occurs 1 to 14 days after ingestion, and can be asymptomatic.

◦ *E. histolytica*—asymptomatic, intestinal symptoms (e.g., colitis and appendicitis), or extraintestinal (e.g., abscess in the liver or lungs, peritonitis, and skin or genital lesions).

LABORATORY STUDIES

• Nematodes.

◦ *E. vermicularis* (pinworm)—microscopic identification of eggs (**Figure 207-1**) collected from perianal area; apply transparent adhesive tape to the unwashed perianal area at the time of presentation or in the morning and then place tape on slide.

◦ *N. americanus* (hookworm)—microscopic identification of eggs in the stool (**Figure 207-2**).

◦ *A. lumbricoides*—microscopic identification of eggs in the stool.

◦ *S. stercoralis*—microscopic identification of larvae in stool (**Figure 207-6**) or duodenal fluid; often requires several samples. Immunologic tests are useful when infection is suspected, but larvae are not seen in several samples. Immunologic tests do not differentiate from past or present infections.

◦ *T. trichiura* (whipworm)—microscopic identification of eggs in stool (**Figure 207-7**).

• Cestodes: *T. solium*—microscopic identification of eggs or proglottids in stool; cysticercus from tissue samples; serologic evaluation may be helpful.

• Protozoa.

◦ *G. lamblia*—microscopic identification of cysts or trophozoites in stool or trophozoites in duodenal fluid or biopsy (**Figure 207-8**). Antigen tests and immunofluorescence are available.

◦ *E. histolytica*—microscopic identification of cysts or trophozoites in stool (difficult to distinguish from nonpathogens). Antibody or antigen detection or molecular tests (PCR) are also available.

DIFFERENTIAL DIAGNOSIS

• Abdominal symptoms seen with several intestinal parasites can also be caused by the following:

◦ Viral or bacterial infections—may present with acute onset of emesis and diarrhea often with fever.

◦ Irritable bowel disease—chronic symptoms of abdominal cramping with diarrhea or loose stools and/or constipation; usually no bloody stools, weight loss, or anemia.

◦ Inflammatory bowel disease—intermittent abdominal pain and bloody stools; diagnosis confirmed by colonoscopy with biopsy.

• Iron-deficiency anemia seen with hookworms can be seen with blood loss from any site from one of many causes. Of course, iron

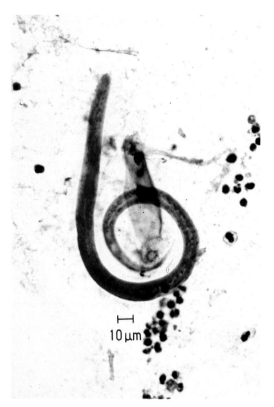

FIGURE 207-6 *Strongyloides stercoralis* ova and parasite in stool. (*Courtesy of James L. Fishback, MD.*)

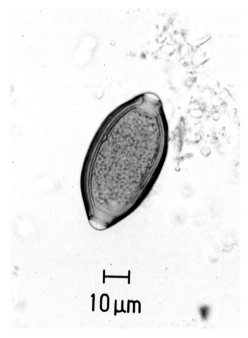

FIGURE 207-7 *Trichuris trichiura* (whipworm) egg in stool. (*Courtesy of James L. Fishback, MD.*)

deficiency can be seen with a diet deficient in iron without having hookworms.

- Gastrointestinal blood loss can be seen with other infections or inflammation, polyps, or masses.

MANAGEMENT

All medication doses are from The Medical Letter[5] and apply to adults and children unless specified.

- Nematodes.
  - *E. vermicularis* (pinworm)—pyrantel pamoate 11 mg/kg once (maximum 1 g), repeat in 2 weeks; or mebendazole 100 mg once, repeat in 2 weeks.
  - *N. americanus* (hookworm)—albendazole 400 mg once; or mebendazole 100 mg twice a day for 3 days 500 mg once or pyrantel pamoate 11 mg/kg (max 1 g) for 3 days.
  - *A. lumbricoides*—albendazole 400 mg once; alternate therapy mebendazole 500 mg once.
  - *S. stercoralis*—ivermectin 200 mcg/kg/d for 2 days; alternate therapy albendazole 400 mg bid for 7 days.
  - *T. trichiura* (whipworm)—mebendazole 100 mg twice a day for 3 days or 500 mg once; alternate therapy albendazole 400 mg once a day for 3 days.
- Cestodes: *T. solinum*—praziquantel 5 to 10 mg/kg once for intestinal stage; brain cysts require seizure prophylaxis and steroids; ophthalmologic examination for eye cysts is recommended.
- Protozoa.
  - *G. lamblia*—metronidazole 250 mg tid for 5–7 days (adults), 15 mg/kg/day divided tid for 5–7 days (children), or tinidazole 2 g once (adults), 50 mg/kg (maximum 2 g) once (children).
  - *E. histolytica*—metronidazole 500–750 tid for 7 to 10 days (adults), 35–50 mg/kg/d divided in three doses for 7 to 10 days (children).

PATIENT EDUCATION

Most intestinal parasites are asymptomatic and easily treatable. Avoid infecting others with good hygiene, including hand washing.

PATIENT RESOURCES

The Center for Disease Control division of parasitic diseases has public information on many parasitic diseases and can be found at www.cdc.gov. Current site is **http://www.cdc.gov/ncidod/dpd/**.

PROVIDER RESOURCES

Information about many parasitic infections can be found through the Center for Disease Control at www.cdc.gov. Current site is **http://www.cdc.gov/ncidod/dpd/**.

The Medical Letter including drugs for parasitic infections is available online at www.medletter.com. The exact URL is **http://www.medletter.com/freedocs/parasitic.pdf**. You will need to register to get it free.

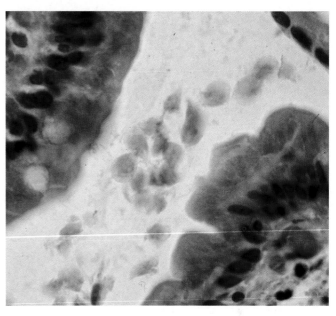

FIGURE 207-8 *Giardia lamblia* in a duodenal biopsy obtained by EGD in a patient with typical symptoms of chronic giardiasis (excessive flatulence and sulfurous belching) that failed to improve on metronidazole. (*Courtesy of Tom Moore, MD.*)

REFERENCES

1. Pinworms. Center for Disease Control, Division of Parasitic Diseases, Professional Information http://www.cdc.gov/ncidod/dpd/professional/default.htm. Accessed September 26, 2007.

2. Hookworm. Center for Disease Control, Division of Parasitic Diseases, Professional Information http://www.cdc.gov/ncidod/dpd/professional/default.htm. Accessed September 26, 2007.

3. Trichuriasis. Center for Disease Control, Division of Parasitic Diseases, Professional Information http://www.cdc.gov/ncidod/dpd/professional/default.htm. Accessed September 26, 2007.

4. Giardiasis. Center for Disease Control, Division of Parasitic Diseases, Professional Information http://www.cdc.gov/ncidod/dpd/professional/default.htm. Accessed September 26, 2007.

5. Drugs for parasitic infections. Treatment Guidelines from The Medical Letter. Vol. 5 (Suppl). 2007, e1–e14.

208 GONOCOCCAL URETHRITIS

Heidi Chumley, MD

PATIENT STORY

A 24-year-old man presents to a skid row shelter clinic with 3 days of dysuria and penile discharge. A heavy purulent urethral discharge is seen (**Figure 208-1**). He admits to using crack cocaine and having multiple female sexual partners. He was diagnosed with gonococcal urethritis by clinical appearance and a urine specimen was sent for testing to confirm the gonorrhea and test for chlamydia. He was treated with 400 mg of oral cefixime for gonorrhea and 1 g of oral azithromycin for possible coexisting chlamydia. He was offered and agreed to testing for other sexually transmitted diseases. He was told to inform his partners of the diagnosis. He was counseled about safe sex, and drug rehabilitation was recommended. On his 1-week follow-up visit, his symptoms were gone and he had no further discharge. His gonorrhea nucleic acid amplification test was positive and his chlamydia, RPR, and HIV tests were negative. His case was reported to the Health Department for contact tracing.

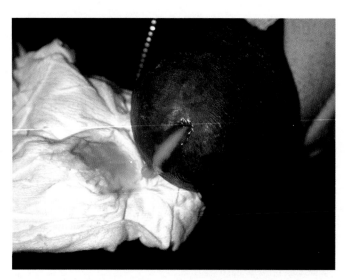

FIGURE 208-1 A 24-year-old man with gonococcal urethritis and a heavy purulent urethral discharge. (*Courtesy of Richard P. Usatine, MD.*)

EPIDEMIOLOGY

- Worldwide, 151 million cases of gonococcal and nongonococcal urethritis are reported annually (**Figures 208-1** and **208-2**).[1]
- Urethritis of all types occurs in 4 million Americans each year.[1]
- The CDC reports 161.1 chlamydia cases and 111.5 gonorrhea cases per 100,000 men.[2]
- The incidence of reported chlamydia in men rose 43% between 2001 and 2005, thought to be caused by increased ease of detection through urine tests.[2]
- Both gonococcal and chlamydial urethritis are probably significantly underreported.

ETIOLOGY AND PATHOPHYSIOLOGY

- Urethritis is urethral inflammation because of infectious or noninfectious causes.
- *Neisseria gonorrhoeae* and *Chlamydia trachomatis* are the most important infectious causes. When transmitted, they can cause other illnesses and complications in men (epididymitis, prostatitis, and Reiter's syndrome) and women (pelvic inflammatory disease and infertility).
- Other infectious agents include *Mycoplasma genitalium*, *Ureaplasma urealyticum*, *Trichomonas vaginalis*, herpes simplex virus 1 and 2, adenovirus, and enteric bacteria.
- Noninfectious causes include trauma, foreign bodies, granulomas or unusual tumors, allergic reactions, or voiding dysfunction (any

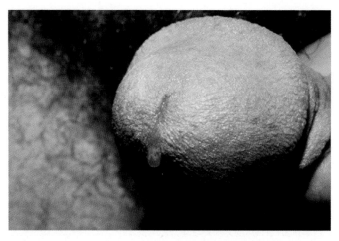

FIGURE 208-2 Nongonococcal urethritis caused by chlamydia. Note the discharge is more clear and less purulent than seen with gonorrhea. (*Courtesy of University of Washington STD/HIV Prevention Training Center.*)

abnormal holding or voiding pattern not caused by an anatomical or a neurological process).

DIAGNOSIS

CLINICAL FEATURES

Male patients with urethritis can be asymptomatic or present with urethral discharge, dysuria, or urethral pruritus.

- Urethritis is diagnosed when one of the following is present:[3]
  - Mucopurulent or purulent discharge (**Figures 208-1** and **208-2**).
  - Gram stain of urethral secretions with ≥5 WBC per oil immersion field. (If Gram-negative intracellular diplococci are seen, gonococcal urethritis is present.)
  - First-void urine with positive leukocyte esterase test or ≥10 WBC per high-power field. (This can also be seen with a urinary tract infection; however, the incidence of UTI in men less than 50 years of age is approximately 50 per 100,000 per year, much lower than the incidence of gonococcal or chlamydial urethritis in this age group.)

LABORATORY STUDIES

- Nucleic acid amplification test (NAAT) is the recommended test for screening asymptomatic at-risk men and testing symptomatic men.[3] Urine is a better specimen than urethral swab and does not hurt.[3,4]
- Gram stain will identify most cases; ≥5 WBCs are seen in 82% of *Chlamydia* and 94% of gonococcal infections.[5] Government regulations concerning in-office laboratory testing have severely curtailed the use of Gram stains in the office.
- Leukocyte esterase test on urine has a good negative predictive value but poor positive predictive value in low prevalence population (NPV 96.4% and PPV 35.4%).[6]
- Urethral culture is less commonly necessary when NAAT is available. Consider culture when tests for gonorrhea and chlamydia are negative, or symptoms persist despite adequate treatment in a patient who is unlikely to have been reinfected by an untreated partner.

DIFFERENTIAL DIAGNOSIS

Dysuria in men can be caused by the following:[7]

- Infections in other sites or the urogenital tract: cystitis, prostatitis with perineal pain or prostate tenderness, or epididymitis with scrotal pain.
- Penile lesions: vesicles of herpes simplex, ulcers of syphilis, chancroid, or lymphogranuloma venereum, and glans irritation from balanitis.
- Mechanical causes: obstruction from BPH causing inflammation without infection, trauma including catheterization, urethral strictures, or genitourinary cancers.
- Inflammatory conditions: spondyloarthropathies, drug reactions, or autoimmune diseases.

MANAGEMENT

- Consider screening the following groups of men for *Chlamydia*, using urine specimen:[3]
  - Men attending an STD clinic.
  - Men attending a national job training program.
  - Men less than 30 years of age who are military recruits.
  - Men less than 30 years of age entering jail.
- Use nucleic acid amplification test for testing and screening.[3] Twelve percent of male patients with chlamydial and 5% with gonococcal infections had no Gram stain evidence of urethral inflammation.[5]
- In patients with dysuria who do not meet criteria for urethritis, test for *N. gonorrhoeae* and *C. trachomatis*; treat if positive and advise sex partners to be evaluated and treated.[2]
- Treat uncomplicated gonococcal urethritis with ceftriaxone 125 mg IM in a single dose or cefixime 400 mg orally in a single dose plus treatment for chlamydia unless ruled out. Avoid fluoroquinolones as drug resistance is too high.[2]
- Treat chlamydia with azithromycin 1 g orally in a single dose or doxycycline 100 mg orally twice a day for 7 days. Acceptable alternate regimens include:
  - Erythromycin base 500 mg four times a day for 7 days or erythromycin ethylsuccinate 800 mg four times a day for 7 days or ofloxacin 300 mg orally twice a day for 7 days or levofloxacin 500 mg orally once daily for 7 days.[2]
- For persistent infection, consider trichomonas vaginalis—culture and treat with metronidazole 2 g single dose.

Consider expedited partner therapy (EPT). EPT is the delivery of medications or prescriptions by persons infected with an STD to their sex partners without clinical assessment of the partners. Legal status by state is available at http://www.cdc.gov/std/ept/legal/default.htm.

PATIENT EDUCATION

The CDC recommends the following for patients diagnosed with gonorrhea or chlamydia:[2]

- Return for evaluation if the symptoms persist or return after therapy is completed.
- Abstain from sexual intercourse until 7 days after starting therapy, symptoms have resolved, and sexual partners have been adequately treated.
- Undergo testing for other STDs including HIV and syphilis.
- Advise sexual partners of the need for treatment and/or take medications directly to them using expedited partner therapy.

FOLLOW-UP

- Reevaluate patients with persistent or recurrent symptoms after treatment. Reexamine for evidence of urethral inflammation and retest for gonorrhea and/or chlamydia.

- Consider chronic prostatitis if symptoms persist for more than 3 months.

PATIENT RESOURCES

The Center for Disease Control has a website at **www.cdc.gov** with CDC fact sheets on sexually transmitted diseases including gonorrhea (**http://www.cdc.gov/std/Gonorrhea/ STDFact-gonorrhea.htm**) and *Chlamydia* (**http://www.cdc.gov/std/chlamydia/STDFact-Chlamydia.htm**), available in English and Spanish.

PROVIDER RESOURCES

The Center for Disease Control has a website at **http://www. cdc.gov/std/default.htm** with the latest epidemiological data and management recommendations.

The newest CDC Treatment Guidelines are at: **http://www.cdc. gov/std/treatment/.**

REFERENCES

1. Terris MK, Sajadi KP. Urethritis from emedicine. Accessed at: http://www.emedicine.com. Accessed June 17, 2007.

2. U.S. Centers for Disease Control and Prevention Division of STD Prevention. Male Chlamydia Screening Consultation, Atlanta, Georgia March 28–29, 2006. Meeting Report May 22, 2007. Available at: http://www.cdc.gov. Accessed June 17, 2007.

3. U.S. Centers for Disease Control and Prevention. http://www. cdc.gov.Accessed June 17, 2007.

4. Sugunendran H, Birley HD, Mallinson H, Abbott M, Tong CY. Comparison of urine, first and second endourethral swabs for PCR based detection of genital *Chlamydia trachomatis* infection in male patients. *Sex Transm Infect.* 2001;77(6):423–426.

5. Geisler WM, Yu S, Hook EW, III. Chlamydial and gonococcal infection in men without polymorphonuclear leukocytes on gram stain: Implications for diagnostic approach and management. *Sex Transm Dis.* 2005;32(10):630–634.

6. Bowden FJ. Reappraising the value of urine leukocyte esterase testing in the age of nucleic acid amplification [Journal Article. Research Support, Non-U.S. Govt]. *Sex Transm Dis.* 1998;25(6): 322–326.

7. Bremnor J, Sadovsky R. Evaluation of dysuria in adults. *Am Fam Physician.* 2002;65(8):1589–1596.

209 SYPHILIS

Richard P. Usatine, MD

PATIENT STORY

A 39-year-old woman presents with a nonhealing ulcer over her upper lip for 1 week and a new-onset rash on her trunk (**Figures 209-1 and 209-2**). The ulcer on her upper lip was misdiagnosed as herpes simplex by the previous physician. Sexual history revealed that the patient had oral sex with a boyfriend who had a lesion on his penis and she suspected that he had been having sex with other women. The examining physician recognized the nonpainful ulcer and rash as a combination of primary and secondary (P&S) syphilis. An RPR was drawn and the patient was treated immediately with IM benzathine penicillin. The RPR came back as 1:128 and the ulcer was healed within 1 week.

EPIDEMIOLOGY

- The rate of P&S syphilis increased between 2001 and 2006. Overall increases in rates between 2001 and 2006 were observed primarily among men (from 3.0 cases per 100,000 population to 5.7 cases per 100,000 population). The rate of P&S syphilis among women increased from 0.8 cases per 100,000 population in 2004 to 1.0 case per 100,000 population in 2006.[1]

- Increases in cases among men who have sex with men (MSM) have occurred and have been characterized by high rates of HIV co-infection and high-risk sexual behavior.

- The estimated proportion of P&S syphilis cases attributable to MSM increased from 4% in 2000 to 62% in 2004.[1]

- The total number of cases of syphilis (all stages: P&S, early latent, late, late latent, and congenital syphilis) reported to CDC increased 11.0% (from 33,288 to 36,935) between 2005 and 2006.[1]

ETIOLOGY AND PATHOPHYSIOLOGY

- Syphilis is caused by the spirochete *Treponema pallidum*.
- It is transmitted sexually and not by toilet seats.

DIAGNOSIS

CLINICAL FEATURES

Primary syphilis is associated with a chancre—usually a nonpainful ulcer. (**Figures 209-1, 209-3, and 209-4**). The presence of pain does not rule out syphilis, and the patient with a painful genital ulcer should be tested for syphilis as well as herpes.

Secondary syphilis occurs when the spirochetes become systemic and may present as a rash with protean morphologies, condyloma lata, and/or mucus patches (**Figures 209-2, 209-5 to 209-11**).

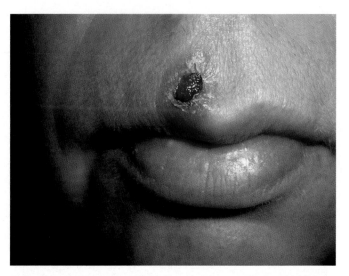

FIGURE 209-1 Primary syphilis with a chancre over the lip of a woman. (*Courtesy of Richard P. Usatine, MD.*)

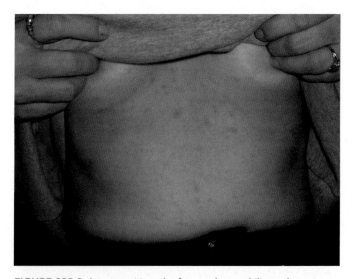

FIGURE 209-2 A nonpruritic rash of secondary syphilis on the abdomen of the patient shown in Figure 209-1. (*Courtesy of Richard P. Usatine, MD.*)

Tertiary syphilis may be visualized with gummas on the skin, but many of the manifestations are internal such as the cardiac and neurological diseases that occur (e.g., aortitis, tabes dorsalis, and iritis) **Figure 209-12** shows a gumma of the scrotum.

TYPICAL DISTRIBUTION

Primary syphilis is usually a single ulcer (chancre) that is not painful in the genital region (**Figures 209-3** and **209-4**). A chancre can be seen on the lip (**Figure 209-1**).

Secondary syphilis may present with the various eruptions are found on the trunk, palms, and soles (**Figures 209-2, 209-5, 209-6,** and **209-8**).

Mucus patches are on the genitals or in the mouth (**Figures 209-7, 209-9,** and **209-10**).

LABORATORY STUDIES

The VDRL and RPR are nontreponemal tests that measure anticardiolipin antibodies. Confirmatory tests measure antibodies to *T. pallidum* and include the FTA-ABS and the MHA-TP. The MHA-TP test is easier to do and interpret because the agglutination can be seen with the naked eye (**Figure 209-13**). The FTA-ABS test requires the use of a fluorescent microscope.

Dark-field microscopy is useful in evaluating moist cutaneous lesions, such as chancre, mucus patches, and condyloma lata (**Figure 209-14**). When dark-field microscopy is not available, direct immunofluorescence staining of fixed smears (direct fluorescent antibody *T. pallidum* [DFA-TP]) is an option. Both procedures detect *T. pallidum* at a rate of approximately 85% to 92%.[2]

DIFFERENTIAL DIAGNOSIS

- Herpes simplex—most common cause of genital ulcers in the United States. These ulcers are painful and often start as vesicles (see Chapter 123, Herpes Simplex).
- Chancroid—painful beefy red ulcers on the penis or vulva, less common than syphilis. Chancroid is also known to cause large painful inguinal adenopathy (bubo) (**Figures 209-15** and **209-16**).
- Drug eruptions—can be on the genital area such as seen in a fixed drug eruption (see Chapter 196, Cutaneous Drug Reactions).
- Erythema multiforme—can look like the rash of secondary syphilis but may have target lesions (see Chapter 170, Erythema Multiforme, Stevens-Johnson Syndrome and Toxic Epidermal Necrolysis).
- Pityriasis rosea—a self-limited cutaneous drug eruption that often begins with a herald patch and may have a Christmas tree distribution on the back (see Chapter 146, Pityriasis Rosea).

MANAGEMENT

Primary, secondary, and early latent:

- Benzathine penicillin G, 2.4 million units IM[3] SOR Ⓐ Penicillin allergy[3] SOR Ⓑ

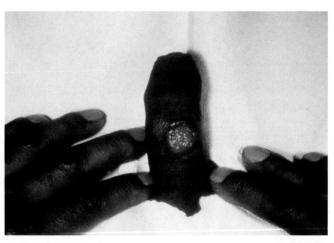

FIGURE 209-3 A painless chancre at the location of treponemal entry. (*Courtesy of the Public Health Image Library, CDC.*)

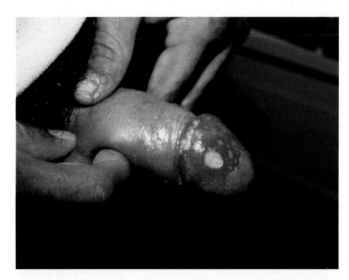

FIGURE 209-4 Primary syphilis with a large chancre on the glands of the penis. The multiple small surrounding ulcers are part of the syphilis and not a second disease. (*Courtesy of Richard P. Usatine, MD.*)

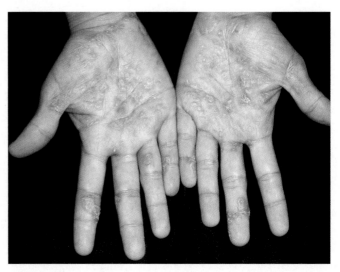

FIGURE 209-5 Papular squamous eruption on the hands of a woman with secondary syphilis. (*Courtesy of Richard P. Usatine, MD.*)

- Doxycycline 100 mg twice daily × 14 days or

- Ceftriaxone 1 g IM/IV daily × 8 to 10 days (limited studies) or

- Azithromycin 2 g single oral dose (preliminary data)

For the management of congenital, latent, tertiary and neurosyphilis, see the Sexually Transmitted Diseases Treatment Guidelines published by the CDC in 2006: http://www.cdc.gov/std/treatment/2006/genital-ulcers.htm#genulc6.

PATIENT EDUCATION

This is a teachable moment to reinforce the importance of safe sex. The IM benzathine penicillin shot is a painful shot in the buttocks, and most patients will not want to repeat this. Condoms can prevent the spread of syphilis. Patients should be advised to get HIV testing and need to know that syphilis is a risk factor for the spread of HIV.

FOLLOW-UP

Reexamine clinically and serologically at 6 and 12 months. Consider treatment failure if signs/symptoms persist or RPR test titer does not decline fourfold within 6 months after therapy. For treatment failures: perform an HIV test along with a lumbar puncture for CSF analysis. If the CSF is positive for neurosyphilis or HIV test is positive treat according to recommendations for these special circumstances. Otherwise, most expert would recommend 2.4 million units of benzathine penicillin IM weekly × 3 wks.[3] SOR **C**

PROVIDER RESOURCE(S)

Sexually Transmitted Diseases Treatment Guidelines published by the CDC in 2006. **http://www.cdc.gov/std/treatment/2006/genital-ulcers.htm#genulc6.**

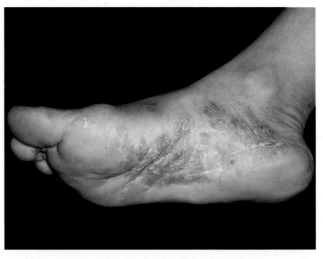

FIGURE 209-6 Papular squamous eruption on the foot of the woman, in **Figure 209-5**, with secondary syphilis. (*Courtesy of Richard P. Usatine, MD.*)

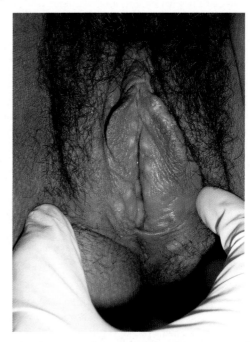

FIGURE 209-7 Mucus patches on the labia of the woman in **Figure 209-5**, with secondary syphilis teeming with spirochetes. (*Courtesy of Richard P. Usatine, MD.*)

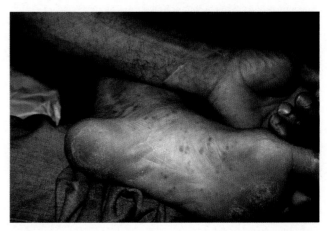

FIGURE 209-8 Pink macules on the feet and wrists of a man with secondary syphilis. (*Courtesy of Richard P. Usatine, MD.*)

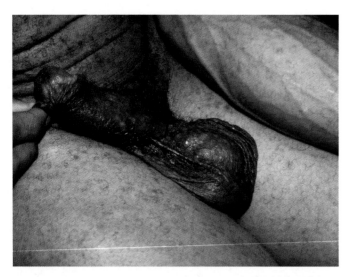

FIGURE 209-9 Mucus patches on the penis and scrotum of the same man with secondary syphilis. (*Courtesy of Richard P. Usatine, MD.*)

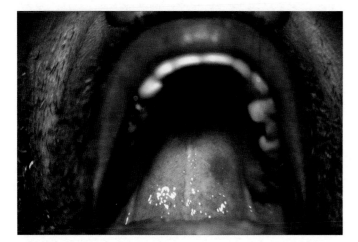

FIGURE 209-10 Oral lesion on the palate of the same man with secondary syphilis. (*Courtesy of Richard P. Usatine, MD.*)

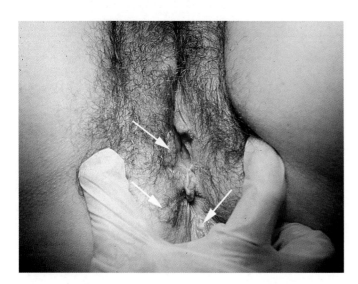

FIGURE 209-11 Condylomata lata (arrows) on the vulva of a woman with secondary syphilis. (*Courtesy of Richard P. Usatine, MD.*)

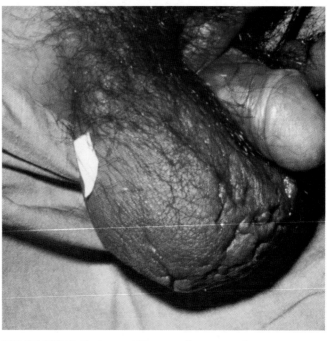

FIGURE 209-12 Tertiary syphilis presenting as a swollen scrotum, which was diagnosed as a syphilitic gumma of the testicle. (*Courtesy of the Public Health Image Library, CDC.*)

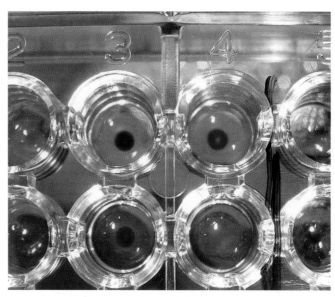

FIGURE 209-13 Microhemagglutination (MHA-TP) test for antibodies to *T. pallidum*. (*Courtesy of Richard P. Usatine, MD.*)

REFERENCES

1. http://www.cdc.gov/std/stats/syphilis.htm. Accessed April 30, 2008.

2. http://www.emedicine.com/ topic=413. Accessed February 19, 2006.

3. Sexually Transmitted Diseases Treatment Guidelines, CDC, 2006. http://www.cdc.gov/std/treatment/2006/genital-ulcers.htm#genulc6. Accessed November 25, 2006.

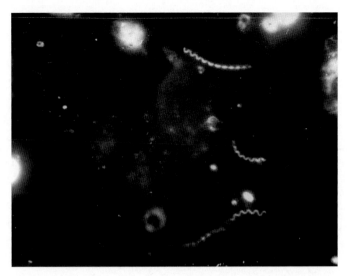

FIGURE 209-14 Live spirochetes of *T. pallidum* seen in a darkfield preparation. (*Courtesy of the Public Health Image Library, CDC.*)

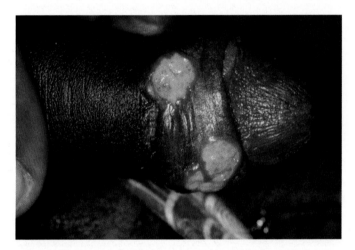

FIGURE 209-15 Culture-proven indurated beefy chancroidal ulcers in an HIV-positive man. (*Courtesy of Professor David Lewis.*)

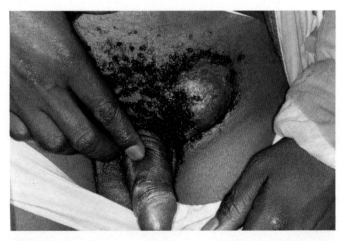

FIGURE 209-16 Left-side inguinal bubo in a patient with a culture proven chancroidal ulcer. (*Courtesy of Professor David Lewis.*)

210 KAPOSI'S SARCOMA

Heidi Chumley, MD

PATIENT STORY

A 35-year-old gay man presented with papular lesions on his elbow (**Figure 210-1**). Shave biopsy demonstrated Kaposi's sarcoma (KS). He subsequently tested positive for HIV and began treatment with antiretroviral combination therapy. The KS resolved with topical Alitretinoin gel treatment.

EPIDEMIOLOGY

- KS can be classic (older Mediterranean men), endemic (young men in sub-Saharan Africa), epidemic (AIDS patients), or post-transplant (organ recipients).[1]

- In the United States, 95% of KS is seen in patients with AIDS (**Figure 210-1**).

- 7.2/1000 person years in HIV-positive patients; 451 times higher than general population.[2]

- 1.4/1000 person years in transplant patients; 128 times higher than general population.[2]

- The prevalence of classic KS in the general population of southern Italy is 2.5/100,00[3] (**Figure 210-2**).

- Male to female ratio for epidemic KS in the United States is approximately 50:1. Male-to-female ratio has been approximately 10:1 for classic and endemic KS but is falling as the prevalence of AIDS increases among women.[4]

- Nearly all patients with KS have antihuman herpes virus antibodies (HHV8). The prevalence of these antibodies varies by geographic region but is less than 5% in the general population of the United States.[1]

- KS is the most common malignancy seen in AIDS patients.

ETIOLOGY AND PATHOPHYSIOLOGY

- KS is an angioproliferative disease, with abnormal proliferation of endothelial cells, myofibroblasts, and monocyte cells.

- Human herpes virus 8 produces a receptor that promotes endothelial cell proliferation.

- Lesions often begin as patches and progress to plaques as proliferation continues.

- Some lesions ulcerate (nodular stage), and lymphedema can occur.

DIAGNOSIS

The diagnosis is often made clinically in a patient who has AIDS and a typical presentation of KS. In atypical presentations, diagnosis is made by biopsy.

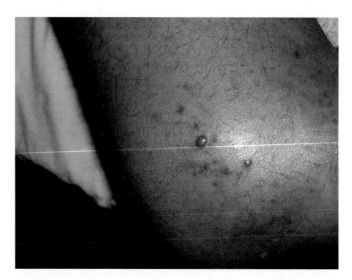

FIGURE 210-1 Several reddish-purple papular lesions of Kaposi's sarcoma on the elbow of a man with HIV/AIDS. (*Courtesy of Heather Goff, MD.*)

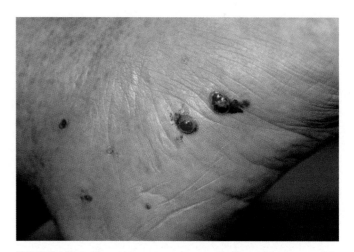

FIGURE 210-2 Classic Kaposi's sarcoma on the foot of an 88-year-old Italian man who does not have HIV/AIDS. These painful purple-red "growths" were present on his left foot for several years before diagnosis. (*Courtesy of John P. Welsh, MD, and Herbert B. Allen, MD.*)

CLINICAL FEATURES

- Cutaneous lesions are usually multifocal, papular, and reddish-purple in color (**Figures 210-1** and **210-2**).
- Plaques or fungating lesions can be seen on the lower extremities including the soles of the feet (**Figure 210-3**).
- Oral cavity lesions can be flat or nodular and are red to purple in color (**Figure 210-4**).
- Gastrointestinal lesions can be asymptomatic or can cause abdominal pain, nausea, vomiting, bleeding, or weight loss.
- Pulmonary lesions can cause shortness of breath or may appear as infiltrates, nodules, or pleural effusions on chest radiographs.

TYPICAL DISTRIBUTION

AIDS-related KS[5]

- Skin lesions are seen mainly on the lower extremities, face, and genitalia. Presence of skin lesions should prompt an oral examination as oral involvement may change prognosis and management.
- Lesions in the oral cavity are common (33%), typically seen on the palate or gingiva (**Figure 210-4**).
- Gastrointestinal involvement is noted in 40% at diagnosis and up to 80% in autopsy studies. GI lesions can occur without skin lesions.
- Pulmonary involvement is also common, and up to 15% may occur without skin lesions. A chest radiograph often demonstrates pulmonary involvement.
- Any organ can be involved.

LABORATORY STUDIES

- Check an HIV test in any person with KS who is not known to be HIV positive.
- CD4+ T lymphocyte count is an important prognostic indicator.

DIFFERENTIAL DIAGNOSIS

Diagnosis often requires a biopsy as several other lesions can mimic early KS.[5]

- Purpura—bleeding under the skin caused by a variety of platelet, vascular, or coagulation disorders; usually not palpable and more widespread.
- Hematomas—localized swelling usually from a break in a blood vessel; history of trauma and usually not palpable.
- Hemangiomas angiomas—benign growths of small blood vessels that blanch with pressure (see Chapter 194, Acquired Vascular Skin Lesions).
- Dermatofibromas—small, firm, red to brown nodules made up of collagen deposit under the skin, often seen on the legs; lesions are usually small (<6 mm) and dimple downward when compressed laterally (see Chapter 153, Dermatofibroma).
- Bacillary angiomatosis—a systemic infectious disease caused by *Bartonella* species. Cutaneous lesions appear as scattered papules and nodules or an abscess. This is seen when the CD4 count is below 200 and is easily treated with antibiotics (**Figure 210-5**).

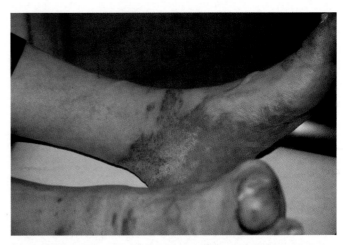

FIGURE 210-3 KS on the foot in a man with AIDS in the 1990s. Note the purple color. (*From Usatine RP, Moy RL, Tobinicak EL, Siegel DM. Skin Surgery: A Practical Guide. 1998, St. Louis: Mosby.*)

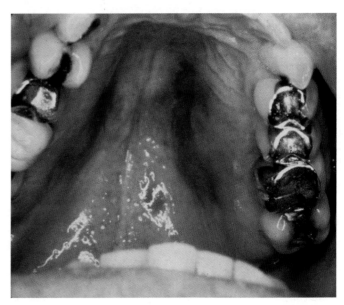

FIGURE 210-4 Early KS on the palate. The color is abnormal but the lesion is still flat. (*Courtesy of Ellen Eisenberg, DMD.*)

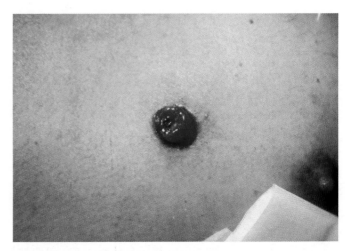

FIGURE 210-5 Cutaneous bacillary angiomatosis in a man with HIV/AIDS. (*From Usatine RP, Moy RL, Tobinicak EL, Siegel DM. Skin Surgery: A Practical Guide. 1998, St. Louis: Mosby.*)

MANAGEMENT

- KS is not curable; treatments include antiretrovirals and chemotherapeutic agents to reduce disease burden and slow progression. High dose steroids can severely aggravate KS, especially pulmonary KS.

AIDS-RELATED KS

- Treat with antiretroviral drugs or refer to a physician with experience initiating and following antiretroviral therapy. Antiretroviral therapy inhibits HIV replication, decreases the response to human herpes virus 8, and has antiangiogenic activity. SOR Ⓐ
- Consider KS-specific therapies
  - Alitretinoin gel 0.1% – patient applies gel to lesions two times a day, increasing to three to four times a day if tolerated, for 4 to 8 weeks (66% response rate).[6] SOR Ⓑ
  - Liposomal doxorubicin 20 mg/m^2 every 3 weeks or liposomal daunorubicin 40 mg/m^2 every 2 weeks (50% response rate).[7] SOR Ⓐ
  - Paclitaxel 100 mg/m^2 every 2 weeks or 135 mg/m^2 every 3 weeks, response rates 60% to 70% in patients who had failed a prior chemotherapy regiment.[8] SOR Ⓐ Premedication with dexamethasone is recommended.[8]
  - Interferon-alpha at 1 million units per day demonstrated the most benefit to patients with KS limited to the skin and CD4+ T-lymphocyte counts more than 200.[9]
  - Intralesional vinblastin (70% response rate)[10] or radiation therapy (80% response rate) are also effective for skin lesions.[11] SOR Ⓑ
- Classic and endemic KS are rare in the United States and are often treated with radiation or surgical excision.
- Removing immunosuppressants or radiation can treat transplant-related KS.

PATIENT EDUCATION

- KS is not curable, but several treatments can result in regression of the lesions for a better cosmetic result.
- KS can affect most parts of the body, commonly the skin, oral cavity, gastrointestinal tract, and lungs.
- During treatment, lesions typically flatten, shrink, and fade.
- Rarely, starting antiretroviral therapy may cause lesions to flare because of an inflammatory reaction as the immune system begins to recover.
- Patients with AIDS-related KS have 5-year survival rates more than 80% when KS is the AIDS-defining illness and the CD4+ T-lymphocyte count is more than 200. Survival rates fall to less than 10% when the patient is more than 50 years old and there is another AIDS-defining illness at the time of presentation.[12]

FOLLOW-UP

KS, particularly AIDS-related KS, is generally treated by physicians with advanced training in HIV/AIDS management and oncology. Follow-up is determined by disease progression and response to therapy.

PATIENT RESOURCES

General information in English or Spanish about the different types of KS and treatment options can be found on the National Cancer Institute website at **http://www.cancer.gov/ cancertopics/pdq/treatment/kaposis/patient/.**

PROVIDER RESOURCES

The National Cancer Institute also has general information for health professionals at **http://www.cancer.gov/cancertopics/ pdq/treatment/kaposis/HealthProfessional.**

REFERENCES

1. Alamartine E. Up-to-date epidemiological data and better treatment for Kaposi's sarcoma. *Transplantation*. 2005;80(12): 1656–1567.

2. Serraino D, Piselli P, Angeletti C, et al. Kaposi's sarcoma in transplant and HIV-infected patients: An epidemiologic study in Italy and France. *Transplantation*. 2005;80(12):1699–1704.

3. Atzori L, Fadda D, Ferreli C, et al. Classic Kaposi's sarcoma in southern Sardinia, Italy. *Br J Cancer*. 2004;91(7):1261–1262.

4. Onyango JF, Njiru A. Kaposi's sarcoma in a Nairobi hospital. *East Afr Med J*. 2004;81(3):120–123.

5. Cheung MC, Pantanowitz L, Dezube BJ. AIDS-related malignancies: emerging challenges in the era of highly active antiretroviral therapy. *Oncologist*. 2005;10(6):412–426.

6. Walmsley S, Northfelt DW, Melosky B, et al. Treatment of AIDS-related cutaneous Kaposi's sarcoma with topical alitretinoin (9-cis-retinoic acid) gel. Panretin Gel North American Study Group. *J Acquir Immune Defic Syndr*. 1999;22:235–246.

7. Cooley HD, Volberding P, Martin F, et al. Final results of a phase III randomized trial of pegylated liposomal doxorubicin versus liposomal daunorubicin in patients with AIDS-related Kaposi's sarcoma. *Proc Am Soc Clin Oncol*. 2002;21:411a; abstract 1640.

8. Gill PS, Tulpule A, Espina BM, et al. Paclitaxel is safe and effective in the treatment of advanced AIDS related Kaposi's sarcoma. *J Clin Oncol*. 1999;17:1876–1883.

9. Krown SE, Li P, Von Roenn JH, et al. Efficacy of low-dose interferon with antiretroviral therapy in Kaposi's sarcoma: a randomized phase II AIDS Clinical Trials Group study. *J Interferon Cytokine Res*. 2002;22:295–303.

10. Boudreaux AA, Smith LL, Cosby CD, et al. Intralesional vinblastine for cutaneous Kaposi's sarcoma associated with acquired immunodeficiency syndrome. A clinical trial to evaluate efficacy and discomfort associated with infection. *J Am Acad Dermatol*. 1993; 28:61–65.

11. Swift PS. The role of radiation therapy in the management of HIV-related Kaposi's sarcoma. *Hematol Oncol Clin North Am*. 1996;10:1069–1080.

12. Stebbing J, Sanitt A, Nelson M, Powles T, Gazzard B, Bower M. A prognostic index for AIDS-associated Kaposi's sarcoma in the era of highly active antiretroviral therapy. *Lancet*. 2006;367(9521): 1495–1502.

211 LYME DISEASE

Thomas J. Corson, DO
Richard P. Usatine, MD

PATIENT STORY

On a warm, summer afternoon a 32-year-old woman presents with low-grade fevers for 5 days and a rash. On physical examination, the physician notes a large, erythematous, annular patch with central clearing on her back (**Figure 211-1**). The patient states that the rash has gotten progressively larger during the last 3 days and she has had a recent onset of intermittent joint pain. She does not recall being bitten by an insect. She denies taking medications within the last month and has no known allergies. When asked about recent travel, she admits to a camping trip in eastern Massachusetts, which she returned from 4 days ago. The patient was diagnosed with Lyme borreliosis and started on doxycycline 100 mg twice daily for 14 days. She responded quickly to the antibiotics and never developed the persistent stage of Lyme disease.

EPIDEMIOLOGY

- In 1977, clusters of patients in Old Lyme, Connecticut, began reporting symptoms originally thought to be juvenile rheumatoid arthritis.[1]

- In 1981, American entomologist, Dr. Willy Burgdorfer, isolated the infectious pathogen responsible for Lyme disease from the midgut of *Ixodes scapularis* (a.k.a., black-legged deer ticks) (**Figure 211-2**), which serve as the primary transmission vector in the United States.[1]

- It was identified as a bacterial spirochete and named *Borrelia burgdorferi* in honor of its founder.

- Based on CDC data reported in 2007, Lyme disease (or Lyme borreliosis) is the most common tick-borne illness in the United States, with an overall incidence of 7.9/100,000 persons.[2]

- Patients living between Maryland and Maine accounted for 93% of all reported cases in the United States in 2005, with an overall incidence of 31.6 cases for every 100,000 persons.[2]

- Over 90% of cases report onset between April and November.[2]

ETIOLOGY AND PATHOPHYSIOLOGY

- *B. burgdorferi* begins to multiply in the midgut of *I. scapularis* ticks upon attaching to humans.

- Migration from midgut to salivary glands of ticks requires 24 to 48 hours.

- Prior to this migration host infection rarely occurs.

- Common hosts include field mice, white-tailed deer, and household pets.

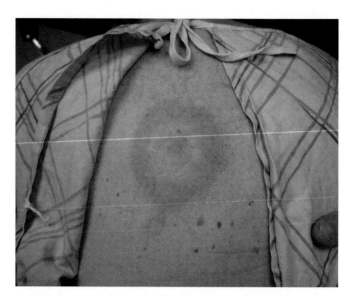

FIGURE 211-1 A 32-year-old woman presents with 5 days of low-grade fevers and the typical eruption of erythema migrans on her upper back. Note the expanding annular lesion with a target-like morphology. (*Courtesy of Thomas Corson, MD.*)

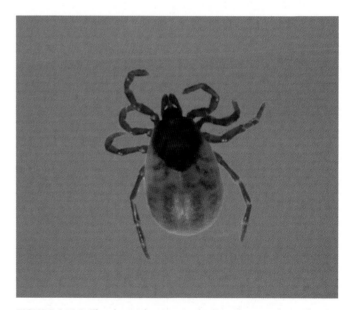

FIGURE 211-2 The deer tick transmits the *Borrelia* spirochete. This is an unengorged female black-legged deer tick. The tick is tiny and can be undetected in its unengorged state. (*Courtesy of Thomas Corson, MD.*)

- Ticks must feed on infested hosts in order to infect humans.
- Thirty percent of infected patients do not recall being bitten.[3]
- Once a human is infected, disease progression is categorized into three stages: localized, disseminated, and persistent.

DIAGNOSIS

CLINICAL FEATURES

Localized (days to weeks)

Erythema migrans (formerly known as erythema chronicum migrans)

This pathognomonic finding occurs in roughly 68% of Lyme disease cases.[3] Described as a "bull's eye" eruption (**Figures 211-1, 211-3 to 211-6**), this nonpruritic, maculopapular lesion typically occurs near the site of infection. The erythematous perimeter migrates outward over several days while the central area clears. Multiple lesions in different sites can develop in some individuals (**Figures 211-3 and 211-4**). Erythema migrans can persist for 2 to 3 weeks if left untreated.

Flu-like symptoms

Roughly 67% of patients will develop flu-like symptoms that can include fever, myalgias, and lymphadenopathy. Symptoms usually subside within 7 to 10 days.

Disseminated (days to months)

Inflammatory arthritis

Typical onset occurs around 3 to 6 months after localized infection. Patients will often present with polyarticular, migratory joint pain with or without erythema, and swelling, which is exacerbated with motion. More than 24 to 48 hours, these symptoms localize to one joint (especially knee, ankle, or wrist) and last approximately 1 week. Recurrence is common and usually happens every few months but typically resolves within 10 years even without treatment.

Cranial nerve palsy

Bell's palsy (seventh cranial nerve) is the most common neurologic manifestation of Lyme disease. However, nearly every cranial nerve has been reported to be involved. Facial nerve palsy is a lower motor neuron lesion that results in weakness of both the lower face and the forehead. Lasting up to 8 weeks, the resolution of symptoms is gradual and begins shortly after initial onset (see Chapter 222, Bell's Palsy).

Atrioventricular blockade

Present in only 1% of patients with Lyme disease, syncope, lightheadedness, and dyspnea are classic symptoms consistent with AV dysfunction.[4] However, patients can be completely asymptomatic. The degree of Lyme-associated blockade varies so that symptoms are generally episodic. Most cases resolve spontaneously within 1 week.[3] Any patient with history and/or examination findings suspicious of Lyme disease should undergo electrocardiogram testing. Hospitalization and continuous monitoring are advisable for symptomatic patients, for patients with second- or third-degree atrioventricular block, as well as for those with first-degree heart block when the PR interval is prolonged to ≥30 milliseconds, because the degree of block may fluctuate and worsen very rapidly in such patients.[5]

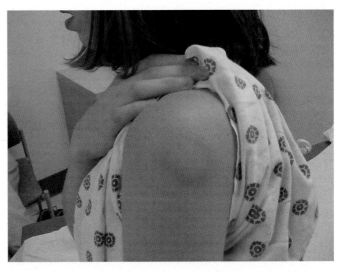

FIGURE 211-3 An 11-year-old girl with erythema migrans eruption on her shoulder. She is febrile and systemically ill. (*Courtesy of Jeremy Golding, MD.*)

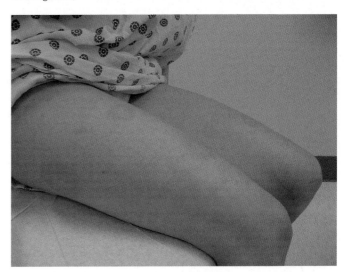

FIGURE 211-4 Same 11-year-old girl in **Figure 211-3** with multiple erythema migrans eruptions on her legs. (*Courtesy of Jeremy Golding, MD.*)

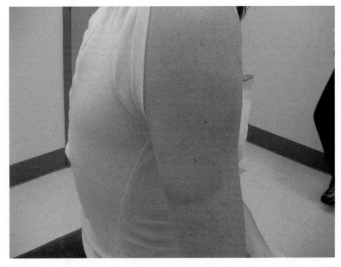

FIGURE 211-5 A 12-year-old girl with erythema migrans eruption on right arm. The annular border is somewhat raised and there is central clearing. (*Courtesy of Jeremy Golding, MD.*)

Aseptic meningitis

Patients may present with complaints similar to bacterial meningitis (photophobia, nuchal rigidity, and headache), but symptoms are generally less severe in nature. This can also occur with or without concomitant cranial nerve palsy.[3]

Fatigue

A depressed level of activity due to fatigue is one of the most common complaints affecting up to 80% of infected patients. Even after adequate treatment, symptoms consistent with chronic fatigue syndrome have developed in patients with known Lyme disease.

Persistent (>1 year)

Chronic arthritis

Generally occurs in the knee, although other sites such as the shoulder, ankle, elbow, or wrist are not uncommon. Approximately 10% of patients with intermittent arthritis will progress to this stage.[3]

Chronic fatigue

Commonly misdiagnosed as fibromyalgia or chronic fatigue syndrome, patients develop debilitating malaise and myalgias that can persist for months or years after infection.

Meningoencephalitis

Symptoms vary from mild (memory loss, mood lability, irritability, or panic attacks) to severe (manic or psychotic episodes, paranoia, and obsessive/compulsive symptoms).[5]

LABORATORY STUDIES

Diagnosing Lyme disease is generally based on pertinent history findings and/or the presence of an EM lesion, especially in endemic areas. In cases where an EM lesion is absent, serological testing may be warranted utilizing the following tests:

- ELISA (sensitivity: 94%, specificity: 97%)[6]—used as a *screening* test in patients lacking physical signs of erythema migrans. Up to 50% of patients with early infection can have false-negative result. If strong suspicion remains, convalescent titers should be obtained in 6 weeks.[6] Prior infection does not indicate immunity. Lyme titers may be falsely positive in patients with mononucleosis, periodontal disease, connective tissue disease, and other less common conditions.[7]

- Western blot (IgM and IgG for *B. burgdorferi*)—if ELISA test yields a positive result, Western blot test is used as a *confirmatory* test. IgM antibodies are detectable between 2 weeks and 6 months after inoculation. IgG may be present indefinitely after 6 weeks, despite appropriate antibiotic therapy. Once it is determined that a person is seropositive for Lyme disease, antibiotic therapy should be initiated promptly.

Empiric antibiotic therapy (no test necessary) should be considered in any of the following clinical presentations: presence of EM rash, flu-like symptoms (in absence of URI or GI symptoms) after known tick bite, Bell's palsy in endemic areas especially between June and September, or tick bites occurring during pregnancy.

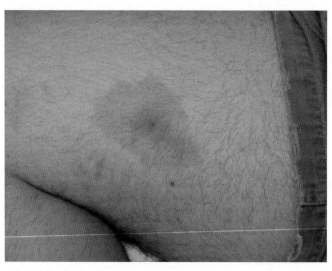

FIGURE 211-6 A 26-year-old man with erythema migrans eruption on right medial thigh. The central papule is the site of the bite, and there has not been much central clearing yet. (*Courtesy of Gil Shlamovitz, MD.*)

Characteristic laboratory findings

- CBC.
  - Leukocytosis (11,000–18,000/μL).
  - Elevated ESR (>20 mm/h).
  - Anemia and thrombocytopenia are rare.

- Liver function tests.
  - Elevated GGT and AST.

- CSF.
  - Pleocytosis and elevated protein levels if CNS is involved. Spirochete antibodies may be detectable.

- Blood culture.
  - Low yield—not recommended.

- Nerve conduction studies and EMG.
  - Useful in patients with paresthesias or radicular pain.

- EKG.
  - To detect AV block and arrhythmias.

DIFFERENTIAL DIAGNOSIS[8]

- Cellulitis—spreads more rapidly than Lyme disease, induration more common, painful and tender, and negative serologic result (see Chapter 114, Cellulitis).

- Urticaria—can resemble erythema migrans when the urticarial lesions are annular. Urticaria is generally more widespread and the wheals come and go over time whereas the lesion of EM is more fixed (see Chapter 143, Urticaria and Angioedema).

- Rocky Mountain spotted fever—associated with *Dermacentor variabilis* (American dog) tick; rash is petechial and the spots are widely distributed over the body. Patients often appear toxic. The endemic range is broader (see Chapter 172, Vasculitis).

- Cutaneous fungal infections—usually pruritic and may be annular; associated with scaling, which is not characteristic of erythema migrans; and spreads slowly if at all. The similarity is that the annular appearance of tinea corporis can mimic EM (see Chapter 132, Tinea Corporis).

- Local reaction to tick bites—tick bites may cause a local reaction in skin and do not expand with time; generally less than 2 cm in diameter, and usually papular.

- Febrile viral illnesses (particularly enteroviruses during summer)—rash, myalgias, arthralgias, and headache; gastrointestinal symptoms; sore throat and/or cough. Perform Lyme serologic test in the absence of erythema migrans.

- Facial nerve palsy—may be bilateral in Lyme disease. This is uncommon in facial nerve palsy not associated with Lyme disease (see Chapter 222, Bell's Palsy).

- Viral meningitis—lymphocytic (aseptic) meningitis caused by viral infection generally results in transient illness that resolves within several days, usually after a monophasic course.

- Heart block—idiopathic conduction system disease (sick sinus syndrome) can present with the same symptoms and signs as Lyme carditis. Use serologic testing and epidemiologic history to discriminate.

- Inflammatory arthritis (reactive arthritis, gout, pseudogout, and rheumatoid arthritis)—acute, large, joint monoarticular or oligoarticular arthritis from multiple causes; may be indistinguishable from acute arthritis associated with Lyme disease at the time of presentation; joint fluid examination, and culture and X-ray may help distinguish from Lyme arthritis (see Chapter 92, Rheumatoid Arthritis).

- Peripheral neuropathy is more often associated with diabetes mellitus, peripheral vascular disease, endocrinopathies, and nerve root impingement syndromes. If Lyme disease is the cause, the serologies should be positive.

- Radiculoneuropathy—dermatomal pain, sensory loss, and/or weakness in a limb or the trunk. Check serologies if Lyme disease is suspected.

- Encephalomyelitis—focal inflammation of the brain or spinal cord. Check serologies if Lyme disease is suspected.

TREATMENT

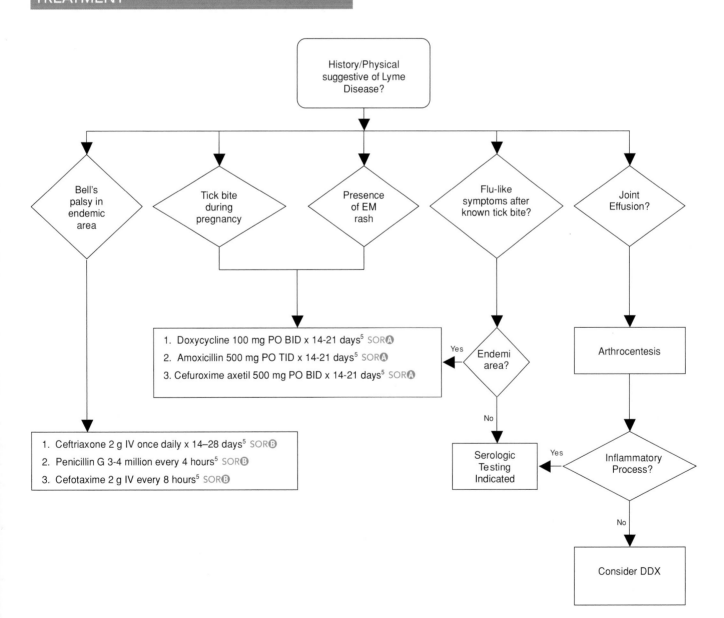

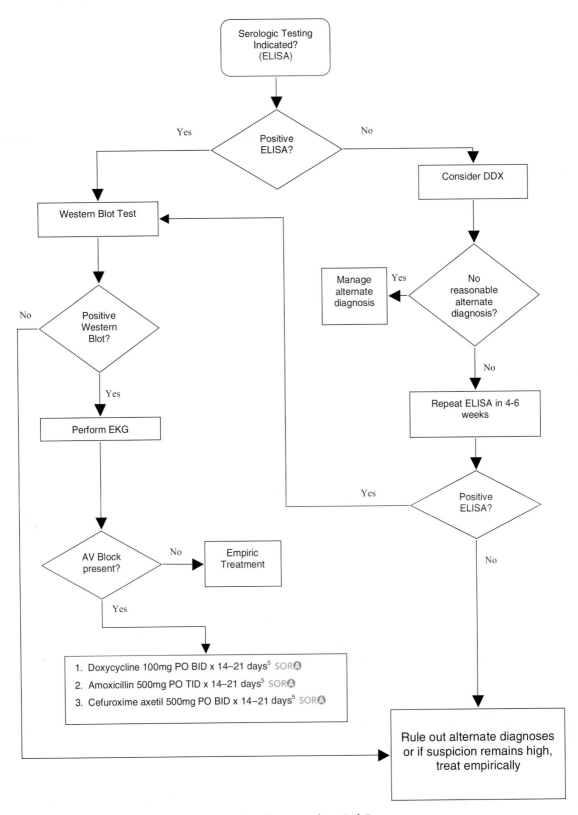

Algorithms designed by Thomas Corson with information from Ref. 5.
Recommendations based on the SORT scale;
A—Recommendation based on consistent and good-quality patient-oriented evidence.
B—Recommendation based on inconsistent or limited-quality patient-oriented evidence.
C—Recommendation based on consensus, usual practice, opinion, disease-oriented evidence,
or case series for studies of diagnosis, treatment, prevention, or screening.

FOLLOW-UP

Most patients respond to appropriate therapy with prompt resolution of symptoms within 4 weeks.

True treatment failures are uncommon and prolonged oral or parenteral antibiotic courses are emphatically discouraged. In patients who continue to present with residual subjective symptoms, providers should seek alternate diagnoses and/or referral to an appropriate specialist.

PATIENT EDUCATION

Prevention is accomplished by reducing exposure to ticks. If you live in an area that has Lyme disease then use tick repellent, tick checks, and other simple measures to prevent tick bites. This is especially important during the high-risk months of April through November. Patients should know the early signs of Lyme disease so that they can get care early when it is most curable. The CDC website is an excellent place to get accurate patient education: http://www.cdc.gov/ncidod/dvbid/lyme/ld_humandisease_symptoms.htm.

If a tick is found on the skin, remove it early using fine-tipped tweezers. See patient resources below.

PATIENT RESOURCES

CDC Lyme disease home page: **http://www.cdc.gov/ncidod/dvbid/lyme/.**

CDC tick information card: Includes information on how to recognize ticks and how to safely remove them using fine-tipped tweezers: **http://www.cdc.gov/ncidod/dvbid/lyme/resources/tick_infocard.pdf.**

PROVIDER RESOURCES

CDC Lyme disease home page: **http://www.cdc.gov/ncidod/dvbid/lyme/.**

MMWR, Lyme disease—United States, 2003–2005. June 15, 2007;56(23):573–576.

REFERENCES

1. Sternbach G. Willy Burgdorfer: Lyme disease. *J Emerg Med*. 1996; 14(5):631–634.

2. Centers for Disease Control and Prevention (CDC). Lyme disease—United States, 2003–2005. *MMWR Morb Mortal Wkly Rep*. 2007;56(23):573–576.

3. www.emedicine.com/med/topic1346.htm. Accessed February 19, 2007.

4. www.cdc.gov/ncidod/dvbid/lyme/index.htm. Accessed February 19, 2007.

5. Wormser GP, et al. Practice guidelines for the treatment of Lyme disease. *Clin Infect Dis*. 2006;43(9):1089–1134.

6. www.harp.org/eng/kaiserslymesummary.htm. Accessed February 26, 2007.

7. www.columbia-lyme.org/flatp/lymeoverview.html. Accessed February 19, 2007.

8. www.acponline.org/journals/news/jun07/critters.pdf. Accessed August 8, 2007.

PART 16

ENDOCRINE

212 ACANTHOSIS NIGRICANS

Mindy A. Smith, MD, MS

PATIENT STORY

An overweight 10-year-old Hispanic girl is brought by her mom to her family physician with concerns about a "dirty area under her arms and on her neck that couldn't be cleaned" (**Figure 212-1**). There is a strong family history of diabetes but the girl's blood sugars are normal. The physician diagnoses it as acanthosis nigricans (AN) and continues to work with the girl and her family on the issues of diet, exercise, and weight loss.

EPIDEMIOLOGY

- AN is a skin lesion usually associated with insulin resistance (IR) and is seen in patients with type 2 diabetes, obesity, and polycystic ovary syndrome.

- AN is present in up to 90% of children with type 2 diabetes.

- AN is sometimes associated with malignancy, primarily adenocarcinoma (60%) of the stomach, colon, ovary, pancreas, rectum, and uterus.[1]

- There is also a familial form of AN.

- A condition of hyperandrogenism (HA), insulin resistance (IR), and AN called HAIR-AN syndrome occurs in approximately 1% to 3% of women with HA.[2] This syndrome may also be seen in patients with autoimmune disorders like Hashimoto's thyroiditis.

ETIOLOGY AND PATHOPHYSIOLOGY

- AN is one of the localized forms of hyperpigmentation that involves epidermal alteration.

- AN results from long-term exposure of keratinocytes to insulin.

- Keratinocytes have insulin and insulin-like growth receptors on their surfaces, and the pathogenesis of this condition may be linked to insulin binding to insulin-like growth receptors in the epidermis.

DIAGNOSIS

The diagnosis of AN is made clinically in a patient with or at risk of IR who has the characteristic lesions.

CLINICAL FEATURES

- AN ranges in appearance from diffuse streaky thickened brown velvety lesions to leathery verrucous papillomatous lesions (**Figures 212-1 to 212-4**).

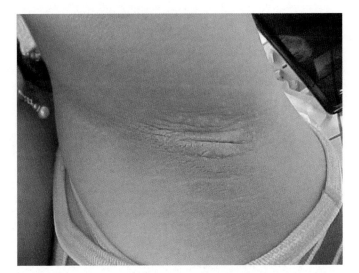

FIGURE 212-1 Acanthosis nigricans in the left axilla of an overweight Hispanic 10-year-old girl. Note areas of dark velvety discoloration and pink filiform hypertrophy. (*Courtesy of Richard P. Usatine, MD.*)

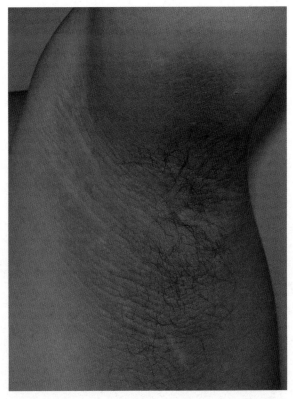

FIGURE 212-2 Acanthosis nigricans in the right axilla of an adult with type 2 diabetes. The skin appears velvety. (*Courtesy of Richard P. Usatine, MD.*)

- Women with HAIR-AN syndrome have evidence of virilization (e.g., increased body hair in male distribution and enlarged clitoris) in addition to AN.

TYPICAL DISTRIBUTION

- Commonly located on the neck (**Figures 212-3** and **212-4**) or skin folds (i.e., axillae (**Figures 212-1** and **212-2**), inframammary folds, groin, and perineum).
- Less often AN can be seen on the nipples or areolae.
- In patients with malignancy, the onset of AN is abrupt and the distribution of lesions is more widespread and may include the palms and soles.[3]

BIOPSY – MAY BE NEEDED IN UNUSUAL CASES

- Histologic examination reveals hyperkeratosis and papillary hypertrophy, although the epidermis is only mildly thickened.[4]

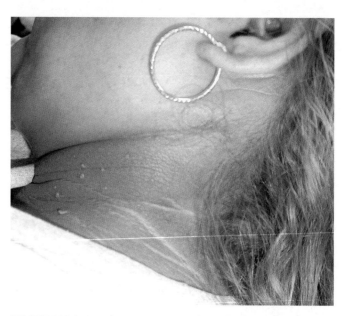

FIGURE 212-3 Acanthosis nigricans on the neck of an obese Hispanic woman with type 2 diabetes. Note that multiple skin tags are also present. (*Courtesy of Richard P. Usatine, MD.*)

DIFFERENTIAL DIAGNOSIS

Other hyperpigmented lesions that may be confused with AN include the following:

- Seborrheic keratosis: Most commonly found on the trunk or the face, these lesions are more plaque-like with adherent, greasy scale and have a "stuck on" appearance (see Chapter 151, Seborrheic Keratosis).
- Pigmented actinic keratosis: Usually in sun-exposed areas, the lesions can be macular or papular with dry, rough adherent scale (see Chapter 159, Actinic Keratosis/Bowen's Disease).

MANAGEMENT

- Weight loss through diet and exercise helps reverse the process probably by reducing both IR and compensatory hyperinsulinemia.
- The use of keratolytic agents (e.g., salicylic acid) may improve the appearance cosmetically.
- Other drugs such as metformin, octreotide, retinoids, and topical cholecalciferol (vitamin D$_3$) analogs[5] and long-pulsed alexandrite laser therapy[6] have also been used to treat AN. SOR Ⓒ
- The use of omega-3-fatty acid and dietary fish oil supplementation has also been reported to treat AN.[7] SOR Ⓒ

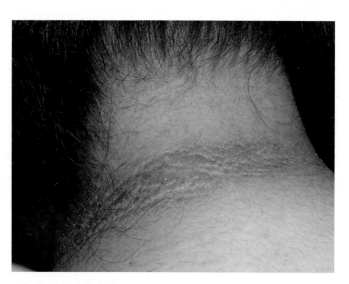

FIGURE 212-4 Acanthosis nigricans on the neck of an obese woman with type II diabetes. Note the hypertrophic thickening of the darker skin. (*Courtesy of Richard P. Usatine, MD.*)

PATIENT EDUCATION

- Patients who are overweight should be encouraged to lose weight through diet and exercise because weight loss can help diminish this condition.

REFERENCES

1. Rendon MI, Cruz PD, Sontheimer RD, Bergstresser PR. Acanthosis nigricans: A cutaneous marker of tissue resistance to insulin. *J Am Acad Dermatol*. 1989;29(3 pt 1):461–469.

2. Elmer KB, George RM. HAIR-AN syndrome: A multisystem challenge. *Am Fam Physician*. 2001;63:2385–2390.

3. Stulberg DL, Clark N. Hyperpigmented disorders in adults: Part II. *Am Fam Physician*. 2003;68:1963–1968.

4. Sibbald RG, Landolt SJ, Toth D. Skin and diabetes. *Endocrinol Metab Clin North Am*. 1996;25(2):463–472.

5. Hermanns-Le T, Scheen A, Pierard GE. Acanthosis nigricans associated with insulin resistance: Pathophysiology and management. *Am J Clin Dermatol*. 2004;5(3):199–203.

6. Rosenbach A, Ram R. Treatment of acanthosis nigricans of the axillae using a long-pulsed (5-msec) alexandrite laser. *Dermatol Surg*. 2004;30(8):1158–1160.

7. Sheretz EF. Improved acanthosis nigricans with lipodystrophic diabetes during dietary fish oil supplementation. *Arch Dermatol*. 1988;124:1094–1096.

213 DIABETIC DERMOPATHY

Mindy A. Smith, MD, MS

PATIENT STORY

A 60-year-old woman with diabetes mellitus for the past 10 years began to notice reddish-colored lesions on both anterior shins that turned brown over the past year (**Figure 213-1**). She reported no pain with the hyperpigmented areas but does have foot pain secondary to neuropathy. The patient is diagnosed with diabetic dermopathy, and she begins working with her physician on achieving better control of her diabetes.

EPIDEMIOLOGY

- Diabetic dermopathy, the most common cutaneous marker of diabetes mellitus, is found in 12.5% to 40% of patients and most often in the elderly. It is less common in women.[1]
- Sometimes seen in persons without diabetes, especially patients with circulatory compromise.

ETIOLOGY AND PATHOPHYSIOLOGY

The cause of diabetic dermopathy is unknown.

- Diabetic dermopathy may be related to mechanical or thermal trauma, especially in patients with neuropathy.
- Lesions have been classified as vascular because histology sections demonstrate red blood cell extravasation and capillary basement membrane thickening.
- There is an association between diabetic dermopathy and the presence of retinopathy, nephropathy, and neuropathy.[2]

DIAGNOSIS

CLINICAL FEATURES

Lesions often begin as pink patches (0.5–1 cm), which become hyperpigmented with surface atrophy and fine scale (**Figures 213-1 to 213-4**).

TYPICAL DISTRIBUTION

Pretibial and lateral areas of the calf (**Figures 213-1 to 213-4**).

BIOPSY

Histology shows epidermal atrophy, thickened small superficial dermal blood vessels, and hemorrhage with hemosiderin deposits.

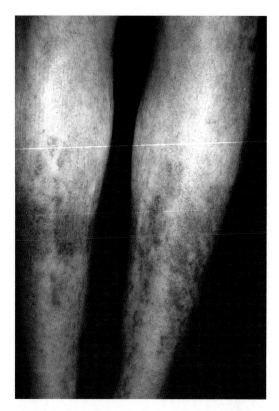

FIGURE 213-1 Lesions of diabetic dermopathy (also called pigmented pretibial papules) on both lower extremities of a 60-year-old woman with diabetes. The skin appears atrophic and the lesions are flat and hyperpigmented. (*Courtesy of the University of Texas Health Sciences Center, Division of Dermatology.*)

DIFFERENTIAL DIAGNOSIS

Consider the following when evaluating patients with similar skin conditions:

- Early lesions of necrobiosis lipoidica diabeticorum—erythematous papules or plaques beginning in the pretibial area, but become larger and darker with irregular margins and raised erythematous borders. Telangiectasias, atropy and yellow discoloration may be seen. The lesion may be painful (see Chapter 214, Necrobiosis Lipoidica).

- Schamberg's disease (pigmented purpuric dermatosis) is a capillaritis that produces brown hemosiderin deposits along with visible pink to red spots like cayenne pepper on the lower extremities. It is not more common in diabetes but may resemble diabetic dermopathy. A biopsy could be used to distinguish between them (see Chapter 172, Vasculitis).

- Stasis dermatitis—the typical site is the medial aspect of the ankle. Early lesions are erythematous, scaly, and sometimes pruritic, becoming progressively hyperpigmented (see Chapter 50, Venous Stasis).

- Traumatic scars—there is no scale, lesions are permanent, and edema is not usually present.

- Pigmentary purpuras—usually more widespread and caused by extravasation of red blood cells into the dermis; associated with many systemic disorders such as thrombocytopenia and amyloidosis (see Chapter 172, Vasculitis).

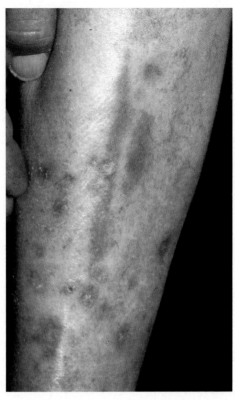

FIGURE 213-2 Diabetic dermopathy on the leg showing pretibial hyperpigmentation and healed ulcers with hypopigmentation. There are also signs of erythema and fine scale. (*Courtesy of the University of Texas Health Sciences Center, Division of Dermatology.*)

MANAGEMENT

- There is no effective treatment, and the lesions may resolve spontaneously.
- It is not known whether the lesions improve with better control of diabetes.
- One informal case report stated that patients may benefit from 15 to 25 mg chelated zinc daily for several weeks.[3] SOR **C**

PATIENT EDUCATION

- Reassure patients that the lesions are asymptomatic and may resolve spontaneously within 1 to 2 years, although new lesions may form.

PATIENT AND PROVIDER RESOURCES

See the following websites for information on diabetic skin conditions for patients and providers:

- American Diabetes Association—**www.diabetes.org.**
- National Institutes of Health—**www.niddk.nih.gov.**
- CDC—**www.cdc.gov/diabetes.**

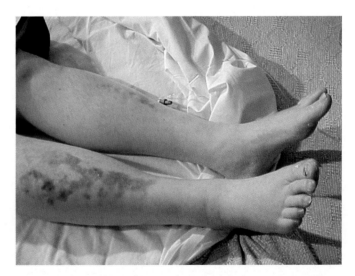

FIGURE 213-3 Diabetic dermopathy on both lower extremities of a middle-aged man with diabetes. The sparse hair is secondary to his vasculopathy. (*Courtesy of Dan Stulberg, MD.*)

REFERENCES

1. Sibbald RG, Landolt SJ, Toth D. Skin and diabetes. *Endocrinol Metab Clin North Am*. 1996;25(2):463–472.

2. Shemer A, Bergnan R, Linn S, et al. Diabetic dermopathy and internal complications in diabetes mellitus. *Int J Dermatol*. 1998; 37(2):113–115.

3. *www.diabetesnet.com/diabetes_complications/diabetes_skin_changes.php*. Accessed March 2, 2006.

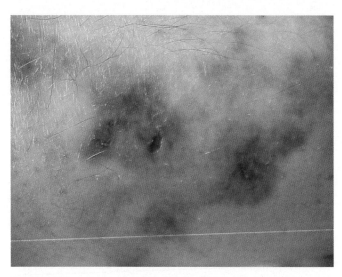

FIGURE 213-4 Close-up of diabetic dermopathy on the right leg showing atrophy, hyperpigmentation, a shallow ulcer, and fine scale. The hyperpigmentation is from hemosiderin deposition. (*Courtesy of Dan Stulberg, MD.*)

214 NECROBIOSIS LIPOIDICA

Mindy A. Smith, MD, MS

PATIENT STORY

A 30-year-old woman presents with discoloration on both lower legs. She has no history of diabetes personally; however, type 2 diabetes does run in her family. Visible inspection of the lesions is highly suggestive of necrobiosis lipoidica (NL) (**Figure 214-1**). There is visible hyperpigmentation, yellow discoloration, atrophy, and telangiectasias. The patient is not overweight and had no symptoms of diabetes. Her blood sugar at this visit is 142 after eating lunch 1 hour prior to testing. The following day, the patient's fasting blood sugar is 121, with a glycosylated hemoglobin of 6.1. The patient is informed of her borderline diabetes, and diet and exercise are prescribed. The NL does not cause her any symptoms, but she is disturbed by its appearance. The patient chooses to try a moderate-strength topical corticosteroid for treatment.

EPIDEMIOLOGY

- NL was previously called necrobiosis lipoidica diabeticorum (NLD) because it was thought to be seen almost exclusively in persons with diabetes. A significant minority of patients with NL do not have diabetes and so the newer name is NL.

- NL is a rare condition that occurs in 0.3% of patients with diabetes.[1,2]

- NL primarily affects women (80%), particularly those with type 1 diabetes mellitus, but it can occur with type 2.[1,2]

- Average age of onset is 34 years.[1,2]

ETIOLOGY AND PATHOPHYSIOLOGY

- The cause of NL remains unknown.

- Patients with NL usually either have or subsequently develop diabetes, but some patients with NL never develop diabetes.

- Angiopathy leading to thrombosis and occlusion of the cutaneous vessels has been implicated in its etiology. However, microangiopathic changes are less common in lesions on areas other than the shins and, therefore, are not necessary for developing the lesions.[2]

- Antibodies and C3 have been found at the dermal–epidermal border, suggesting vasculitis.

- The presence of fibrin in these lesions associated with palisading histiocytes may indicate a delayed hypersensitivity reaction.

DIAGNOSIS

CLINICAL FEATURES

- The lesions are usually located on the shins (90%) (**Figures 214-1** to **214-4**).

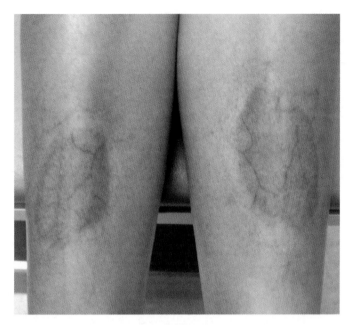

FIGURE 214-1 Necrobiosis lipoidica in a 30-year-old woman with impaired glucose tolerance (borderline diabetes). Note the brown pigmentation and prominent blood vessels. (*Courtesy of Suraj Reddy, MD.*)

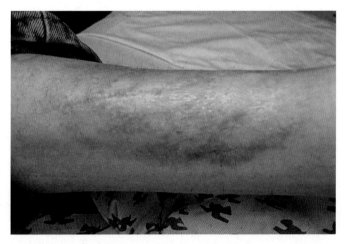

FIGURE 214-2 Necrobiosis lipoidica in a patient with type 1 diabetes. Note the pink area at the site of a healed superficial ulcer. (*Courtesy of Amber Tully, MD.*)

- They begin as erythematous papules or plaques in the pretibial area and become larger and darker with irregular margins and raised erythematous borders. The lesion's center atrophies and turns yellow in color (**Figures 214-3** and **214-4**).

- There is often a prominent brown color or hyperpigmentation visible (**Figures 214-1** to **214-4**).

- The lesions may ulcerate (occurs in approximately one-third) and become painful.

- Telangiectasias and prominent blood vessels may be seen within the lesions (**Figures 214-1** to **214-4**).

- The yellow color may be because of lipid deposits or beta-carotene.

BIOPSY

- Biopsy is usually not needed as the clinical picture is usually clear. The dangers of a biopsy include delayed healing and infection in a patient who often has diabetes. The shin region of the leg is notorious for delayed healing even in healthy persons and so biopsy should be avoided in most cases.

- If the diagnosis is uncertain, a punch biopsy will show a thin atrophic epidermis with dermal granulomatous inflammation and obliterative endarteritis. The dermal change shows increased necrobiosis or degeneration of collagen with absence of elastic tissue.

DIFFERENTIAL DIAGNOSIS

NL may be confused with the following conditions:

- Erythema nodosum (EN) is an inflammatory panniculitis that occurs in the same areas (especially shins) as NL. These nodules are pink in color and the skin is smooth above them. The color and lack of epidermal changes should differentiate EN from NL (see Chapter 171, Erythema Nodosum).

- Granuloma annulare—appears as asymmetric annular red plaques on the dorsum of the hands, extensor surface of the extremities, or posterior neck. They lack the yellow discoloration of NL. These lesions are so visibly like red raised rings that they should appear different from NL. If biopsy is needed, the presence of abundant mucin deposits helps to distinguish these lesions from NL (see Chapter 166, Granuloma Annulare).[2]

- Lichen simplex chronicus—a chronic pruritic eczematous lesion. The lesions are well-circumscribed plaques or papules with lichenified or thickened skin caused by chronic scratching or rubbing. Lesions are commonly located on the ankles, wrists, or posterior nuchal region. The prominent scale and lichenification should help differentiate these lesions from NL (see Chapter 139, Atopic Dermatitis).

- Sarcoidosis skin lesions—including EN, maculopapular eruptions on the face, nose, back and extremities, skin plaques that are often purple and raised, and broad macules with telangiectasias that are most commonly seen on the face or hands . Punch biopsy will distinguish between sarcoidosis and NL (see Chapter 168, Sarcoidosis).

- Stasis dermatitis—occurs on the lower extremities secondary to venous incompetence and edema. Affected patients are usually older, and the typical site is the medial aspect of the ankle. Early

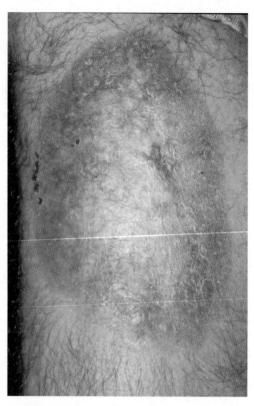

FIGURE 214-3 Necrobiosis lipoidica on the leg of a man with type 2 diabetes. Note the central atrophy and yellow discoloration with a well-demarcated brown border. (*Courtesy of the University of Texas Health Sciences Center, Division of Dermatology.*)

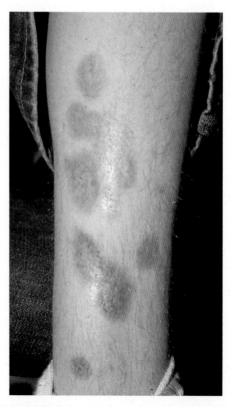

FIGURE 214-4 Multiple lesions of necrobiosis lipoidica in a young adult with type 1 diabetes. Note the central yellow discoloration and well-circumscribed brown borders. (*Courtesy of the University of Texas Health Sciences Center, Division of Dermatology.*)

lesions are erythematous, scaly, and sometimes pruritic that progressively become hyperpigmented. These lesions are rarely well circumscribed, as seen in NL (see Chapter 50, Venous Stasis).

MANAGEMENT

Evaluate patients not previously diagnosed with diabetes mellitus for diabetes. Even though glycemic control does not correlate with progression of these lesions, diabetes mellitus should be treated to decrease the risk of macro- and microvascular complications.

Spontaneous resolution occurs in 10% to 20% of cases. Necrobiosis lesions may respond to the following treatments:

- Local application of potent steroids or intralesional injections of 2.5 mg/mL of triamcinolone.[2] SOR Ⓒ The major risk of these treatments includes increasing the existing atrophy, so patients should be informed of risks and benefits before initiating steroid treatments.
- Pentoxiphylline (400 mg two to three times daily), an agent that improves blood flow and decreases red cell and platelet aggregation, was shown in two case reports to completely resolve the lesions at 8 weeks in one[3] and at 6-month follow-up in the other.[4] The latter patient continued therapy and remained in remission at a 2-year follow-up. SOR Ⓒ

PATIENT EDUCATION

Patients with NL without diabetes mellitus should be advised about the increased risk of developing the disease and counseled about symptoms and periodic surveillance.

NL may resolve spontaneously and does respond to several treatments.

PATIENT RESOURCES

- American Diabetes Association—**www.diabetes.org; http://www.diabetes.org/for-parents-and-kids/ what-is-diabetes/skin-complications.jsp**
- National Institutes of Health—**www.niddk.nih.gov**
- CDC—**www.cdc.gov/diabetes**

PROVIDER RESOURCES

- **http://www.aocd.org/skin/dermatologic_diseases/ necrobiosis_lipoid.html**
- **http://www.aocd.org/skin/dermatologic_diseases/ necrobiosis_lipoid.html**

REFERENCES

1. Noz KC, Korstanje MJ, Vermeer BJ. Cutaneous manifestations of endocrine disorders: a guide for dermatologists. *Am J Clin Dermatol*. 2003;4(5):315–331.

2. Sibbald RG, Landolt SJ, Toth D. Skin and diabetes. *Endocrinol Metab Clin North Am*. 1996;25(2):463–472.

3. Noz KC, Korstanje MJ, Vermeer BJ. Ulcerating necrobiosis lipoidica effectively treated with pentoxifylline. *Clin Exp Dermatol*. 1993;18(1):78–79.

4. Basaria S, Braga-Basaria M. Necrobiosis lipoidica diabeticorum: Response to pentoxiphylline. *J Endocrinol Invest*. 2003;26(10): 1037–1040.

215 XANTHOMAS

Mindy A. Smith, MD, MS

PATIENT STORY

A 27-year-old Hispanic man reported new painful nonpruritic bumps, which started 6 months ago, over his entire body. The patient had not seen a physician for 10 months and had run out of his oral medicines for type 2 diabetes. His grandmother had some milder version like this years ago. These firm yellowish papules were present all over his body from the neck down (**Figures 215-1** to **215-3**). Laboratory evaluation revealed a random blood sugar of 203, a fasting triglyceride level of more than 7000 mg/dL, and total cholesterol more than 700 mg/dL. High-density lipoproteins were 32 mg/dL, and there were no chylomicrons present. The patient was diagnosed with xanthomas, poorly controlled diabetes mellitus, and hyperlipidemia and was started on metformin, gemfibrozil, and an HMG-CoA-reductase inhibitor.

EPIDEMIOLOGY

Xanthomas are skin manifestation of familial or severe secondary hyperlipidemia.

- Patients with homozygous familial hypercholesterolemia (FH) (one in 1 million persons worldwide) present in childhood with cutaneous xanthomas on the hands, wrists, elbows, knees, heels, or buttocks.[2]
- Patients with heterozygous FH (one in 500 persons worldwide) present as adults with tendon xanthomas in 75%.

ETIOLOGY AND PATHOPHYSIOLOGY

- Lipoproteins are complexes of lipids and proteins essential for transporting cholesterol, triglycerides, and fat-soluble vitamins.
- Xanthomas are usually a consequence of primary or secondary hyperlipidemia. There are five basic types of xanthomas:
  - Eruptive xanthomas (also called tuberoeruptive) are the most common form. These appear as crops of yellow or hyperpigmented papules with erythematous halos in white persons (**Figures 215-1** to **215-3**), appearing hyperpigmented in black persons (**Figures 215-4** and **215-5**).
  - Tendon xanthomas are frequently seen on the Achilles and extensor finger tendons.
  - Plane xanthomas are flat and commonly seen on the palmar creases, face, upper trunk, and on scars.
  - Tuberous xanthomas are found most frequently on the hand or over large joints.
  - Xanthelasma are yellow papules found on the eyelids (**Figure 215-6**). Fifty percent of individuals with xanthelasmas have normal lipid profiles.

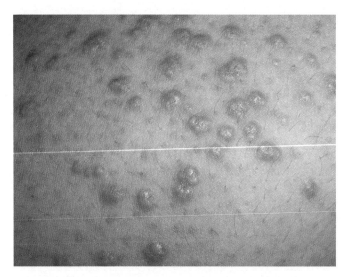

FIGURE 215-1 Close-up of eruptive xanthomas on the arm of a 27-year-old man with untreated hyperlipidemia and diabetes.[1] (*Courtesy of Richard P. Usatine, MD.*)

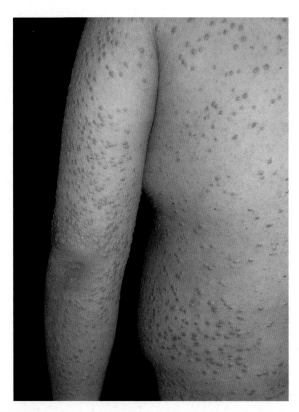

FIGURE 215-2 Eruptive xanthomas on the arm and trunk of the man in **Figure 215-1**. (*Courtesy of Richard P. Usatine, MD.*)

DIAGNOSIS

CLINICAL FEATURES

- Xanthomas are deposits of lipid in the skin or subcutaneous tissue that manifest clinically as yellowish papules, nodules, or tumors (**Figures 215-1**).
- Eruptive xanthomas (**Figures 215-2** to **215-5**) begin as clusters of small papules on the elbows, knees, and buttocks that can grow to the size of grapes.

TYPICAL DISTRIBUTION

Xanthomas are most commonly found in superficial soft tissues such as skin and subcutis or on tendon sheaths.

BIOPSY

Biopsy is rarely needed and shows collections of lipid-filled macrophages.

DIFFERENTIAL DIAGNOSIS

Other skin papules that can be mistaken for xanthomas include the following:

- Gouty tophi—deposits of monosodium urate that are usually firm and occasionally discharge a chalky material (see Chapter 94, Gout).
- Pseudoxanthoma elasticum—a disorder caused by abnormal deposits of calcium on the elastic fibers of the skin and eye.
- Molluscum contagiosum—caused by a virus; lesions can be papular and widespread but generally have a central depression (see Chapter 124, Molluscum Contagiosum). The patient in **Figures 215-1** to **215-3** was originally misdiagnosed with molluscum.

MANAGEMENT

- Initial treatment should target the underlying hyperlipidemia (when present) because hypolipidemic drug treatment often results in regression of the lesions. SOR Ⓒ
- When standard therapy fails, LDL apheresis has lowered lipid levels with subsequent regression of tendon xanthomas.[3] SOR Ⓒ
- Xanthelasma lesions may be treated for cosmetic purposes. Methods of treatment include surgery, electrosurgery, cryotherapy, and laser therapy. In a case report of 24 patients, argon laser coagulation was well tolerated and the cosmetic outcome was considered to be good in 85%.[4] SOR Ⓒ

PATIENT EDUCATION

- Patients with hyperlipidemia and/or diabetes mellitus should be encouraged to establish and maintain good control of these diseases, as this often results in regression of the lesions.

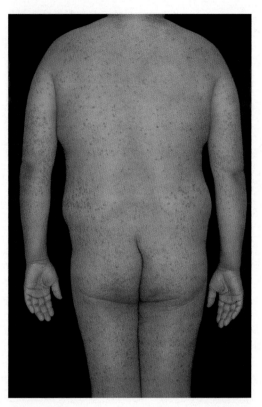

FIGURE 215-3 Eruptive xanthomas covering most of the body of the man in **Figure 215-1**. (*Courtesy of Richard P. Usatine, MD.*)

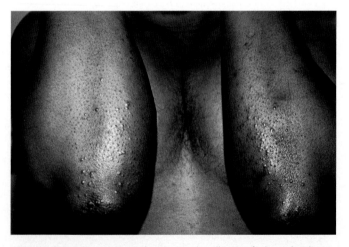

FIGURE 215-4 Eruptive xanthomas on the elbows of a hyperlipidemic black man with type 2 diabetes. His triglycerides and total cholesterol levels were high.[1] (*From the Western Journal of Medicine.*)

REFERENCES

1. Usatine RP. A cutaneous manifestation of a systemic disease. *West J Med*. 2000;172(2):84.

2. Rader DJ, Hobbs HH. Disorders of lipoprotein metabolism. In: Kasper DL, Braunwald E, Fauci AS, Hauser SL, Longo DL, Jameson JL eds. *Harrison's Principles of Internal Medicine*. New York, NY: McGraw-Hill Companies Inc., 2005:2286–2298.

3. Scheel AK, Schettler V, Koziolek M, et al. Impact of chronic LDL-apheresis treatment on Achilles tendon affection in patients with severe familial hypercholesterolemia: A clinical and ultrasonographic 3-year follow-up study. *Atherosclerosis*. 2004;174(1):133–139.

4. Basar E, Oguz H, Ozdemir H, et al. Treatment of xanthelasma palpebrarum with argon laser photocoagulation. Argon laser and xanthelasma palpebrarum. *Int Ophthalmol*. 2004;25(1):9–11.

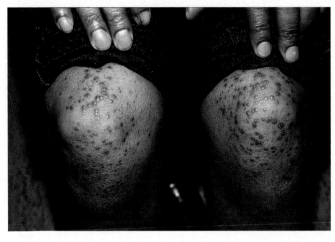

FIGURE 215-5 Eruptive xanthomas on the knees in the patient in **Figure 215-4**. (*From the Western Journal of Medicine*.)

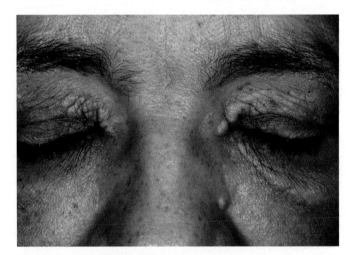

FIGURE 215-6 Xanthelasma around the eyes (xanthoma palpebrarum); most often seen on the medial aspect of the eyelids, with upper lids being more commonly involved than lower lids. (*Courtesy of Richard P. Usatine, MD*.)

216 GOITER AND HYPOTHYROIDISM

Mindy A. Smith, MD, MS

PATIENT STORY

A 55-year-old woman presented with a several-month history of fatigue and weight gain. She reported that she felt puffy and swollen. She had difficulty buttoning the top button of her blouse because her neck was so large, but she reported no neck pain. Review of systems was positive for constipation, dry skin, and cold intolerance. On physical examination, a large goiter was found (**Figure 216-1**). Laboratory testing revealed an elevated thyroid-stimulating hormone (TSH) and a low free thyroxine (FT_4) level confirming hypothyroidism. The patient was started on levothyroxine and further workup for etiology of the hypothyroidism was initiated.

EPIDEMIOLOGY

- Worldwide, goiter is the most common endocrine disorder with rates of 4% to 15% in areas of adequate iodine intake and more than 90% where there is iodine deficiency.[1] Endemic goiter is defined as goiter that affects more than 5% of the population.

- Most goiters are not associated with thyroid dysfunction.

- The prevalence of goitrous hypothyroidism varies from 0.7% to 4% of the population.

- The female-to-male ratio of goiter is 3:1, and 6:1 for goitrous hypothyroidism.

- The annual incidence of autoimmune hypothyroidism is 4/1000 women and 1/1000 men, with a mean age at diagnosis of 60 years.[2]

ETIOLOGY AND PATHOPHYSIOLOGY

Goiter is actually a spectrum of changes in the thyroid gland ranging from diffuse enlargement to nodular enlargement depending on the cause. In the United States, the most common etiology of goiter with normal thyroid function or transient dysfunction is thyroiditis. Contributing factors for goiter:

- Iodine deficiency or excess.

- TSH stimulation.

- Drugs including lithium, amiodarone, and interferon alpha.

- Autoimmunity/heredity.

  Hypothyroidism develops as a result of thyroid failure. The most common cause of goitrous hypothyroidism is chronic lymphocytic (Hashimoto's) thyroiditis.

- Hashimoto's thyroiditis is caused by thyroid peroxidase (TPO) antibodies.

- HLA-DR and CTLA-4 are the best documented genetic risk factors for this disorder.[2]

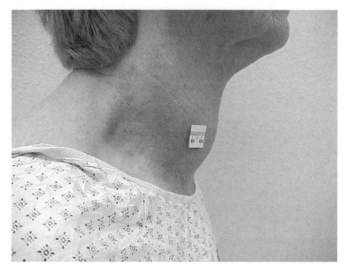

FIGURE 216-1 Goiter that extends approximately 2 cm forward when viewed from the patient's side. (*Courtesy of Dan Stulberg, MD.*)

- There is marked lymphocytic infiltration of the thyroid in Hashimoto's thyroiditis; the infiltrate is composed of activated CD4+ and CD8+ T cells as well as B cells.

- Thyroid destruction in Hashimoto's thyroiditis is believed to be primarily mediated by CD8+ cytotoxic T cells.

DIAGNOSIS

CLINICAL FEATURES

The history can be the key to the diagnosis:

- A painful neck mass is usually a form of thyroiditis.

- Large goiters are easily visible before palpating the neck (**Figures 216-1 to 216-3**).

- Asymmetric goiters can shift the trachea away from the midline (**Figure 216-4**).

- Common signs and symptoms of hypothyroidism are
  - Fatigue/weakness,
  - Dry and cool skin,
  - Diffuse hair loss,
  - Difficulty concentrating,
  - Puffy face/hands/feet from myxedema (**Figure 216-5**),
  - Bradycardia,
  - Delayed deep tendon reflex relaxation,
  - Weight gain despite poor appetite, and
  - Constipation.

- The most useful signs for diagnosing hypothyroidism are puffiness (likelihood ratio positive (LR+) 16.2) and delayed ankle reflex (LR+ 11.8).[3]

    Physical examination maneuvers that help detect goiter are[4]

- Neck extension,

- Observation from the side,

- Palpation by locating the isthmus first, and

- Having the patient swallow.

LABORATORY STUDIES

Laboratory tests include a sedimentation rate (ESR) if thyroiditis is suspected, and a TSH and free thyroxine (FT_4) level.

- In acute granulomatous thyroiditis, ESR is >50 (LR+ 95) and the TSH and free T_4 are usually normal.

- In primary hypothyroidism, the TSH is >10 mU/L (LR+ 16) and FT_4 is <8 (LR+ 11).

- The presence of antibodies to TPO and thyroglobulin help establish the diagnosis of Hashimoto's thyroiditis but is unnecessary for treatment. TPO antibodies will be positive in 90% to 95% of patients.[2]

DIFFERENTIAL DIAGNOSIS

Goiter presenting as a painful neck mass is most commonly caused by subacute granulomatous (de Quervain's) thyroiditis (likely viral) or

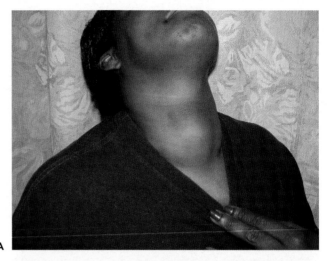

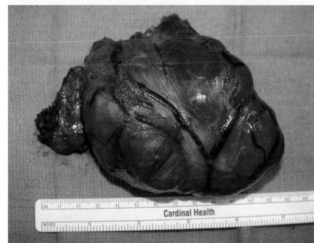

FIGURE 216-2 (A) A 36-year-old woman with large goiter. (B) The resected goitrous thyroid gland. (*Courtesy of Frank Miller, MD.*)

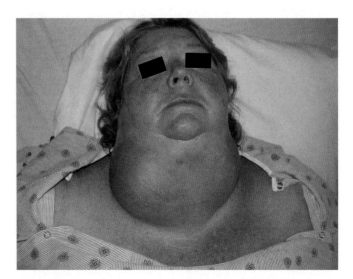

FIGURE 216-3 Massive multinodular goiter before surgery. (*Courtesy of Frank Miller, MD.*)

hemorrhage into a thyroid cyst or adenoma. Other causes include the following:

- Painful Hashimoto's thyroiditis—hypothyroidism with the presence of antibodies helps to confirm this diagnosis.

- Infected thyroglossal duct or branchial cleft cyst—mass palpates as cystic and may be fluctuant; focal (e.g., erythema and warmth) and systemic symptoms of infection (e.g., fever) may be present. Even a noninfected thyroglossal duct cyst can be confused for an enlarged thyroid (**Figure 216-6**).

- Acute suppurative thyroiditis (microbial)—focal (e.g., erythema and warmth) and systemic symptoms of infection (e.g., fever) are usually present.

- Thyroid carcinoma—hard mass within thyroid gland (**Figure 216-7**).

Painless goiter and hypothyroidism are most often caused by Hashimoto's thyroiditis but may also be caused by the following:

- Environmental goitrogens (e.g., excess iodine, foods such as cassava, cabbage, and soybeans)

- Iodine deficiency

- Pharmacologic inhibition (rare)—drugs include lithium, amiodarone, and interferon alpha

Painless goiter and hyperthyroidism may be caused by the following:

- Graves' disease (common, 0.5%–2.5% of the population)—symptoms of nervousness, fatigue, weight loss, heat intolerance, palpitations, and exophthalmus (see Chapter 217, Graves Exophthalmos and Goiter).

- Postpartum thyroiditis (2%–16% within 3–6 months of delivery)—recent delivery.

- Toxic nodular goiter (uncommon)—usually in the elderly; thyroid gland feels nodular (**Figure 216-4**) and thyroid scan shows multiple foci of increased uptake.

MANAGEMENT

Patients with endemic goiter should be provided with iodine. For nonendemic goiter, consider the following:

- Removal of goitrogens

- TSH suppression with levothyroxine (1–2.2 mg/kg/d) (variable but limited effect on goiter size and can cause hyperthyroidism).[5] SOR **B**

- Subtotal thyroidectomy (recurrence rates can be high).[6] SOR **A**

- Radioactive iodine treatment if enough functioning tissue is present. SOR **C**

Treat patients with acute microbial thyroiditis with antibiotics against the most common pathogens (i.e., *Staphylococcus aureus, Streptococcus pyogenes,* and *Streptococcus pneumoniae*). Alternative agents, used for 7 to 10 days, include: SOR **C**

- Amoxicillin/clavulanate (500 mg three times daily),

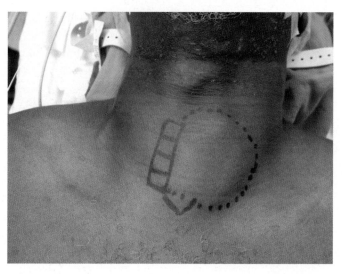

FIGURE 216-4 Asymmetric multinodular goiter causing trachea to deviate from the midline prior to resection. (*Courtesy of Frank Miller, MD.*)

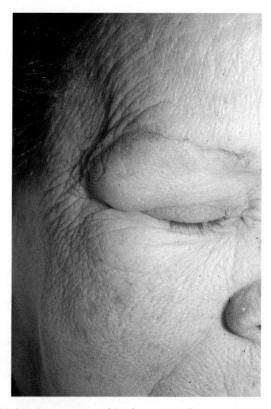

FIGURE 216-5 Myxedema of the face with puffiness around the eye. (*Courtesy of the University of Texas Health Sciences Center, Division of Dermatology.*)

- A first- or second-generation cephalosporin (e.g., cephalexin 500 mg four times daily), and

- Penicillinase-resistant penicillin (e.g., dicloxacillin 500 mg four times daily).

In patients with subacute thyroiditis:

- Oral corticosteroids can reduce pain and swelling. SOR Ⓒ

- Symptoms of hyperthyroidism can be treated with beta-blockers or calcium channel blockers.[7] SOR Ⓑ

- Symptoms of hypothyroidism can be treated with levothyroxine.[7] SOR Ⓑ

Patients with Hashimoto's thyroiditis and low FT4 are treated with levothyroxine as follows:

- Younger patients start with 50 to 100 μg/d increasing by 25 to 50 μg/d at 6-week intervals until the TSH is normal (approximately 1.6 μg/kg/d of levothyroxine).[7] SOR Ⓑ

- Older patients or those with cardiac disease start with 25 μg/d and advance slowly to normalize the TSH (approximately 1 μg/kg/d of levothyroxine). SOR Ⓒ

- Large goiters that impinge upon the trachea or do not respond to medications may be treated with surgery (**Figure 216-4**).

FOLLOW-UP

- In the most extensive community survey on goiter (Whickham, England), goiter was present in 15.5% of the population.[1] At the 20-year follow-up, 20% of women and 5% of men no longer had goiter and 4% of women and no men had acquired one.

- Suppression of TSH with levothyroxine effectively reduces the goiter of Hashimoto's thyroiditis and should be continued indefinitely. In one study, withdrawal of medication after 1 year resulted in only 11.4% remaining euthyroid.[8]

- Large goiter, TSH >10 mU/L, and a family history of thyroid disease are associated with failure to recover normal thyroid function and treatment should continue indefinitely.

PATIENT RESOURCES

- Booklet from the American Thyroid Association: **http://www.thyroid.org/patients/brochures/Hypo_brochure.pdf.** (Accessed February 27, 2006.)

- Web-based resources: **http://www.nlm.nih.gov/medlineplus/thyroiddiseases.html.** (Accessed February 27, 2006.)

PROVIDER RESOURCES

- Guideline: AACE Thyroid Task Force. American Association of Clinical Endocrinologists medical guidelines for clinical practice for the evaluation and treatment of hyperthyroidism and hypothyroidism. *Endocr Pract*. 2002;8(6):457–469.

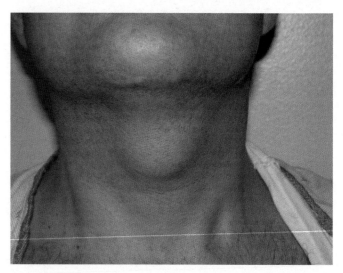

FIGURE 216-6 Thyroglossal duct cyst in the midline superior to the thyroid. (*Courtesy of Frank Miller, MD.*)

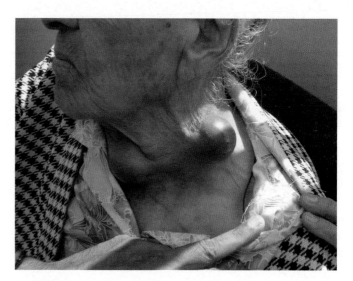

FIGURE 216-7 A 93-year-old woman with thyroid cancer that went untreated for 3 years. Two large firm masses are visible in the neck. (*Courtesy of Dustin Williams, MD.*)

REFERENCES

1. Wang C, Crapo LM. The epidemiology of thyroid disease and implications for screening. *Endorinol Metab Clin North Am*. 1997;26(1):189–218.

2. Jameson JL, Weetman AP. Disorders of the thyroid gland. In: Kasper DL, Braunwald E, Fauci AS, Hauser SL, Longo DL, Jameson JL eds. *Harrison's Principles of Internal Medicine*. New York, NY: McGraw-Hill, 2005:2109–2113.

3. Zulewski H, Müller B, Exer P, et al. Estimation of tissue hypothyroidism by a new clinical score: Evaluation of patients with various grades of hypothyroidism and controls. *J Clin Endocrinol Metab*. 1997;82:771–776.

4. Siminoski K. Does this patient have a goiter? *JAMA*. 1995;273(10):813–819.

5. Zelmanovitz F, Genro S, Gross JL. Suppressive therapy with levothyroxine for solitary thyroid nodules: A double-blind controlled clinical study and cumulative meta-analyses. *J Clin Endocrinol Metab*. 1998;83:3881–3885.

6. Rojdmark J, Jarhult J. High long term recurrence rate after subtotal thyroidectomy for nodular goitre. *Eur J Surg*. 1995;161:725–727.

7. Singer PA, Cooper DS, Levy EG, et al. Treatment guideline for patients with hyperthyroidism and hypothyroidism. *JAMA*. 1995;273(10):808–812.

8. Comtois R, Faucher L, Lafleche L. Outcome of hypothyroidism cause by Hashimoto's thyroiditis. *Arch Intern Med*. 1995;155(13):1404–1408.

217 GRAVES' EXOPHTHALMUS AND GOITER

Mindy A. Smith, MD, MS

PATIENT STORY

A 32-year-old woman presents with fatigue and "eye strain" (**Figure 217-1**). She had been working as a secretary and noticed difficulty focusing her eyes. She said she was anxious and was having difficulty in writing. She reported that her sister was taking medication for "thyroid trouble." A low thyroid-stimulating hormone (TSH) and an elevated free thyroxin level (T_4) were found on laboratory testing, and the patient was diagnosed with Graves' disease (GD). Her thyroid scan showed an enlarged thyroid with increased uptake (**Figure 217-2**). The patient chose radioactive iodine (RAI) as her treatment and her symptoms resolved. One year later she ended up needing levothyroxine treatment.

EPIDEMIOLOGY

- GD is a common disorder affecting 0.5% to 2.5% of the population.
- There is a female-to-male ratio of 7–10:1.
- Among patients with hyperthyroidism, 60% to 80% have GD; younger patients (<64 years) with hyperthyroidism are more likely to have GD than older patients.
- Graves' ophthalmopathy (see "Clinical features" below) occurs in more than 80% of patients within 18 months of diagnosis of GD.
- Goiter is present in 90% of patients aged <50 years (vs. 75% in older patients with GD).[1]

ETIOLOGY AND PATHOPHYSIOLOGY

- GD is an autoimmune disorder characterized by circulating antibodies that stimulate the TSH receptor.[2] These antibodies are synthesized in the thyroid gland, bone marrow, and lymph nodes.
- The etiology is seen as a combination of genetic (HLA-DR and CTLA-4 polymorphisms) and environmental factors including stress and smoking (a strong risk factor for Graves' ophthalmopathy).[2] Siblings have higher incidence of both GD and Hashimoto's thyroiditis.
- The ophthalmopathy is believed to result from an autoimmune response directed toward an antigen shared by the thyroid and the eye's orbit. There is infiltration of the extraocular muscles by activated T cells, which release cytokines, activating fibroblasts (fibrosis can lead to diplopia) and increasing the synthesis of glycosaminoglycans (water trapping causes swelling).[2]

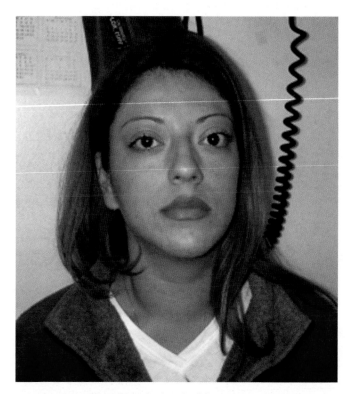

FIGURE 217-1 This patient displays the following common findings of Graves' disease (GD): Lid retraction and mild proptosis (exophthalmus), particularly evident on the left eye, and goiter. (*Courtesy of Dan Stulberg, MD.*)

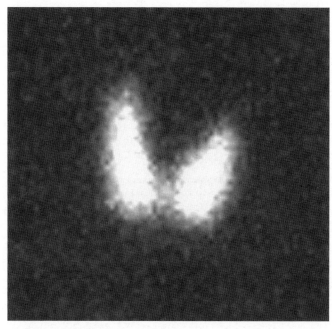

FIGURE 217-2 Nuclear scan of the thyroid in Graves' disease showing increased uptake (61%). (*Courtesy of Michael Freckleton, MD.*)

DIAGNOSIS

CLINICAL FEATURES

Symptoms depend on the severity of thyrotoxicosis, duration of disease, and age (findings are more subtle in the elderly). More than half of patients diagnosed with GD have these common symptoms:

- Nervousness.

- Fatigue.

- Weight loss.

- Heat intolerance.

- Palpitations.

- Skin and nail changes include:
  - Warm, erythematous, moist skin (from increased peripheral circulation).
  - Palmer erythema.
  - Pretibial myxedema—occurring in a small percentage of patients (0.5–4%), it consists of nonpitting scaly thickening and induration of the skin usually on the anterior shin and dorsa of the feet (**Figures 217-3** and **217-4**).[3] It can also appear as a few well-demarcated pink, flesh-colored, or purple-brown papules or nodules.
  - Nails are soft and shiny and may develop onycholysis (distal separation of the nail plate from the underlying nail bed).

Eye involvement may occur before hyperthyroidism (in 20% of patients) and gradually progresses with only mild discomfort (a gritty sensation with increased tearing is the earliest manifestation). The eye findings in GD[1,2] are:

- Lid retraction (drawing back of the eyelid allowing more sclera to be visible) (**Figures 217-1** and **217-5**)

- Frank proptosis (displacement of the eye in the anterior direction): occurs in one-third (**Figures 217-1** and **217-5**)

- Extraocular muscle dysfunction (e.g., diplopia)

- Corneal exposure keratitis or ulcer

- Periorbital edema, chemosis, and scleral injection

LABORATORY STUDIES AND IMAGING

- With typical symptoms, you can confirm the diagnosis of GD with a low or undetectable sensitive assay for TSH and an elevated free thyroxin level (T_4).

- The presence of TSH receptor antibodies (present in 70% to 100% of patients at diagnosis) has a positive and negative likelihood ratio of 247 and 0.01, respectively.[4]

- If the clinical picture is uncertain, obtain a radioactive iodine scan and uptake. Elevated uptake (>30%) and a homogeneous pattern on scan are diagnostic (**Figure 217-2**).

DIFFERENTIAL DIAGNOSIS

Other causes of hyperthyroidism:

- Autonomous functioning nodule—this is an uncommon cause of thyrotoxicosis (present in 1.6%–9%),[5] and most nodules do not

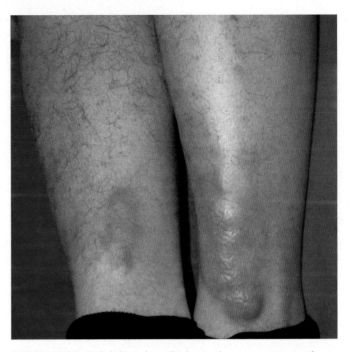

FIGURE 217-3 Early bilateral pretibial myxedema in a patient with Graves' eye disease. These asymmetrical erythematous plaques and nodules are firm and nonpitting. (*Courtesy of the University of Texas Health Sciences Center, Division of Dermatology.*)

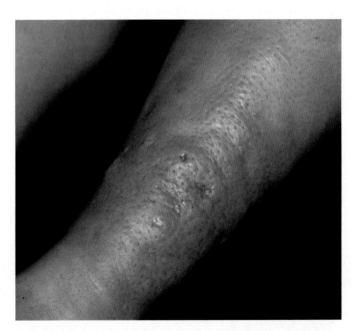

FIGURE 217-4 Pretibial myxedema in a patient with Graves' ophthalmopathy. Hair follicles are prominent, giving a peau d'orange appearance. (*Courtesy of the University of Texas Health Sciences Center, Division of Dermatology.*)

cause hyperthyroidism. These would present as a discrete swelling in an otherwise normal thyroid gland, and thyroid scan would show a discrete nodule.

- Toxic multinodular goiter—more common cause of hyperthyroidism in the elderly; thyroid scan shows multiple foci of increased uptake.

- Thyrotropin-secreting pituitary adenoma (rare)—adenomas may cause visual disturbance (in the absence of exophthalmus), and other hormonal stimulation may occur (e.g., elevated serum prolactin).

The differential diagnoses for the eye findings include the following:

- Metastatic disease to the extraocular muscles.

- Pseudotumor—this condition's rapid onset and pain differentiate it from Graves' ophthalmopathy.

MANAGEMENT

- Symptoms of hyperthyroidism can be controlled with beta-adrenergic blockers (e.g., propranolol, 10–40 mg BID–QID) or calcium channel blockers (e.g., diltiazem, 30–90 mg BID). SOR **B**

- Supportive measures for eye symptoms include dark glasses, artificial tears, propping up the head and taping the eyelids closed at night.

- Three options are available to treat the hyperthyroidism SOR **A**[1,2]:
  - Antithyroid drugs (propylthiouracil (PTU), 100–200 mg q8h or methimazole 10–20 mg/d).
    - The drugs may be reduced after the patient is euthyroid (typically PTU 50–100 mg/d and methimazole 2.5–10 mg/d).
    - Antithyroid drugs are preferred during pregnancy and can be considered in patients with mild disease, small goiter, and lower antibody levels.
    - Remission rates following antithyroid drugs vary from 37% to 70% and occur within 6 to 8 weeks; relapse rates are high (30%–50%), especially in black patients.
    - The optimal duration of titrated antithyroid drug therapy is 12 to 18 months to minimize relapse.[6] SOR **A**
  - Radioactive iodine (RAI): It is the most commonly prescribed treatment in the United States but is contraindicated in pregnancy or with breastfeeding and should be used with caution in patients with cardiovascular disease.
    - One concern is that radiation-induced thyroiditis can aggravate ophthalmopathy. This side effect can be minimized by early levothyroxine replacement and prednisone (60–80 mg/d starting at the time of RAI treatment and tapering, after 2 to 4 weeks, over the next 3 to 12 months).[7]
    - Following RAI, 50% to 75% of patients become euthyroid after 5 to 8 weeks, but 50% to 90% of patients with GD eventually become hypothyroid (10% to 20% in year 1 and 5% per year afterward).
  - Subtotal thyroidectomy:
    - Indications for surgery are very large goiters, presence of suspicious nodules, and allergy or failure of other therapies.

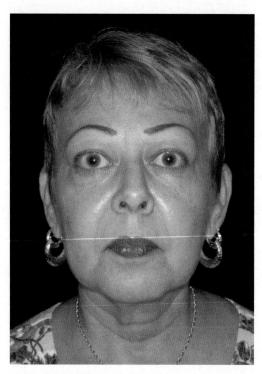

FIGURE 217-5 Bilateral exophthalmus that has been present for 5 years since patient was diagnosed with Graves' disease. While the radioactive iodine returned her thyroid function to normal, the exophthalmus continues to bother the patient. (*Courtesy of Richard P. Usatine, MD.*)

- Following surgery, small remnants of thyroid tissue (<4 g) result in rates of hypothyroidism of >50% and large remnants (>8 g) have higher rates of recurrent hyperthyroidism (15%).

- With respect to the eye findings, most symptoms except for proptosis improve with control of the hyperthyroidism. In one study, 64% of the patients spontaneously improved, 22% stabilized, and 14% progressed.[7]

- Treatment options for the persistent severe ophthalmopathy include high-dose systemic steroids (40–80 mg/d), orbital radiotherapy, and orbital decompression surgery.[8] SOR **B**

PATIENT EDUCATION

- Patients should be told that the goals of therapy are to resolve the symptoms of thyroid excess and to restore the thyroid function to normal.

- The treatment choices should be discussed as each has advantages and disadvantages; treatment should be individualized.

- Regardless of the therapy chosen, long-term follow-up is needed to monitor thyroid status; there is a high risk of becoming hypothyroid in the future or to relapse again into hyperthyroidism. Patients should be made aware of symptoms to watch for and to report any recurrent symptoms.

- Ophthalmopathy usually runs its own course independent of the thyroid function. Additional treatment may be needed in consultation with an ophthalmologist.

- Smoking cessation may have a beneficial effect on the course of ophthalmopathy.

- Siblings and children should be made aware of their increased risk of developing this or associated disorders and should monitor themselves for symptoms.

FOLLOW-UP

- The goals of therapy are to resolve hyperthyroid symptoms and to restore the euthyroid state. Close follow-up is needed in the initial treatment period; medications for symptoms of hyperthyroidism may be withdrawn slowly following treatment.
  - Antithyroid drug dosages may be reduced after the patient is euthyroid (typically PTU 50-100 mg/d and methimazole 2.5–10 mg/d), but drugs should be continued for 12–18 months to minimize relapse. SOR **A**
  - Following treatment with RAI, most patients eventually become hypothyroid (20% within the first year) and so periodic monitoring of thyroid function is important.

- Following surgery, patients may become hypothyroid or have a recurrence of hyperthyroidism, depending on the size of the remnant remaining; patients should be monitored with periodic blood tests and for symptoms.

PATIENT RESOURCE

- Patient/Family Resource: National Graves' Disease Foundation: **www.ngdf.org.**

PROVIDER RESOURCE

- Guideline: AACE Thyroid Task Force. American Association of Clinical Endocrinologists medical guidelines for clinical practice for the evaluation and treatment of hyperthyroidism and hypothyroidism. *Endocr Pract.* 2002;8(6):457–469.

REFERENCES

1. Weetman AP. Graves' disease. *N Engl J Med.* 2000;343(17): 1236–1248.

2. Jameson JL, Weetman AP. Disorders of the thyroid gland. In: Kasper DL, Braunwald E, Fauci AS, Hauser SL, Longo DL, Jameson JL eds. *Harrison's Principles of Internal Medicine.* New York, NY: McGraw-Hill, 2005:2109–2113.

3. Jabbour SA. Cutaneous manifestations of endocrine disorders. *Am J Clin Dermatol.* 2003;4(5):315–331.

4. Costagliola S, Marganthaler NG, Hoermann R, et al. Second generation assay for thyrotropin receptor antibodies has superior diagnostic sensitivity for Graves' disease. *J Clin Endocrinol Metab.* 1999; 84:90–97.

5. Siegel RD, Lee SL. Toxic nodular goiter—toxic adenoma and toxic multinodular goiter. *Endocrinol Metab Clin North Am.* 1998;27(1): 151–166.

6. Abraham P, Avenell A, Watson W, et al. Antithyroid drug regimen for treating Graves' hyperthyroidism. *Cochrane Database Syst Rev.* 2005;2:CD003420.

7. Kaplan MM, Meier DA, Dworkin HJ. Treatment of hyperthyroidism with radioactive iodine. *Endocrinol Metab Clin North Am.* 1998;27(1):205–222.

8. Boulos PR, Hardy I. Thyroid-associated orbitopathy: A clinicopathologic and therapeutic review. *Curr Opin Ophthalmol* 2004;15(5): 389–400.

218 ACROMEGALY

Mindy A. Smith, MD, MS

PATIENT'S STORY

A 60-year-old man presents to his family physician with severe headache and weakness (**Figure 218-1**). He has noted enlargement of his hands (**Figure 218-2**), which made him remove his wedding ring when it became too tight, and feet (his shoe size had increased). He said his voice seemed to be deeper and his hands feel doughy and sweaty. Laboratory testing reveals an elevated insulin-like growth factor (IGF-I), and there is a failure of GH suppression following an oral glucose load confirming the diagnosis of acromegaly. A CT scan of the head demonstrates a pituitary adenoma.

EPIDEMIOLOGY

- Rare (6/100,000 adults), debilitating condition usually caused by autonomous growth-hormone (GH) hypersecretion.

- Most typically caused by a pituitary somatotrope macroadenoma. It may also be caused by growth hormone releasing hormone (GHRH) excess from lesions of the pancreas, lung, or ovaries or from a chest or abdominal carcinoid tumor.

- The disorder is usually sporadic but may be familial (rare) and has been associated with other endocrine tumors (e.g., multiple endocrine neoplasia type I).

- In a Spanish multicenter epidemiologic study, the reported mean age at diagnosis was 45 years.[1]

- The occurrence of GH hypersecretion in children and adolescents, prior to epiphyseal closure, causes gigantism.

ETIOLOGY AND PATHOPHYSIOLOGY

- The clinical signs and symptoms of acromegaly result from GH excess, which stimulates linear and organ growth (through IGF-I) and chondrocyte action.

- Acromegaly is also associated with insulin resistance and an increased risk of cardiovascular disease.

- An increased risk for several cancers among these patients may be because of the proliferative and antiapoptotic activity associated with increased circulating levels of IGF-I.

DIAGNOSIS

The diagnosis of acromegaly is established by documenting autonomous GH hypersecretion and by imaging the pituitary.[2]

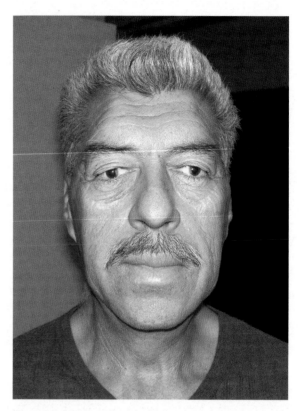

FIGURE 218-1 A 60-year-old man with acromegaly. Note the coarse facial features and moderate prognathism (protrusion of the lower jaw). (*Courtesy of Richard P. Usatine, MD.*)

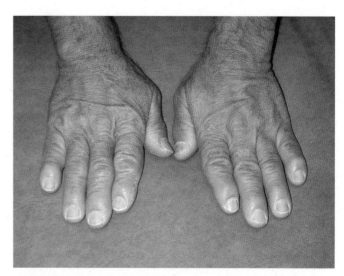

FIGURE 218-2 The man in **Figure 218-1** with acromegaly producing hands that are large and doughy with widened fingers. (*Courtesy of Richard P. Usatine, MD.*)

CLINICAL FEATURES

The clinical manifestations of acromegaly are often subtle and may not be noticed for many years (**Figure 218-1**). Gigantism occurs if excessive GH exposure occurs *before* closure of the epiphyses; acromegaly develops *after* closure of the epiphyses. Clinical features of acromegaly include the following:[3]

- Soft-tissue swelling, resulting in hand and foot enlargement (**Figure 218-2**).
- Coarse facial features and a large fleshy nose (**Figures 218-1** and **218-4**).
- Hyperhidrosis and oily skin.
- Acanthosis nigricans (see Chapter 212, Acanthosis Nigricans).
- Other common features are deep voice, arthropathy, carpel tunnel syndrome, kyphosis, proximal muscle weakness, and fatigue.
- Associated medical conditions include sleep apnea (60%), coronary heart disease (30%), and diabetes mellitus (25%).

LABORATORY STUDIES

- An elevated serum IGF-I concentration (age and gender matched) is extremely useful in the diagnosis of acromegaly.[3]
- Failure of GH suppression to <1 µg/L within 1 to 2 hours of an oral glucose load (75 g) can confirm the diagnosis, although 20% of patients exhibit a paradoxical increase in GH.
- A single measure of GH is not helpful because of its pulsatile secretion.

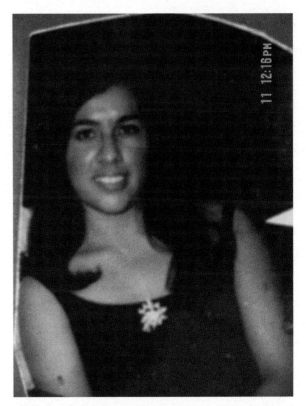

FIGURE 218-3 A 26-year-old attractive woman prior to acromegaly changes. (*Courtesy of Vernon Burke, DMD, MD.*)

MANAGEMENT

- Surgical resection (adenomectomy) is the cornerstone of treatment. SOR Ⓐ
- Medical therapy with somatostatin analogs can be considered instead of surgery.[2] SOR Ⓑ Even if surgical resection is performed some patients will still need adjunctive medical therapy to normalize GH and IGF-1 levels as described below.[2] SOR Ⓑ
- Although GH reduction may alleviate symptoms, attempts to normalize levels of GH and its target growth factor (i.e., IGF-I) should be made because persistent secretion of excess GH and IGF-I may pose significant long-term health risks (see below).
- Adjunctive therapies include the following:
  ○ Somatostatin analogues—these have been shown to improve clinical symptoms of acromegaly, decrease hypersecretion of GH and IGF-I, and reduced tumor volume.
    ▪ Subcutaneous octreotide (50 µg TID to 1500 µg/d) has been shown to suppress GH secretion (70% to <5 µg/L) and normalizes IGF-I in 75% of patients.[3] SOR Ⓑ
    ▪ It is of particular benefit to patients with persistently high levels of GH and IGF-I that cannot be suppressed by other means or until the long-term effects of radiation occur.
    ▪ Side effects are related to suppression of gastrointestinal motility and secretion and include nausea, abdominal pain, diarrhea, and flatulence (one-third of patients with improvement in the first 2 weeks) and gallstones or sludge (20%–30%).

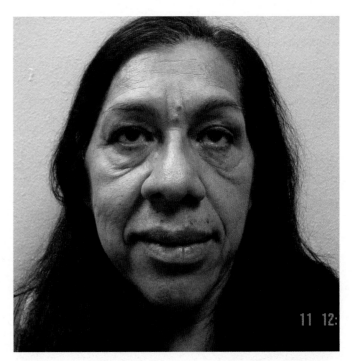

FIGURE 218-4 Facial changes 20 years later in the woman in **Figure 218-3**. Note the coarse facial features with large nose, lips, and chin. Protrusion of the lower jaw is visible. (*Courtesy of Vernon Burke, DMD.*)

- Two long-acting somatostatin depot formulations, octreotide and lanreotide, are available.
○ Dopamine agonists, like bromocriptine, bind to the D2 receptor and suppress GH hypersecretion in some patients with acromegaly.
  - Clinical effectiveness is modest (20% reach GH <5 μg/L and IGF-I normalizes in approximately 10%).[3]
  - Two long-acting agents, quinagolide and cabergoline, are being tested.
○ Subcutaneous pegvisomant, a GH receptor antagonist, is a relatively new agent for the medical management of acromegaly.
  - It was shown, in a small trial, to be better than placebo in clinical improvement and reduction in serum IGF-I levels.[4]
  - Liver enzymes should be monitored.
○ Radiation therapy, conventional and stereotactic procedures, is also effective in decreasing GH levels but takes years to work and carries a risk of hypopituitarism.

PATIENT EDUCATION

- Patients should be advised that, if untreated, one's lifespan is decreased by an average of 10 years. Survival improves greatly if GH and IGF-I can be normalized.

FOLLOW-UP

- After surgical resection, 70% of patients with microadenomas, but less than 50% of patients with macroadenomas, have persistent GH hypersecretion.[5]
  ○ Irradiation of adenomas results in attenuation of GH secretion in 50% of subjects after 12 years; the effect of these treatments on IGF-I levels is less certain.
  ○ Approximately 60% to 75% of patients receiving somatostatin analogs achieve normal IGF-I levels.[3,5]
- Based on a cohort study of patients hospitalized for acromegaly (Denmark, 1977–1993; Sweden, 1965–1993) linked to tumor registry data for up to 15 to 28 years of follow-up, individuals with acromegaly have higher rates of small intestine, colon, rectal, kidney, and bone cancer.[6] The researchers also found that these patients had elevated rates for cancers of the brain and thyroid, which may be related to pituitary irradiation.
- Options for monitoring treatment success postoperatively or following radiation therapy include serum insulin-like growth factor-binding protein-3 (IGFBP-3), serum leptin, and plasma IGF-I.
  ○ In one study, plasma IGF-I measurement had the best discriminatory power to differentiate patients with postsurgically active acromegaly from healthy people.[7]

PATIENT AND PROVIDER RESOURCES

- **http://www.endocrine.niddk.nih.gov/pubs/acro/acro. htm.** (Accessed on February 27, 2006.)
- **http://patients.uptodate.com/topic.asp?file= endo_hor/4528&title=Acromegaly.** (Accessed on February 27, 2006.)

REFERENCES

1. Mestron A, Webb SM, Astorga R, et al. Epidemiology, clinical characteristics, outcome, morbidity and mortality in acromegaly based on the Spanish Acromegaly Registry (Registro Espanol de Acromegalia, REA). *Eur J Endocrinol*. 2004;151(4):439–446.

2. Ezzat S, Wilkins GE, Patel Y, et al. The diagnosis and management of acromegaly: A Canadian consensus report. *Clin Invest Med*. 1996;19(4):259–270.

3. Melmed S, Jameson JL. Disorders of the anterior pituitary and hypothalamus. In: Kasper DL, Braunwald E, Fauci AS, Hauser SL, Longo DL, Jameson JL eds. *Harrison's Principles of Internal Medicine*. New York, NY: McGraw-Hill, 2005:2090–2092.

4. Trainer PJ. Lessons from 6 years of GH receptor antagonist therapy for acromegaly. *J Endocrinol Invest*. 2003;26(10 Suppl): 44–52.

5. Diez JJ, Iglesias P. Current management of acromegaly. *Expert Opin Pharmacother*. 2000;1(5):991–1006.

6. Baris D, Gridley G, Ron E, et al. Acromegaly and cancer risk: A cohort study in Sweden and Denmark. *Cancer Causes Control*. 2002;13(5):395–400.

7. Paramo C, Fluiters E, de la Fuente J, et al. Monitoring of treatment success in patients with acromegaly: The value of serum IGFBP-3 and serum leptin measurements in comparison to plasma insulin-like growth factor I determination. *Metabolism*. 2001;50(9): 1117–1121.

PART 17

NEUROLOGY

219 CEREBRAL VASCULAR ACCIDENT

Heidi Chumley, MD

PATIENT STORY

A 65-year-old hypertensive black man presented to the emergency department with onset of right face, arm, and hand paralysis and difficulty communicating. Rapid diagnostic testing using MRI revealed an ischemic infarct in the left middle cerebral artery (**Figure 219-1**). He was evaluated by a stroke response team and was found to be a candidate for tissue plasminogen activator (TPA). After the stroke, he was treated with aspirin, antihypertensives, and cholesterol-lowering medication. He recovered 80% of his neurological deficit over the next 3 months. A noncontrast CT image of this patient two weeks later is shown in **Figure 219-2**.

EPIDEMIOLOGY

- Cerebral vascular accident (CVA or stroke) affects approximately 700,000 people per year in the United States, most being older than 65 years.[1]
- Ischemic (66%) and hemorrhagic (10%) strokes account for most strokes.[1]
- Prevalence of stroke and mortality are higher in blacks than in whites. Prevalence is 753 vs. 424/100,000 and mortality is 95.8 vs. 73.7/100,000 for black and white men, respectively.[1]
- The 30-day mortality rate after a first or second stroke is 22% and 41%, respectively.[2]
- Following are the risk factors for stroke or CVA:
  - Hypertension (HTN): the predominant risk factor for more than 50% of all strokes. Prehypertension (blood pressure in the range of 130–139/85–89) carries a hazard ratio of 2.5 for women and 1.6 for men.[2]
  - Cigarette smoking: increases the risk of having a stroke by 50%.[2]
  - Type 2 diabetes mellitus (DM) increases the risk of having a stroke sixfold.[2]
  - Atrial fibrillation increases the risk of stroke. The CHADS2 (CHF, HTN, age >75, DM, stroke) scoring system (see below) separates patients into low risk (stroke rate 1%–1.5% per year), moderate risk (2.5%), high risk (4%), and very high risk (7%).[2]
  - Homocysteine level >15 mg/dL; however, lowering homocysteine has not been demonstrated to lower stroke risk.

ETIOLOGY AND PATHOPHYSIOLOGY

- CVAs are typically classified into cardioembolic (15%–22%), large vessel (10%–12%), small vessel (15%–18%), other known cause (2%–4%), and undetermined cause (46%–51%).[3]

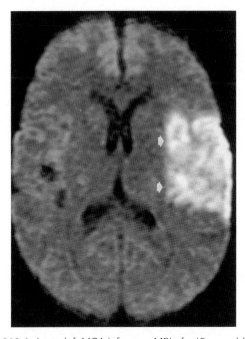

FIGURE 219-1 Acute left MCA infarct on MRI of a 65 year-old hypertensive man. The MRI demonstrates increased signal intensity (arrows). Abnormalities in MRI occur before those seen on CT during ischemic strokes. (*From Chen MYM, Pope TL, Ott DJ. Basic Radiology. New York: McGraw-Hill. 2004, p. 338.*)

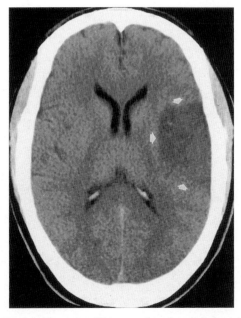

FIGURE 219-2 Noncontrast CT image of a subacute left middle cerebral artery infarct (arrows). This was done 2 weeks after the stroke in the same patient as previous figure. CT findings occur later than MRI findings in ischemic strokes (*From Chen MYM, Pope TL, Ott DJ. Basic Radiology. New York: McGraw-Hill. 2004, p. 338.*)

- Ischemic CVAs occur when atherosclerosis progresses to a plaque, which ruptures acutely. Each step of this process is mediated by inflammation.[4]

- Hemorrhagic CVAs occur when vessels bleed into the brain, usually as the result of elevated blood pressure.

- Other known causes of CVAs include inflammatory disorders (giant cell arteritis, SLE, polyarteritis nodosa, granulomatous angiitis, syphilis, and AIDS), fibromuscular dysplasia, drugs (cocaine, amphetamines, and heroin), hematologic disorders (thrombocytopenia, polycythemia, and sickle cell), and hypercoagulable states.

DIAGNOSIS

Diagnosis of CVA must be made expediently to minimize mortality and morbidity.

CLINICAL FEATURES

- History of risk factors including older age, hypertension, cigarette smoking, type 2 DM, or previous transient ischemic attack (TIA) or stroke.

- Acute onset of neurological signs and symptoms based on the site of the CVA (see typical distribution).

TYPICAL DISTRIBUTION

TIA or stroke can occur in any area of the brain; common areas with typical symptoms include the following:

- Middle cerebral artery is the most common ischemic site (**Figure 219-3**):
  - Superior branch occlusion causes contralateral hemiparesis and sensory deficit in face, hand, and arm, and an expressive aphasia if the lesion is in the dominant hemisphere.
  - Inferior branch occlusion causes a homonymous hemianopia, impairment of contralateral graphesthesia and stereognosis, anosognosia and neglect of the contralateral side, and a receptive aphasia if the lesion is in the dominant hemisphere.

- Internal carotid artery (approximately 20% of ischemic strokes) occlusion causes contralateral hemiplegia, hemisensory deficit, and homonymous hemianopia; aphasia is also present with dominant hemisphere involvement.

- Posterior cerebral artery occlusion causes a homonymous hemianopia affecting the contralateral visual field.

LABORATORY STUDIES

These tests may be helpful in the context of an acute stroke, particularly when the cause of the stroke is not immediately evident:

- Complete blood count (CBC) for thrombocytosis or polycythemia.

- Erythrocyte sedimentation rate (ESR) for diseases such as giant cell arteritis or systemic lupus erythematosis.

- Venereal Disease Research Laboratory (VDRL) slide test for syphilis.

- Serum glucose to eliminate hypoglycemia as the cause of the neurological symptoms.

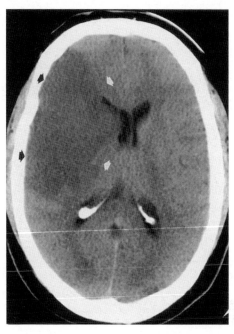

FIGURE 219-3 CT image of right middle cerebral artery infarct: the hypodense (darker) area (arrows) indicates the infarct. The midline structures are shifted to the left. (*From Chen MYM, Pope TL, Ott DJ. Basic Radiology. New York: McGraw-Hill. 2004, p. 335.*)

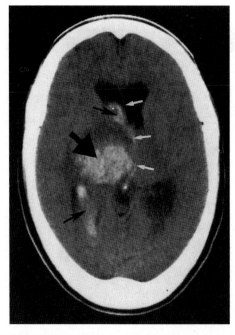

FIGURE 219-4 CT image demonstrates bleeding in the right basal ganglia (large black arrow) into the ventricles (small black arrows). Blood appears white on the CT scan. The white arrows illustrate midline shift. (*From Chen MYM, Pope TL, Ott DJ. Basic Radiology. New York: McGraw-Hill. 2004, p. 337.*)

IMAGING

CT or MRI can distinguish ischemic from hemorrhagic and localize the lesion (**Figure 219-4**).

DIFFERENTIAL DIAGNOSIS

Other causes of acute neurological dysfunction include the following:

- TIA: this precursor to a CVA can appear identical; however, no lesion is seen on imaging, and symptoms resolve within 48 hours.
- Multiple sclerosis: multiple anatomically distinct neurological signs and symptoms that occur over time and resolve; vision is often affected. MRI findings should help to distinguish between multiple sclerosis.
- Brain mass: more common presentation is headache or seizure; however, may present with focal neurological signs based on location. CT or MRI will help to diagnose a brain mass and differentiate this from stroke.
- Migraines: throbbing, unilateral headache with photophobia, and nausea; hemiparesis or aphasia may be part of the aura.
- Vertigo from benign positional vertigo or acute labyrinthitis: can mimic a CVA in the posterior circulation; however, symptoms such as dysarthria, dysphagia, and diplopia are typically absent.
- Hypoglycemia: confused state is similar to large stroke syndromes but is easily differentiated by a blood glucose measurement.

MANAGEMENT

ACUTE STROKE (WITHIN THE FIRST 3 HOURS)

- Rapidly evaluate or consult specialists to identify candidates for TPA. Odds for a favorable 3-month outcome for TPA compared to no TPA are 2.8 (95% CI 1.8–4.5) for 0–90 minutes, 1.6 (1.1–2.2) for 91 to 180 minutes.[5] SOR **A**
- Currently, only 3% of patients who meet the criteria receive TPA.[2]
- Preliminary studies raised caution about using TPA in community settings; however, recent studies indicate several options to improve outcomes including telephone consultation with a regional stroke center.[6]
- Acutely elevated blood pressure should not be aggressively treated in most cases.

  After stabilization, treat ischemic strokes with antithrombotic, antihypertensives, statins, and lifestyle changes.

- Prescribe 81 or 325 mg aspirin for secondary stroke prevention in patients with prior ischemic stroke or TIA (RR reduction 28%; NNT to prevent one stroke/y = 77).[2] SOR **A**
- Lower blood pressure (RR reduction 28%; NNT to prevent one stroke/y = 51).[2] Current data demonstrate that thiazide-type diurectic and ACE-I (or ARB) may provide additional risk reduction beyond BP control and should be used first. ACE and ARB may not be as effective in black populations.[2] SOR **A**

- Lower LDL cholesterol to <100 mg/dL for patients with a prior stroke or at high risk of stroke using a statin (RR reduction 25%; NNT to prevent one stroke/y = 57).[2] SOR **A**
- Assist patients to stop smoking (RR reduction 33%; NNT to prevent one stroke/y = 43).[2] SOR **A**
- Advise patients to adopt a health lifestyle increase fruits and vegetables, lose weight, and start a physical exercise program. SOR **B**

  Consider the following to further decrease morbidity and mortality.

- Avoid indwelling urinary catheters to reduce the risk of urinary tract infection.
- Encourage early ambulation to reduce the risk of a deep venous thrombosis.
- Use antiembolism stockings to reduce the risk of a deep venous thrombosis.
- Consider a swallowing study to identify patients at risk of aspiration.

SPECIAL SITUATIONS

- Hemorrhagic stroke:
  - Acutely: do not aggressively lower blood pressure. Some authorities recommend lowering blood pressure only when mean arterial pressure (MAP) is more than 130 mm Hg (MAP = [(2 × diastolic BP) + systolic BP]/3).
  - After the hemorrhagic stroke is over, treat blood pressure aggressively; modest decreases (12/5 mm Hg) from one of many classes of hypertensive drugs lower recurrent stroke risk by 50% to 75%.[2]
- Nonvalvular atrial fibrillation (AF): use the CHADS2 scoring system to identify patients with AF who can be managed with aspirin or should be anticoagulated with coumadin.[2]
- The CHADS/CHADS2 scoring table is shown below[3]:

C: Congestive heart failure	= 1 point
H: Hypertension (or treated hypertension)	= 1 point
A: Age >75 years	= 1 point
D: Diabetes	= 1 point
S: Prior Transient ischemic attack or Stroke	= 2 points

  - For 0–1 point, use aspirin; 2 points, weigh risk of bleeding, adequacy of follow-up vs. benefit; 3 or greater, use coumadin if at all possible.
- Patients with symptomatic carotid stenosis: refer for carotid endarterectomy patients with ≥70% carotid stenosis with ipsilateral focal neurological signs (RR reduction 44%; NNT to prevent one stroke/y = 26).[2] Consider referring symptomatic patients with moderate stenosis of 50% to 70%. SOR **A**
- Patients with asymptomatic carotic artery stenosis >60%. Consider referral for carotid endarterectomy in patients less than the age of 75 years (NNT = 20 to prevent one stroke in 5 years).[2]

PATIENT EDUCATION

Educate patients who have had a stroke about the high risk of having a second stroke, the high morbidity and mortality associated with a recurrent stroke, and the need for lifestyle modifications and medications to reduce this risk.

FOLLOW-UP

- Patients with symptoms of an acute stroke should be hospitalized, evaluated immediately for appropriateness of TPA and treatment of reversible causes, and managed, if possible, in a stroke unit or using the "best practices" associated with these units.
- After a stroke and rehabilitation, patients should be followed at regular intervals to evaluate risk reduction strategies.

PATIENT RESOURCES

- The National Stroke Association has patient information including signs of a stroke and HOPE: The stroke recovery guide at **www.stroke.org.**
- The Internet Stroke Center has a section for patients and families with patient education about signs of a stroke and living after a stroke at **www.strokecenter.org.**
- The National Institute of Neurological Diseases and Stroke has a number of patient handouts at **www.ninds.nih.gov.**

PROVIDER RESOURCES

The Internet Stroke Center has a large collection of stroke scales and clinical assessment tools, a neurology image library, listings of professional resources, and evidence-based diagnosis and management strategies at **www.strokecenter.org.**

REFERENCES

1. Stansbury JP, Jia H, Williams LS, Vogel WB, Duncan PW. Ethnic disparities in stroke: Epidemiology, acute care, and postacute outcomes [see comment] [review] [91 refs]. *Stroke.* 2005;36(2): 374–386.

2. Sanossian N, Ovbiagele B. Multimodality stroke prevention [review] [179 refs]. *Neurologist.* 2006;12(1):14–31.

3. Schneider AT, Kissela B, Woo D, et al. Ischemic stroke subtypes: A population-based study of incidence rates among blacks and whites. *Stroke.* 2004;35(7):1552–1556.

4. Elkind MS. Inflammation, atherosclerosis, and stroke [review] [72 refs]. *Neurologist.* 2006;12(3):140–148.

5. Tonarelli SB, Hart RG. What's new in stroke? The top 10 for 2004/05 [review] [25 refs]. *J Am Geriatr Soc.* 2006;54(4):674–679.

6. Frey JL, Jahnke HK, Goslar PW, Partovi S, Flaster MS. TPA by telephone: Extending the benefits of a comprehensive stroke center. *Neurology.* 2005;64(1):154–156.

220 SUBDURAL HEMATOMA

Heidi Chumley, MD

PATIENT STORY

A 34-year-old driver was hit from behind at approximately 25 miles/h. He hit his head but did not lose consciousness and did not seek care. Approximately 12 hours later, he developed a headache and confusion and was taken to the emergency department by a family member. He was found to have an acute subdural hematoma (**Figure 220-1**). He was hospitalized, and a neurosurgeon was consulted for surgical management.

EPIDEMIOLOGY

- Subdural hematomas occur at all ages.

- Eight percent of asymptomatic newborns can have a subdural hematoma.[1]

- 24/100,000 infants age 0 to 1 year in United Kingdom population studies.[2]

- Incidence or prevalence in older children, adults, and geriatric patients are unknown.

- Mortality rates in treated older adults are approximately 8% for patients younger than 65 years and 33% for patients older than 65 years.[3]

ETIOLOGY AND PATHOPHYSIOLOGY

- Most subdural hematomas are caused by trauma, either accidental or intentional, from a direct injury to the head or shaking injury in an infant.

- Subdural hematomas have been reported from chronic jarring from rapid walking in older patients and can occur during a nontraumatic birth.

- Motion of the brain within the skull causes a shearing force to the cortical surface and interhemispheric bridging veins.[2]

- This force tears the weakest bridging veins as they cross the subdural space, resulting in an acute subdural hematoma as seen in **Figure 220-1**.[2]

- Three days to 3 weeks after the injury, the body breaks down the blood in a subdural hematoma; water is drawn into the collection causing hemodilution, which appears less white and more grey on noncontrast CT.[2]

- If the hematoma fails to resolve, the collection has an even higher content of water and appears darker on a noncontrast CT; it may have fresh bleeding or may calcify (chronic subdural hematoma, **Figure 220-2**).[2] This is often of the same color as brain parenchyma on noncontrast CT.

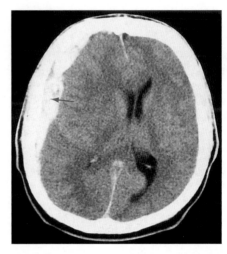

FIGURE 220-1 CT scan of an acute subdural hematoma (arrow) seen as a hyperdense clot with an irregular border. There is a midline shift from the mass effect of the accumulated blood. (*From Kasper DL, Braunwald E, Fauci, AS, Hauser SL, Longo DL, Jameson JL. Harrison's Principles of Internal Medicine, 16th ed. New York: McGraw-Hill. 2005, p. 2450.*)

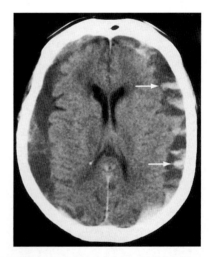

FIGURE 220-2 CT scan of chronic bilateral subdural hematomas. As subdural hematomas age, these become isodense grey and then hypodense (darker grey to black) compared to the brain. Some resolving blood is still visible on the left (arrows). (*From Kasper DL, Braunwald E, Fauci, AS, Hauser SL, Longo DL, Jameson JL. Harrison's Principles of Internal Medicine, 16th ed. New York: McGraw-Hill. 2005, p. 2450.*)

- Nontraumatic causes reported in the literature include spontaneous bleeding because of bleeding disorders or anticoagulation, meningitis, and complications of neurological procedures including spinal anesthesia.

DIAGNOSIS

CLINICAL FEATURES

The clinical features are often nonspecific, making the diagnosis difficult in the absence of known trauma.

- Infants may present with drowsiness, irritability, poor tone, poor feeding, or new seizures.[2]
- Older adults may present with headaches, confusion, subtle changes in mental status, gait disturbances, hemiparesis, or other focal neurologic signs.[4]

TYPICAL DISTRIBUTION

Subdural hematomas by definition occur in the subdural space, most commonly seen in the parietal region.

RADIOGRAPHIC STUDIES

Acute subdural hematomas are seen easily on a noncontrast CT scan (**Figure 220-1**). Subacute and chronic subdural hematomas (**Figure 220-2**) can be similar in color to the brain parenchyma and may be easier to see on a contrast CT or an MRI.

DIFFERENTIAL DIAGNOSIS

Other causes of nonspecific symptoms seen with subdural hematoma can be differentiated by neuroimaging and include the following:

- Infections such as sepsis or meningitis—fever, elevated white blood cells, positive blood cultures, and cerebral spinal fluid consistent with meningitis.
- Hemorrhagic (**Figure 220-3**) or ischemic stroke or transient ischemic attacks—consider risk factors for stroke such as hypertension, diabetes, atrial fibrillation and smoking (see Chapter 219, Cerebral Vascular Accident).
- Dementia or depression—less acute onset, advanced age, and other symptoms consistent with depression.
- Primary or metastatic brain neoplasms—history of cancer and risk factors for cancer.

Other causes of intracranial bleeding can also be differentiated by neuroimaging and include the following:

- Epidural hematoma (**Figure 220-4**)—well-defined biconvex bright white density that resembles the shape of the lens of the eye.
- Subarachnoid hemorrhage (**Figure 220-5**)—bright white blood outlines cerebral sulci.
- Hemorrhage in brain parenchyma—bright white lesion apart from dura.

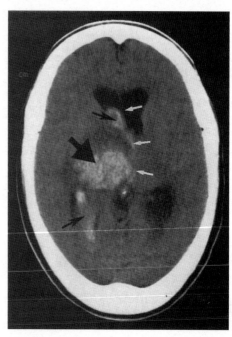

FIGURE 220-3 Hemorrhagic stroke seen on CT. The CT image demonstrates bleeding in the right basal ganglia (large black arrow) into the ventricles (small black arrows) with midline shift (white arrows). (*From Chen MYM, Pope TL Jr., Ott, DJ. Basic Radiology. New York: McGraw-Hill. 2004, p. 337.*)

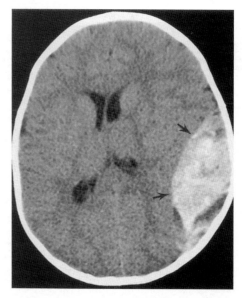

FIGURE 220-4 This head CT demonstrates an epidural hematoma, with the typical biconvex appearance (arrows). Note how the biconvexvex appearance resembles the lens of an eye. (*From Chen MYM, Pope TL Jr., Ott, DJ. Basic Radiology. New York: McGraw-Hill. 2004, p. 346.*)

MANAGEMENT

Most subdural hematomas are managed surgically, and there is little evidence about conservative management.

- Determine the Glasgow Coma Scale in patients with serious head trauma and consider airway protection in patients with a score less than 12.

- Obtain an urgent noncontrast CT scan on any patient suspected of having a subdural hematoma.

- If the noncontrast CT scan is nonrevealing, obtain a contrast CT or MRI, particularly if the traumatic event occurred 2 to 3 days prior.

- Emergently refer patients with a subdural hematoma and deteriorating neurologic status or evidence of brain edema or midline shift to a hospital with neurosurgeons.

- Consult a neurosurgeon expediently in patients with a subdural hematoma and stable focal neurological signs.

- Consider neurosurgical consultation in asymptomatic patient or patients with only a headache and a small acute subdural hematoma without brain edema or midline shift. These patients may be followed by serial CT scans without surgical treatment, but this should be done in consultation with experts in CT interpretation and management of subdural hematomas.[4] SOR **C**

- Evaluate any infant with a subdural hematoma for child abuse or neglect.[2] SOR **C**

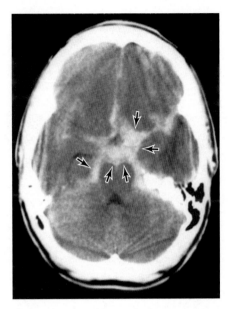

FIGURE 220-5 A subarachnoid hemorrhage appears as areas of high density (more white like bone rather than the darker grey of brain tissue) in the subarachnoid space (arrows). (*From Aminoff MJ, Greenberg DA, Simon RP. Clinical Neurology, 6th ed. New York: McGraw-Hill. 2005, p. 77.*)

PATIENT EDUCATION

- Advise patients to seek medical care immediately for head trauma, which can cause several emergencies including a subdural hematoma.

- Discuss with parents or guardians the need for a thorough evaluation for child abuse and neglect in infants with a subdural hematoma.

FOLLOW-UP

Appropriate follow-up is dictated by the extent of the subdural hematoma and initial treatment. Subdural hematomas treated surgically should be monitored in a hospital setting with neurosurgical resources available, as complications such as rebleeding are common. In patients treated conservatively, follow with serial CT scans until the hematoma has resolved. This typically takes several days and may require up to 2 to 3 weeks. After 3 weeks, the subdural hematoma is considered chronic and is unlikely to resolve spontaneously.

PATIENT RESOURCES

MedlinePlus has patient education on subdural hematoma at **http://www.nlm.nih.gov/medlineplus.**

REFERENCES

1. Whitby EH, Griffiths PD, Rutter S, et al. Frequency and natural history of subdural haemorrhages in babies and relation to obstetric factors [see comment]. *Lancet*. 2004;363(9412):846–851.

2. Minns RA. Subdural haemorrhages, haematomas, and effusions in infancy [comment] [review] [9 refs]. *Arch Dis Child*. 2005;90(9): 883–884.

3. Munro PT, Smith RD, Parke TR. Effect of patients' age on management of acute intracranial haematoma: Prospective national study. *BMJ*. 2002;325(7371):1001.

4. Karnath B. Subdural hematoma. Presentation and management in older adults. *Geriatrics*. 2004;59(7):18–23.

221 NORMAL PRESSURE HYDROCEPHALUS

Heidi Chumley, MD

PATIENT STORY

A 68-year-old man presented with a gradual onset of difficulty with his gait, increased urinary incontinence, and difficulty with his memory during the past several months. His gait was wide-based and slow, with decreased step height and length. His mini-mental status examination was consistent with impaired cognition. As part of his workup, he had a noncontrast head CT, which demonstrated dilated ventricles (**Figure 221-1**) without extensive cortical atrophy. He had normal cell counts and opening pressure on a spinal tap. He was diagnosed with normal pressure hydrocephalus (NPH) and referred to a neurosurgeon to be evaluated for a ventricular shunt. The patient had the shunt placed (**Figure 221-2**). His gait and urinary incontinence problem improved. Unfortunately, his cognitive impairments did not improve as is often the case.

EPIDEMIOLOGY

- Prevalence: 1 in 250 in those older than 65 years; determined in a door-to-door survey in Germany.[1]

- Incidence: 1–2/100,000/y; determined by number of surgeries in Sweden.[2]

- Most common in ages 60 to 70 years.

- Less than 5% of dementias are caused by NPH.[3]

ETIOLOGY AND PATHOPHYSIOLOGY

- Cerebral spinal fluid (CSF) is produced by the choroid plexus, circulates through the ventricles, exits into the subarachnoid space, and is reabsorbed by the arachnoid granulations at the top of the brain.[3]

- NPH is thought to be due to of impaired reabsorption and can be idiopathic or secondary to meningitis, subarachnoid hemorrhage, or head trauma.

DIAGNOSIS

NPH is a clinical diagnosis based on signs and symptoms, cerebral spinal fluid studies, radiographic imaging, and a clinical response to ventriculoperitoneal (VP) shunting.

CLINICAL FEATURES

Classic triad is gait disturbance, incontinence, and cognitive impairment:

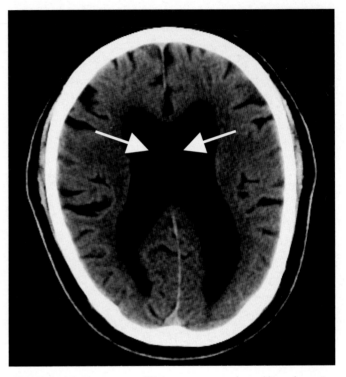

FIGURE 221-1 Noncontrast CT demonstrates enlarged lateral ventricles (white arrows) without significant cerebral atrophy. (*Courtesy of Reginald Dusing, MD.*)

- Gait disturbances typically occur first—wide-based stance; slow, shuffling steps; difficulty with initiation[3]
- Urinary incontinence usually with urgency; abnormal detrusor contractions on urodynamic studies[3]
- Cognitive impairment—difficulty with attention and concentration (digit span, arithmetic) with sparing of orientation and general memory.[4]

CSF STUDIES

- Normal cell counts and opening pressure less than 200 mm Hg.[3]
- High-volume spinal tap (removal of 30 to 66 cc of CSF) or prolonged CSF drainage (3–5 days via an indwelling catheter) followed by clinical improvement can be helpful in selecting patients more likely to respond to VP shunting.[5]
- Prolonged CSF drainage—continual drainage followed by clinical improvement.
- Continuous monitoring of intracranial pressure demonstrates characteristic waves of NPH; however, this is done only in specialized centers.

RADIOGRAPHIC STUDIES

- Enlarged ventricles without substantial cerebral atrophy can be seen on CT or MRI.
- Cysternography, a nuclear medicine test, can demonstrate impaired clearing of CSF from the lateral ventricles at 48 hours (**Figure 221-3**).

DIFFERENTIAL DIAGNOSIS

- Alzheimer's disease—impaired orientation and memory, which are often spared in NPH; cortical atrophy.
- Parkinson's disease—tremor and rigidity in addition to bradykinesia and gait disturbances; normal neuroimaging.
- Chronic alcoholism—history of alcohol use, memory and learning difficulties; cortical atrophy.
- Multi-infarct dementia, atherosclerotic disease, subdural hematomas, and tumors—identifiable on neuroimaging.
- Intercranial infections or carcinomatous meningitis—abnormal CSF findings.
- Hypothyroidism—has other symptoms such as fatigue, weakness, dry and cool skin, diffuse hair loss, cold-intolerance, constipation and difficulty concentrating. The TSH is elevated and there is no urinary incontinence (see Chapter 216, Goitrous Hypothyroidism).

MANAGEMENT

- Refer to a neurosurgeon to evaluate for VP shunting (**Figure 221-2**).
- VP shunting is the only known effective treatment (**Figure 221-2**). In larger retrospective studies, 39% to 75% of patients demonstrated improvement by 24 months.[5,6] Predictors of improvement were shorter duration of symptoms and primary symptom of gait disturbance.[5]

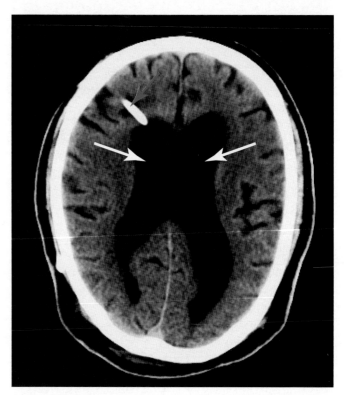

FIGURE 221-2 Noncontrast CT shows ventricular shunt (red arrow) in place. Lateral ventricles remain enlarged after shunting (white arrows). (*Courtesy of Reginald Dusing, MD.*)

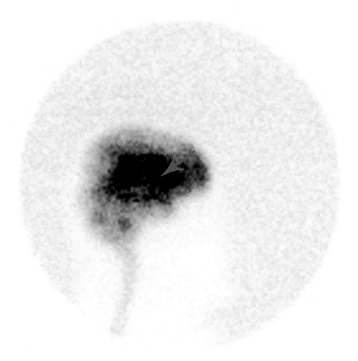

FIGURE 221-3 Lateral view on cysternography demonstrates increased uptake in the lateral ventricle (red arrow). In this nuclear medicine study, indium is injected into the cerebral spinal fluid at the lower lumbar spine and a scan is done 48 hours later. Normally, the indium-tagged spinal fluid has been reabsorbed at 48 hours, and the lateral ventricle does not have increased uptake. (*Courtesy of Reginald Dusing, MD.*)

- Cognitive improvement occurs less commonly, in approximately one-third of patients. Predictors of better cognitive improvement include younger age and female gender.[7]
- The risks of VP shunting can be substantial; moderate to severe complications occurred in 28% of patients in one study.[6]

PATIENT EDUCATION

Advise patients that improvements from VP shunting

- Do not occur for all patients.
- Appear slowly over several months.
- May last several years.
- Are more likely to involve gait disturbances rather than cognitive deficits.

Advise patients to inform any health care provider they see about their VP shunt.

FOLLOW-UP

Long-term multidisciplinary follow-up can facilitate gait and bladder retraining and early recognition of signs of shunt malfunction including vomiting, headache, fever, or seizures.

PATIENT RESOURCES

The American Academy of Family Physicians has a patient handout: Normal pressure hydrocephalus: What is it and how is it treated? **www.aafp.org.** (Accessed October 24, 2006.)

The National Institute of Neurological Disorders and Stroke has an information handout at: **http://www.ninds.nih.gov.** (Accessed October 24, 2006.)

PROVIDER RESOURCES

An international expert panel devised diagnostic guidelines for NPH, which can be found in the journal Neurosurgery. (Diagnosing Idiopathic Normal-pressure Hydrocephalus, Vol. 57(3), Supplement: S2-4–S2-16, 2005).

REFERENCES

1. Trenkwalder C, Schwarz J, Gebhard J, et al. Starnberg trial on epidemiology of Parkinsonism and hypertension in the elderly. Prevalence of Parkinson's disease and related disorders assessed by a door-to-door survey of inhabitants older than 65 years. *Arch Neurol.* 1995;52(10):1017–1022.

2. Tisell M, Hoglund M, Wikkelso C. National and regional incidence of surgery for adult hydrocephalus in Sweden. *Acta Neurol Scand.* 2005;112(2):72–75.

3. Verrees M, Selman WR. Management of normal pressure hydrocephalus [summary for patients in *Am Fam Physician.* 2004 Sep 15;70(6):1085–1086; PMID: 15456117]. *Am Fam Physician.* 2004;70(6):1071–1078.

4. Ogino A, Kazui H, Miyoshi N, et al. Cognitive impairment in patients with idiopathic normal pressure hydrocephalus. *Dement Geriatr Cogn Disord.* 2006;21(2):113–119.

5. McGirt MJ, Woodworth G, Coon AL, Thomas G, Williams MA, Rigamonti D. Diagnosis, treatment, and analysis of long-term outcomes in idiopathic normal-pressure hydrocephalus. *Neurosurgery.* 2005;57(4):699–705; discussion 699–705.

6. Vanneste J, Augustijn P, Dirven C, Tan WF, Goedhart ZD. Shunting normal-pressure hydrocephalus: Do the benefits outweigh the risks? A multicenter study and literature review [review] [46 refs]. *Neurology.* 1992;42(1):54–59.

7. Chang S, Agarwal S, Williams MA, Rigamonti D, Hillis AE. Demographic factors influence cognitive recovery after shunt for normal-pressure hydrocephalus. *Neurologist.* 2006;12(1):39–42.

222 BELL'S PALSY

Heidi Chumley, MD

PATIENT STORY

Five years ago, a young woman awoke with the inability to move the left side of her face. She was pregnant at that time. On examination it was found that she had absent brow furrowing, weak eye closure, and dropping of her mouth angle. She was diagnosed with Bell's palsy and was provided eye lubricants and guidance on keeping her left eye moist. Her physician discussed the available evidence about treatment with steroids and antivirals. She chose not to take medications because of her pregnancy. Some improvement occurred after her delivery, but 5 years later, she continues to have the Bell's palsy (**Figure 222-1**).

EPIDEMIOLOGY

- 13.1 to 15.2/100,000 in a Canadian study.[1]
- 42.77/100,000 in a study of United States military members, with higher incidence in females, blacks, and Hispanics; arid climate and cold months were independent predictors of risk with adjusted relative risk ratios of 1.34 and 1.31, respectively.[2]
- Women who develop Bell's palsy in pregnancy have a fivefold increased risk over national average of preeclampsia or gestational hypertension.[3]
- Seventy percent of cases of acute peripheral facial nerve palsy are idiopathic (Bell's palsy); 30% have known etiologic factors such as trauma, diabetes mellitus, polyneuritis, tumors, or infections such as herpes zoster or borrelia.[4]

ETIOLOGY AND PATHOPHYSIOLOGY

- Etiology is currently unknown and under debate; the prevailing theory suggests a viral etiology from the herpes family.
- The facial nerve becomes inflamed, resulting in nerve compression.
- Compression of the facial nerve compromises muscles of facial expression, taste fibers to the anterior tongue, pain fibers, and secretory fibers to the salivary and lacrimal glands.
- This is a lower motor neuron lesion; the upper and lower portions of the face are affected (**Figure 222-1**). In upper motor neuron lesions (e.g., cortical stroke), the upper third of the face is spared, while the lower two-thirds are affected as a result of the bilateral innervation of the orbicularis, frontalis, and corrugator muscles, which allows sparing of upper face movement.

DIAGNOSIS

CLINICAL FEATURES

- Weakness of all facial muscles on the affected side: loss of brow furrowing, weak eye closure, and dropped angle of mouth.

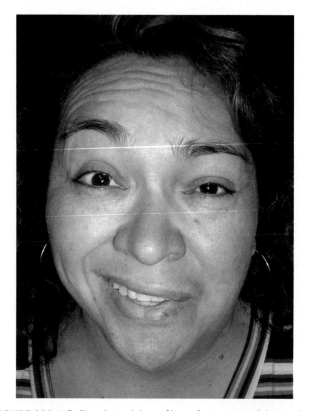

FIGURE 222-1 Bell's palsy with loss of brow furrowing and dropped angle of the mouth on the affected left side of her face demonstrated during a request to smile and raise her eyebrows. The Bell's palsy has been present for 5 years and the patient is being evaluated by ENT for surgery to restore facial movement. (*Courtesy of Richard P. Usatine, MD.*)

- Postauricular pain.
- Dry eyes.
- Involuntary tearing.
- Hyperacusis.
- Altered tastes.

  Other testing is not usually indicated:

- Herpes virus titers are not usually helpful.
- Consider serological tests for Lyme disease in endemic areas.
- Consider MRI to look for a space-occupying lesion with atypical presentations.

DIFFERENTIAL DIAGNOSIS

- Upper motor neuron diseases including stroke—normal brow furrowing, eye closure, and blinking.
- Space-occupying lesion—symptoms are dependent on the location of the mass; consider with an isolated facial nerve palsy that does not affect all three branches of the facial nerve.
- Lyme disease—occurs in endemic area with skin rash, joint inflammation, and flu-like symptoms. Bell's palsy is the most common neurologic manifestation of Lyme disease (see Chapter 211, Lyme Disease).
- Suppurative ear disease—ear pain, abnormal tympanic membrane, and more common in children.
- Facial nerve damage from microvascular disease—most commonly in diabetes mellitus.
- Facial nerve damage from trauma—history of trauma differentiates this from Bell's palsy that is idiopathic or from an infectious etiology.
- Isolated third nerve palsy—manifestations include diplopia and drooping of the upper eyelid (ptosis) (**Figure 222-2**). The affected eye may deviate out and down in straight-ahead gaze; adduction is slow and cannot proceed past the midline. Upward gaze is impaired. When downward gaze is attempted, the superior oblique muscle causes the eye to adduct. The pupil may be normal or dilated; its response to direct or consensual light may be sluggish or absent (efferent defect). Pupil dilation (mydriasis) may be an early sign.

MANAGEMENT

- Provide eye protection with artificial tears, lubricants, or closing of the eyelid. SOR **C**
- Steroids are controversial and have not been demonstrated to improve facial nerve function, although the latest Cochrane review contained only four studies with 179 patients.[5]
- Acyclovir or valacyclovir have conflicting results in studies, and the latest Cochrane review recommended further study before making a recommendation.[6]
- Acupuncture alone improved Bell's palsy, as measured by an accepted scoring system when compared to acupuncture plus steroids or steroids alone in a multicenter trial of 439 cases.[7] SOR **B**

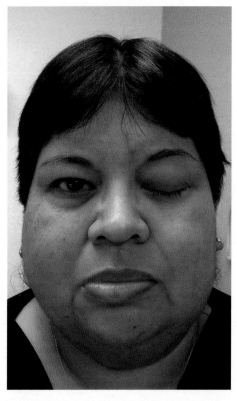

FIGURE 222-2 Ptosis from an isolated third nerve palsy in a patient with diabetes. Note the symmetry of the facial creases, which would be absent in Bell's palsy. This patient would also have abnormal eye movements. The eye would deviate down and out, adduction would not pass the midline, and upward gaze would be impaired. (*Courtesy of Richard P. Usatine, MD.*)

- Electrical stimulation may be useful in determining prognosis, but more research is needed to determine if electrical stimulation has beneficial therapeutic effects.[8]

- It is possible to restore some facial movement with specialized surgical procedures including regional muscle transfer and microvascular free tissue transfer.[9] SOR **C** In longstanding facial paralysis, consider referral to an ENT surgeon or plastic surgeon with experience in these procedures.

PATIENT EDUCATION

- Most patients recover spontaneously without treatment with steroids or antiviral medications.

- Ninety-five percent of children recover; 70% recover within 3 weeks.

FOLLOW-UP

Consider seeing patients in 2 to 3 weeks to evaluate recovery and to reconsider diagnosis if there has been no recovery, particularly in children.

PATIENT RESOURCES

The National Institute of Neurological Disorders and Stroke has a patient information page available at **http://www.ninds.nih.gov.** (Accessed October 21, 2006.)

PROVIDER RESOURCES

The Cochran Collaborative contains updated systematic reviews of steroid and/or antiviral treatment of Bell's palsy at **www.cochran.org.**

REFERENCES

1. Morris AM, Deeks SL, Hill MD, et al. Annualized incidence and spectrum of illness from an outbreak investigation of Bell's palsy. *Neuroepidemiology*. 2002;21(5):255–261.

2. Campbell KE, Brundage JF. Effects of climate, latitude, and season on the incidence of Bell's palsy in the US Armed Forces, October 1997 to September 1999. *Am J Epidemiol*. 2002;156(1):32–39.

3. Shmorgun D, Chan WS, Ray JG. Association between Bell's palsy in pregnancy and pre-eclampsia. *QJM*. 2002;95(6):359–362.

4. Berg T, Jonsson L, Engstrom M. Agreement between the Sunnybrook, House-Brackmann, and Yanagihara facial nerve grading systems in Bell's palsy. *Otol Neurotol*. 2004;25(6):1020–1026.

5. Salinas RA, Alvarez G, Ferreira J. Corticosteroids for Bell's palsy (idiopathic facial paralysis) [update of *Cochrane Database Syst Rev*. 2002;(1):CD001942; PMID: 11869613] [review] [29 refs]. *Cochrane Database Syst Rev*. 2004;4:CD001942.

6. Allen D, Dunn L. Aciclovir or valaciclovir for Bell's palsy (idiopathic facial paralysis) [update of *Cochrane Database Syst Rev*. 2001;(4):CD001869; PMID: 11687127] [review] [26 refs]. *Cochrane Database Syst Rev*. 2004;3:CD001869.

7. Liang F, Li Y, Yu S, et al. A multicentral randomized control study on clinical acupuncture treatment of Bell's palsy. *J Trad Chin Med*. 2006;26(1):3–7.

8. May M, Blumenthal F, Klein SR. Acute Bell's palsy: prognostic value of evoked electromyography, maximal stimulation, and other electrical tests. *Am J Otol*. 1983;5(1):1–7.

9. Chuang DC. Free tissue transfer for the treatment of facial paralysis. *Facial Plast Surg*. 2008;24(2):194–203.

223 NEUROFIBROMATOSIS

Heidi Chumley, MD

PATIENT STORY

A 44-year-old Hispanic man has neurofibromatosis, type 1 (NF-1). He has typical features of NF-1, including eight café au lait spots, axillary freckling, and neurofibromas all over his body (**Figures 223-1** to **223-4**). He states that he is used to having the neurofibromatosis and it does not currently affect his work or life. He is happily married but never had children. No intervention is necessary at this time other than recommending yearly visits to the ophthalmologist and his family physician.

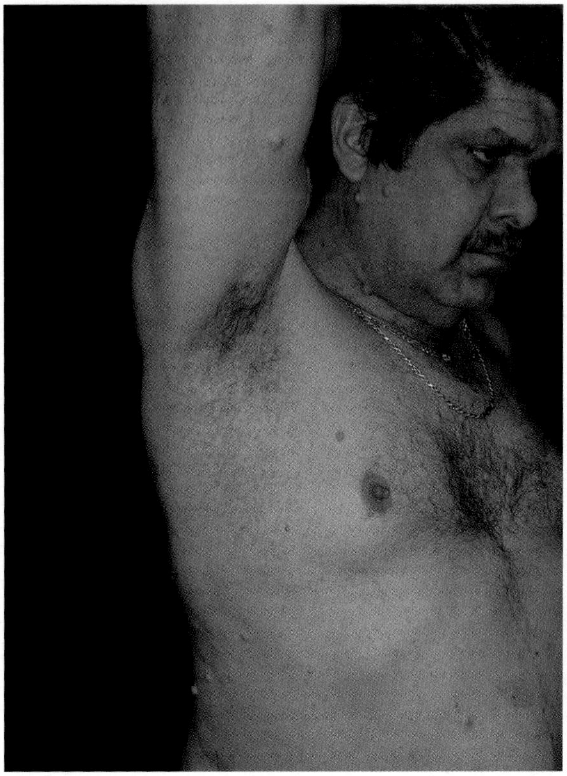

EPIDEMIOLOGY

- Neurofibromatosis type 1 is relatively common: birth incidence is one in 3000 and prevalence in the general population is one in 5000.[1]

- Autosomal-dominant inheritance; however, up to 50% of cases are sporadic.[1]

- Diagnosis is typically made during childhood.

ETIOLOGY AND PATHOPHYSIOLOGY

- Mutations in the NF-1 gene (on the long arm of chromosome 17) result in loss of function of neurofibromin, which helps keep proto-oncogene ras (which increases tumorigenesis) in an inactive form.

- Loss of neurofibromin results in increased proto-oncogene ras activity in neurocutaneous tissues, leading to tumorigenesis.[1]

DIAGNOSIS

For a diagnosis of NF-1, patients need to have at least two of the following:[2]

- Two or more neurofibromas or one or more plexiform neurofibromas (**Figures 223-1** to **223-6**).

- Six or more café au lait spots, 0.5 cm or larger before puberty and 1.5 cm or larger after puberty (**Figures 223-3** and **223-4**).

- Axillary or inguinal freckling (**Figures 223-1** and **223-4**).

- Optic glioma.

- Two or more Lisch nodules (melanotic iris hamartomas) (**Figure 223-7**).

- Dysplasia of the sphenoid bone or dysplasia/thinning of long bone cortex.

- A first-degree relative with NF-1.

FIGURE 223-1 A 44-year-old Hispanic man with neurofibromatosis-1 showing all the typical findings including neurofibromas, café au lait spots, and axillary freckling. (*Courtesy of Richard P. Usatine, MD.*)

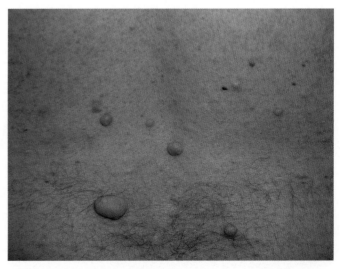

FIGURE 223-2 Close-up of neurofibromas on the back of the man in **Figure 223-1**. These are soft and round. (*Courtesy of Richard P. Usatine, MD.*)

CLINICAL FEATURES

- Ninety-five percent have café au lait macules, mostly before the age of 1 year.
- Ninety percent have axillary or inguinal freckling (**Figures 223-1** and **223-4**).
- Eighty-one percent have cognitive dysfunction manifest as learning disorder, attention-deficit hyperactivity disorder, or mild cognitive impairment.[3]
- Nerve sheath, intracranial, or spinal tumors.
- Cutaneous or subcutaneous neurofibromas (**Figures 223-1** to **223-6**).
- Other bony pathology including dysplasia of the sphenoid or long bones, scoliosis, or short stature.
- Eye abnormalities including Lisch nodules or early glaucoma (**Figure 223-7**).

DIFFERENTIAL DIAGNOSIS

NF-1 is the predominant cause of café au lait spots, which can also be seen in the following cases:

- Normal childhood: 13% to 27% of children younger than 10 years of age have at least one spot.
- Neurofibromatosis type 2: vestibular schwannomas, family history of NF-2, meningioma, glioma, schwannoma, juvenile posterior subcapsular lenticular opacities, or juvenile cortical cataracts.
- Tuberous sclerosis: angiofibromas (skin-colored telangiectatic papules most commonly in the nasolabial folds, cheek, or chin; **Figure 223-8**) and hypopigmented ovoid or ash leaf-shaped macules.
- McCune Albright syndrome: fibrous dysplasia of bone and endocrine gland hyperactivity.
- Fanconi anemia: decreased production of all blood cells, short stature, upper limb anomalies, genital changes, skeletal anomalies, eye/eyelid anomalies, kidney malformations, ear anomalies/deafness, and gastrointestinal/cardiopulmonary malformations.
- Segmental neurofibromatosis: cutaneous neurofibromas limited to specific dermatome(s); very rare.
- Bloom syndrome: growth delay and short stature, increased risk of cancer, telangiectatic erythema on the face, cheilitis, narrow face, prominent nose, large ears, and long limbs.
- Ataxia telangiectasia: progressive neurologic impairment, cerebellar ataxia, immunodeficiency, impaired organ maturation, ocular and cutaneous telangiectasia, and a predisposition to malignancy.
- Proteus syndrome: very rare condition with hamartomatous and multisystem involvement. Joseph Merrick (also known as "the elephant man") is now, in retrospect, thought by clinical experts to have had Proteus syndrome and not neurofibromatosis.

MANAGEMENT

Management focuses on early recognition and treatment of manifestations.

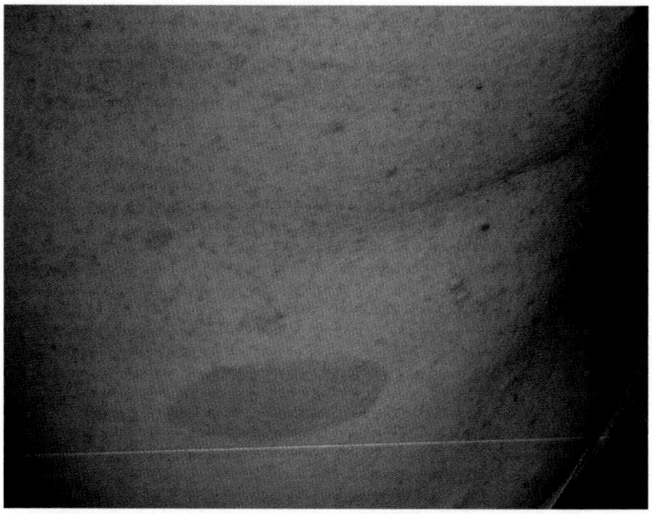

FIGURE 223-3 Large café au lait spot on the back of the man in **Figure 223-1**. Café au lait spots are ovoid hyperpigmented macules, 10 to 40 mm in diameter, with smooth borders. (*Courtesy of Richard P. Usatine, MD.*)

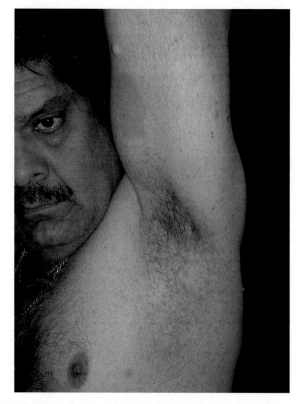

FIGURE 223-4 Close-up of axillary freckling (Crow's sign) with large café au lait spot on arm. (*Courtesy of Richard P. Usatine, MD.*)

- Evaluate children twice a year and adults annually. SOR **C**

- Screen for cognitive impairment and refer early for intervention. SOR **C**

- Screen for scoliosis and treat accordingly.

- Refer patients annually for ophthalmologic evaluation.

- Consider treatment or referral for treatment of café au lait spots if desired by the patient. Topical vitamin D$_3$ analogs (calcipotriene) and laser therapy independently may improve the appearance of café au lait spots.[4,5] SOR **B** One small study suggests that intense pulsed–radio frequency (IPL-RF) in combination with topical application of vitamin D$_3$ ointment may lighten small-pigmented lesions in patients with NF1.[6] SOR **B** While calcipotriene (Dovonex) is approved for use in psoriasis it can be prescribed off-label to patients disturbed by their hyperpigmented macules.[4,6] SOR **B**

- Examine other undiagnosed first-degree relatives. SOR **C**

- Surgical excision of tumors is required for tumors pressing on vital structures (i.e., spinal cord impingement) or when characteristics such as rapid enlargement are worrisome for malignant transformation.

PATIENT EDUCATION

- Recommend that family members get evaluated. NF-1 is an autosomal genetic disorder, although, up to 50% of the time, the disease may arise from a spontaneous mutation.

- Regular follow-up with primary-care physicians and specialists is recommended to identify complications of the disease and treat them as early as possible.

FOLLOW-UP

- Primary-care evaluation biannually for children; annually for adults.

- Ophthalmologic examination annually for children and adults.

PATIENT RESOURCES

- Neurofibromatosis, Inc has a variety of patient education materials, information about local support groups, ongoing clinical trials, and camp New Friends for children with NF at **www.nfinc.org.**

- The National Institute of Neurological Diseases and Stroke has patient information at **www.ninds.nih.gov.**

PROVIDER RESOURCES

Neurofibromatosis, Inc has a variety of resources including NF specialists by location at **www.nfinc.org.**

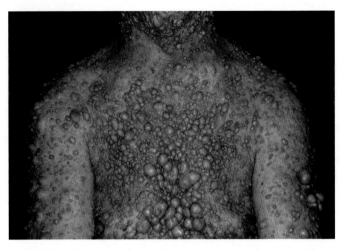

FIGURE 223-5 A man with neurofibromatosis covered with neurofibromas. (*Courtesy of Jack Resneck, Sr., MD.*)

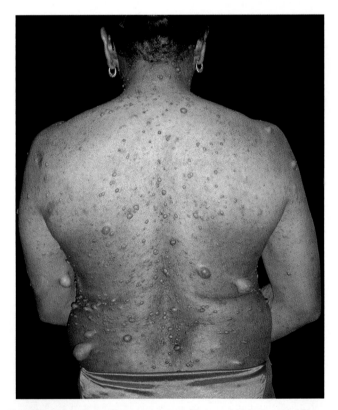

FIGURE 223-6 Neurofibromatosis in a 62-year-old black woman. Note how large some the neurofibromas can become. (*Courtesy of Richard P. Usatine, MD.*)

REFERENCES

1. Yohay K. Neurofibromatosis types 1 and 2 [review] [65 refs]. *Neurologist*. 2006;12(2):86–93.

2. Hirsch NP, Murphy A, Radcliffe JJ. Neurofibromatosis: clinical presentations and anaesthetic implications [review] [114 refs]. *Br J Anaesth*. 2001;86(4):555–564.

3. Hyman SL, Shores A, North KN. The nature and frequency of cognitive deficits in children with neurofibromatosis type 1. *Neurology*. 2005;65(7):1037–1044.

4. Nakayama J, Kiryu H, Urabe K, et al. Vitamin D3 analogues improve cafe au lait spots in patients with von Recklinghausen's disease: Experimental and clinical studies. *Eur J Dermatol*. 1999; 9(3):202–206.

5. Shimbashi T, Kamide R, Hashimoto T. Long-term follow-up in treatment of solar lentigo and cafe-au-lait macules with Q-switched ruby laser. *Aesthetic Plast Surg*. 1997;21(6):445–448.

6. Yoshida Y, Sato N, Furumura M, Nakayama J. Treatment of pigmented lesions of neurofibromatosis 1 with intense pulsed-radio frequency in combination with topical application of vitamin D$_3$ ointment. *J Dermatol*. 2007;34(4):227–230.

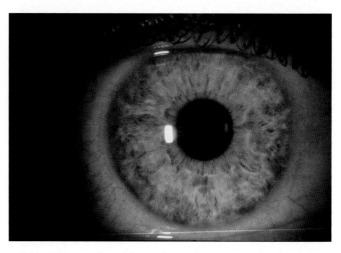

FIGURE 223-7 Lisch nodules (melanotic hamartomas of the iris) are clear yellow-to-brown, dome-shaped elevations that project from the surface of this blue iris. These hamartomas are the most common type of ocular involvement in NF-1 and do not affect vision. (*Courtesy of Paul Comeau.*)

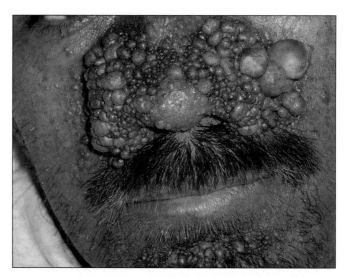

FIGURE 223-8 Angiofibromas (previously called adenoma sebaceum) on the face of a patient with tuberous sclerosis. The patient was originally thought to have neurofibromatosis. He also has epilepsy and cognitive impairment, which goes with tuberous sclerosis. (*Courtesy of Natalie Norman, MD.*)

PART 18

SUBSTANCE ABUSE

224 SUBSTANCE ABUSE DISORDER

Richard P. Usatine, MD
Kelli Hejl, MA

PATIENT STORY

A 21-year-old mother and her four children are being seen in a free clinic within a homeless shelter for various health reasons (**Figure 224-1**). The woman is currently clean and sober, but has a long history of cocaine use and addiction (**Figure 224-2**). Her children span the ages of 3 months to 5 years. She was recently living with her mother after the birth of her youngest child, but was kicked out of her mother's home when she went out to use cocaine once again. The patient gave written consent to the photograph and when she was shown the image on the digital camera she noted how depressed she looked. She asked for me to tell the viewers of this photograph that these can be the consequences of drug abuse—being depressed, homeless, and a single mom.

EPIDEMIOLOGY

- An estimated 71.5 million Americans aged 12 years or older were current users of a tobacco product in 2005. This represents 29.4% of the population in that age range. In addition, 60.5 million persons (24.9% of the population) were current cigarette smokers, 13.6 million (5.6%) smoked cigars, 7.7 million (3.2%) used smokeless tobacco, and 2.2 million (0.9%) smoked tobacco in pipes.[1]

- An estimated 19.7 million Americans aged 12 years or older were current illicit drug users in 2005. This represents 8.1% of the population aged 12 years old or older.[1]

- Marijuana was the most commonly used illicit drug (14.6 million users) (**Figures 224-3** and **224-4**). It was used by 74.2% of current illicit drug users. Among current illicit drug users, 54.5% used only marijuana, 19.6% used marijuana and another illicit drug, and the remaining 25.8% used only an illicit drug other than marijuana.[1]

- There were 2.4 million persons who were current cocaine users in 2005.[1]

- The number of current crack users increased from 467,000 in 2004 to 682,000 in 2005.[1]

- There were 512,000 persons using methamphetamine in 2005 (**Figure 224-5**).[1]

- Hallucinogens were used by 1.1 million persons (0.4%) in 2005, including 502,000 (0.2%) who had used Ecstasy (**Figure 224-6**).[1]

- Current heroin users in 2005 were 136,000 persons (0.1%) (**Figure 224-7**).[1]

- There were 9.0 million people aged 12 or older (3.7%) who were current users of illicit drugs other than marijuana in 2005. Most

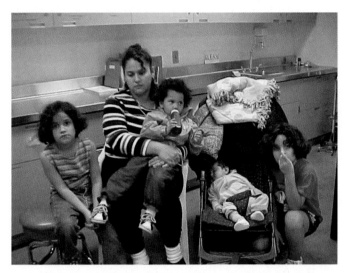

FIGURE 224-1 A cocaine-addicted mother with her children in a homeless shelter. Her drug addiction resulted in their homelessness. (*Courtesy of Richard P. Usatine, MD.*)

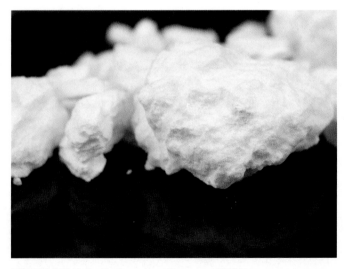

FIGURE 224-2 Purified cocaine. (*Courtesy of DEA.*)

(6.4 million, 2.6%) used psychotherapeutic (including prescription drugs) drugs nonmedically. Of these, 4.7 million used pain relievers, 1.8 million used tranquilizers, 1.1 million used stimulants (including 512,000 using methamphetamine), and 272,000 used sedatives.[1]

- The rate of current use of sedatives declined from 0.2% in 2002 to 0.1% in 2005.[1]

- In 2005, the most prevalent source from which recently used drugs were obtained among nonmedical users of prescription-type drugs was "from a friend or relative for free."[1]

- Among persons aged 12 years or older who used pain relievers nonmedically in the past 12 months, 59.8% reported that the source of the drug the most recent time they used was from a friend or relative for free. Another 16.8% reported that they got the drug from some physician. Only 4.3% got the pain relievers from a drug dealer or other stranger, and only 0.8% reported buying the drug on the Internet.[1]

- More than half (57.6%) of past year nonmedical users of stimulants aged 12 years or older reported getting the drug from a friend or relative for free. Also, 6.5% bought the drug from a drug dealer or other stranger and 7.2% bought it on the Internet.[1]

ASSOCIATION WITH CIGARETTE AND ALCOHOL USE

- In 2005, the rate of current illicit drug use was approximately eight times higher among youths aged 12 to 17 years who smoked cigarettes in the past month (46.7%) than it was among youths who did not smoke cigarettes in the past month (5.5%).[1]

- Past month illicit drug use was also associated with the level of past month alcohol use. Among youths aged 12 to 17 years in 2005 who were heavy drinkers (i.e., drank five or more drinks on the same occasion [i.e., at the same time or within a couple of hours] on each of 5 or more days in the past 30 days), 59.9% were also current illicit drug users, which was higher than among nondrinkers (5.0%).[1]

- Among youths aged 12 to 17 years who were both smokers and heavy drinkers in the past month in 2005, 70.9% used illicit drugs in the past month, higher than the 3.5% among youths who did not drink or smoke in the past month.[1]

ETIOLOGY AND PATHOPHYSIOLOGY

- "Drug addiction is a brain disease. Although initial drug use might be voluntary, drugs of abuse have been shown to alter gene expression and brain circuitry, which in turn affect human behavior. Once addiction develops, these brain changes interfere with an individual's ability to make voluntary decisions, leading to compulsive drug craving, seeking and use."[2]

- The medical consequences of addiction are far reaching and very costly to society. Cardiovascular disease, stroke, cancer, HIV/AIDS, hepatitis, and lung disease can all be increased by drug abuse. Some of these effects occur when drugs are used at high doses or after prolonged use. Some consequences occur after just one use.[2]

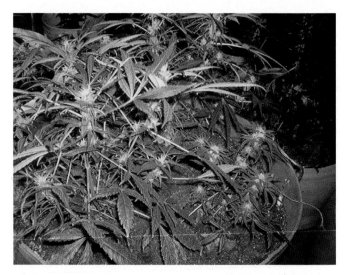

FIGURE 224-3 Home-grown marijuana plant. (*Courtesy of DEA.*)

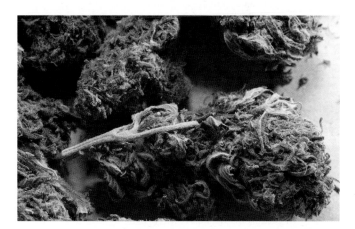

FIGURE 224-4 Marijuana ready to be smoked. (*Courtesy of DEA.*)

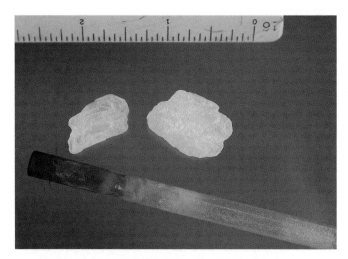

FIGURE 224-5 Methamphetamine ice with pipe. (*Courtesy of DEA.*)

- Familial pattern—both genetics and learned behaviors can increase a person's risk for substance abuse.
- Family, twin, and adoption studies have convincingly demonstrated that genes play an important role in the development of alcohol dependence, with heritability estimates in the range of 50% to 60% for both men and women. A number of studies are under way to identify specific genes involved in the predisposition toward alcohol dependence. These include genes involved in alcohol metabolism, as well as genes involved in gamma-aminobutyric acid (GABA), endogenous opioid, dopaminergic, cholinergic, and serotonergic transmission.[3]
- A wealth of literature supports the role of GABA in neurobiological pathways contributing to alcohol dependence and related phenotypes. Dick et al. found evidence of association with several drinking behaviors, including alcohol dependence, history of blackouts, age at first drunkenness, and level of response to alcohol with single-nucleotide polymorphisms (SNPs) within one of four GABA receptor genes on chromosome 5q.[4] Much work still needs to be done to elucidate the genetics of alcoholism and other addictions.
- Comorbid mental health issues and chronic pain disorders are highly prevalent among persons with substance abuse disorders. Addicts use drugs to self-treat feelings of depression and symptoms of pain.
- Classes of substances that are frequently abused and involved in addiction include:
  - Depressants: alcohol, sedatives, hypnotics, opioids, and anxiolytics.
  - Stimulants: cocaine, amphetamines, and nicotine.
  - Hallucinogens: cannabis, PCP, and LSD.
  - Toxic inhalants.
- The onset of drug effects is approximately:
  - 7 to 10 seconds for inhaling or smoking.
  - 15 to 30 seconds for intravenous injection.
  - 3 to 5 minutes for intramuscular or subcutaneous injection.
  - 3 to 5 minutes for intranasal use (snorting).

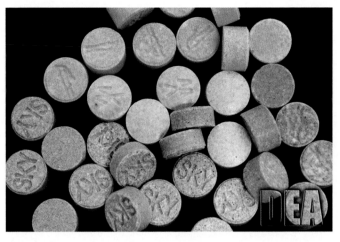

FIGURE 224-6 Ecstasy tablets used at raves where people dance all night long and some collapse in dehydration. (*Courtesy of DEA.*)

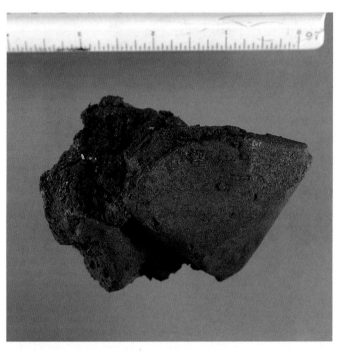

FIGURE 224-7 Black tar heroin for injection. (*Courtesy of DEA.*)

DIAGNOSIS

It helps to make the distinction between substance abuse and substance dependence to understand how to provide help for the patient.

DSM IV CRITERIA FOR SUBSTANCE ABUSE[5]

Substance abuse is defined as a maladaptive pattern of substance use leading to clinically significant impairment or distress, as manifested by one (or more) of the following, occurring within a 12-month period:

- Recurrent substance use resulting in a failure to fulfill major role obligations at work, school, or home (such as repeated absences or poor work performance related to substance use; substance-related absences, suspensions, or expulsions from school; or neglect of children or household).

- Recurrent substance use in situations in which it is physically hazardous (such as driving an automobile or operating a machine when impaired by substance use).

- Recurrent substance-related legal problems (such as arrests for substance-related disorderly conduct).

- Continued substance use despite having persistent or recurrent social or interpersonal problems caused or exacerbated by the effects of the substance (for example, arguments with spouse about consequences of intoxication and physical fights).

DSM IV CRITERIA FOR SUBSTANCE DEPENDENCE[5]

A maladaptive pattern of substance use leading to clinically significant impairment or distress, as manifested by three (or more) of the following, occurring at any time in the same 12-month period:

- Substance is often taken in larger amounts or over longer period than intended.

- Persistent desire or unsuccessful efforts to cut down or control substance use.

- A great deal of time is spent in activities necessary to obtain the substance (e.g., visiting multiple physicians or driving long distances), use the substance (e.g., chain smoking), or recover from its effects.

- Important social, occupational, or recreational activities given up or reduced because of substance abuse.

- Continued substance use despite knowledge of having a persistent or recurrent psychological or physical problem that is caused or exacerbated by use of the substance.

- Tolerance, as defined by either
  - need for markedly increased amounts of the substance in order to achieve intoxication or desired effect; or
  - markedly diminished effect with continued use of the same amount.

- Withdrawal, as manifested by either
  - characteristic withdrawal syndrome for the substance; or
  - the same (or closely related) substance is taken to relieve or avoid withdrawal symptoms.

CLINICAL FEATURES VISIBLE WITH SUBSTANCE ABUSE

- With intoxication, the following signs may be visible:
  - Via stimulants—dilated pupils and increase in blood pressure, respiratory rate, pulse, and body temperature.
  - Via depressants—decrease in blood pressure, respiratory rate, pulse, and body temperature. Opioids produce pinpoint pupils. Alcohol intoxication produces dilated pupils.

- Withdrawal develops with decline of substance in the CNS. Withdrawal reactions vary by the substance used. Alcohol withdrawal is one of the most deadly and dangerous types of withdrawal.

LABORATORY STUDIES

- All injection drug users and persons engaged in high-risk sexual activities should be screened for HIV (with consent), Hepatitis B and C, and syphilis (RPR).

- Women should have Pap smears performed and be screened for chlamydia and gonorrhea based on age, risk factors and previous history of screening. Unfortunately women who are addicted to substances often neglect their routine health care and may be long overdue for their Pap smears. If women are sexually promiscuous while using drugs or are having sex for drugs, they are at high risk for STDs.

- Purified protein derivative (PPD) test to screen for tuberculosis (especially if the patient is homeless or HIV positive).

- Electrocardiogram is warranted if there are any cardiac symptoms or if the physical examination reveals signs of cardiac disease.

- Urine screen for common drugs of abuse may reveal other drugs not admitted to in the history. Substances have different physiological half-lives in the body and show up for varying amounts of time in the urine. Marijuana has a long excretion half-life and may be detectable for 1 month after its use. Other substances may last for only days.

DIFFERENTIAL DIAGNOSIS

Substance abuse disorders are commonly comorbid with and complicate the course and treatment of numerous psychiatric conditions.

- Mood/anxiety disorders—especially depression, bipolar affective disorder, panic disorder, and generalized anxiety disorder. Persons with addictions can develop the symptoms of these disorders from the drugs of abuse. However, mood and anxiety disorders can predate the use of drugs, and some of the motivation for drug use can stem from the desire to self-treat the pain and suffering from these psychological conditions. It is best to evaluate persons when they are off the drugs whenever possible.

- Schizophrenia—while drugs can cause temporary psychosis and paranoia, if these symptoms persist after the drugs are stopped for some time, consider schizophrenia and other causes of psychosis.

- Personality disorders—these are a complicated set of disorders that can coexist and be confused with substance abuse disorder. An addict may appear to have an antisocial personality disorder when committing crimes to get money for expensive drugs. It is best to not use this diagnosis unless the behaviors continue when the person is off the drugs.

MANAGEMENT

- Recognize addiction (referred to as dependence in the DSM-IV criteria). One simple mnemonic device is the "three C's of addiction":
  - **C**ompulsion to use.
  - Lack of **C**ontrol.
  - **C**ontinued use despite adverse consequences.
- Use the "5 As"—ask, advise, assess, assist, and arrange—to help smokers who are willing to quit. This model can be applied to any substance of abuse.[6]
- Offer counseling and pharmacotherapy to aid your patients to quit smoking.

- Use the CAGE[7] questionnaire when asking about alcohol use:
  - Cut down (Have you ever felt you should *cut* down on your drinking?).
  - Annoyed (Have people *annoyed* you by criticising your drinking?).
  - Guilty (Have you ever felt bad or *guilty* about your drinking?).
  - Eye opener (Have you ever had a drink first thing in the morning to steady your nerves or get rid of a hangover (eye-opener)?).

Interpreting the results: one positive suggests at risk, two positives suggest abuse, and three or four positives suggest dependence. This is just a screening tool, and further evaluation is always needed.

- Recommend the 12-step programs to your patients. These have been very effective for millions of people worldwide.

- Refer to substance abuse programs. Such programs include hospital- and community-based programs. Some programs include detox and others require the patient to have gone through detox before starting the program. There are residential treatment units, outpatient programs, and ongoing self-help programs. Learn about the programs in your community and work with them.

- When prescribing opioid analgesics for chronic pain consider the outcomes in four domains, or the "four *A*s." Is the patient
  - Receiving adequate Analgesia?
  - Experiencing improvements in Activities of daily life?
  - Experiencing any Adverse effects?
  - Demonstrating Aberrant medication-taking behaviors that may be linked to addiction?[7]

- When patients are exhibiting aberrant drug-taking behaviors, consider the following
  - They may have an addiction.
  - They may not be getting adequate pain relief taking the drug as prescribed.
  - They may have a comorbid mental illness.
  - They may intend to distribute pain medications illegally.[8]

- Help your patients acknowledge that they have a problem and offer them help in a nonjudgmental manner.

- Enlist family members to help whenever the patient gives your permission to do so.

- Demonstrate genuine concern and care; suspend judgment and you will have a higher chance of succeeding to help your patients overcome addiction.

- Advanced brain imaging and genetic tests are helping us to understand the physiological basis of addiction and will ultimately provide us with better treatments for the medical disease of addiction.

PERSONS IN RECOVERY

Be careful how you prescribe medications to persons in recovery. A "simple" prescription for hydrocodone (Vicodin) postoperatively can start a recovered person down the road of active addiction. This does not mean that you can never prescribe pain medications or anxiolytics to a patient in recovery. Avoid giving opioids and benzodiazepines whenever there are good alternatives. Stick with NSAIDs for pain if possible. Use SSRIs, other antidepressants, or buspirone for anxiety if a medication is needed. If an opioid is needed, work with the patient to monitor the amount and manner of use. Involving a third person or sponsor to help meter out the dose may prevent relapse. Be upfront and honest about a shared goal to avoid relapse. This can save an addict's life because addiction is a lifelong disease that can be lethal.

PATIENT EDUCATION

Explain to patients that addiction is a disease and not a failing of their moral character. Inform patients about the existing treatment programs in their community and offer them names and phone numbers so that they may get help. If your patient is not ready for help today give the numbers and names for tomorrow. Speak about the value of 12-step programs because these are effective and everyone can afford a 12-step program (these are free). There are 12-step programs in the community for everyone including nonsmokers and agnostics.

FOLLOW-UP

Follow-up is important for the treatment of all types of substance abuse. While we standardly set up follow-up appointments for hypertension and diabetes we do not always remember to follow our patients with substance abuse and addiction. These are also chronic (and relapsing) conditions and merit long-term follow-up. Whether the addiction is tobacco, alcohol, pain medications, or illicit substances, your intervention and caring attitude can help the patient overcome addiction to live a sober and drug-free life. Do not give up on patients who relapse because it often takes more than one attempt before long-term cessation can be achieved.

The frequency and intensity of follow-up depends on the substance, the addiction, and the patient.

PATIENT RESOURCES

- Alcoholics Anonymous (AA): **http://www.alcoholics-anonymous.org/**—meetings and the Big Book are free. The Big Book is online for free in three languages.
- Narcotics Anonymous (NA): **http://www.na.org/index.htm**—meetings are free. The "Basic Text" costs $10—it is similar to the AA big book, but the language is more up to date and readable.
- Cocaine Anonymous (CA): **http://www.ca.org/**—meetings are free. Their first book "Hope, Faith and Courage: Stories from the Fellowship of Cocaine Anonymous" was published in 1994 and sells for $10.
- Crystal Meth Anonymous (12-step meetings): **http://www.crystalmeth.org/**.
- Drugstory.org: **http://www.drugstory.org/**.

PROVIDER RESOURCES

- The National Institute on Drug Abuse (NIDA), **http://www.nida.nih.gov/consequences/**.
- Substance Abuse and Mental Health Services Administration, **http://www.samhsa.gov/**.
- Drugstory.org: **http://www.drugstory.org/**.
- Drug Enforcement Agency website: **http://www.usdoj.gov/dea/multimedia.html**.

REFERENCES

1. Substance Abuse and Mental Health Services Administration. *Results from the 2005 National Survey on Drug Use and Health: National Findings* (Office of Applied Studies, NSDUH Series H-30, DHHS Publication No. SMA 06-4194). Rockville, MD, 2006. Report online at: http://www.oas.samhsa.gov/nsduh.htm.

2. The National Institute on Drug Abuse (NIDA). Medical Consequences of Drug Abuse. http://www.nida.nih.gov/consequences/. Accessed May 27, 2007.

3. Dick DM, Bierut LJ. The genetics of alcohol dependence. *Curr Psychiatry Rep*. 2006;8:151–157.

4. Dick DM, Plunkett J, Wetherill LF, et al. Association between GABRA1 and drinking behaviors in the collaborative study on the genetics of alcoholism sample. *Alcohol Clin Exp Res*. 2006;30: 1101–1110.

5. The American Psychiatric Association. *Diagnostic and Statistical Manual of Mental Disorders*. 4th edn (DSM-IV). Washington: The American Psychiatric Association, 1994.

6. Fiore MC, Bailey WC, Cohen SJ, et al. *Treating Tobacco Use and Dependence. Quick Reference Guide for Clinicians*. Rockville, MD: U.S. Department of Health and Human Services, Public Health Service, October 2000.

7. Ewing JA. Detecting alcoholism: the CAGE questionnaire. *JAMA* 1984;252:1905–1907.

8. Passik SD, Kirsh KL, Whitcomb L, et al. A new tool to assess and document pain outcomes in chronic pain patients receiving opioid therapy. *Clin Ther*. 2004;26: 552–561.

225 METHAMPHETAMINE

Michelle Rowe, DO
Andrew Schechtman, MD

PATIENT STORY

A 40-year-old woman with diabetes comes to the clinic with blood sugar in the 400s because she ran out of insulin a few weeks ago. She appears poorly groomed and has nicotine stains on her fingertips. Excoriated lesions (**Figure 225-1**) are noted on her forearms and face. She reports no itching at this moment, but when asked confirms that she regularly smokes methamphetamine. The diagnosis of her skin condition is meth mites. She acknowledges that she picks at her skin when she is high on meth. The physician asks her if she wants help to get off the meth so she can care for her health and well-being. She breaks down in tears and says that her craving for meth is very strong, but she is willing to try something because she knows the meth is ruining her body and life.

EPIDEMIOLOGY

- Worldwide, compared to other drugs of abuse, only marijuana is used more often than amphetamine/methamphetamine.[1]
- The lifetime prevalence ("ever-used") rate for methamphetamine was 4.4% for 12th graders in the 2006 Monitoring the Future study, which surveys 50,000 students in eighth, 10th, and 12th grades in 400 schools nationwide annually. This has decreased from 1999 when the lifetime prevalence for methamphetamine use in 12th graders was 8.2%. For comparison, marijuana/hashish had a lifetime prevalence in 12th graders of 42.3% and 49.7% in 2006 and 1999, respectively.[2]
- Stimulants (methamphetamine and amphetamine) accounted for 5% of nationwide emergency department visits in 2004, with the highest incidence in those from 18 to 44 years old.[3]
- Of 14,322 respondents aged 18 to 26 years surveyed in 2001–2002, 2.8% had used crystal methamphetamine in the past year. Crystal methamphetamine use was associated with white or Native American race, residence in the west or south, having an ever-incarcerated father, marijuana, cocaine, intravenous drug use and high novelty seeking behavior.[4]
- The Community Epidemiology Work Group (CEWG), a drug surveillance system monitoring usage trends involving 21 US cities/regions, reported data in June 2006 that methamphetamine use continues to be most prevalent in Hawaii and the Western United States (San Diego, LA County, Seattle, and Phoenix). However, methamphetamine use has been spreading eastward, as demonstrated by the pockets of high abuse in Minneapolis/St. Paul, Atlanta, and Texas.[5]
- The number of admissions to treatment in which methamphetamine was the primary drug of abuse increased from 47,695 in 1995 to 152,368 in 2005. The methamphetamine admissions

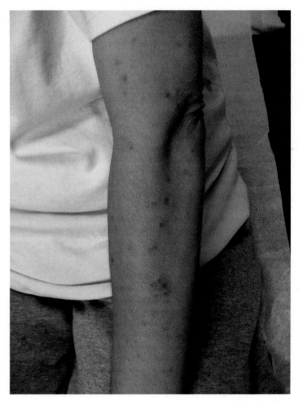

FIGURE 225-1 A 40-year-old woman with sores on her arm caused by picking at her skin while using methamphetamine. Also called meth mites, although there are no mites. (*Courtesy of Andrew Schechtman, MD.*)

represented 2.8% of the total drug/alcohol admissions to treatment during 1995 and 8.2% of the treatment admissions in 2005.[6]

- Methamphetamine is a Schedule II stimulant with legitimate medical uses including the treatment of narcolepsy and attention-deficit hyperactivity disorder.

- Methamphetamine is known on the street as meth, crank, ice (**Figure 225-2**), and crystal. It is abused by smoking, injecting, snorting, or oral ingestion. Smoking or injecting the drug gives an intense, short-lived "flash" or rush. Snorting or oral ingestion creates euphoria but no rush.

- Methamphetamine can be manufactured from inexpensive, readily available chemicals using recipes easily found on the Internet and in books (**Figure 225-3**).

- Common industrial and household chemicals used to make methamphetamine include isopropyl (rubbing) alcohol, toluene (brake cleaner), ether (engine starter), sulfuric acid (drain cleaner), red Phosphorus (matches/road flares), salt (table/rock), iodine (teat dip or flakes/crystal), lithium (batteries), trichloroethane (gun scrubber), MSM (cutting agent), sodium metal, methanol (gasoline additives), muriatic acid (used in swimming pools), anhydrous ammonia (farm fertilizer), sodium hydroxide (lye), pseudoephedrine and ephedrine (cold tablets), acetone, and cat litter.[7]

- The "meth laboratory," the site of small-scale methamphetamine production (**Figure 225-4**), brings with it many hazards, including exposure to toxic chemicals for the meth cooks themselves, their children, and law enforcement, medical, and fire personnel entering the laboratory in the course of their duties. Explosions and fires at meth laboratories are common. Improper disposal of the toxic chemicals used in the laboratories frequently leads to environmental contamination.[8]

- Effects of methamphetamine such as euphoria, increased libido, and impaired judgment may lead to increased high-risk sexual behaviors such as unprotected sexual intercourse and contact with multiple sexual partners. As a result, methamphetamine users are at increased risk of contracting sexually transmitted infections including HIV.

ETIOLOGY AND PATHOPHYSIOLOGY

- Methamphetamine acts as a central nervous system stimulant by blocking presynaptic reuptake of dopamine, norepinephrine, and serotonin.

- Compared to amphetamines, methamphetamine has an increased ability to cross the blood–brain barrier and prolonged half-life (10–12 hours). This leads to faster-onset, more intense, and longer-lasting effects when compared to amphetamine.

- Intended effects of methamphetamine use include euphoria, increased energy, a heightened sense of alertness, and increased libido.

- Unintended effects include increased heart rate, blood pressure, and body temperature; headaches; nausea; anxiety; aggression; paranoia; visual and auditory hallucinations; insomnia; tremors; and cardiac arrhythmias.

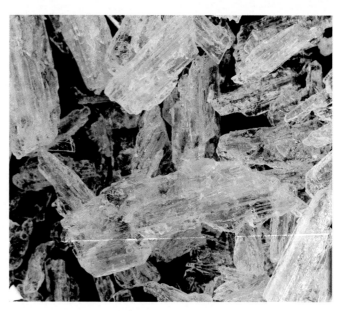

FIGURE 225-2 Methamphetamine in its ice format. (*Courtesy of DEA.*)

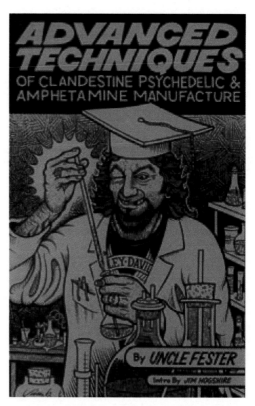

FIGURE 225-3 One of many books by Uncle Fester that can be purchased on the Internet. The information to manufacture methamphetamine is readily available. (*Reproduced with permission from Uncle Fester, www.unclefesterbooks.com*)

- With chronic abuse, confusion, poor concentration, paranoia, depression, weight loss, and dental decay can occur. The face and body become atrophic and gaunt, making the chronic methamphetamine user appear older than their stated age.

- Methamphetamine users may experience formication, the hallucination that bugs are crawling under the skin. The skin excoriations resulting from picking at the imagined bugs are known as "meth mites (**Figures 225-1, 225-5** and **225-6**)."

- The rampant dental caries and gingivitis commonly seen in methamphetamine users is known as "meth mouth" (**Figures 225-7** and **225-8**). The causes of meth mouth are multiple. Vasoconstriction leads to decreased saliva production and dry mouth, which often result in consumption of large amounts of sugar-containing beverages. Methamphetamine users often neglect their oral hygiene when preoccupied with obtaining and using the drug. Methamphetamine-induced bruxism also damages the teeth. Neglect of early symptoms and lack of access to or failure to seek dental care often lead to unsalvageable teeth that can only be extracted.[9–11]

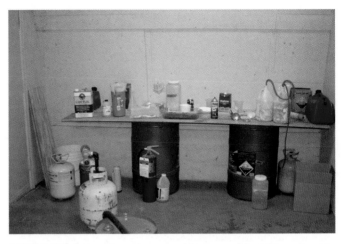

FIGURE 225-4 A methamphetamine laboratory with visible toxic and flammable substances. (*From www.streetdrugs.org.*)

DIAGNOSIS

ACUTE INTOXICATION

This can lead to tachycardia, hypertension, chest pain, hyperthermia, mydriasis, agitation, irritability, hypervigilance, paranoia, hallucinations, and tremor.

CHRONIC USE

Chronic use of methamphetamine can cause violent behavior, anxiety, depression, confusion, insomnia, and psychotic symptoms (paranoia, auditory hallucinations, delusions, and formication).[12,13]

WITHDRAWAL SYMPTOMS

The symptoms include drug cravings, depressed mood, disturbed sleep patterns, increased appetite, and fatigue.

COMPLICATIONS

Complications arising from using methamphetamine include neurologic (seizures, stroke caused by intracerebral hemorrhage or vasospasm), cardiovascular (myocardial ischemia or infarction, dilated cardiomyopathy, and cardiac arrhythmias), hyperthermia (potentially fatal), rhabdomyolysis, consequences of injection drug abuse (skin infections and abscesses, endocarditis), and high-risk sexual behavior increasing risks of contracting sexually transmitted infections including hepatitis B, hepatitis C, and HIV.

LABORATORY STUDIES

- Urine drug screening is commonly done with immunoassays. These tests are highly cross-reactive and may give false-positive results for methamphetamine or amphetamine caused by the presence of other sympathomimetic amines such as pseudoephedrine or ephedrine. Unexpected positive results on a screening test can be confirmed with more specific tests such as gas chromatography/mass spectrometry (GC/MS) and stereospecific chromatography.[14] One limitation of urine drug testing for methamphetamine is that the drug may only be detectable for 1 to 2 days after use.

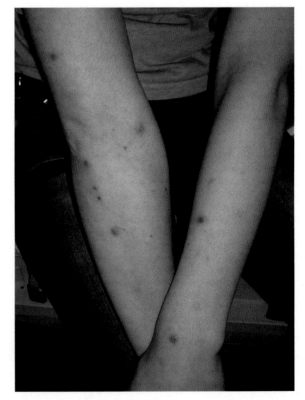

FIGURE 225-5 A 19-year-old woman with sores on her arms from picking at her skin while using methamphetamine. Also called meth mites. (*Courtesy of Richard P. Usatine, MD.*)

Hair testing is available and remains positive for up to 90 days after drug use.

- Methamphetamine users are at increased risk of sexually transmitted diseases and diseases transmitted through the use of shared needles. Consider screening for HIV, hepatitis B & C, and other sexually transmitted infections.

- For patients with signs and symptoms of acute intoxication, consider excluding complications of methamphetamine abuse by ordering creatinine phosphokinase (CK), CBC, and Chem panel. If chest pain is present, cardiac enzymes and ECG are indicated.

DIFFERENTIAL DIAGNOSIS

ACUTE METHAMPHETAMINE INTOXICATION

- Intoxication with other substances of abuse causing sympathetic stimulation and/or altered mental status (cocaine, ecstasy, and LSD).

- Psychiatric disorders (bipolar disorder, panic attack, and schizophrenia).

- Hyperthyroidism and thyroid storm (see Chapter 217, Greaves Exophthalmos and Goiter).

METHAMPHETAMINE-INDUCED SKIN LESIONS (METH MITES)

- Scabies—burrows may be present; located on wrists, fingers, genital region, and spares face; very pruritic. Family members may be infected too (see Chapter 137, Scabies).

- Atopic dermatitis—is very pruritic as is meth mites. In most cases there is a long history of the dermatitis before the meth use had begun (see Chapter 139, Atopic Dermatitis).

- Contact dermatitis is pruritic but is generally localized to the area in which the contact allergen has touched the skin. A good history should allow this to be differentiated from meth mites (see Chapter 140, Contact Dermatitis).

- Neurodermatitis and prurigo nodularis—persistent complaints of severe pruritus. In many ways there are similar to meth mites in that the stimulus to scratch is from the brain not just the skin. Absence of meth use should be present in these self-inflicted dermatoses to distinguish them from meth mites (see Chapter 142, Self-Inflicted Dermatoses).

MANAGEMENT

- Acute methamphetamine intoxication is treated with supportive measures. Sedation with haloperidol, droperidol, or benzodiazepines (diazepam and lorazepam) can be used for agitated patients. Methamphetamine-induced cardiac ischemia is treated with oxygen, nitrates, and beta blockers. Seizures and rhabdomyolysis are treated in the standard fashion.[15] SOR **B**

- Treatment of methamphetamine dependence and addiction is challenging. Inpatient detoxification may be required initially, followed by a long-term program of behavioral interventions. SOR **C**

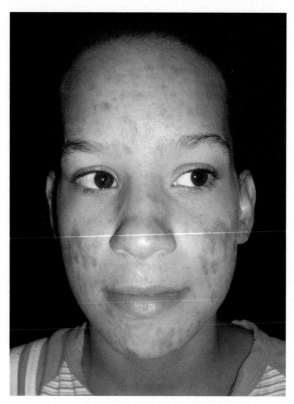

FIGURE 225-6 Postinflammatory hyperpigmentation in a young woman who has picked at her skin while addicted to methamphetamine. (*Courtesy of Richard P. Usatine, MD.*)

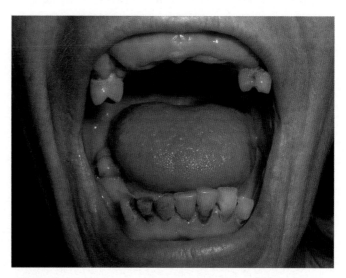

FIGURE 225-7 Methamphetamine mouth (meth mouth) in a 42-year-old woman with 20 years of methamphetamine use. The meth has completely destroyed her teeth. (*Courtesy of Richard P. Usatine, MD.*)

- Refer patients to 12-step programs, which are valuable and free. Crystal Meth Anonymous is a 12-step program modeled on the 12 steps of Alcoholics Anonymous and the White Book of Narcotics Anonymous. If Crystal Meth Anonymous meetings are not available, any 12-step program can be of help in recovery and maintaining sobriety. SOR **B**

- The Matrix model, a behavioral treatment method initially developed for treatment of cocaine addiction, has been used successfully to treat methamphetamine addiction. It consists of a 16-week program including group and individual therapy, relapse prevention, family involvement, participation in a 12-step program or other spiritual group, and weekly drug testing.[16] SOR **C**

- In the context of outpatient behavioral treatment programs, providing small incentives for drug-free urine samples can help promote abstinence. One study found that 19% of incentivized patients achieved 12 weeks of continuous abstinence while only 5% of non-incentivized patients did so (NNT = 7.1) at a cost of only $2.42 per day per participant.[17] SOR **B**

- While there are currently no FDA-approved medications to help treat methamphetamine dependence, several medications under study have shown favorable early results, including modafinil, buproprion, and some antiepileptic drugs.[18] SOR **B**

- Methamphetamine-related skin excoriation should heal without treatment if the picking behavior stops. However, post-inflammatory hyperpigmentation may never resolve (**Figure 225-6**). Antibiotic treatment with an antistaphylococcal agent such as cephalexin or dicloxacillin is indicated if the excoriations become infected. If MRSA is suspected, choose an antibiotic that covers MRSA (see Chapter 110, Impetigo).

- Referral for dental care is indicated for patients with gingivitis and dental caries caused by chronic methamphetamine use. Recommend daily use of a soft-bristled tooth brush and dental floss for treatment and prevention of oral pathology. SOR **A** Rinsing with a chlorhexidine-containing mouthwash may be a reasonable alternative for patients who find it too painful to floss. SOR **C** (see Chapters 38, Gingivitis and Periodonted Disease and 44, Adult Dental Caries).

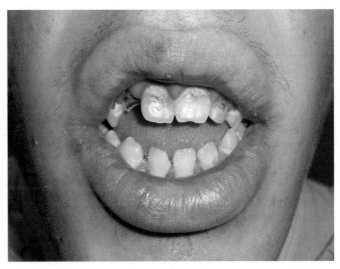

FIGURE 225-8 "Meth mouth" in a 17-year-old man actively using methamphetamine. (*Courtesy of Michelle Rowe, MD.*)

PATIENT EDUCATION

- Encourage patients to stop using methamphetamine. Offer referral to a treatment program in the community.

- Inform patients that methamphetamine use carries risks of heart attack, stroke, and death that can result from a single dose. There is no safe level of methamphetamine use.

- Counsel patients who have sex while using methamphetamine that this combination increases the likelihood of unsafe sexual practices and their risk of getting a sexually transmitted infection.

- Advise users who inject methamphetamine to use clean needles and to avoid sharing needles to decrease their risk of contracting hepatitis B, hepatitis C, and HIV.

FOLLOW-UP

- Methamphetamine users who have recently quit are at high risk of relapse. Close follow-up is indicated to identify relapses and to reinitiate treatment.
- Maintenance of abstinence can be aided by participation in an outpatient treatment program and 12 step programs.
- Methamphetamine-induced skin lesions should heal when the picking behavior ceases. Resolution is unlikely if methamphetamine abuse continues.

PATIENT RESOURCES

- Crystal Meth Anonymous (12-step meetings): **http://www. crystalmeth.org/**.
- Meth Stories: Affecting your community. **http://www. drugfree. org/Portal/DrugIssue/Meth/index.html**.
- "Methamphetamine Use and Oral Health" from Journal of American Dental Association's For the Dental Patient series (*JADA*. 2005;136(10):1491). Available at: **http://www.ada. org/prof/ resources/pubs/jada/patient/ patient_55.pdf**.
- Frontline: The meth epidemic: How meth destroys the body; PBS. Available at: **http://www.pbs.org/wgbh/pages/ frontline/ meth/body/**.

PROVIDER RESOURCES

- National Institute on Drug Abuse website: **http://www.nida. nih.gov/DrugPages/Methamphetamine.html**.
- Rawson R. SAMHSA/CSAT Treatment Improvement Protocols 33: Treatment for Stimulant Use Disorders. 1999. **http://www.ncbi. nlm.nih.gov/books/bv.fcgi?rid= hstat5.chapter.57310**.

REFERENCES

1. United Nations Office of Drugs and Crime (UNODC). *2005 World Drug Report*. Vienna, Austria: UNODC; 2005.

2. Monitoring the Future. Trends in lifetime prevalence of use of various drugs for eight, tenth and twelfth graders. Available at: http://monitoringthefuture.org/data/06data/pr06t1.pdf. Accessed June 24, 2007.

3. Drug Abuse Warning Network. *2004: National Estimates of Drug-Related Emergency Department Visits*. DAWN Series D-28, DHHS Publication No. (SMA) 06-4143. Rockville, MD; April 2006.

4. Iritani BJ, Hallfors DD, Bauer DJ. Crystal methamphetamine use among young adults in the USA. *Addiction*. 2007;102:1102–1113.

5. Community Epidemiology Working Group. Epidemiologic trends in drug abuse: Advance report. June 2006. Available at: http://www.drugabuse.gov/PDF/CEWG/AdvReport606.pdf. Accessed June 24, 2007.

6. Office of National Drug Control Policy. Drug facts – methamphetamine. Available at: http://www.whitehousedrugpolicy. gov/drugfact/methamphetamine/index.html. Accessed June 24, 2007.

7. Street Drugs University. Available at: http://www.streetdrugs-university.org/amember/sduniversity%20secure/index_files/ Page1889.htm. Accessed June 24, 2007.

8. Lineberry TW, Bostwick JM. Methamphetamine abuse: A perfect storm of complications. *Mayo Clin Proc*. 2006;81(1):77–84.

9. American Dental Association. Methamphetamine use (meth mouth). Available at: http://www.ada.org/prof/resources/ topics/methmouth.asp. Accessed June 24, 2007.

10. Klasser G, Epstein J. Methamphetamine and it's impact on dental care. *J Can Dental Assoc*. 2005;71(10):759–762.

11. Shaner JW, Kimmes N, Saini T, Edwards P. "Meth mouth": Rampant caries in methamphetamine abusers. *AIDS Patient Care STD*. 2006;20(3):146–150.

12. Rawson RA, Condon TP. Why do we need an Addiction supplement focused on methamphetamine? *Addiction*. 2007; 102(Suppl 1):1–4.

13. Volkow ND. Methamphetamine abuse – testimony before the Senate Subcommittee on Labor, Health and Human Services, Education, and Related Agencies – Committee on Appropriations. April 21, 2005. Available at: http://www.nida.nih.gov/ Testimony/4-21-05Testimony.html. Accessed June 24, 2007.

14. Gourlay DL, Heit HA, Caplan YH. Urine drug testing in clinical practice. California Academy of Family Physicians Monograph Edition 3, 2006. Available at: http://www.familydocs.org/files/ UDTmonograph.pdf. Accessed June 24, 2006.

15. Derlet R, Albertson T. Methamphetamine toxicity. eMedicine. Available at: http://www.emedicine.com/EMERG/topic859. htm. Accessed June 24, 2007.

16. Rawson RA, Gonzales R, Brethen P. Treatment of methamphetamine use disorders: An update. *J Substance Abuse Treat*. 2002;23(2): 145–150.

17. Petry NM, Peirce JM, Stitzer ML, et al. Effect of prize-based incentives on outcomes in stimulant abusers in outpatient psychosocial treatment programs: A National Drug Abuse Treatment Clinical Trials Network Study. *Arch Gen Psychiatry*. 2005;62(10):1148–1156.

18. Volkow ND. Availability and effectiveness of programs to treat methamphetamine abuse – testimony before the Subcommittee on Criminal Justice, Drug Policy, and Human Resources – Committee on Government Reform – United States House of Representatives. June 28, 2006. Available at: http://www.nida. nih.gov/Testimony/6-28-06Testimony.html. Accessed June 24, 2007.

226 COCAINE

Mindy A. Smith, MD

PATIENT STORY

A 26-year-old man is brought into the emergency department in status epilepticus by his "friends," who promptly flee the scene. His seizures spontaneously cease, and he is noted to have an altered mental status. Intravenous (IV) access is obtained and he is stabilized. A urine toxicology screen is positive for cocaine and his creatinine phosphokinase is markedly elevated. He is admitted for cocaine-induced seizures and rhabdomyolysis. He survives the hospitalization and consents to a photograph of his eyes before discharge. **Figure 226-1** shows the bilateral subconjunctival hemorrhages that occurred during his seizures. The patient states that he understands the gravity of the situation and will enter a drug rehabilitation program when he leaves the hospital.

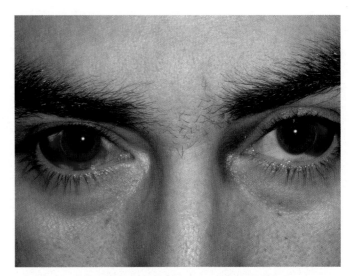

FIGURE 226-1 Bilateral subconjunctival hemorrhages after severe cocaine-induced seizures in a young man. This patient also developed rhabdomyolysis and was hospitalized. (*Courtesy of Beau Willison, MD.*)

EPIDEMIOLOGY

- Based on the National Comorbidity Survey Replication (NCS-R) using interviews with a nationally representative sample of 9282 English-speaking respondents aged 18 years and older (conducted in 2001–2003), the cumulative incidence of cocaine use was 16%.[1]
- Similar numbers were reported from the National Survey on Drug Use and Health in 2004[2]:
  - A total of 34.2 million Americans aged 12 years and older reported lifetime use of cocaine, and 7.8 million reported using crack cocaine.
  - An estimated 2 million Americans reported current use of cocaine (467,000 of whom reported using crack).
  - Of the estimated 1 million new users of cocaine in 2004, most were aged 18 years or older, with the average age of first use being 20 years.
  - The percentage of youth aged 12 to 17 years reporting lifetime use of cocaine was 2.4%, and among young adults aged 18 to 25 years the rate was 15.2%.
- For both men and women cocaine users, the estimated risk for developing cocaine dependence, based on data from the NCS-R, was 5% to 6% within the first year after first use.[3] Thereafter, the estimated risk decreased from the peak value, with a somewhat faster decline for women in the next 3 years after first use.
  - Women may be more susceptible to crack/cocaine dependence; in a study of 152 individuals (37% women) in a residential substance-use treatment program, women evidenced greater use of crack/cocaine (current and lifetime heaviest) and were significantly more likely to show crack/cocaine dependence than men.[4]
- In one study, siblings of cocaine-dependent individuals had an elevated risk of developing cocaine dependence (RR = 1.71).[5]

ETIOLOGY AND PATHOPHYSIOLOGY

- Cocaine is a stimulant and local anesthetic that causes potent vasoconstriction.
  - It produces its stimulant effects by causing increasing synaptic concentration of monoamine neurotransmitters (i.e., dopamine, norepinephrine, and serotonin).[6]
  - Similar to other local anesthetics, cocaine blocks the generation and conduction of electrical impulses in excitable tissues (e.g., neurons and cardiac muscle) blocking the voltage-gated fast sodium channels in the cell membrane and abolishing the ability of the tissue to generate an action potential.[7]
- Effects are seen following oral, intranasal (as a powder; [**Figure 226-2**]), IV, and inhalation administration (as crack cocaine [**Figure 226-3**], coca paste, and free-base).
- In a study of inner-city incarcerated male adolescents (23% of whom had used cocaine or crack in the month before arrest and 32% had used cocaine at least once), current cocaine/crack users were more likely to have the following characteristics[8]:
  - Alcohol, marijuana, and intranasal heroin use.
  - Multiple previous arrests.
  - To be out of school.
  - To be psychologically distressed.
  - To have been sexually molested as a child.
  - To have substance-abusing parents.
  - To have frequent sex with girls, to be gay or bisexual, and to engage in anal intercourse.
- Among those who died from an accidental drug overdose in New York City, those dying from cocaine-only vs. opiates were more likely to be men, black or hispanic have alcohol detected at autopsy, and to be of older age.[9]

DIAGNOSIS

CLINICAL FEATURES

- Acute effects occur within 3 to 5 minutes with intranasal administration (8–10 seconds with free base) and last approximately 1 hour, after which there is an abrupt disappearance of the effects.[6] When used IV or smoked as crack cocaine, the onset of action is immediate and the peak effect occurs 3 to 5 minutes later, lasting for 20 to 30 minutes.[7]
  - The acute effects include:[6,7]
    - Elevated heart rate, increased blood pressure, and usually increased temperature;
    - Increased respiratory rate and/or dyspnea followed by decreased respiratory rate;
    - Mood changes including enhanced mood/euphoria, hyperactivity, irritability and anxiety, excessive talking, and long periods without eating or sleeping;
    - Involuntary movements (e.g., tremors, chorea, and dystonic reactions).
  - Additional findings on physical examination can include:
    - Dilated pupils, nystagmus, and/or retinal hemorrhages;
    - Nasal septum perforation (**Figure 226-4**), epistaxis, and/or cerebrospinal fluid (CSF) rhinorrhea;

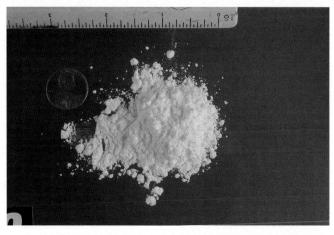

FIGURE 226-2 Cocaine in a powder form used for snorting and injecting. (*Courtesy of The Drug Enforcement Agency.*)

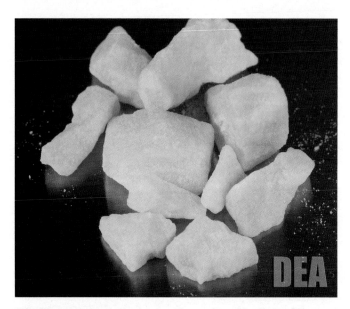

FIGURE 226-3 Crack cocaine used for smoking. (*Courtesy of The Drug Enforcement Agency.*)

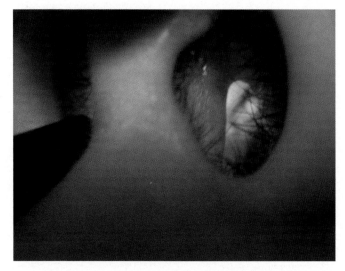

FIGURE 226-4 Shining a light through a hole in the nasal septum caused by 10 years of snorting cocaine. (*Courtesy of Richard P. Usatine, MD.*)

- Wheezing, rales, and/or pneumothorax;
- Absent bowel sounds (mesenteric ischemia) and/or right upper quadrant tenderness (hepatic necrosis).
- Skin tracking from IV use (**Figure 226-5**).
  - Acute effects may be altered by concomitant use of other drugs or alcohol.

- Adverse effects of cocaine use can include:[6]
  - Respiratory depression that may result in death;
  - Cardiac arrhythmias, chest pain, and myocardial infarction (MI);
  - Neurologic symptoms including headache, tonic-clonic seizures, ischemic or hemorrhagic stroke, and subarachnoid hemorrhage;
  - Myalgias and rhabdomyolysis;
  - Severe pulmonary disease (e.g., alveolar hemorrhage and pulmonary edema) and hepatic necrosis caused by crack cocaine;
  - Exacerbation of existing hypertension, cardiac, and cerebrovascular disease;
  - Recurrent diabetic ketoacidosis.[10]

- Chronic use is associated with decreased libido and impaired reproductive function.[1]
  - In men, cocaine can cause impotence and gynecomastia.
  - In women, cocaine can cause galactorrhea, amenorrhea, and infertility.
  - In pregnant women, crack cocaine is associated with an increase in placental abruption, miscarriage, and congenital malformation.

- Protracted use can cause paranoid ideation and visual and auditory hallucinations. Severe depression can follow recovery from cocaine intoxication (called "crashing").[1]

- Withdrawal from chronic cocaine use can cause depression, insomnia, and anorexia.

LABORATORY STUDIES

- Urine toxicology screen (using immunoassays) for common drugs of abuse (e.g., cocaine, marijuana, and opiates) is the gold standard.
  - Cocaine may be detected in the urine for 24 hours after use and the metabolite of cocaine, benzoylecgonine, may be detected as long as 60 hours after a single use.[7]
  - In chronic cocaine users, benzoylecgonine may be detected for up to 22 days.[7]
  - A rapid urine test, OnTrak Testcup-5, was reported in a manufacturer-supported study to be accurate and reproducible for marijuana, cocaine, and heroin.[11]

- Saliva and hair tests are also available but may not be as accurate for all drugs of interest.

- All injection drug users should be screened for human immunodeficiency virus (HIV) (with consent) and hepatitis B and C.

- If there is a history of multiple sexual partners, unsafe sex and/or sex for drugs, cocaine users should be screened for STDs. This might include chlamydia, gonorrhea, hepatitis B and C, HIV (with consent) and syphilis (**Figure 226-6**).

- In an unconscious patient and in patients denying cocaine use, the following laboratory tests can be considered to rule out other diseases with similar symptoms[7]:
  - Serum glucose, magnesium, and phosphorus
  - Serum electrolytes

- Laboratory tests that can be completed to detect or monitor acute complications of cocaine overdose include[7]

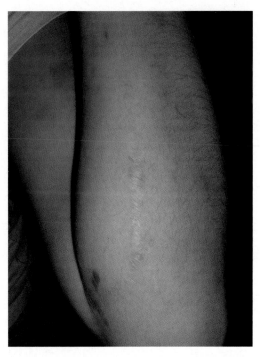

FIGURE 226-5 An injection track along the vein of a young woman in recovery from IV cocaine use and addiction. (*Courtesy of Richard P. Usatine, MD.*)

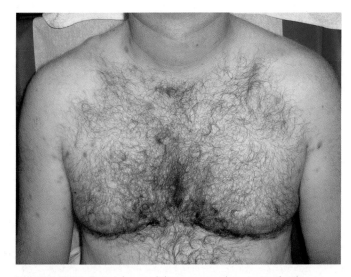

FIGURE 226-6 Secondary syphilis in a man who was involved in unsafe sex while addicted to cocaine. The papulonodular eruption is an unusual presentation of secondary syphilis that was diagnosed with a skin biopsy and confirmed with an RPR titer of 1:512. The specific treponemal blood test was also positive. (*Courtesy of Richard P. Usatine, MD.*)

- ○ Arterial blood gas (respiratory acidosis or alkalosis)
- ○ BUN and/or creatinine (renal infarction)
- ○ Creatinine kinase (CK) (rhabdomyolysis) and isoenzyme of creatine kinase (CK-MB) (MI)
- ○ Liver function tests (liver necrosis)
- ○ Urine dipstick (rhabdomyolysis)

IMAGING AND OTHER TESTS

- Plain films of the abdomen (supine and upright) can be useful in the diagnosis of body packing or stuffing of cocaine (swallowing or inserting packets of cocaine into a body orifice), but false-negative results may occur. Serial abdominal roentgenograms may be useful in detecting the passage of drug packages.[7]
- A chest x-ray and head CT can be considered for respiratory and neurologic symptoms, respectively.

DIFFERENTIAL DIAGNOSIS

- Adrenal hyperplasia or adenoma—produces excess cortisol causing signs and symptoms of Cushing's syndrome, including hypertension and emotional changes (ranging from irritability to severe depression and psychosis). Distinguishing features are increased body weight with adipose deposition in the upper face ("moon" faces) and interscapular area ("buffalo" hump), hirsutism, violaceous cutaneous striae, and proximal myopathy. A 24-hour urine test for free cortisol or overnight dexamethasone suppression test is recommended for diagnosis.

- Hyperthyroidism—in addition to tachycardia and nervousness/agitation, patients can report fatigue, weight loss, and heat intolerance. Exophthalmus and pretibial myxedema may be seen, and laboratory testing reveals a low or undetectable thyroid-stimulating hormone (TSH) and an elevated free thyroxin level (T_4) (see Chapter 217, Graves Exophthalmous and Goiter).

- Delirium—defined as a state of confusion accompanied by agitation, hallucinations, tremor and illusions, delirium can be caused by drug toxicity or withdrawal, seizure, head injury, systemic infections, metabolic disorders, or a chronic dementing condition. The history, physical examination, and laboratory tests (many noted above) can help to identify the etiology.

- Hypoglycemia—low blood sugar most commonly caused by taking insulin or oral drugs used to treat diabetes mellitus. Symptoms include confusion, fatigue, seizures, and loss of consciousness. Autonomic responses to hypoglycemia include palpitations, sweating, tremor, and anxiety. Laboratory testing for serum glucose will document the condition, and symptoms resolve with administration of oral or IV glucose.

- Meningitis—acute infection within the subarachnoid space presenting within hours or days with fever, headache, and stiff neck (more than 90% of patients); additional potential signs are change in mental status (e.g., confusion and decreased consciousness), seizures, increased intracranial pressure, and stroke. The appearance of a rash/petechiae can aid in the diagnosis (meningococcemia). Diagnosis is made with examination of the CSF following lumbar puncture (LP).

- Encephalitis—acute infection of the central nervous system that involves the brain parenchyma usually caused by viruses. The clinical features include fever, altered level of consciousness, and focal (e.g., aphasia, ataxia, hemiparesis, and involuntary movements) or diffuse (e.g., agitation, hallucinations, and personality change) symptoms. Diagnosis is established with examination of the CSF following LP.

MANAGEMENT

- Acute overdose is a medical emergency best managed in the intensive care unit because of the hyperadrenergic state and seizures.
  - Hyperthermia and severe psychomotor agitation are the most immediately life-threatening complications of cocaine poisoning.[7] Temperatures as high as 114°F have been recorded. Rapid physical cooling with sponging, fans, ice baths, and cooling blankets can be used and gastric or peritoneal lavage with iced saline is considered if persistent.
  - IV diazepam up to 0.5 mg/kg given over 8 hours is used to control psychomotor agitation and seizures.
    - Hypertension may also respond to benzodiazepines. Beta-blockers should not be used in the setting of cocaine toxicity (except to control ventricular arrhythmia, as below) because they may result in unopposed alpha effects of cocaine.[7]
    - Avoid the use of neuroleptic agents because they can interfere with heat dissipation and, perhaps, lower the seizure threshold.[7]
  - Propranolol (0.5–1 mg IV) can be used to control ventricular arrhythmia.
    - Perform defibrillation in all patients with pulseless ventricular tachycardia.[7]
    - Consider electrical cardioversion in all unstable patients.[7]
    - Beta-blockers should not be used in cocaine-induced cardiac ischemia.[12]
  - Administer activated charcoal to patients with oral ingestions of cocaine (i.e., body stuffers and body packers) to reduce absorption. Whole bowel irrigation may be used to reduce transit time in these patients.[7]
- Medical providers should be prepared to manage multiple drug effects, especially heroin.
- Cognitive behavioral therapy is effective in the treatment of cocaine-dependent outpatients.[13]
- There is no current evidence supporting the clinical use of carbamazepine, antidepressants, dopamine agonists, disulfiram, mazindol, phenytoin, nimodipine, lithium, and NeuRecover-SA in the treatment of cocaine dependence.[14]
- Antidepressant medication exerts a modest beneficial effect for patients with combined depressive and substance-use disorders but should be used as part of a program to directly target the addiction.[15]

PATIENT EDUCATION

- Encourage patients to quit cocaine use and offer assistance.
- Recommend 12-step programs including cocaine anonymous.

- Patients should be made aware of the potential complications associated with use of cocaine, including its powerful psychologically addictive properties.
- Instruct patients about seeking help in the emergency department for any of the following[16]:
  - Facial pain or headache with a fever.
  - Severe chest pain, difficulty breathing, or shortness of breath.
  - If pregnant, vaginal bleeding or premature labor pains.
  - Significant swelling, pain, redness, and red lines leading from the injection site and accompanied by fever.
  - Severe abdominal pain, persistent vomiting, and vomiting blood.
  - If you think that one of your packets you have swallowed or stuffed in a body orifice (vagina and rectum) is leaking or has broken.
- Instruct IV drug users who continue to use not to reuse or share needles or syringes; cleaning the skin before injection can also decrease risk of infection. Harm reduction programs exist that help addicts obtain and maintain clean needles and syringes.

FOLLOW-UP

- Following withdrawal from chronic cocaine use, patients may benefit from individual, group, and/or family therapy and peer assistance.[6]
- Patients and their families may need ongoing support, home health care, and physical and occupational therapy to address long-term neurologica and cardiovascular complications of cocaine including anoxic encephalopathy, stroke, intracerebral hemorrhage, congestive heart failure, and cardiomyopathy.
- Referral to specialists may be needed to assist patients with upper respiratory tract (e.g., CSF rhinorrhea and nasal septum perforation) or ophthalmologic complications (e.g., central retinal artery occlusion).
- Physicians should closely monitor and assist patients in managing depression, insomnia, and anorexia that may follow cessation of chronic cocaine use.[6]
- Among individuals leaving residential detoxification, chronic pain is a common problem and is associated independently with long-term substance use after detoxification; management of pain may improve long-term outcomes.[17]

PATIENT RESOURCES

http://www.emedicinehealth.com/cocaine_abuse/page3_em.htm.

Treatment referral: 1-800-662-HELP or findtreatment.samhsa.gov.

For parents: http://www.drugabuse.gov/prevention/prevopen.html.

Cocaine Anonymous (CA) http://www.ca.org/—meetings are free. Their first book "Hope, Faith and Courage: Stories from the Fellowship of Cocaine Anonymous" was published in 1994 and sells for $10.

REFERENCES

1. Degenhardt L, Chiu WT, Sampson N, et al. Epidemiological patterns of extra-medical drug use in the United States: Evidence from the National Comorbidity Survey Replication, 2001–2003. *Drug Alcohol Depend*. 2007;90(2–3):210–223.

2. National Survey on Drug Use and Health. Substance Abuse and Mental Health Services Administration. www.samhsa.gov. Accessed June 1, 2007.

3. Wagner FA, Anthony JC. Male-female differences in the risk of progression from first use to dependence upon cannabis, cocaine, and alcohol. *Drug Alcohol Depend*. 2007;86(2–3):191–198.

4. Lejuez CW, Bornovalova MA, Reynolds EK, et al. Risk factors in the relationship between gender and crack/cocaine. *Exp Clin Psychopharmacol*. 2007;15(2):165–175.

5. Bierut LJ, Dinwiddie SH, Begleiter H, et al. Familial transmission of substance dependence: Alcohol, marijuana, cocaine, and habitual smoking: A report from the Collaborative Study on the Genetics of Alcoholism. *Arch Gen Psychiatry*. 1998;55(11):982–988.

6. Mendelson JH, Mello NK. Cocaine and other commonly abused drugs. In: Kasper DL, Braunwald E, Fauci AS, Hauser SL, Longo DL, Jameson JL eds. *Harrison's Principles of Internal Medicine*, 16th ed. New York, NY: McGraw-Hill, 2005:2570–2573.

7. Roldan CJ, Habal R. Toxicity, cocaine. http://www.emedicine.com/med/topic400.htm. Accessed January 6, 2007.

8. Kang SY, Magura S, Shapiro JL. Correlates of cocaine/crack use among inner-city incarcerated adolescents. *Am J Drug Alcohol Abuse*. 1994;20(4):413–429.

9. Bernstein KT, Bucciarelli A, Piper TM, et al. Cocaine- and opiate-related fatal overdose in New York City, 1990–2000. *BMC Public Health*. 2007;7:31.

10. Nyenwe EA, Loganathan RS, Blum S, et al. Active use of cocaine: an independent risk factor for recurrent diabetic ketoacidosis in a city hospital. *Endocr Pract*. 2007;13(1):22–29.

11. Yacoubian GS Jr, Wish ED, Choyka JD. A comparison of the OnTrak Testcup-5 to laboratory urinalysis among arrestees. *J Psychoactive Drugs*. 2002;34(3):325–329.

12. Sen A, Fairbairn T, Levy F. Best evidence topic report. Beta-Blockers in cocaine induced acute coronary syndrome. *Emerg Med J*. 2006;23(5):401–402.

13. Carroll KM, Onken LS. Behavioral therapies for drug abuse. *Am J Psychiatry*. 2005;162(8):1452–1460.

14. de Lima MS, de Oliveira Soares BG, Reisser AA, Farrell M. Pharmacological treatment of cocaine dependence: A systematic review. *Addiction*. 2002;97(8):931–949.

15. Nunes EX, Levin FR. Treatment of depression in patients with alcohol or other drug dependence: A meta-analysis. *JAMA*. 2004;291(15):1887–1896.

16. Arkangel C Jr. http://www.emedicinehealth.com/cocaine_abuse/article_em.htm. Accessed January 6, 2007.

17. Larson MJ, Paasche-Orlow M, Cheng DM, et al. Persistent pain is associated with substance use after detoxification: A prospective cohort analysis. *Addiction*. 2007;102(5):752–760.

227 INJECTION DRUG USE

Richard P. Usatine, MD

PATIENT STORY

A 23-year-old woman is seen for her intake physical in a residential treatment program for women recovering from substance abuse. She has not injected heroin for 2 days now, but her tracks are still visible (**Figure 227-1**). Her parents were both addicted to heroin, and she admits to having been born addicted to heroin herself. She began using heroin on her own in her early teens and has been on and off heroin since that time. She acknowledges a history of physical and sexual abuse as a child. She has had many suicide attempts and has cut herself with a knife across her arm many times. She has traded sex for money to buy heroin. Her two children are in foster care after having been removed by child protective services. She is an attractive young woman looking for help and is thankful to have been admitted to this program. She does not know whether she has acquired hepatitis B, hepatitis C, or HIV but wants to get tested.

EPIDEMIOLOGY

- From 1999 to 2001, an annual average of 338,000 persons in the United States aged 12 years or older used a needle to inject cocaine, heroin, or stimulants during the past year.[1]

- Young adults aged 18 to 25 years were more likely to have injected drugs in the past year compared with youths aged 12 to 17 years or adults aged 26 years or older.[1]

- The last time injection drug users used a needle for injecting drugs, 14% of past year injection drug users knew or suspected someone else had used the needle before them and 16% used a needle that someone used after them.[1]

- There were 237,000 substance-abuse treatment admissions for injection drug use (13% of all admissions reported to Substance Abuse and Mental Health Services Administration's (SAMHSA) Treatment Episode Data Set for 2003).[1]
  - Opiates accounted for 77% of admissions for injection drug use, followed by stimulants (16%) and cocaine (6%).[1]

- The most commonly injected drugs are heroin and cocaine. Amphetamines, buprenorphine, benzodiazepines, and barbiturates also are injected.[2]

- In 2005, the estimated number of cases of HIV/AIDS in the 33 states and four dependent areas with confidential name-based HIV infection reporting was 38,133. Of these cases, 8985 were from injection drug use alone and 2190 involved male-to-male sexual contact and injection drug use.[3]

- The 2005 Monitoring the Future Survey showed that 1.5% of 12th graders in the United States were using anabolic steroids[4] (**Figure 227-2**).
  - Anabolic steroid abuse among athletes may range between 1% and 6%.[4]

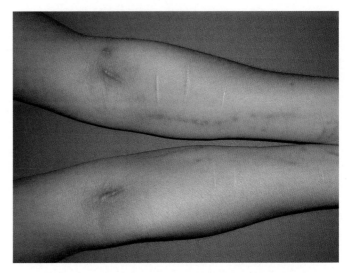

FIGURE 227-1 A 23-year-old woman with visible tracks on her arms from intravenous heroin use. She also has visible scars from self-mutilation with a knife. (*Courtesy of Richard P. Usatine, MD.*)

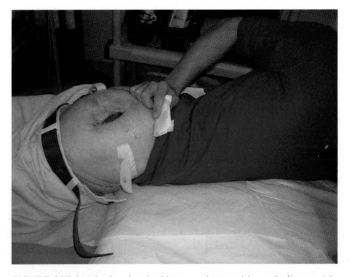

FIGURE 227-2 A high-school athlete used injectable anabolic steroids for muscle building and developed a large abscess in his buttocks. This photograph was taken 2 months after the original abscess was drained and the wound is healing by secondary intention. (*Courtesy of William Rodney, MD.*)

○ Some adolescents abuse steroids as part of a pattern of high-risk behaviors. These adolescents also take risks such as drinking and driving, carrying a gun, driving a motorcycle without a helmet, and abusing other illicit drugs.[4]

ETIOLOGY AND PATHOPHYSIOLOGY

- Most injecting drug users inject drugs intravenously, but subcutaneous injection (skin-popping) also is common.[2]

- Injected, snorted, or smoked heroin causes an almost immediate "rush" or brief period of euphoria that wears off very quickly, terminating in a "crash." The user then experiences an intense craving to use more heroin to stop the crash and bring back the euphoria. The cycle of euphoria, crash, and craving—repeated several times a day—leads to a cycle of addiction.

- Injection drug users are at increased risk of HIV/AIDS as well as other infectious diseases like hepatitis, tuberculosis, and sexually transmitted infections. For these individuals and the community at large, drug addiction treatment is disease prevention.

- A heroin overdose can lead to death from respiratory depression, coma, and pulmonary edema. Death from the direct effects of cocaine is usually associated with cardiac dysrhythmias and conduction disturbances, leading to myocardial infarction and stroke.[2]

- Anabolic steroids can lead to early heart attacks, strokes, liver tumors, kidney failure, and serious psychiatric problems. In addition, because steroids are often injected, users who share needles or use nonsterile techniques when they inject steroids are at risk of contracting dangerous infections, such as HIV/AIDS and hepatitis B and C.[4]

- Injecting drug users are at high risk of developing abscesses of the skin. Skin abscesses can occur at the site of injection or elsewhere (**Figures 227-2** and **227-3**) (see Chapter 115, Abscess).

- Injecting drug users are at risk of endocarditis, osteomyelitis (**Figures 227-4** and **227-5**), and an abscess of the epidural region. These infections can lead to long hospitalizations for intravenous antibiotics (see Chapter 48, Endocarditis).

DIAGNOSIS

CLINICAL FEATURES

Heroin use produces the following clinical appearances:

- Pinpoint pupils and no response of pupils to light.
- A rush of pleasurable feelings.
- Cessation of physical pain.
- Lethargy and drowsiness.
- Slurred speech.
- Shallow breathing.
- Sweating.
- Vomiting.
- A drop in body temperature.

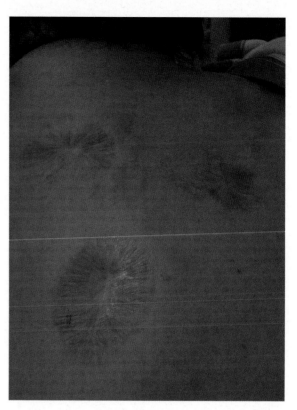

FIGURE 227-3 A 32-year-old woman with type 1 diabetes and injection drug use, leading to large abscesses all over her body. Her back shows the large scars remaining after the healing of these abscesses. (*Courtesy of Richard P. Usatine, MD.*)

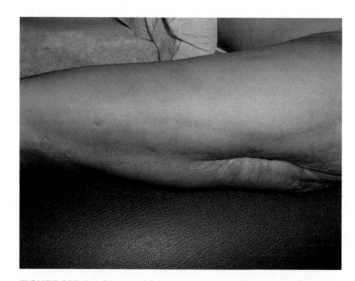

FIGURE 227-4 A 24-year-old woman with an 8-year history of injection drug use. She has a large deep linear scar from osteomyelitis of the ulnar bone and smaller round scars from skin popping. A track is also visible above the deep scar. (*Courtesy of Richard P. Usatine, MD.*)

- Sleepiness.
- Loss of appetite.[5]

Cocaine (by injection) can produce the following signs, symptoms, and adverse effects:

- Dilated pupils.
- Hyperactivity.
- Euphoria.
- Irritability and anxiety.
- Excessive talking.
- Depression or excessive sleeping.
- Long periods without eating or sleeping.
- Weight loss.
- Dry mouth and nose.
- Paranoia.
- Cardiac—arrhythmias, chest pain, MI, and CHF.
- Strokes and seizures.
- Respiratory failure.[5]

COMPLICATIONS OF INJECTING DRUG USE

- Local problems: abscess, cellulitis, septic thrombophlebitis, local induration, necrotizing fascitis, gas gangrene, pyomyositis, mycotic aneurysm, compartmental syndromes, and foreign bodies (e.g., broken needle parts) in local areas[2]
  - Injection drug users are at higher risk of getting MRSA skin infections that the patient may think is spider bites (**Figure 227-6**).
  - Some injection drug users give up trying to inject into their veins and put the cocaine directly into the skin. This causes local skin necrosis that produces round atrophic scars (**Figure 227-7**).
- Systemic complications: HIV infection, hepatitis B or C, pneumonia or lung abscess from septic emboli to the lung, acute and subacute bacterial endocarditis, group A beta-hemolytic streptococcal septicemia, osteomyelitis, septic arthritis, and candidal and other fungal infections. The endocarditis that occurs in injection drug users involves the right-sided heart valves.[2]

LABORATORY STUDIES

- All injection drug users should be screened for HIV (with consent) and Hepatitis B and C.
- If there is a history of high-risk sexual behavior, screen for syphilis (RPR), chlamydia and gonorrhea.
- Purified protein derivative (PPD) test to screen for tuberculosis (especially if the patient is homeless or HIV positive).
- Urine screen for common drugs of abuse may reveal other drugs not admitted to in the history.
- Electrocardiogram is warranted if there are any cardiac symptoms or if the physical examination reveals signs of cardiac disease.

MANAGEMENT

- Addiction is similar to other chronic illnesses because:
  - Recovery from it is often a long-term process requiring repeated treatments.

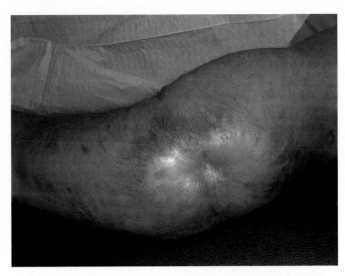

FIGURE 227-5 The other arm of the woman in **Figure 227-4** with deep scar from osteomyelitis secondary to injecting drugs that destroyed the bones in her left forearm. Her arm is deformed and poorly functional. (*Courtesy of Richard P. Usatine, MD.*)

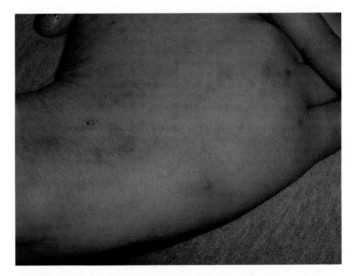

FIGURE 227-6 A young woman with MRSA infection from injection drug use. Track visible on hand with pustule from MRSA. (*Courtesy of Richard P. Usatine, MD.*)

○ Relapses to drug abuse can occur during or after successful treatment episodes.

• Participation in self-help support programs during and following treatment can be helpful in sustaining long-term recovery.[6]

• Treating criminal justice-involved drug abusers and addicts: drug abusers may come into contact with the criminal justice system earlier than with other health or social systems. Thus, the period of involvement with the criminal justice system may offer an opportunity to engage individuals in a treatment that can shorten a pattern of drug abuse and related crime. Research supports the efficacy of combining criminal justice sanctions and drug abuse treatment.[6]

• Drug abuse treatment is less expensive than alternatives, such as not treating addicts or incarcerating them. The average cost for 1 full year of methadone maintenance treatment is approximately $4700 per patient, whereas 1 full year of imprisonment costs approximately $18,400 per person. According to several conservative estimates, every $1 invested in addiction treatment programs yields up to $7 in savings, much of which results from reduced drug-related crime and criminal justice costs.[6] While methadone maintenance is not as desirable as full abstinence, the comparative costs are in favor of drug treatment over incarceration.

• Recovery from drug addiction has two key components: treatment and continuing care. The clinical practices that make up the treatment phase (e.g., residential/outpatient treatment) must be followed up by management of the disorder over time (e.g., drug abuse monitoring, booster sessions, and reevaluation of treatment needs).[6]

• Research has shown that treatment must last, on average, at least 3 months to produce stable behavior change.[6] This accounts for the existence of 90 day residential treatment programs.

• A comprehensive assessment is the first step in the treatment process and includes identifying individual strengths to facilitate treatment and recovery. In addition, drug abuse cannot be treated in isolation from related issues and potential threats, such as criminal behavior, mental health status, physical health, family functioning, employment status, homelessness, and HIV/AIDS.[6]

• Treatments that utilize cognitive behavioral therapies, residential treatment, contingency management, and medications have demonstrated effectiveness in reducing drug abuse and criminal behavior.[6]

• Medications are a key treatment component for drug abusers and can stabilize the brain and help return it to normal functioning. Methadone and buprenorphine are effective in helping individuals addicted to heroin or other opiates reduce their drug abuse. Naltrexone is also an effective medication for some opiate-addicted patients and those with co-occurring alcohol dependence.[6]

• Self-help groups can complement and extend the effects of professional treatment. The most prominent self-help groups are those affiliated with Alcoholics Anonymous (AA), Narcotics Anonymous (NA), and Cocaine Anonymous (CA), all of which are based on the 12-step model, and Smart Recovery®. Most drug addiction treatment programs encourage patients to participate in a self-help group during and after formal treatment.[6]

• Family and friends can play critical roles in motivating individuals with drug problems to enter and stay in treatment. Family therapy is important, especially for adolescents. Involvement of a family

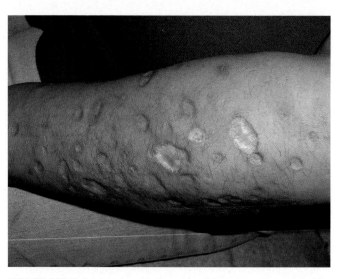

FIGURE 227-7 A young woman in residential treatment program with multiple scars from skin popping cocaine. She gave up trying to inject into her veins and put the cocaine directly into the skin. Note how the local skin necrosis caused round atrophic scars. (*Courtesy of Richard P. Usatine, MD.*)

member in an individual's treatment program can strengthen and extend the benefits of the program.[6]

- Drug injectors who do not enter treatment are up to six times more likely to become infected with HIV than injectors who enter and remain in treatment. Drug users who enter and continue in treatment reduce activities that can spread disease, such as sharing injection equipment and engaging in unprotected sexual activity. Participation in treatment also presents opportunities for screening, counseling, and referral for additional services. The best drug abuse treatment programs provide HIV counseling and offer HIV testing to their patients.[6]

- Buprenorphine, a partial opioid agonist, is also used for opioid detoxification and for opioid replacement therapy.[2] In the United States, physicians who wish to prescribe buprenorphine must take a certification course.
  - Opioid replacement therapy reduces injecting drug use and thus reduces the mortality and morbidity associated with injecting drug use, including the transmission of HIV and HCV.[2]
  - Buprenorphine (Subutex or, in combination with naloxone, Suboxone) is demonstrated to be a safe and acceptable addiction treatment. Congress passed the Drug Addiction Treatment Act (DATA 2000), permitting qualified physicians to prescribe narcotic medications (Schedules III–V) for the treatment of opioid addiction. This legislation created a major paradigm shift by allowing access to opiate treatment in a medical setting rather than limiting it to specialized drug treatment clinics. Approximately 10,000 physicians have taken the training needed to prescribe these two medications, and nearly 7000 have registered as potential providers.

- Methadone and Levo-Alpha Acetyl Methadol (LAAM) have more gradual onsets of action and longer half-lives than heroin. Patients stabilized on these medications do not experience the heroin rush. Both medications wear off much more slowly than heroin, so there is no sudden crash, and the brain and body are not exposed to the marked fluctuations seen with heroin use. Maintenance treatment with methadone or LAAM markedly reduces the desire for heroin.
  - If an individual maintained on adequate, regular doses of methadone (once a day) or LAAM (several times per week) tries to take heroin, the euphoric effects of heroin will be significantly blocked. According to research, patients undergoing maintenance treatment do not suffer the medical abnormalities and behavioral destabilization that rapid fluctuations in drug levels cause in heroin addicts.

PATIENT EDUCATION

- For patients not ready to stop their injecting drug use there are still harm reduction programs and counseling that can be helpful. Encourage patients to use clean and sterile needles and not to share their needles with anyone. Bleach can be used to clean and sterilize needles and prevent the spread of HIV and hepatitis.

- Refer continuing drug users to needle exchange programs that exist to help injection drug users use clean needles and avoid infectious diseases. These programs can also be helpful if they give out condoms to encourage safe sex.

- Encourage patients to get help to become drug-free and abstinent. There is no safe level of injecting drug use.

- Explain to patients that addiction is a disease and not a failing of their moral character.

- Inform patients about the existing treatment programs in their community and offer them names and phone numbers so that they may get help.

- If your patient is not ready for help today give the numbers and names for tomorrow.

- Speak about the value of 12-step programs including NA and CA because everyone can afford a 12-step program. There are 12-step programs in the community for everyone including nonsmokers and agnostics.

FOLLOW-UP

Follow-up is important for the treatment of injection drug users. Addiction is a chronic (and relapsing) condition and requires long-term follow-up. Your intervention and caring attitude can help the patient to overcome addiction and to live a sober and drug-free life. Do not give up on patients who relapse because it often takes more than one attempt before long-term cessation can be achieved. The frequency and intensity of follow-up depend upon the substance, the addiction, and the patients and their complications.

PATIENT RESOURCES

- Narcotics Anonymous (NA) **http://www.na.org/index.htm**—meetings are free. The "Basic Text" costs $10—it is similar to the AA big book but the language is more up to date and readable.

- Cocaine Anonymous (CA) **http://www.ca.org/**—meetings are free. Their first book "Hope, Faith and Courage: Stories from the Fellowship of Cocaine Anonymous" was published in 1994 and sells for $10.

- Drugstory.org: **http://www.drugstory.org/.**

PROVIDER RESOURCES

- The National Institute on Drug Abuse (NIDA), **http://www.nida.nih.gov/consequences/.**

- Substance Abuse and Mental Health Services Administration, **http://www.samhsa.gov/.**

- Drugstory.org: **http://www.drugstory.org/.**

- Drug Enforcement Agency website: **http://www.usdoj.gov/dea/multimedia.html.**

REFERENCES

1. Substance Abuse and Mental Health Services Administration. *Results from the 2005 National Survey on Drug Use and Health: National Findings.* NSDUH Series H-30, DHHS Publication No. SMA 06-4194. Rockville, MD: Office of Applied Studies, 2006. Report online at: http://www.oas.samhsa.gov/nsduh.htm

2. Baciewicz, GJ. Injecting drug use. eMedicine. updated June 2005. http://www.emedicine.com/med/topic586.htm. Accessed May 27, 2007.

3. HIV/AIDS Surveillance report: HIV Infection and AIDS in the United States and dependent areas, 2005. http://www.cdc.gov/hiv/topics/surveillance/basic.htm#exposure. Accessed May 27, 2007.

4. NIDA Research report—steroid abuse and addiction: NIH Publication No. 00-3721, Printed 1991, Reprinted 1994, 1996. Revised April, 2000, and September 2006 online at: http://www.drugabuse.gov/ResearchReports/Steroids/. Accessed May 27, 2007.

5. Street drugs university. http://www.streetdrugs-university.org/amember/sduniversity%20secure/index_files/Page724.htm. Accessed May 27, 2007.

6. *Principles of Drug Abuse Treatment for Criminal Justice Populations—A Research-Based Guide*. http://www.drugabuse.gov/drugpages/cj.html. Accessed May 27, 2007.

APPENDIX

APPENDIX A INTERPRETING EVIDENCE-BASED MEDICINE (EBM)

Mindy A. Smith, MD, MS

"Evidence-based medicine—is this something new?" asked my father, incredulously, "what were you practicing before?"

Like my father, our patients assume that we provide recommendations to them based on scientific evidence. The idea that there might not be relevant evidence or that we might not have access to that evidence has not even occurred to most of them. This is certainly not to imply that such evidence is the be-all and end-all of medical practice or that our patients would follow such recommendations blindly—rather, for me, it is a starting point from which to begin rational testing or outline a possible therapeutic plan.

The first time that I recall the term "evidence-based medicine" being discussed was in the early 90's.[1,2] It seemed that we would need to develop skills in evaluating the published literature and determining its quality, validity, and relevance to the care of our patients. As a teacher and researcher, I was intrigued by the challenges of critically appraising articles and teaching this newfound skill to others. As a clinician, however, I was most interested in answering clinical questions and doing so in a compressed timeframe. I needed rapid access to tools or sources that provided summary answers to those questions tagged to information about the quantity and quality of the evidence and the consistency of information across studies.

There seemed to be many systems for rating literature but few that met the needs of the busy practitioner trying to make sense of individual clinical trials and the hundreds of both evidence-based and consensus-based guidelines that seemed to spring up overnight. In 2004, the editors of the U.S. family medicine and primary care journals and the Family Practice Inquiries Network published a paper on a unified taxonomy called Strength of Recommendation (SOR) Taxonomy that seemed to fit the bill (**Figure A-1**).[3] This taxonomy made use of existing systems for judging study quality while incorporating the concept of patient-oriented (e.g., mortality, morbidity, symptom improvement) rather than disease-oriented (e.g., change in blood pressure, blood chemistry) outcomes as most relevant SOR **Ⓐ** recommendation is one based on consistent, good-quality patient-oriented evidence; SOR **Ⓑ** is a recommendation based on inconsistent or limited-quality patient-oriented evidence; and SOR **Ⓒ** is a recommendation based on consensus, usual practice, opinion, disease-oriented evidence, or case series (**Figures A-1** and **A-2**).

In this book, we made a commitment to search for patient-oriented evidence to support the information that we provided in each of the chapter sections (i.e., epidemiology, etiology/pathophysiology, making the diagnosis, differential diagnosis, management, and follow-up) and to provide a SOR rating for that evidence whenever possible. The bulleted format within these divisions would allow the practitioner to quickly find answers to their clinical questions while providing some direction about how confident we were that each recommendation had high-quality patient-oriented evidence to support it.

For example, a practitioner asks, "What is the best antithyroid drug regimen for treating Graves' hyperthyroidism?" Fortunately, there is a Cochrane Database Systematic Review to answer that question with SOR at the A level.[4] If you want to know the optimal duration of titrated antithyroid drug therapy, an answer can be found in Management section of Chapter 217, Graves Exophthalmos and Goiter. The optimal duration is 12 to 18 months to minimize relapse.[4] SOR **Ⓐ** However, the treatment options for persistent severe ophthalmopathy can only be rated with a SOR **Ⓑ** (Management section of Chapter 217, Graves Exophthalmos). These include high-dose systemic steroids (40–80 mg/d), orbital radiotherapy, and orbital decompression surgery.[5] SOR **Ⓑ** While these are accepted therapies, the evidence is less rigorous and patients need to know this before embarking on any one of these options. Particularly in this case, the clinician's experience and the patient preferences are important aspects of shared decision making. One definition of EBM is "The integration of best research evidence with clinical expertise and patient values."[6]

Several other concepts are used throughout the book that can assist practitioners in using evidence-based information and explaining that information to patients. Risk reductions from medical treatments are often presented in relative terms—the relative risk reduction or the difference in the percentage of adverse outcomes between the intervention group and the control group divided by the percentage of adverse outcomes in the control group. These numbers are often large and use of them not only causes us to overestimate the importance of a treatment but misses its clinical relevance. A more meaningful term is the absolute risk reduction (ARR)—the risk difference between the two groups. This number can then be used to obtain a number needed to treat (NNT)—the number of patients that would need to be treated (over the same time as used in the treatment trial) to prevent one bad outcome. This is calculated as 100% divided by the ARR. NNT is more easily understood by us and our patients.

Using the same Cochrane Review cited above, patients on longer duration antithyroid drug therapy (18 mo vs. 6 mo) had significantly fewer relapses (37% vs. 58%).[4] The relative risk reduction is (58%–37%)/58% or a 36% relative risk reduction. The difference in outcome or the ARR, however, is somewhat smaller (58%–37%) or 21% ARR. From this number we can tell our patients the NNT (100%/21% or 4.76); about five patients would need to be treated with the longer therapy to prevent one relapse.

Another term that is used in this book is the likelihood ratio (LR). This number, based on the sensitivity and specificity of a diagnostic test, is used to determine the probability of a patient with a positive test (LR+) having the disease or the probability of the patient with a negative test (LR−) not having the disease in question. The LR is defined as the likelihood that a given test result would be expected in a patient with the target disorder compared to the likelihood that that same result would be expected in a patient without the target disorder.[6] The number obtained for the LR+ [Sensitivity/(100 − Specificity)] or the LR− [(100 − Sensitivity)/Specificity] can be multiplied by the pretest probability of disease to determine the post-test probability of disease. A nomogram (one can be found by visiting the Web site mentioned in Ref. 6) can be used to more easily work with these numbers to convert a pretest probability into a post-test probability. A LR+ over 10 is considered strong evidence to rule in disease while a LR− of less than 0.1 is strong evidence to rule out disease.

We both are privileged and cursed with practicing medicine in an information-rich environment. We have designed our Color Atlas to link evidence to clinical recommendations so that we can provide our patients the best science available. When the evidence is lacking, we make that clear and encourage you to engage in frank and honest discussions that lead to the shared responsibility for decisions. Our patients are justified in expecting science along with humanism—can we give them anything less?

Figure A-1

How recommendations are graded for strength, and underlying individual studies are rated for quality

In general, only key recommendations for readers require a grade of the "Strength of Recommendation." Recommendations should be based on the highest quality evidence available. For example, vitamin E was found in some cohort studies (level 2 study quality) to have a benefit for cardiovascular protection, but good-quality randomized trials (level 1) have not confirmed this effect. Therefore, it is preferable to base clinical recommendations in a manuscript on the level 1 studies.

Strength of recommendation	Definition
A	Recommendation based on consistent and good-quality patient-oriented evidence.*
B	Recommendation based on inconsistent or limited-quality patient-oriented evidence.*
C	Recommendation based on consensus, usual practice, opinion, disease-oriented evidence,* or case series for studies of diagnosis, treatment, prevention, or screening

Use the following scheme to determine whether a study measuring patient-oriented outcomes is of good or limited quality, and whether the results are consistent or inconsistent between studies.

Study quality	Type of Study		
	Diagnosis	Treatment/prevention/ screening	Prognosis
Level 1— good-quality patient-oriented evidence	Validated clinical decision rule SR/meta-analysis of high-quality studies High-quality diagnostic cohort study[†]	SR/meta-analysis of RCTs with consistent findings High-quality individual RCT[‡] All-or-none study[§]	SR/meta-analysis of good-quality cohort studies Prospective cohort study with good follow-up
Level 2— limited-quality patient-oriented evidence	Unvalidated clinical decision rule SR/meta-analysis of lower-quality studies or studies with inconsistent findings Lower-quality diagnostic cohort study or diagnostic case-control study[§]	SR/meta-analysis lower-quality clinical trials or of studies with inconsistent findings Lower-quality clinical trial[‡] or prospective cohort study Cohort study Case-control study	SR/meta-analysis of lower-quality cohort studies or with inconsistent results Retrospective cohort study with poor follow-up Case-control study Case series
Level 3— other evidence	Consensus guidelines, extrapolations from bench research, usual practice, opinion, other evidence disease-oriented evidence (intermediate or physiologic outcomes only), or case series for studies of diagnosis, treatment, prevention, or screening		

Consistency across studies	
Consistent	Most studies found similar or at least coherent conclusions (coherence means that differences are explainable); *or* If high-quality and up-to-date systematic reviews or meta-analyses exist, they support the recommendation
Inconsistent	Considerable variation among study findings and lack of coherence; *or* If high-quality and up-to-date systematic reviews or meta-analyses exist, they do not find consistent evidence in favor of the recommendation

*Patient-oriented evidence measures outcomes that matter to patients: morbidity, mortality, symptom improvement, cost reduction, and quality of life. Disease-oriented evidence measures intermediate, physiologic, or surrogate end points that may or may not reflect improvements in patient outcomes (ie, blood pressure, blood chemistry, physiologic function, and pathologic findings).

† High-quality diagnostic cohort study: cohort design, adequate size, adequate spectrum of patients, blinding, and a consistent, well-defined reference standard.

‡ High-quality RCT: allocation concealed, blinding if possible, intention-to-treat analysis, adequate statistical power, adequate follow-up (greater than 80 percent).

§ In an all-or-none study, the treatment causes a dramatic change in outcomes, such as antibiotics for meningitis or surgery for appendicitis, which precludes study in a controlled trial.

SR, systematic review; RCT, randomized controlled trial

FIGURE A-1 (With permission from Ebell MH, Siwek J, Weiss BD, et al. Simplifying the language of evidence to improve patient care: Strength of recommendation taxonomy (SORT). *J. Fam Pract.* 2004 Feb;53(2):110-20. Dowden Health Media.)

Strength of Recommendation Based on a Body of Evidence

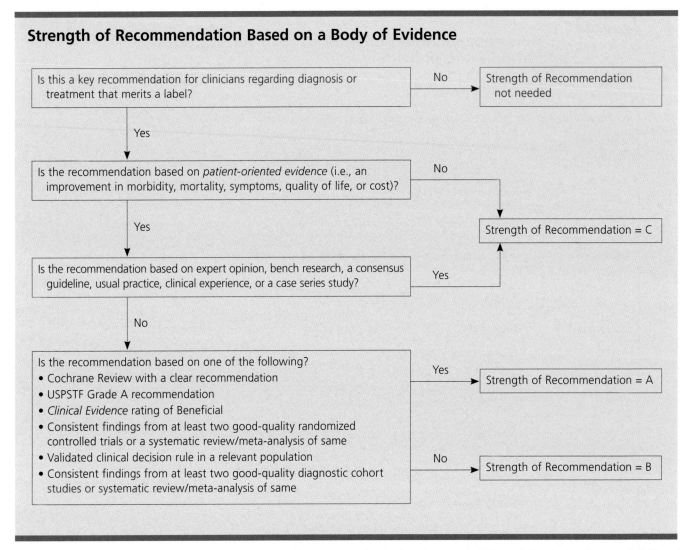

FIGURE A-2 Assigning a Strength-of-Recommendation grade based on a body of evidence. (USPSTF = U.S. Preventive Services Task Force.) (With permission from Ebell MH, Siwek J, Weiss BD, et al. Simplifying the language of evidence to improve patient care: Strength of recommendation taxonomy (SORT). *J. Fam Pract.* 2004 Feb;53(2):110-20. Dowden Health Media.)

REFERENCES

1. Evidence-Based Medicine Working Group. Evidence-based medicine. A new approach to teaching the practice of medicine. *JAMA.* 1992;268:2420–2425.

2. Shaughnessy AF, Slawson DC, Bennett JH. Becoming an information master: A guidebook to the medical information jungle. *J Fam Pract.* 1994; 39:489–499.

3. Ebell MA, Siwek J, Weiss BD, et al. Strength of Recommendation Taxonomy (SORT): A patient-centered approach to grading evidence in the medical literature. *J Fam Pract.* 2004 Feb; 53(2):111–20.

4. Abraham P, Avenell A, Watson W, et al. Antithyroid drug regimen for treating Graves' hyperthyroidism. *Cochrane Database Syst Rev.* 2005;2:CD003420.

5. Boulos PR, Hardy I. Thyroid-associated orbitopathy: A clinico-pathologic and therapeutic review. *Curr Opin Ophthalmol.* 2004; 15(5):389–400.

6. Center for Evidence-Based Medicine. http://www.cebm.net/index.aspx?o=1162. Accessed June 30, 2008.

APPENDIX B USE OF TOPICAL AND INTRALESIONAL CORTICOSTEROIDS

TABLE B-1 Carticosteroid Potency Chart

Generic Name	Trade Name and Strength
Class 1—Superpotent	
Betamethasone dipropionate	Diprolene lotion/gel/ointment, 0.05%
Diflorasone diacetate	Psorcon ointment, 0.05%
Clobetasol propionate	Temovate cream/ointment, 0.05%; Cormax cream/ointment, 0.05%
Halobetasol propionate	Ultravate cream/ointment, 0.05%
Class 2—Potent	
Amcinonide	Cyclocort ointment, 0.1%
Betamethasone dipropionate	Diprosone ointment, 0.05%
Desoximetasone	Topicort cream/ointment, 0.25%; gel, 0.05%
Diflorasone diacetate	Florone ointment, 0.05%; Maxiflor ointment, 0.05%
Fluocinonide	Lidex cream/ointment, 0.05%
Halcinonide	Halog cream, 0.1%
Class 3—Upper mid-strength	
Betamethasone dipropionate	Diprosone cream, 0.05%
Betamethasone valerate	Valisone ointment, 0.1%
Diflorasone diacetate	Florone, Maxiflor creams, 0.05%
Mometasone furoate	Elocon ointment, 0.1%
Triamcinolone acetonide	Aristocort cream, 0.5%
Class 4—Mid-strength	
Desoximetasone	Topicort LP cream, 0.05%
Fluocinolone acetonide	Synalar-HP cream, 0.2%; Synalar ointment, 0.025%
Flurandrenolide	Cordran ointment, 0.05%
Triamcinolone acetonide	Aristocort, Kenalog ointments, 0.1%
Class 5—Lower mid-strength	
Betamethasone dipropionate	Diprosone lotion, 0.05%
Betamethasone valerate	Valisone cream/lotion, 0.1%; Betatrex 0.1%
Fluocinolone acetonide	Synalar cream, 0.025%
Flurandrenolide	Cordran cream, 0.05%
Hydrocortisone butyrate	Locoid cream, 0.1%
Hydrocortisone valerate	Westcort cream, 0.2%
Prednicarbate	Dermatop emollient cream, 0.1%
Triamcinolone acetonide	Kenalog cream/lotion, 0.1%
Class 6—Mild	
Alclometasone dipropionate	Aclovate cream/ointment, 0.05%
Triamcinolone acetonide	Aristocort cream, 0.1%
Desonide	DesOwen cream, 0.05%
Fluocinolone acetonide	Synalar cream/solution, 0.01%; Capex shampoo, Dermasmooth, 0.01%
Desonide	Tridesilon cream, 0.05%
Betamethasone valerate	Valisone lotion, 0.1%
Class 7—Least potent	
Hydrocortisone	Hyton, Cortate, Unicort, other OTC cream/lotion/foam

TABLE B-2 Common Side Effects of Topical Corticosteroids

Skin atrophy	Most common adverse effect Epidermal thinning may begin after only a few days Dermal thinning usually takes several weeks to develop Usually reversible within 2 months after stopping the corticosteroid
Telangiectasia	Most often occurs on the face, neck, and upper chest Tends to decrease when steroid discontinued, but may be irreversible
Striae	Usually occur around flexures (groin, axillary, and inner thigh areas) Usually permanent, but may fade with time
Purpura	Frequently occurs after minimal trauma Attributed to loss of perivascular supporting tissue in the dermis
Hypopigmentation	Reversible upon discontinuing the corticosteroid
Acneform eruptions	Particularly common on the face, especially with the "potent" and "very potent" corticosteroids Usually reversible
Fine hair growth	Reversible upon discontinuation of the corticosteroid
Infections	May worsen viral, bacterial, or fungal skin infections May cause tinea incognito
Hypothalamic-pituitary- adrenal axis suppression	Rare with topicals >30 g/wk of "very potent" corticosteroids should be limited to 3–4 wk Children (>10 g/wk) and elderly are at higher risk because of thinner skin

TABLE B-3 Intralesional Steroids—Concentrations for Injection

Condition	Concentration of Triamcinolone Acetonide Solution (mg/cc)
Acne	2–2.5
Alopecia areata	5–10
Granuloma annulare	5–10
Psoriasis	5–10
Hypertrophic lichen planus	5–10
Prurigo nodularis	10
Hidradenitis suppurativa	10
Keloids	10–40

C DERMOSCOPY

Ashfaq A. Marghoob, MD

APPENDIX C: DERMOSCOPY DIAGNOSIS (EXCLUDING LESIONS ON PALMS, SOLES AND FACE)

Dermoscopy allows the clinician to visualize structures below the level of the stratum corneum. These structures are not routinely discernable without dermoscopy. The presence or absence of specific dermoscopic structures, their location and their distribution can assist the clinician in making a diagnosis or at least in narrowing the differential diagnosis.

Dermoscopic diagnosis is based on the 2-step dermoscopy algorithm. Step one requires the observer to decide whether the lesion in question is of melanocytic origin. If the lesion is deemed to be a melanocytic lesion then the observer proceeds to step 2. In this phase of the evaluation the observer needs to decide whether the lesion is a benign nevus or a melanoma. However, if during step 1 analysis the lesion does not display any features of a melanocytic lesion then the observer needs to decide if the lesion possesses any criteria for a basal cell carcinoma, seborrheic keratosis, hemangioma, or dermatofibroma. If the lesion does not display any structures common to the aforementioned lesions then the lesion is considered nondescript or featureless. The index of suspicion needs to remain high for all featureless lesions since amelanotic melanoma can present as a completely structureless lesion. These featureless lesions sometimes do reveal blood vessels and, if present, their morphology can often help in narrowing the differential diagnosis.

Except for figure 17 all dermoscopic images were obtained via a contact non-polarized dermoscope. The lesion in figure 17 was obtained with a polarized dermoscope.

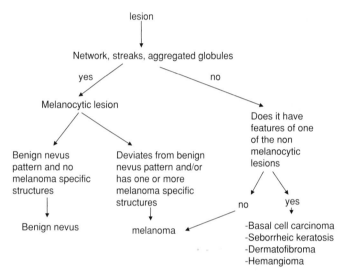

FIGURE 1.

STEP 1

- A melanocytic lesion usually will display one of the following structures:
  - Network (figure 2)
  - Streaks or pseudopods
  - Aggregated globules (figure 3)
- Melanocytic lesions can also be completely structureless. One should always consider melanoma in the differential diagnosis of structureless lesions (figure 5).

This lesion has a typical network and a negative network. The presence of a network indicates that the lesion is of melanocytic origin.

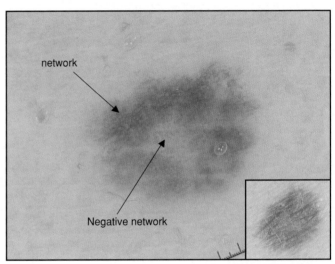

Diagnosis: Melanoma

FIGURE 2.

This lesion has aggregated globules. The presence of these globules indicates that the lesion is of melanocytic origin.

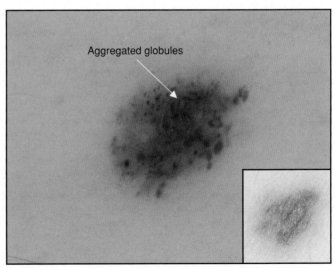

Diagnosis: Spitz nevus

FIGURE 3.

This lesion has streaks/pseudopods. This structure helps identify the lesion as being of melanocytic origin. In addition, the lesion has a network which is another melanocytic specific structure. The lesion also has structureless blotches.

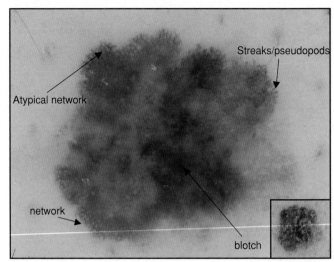

Diagnosis: Melanoma

FIGURE 4.

This lesion does not display any of the structures commonly seen in melanocytic lesions (i.e., network, streaks, globules). It also does not have any features of a basal cell carcinoma, seborrheic keratosis, dermatofibroma, or hemangioma. Thus, this is a featureless lesion. However, it does display many irregular tortuous blood vessels, which may be a sign of neoangiogenesis. The possibility of melanoma needs to be entertained for such featureless lesion.

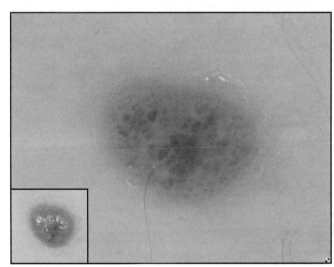

Diagnosis: Melanoma

FIGURE 5.

STEP 2

- If the lesion is deemed to be of melanocytic origin then one needs to decide whether the lesion is a benign nevus or a melanoma.

- Nevi tend to manifest one of the following benign patterns: diffuse or patchy network (figures 6 and 7), peripheral network with central hypopigmented (figure 8) or hyperpigmented area (figure 9), peripheral network with central globules (figure 10), globules only (figure 11), or peripheral globules with central network (figure 12).

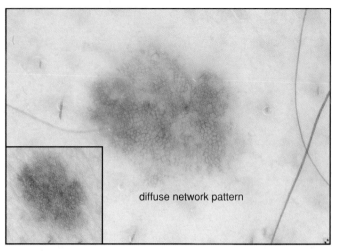

diffuse network pattern

Diagnosis: Benign nevus

FIGURE 6.

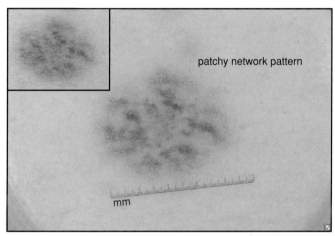

patchy network pattern

mm

Diagnosis: Benign nevus

FIGURE 7.

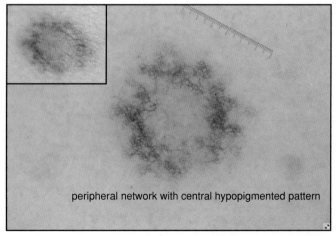

peripheral network with central hypopigmented pattern

Diagnosis: Benign nevus

FIGURE 8.

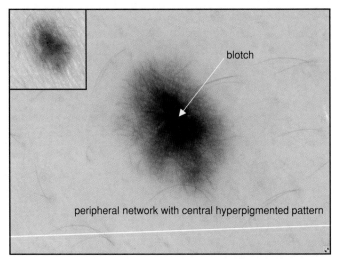

Diagnosis: Benign nevus

FIGURE 9.

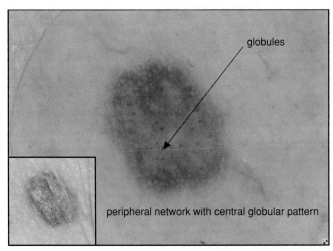

Diagnosis: Benign nevus

FIGURE 10.

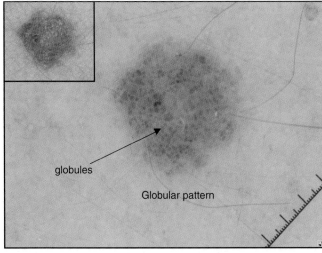

Diagnosis: Benign nevus

FIGURE 11.

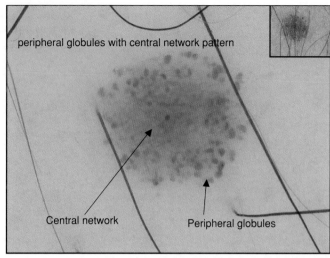

Diagnosis: Benign enlarging nevus

FIGURE 12.

STEP 2

In contrast, melanomas tend to deviate from the benign pattern described above. Furthermore, the structures in a melanoma are often distributed in an asymmetric fashion. Most melanomas will also reveal one or more of the melanoma specific structures:

MELANOMA SPECIFIC STRUCTURES

- Atypical network (figures 4,14)
- Streaks (figure 4)
- Negative network (figure 2)
- Chrysalis structures (figure 17)
- Atypical dots and/or globules (figures 14, 15, 16)
- Off center blotch (figure 4)
- Blue white veil over raised portion (figure 14)
- Blue white veil over flat portion (peppering)(figure 13)
- Peripheral tan-brown structureless areas (figure 14)
- Atypical blood vessels (figures 5, 16)

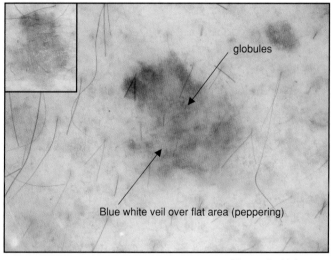

Diagnosis: Melanoma

FIGURE 13.

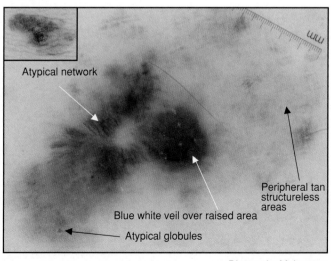

Diagnosis: Melanoma

FIGURE 14.

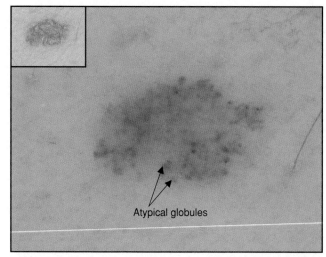

Atypical globules

Diagnosis: Melanoma

FIGURE 15.

Figure 16 was obtained via a contact non-polarized dermoscope.

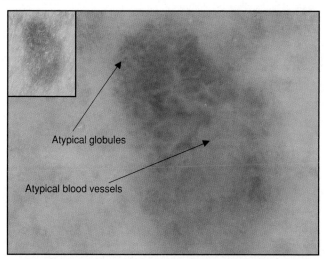

Atypical globules

Atypical blood vessels

Diagnosis: Melanoma

FIGURE 16.

This is the same lesion as depicted in the previous slide. However, this image was captured using polarized light dermoscopy. Polarized light allows one to appreciate the chrysalis like structures (shiny white stellate streaks) as can be seen within the dotted circle on the image.

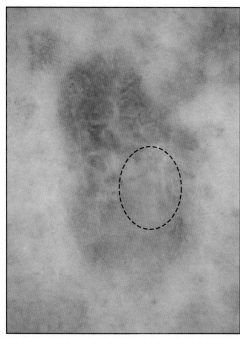

FIGURE 17.

STEP 1

- If the lesion is not of melanocytic origin then one needs to look for structures seen in:
  - ○ Basal cell carcinoma
  - ○ Seborrheic keratosis
  - ○ Dermatofibroma
  - ○ Hemangioma

BASAL CELL CARCINOMA

- Blue gray ovoid nests/globules
- Leaf like structures
- Spoke wheel like structures
- Arborizing telangiectasias
- Ulceration
- Shiny white areas

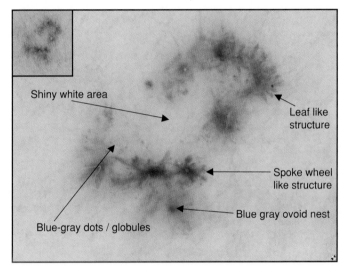

Diagnosis: Basal cell carcinoma

FIGURE 18.

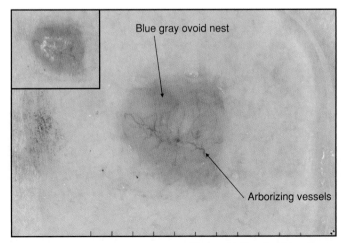

Diagnosis: Basal cell carcinoma

FIGURE 19.

SEBORRHEIC KERATOSIS

- Milia like cysts
- Comedo like openings
- Fissures and ridges giving a cerebriform pattern
- Fat finger like structures
- Sharp demarcation
- Fingerprint like structures
- Moth eaten borders
- Hairpin vessels with white halo

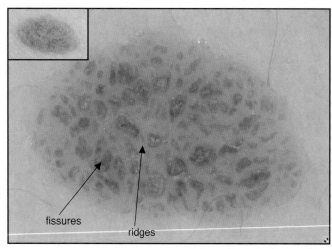

Diagnosis: Seborrheic keratosis

FIGURE 20.

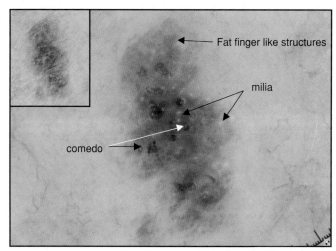

Diagnosis: Seborrheic keratosis

FIGURE 21.

DERMATOFIBROMA

- Peripheral delicate fine network
- Central scar like area
- Blood vessels within the scar like area
- Ring-like globular structures

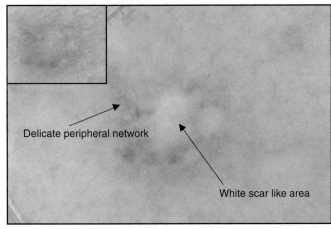

Diagnosis: Dermatofibroma

FIGURE 22.

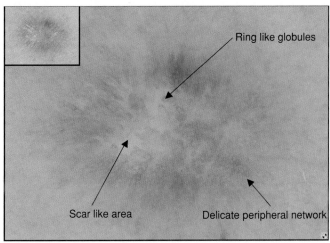

Diagnosis: Dermatofibroma

FIGURE 23.

HEMANGIOMA

- Red to maroon lacunae = cherry hemangioma
- Black lacunae = angiokeratoma

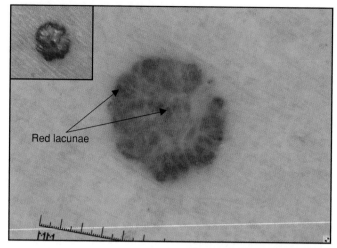

Red lacunae

Diagnosis: Cherry hemangioma

FIGURE 24.

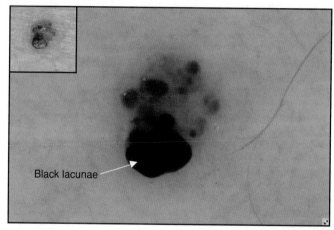

Black lacunae

Diagnosis: Angiokeratoma

FIGURE 25.